D0929564

PRINCIPLES AND PRACTICE OF
PAIN
MANAGEMENT

PRINCIPLES AND PRACTICE OF
PAIN
MANAGEMENT

Editor
CAROL A. WARFIELD, M.D.
Assistant Professor of Anesthesia
Harvard Medical School, Boston, Massachusetts

Director, Pain Management Centre
Beth Israel Hospital, Boston, Massachusetts

McGRAW-HILL, INC.
Health Professions Division
New York   St. Louis   San Francisco   Auckland   Bogotá   Caracas
Lisbon   London   Madrid   Mexico   Milan   Montreal   New Delhi
Paris   San Juan   Singapore   Sydney   Tokyo   Toronto

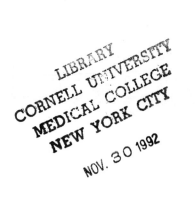

PRINCIPLES AND PRACTICE OF PAIN MANAGEMENT

1234567890 HAL HAL 98765432

ISBN 0-07-068291 -7

This book was set in Times Roman by Kachina Typesetting, Inc.

The editors were Michael J. Houston and Susan Finn.

The production supervisor was Richard Ruzycka.

The cover was designed and the project was supervised by M 'N O Production Services, Inc.

Arcata Graphics/Halliday was the printer and binder.

Library of Congress Cataloging-in-Publication Data

Principles and practice of pain management / editor, Carol A. Warfield.
    p. cm.
  Includes bibliographical references and index.
  ISBN 0-07-068291-7
  1. Pain—Treatment. 2. Analgesia. I. Warfield, Carol A.
RB127.P754 1993   92-20392
616'.0472—dc20   CIP

This book is dedicated to my family for their patience, support, and understanding.

Contents

Contributors

Peter J. Armstrong, M.B., B.S., F.F.A.R.A.C.S.
Department of Anaesthesia, Newcastle Mater Misericordiae Hospital, Waratah, Australia

Gerald M. Aronoff, M.D.
Assistant Clinical Professor, Tufts University School of Medicine, Boston, Massachusetts
Director, Boston Pain Center, Melrose, Massachusetts

Francis J. Balestrieri, M.D.
Former Professor, Department of Anesthesia, Bowman Gray School of Medicine, Wake Forest University, Winston-Salem, North Carolina
Currently in private practice, Arlington, Virginia

Dhirendra S. Bana, M.D.
The John R. Graham Headache Center, The Faulkner Hospital, Boston, Massachusetts
Clinical Instructor in Medicine, Tufts University School of Medicine, Boston, Massachusetts

Robert Bengston, M.S., P.T.
Former Director of Physical Therapy, Beth Israel Hospital, Boston, Massachusetts
Currently Clinical Director, Worker's Comprehensive, Woburn, Massachusetts

Herbert Benson, M.D.
Chief, Division of Behavioral Medicine, New England Deaconess Hospital, Boston, Massachusetts
Associate Professor of Medicine, The Mind/Body Medical Institute, Harvard Medical School, Boston, Massachusetts
President, The Mind/Body Medical Institute, New England Deaconess Hospital, Boston, Massachusetts

Charles B. Berde, M.D.
Assistant Professor of Anesthesiology, Harvard Medical School, Boston, Massachusetts
Department of Anesthesiology, Children's Hospital, Boston, Massachusetts

Stuart Berger, M.D., M.P.H., P.C.
Deparment of Psychiatry, New York University, New York, New York (1977–1979)
Pritkin Professor of Nutrition, Mercy College, New York, New York (1985–1986)
Private practice and author, New York, New York

Charles D. Boucek, Ph.D.
Clinical Associate Professor, Anesthesiology and Assistant Professor, Internal Medicine, University of Pittsburgh Medical Center, Pittsburgh, Pennsylvania

Steven F. Brena, M.D.
Chairman of the Board, Pain Control and Rehabilitation Institute of Georgia, Decatur, Georgia
Clinical Professor of Rehabilitation Medicine, Emory University, Atlanta, Georgia

Burnell R. Brown, Jr., M.D., Ph.D.
Professor and Head, Department of Anesthesiology, University of Arizona Health Sciences Center, Tucson, Arizona

Leonard S. Bushnell, M.D.
Associate Professor of Anesthesia, Harvard Medical School, Boston, Massachusetts
Director, Acute Pain Service, Beth Israel Hospital, Boston, Massachusetts

René Cailliet, M.D.
Professor Emeritus, University of Southern California School of Medicine, Los Angeles, California

Lena E. Dohlman, M.D.
Instructor in Anesthesia, Harvard Medical School, Boston, Massachusetts
Assistant Anesthetist, Beth Israel Hospital, Boston, Massachusetts

Alice D. Domar, Ph.D.
Staff Psychologist, New England Deaconess Hospital, Boston, Massachusetts
Instructor in Medicine, Harvard Medical School, Boston, Massachusetts
Senior Staff Scientist, The Mind/Body Medical Institute, Boston, Massachusetts

David Dubuisson, M.D., Ph.D.
Assistant Professor of Neurosurgery, Harvard Medical School, Boston, Massachusetts
Assistant Neurosurgeon, Beth Israel Hospital, Boston, Massachusetts

Ashley M. Duthie, M.D., F.F.A.R.C.S.
Consultant in Pain Relief, Norfolk and Norwich Hospital, Norwich, England

W. Thomas Edwards, Ph.D., M.D.
Associate Professor of Anesthesiology and Director, Pain Relief Services, University of Washington, Harborview Medical Center, Seattle, Washington

John H. Eichhorn, M.D.
Professor and Chairman, Department of Anesthesiology, University of Mississippi, Jackson, Mississippi

H. Elliot Fives, R.N., B.S.N.
Affiliated with William Douglass, M.D., Little Company of Mary, Pavilion Hospital, Torrance, and Center for Behavioral Medicine, Los Angeles, California

Richard Friedman, Ph.D.
Associate Professor of Psychiatry and Psychology, State University of New York at Stonybrook, Stonybrook, New York
Director, Division of Behavioral Medicine, State University of New York at Stonybrook, Stonybrook, New York
Director of Research, The Mind/Body Medical Institute, Boston, Massachusetts
Lecturer in Medicine, Harvard Medical School, Boston, Massachusetts

Tobin Gerhart, M.D.
Assistant Clinical Professor of Orthopedic Surgery, Harvard Medical School, Boston, Massachusetts
Beth Israel Hospital, Boston, Massachusetts

Richard L. Gilbert, M.D.
Chairman, Department of Anesthesia and Director, Southeast Pain Care, Carolinas Medical Center, Charlotte, North Carolina

John R. Graham, M.D. (deceased)
Former Director, The Headache Research Foundation, Faulkner Hospital, Boston, Massachusetts

Nelson H. Hendler, M.D.
Clinical Director, Mensana Clinic, Stevenson, Maryland
Assistant Professor of Neurosurgery, Johns Hopkins University School of Medicine, Baltimore, Maryland
Associate Professor of Physiology, University of Maryland School of Dental Surgery, Baltimore, Maryland

Subhash Jain, M.D.
Clinical Assistant Professor of Anesthesiology, Cornell University Medical College, New York, New York
Director, Nerve Block Service, Memorial Sloan-Kettering Cancer Center, New York, New York

David A. Keith, B.D.S., F.D.S.R.C.S., D.M.D.
Associate Professor of Oral and Maxillofacial Surgery, Harvard School of Dental Medicine, Boston, Massachusetts
Visiting Oral and Maxillofacial Surgeon, Massachusetts General Hospital, Boston, Massachusetts
Chief of Oral and Maxillofacial Surgery, Harvard Community Health Plan, Boston, Massachusetts

Garrett D. Kine, M.D.
Spinal Diagnostics, Spine Care Medical Group, San Francisco, California

Babu V. Koka, M.D.
Assistant Professor of Anesthesiology, Harvard Medical School, Boston, Massachusetts
Department of Anesthesiology, Children's Hospital, Boston, Massachusetts

Scott P. Laff, B.A.
Research Assistant, Department of Obstetrics and Gynecology, Beth Israel Hospital, Boston, Massachusetts

Michael H. Levy, M.D., Ph.D.
Co-director, Pain Management Center, Fox Chase Cancer Center, Philadelphia, Pennsylvania
Assistant Professor of Medicine, Temple University School of Medicine, Philadelphia, Pennsylvania

Eric D. Lichter, M.D.
Instructor in Obstetrics and Gynecology, Harvard Medical School, Boston, Massachusetts
Director of Emergency Services, Department of Obstetrics and Gynecology, Beth Israel Hospital, Boston, Massachusetts

Anthony M. Lin, M.D.
Former Instructor in Anesthesia, Harvard Medical School, Boston, Massachusetts
Currently Staff Anesthesiologist, Community Hospital, Los Gatos, California

Sampson Lipton, M.D., O.B.E., F.F.A.R.C.S.
Medical Director, Pain Research Institute, Walton Hospital, Liverpool, England

Elizabeth Bowyer Malacoff, R. N., B.S.N., J.D.
Former Risk Manager, Risk Management Foundation of the Harvard Medical Institutions, Cambridge, Massachusetts
Currently in private practice of health care law, Bethlehem, Pennsylvania

Bonnie McLean, O.M.D., L.Ac., M.A., R.N.
Affiliation with Murray Susser, M.D. and Michael Turek, M.D., Pine Grove Hospital, Canoga Park, California, and Woodview Calabasas Hospital, Calabasas, California

Charles H. McLesky, M.D.
Professor and Director of Academic Affairs, Department of Anesthesiology, University of Colorado Health Sciences Center, Denver, Colorado

Mark Mehta, M.D., F.F.A.R.C.S.
Consultant in Pain Management, King Edward VIII Hospital, Midhurst, West Sussex, England
Honorary Fellow, University of Murcia, Murcia, Spain
Special awards: Murcia (Spain), Triesie and Conversano (Italy), Moscow (Russia)

Terence M. Murphy, M.B., Ch.B., F.F.A.R.C.S.

Professor of Anesthesiology, University of Washington, Seattle, Washington

Ann-Marie E. Nehme, M.S., M.D.

Instructor in Anesthesia, Harvard Medical School, Boston, Massachusetts

Associate Anesthetist, Beth Israel Hospital, Boston, Massachusetts

Christine Peeters-Asdourian, M.D.

Assistant Professor of Anesthesiology and Director, Pain Control Center, University of Massachusetts Medical Center, Worcester, Massachusetts

Prithvi Raj, M.D.

Professor, Department of Anesthesiology, Medical College of Georgia, Augusta, Georgia

Executive Medical Director, Southeast Pain Institute, Atlanta, Georgia

John C. Rowlingson, M.D.

Professor of Anesthesiology and Director, Pain Management Center, Department of Anesthesiology, University of Virginia, Health Sciences Center, Charlottesville, Virginia

Thomas E. Rudy, Ph.D.

Associate Professor, Anesthesiology, Psychiatry, and Behavioral Sciences, and Associate Director, Pain Evaluation and Treatment Institute, University of Pittsburgh Medical Center, Pittsburgh, Pennsylvania

Norma J. G. Sandrock, M.D.

Instructor in Anesthesia, Harvard Medical School, Boston, Massachusetts

Assistant Anesthetist, Beth Israel Hospital, Boston, Massachusetts

Ivor G. Schraibman, M., Ch., F.R.C.S. (Ed) F.R.C.S.

Consultant Surgeon, Rochdale District Health Authority, Rochdale, England

Navil Sethna, M.B., Ch.B.

Instructor in Anesthesia, Harvard Medical School, Boston, Massachusetts

Department of Anesthesiology, Children's Hospital, Boston, Massachusetts

Shulim Spektor, M.D.

Physiatrist, Clinical Assistant Professor, Rehabilitation Medicine, Emory University, Atlanta, Georgia

Pain Control and Rehabilitation Institute of Georgia, Decatur, Georgia

Michael J. Stabile, M.D.

Former Instructor in Anesthesia, Harvard Medical School, Boston, Massachusetts

Former Assistant Anesthetist, Beth Israel Hospital, Boston, Massachusetts

Currently Anesthesiologist, Centennial Medical Center, Nashville, Tennessee

Mark Swerdlow, M.D., M.Sc., F.F.A.R.C.S., D.A.

Former Director, North West Regional Pain Relief Centre, Hope Hospital and University of Manchester School of Medicine, Manchester, England

R. R. Tasker, M.D., F.R.C.S.(C)

Professor, Department of Surgery, University of Toronto, Division of Neurosurgery, The Toronto Hospital, Toronto, Canada

Edwin M. Todd, M.D., J.D., Ph.D.

Clinical Professor of Neurosurgery, University of Southern California, Los Angeles, California

Co-sponsor Todd-Wells Chair in Neurosurgery, University of Southern California, Los Angeles, California

Yvona Trnka, M.D.

Instructor in Medicine, Harvard Medical School, Boston, Massachusetts

Director, Gastroenterology, Harvard Community Health Plan, Boston, Massachusetts

Dennis C. Turk, Ph.D.

Professor of Psychiatry, Anesthesiology, and Behavioral Sciences, and Director, Pain Evaluation and Treatment Institute, University of Pittsburgh School of Medicine, Pittsburgh, Pennsylvania

Jeffrey Uppington, M.D.

Instructor in Anesthesia, Harvard Medical School, Boston, Massachusetts

Assistant Anesthetist, Beth Israel Hospital, Boston, Massachusetts

Carol A. Warfield, M.D.

Assistant Professor of Anesthesia, Harvard Medical School, Boston, Massachusetts

Director, Pain Management Centre, Beth Israel Hospital, Boston, Massachusetts

Duke B. Weeks, M.D.

Professor, Department of Anesthesia, Bowman Gray School of Medicine, Wake Forest University, Winston-Salem, North Carolina

Peter White, M.D., F.F.A.R.C.S.

Instructor in Anesthesia, Harvard Medical School, Boston, Massachusetts

Director of Regional Anesthesia, Beth Israel Hospital, Boston, Massachusetts

Preface

Pain is an almost universal aftermath of injury. In this context, it serves a useful purpose as a warning system, alerting the individual to seek treatment of the underlying pathology. It is now well accepted that pain can occur without any discernable trauma at all, or can persist beyond the expected healing period. This knowledge prompted the taxonomy committee of the International Association for the Study of Pain to define pain as "an unpleasant sensory and emotional experience associated with actual or potential tissue damage, or described in terms of such damage."

Pain takes its toll, not only in human suffering, but also causes relationship and job disruption and has a tremendous economic impact on society. In 1980, it was estimated that approximately 65,000,000 Americans suffered from chronic pain and that of these, 50,000,000 were partially or totally disabled. Their pain resulted in over 70,000,000 lost work days and cost Americans nearly 60 billion dollars annually.[1] In 1991, Frymoyer[2] estimated that 50–100 billion dollars were spent each year on the direct and indirect costs of low back pain alone and that 75 percent of these costs could be attributed to the 5 percent of patients who become disabled because their pain has not been adequately treated.

Despite these startling statistics, pain still remains inappropriately or inadequately treated. Although tremendous scientific and technological advances have been made in recent years, the knowledge and techniques available are widely underutilized. This is due in great part to a lack of dissemination of information to clinicians. Formal medical education and training has long considered pain treatment a discipline of little importance. This is evidenced by the lack of formal training in pain management in most residency programs today, even in such disciplines as anesthesiology, neurology, neurosurgery, psychiatry, and orthopedic surgery.

On the other hand, anesthesiologists in particular are called upon more and more frequently to treat chronic painful syndromes.[3] Since the first pain clinics were established in the 1940s, the number of pain clinics has risen dramatically. Today there are hundreds of pain clinics in the United States, over 60 percent of which are directed by anesthesiologists.[4] The field of pain management is finally gaining recognition as a subspecialty as is evidenced by the International Association for the Study of Pain's publication of standards for physician fellowships in pain management.[5] In addition, the American Board of Anesthesiology is making plans for the first examination to grant anesthesiologists board certification in pain management.

In the 1960s, the idea of a multidisciplinary approach to pain management was born. Although many pain clinics today are multidisciplinary in nature, many others rely upon one type of treatment or discipline and yet others treat only a particular type of pain (such as headaches).

For most, however, it has become obvious that pain specialists cannot practice pain management in a vacuum. They must rely upon their colleagues in other disciplines to lend their expertise and in this regard must have a solid knowledge of the other techniques available to treat pain and their physiological and pharmacological basis.

Most anesthesiologists have been trained to deal exclusively with acute pain. Once its function as a warning system has served its purpose to define the underlying pathology, acute pain should be swiftly and aggressively treated to prevent the untoward physiological and emotional effects of pain. Chronic pain, however, is not the same as acute pain and should not be treated as such. Not only is the pathophysiology distinct, but the patient will experience different physiological and psychological responses to chronic pain than to acute pain.

Chronic pain has often been arbitrarily defined as pain persisting for longer than six months. This distinction is not always correct, however, and chronic pain can better be defined as pain persisting for longer than the expected time for an injury to heal. Chronic pain may be caused by chronic somatic or visceral pathology, by a dysfunction of the peripheral or central nervous system, or by psychological or environmental factors. The physiological changes associated with acute pain (tachycardia, diaphoresis, etc.) are often lacking and in their place affective disorders are more common.

[1]Bonica JJ. Pain research and therapy: Past and current status and future needs. In: Ng LKY and Bonica JJ, eds. *Pain, Discomfort and Humanitarian Care*. New York: Elsevier; 1980:1–46.

[2]Frymoyer JM. Cats-Baril WL: An overview of the incidences and costs of low back pain. *Orthop Clin North Am* 1991; 22(2)263–271.

[3]Carron H. The changing role of the anesthesiologist in pain management. *Reg Anesth* 1989; 14(1),4–9.

[4]American Society of Anesthesiologists. *Pain Center/Clinic Directory*. Park Ridge, IL: American Society of Anesthesiologists; 1979.

[5]International Association for the Study of Pain Newsletter; January–February 1991:1.

The clinician must learn to make the distinction between acute and chronic pain before embarking upon treatment. The skills of proper pain management lie not in the ability to perform technically difficult nerve blocks but in the determination of appropriate diagnostic and therapeutic modalities.

In recent years several texts have been written on the subject of pain management. This text is intended specifically for the pain specialist who is called upon to manage painful syndromes. Part I provides the basic knowledge needed for the initial diagnostic approach to the patient. Part II deals with pain by anatomic location, since most patients will present to the clinician with a complaint of pain in some general location. This section is intended to provide the physician with a differential diagnosis of potential causes of pain in the area of the patient's complaints. In Part III, a comprehensive discussion of the diagnosis and treatment of common painful syndromes is presented. Part IV includes a detailed explanation of the mechanisms of action and indications for the various treatments used in pain management. The last chapter deals with the clinician's legal obligations and rights in the practice of pain management.

Since this text was not intended as an atlas of regional anesthesia, techniques of specific nerve blocks were not included in the chapters. The Appendix include guidelines and illustrations of the technical aspects of blocks commonly utilized in pain management. It also contains an example of a pain unit chart that has incorporated space for recording anesthetic procedures. A table of commonly used local anesthetics is also included.

The glossary provides definitions of some of the confusing terminology associated with pain treatment. It also contains a listing of commonly used abbreviations.

I hope the readers find this text a useful guide in their treatment of pain.

PRINCIPLES AND PRACTICE OF
PAIN
MANAGEMENT

Pain: Historical Perspectives

Edwin M. Todd

Pain is timeless, ineluctable, and disconcertingly indefinable. The anguished cry of the newborn infant is a reverberating echo of our primordial roots in pain. In the listener, it strikes the deepest reaches of the sensibilities, where it is perceived as a paradox of curse and blessing imposed ineradicably upon the human trinity of birth, existence, and death. We are put in awe by the wonder of creation, and the awe is conditioned in the first instance by the shattering impact of release from the womb. It is the pervading essence that marks and mocks our journey from cradle to grave, discoloring our thinking and evoking groping heuristic efforts to express its influence on evolving and passing civilizations.

When people began to think, preeminent among the perplexities and problems that weighed upon us was the irksome nature of pain, and this concern has traveled with us through time. We must have sensed that pain was our protector, but even as it happened, we could hardly have recognized it as the central core of our feelings of compassion, sympathy, and forgiveness that served to bond our fellowship with other creatures in the humblest origins of social intercourse. Without it, life could have been nothing for human beings but a flat complacency, and the species would not have survived. But humans did survive, and they must have puzzled over the nature of this noxious benefactor even as we now speculate on its historical associations, courteously respectful in the awareness of our own interpretive inadequacies.

Somewhere within us, say the pundits, there is a *sensorium commune,* an undetermined site wherein the nature of pain is revealed. More elusive than the Holy Grail for which medieval men sought widely and in vain, the sensorium commune has preoccupied and frustrated thinking people since time immemorial. To find it, and to define it, may resolve the problem of dealing with it, but so far biopsychosocial research has only given new insights into the complexity of the quest. Its epistemological orientations are only vaguely perceived in anthropological suggestions, and its ontological essences are shrouded in confused psychological inferences.

Reprinted by permission of the publisher from pages 39–56, Chapter 4 in *Chronic Pain: Further Observations from City of Hope National Medical Center* by Benjamin L. Crue, Jr., ed. Copyright 1978, Spectrum Publications, Inc. Jamaica, New York.

In all ages, pain has been a very real and immediate concern, but, always, the attitudes and beliefs of people have been shaped by magical, demonological, theological, philosophical, and practical influences in varying degrees and with shifting emphasis. It is our purpose to capture and examine some of these changing patterns of thought in our spotty passage through time.

PRIMITIVE SOCIETY

The human race took a giant step forward seven thousand years ago when it emerged from obscurity with the discovery of a written means of recording its activities. Beyond this curtain lay many thousands of years of intelligent existence about which we can only speculate, but there is evidence in fossil remains, in surviving tools, in paintings and carvings, and in the study of primitive cultures throughout the modern world from which we can form reasonable hypothetical constructs of human behavior and beliefs.

It is reasonable to suppose that early people found rational means of dealing with minor ills and obvious wounds, just as we see cultures, untouched by modern civilization using heat and cold, mud packs and poultices, intoxicants and analgesics, simple techniques of extracting foreign bodies, and bone-setting procedures. Trephinations and ceremonial mutilations such as circumcisions, castrations, and piercing operations bear witness to very old surgical skills.[1] In contrast, internal pain most certainly had supernatural connotations. Causation was steeped in superstition, as life itself was a strange and magical process and management necessarily entailed supernatural means. The source of pain was thought to be external, something magical and insidious acting upon the body by an "intrusion" of objects and spirits or by a life-sapping "withdrawal" of vital substance. Active pain states were instances of intrusion such as the "ghost shot" of medicine men in New Guinea tribes, whereas wasting and death were extraction processes manipulated by sinister outside forces. The concept of intrusion reaches through time and is preserved in Welsh superstition as the "shot of the elf" and in the German *Hexenschuss,* or "witches shot," for lumbago.[2] This remote, external cause of pain in primitive human thought found its site in mysterious hovering spirits seeking a body to inhabit. Treatment was directed toward extracorporeal

1

flights of fancy, and physiology had not yet awakened in the Stone Age mentality.[3]

ANCIENT KINGDOMS

As we became more civilized we settled in fertile valleys at the mouths of great waterways and founded thriving communities where our sophistication increased. Under the growing stimulus of accumulating knowledge and technology medicine flourished in early settlements along the Nile, the Indus, the Yangtze and Hwang Ho, and in the fertile crescent between the Euphrates and the Tigris.

Egypt

Owing to a combination of fortuitous circumstances, including a dry climate, an ideal reed growing abundantly in the deltas, and a talent for concocting stable dyes and inks, some notion of the lost art of ancient Egyptian medicine has come down to us through the Ebers, Berlin, and Edwin Smith papyri.[4] It is only a fragmented glimpse, but it is quite revealing in many respects in which it establishes precedents and preserves precious little cameos of medical practice. A surprisingly rational empiricism is exhibited in the therapeutic decisions of the Edwin Smith papyrus, copied by scribes in the sixteenth century B.C. from earlier medical writings ascribed to the era of Imhotep of the Third Dynasty. It was Imhotep, builder of pyramids, architect, astronomer, and "blameless physician," whose apotheosis later served as the prototype for the Greek deification of Asclepios.[5]

Unfortunately, the high level of clinical competence shown by the Smith Papyrus and the amazing spectrum of pharmaceutical knowledge of the Ebers manuscript were not sustained in later periods as Egyptian medicine declined under the growing influences of religious mysticism and demonology.

A priceless legacy of Egyptian civilization is the absence of proscriptions against human dissection. We consequently have a wealth of surviving material for study in mummies and in descriptive accounts of anatomical dissection. Regrettably, the art reached its highest expression in the masterful works of morticians rather than physicians, and the former were a secretive lot who did not broadcast their marvelous techniques but left only their products for our edification. Nevertheless, there are numerous references in the papyri from which we may draw reasonable assumptions. It is clear that their anatomical knowledge was poorly organized, their physiology crude and inconsistent. Their concepts of pain were muddied by magical-religious influences differing little from primitive beliefs except in imaginative complexity. Anthromorphic spirits of the dead with sinister intent to cause pain were dispatched by the gods and other forces of darkness into human orifices or through pores to wreck havoc within. The left nostril was a

favorite portal of entry. Yet for all the mystical aberrations there was a groping effort to provide rational explanations in anatomical and physiological terms.

The brain was totally ignored as a vital organ although paresis of the opposite side of the body due to head injury is described in the Smith papyrus.[4] The brain was the one organ destroyed or discarded in the embalming process, which more or less signifies the esteem it engendered. The Egyptians elevated the heart to a status of preeminence over all organs, and with its vessels reaching out into all areas it was credited with being the seat of all motor and sensory activity. There was no knowledge of a nervous system; the heart and its vessels were believed to serve all these functions. These included the appreciation of pain from obvious causes such as gross injury, although the anatomical references are often intermingled with confusing mystical associations.[6] With the passage of centuries the rational practices and astute clinical observations of the early Egyptians were replaced by sorcery and incantation, offering nothing of value to medicine or our review of pain concepts. Nevertheless, the influences of the early physicians were to have profound and enduring effects on subsequent civilizations.[3]

India

Unlike other ancient civilizations that rose to enjoy a lusty moment in history and then faded into obscurity, those crystallized along the murky waters of the Indus and the lazy river valleys of China endured and projected their ancient medical practices almost intact into the living present. In both countries anesthetic techniques and drugs to relieve pain were old when civilization was new.

The oldest of the sacred books of India, the Rig-Veda, reputedly written as far back 4000 years B.C., describes hundreds of methods deriving from mineral, plant, and animal sources, including anesthetics and analgesics still in use. Practical healing and vigorous therapeutic measures ranging through a versatile surgical repertory culminated in Susruta, the great physician and surgeon who lived about 600 B.C. It was a time when disease had a locus in anatomy, and physiological explanations aided in the diagnosis of disturbed function. A crude concept of the nervous system centered on the heart, from which ducts radiated to all sensory organs and all excitable parts. Susruta's writings reflect some awareness of pain pathways connected with this misconceived center.[7] The advent of Buddhism in the fifth century B.C. cast a pall over scientific discovery and directed medical thinking into spiritual channels, where the sensorium commune became illusory. Physiological phenomena were unreal and pain was denied existence. The slow, steady crawl of scientific progress in anatomical matters was abruptly arrested by religious dogma just as it seemed poised on the threshold of new adventure, and the creative energies of Indian medicine were diverted to other interests.[8]

Mesopotamia

No place on earth holds deeper significance for the history of human progress than the fertile crescent of land lying between the Euphrates and Tigris rivers, aptly designated as the Cradle of Civilization. It was here that a practical system of writing was first invented to initiate a cultural and intellectual metamorphosis in human relations. A stable and well-organized society is portrayed in the Code of Hammurabi, but medical practice failed to achieve the high standard of the legal system. Rational practitioners competed at a disadvantage with exorcist-priests who dealt in omens, divination, astrology, and magic arts. It was eminently safer to diagnose and treat in accordance with revelations conjured out of livers and other entrails of sacrificed animals than to rely on surgical skills, for it was expressly stated in the Code: "If a surgeon has opened an eye infection with a bronze instrument and so saved the man's eye, he shall take ten shekels. If a surgeon has opened an eye infection with a bronze instrument and thereby destroyed the man's eye, they shall cut off his hand." Scientific medicine at best was a descriptive art singularly unencumbered by physiological considerations that might conflict with dominant magical-religious dictates, designating the heart as the seat of intelligence, the liver of emotion, the uterus of compassion, and the stomach, curiously, of cunning.[9] Little stimulus was afforded for rational investigation of painful afflictions when disease was regarded as a punishment for sin and the gods demanded homage in the form of sacrifice and prayer for these transgressions.[8] The pregnant promises of early ingenuity in writing, art, architecture, law, and astronomy never quite extended into the medical arts, which remained unexceptional and uninspiring to future scientific interests.

China

From very early times the Chinese viewed the human predicament as a microcosm of the harmonious universe. Harmony prevailed in life when the polarity of Yang and Yin was in proper balance. Nei Ching, the Chinese canon of medicine, reflects the very ancient concern with maintaining a state of equilibrium between opposing forces. There is no clear distinction between mythology and historical reality in these writings, and mystical numerology, remindful of Pythagorean precepts, strongly influences an over-systematized medical taxonomy.[10] Yang represents maleness, light, heat, aggressiveness, and strength, while Yin exemplifies femaleness, darkness, cold, passivity, and weakness. There are five elements in nature (earth, water, fire, wood, and metal), five organs in the body (heart, lungs, liver, spleen, and kidneys), and five winds that inhabit the arteries. Natural laws regulating the universe also participate in the functioning of human physiology as reflected in the forces of Yang and Yin. The brain is simply the marrow of the skull, playing no part in vital activities. The heart is the majordomo of organs as the storehouse of the blood and airs; these contain the vital energy and intelligence that circulate to all areas, announcing the state of health of the body in a variety of pulses. Clinical practice depends upon an astute appreciation of subtle messages conveyed in these pulsations. There are 365 parts of the body, and each has a precise focal representation so important to the therapeutic arts of acupuncture and moxibustion,[2] each of which has been sporadically popular.

Pain has no particular center, but disturbance in Yang or Yin, especially excesses of heat or cold, usually relate to the heart and vessels. Emotional overindulgence upsets Yang or Yin and begets pain in the particular organ allotted the psychological function involved. Rage upsets Yin in the liver, and violent joy is hurtful to Yang in the heart. Excessive grief disturbs the lung, and evil thoughts provoke the spleen. Obviously, "moderation in all things," was as important to Yang and Yin as it was to healthy coexistence of mind and body in Hellenic Greece.[6] The anatomy of pain had multifocal, situational orientation for ancient China, evoking therapeutic responses that still prevail but remain for the most part oriental.

HELLENIC GREECE

The miracle of the Greek achievement is exemplified, rather than explained, by the enduring enchantment it continues to exert over the human imagination. Greek ideas in medicine, as in art, architecture, astronomy, literature, and philosophy, still excite and exalt us. Pain-relieving drugs and healing arts are woven into the fabric of Homeric legend and Greek mythology, from which Greek medicine originated. Mythology and legend provided a strong base for early medical practice in other ancient societies as well, but Greek emphasis on individual achievement allowed the creative thinkers to emerge from anonymity, and the line between mythology and history is made more distinct by biographical knowledge of their great figures.[6]

We know little about the birth of Greek science in the sixth century B.C. in Ionia, but we all share the wealth of the intellectual revolution that was fostered when the veils of myth and religious dogma were swept aside to reveal a wondrous world operating in an orderly manner in accordance with rational, ascertainable natural laws. The legacy of Thales (624–545 B.C.) and his philosophical colleagues was a new, open-minded world view that filtered down from philosophy to science and ignited an intellectual explosion that reverberated through time and space into every aspect of human inquiry. The first great medical figure to surface was Alcmaeon (c. 500 B.C.) of Croton. Alcmaeon was a student and disciple of Pythagoras (566–497 B.C.), the mystic numerologist and patron saint of theoretical science. Pythagoras had already established a brotherhood and center for the arts and sciences in this ancient Greek colony at the southern tip of the Italian peninsula, when Alcmaeon added his medical school. Relying upon the findings of animal dissection, Alcmaeon elaborated a theory of sensory appreciation that comprehended the brain as the center for sensation. He postulated a mechanism of consciousness dependent upon variations in cerebral circulation for sleep and wakefulness. His concept of the nervous system consisted of a network of ducts and vessels carrying sensation in the form of particles of elements that invaded the body through several sensory organs to the sensorium in the brain.[8] The views of Alcmaeon, the lonely empiricist, fell on the deaf ears of a rationalist society that eschewed vulgar dissection for more noble mental gymnastics in physiological matters.

Democritus (460–362 B.C.), who taught that all matter was composed of ever changing atoms of the elements of fire, air, earth, and water, applied his atomic theory to sensation and pain. Sensation was a state of awareness in the soul atoms, occasioned when elementary particles invaded the body's pores and ducts. The size, shape, and movement of particles determined the nature of the perception. Thus, pain was an intrusion of sharp-hooked particles in a state of agitated motion disturbing the normal calm of the soul atoms. Democritus scattered his body and soul atoms over a universe in which life and death did not exist, where everything was always changing and only the total quality of matter remained constant; he did, however, make reluctant concessions to materialism by placing the center of consciousness and reason in the brain, emotions in the heart, and lust in the liver.[2]

The Hippocratic Corpus reflects the medical spirit and methods of the venerated physician Hippocrates (c. 460–360 B.C.) of Cos. Hippocratic medicine was practical and rational, stressing an expectant attitude while trusting in the marvelous healing power of nature.[9] Anatomy was rudimentary, and physiology was based upon a proper balance of the four elements, the four qualities (hot, cold, moist, dry), and the four humors present in every body. Pain was a manifestation of conditions disturbing the natural state of equilibrium in a healthy body. The brain was regarded as a gland of sorts, excreting mucous matter that played a part in regulating body heat. With his disciples, Hippocrates paid considerable attention to the problem of pain, continually seeking effective measures for easing human suffering at the clinical level. They experimented with drugs, including opium, mandrake, and hemlock, and actively employed cooling techniques and physiotherapy. To ease the pain of surgery, they sometimes produced unconsciousness by compressing the carotid arteries, the name carotid deriving from *Karoun,* the Greek word for deep sleep. Always stressing moderation, Hippocrates cautioned his students and colleagues to observe carefully, proceed slowly, and exercise restraint in treatment, a philosophy admirably expounded in his aphorism "First do no harm."[6,11,12]

That the Greeks were independent and original thinkers we have no doubt. The magnitude of their minds stunned subsequent generations to the extent that the gross errors of the Greeks became indistinguishable from their magnificent triumphs, slavishly accepted as irrefutable law. The astonishing physiological inaccuracies of Plato and Aristotle stem from a common ignorance of human anatomy. We can only admire the fanciful flights of their richly speculative minds when they strayed. If we must condemn, the blame should be placed where it belongs, in gullible, locked-in-lesser minds that bought the packages without question.

The speculative physiology of Plato (427–347 B.C.), lacking the necessary substratum of anatomy, as with all Greeks since Alcmaeon, frequently becomes unintelligible to the modern reader. In *Timaeus,* Plato aspires to present a comprehensive account of the nature of man. The fundamental blending of mortal body with immortal soul entails a rather complicated commotion of atoms and elements in relation to a percipient soul scattered among a multiplicity of organs.[6] Pain is perceived by the soul in its several sites from the intrusion of the four elements, streaming into the body from without in disharmonious and violent motions. In Plato's system, the heart became the receiving and distribution center for sensory input. In deference to Alcmaeon, perhaps, the brain was allotted memory and reasoning. The liver harbored lust and other lower-level appetites. Sensations, entering the body as atoms in motion, were conveyed to the heart and somehow distributed in accordance with protocol to the souls residing in the various organs: To the brain went those sensations affecting mental processes and to the liver those likely to stir baser instincts. Retained in the heart were those related to love, pleasure, and nobler emotions. The size and shape of particles and the violence of the intruding motion graded the level of awareness by which they were perceived in the respective souls as pleasure or pain.[2]

Aristotle (384–322 B.C.), son of a physician, was surprisingly uninterested in medicine, but in biological matters he was superbly knowledgeable. The astonishing wealth of detail in his writings never restricts the broadness and complexity of his outlook. There is no reference to human dissection in his works, which deal exclusively with the comparative anatomy of animals. A teleological point of view permeates his thinking on structure and function. *De Partibus Animalius,* his major physiological treatise, reiterates the premise that everything has a design or purpose, as "nature never makes anything that is superfluous." It is sometimes difficult to reconcile the exquisitely detailed differentiations of form and function in his comparative anatomy with his completely erroneous ideas concerning the brain and heart. For Aristotle the heart was the seat of intelligence, emotion, and sensation; the brain was relegated to the specious role of thermostatic sponge for cooling the heart to prevent overheating. Vital heat in the heart's blood controlled sensitivity to pain. Flesh was the end organ from which pain sensation was conveyed by blood vessels to the heart, where it was perceived and dealt with in accordance with the heart's enormous proclivities for regulating reception and response. The irony of mistaken identification is compounded by the fact that it was Aristotle who coined the term *sensorium commune,* and the powerful effects of his prodigious output in all fields of knowledge gave his works a force of dogma that misdirected physiological research for 2000 years.[2,6,8]

With the death of Alexander in 323 B.C., and of Aristotle, his tutor, the following year, the glorious era of Hellenic Greece quietly faded from the center stage of history. The spotlight casually shifted across the Mediterranean Sea to a new and vigorously creative scientific community rising like a phoenix from the germinal ashes of a reawakening ancient culture.

ALEXANDRIAN INTERLUDE

For a brief moment in history the restraints imposed by dogma and tabu on scientific investigation were lifted to allow an unprecedented breath of fresh air for intellectual debate and expansion. This exciting interlude occurred in Alexandria, fertile culture and thriving crossroad for international commerce and learning. Under the enlightened suzerainity of Ptolemy, following the fragmentation of the Greek empire, a free spirit of inquiry acted as a magnet to attract bright young minds to long dormant problems in anatomy and physiology. Greek disdain for work with the hands was temporarily abandoned, as mind and technical skills were united for intensive study of the human body in health and disease. Inchoate dabbling at human dissection in preconfucian China and prebuddhist India had never really progressed to a level of fruitful revelation. Meaningful study of pain and discovery of a functioning nervous system were now possible under conducive circumstances.

Irresistibly drawn to Alexandria by the inviting intellectual climate, Herophilus (315–280 B.C.) of Chalcedon was the first great talent to address these problems. His extensive anatomical dissections on human cadavers identified the brain as the seat of motor and sensory function. He clearly distinguished between nerves and arteries and traced the course of nerves to and from the brain and spinal cord. Moreover, he recognized the function of these nerves in motor and sensory activities. His laboratory findings led him to speculate on the site of the soul; he placed it in the fourth ventricle.[12–14] These original observations were first challenged, then brilliantly expanded, a generation later by Erasistratus (310–250 B.C.) of Cheos. Erasistratus went into great detail describing and differentiating the cerebrum and cerebellum with their deep-lying system of ventricles and connecting foramina. Curiously, he chose to differ with Herophilus on the proper dwelling for the soul, ensconcing it somewhere in the cerebellum. He commented on the rich convolutional development of the human brain and hypothesized an association with intellectual capacity. He noted the constant tripartite company of artery, vein, and nerve along pathways subserving organs and other discrete anatomical parts. He identified the heart as a central pump propelling blood and air to all parts of the body and discredited it as a sensory organ.

All the original texts of these great contributions have disappeared in wars, fires, and cultural dissolutions, but medical historians have pieced together enough fragmentary accounts from Galen and other diverse sources to amply justify our recognition of Herophilus as the father of human anatomy and of Erasistratus as the founder of experimental physiology.[2,8,14] Celsus, the elegant translator and encyclopedic compiler of first century A.D. Rome, for reasons not disclosed, chose to ignore their work on the nervous system. However, in *De Re Medicina* he establishes their lofty status in other areas and specifically recounts their important practical interests in pain:[2,8]

> Moreover, as pain and also various kinds of disease arise in the internal parts, they hold that no one can apply remedies for these who are ignorant of the parts themselves: hence it becomes necessary to lay open bodies of the dead and to scrutinize their viscera and intestines . . . for when pain occurs internally, it is not possible for one to learn what hurts the patient unless he has acquainted himself with the position of each organ or intestine; nor can a diseased portion of the body be treated by one who does not know what that part is.

Centuries would pass before the fickle vehicle of human progress could renegotiate the brightly lighted pathways consummately laid out for us by our distant Alexandrian colleagues.

ROME

During the years when Rome evolved from a scattered assortment of tribal colonies to an orderly society, these sober, practical people remained remarkably unimpressed by the development of medical science in other parts of the world. Pain was something to be borne with magnanimity and stoic indifference, as is usually characteristic of the warrior mentality. For hundreds of years, ancient herbal lore and prayers or incantations to a variety of household gods served the Romans' unpretentious medical requirements. As waves of Roman legions spread out over the known world, the culture and finer representations of the conquered were preserved and absorbed. Greek medical arts were part of the bounty, and although the Romans never exhibited an enthusiasm to participate, they did often encourage and actively patronize some of the more gifted Greek practitioners. In a long poem, "De Rerum Natura," Lucretius (97–54 B.C.) an Epicurean disciple, brought a wide spectrum of Greek science to the attention of literate Romans. His physiology of pain, based upon the atomic theories of Democritus, stimulated considerable interest, but the Romans were doers, with an innate distrust for fanciful theorizing.[14] They were content with compilation and commentary as so admirably demonstrated by the works of Celsus (first century A.D.) and Pliny the elder (A.D. 23–79). It remained for Galen (A.D. 130–200), a Greek physician from Pergamon, to rescue the great achievements of the Alexandrians and to restore the concept of a central nervous system to explain the physiology of sensation.

Animal dissection supplemented by practical observations in his role as surgeon to the gladiators led Galen to much personal theorizing about psychological mechanisms. It is not possible to distinguish his own opinions from the knowledge he acquired of Herophilus and Erasistratus, but his systematized organization of data had a compelling ring of authority that appealed to church fathers, who later attached the stamp of dogma to his work. Galen's experiments on the spinal cord and peripheral nerves were richly rewarding in providing new information about motor and sensory enervation. He concluded that pain was the lowest form of conscious sensation, caused either by dissolution of continuity in tissues (cuts, burns, overdistention of hollow viscera) or by sudden violent commotion in the humors (pressure and tension). Unfortunately, Galen's physiology was contaminated by Aristotelian teleological influences. Instead of attempting to ascertain how organs and systems functioned, he sought to determine why, and this led his reasoning off on bizarre tangents at times. His doctrine of Vitalism, his belief in the transmission of blood from right to left heart through invisible pores, and his concept of suppuration as an essential part of healing sent medical theory off on senseless wild goose chases for centuries, yet his fruitful experimental physiology, his excellent anatomical descriptions, and his encyclopedic records of the knowledge of his time far outweighed his errors. Roman medicine died with Galen.[11,14,15]

DARK AGES

The Dark Ages between the fall of Rome and the Renaissance were truly dark, sterile, and regressive years for medicine. Crushed and devastated beneath succeeding ravages of war, famine, plagues, and economic chaos, the human spirit sank to unaccustomed depths of despair, mirroring the desolation of European civilization.[16] Christianity was the rallying force that restored some promise of salvation, but its triumph was a defeat for science. Physiological experimentation was dead under the oppressive weight of Church dogma that brooked no threat of challenge or contradiction. Pain was to be perceived in the light of Christian doctrine as a means of purification and redemption, for had not the sufferings of Christ endowed it with a touch of divinity? Mystical attitudes toward pain promoted martyrdom and gave voluntary suffering an exalted aura of spiritual beauty. Nature could never be questioned for her secrets. Medieval thinkers were restricted under the ban of authority to seek truth through logical deduction. The library replaced the laboratory as the source of discovery. It was a tedious period of scientific and intellectual decadence when Western concepts of medicine and pain deteriorated to primitive levels.[17-20]

ISLAMIC BRIDGE OF CULTURE

As the imperial majesty of Rome crumbled, and Western European civilization sank into the obscurity of the Dark Ages, a fresh spring of intellectual inspiration was flooding the arid lands of distant Persia. To Jundishapur and other Persian centers fled refugee scholars attracted by an unprejudiced climate for learning and the generous patronage of the ruling class. Hindu, Chinese, and native Persian influences blended with surviving vestiges of ancient Near Eastern cultures gathered by Jewish and Syrian scholars. This selective corpus of knowledge was richly expanded by Greek and Roman remnants brought by the Nestorians after their expulsion from Edessa in 489. In 529, the year of the founding of Monte Cassino, the Greek Academy was closed by Justinian because of its perverse pagan teachings. Many of its teachers escaped to Persia with priceless treasures of Greek learning that otherwise most certainly would have been destroyed. Far from the chaos and desolation of decadent Europe, a desert oasis had collected a colony of learned exiles who in their meager baggage but retentive minds had preserved the major sources of our visions of the ancient worlds. Most of what we know about the anatomy and physiology of pain we owe to the miraculous coincidences of time and place that made such a magnificent reservoir possible. The wonder is awesomely compounded by the subsequent course of events.

Following the death in 632 of Muhammad, Arab prophet and founder of Islam, Muslim hordes poured out of the Saudi Arabian desert, conquering all before them and proclaiming that "there is no god but God, and Muhammad is the messenger of God." These fanatical warriors carried their message triumphantly into Persia and India, and in one of the great paradoxes of all history, exhibited a tender and merciful regard for preserving the culture and properties of the conquered in deference to the veneration for knowledge and learning preached by their prophet. The true greatness of Muhammad is best exemplified in the Islamic doctrine "Science lights the path to paradise. Take ye knowledge even from the lips of the infidel. The ink of the scholar is more holy than the blood of the martyr." For this we are profoundly grateful; it was the guiding precept in the preservation of antiquity. Islamic centers of learning gathered scholars of all faiths and ethnic backgrounds. The school of medicine founded by the Nestorians in Jundishapur was the first of many spread out over the Arab world, and science flourished. Ancient Greek and Latin texts were translated by Jewish and Syriac philologists into Syriac and Hebrew, later into Arabic.

Persian centers dominated in the early years of Islam with new developments in chemistry and pharmacology and with the emergence of great medical writers. Al Rhazi (860–932) wrote extensively, elaborating on ancient ideas and contributing new ones. The most influential physician was another Persian: Avicenna, or Ibn Sina (980–1063).

His medical textbook, the *Canon,* exercised a persuasive influence over medical practice for centuries. Avicenna's notions of pain were drawn from his encyclopedic knowledge of Hippocrates, Aristotle, Galen, and Nemesius, a fourth-century Syrian. He recognized 15 varieties of pain produced by humoral changes that disturbed the natural state of things in the body. Not satisfied with the vague cerebral sensory centers of Galen, he followed the lead of Herophilus, who advocated a fourth-ventricle localization, but Avicenna distributed the sites more generously through the ventricles as suggested by Nemesius. From an extensive Arab pharmaceutical lore he extracted three groups of medicinals for relief of pain: those contrary to the cause, those that exert a soothing effect, and those that have anesthetic properties. Opium, herbane, and mandrake were liberally prescribed.

By the eleventh century the scientific and medical leadership had shifted westward to the Moorish capitals on the Iberian peninsula, largely dominated by Jewish scholars who reached great heights in medicine and philosophy under Islam. Jewish medicine, and pain treatment in particular, was basically rational, practical, and highly effective. With the creative energies of Islam exhausted, their decline coincided with a corresponding reawakening of long-slumbering cultural interests in Western Europe.[2,8,21,22] The priceless treasures of ancient learning, incubated in Persia and assiduously nurtured with loving care by their serendipitous conservators, had been borne across the Islamic bridge of culture to a revitalized Europe, eager to reclaim its lost heritage.

THE RENAISSANCE

In a growing spirit of confidence the minds of Renaissance men were awakened with a sense of excitement of two great discoveries: classical antiquity and themselves. These new-found interests produced an explosion of creativity and achievement in which medicine and science were bountiful participants. It was all made possible by a fruitful chemistry of unrelated, extraordinary interacting events, strategically centered, and affecting Western civilization at this particular time. The invention of printing most advantageously facilitated communication, as navigation broadened geographical perspectives and the idea of a heliocentric universe awesomely exposed a new universe. Gunpowder demolished the last strongholds of feudalism, and following the fall of Constantinople in 1453 a wave of fleeing Greek scholars fanned out over Europe to give the humanist movement the necessary impetus. A closer intermingling of the arts and sciences provided mutual benefits. Interest of the legal profession in autopsies spurred the revival of human dissection, which in turn was raised to a higher plane by the involvement of physicians in art and of artists in dissection. Berengarius, Vesalius, and Eustachius were notable anatomists with uncommon artistic skills, and of course, the

sublime Leonardo da Vinci was a skilled dissector whose great original anatomical discoveries and physiological speculations were mislaid for centuries.[17,23,24] Leonardo's extensive dissections on cadavers were conducted in secrecy for a very practical reason: survival. It was not selfishness or the need for further experimental proofs that led Da Vinci to devise mirror image note taking, nor devious purposes that caused him to conceal his findings. The specter of heresy still muted the creative urge. Church dogma and stultifying tradition dictated an attitude of caution for those adventurous souls who would peek beyond the curtain of authority to view the unknown. Leonardo's dissections focused on the ventricles, brainstem, and spinal cord, but there are voluminous notes on peripheral nerves and their functions. He described but did not recognize the significance of the sympathetic nervous system or the reflex arc. Experimenting with frogs, he found persisting sensation and motion after decerebration, but almost instant death when he pithed the medulla. He concluded that this must be the site of the soul. He regarded pain as a component or particularly intense aspect of the sensation of touch. His animal experiments included sensory mapping of anesthetic areas produced by cutting specific nerves. From these investigations he was motivated to speculate on the selective protectiveness of pain in vital areas for man's preservation.[2]

A more open and audacious anatomist was Vesalius, a Belgian lured to Padua by its superior facilities and academic opportunities, whose masterful technique and original inquiring mind unmasked the absurdities of Galenic animal dissections. His great work *De Humani Corporis Fabrica* (1543), brilliantly illustrated by woodcuts of Von Kalcar and possibly Titian and superbly printed by Oporinus at Basle, is one of the priceless treasures of the Renaissance. He brazenly refuted many established anatomical misconceptions and paid the price in character assassination and exile.[15,17,24] No less beautiful in design or accurate in detail are the exquisite copper plates of Eustachius, which, possibly because of the fate of Vesalius, remained unprinted until recovered from the Vatican library 162 years later.[18]

Religious proscriptions put an effective damper on the employment of pain-relieving drugs, although sporadic accounts of their use appear in the literature. Paracelsus rediscovered ether, the "sweet vitriol" of Ramon Lullus, when he mixed sulfuric acid and alcohol, and he was aware of its sleep-inducing qualities. Surgeons were known to use soporific sponges and physicians were well acquainted with the narcotic effects of opium, but these were dangerous times, when pain was considered an instance of God's will and the stake loomed as a threat to those who would ally themselves with the devil's work. Kings could "lay on hands" to accomplish miraculous cures; the lowly practitioner had to avoid the inquisitors of witchcraft and heresy. Nevertheless, carotid compression anesthesia was used by Ambroise Paré. Snow packs and other cold applications were used for local anesthesia, and a small body of rebellious free spirits, taking courage from the writings and example of Paracelsus, used atropine, belladonna, mandrake, and a host of medicinals for pain, as described in the splendid pharmaceutical books of Cordus and others.[2,8]

The inexorable march of progress gradually eroded the shackles of dogma and blind authority, but the process was slow and the course quite dangerous for those enlightened physicians and scientists who persisted in the struggle to conquer pain. Fortunately, the Renaissance had its share of courageous scientists to accept the challenges, and we are ever in their debt.

EARLY MODERN ERA

In the seventeenth century the chain of events initiated by Copernicus and substantially implemented by Kepler and Galileo culminated in the synthesis of Newton to complete the scientific revolution. This brought forth a rash of attempts to systematize all fields of knowledge. Efforts to demonstrate a system of medicine reflecting the same order as Newton's universe approached the ludicrous. Fanciful preoccupation with systems orientation diverted some of the better minds, and the mysteries of the central nervous system remained unresolved, but random individual contributions of enormous consequence were made in anatomy and physiology. However, it was not until 1800, when Bell and Magendie defined the roles of the anterior and posterior nerve roots, that pain physiology could step beyond the advances made by the Ancient Alexandrians. Meanwhile, scientific discovery was furnishing patchy pieces for the puzzle of pain as certain developments such as the birth of scientific societies and journals, the invention of the microscope, and a technological explosion were helping to organize and consolidate a solid foundation from which modern biological concepts could evolve.[23] Publication of William Harvey's (1578–1657) *De Motu Cordis* in 1628 did for physiology what the *Fabrica* had done for anatomy. Not only was the circulation of the blood proven by morphological, experimental, and mathematical arguments, but physiology itself was elevated on the strength of this discovery to the status of a dynamic science. Harvey's genius for inductive reasoning did not sustain him when he ventured into the realm of sensation, where his Aristotelian indoctrination misled him to view the circulating blood as the abode of the soul and the heart as the center of sensation and the seat of all natural motion.

Medieval mysticism continued to exert a crippling influence on scientific thought well into the nineteenth century. Iatrochemists made notable contributions to physiology and added to our comprehension of pain while introducing considerable confusion with their mysterious *archeus*, or spirit forces that governed bodily functions. Von Helmont (1577–1649), a follower of Paracelsus, was so fascinated by the stomach in his original studies on digestion that he made it the dominant organ of the body and resting place of the soul, holding dominion over consciousness, emotion,

and pain. Despite the confusing superimposition of circulating spirits on physiological systems, the iatrochemists were the first to introduce the idea of a physical transmission of nerve impulses in motor and sensory processes.[2]

In contrast to the carefully documented experimentation and inductive proofs of Harvey, the Frenchman René Descartes (1596–1650) developed his concepts of man as a machine out of pure deductive reasoning. Man functioned as any other machine, differing only in sensitivity and reasoning capacity. Descartes derived his physiology from Galen. Impressed by the delicately poised central position of the pineal gland he imbued it with a soul and imagined a sensory-motor response mechanism operating from the pineal gland that fits our concept of the reflex arc (*De Homine*, 1662).

With the passage of time, piece by piece, the knowledge of pain and effective means for its alleviation increased quantitatively. A somewhat amorphous mass of seemingly unrelated data awaited unscrambling and reorganization into a coherent theoretical structure for modern debate and methodical application to the problems of our times. Other chapters in this book deal with these problems, standing on the shoulders of the past to recapitulate the great progress that science has made to achieve our present sophistication in these matters. Still, the puzzle is far from solved. The enigma of pain is still with us. To cast a retrospective glance at the remote past is a pause that refreshes and assures us that we are not alone in our frustration. The task has always been arduous, and we must press on in the noble tradition of the great minds that have laid the groundwork for us.

References

1. Gurdjian ES. *Head Injury from Antiquity to Present with Special Reference to Penetrating Head Wounds.* Springfield, IL: Charles C Thomas; 1973.
2. Keele KD. *Anatomies of Pain.* Springfield, IL: Charles C Thomas; 1957.
3. Margotta R. In: Lewis P, ed. *The Story of Medicine.* New York: Golden Press; 1968.
4. Breasted JH. *The Edwin Smith Surgical Papyrus.* Chicago: University of Chicago Press; 1930.
5. Camac CNB. *From Imhotep to Harvey.* New York: Paul B. Hoeber; 1931.
6. Sarton G. *A History of Science: Ancient Science Through the Golden Age of Greece.* New York: Norton; 1952.
7. Methu DC. *The Antiquity of Hindu Medicine and Civilization.* New York: Paul B. Hoeber; 1931.
8. Seeman B. *Man Against Pain.* Philadelphia and New York: Chilton Company; 1962.
9. Agnew LRC. Medicine, history of. In: *The New Catholic Encyclopedia.* New York: McGraw-Hill; 1967.
10. Morse WR. *Chinese Medicine.* New York: Paul B. Hoeber; 1929.
11. Gordon BL. *Medicine Throughout Antiquity.* Philadelphia: F.A. Davis; 1949.
12. Singer CJ. *Greek Biology and Greek Medicine.* London: Oxford University Press; 1922.

13. Asimov I. *A Short History of Biology*. Garden City, NY: The Natural History Press; 1964.

14. Sarton G. *A History of Science: Hellenistic Science and Culture in the Last Three Centuries B.C.* New York: Norton; 1959.

15. Cumston CG. *An Introduction to the History of Medicine*. London: Dawson of Pall Mall; 1968.

16. Clark K. *Civilization: A Personal View*. New York: Harper & Row; 1969.

17. Ackerknecht EH. *A Short History of Medicine*. New York: The Ronald Press; 1968.

18. Garrison FH. *An Introduction to the History of Medicine*. 4th ed. Philadelphia: Saunders; 1929.

19. Reisman D. *The Story of Medicine in the Middle Ages*. New York: Paul B. Hoeber; 1935.

20. Walsh JJ. *Medieval Medicine*. New York: Macmillan; 1920.

21. Browne EG. *Arabian Medicine*. Cambridge, England: Cambridge University Press; 1921.

22. Simpson MWH. *Arab Medicine and Surgery*. London: Oxford University Press; 1922.

23. Boas M. *The Scientific Renaissance* 1450–1630. New York: Harper & Row; 1962.

24. Castiglione A. *The Renaissance of Medicine in Italy*. Baltimore, MD: Johns Hopkins Press; 1934.

PART ONE

Understanding Pain

CHAPTER 1

Pathophysiology of Pain

David Dubuisson

It seems reasonable to think that the best treatment of a given individual's chronic pain would depend on our most fundamental understanding, at a physiological level, of the source of discomfort. Too often, we try to mask pain with our treatments rather than trying to envision its source in the nervous system, and that is not logical. Seldom is it entirely clear whether the peripheral nervous system is responsible, or the central nervous system, or the autonomic system. Many clinicians continue to await modern diagnostic techniques and neuroscientific revelations that will make these distinctions clear, but the disheartening fact emerging from experimental pain research is that any damage or manipulation of one part of the nervous system may have profound effects on the rest.

The discussion that follows attempts to condense information from several well-established areas of pain research. It reviews some neuroanatomical and physiological topics relevant to pain, beginning with peripheral nerves and afferent channels and continuing through spinal cord, ascending and descending systems, neurotransmitters and neuropeptides, and conditions that produce analgesia. Finally, the topic of abnormal neuronal discharges after damage to the peripheral or central nervous system is discussed.

There is no single pain pathway. Instead there are many interlocking ascending, descending, and segmental neuronal systems that may transmit, block, or otherwise modify information relevant to pain.[1] These interactions may take place with a time course of milliseconds or days, depending on the circumstances, with remarkable plasticity of the accompanying physiological responses. After a painful injury, neuronal function appears to be quite disordered, not only within peripheral nerves but at high levels of the central nervous system. It is the physiologist's lot to try to find order amid this chaotic state.

DERMATOMES, RADICULAR PAIN, AND REFERRED PAIN

A clear idea of the source of chronic pain often requires some consideration of the organization of the spinal cord segments and the parts of the body to which they correspond.

The body surface is divided into overlapping sensory territories of the spinal and cranial nerve roots, called *dermatomes*. Several rather arbitrary charts of the dermatomes are available, but these charts do not agree in all details. Clearly, we need to know the amount of overlap of these nerve root territories and the extent of their variability among different individuals. We also need to know the extent of their plasticity, that is, whether they may change their shapes and locations over time, especially after trauma to the nervous system.

The body surface is mapped in a highly organized fashion within the gray matter of the spinal cord. Within each segment of the cord, it is possible to find a somatotopic representation of some portion of the body. For instance, in the lumbar segments, proximal parts of the limb are represented laterally in the gray matter, and distal parts of the limb are represented medially. Under some circumstances, this somatotopic organization may be disrupted. In the rat, when peripheral nerves to the foot are sectioned, cord neurons originally representing the foot take on new receptive fields in a more proximal territory.[2] Therefore it is quite likely that in some cases of chronic peripheral nerve damage, the spinal cord's representation of the body surface is no longer organized in a normal fashion.

The consistency of the profile of one dermatome on the body surface in the absence of injury is not known, but it is clear from the work of Foerster[3] that the dermatomes may vary tremendously from one individual to another. In addition, one dermatome may have two superficial territories, proximal and distal, which do not appear to be connected, as shown in Figure 1-1. Foerster's dermatomal diagrams were made by cutting several dorsal roots above and below the chosen cord segment, leaving only one intact.

An old rule of clinical neurology stated that each point on the body is represented by three overlapping dermatomes, but neural recordings in monkeys made it clear that the territory of each dermatome was sometimes even wider than this, and quite variable.[4] Moreover, the apparent size of a dermatome was shown to vary depending on the integrity of neighboring nerve roots and of superficial portions of the cord such as the Lissauer tract.[5,6]

Dermatome charts differ partly because observers have used different human subjects to compile the charts, and partly because observers have chosen different methods to determine the dermatomes. The charts by Head and

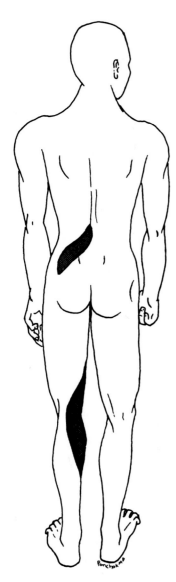

FIGURE 1-1. Completely separate proximal and distal portions of the third lumbar dermatome, by the method of remaining sensation after multiple nerve root section excluding the L3 root (after Foerster,[3]). (Illustration: Stephen Ponchak, M.D.)

Campbell[7] were based on the appearance of skin lesions in herpes zoster infections, which were thought to be restricted to the territories of single nerve roots. This was an unsafe assumption because the viral infection might have involved the adjacent roots or spinal cord. The dermatome charts by Keegan and Garrett[8] were designed from observations of many patients with disk protrusions. It was assumed that the zones of skin sensory loss were due to discrete compression of single nerve roots, which may not have been true in all cases. In this author's experience, it is unusual to see a long, continuous zone of sensory loss due to compression of a single nerve root. Instead, numbness may appear in only a small portion of the dermatome, such as the lateral aspect of the foot with first sacral root compression. It is also unusual to see actual pain in the hand or foot due to nerve root compression. Rather, the radicular pain is proximal while only numbness is felt distally.

For the reason just mentioned, it would be unwise to assume that pain in the foot or in the hand was due to nerve root compression. Likewise, it would be unwise to try to deny that a patient's pain in the back, neck, hip, shoulder, or scapular region could be due to a nerve root lesion simply because the location of pain did not look like a textbook dermatome. Only part of the dermatome might be involved, often the proximal part, or else muscles, joints, or ligaments innervated by the same root might be a location of referred pain due to the root lesion. These areas do not usually underlie the dermatome directly, so that pain due to cervical root compression can spread not only to the arm but also to the pectoral muscles, shoulder muscles, and scapular muscles (Fig. 1-2).

In the common event of disk protrusion, it is known that the constant dull aching pain in the neck or lower back may be due to stress in the annulus of the disk, where there are sensory nerve endings. The tiny nerve branches giving rise to these endings originate from the area of the dorsal root ganglion or just distal to it, and they pass retrogradely through the intervertebral foramen to reach the disk and surrounding ligamentous structures. In some cases, radicu-

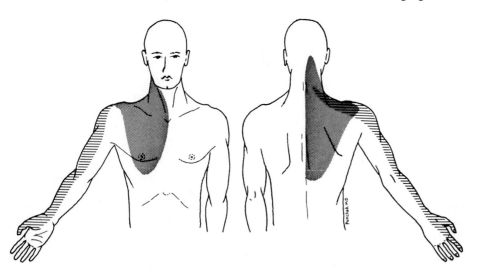

FIGURE 1-2. Distribution of referred pain (shaded area) in a case of C6 nerve root compression. Note that the pain in neck, back, and chest muscles does not correspond to the cutaneous distribution (cross-hatched area) of the nerve. (Illustration: Stephen Ponchak, M.D.)

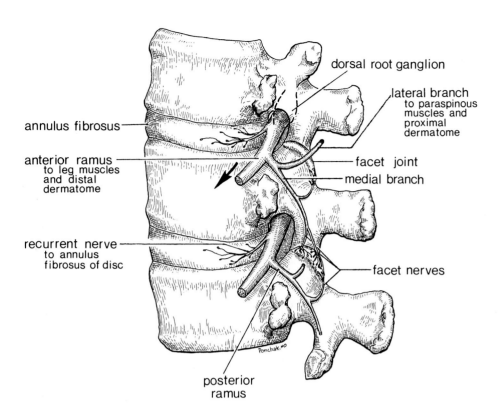

annulus fibrosus

anterior ramus
to leg muscles
and distal
dermatome

recurrent nerve
to annulus
fibrosus of disc

dorsal root ganglion

lateral branch
to paraspinous
muscles and
proximal
dermatome

facet joint

medial branch

facet nerves

posterior
ramus

FIGURE 1-3. Anatomical features of a typical lumbar nerve root. Branches to the spinal facet joints, disk annulus, and back muscles are present and may be sources of pain referred to the leg as sciatica. (Illustration: Stephen Ponchak, M.D.)

lar pain may occur despite the lack of myelographic evidence of root compression, suggesting that the pain is referred or falsely localized to the distal part of the dermatome (Fig. 1-3).

It appears very likely from the cumulative experience with local anesthetic injections in myofascial trigger zones, from acupuncture and related techniques, and from percutaneous procedures directed at the nerve supply of the spinal facet joints, that many cases of sciatica and radiating arm pain may in fact be due to local factors such as arthritis, tendon inflammation, or ligament strain causing sensitization or activation of sensory afferents and referred pain in the corresponding dermatome. Clearly it is important to search for such factors before choosing a treatment.

It is also known that local anesthetic blockade of a nerve or root distal to the cause of radiculopathy may nevertheless reduce pain.[9] This phenomenon is commonly seen in cases of trigeminal neuralgia where local block of a peripheral nerve branch temporarily relieves facial pain presumed to be due to a lesion at the root or ganglion level.

Presumably, local blockade of a root or peripheral nerve can reduce pain due to a lesion of an adjacent root or nerve because afferent fibers of adjacent nerve roots have synapses upon many cord neurons and some degree of summation must be required to activate dorsal horn cells (Fig. 1-4). Therefore we must be cautious about interpreting the results of root block or even peripheral nerve block. The range of spread of primary afferents from a single nerve root entering the cord is far wider than previously supposed. Wall and

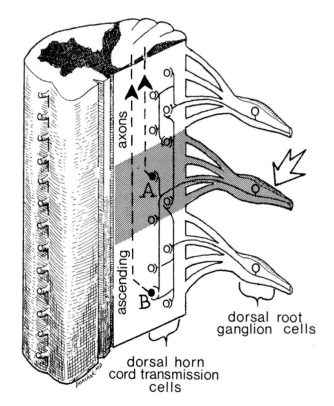

axons

ascending

A

B

dorsal root
ganglion cells

dorsal horn
cord transmission
cells

FIGURE 1-4. The concept of facilitation in the dorsal horn of the spinal cord. Application of a local anesthetic nerve root block (open arrow) decreases the synaptic input to cord transmission neuron in same cord segment (A) and also to cord cell in a neighboring segment (B) by means of long-ranging afferent branches. (Illustration: Stephen Ponchak, M.D.)

Werman[10] showed that afferents range over many segments of the cord. When the afferent inputs that usually drive a dorsal horn cell are removed, the cell may respond to afferent volleys in distant roots. It appears from the studies of Wall[11] that there are normally many ineffective synapses upon dorsal horn cells, and under appropriate circumstances they may become effective.

These physiological phenomena clearly illustrate that segmental pain need not involve an entire nerve root territory, that a root lesion may lead to referred pain in structures at some distance from the cutaneous zone of the root, and that stimuli anywhere within the broad territory of the segment concerned may influence the perception of pain in other parts of that territory, or perhaps even in other territories.

THE DORSAL HORN AND PRIMARY AFFERENT FIBERS

Our understanding of the detailed anatomical structure and of the physiology of the dorsal horn of the spinal cord has grown considerably in the last twenty years. In 1965, Melzack and Wall[12] proposed the gate control theory of pain, which hypothesized that a mechanism within the dorsal horn could act as a gate to admit or block afferent information from the periphery. It was suggested that activity in small afferent nerve fibers entering the dorsal horn tended to open the gate whereas activity in large fibers tended to close it. In this way, the discharge of large sensory transmission neurons in the cord gray matter could be regulated so that stimuli were perceived as noxious or innocuous. The precise synaptic arrangement responsible for this gate was a matter of some speculation at that time, but reasons were given to support the concept that smaller neurons in the substantia gelatinosa region of the dorsal horn acted as interneurons to adjust the gate.

When the gate control theory was published, electrophysiological recordings from neurons of the substantia gelatinosa had not been made. Now there is a great deal of information about these cells and about the primary afferent fibers which enter the dorsal horn, the ascending systems which leave the dorsal horn, and the descending systems which reach it from the brain stem.

Entering the dorsal horn from each dorsal rootlet are the terminations of numerous primary afferent fibers whose cell bodies are in the dorsal root ganglion. Some of these afferents are thickly myelinated and originate in hair follicles and other cutaneous end organs that detect innocuous stimuli.[13] Others are of small caliber, unmyelinated or thinly myelinated, and originate from receptors that respond primarily to intense stimuli such as heat, pressure, or noxious chemical substances.[14,15] Of these, there are two main cutaneous afferent fiber types which qualify as specific nociceptors. One is the high threshold mechanoreceptor with a small, thinly myelinated axon in the A delta range.

The other is the polymodal nociceptor in the C fiber range. The A delta axon responds to intense pressure over many points comprising a receptive field of perhaps a square centimeter, whereas the polymodal nociceptor responds to a variety of noxious stimuli such as pressure, heat, and irritant chemicals applied in a single punctate area. The substances that excite these C fiber nociceptors include bradykinin, histamine, serotonin, and sometimes substance P.[16] Responses to heat and to bradykinin are enhanced by prostaglandin (PGE_1.)[17]

These substances may be released by inflammation and tissue damage. Prior skin stimulation may sensitize the polymodal nociceptors to further stimulation. Sensitization occurs within minutes for heat, intense pressure stimuli, or skin injury, and may contribute to the development of cutaneous hyperalgesia after injury.[18] Polymodal nociceptors have been described in humans and may in fact make up 96 percent of the afferent C fiber population according to microneurography experiments.[19] Additional types of cutaneous afferent units have been described in laboratory animals and humans, but they are not considered here.

The substance capsaicin, derived from hot peppers, selectively destroys unmyelinated afferent fibers as well as some fine, thinly myelinated fibers if given to neonatal rats or mice.[20] This destruction is accompanied by analgesia in certain experimental tests of pain sensitivity. If capsaicin is applied to peripheral nerves of adult animals, it does not destroy these small fibers, but the excitatory effect of impulses traveling in them to the spinal cord is diminished.[21] Moreover, the peripheral receptive fields of neurons supplied directly or indirectly by these afferents are disorganized.[22] In addition to signaling acute noxious events, these fibers may somehow provide long-term information about the presence of tissue damage in the periphery.

In recent years there has been considerable interest in unmyelinated nociceptive afferents in the ventral roots of the spinal cord. Some of these fibers are known to have their cells of origin in the dorsal root ganglion. The axons may travel in the ventral root for some distance before looping back to enter the spinal cord through the dorsal root, or else some of them may carry sensory information from endings in the meninges around the spinal cord.[23]

The dorsal horn also receives central terminations of a variety of receptors in muscle, joints, and viscera.[24,25] Joint tissues have both myelinated and unmyelinated fibers, some of which respond selectively to noxious stresses.

It has been known for several decades that the neurons of the dorsal horn form laminar arrangements, with cells of a particular morphology tending to reside in particular layers of the gray matter.[26] We now know that different types of afferent fibers entering the dorsal horn also end in laminar zones so that they may contact only certain types of cord neurons. Nociceptive afferents terminate primarily in the superficial layers of the dorsal horn, and also in lamina 5.[27] The structure of the dorsal horn in the most caudal portion of the medulla, where it forms the nucleus caudalis of the trigeminal system, is comparable to that of the spinal cord.[28]

THE SUBSTANTIA GELATINOSA AND MARGINAL ZONE

The superficial layers of the dorsal horn are translucent in light microscopic sections, mainly because they lack myelinated afferent fibers. Rexed's lamina 2 and perhaps also lamina 1 are the equivalent of the substantia gelatinosa. These layers, and to some extent the deeper layers of the dorsal horn, contain numerous tiny neurons that appear to synapse locally. Some of them send axons into the nearby Lissauer tract where they mingle with fine afferent fibers before reentering the substantia gelatinosa.[29] These cells receive a mixture of afferent inputs including the terminations of nociceptive fibers from the periphery.

Some of the lamina 1 neurons project to the thalamus and respond only to noxious inputs.[30] They may include the majority of large, flat Waldeyer cells which characterize the marginal layer of the dorsal horn. Other lamina 1 cells are thought to have axons that ramify and terminate locally and do not project for long distances. Many lamina 1 cells contain opioid peptides such as enkephalin or dynorphin,[31] which is surprising given these cells' suspected role as pain transmission neurons.

In lamina 2 are two main cell types defined by Golgi stains and intracellular marking techniques: the stalked cells at the lamina 1–2 border, and the islet cells within layer 2.[32] The role of the substantia gelatinosa neurons that do not transmit information to rostral portions of the nervous system remains to be demonstrated, but it is already clear that some of these cells have unusual properties. Their receptive fields on the skin surface are frequently variable, and they may show spontaneous activity in the apparent absence of sensory stimuli.[29,33] Some cells of the substantia gelatinosa have peripheral receptive fields that may migrate to include a new cutaneous injury.[34] The smallest neurons may possibly transmit information to neighboring layers of the cord, lamina 1 or laminae 3 to 5. We do not know if the receptive fields of large neurons that project their axons to the brain stem or thalamus are composites of smaller fields of substantia gelatinosa neurons. It is increasingly evident that both large and small dorsal horn neurons may receive inputs not only from primary afferent fibers, which are predominantly excitatory, but also from neighboring dorsal horn neurons, which may be excitatory, inhibitory, or both.

The evidence that many of these neurons contain enkephalin and other neurally active peptides[35] suggests that they may form a network of local interneurons which act at the junction of the primary afferent fibers and the larger cord neurons which send their axons to the brain. Some lamina 2 cells are known to contain γ-aminobutyric acid (GABA), a known inhibitory neurotransmitter; others contain the peptide neurotensin.[36] The role of these substances in sensation is still entirely conjectural.

It has also been shown that the primary afferent fiber terminals within the substantia gelatinosa contain peptides such as substance P, vasoactive intestinal polypeptide, somatostatin, and an octapeptide similar to cholecystokinin.[37,38] These substances are depleted from the region by section of the peripheral nerve or root. Although there is a popular notion that these peptides may simply be neurotransmitters, it was shown that the central excitatory effect of a volley of nerve impulses in an intact nerve is the same as that produced by a similar volley in a cut nerve. This was true even at a time when peptides, including substance P, were depleted from afferent fiber terminals in the dorsal horn.[39]

Opiate receptors labeled by autoradiographic methods disappear from the substantia gelatinosa after root section,[40] which makes it tempting to speculate that a natural source of opioid peptides is the population of neurons in this region, and that enkephalin or a similar molecule could be released to fit the receptors on afferent fiber terminals. Some laboratory findings that are not inconsistent with this hypothesis are the effectiveness of opiate analgesics administered intrathecally[41] and the diminished release of substance P from afferent terminals after treatment of rat trigeminal nucleus with opiates in vitro.[42] There is also some evidence that microiontophoresis of morphine into the substantia gelatinosa can reduce the response of large transmission neurons deeper in the dorsal horn.[43]

The complex synaptic structures of the substantia gelatinosa include terminals of primary afferent fibers, terminals of local axons and dendrites, and terminals of brain stem neurons which descend to all levels of the cord. The substantia gelatinosa of the trigeminal nucleus caudalis in the medulla is very similar to the spinal cord substantia gelatinosa.

ASCENDING PROJECTIONS FROM THE DORSAL HORN

Two neuroanatomical techniques have given us new information about the morphology and laminar location of dorsal horn neurons, many of which give rise to long axons traveling rostrally in the ascending sensory tracts to reach the brain stem or thalamus. The first of these techniques is transport of horseradish peroxidase (HRP) retrogradely along the axons to label and visualize their cell bodies of origin. When HRP is injected into the thalamic sensory nuclei, it eventually labels cell bodies in the dorsal horn. The second technique is combined intracellular recording and dye labeling of single neurons. The target of a projecting axon can be identified by electrical stimulation, which sends impulses antidromically to the cell body where intracellular recording is taking place. Then dye is microinjected into the cell and appropriate histological methods demonstrate its individual morphology. Ascending axons relevant to pain sensation travel in nearly all portions of the spinal cord white matter, in several discrete systems. (Fig. 1-5).

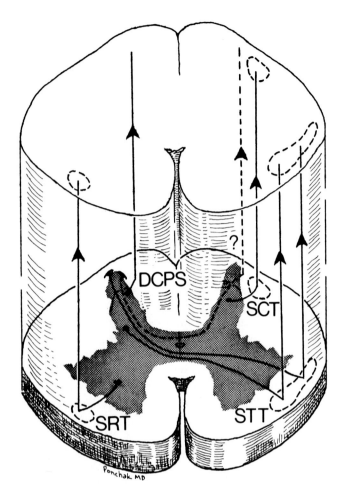

FIGURE 1-5. Axonal systems ascending the spinal cord in different quadrants. SCT = spinocervical tract. DCPS = dorsal column postsynaptic system. STT = spinothalamic tract. SRT = spinoreticular tract. Some lamina 1 cells may send axons into the opposite dorsolateral quadrant in an unnamed pathway. (Illustration: Stephen Ponchak, M.D.)

It is highly erroneous to assume that the transmission of all information about painful events takes place in the spinothalamic tract, although this still seems to be taught or implied in some major textbooks of medicine and neurology. Instead, we now know that some information about noxious stimuli travels rostrally in the spinocervical tract,[44] in the dorsal columns where some 15 percent of axons originate from dorsal horn neurons forming a second-order pathway,[45] and also in the crossed and uncrossed spinoreticular pathways which transmit from the dorsal horn to the brain stem reticular formation. In the rat, an additional pathway has been identified which leaves lamina 1 of the dorsal horn to travel in the opposite dorsolateral funiculus of the cord, transmitting information about a wide range of stimuli.[46] Some information about painful events may also ascend through the spinal gray matter in polysynaptic chains of neurons that do not form a discrete tract.[47]

In primates, dorsal horn neurons giving rise to spinothalamic tract fibers are situated mainly in laminae 1 and 5 to 8.[48] It appears that axons reaching the lateral thalamus, including the ventral posterolateral nucleus, tend to originate from layers 1 and 5 of the spinal cord. Axons projecting to some of the medial thalamic nuclei, including the intralaminar nuclei, are more likely to originate from layers 6 to 8.[48] This finding is in keeping with the concept that the intralaminar complex of the thalamus is related to the brain stem reticular formation, which receives axons of spinoreticular tract neurons situated mainly in laminae 7 and 8.[49] Some of the spinoreticular tract projections are ipsilateral, whereas the spinothalamic tract is predominantly a crossed pathway.

Dorsal horn neurons that project through the dorsal half of the spinal cord are seldom located outside laminae 3 to 5.[13] Spinocervical tract neurons, which send their axons rostrally to the lateral cervical nucleus at the cord–brain stem junction, are typically situated in layer 4 with dendrites extending dorsally. Cells of the dorsal column postsynaptic system (DCPS) are often located in laminae 3 and 4.[45] Their axons reach the dorsal column nuclei. Cells of the lateral cervical nucleus and the dorsal column nuclei project to the thalamus.

The brain stem and thalamic regions which receive information from these ascending systems project extensively to other diencephalic and forebrain structures, including the cerebral cortex[50] and the limbic system. In addition to their alerting function, these ascending systems may in turn trigger descending controls.

CONTROL OF SPINAL SENSORY NEURONS BY THE BRAIN STEM

The finding by Reynolds[51] that stimulation of certain discrete regions of the brain stem in rats produces analgesia was the beginning of an extensive line of research. In laboratory animals and in humans, electrical stimulation of the midbrain periaqueductal gray matter can produce impressive analgesia.[52–54] Electrophysiological studies in cats demonstrated that this type of stimulation directly activates medullary neurons which project axons to all levels of the spinal cord[55] and that it suppresses the responses of spinothalamic tract neurons in the cord.[56,57] Stimulation of brain stem analgesia-producing areas and of the dorsolateral funiculus where the brain stem neurons send their axons enhances the activity of some neurons in the substantia gelatinosa.[58–60] The analgesic effects of brain stem stimulation may outlast the actual period of stimulation in animals and in humans, and this phenomenon is sometimes matched by a similar prolonged period of alteration of cord cell activity. The existence of inhibitory interneurons in the dorsal horn has not been proven, nor has it been excluded.

In the animal model of stimulation-produced analgesia, it was shown that pharmacological agents that deplete serotonin from the central nervous system could interfere with the analgesic effect of brain stem stimulation.[61] In some of the regions in the medulla where this type of stimulation is quite effective, there are prominent cell groups that contain serotonin.[62] It has been demonstrated experimentally that the analgesic effect of brain stem stimulation depends upon the integrity of the midline raphe nuclei of the medulla and the adjacent reticular formation of the medulla where cell groups containing serotonin give rise to descending axons to the cord and trigeminal nucleus. In animals, after sectioning of the dorsolateral white matter of the cord, thereby interrupting descending aminergic pathways, analgesia is no longer produced in regions of the body caudal to the lesion.[63] Norepinephrine pathways have also been implicated in stimulation-produced analgesia, but their predominant effect is controversial. Tryptophan, the dietary precursor of serotonin, has been given to human patients as an adjunct to other treatments of pain. King[64] reported reexpansion of gradually diminishing zones of cutaneous sensory deficit following rhizotomy or cordotomy in five patients given tryptophan.

In light of the foregoing information, it is interesting to consider the possible relationship of endogenous depression and chronic pain. It is known that catecholamine and serotonin levels in the central nervous system may be depleted in cases of clinical depression. Since many patients experiencing chronic pain are also depressed, it is tempting to conclude that depletion of serotonin or another catecholamine neurotransmitter might contribute to both the depression and the failure of the patient's own brain stem analgesia-producing system to reduce pain. This provides a rationale for the use of antidepressant drugs such as amitriptyline in the treatment of chronic pain, since these drugs can augment catecholamine and indoleamine levels in the brain stem and spinal cord.

ENDOGENOUS OPIOID SUBSTANCES AND OPIATE RECEPTORS

Closely related to the descending analgesia-producing network are a group of endogenous opioid peptides. They include β-endorphin; leucine and methionine enkephalin; dynorphin and α-neoendorphin. These peptides have been identified by neuroanatomical methods in cells at all levels of the analgesia-producing system from the periaqueductal gray matter to the spinal cord. In all, over 20 different opioid peptides have been identified by biochemical techniques.[65] These peptides are derived from three types of larger prohormones, called proopiomelanocortin, proenkephalin A, and proenkephalin B, which are biologically inactive precursors. These large protein molecules are cleaved by proteolytic enzymes within the peptide neuron to form mixtures of smaller peptides. The enkephalins, which are the smallest known opioid peptides, are derived from proenkephalin A. The dynorphins, including α-neoendorphin, are formed from proenkephalin B and are intermediate in size. β-Endorphin, which is the largest opioid peptide, is formed from the proopiomelanocortin molecule. All of the opioid peptides contain N-terminal amino acid se-

quences identical to those of either met-enkephalin (tyr-gly-gly-phen-met) or leu-enkephalin (tyr-gly-gly-phen-leu). The three classes of opioid peptides (enkephalins, dynorphins, and β-endorphin) are genetically distinct and have different regional localizations within the central nervous system as well as different affinities for the various subclasses of opiate receptors.

Opiate drugs and opioid peptides exert their effects by interacting with receptors on the cell surfaces of neurons. The many peptides and opiate drugs are bound to the different subclasses of receptors with varying selectivities so that no one drug or peptide can be considered a perfect match for any particular receptor. Instead, a given opiate analgesic drug has a characteristic profile consisting of many different pharmacological actions mediated by subclasses of opiate receptors.

Opiate receptors are classified according to the drugs or endogenous peptides that bind to them strongly (Table 1-1). Morphine interacts strongly with μ-receptors; its antagonist naloxone also has high affinity for μ-receptors and far less affinity for other subclasses. One of the endogenous opioid peptides, methorphamide, derived from the proenkephalin A system, also binds selectively to μ-receptors. The enkephalins do bind to μ-receptors but are more selective for δ-receptors.[66] The endogenous ligand for κ-receptors is dynorphin: α-neoendorphin is also fairly selective for this receptor subclass.[67] β-Endorphin is selective for ϵ-receptors. Unfortunately, there is no simple relationship of opioid peptide precursor systems to opiate receptors, since the individual products of each precursor system activate several receptors with varying degrees of selectivity.[68]

Analgesia produced by opiates and opioid peptides is produced at many levels of the central nervous system. For the sake of simplicity, it is useful to consider actions at the level of the spinal cord and actions within the brain stem or at higher levels. There is much experimental evidence in support of a direct spinal analgesic effect of opiates, and this effect is probably mediated predominantly by δ-receptors. In animal studies, the selective δ-receptor agonist DADL (D-Ala, D-Leu-enkephalin) is a potent analgesic when given intrathecally, even to morphine-tolerant an-

Table 1-1

Opiate/Opioid Receptor Subtypes and Substances That Typically Bind to Them

Receptor Subtype	Ligand
μ	μ_1 = Opiate drugs; enkephalins μ_2 = Morphine
κ	Ketocyclazocine; dynorphin
δ	Enkephalins; DADL
σ	SKF 10,047
ϵ	β-endorphin

imals.[69] The same substance has been shown to be highly effective when given intrathecally to cancer patients with chronic pain.[70]

Morphine and other opiate drugs given systemically may act predominantly at supraspinal levels, via μ-receptors. This receptor type has been identified in the dorsal horn, but it is widespread in the periaqueductal gray matter, other regions of brain stem, and the limbic system. Several lines of evidence indicate that the induction of analgesia by electrical stimulation of brain stem structures involves one or more of the opioid peptides acting as a neurotransmitter or neuromodulatory agent. The analgesia produced by stimulation of the ventral medulla can be reversed by intraspinal injection of naloxone.[71] Microinjections of morphine into the brain stem can produce potent analgesia which is also blocked by naloxone.[72]

Some neuronal cell bodies in the periaqueductal gray matter contain dynorphin or enkephalin, and some axon terminals in the same region contain β-endorphin thought to be derived from more rostral cells of the hypothalamus.[73] Descending inputs to the periaqueductal gray matter from the hypothalamus have been demonstrated anatomically.[74] These inputs probably travel through the periventricular area where electrical stimulation in human patients is known to be effective in controlling chronic pain. Stimulation of the periventricular gray matter in human pain patients raises the levels of immunoreactive β-endorphin in the cerebrospinal fluid.[75] It is possible that the endogenous analgesia system is tonically active. If so, it appears that its action pertains mainly to prolonged noxious stimuli rather than to brief acute pain. For instance, the hyperanalgesic effect of naloxone in a rat model using the hot plate test was most evident at lower temperatures that is, when the baseline latency for the animal's response was prolonged.[76]

Certain stressful stimuli can induce analgesia. Among them are electric shock, rapid rotation, and perhaps needling or acupuncture. In a study of analgesic effects produced in rats by foot shock, it was shown that naloxone could block the analgesia only after prolonged stimulation.[77] This again suggests that the endogenous opioid system is involved only in chronic pain and not in instances of acute noxious stimuli. If narcotic drugs such as morphine share the receptors of this system, then these findings would be relevant to the failure of narcotics to prevent behavioral reactions to needles and other acute stimuli even when severe chronic pain is helped. The delayed and prolonged actions of opiates and opioid peptides may be appropriate for a role in chronic pain rather than acute responses, because of the slow natural process of peptide production. This involves gene transcription of large prohormone precursors in the neuronal cell body, secretion in granules by the Golgi apparatus, axonal transport, and processing of the precursor to yield active peptide fragments. Such a prolonged mechanism lasting hours or days would not be needed for immediate reactions to stimuli, but it might be very useful for long-term modulation of neuronal activity.

By this model, the opioid peptides might set the threshold of neuronal response in a sensory neuron or in its neighbors, while a classic neurotransmitter substance within the same cell could exert immediate effects at synapses to guarantee transmission of nociceptive information to the rest of the nervous system.

CONTROL BY LOW- AND HIGH-INTENSITY AFFERENT INPUTS

The gate control theory proposed by Melzack and Wall[12] gave impetus to the idea that pain could be reduced or suppressed by innocuous stimuli reaching the same spinal cord segment. It was hypothesized that activity induced mechanically or electrically in large diameter, low-threshold afferent fibers could interfere with the transmission of neural information relevant to pain.

Two major developments came about as a result of this hypothesis: the use of low-intensity transcutaneous electrical nerve stimulation (TENS) and trials of electrical stimulation of the dorsal columns of the spinal cord, from which abundant low-threshold primary afferent fiber collaterals reach the dorsal horn of the cord. The latter might be thought of as a type of massive afferent stimulus inducing a barrage of impulses in large-diameter fibers. In both cases, the interaction with small diameter, high-threshold afferents was thought to occur at the level of the dorsal horn, where the first of an ascending chain of synapses occurred. Both TENS and dorsal column stimulation were effective in relieving a wide variety of chronic pains,[78,79] and they continue to be used although technical failures and intolerance of these treatments by patients have limited their effectiveness.

It is known that low-intensity stimulation of afferent nerves in animals can produce analgesia[80] and inhibit large dorsal horn neurons.[81] Dorsal column stimulation inhibits spinocervical tract cells[82] while exciting units in the substantia gelatinosa.[34] Since these effects may occur in distant cord segments as well, a theoretical explanation for the clinical benefits of such treatments as massage, exercise, and ultrasound is available. These treatments may excite impulses in low-threshold afferent fibers, possibly blocking transmission through the dorsal horn.

A variety of pain remedies including acupuncture, dry needling, heat application, and brief intense electrical stimulation rely on the aftereffects of moderate or frankly noxious sensory inputs.[83] These may be applied to the body at a great distance from the painful area in some cases. There is ample evidence that intense stimuli such as high-threshold electrical stimulation can inhibit dorsal horn neurons even in distant cord segments.[84] The mechanism of this diffuse inhibitory effect is not fully known. Some of the effect may be mediated through brain stem circuits and some through local cord circuits. Whether opioid peptides are involved in the production of acupuncture analgesia is still debated. Naloxone was reported to reverse acupuncture analgesia[85] but not the analgesia produced by intense peripheral electrical stimuli.[86] The analgesic effect of high-intensity stimulation may outlast the period of stimulation for a long time, in some cases even for days. The mechanism of this prolonged effect is unknown.

ECTOPIC NEURONAL ACTIVITY AND LOSS OF CONNECTIONS

Several animal models have demonstrated that abnormal ectopic neuronal discharges may arise in peripheral nerves, roots, or ganglia, and in the central nervous system, when the afferent pathways are damaged. It is important to keep in mind that normal axons in the midportion of a nerve are not specialized to generate nerve impulses. Instead, normal nerve impulse generation occurs at receptors. When a normal nerve is distorted or cut, there is a brief injury discharge followed by electrical silence. Here we are considering abnormal, repetitive discharges which originate in axons or in central neurons that would normally be silent most of the time.

It has long been known that nerve injuries in humans can lead to severe chronic pain, often accompanied by unusual sensations (paresthesias). In the event of causalgia, which may follow injury of nerves such as the sciatic, median, and digital, there is often a burning sensation. The skin becomes oversensitive to touch in the territory of the damaged peripheral nerve,[87,88] and color changes may occur. Excitement and emotions may cause an exacerbation of pain. Inactivation of the efferent sympathetic nerve supply to the involved area, by sympathetic ganglion block, by regional perfusion of an extremity with reserpine or guanethidine, or by surgical sympathectomy, almost always relieves the pain.

Experimental neuromas of the rat sciatic nerve serve as a model of nerve injury in humans. When the rat sciatic nerve is sectioned and a neuroma is allowed to form, the animal typically begins to show behavior suggestive of abnormal sensation in the deafferented portion of the limb. Wall and Gutnick[89] demonstrated spontaneous activity arising from nerve fiber sprouts in such neuromas. This ectopic discharge occurred at a time when foot-biting behavior was evident.[90] Furthermore, discharges originating from a neuroma could be produced, or their frequency increased, by slight mechanical stimuli[91] and by application of adrenaline, noradrenaline, or phenylephrine.[92] These effects appear to be mediated by α-adrenergic receptors and support the idea that sympathetic outflow reaches the neuroma and triggers ectopic activity in sprouts of sensory afferents which have developed adrenergic chemosensitivity.[93] This sequence of events might take place in causalgia. Corticosteroids have been shown to decrease the amount of ectopic impulse generation in experimental neuromas of the rat sciatic nerve.[94] This finding may be relevant to the improvement of pain noted in humans following local steroid injection.

Dorsal root ganglia also develop sensitivity to mechanical stimuli and a tendency to generate ectopic afferent impulses after peripheral nerve injury.[95,96] This abnormal activity in dorsal root ganglia appears more likely to arise after chronic damage and scarring of the adjacent root or of the ganglion itself, which helps to explain the common occurrence of relentless sciatica and paresthesias related to radiculopathy in humans who have undergone repeated surgery for an entrapped spinal nerve root. Disk protrusion, facet joint enlargement, trauma, arachnoiditis, and epidural scar formation may all contribute.

We do not yet know whether abnormal afferent discharges originate from sites of nerve injury in humans with phantom limb pain, trigeminal neuralgia, or anesthesia dolorosa following nerve injury. The technique of percutaneous recording of single-fiber activity in injured human nerves has demonstrated ongoing spontaneous discharges at times when pain was felt,[97,98] so it does appear likely that the sort of ectopic activity seen in experimental preparations also occurs in humans. We do know that chronic, focal mechanical compression of the root of the trigeminal nerve by a tortuous artery or vein, a tumor, or a band of scarred arachnoid may lead to attacks of trigeminal neuralgia. It is quite likely that bursts of afferent discharges in the root originate near the site of pressure, where a zone of demyelination may occur. We do not know how innocuous stimuli such as washing the face might trigger such an afferent barrage.

Ectopic activity has also been reported in spinal cord neurons following deafferentation by dorsal root section.[99] Spontaneous activity may also originate at sites of focal demyelination in peripheral nerve.[100,101] Since many pathological processes may lead to loss of myelin, these experimental findings suggest that various types of peripheral nerve lesions may, even in the absence of frank axon transection, lead to abnormal neuronal discharges and perhaps pain. Further evidence in support of this concept is the finding that thalamic sensory neurons begin to show abnormal spontaneous discharges following deafferentation of a portion of the spinal cord.[102]

Some authors report high-frequency bursting discharge patterns of deafferented central neurons, in a fashion resembling that of cerebral cortical neurons in epilepsy. These findings are pertinent to the cases of chronic pain that respond to anticonvulsant drugs such as phenytoin and carbamazepine. These drugs are sometimes effective in cases of painful peripheral neuropathy, suggesting that abnormal generators of nerve impulses may be present. Perhaps the greatest use of anticonvulsants has been in cases of trigeminal neuralgia. Although the mode of action of anticonvulsant drugs in these cases may be partly to suppress a central discharge, we know that in many of these cases, a tortuous blood vessel or other lesion compressing the trigeminal nerve root can be identified. As mentioned above, it is quite possible that lesions such as this cause focal demyelination of the trigeminal root, and that the demyelinated segment of nerve acts as a source of ectopic discharge. It has been postulated that anticonvulsants may also suppress this abnormal peripheral discharge.

Deafferentation pain may also arise from lesions within the central nervous system, at any level of the neuraxis, usually after a delay, and often with unusual sensory qualities and poor somatic localization.[103] The chronic pain syndromes associated with deep cerebral hemisphere infarctions (thalamic syndrome) and cavitation of the spinal cord (syringomyelia) are well-known examples which are particularly difficult to treat. Pain is a frequent problem in cases of paraplegia due to spinal cord injury, in which the afferent pathways of the cord are totally disrupted, yet pain occurs at the level of injury and below it. The success of the radiofrequency dorsal root entry zone lesion technique for this condition[104] indicates that the damaged part of the cord and the partially deafferented segments just above it may serve as sources of abnormal neuronal discharge.

Some central lesions produce demyelinative changes. Indeed, a variety of pain syndromes may occur in cases of multiple sclerosis. They include burning dysesthesias, radicular pains, and tic douloureux indistinguishable from the pain of idiopathic trigeminal neuralgia. Anticonvulsant drugs are equally effective for the neuralgia associated with multiple sclerosis. In many of these cases, demyelinative plaques have been identified at the entry zone of the trigeminal nerve. It has been shown experimentally that spinal cord axons in a zone of focal demyelination may discharge spontaneously during mild mechanical stresses.[105] It is not unreasonable to suppose that ectopic discharges may originate centrally in demyelinative lesions, not only in the plaques of multiple sclerosis but in the vicinity of certain types of cavities, ischemic zones, and infarcts of the brain or spinal cord. If these discharges originated in sensory systems transmitting information relevant to tissue damage or other intense peripheral stimuli, falsely localized pain might occur.

CONCLUSION

Our comprehension of pain relies increasingly on the current state of knowledge of the structure and function of all parts of the nervous system. Clearly, there are substantial differences in the physiology of simple nociception and that of chronic deafferentation. Since the nervous system appears to have diverse intrinsic mechanisms of controlling sensory input, our goal must be to understand the efferent mechanisms of pain as well as the afferent.

Even though the appearance of ectopic activity at multiple levels after injury to the nervous system may suggest that our treatments of chronic pain are futile, the plasticity of responses and of receptive fields of central neurons, and the variety of neurotransmitters and other substances relevant to pain and analgesia make it likely that as our understanding of basic physiology advances, many new means of controlling pain will be found.

References

1. Helme RD, Gibson S, Khalil Z. Neural pathways in chronic pain. *Med J Aust* October 1, 1990; 153(7):400–406.
2. Devor M, Wall PD. Plasticity in the spinal cord sensory map following peripheral nerve injury in rats. *J Neurosci* 1981; 1:679–684.
3. Foerster O. The dermatomes in man. *Brain* 1933; 56:1–39.
4. Dykes RW, Terzis JK. Spinal nerve distribution in the upper limb: the organization of the dermatome and afferent myotome. *Philos Trans R Soc Lond* [Biol] 1981; 293:509–554.
5. Kirk EJ, Denny-Brown D. Functional variation in dermatomes in the macaque monkey following dorsal root lesions. *J Comp Neurol* 1970; 139:307–320.
6. Denny-Brown D, Kirk EJ, Yanagisawa M. The tract of Lissauer in relation to sensory transmission in the dorsal horn of the spinal cord of the macaque monkey. *J Comp Neurol* 1973; 151:175–200.
7. Head H, Campbell AW. The pathology of herpes zoster and its bearing on sensory localization. *Brain* 1900; 23:353–523.
8. Keegan JJ, Garrett FD. The segmental distribution of the cutaneous nerves in the limbs of man. *Anat Rec* 1948; 102:409–437.
9. Kibler RF, Nathan PW. Relief of pain and paresthesiae by nerve block distal to the lesion. *J Neurol Neurosurg Psychiatry* 1960; 23:91–98.
10. Wall PD, Werman R. The physiology and anatomy of long ranging afferent fibers within the spinal cord. *J Physiol* 1976; 255:321–334.
11. Wall PD. The presence of ineffective synapses and the circumstances which unmask them. *Philos Trans R Soc Lond* [Biol] 1977; 278:361–372.
12. Melzack R, Wall PD. Pain mechanisms: a new theory. *Science* 1965; 150:971–979.
13. Brown AG: *Organization in the Spinal Cord*. New York: Springer-Verlag; 1981.
14. Bessou P, Perl E. Response of cutaneous sensory units with unmyelinated fibers to noxious stimuli. *J Neurophysiol* 1969; 32:1025–1043.
15. Light AR, Perl E. Spinal termination of functionally identified primary afferent neurons with slowly conducting myelinated fibers. *J Comp Neurol* 1979; 186:133–150.
16. Fitzgerald M, Lynn B. The weak excitation of some cutaneous receptors in cats and rabbits by synthetic substance P. *J Physiol* 1979; 293:66–67P.
17. Handwerker HO. Influences of algogenic substances and prostaglandins on the discharges of unmyelinated cutaneous nerve fibers identified as nociceptors. *Adv Pain Res Ther* 1976; 1:41–45.
18. Lynn B. Cutaneous hyperalgesia. *Br Med Bull* 1977; 33:103–108.
19. Torebjork HE. Afferent C units responding to mechanical, thermal and chemical stimuli in human non-glabrous skin. *Acta Physiol Scand* 1974; 92:374–390.
20. Lynn B. Capsaicin: actions on nociceptive C-fibres and therapeutic potential. *Pain* April 1990; 41(1):61–69.
21. Wall PD, Fitzgerald M. Effects of capsaicin applied locally

to adult peripheral nerve. I. Physiology of peripheral nerve and spinal cord. *Pain* 1981; 11:363–377.

22. Wall PD, Fitzgerald M, Nussbaumer JC, Van der Loos H, Devor M. Somatotopic maps are disorganized in adult rodents treated with capsaicin as neonates. *Nature* 1982; 295:691–693.

23. Chung JM, Lee KH, Coggeshall RE. Nociceptive role of ventral root afferents. In: Fields HL, Dubner R, Cervero F, eds. *Advances in Pain Research and Therapy,* vol 9. New York: Raven Press; 1984:103–109.

24. Mesulam M-M, Brushart TM. Transganglionic and anterograde transport of horseradish peroxidase across dorsal root ganglia: a tetramethyl benzidine method for tracing central sensory connections of muscles and peripheral nerves. *Neuroscience* 1979; 4:1107–1117.

25. Mense S, Light AR, Perl ER. Spinal terminations of high threshold mechanoreceptors. In: Brown AG, Rethelyi M, eds. *Spinal Cord Sensation.* Edinburgh: Scottish Academic Press; 1981:79–85.

26. Rexed B. The cytoarchitectonic organization of the spinal cord in the cat. *J Comp Neurol* 1952; 96:415–466.

27. Fitzgerald M. The course and termination of primary afferent fibers. In: Wall PD, Melzack R, eds. *Textbook of Pain.* London: Churchill-Livingstone; 1984:34–48.

28. Gobel S, Falls WM, Hockfield S. The division of the dorsal and ventral horns of the mammalian caudal medulla into eight layers using anatomical criteria. In: Anderson DJ, Matthews B, eds. *Pain in the Trigeminal Region.* Amsterdam: Elsevier; 1977:443–453.

29. Wall PD, Merrill EG, Yaksh TL. Responses of single units in laminae 2 and 3 of cat spinal cord. *Brain Res.* 1979; 160:245–260.

30. Perl ER. Afferent basis of nociception and pain: evidence from the characteristics of sensory receptors and their projections to the spinal dorsal horn. In: Bonica JJ, ed. *Pain.* New York: Raven Press; 1980:19–45.

31. Basbaum AI. Functional analysis of the cytochemistry of the spinal dorsal horn. In: Fields HL, Dubner R, Cervero F., eds. *Advances in Pain Research and Therapy,* vol 9. New York: Raven Press; 1985:149–175.

32. Gobel S. Golgi studies of the neurons in layer 2 of the dorsal horn of the medulla (trigeminal nucleus caudalis). *J Comp Neurol* 1978; 180:395–414.

33. Dubuisson D, Fitzgerald M, and Wall PD. Ameboid receptive fields of cells in laminae 1, 2 and 3. *Brain Res* 1979; 177:376–378.

34. Gibson SJ, Polak JM, Wall PD, Bloom SR. The distribution of nine peptides in rat spinal cord, with special emphasis on the substantia gelatinosa and on the area around the central canal (lamina X). *J Comp Neurol* 1981; 201:65–79.

34. Dubuisson D. *The Descending Control of Substantia Gelatinosa.* London: University of London; 1981. Ph.D. Dissertation.

35. Otsuka M, Yanagisawa M. Pain and neurotransmitters. *Cell Mol Neurobiol* September 1990; 10(3):293–302.

36. Hunt SP. Cytochemistry of the spinal cord. In: Emson PC, ed. *Chemical Neuroanatomy.* New York: Raven Press; 1983:53–84.

37. Tiseo PJ, Adler MW, Liu-Chen LY: Differential release of substance P and somatostatin in the rat spinal cord in response to noxious cold and heat; effect of dynorphin

A(1–17). *J Pharmacol Exp Ther* February 1990; 252(2):539–45.

38. Carr DB, Lipkowski AW. Neuropeptides and pain. *Agressologie* April 1990; 31(4):173–177.

39. Wall PD, Fitzgerald M, Gibson SJ. The response of rat spinal cord cells to unmyelinated afferents after peripheral nerve section and after changes in substance P levels. *Neuroscience* 1981; 6:2205–2215.

40. Lamotte C, Pert CB, Snyder SH: Opiate receptor binding in primate spinal cord. Distribution and changes after dorsal root section. *Brain Res* 1976; 112:407–412.

41. Yaksh TL, Rudy TA: Analgesia mediated by a direct spinal action of narcotics. *Science.* 1976; 192:1357–1358.

42. Jessell TM, Iverson LL. Opiate analgesics inhibit substance P release from rat trigeminal nucleus. *Nature* 1977; 268:549–551.

43. Duggan AW, Hall JG, Headley PM. Suppression of transmission of nociceptive impulses by morphine: selective effects of morphine administered in the region of substantia gelatinosa. *Br J Pharmacol* 1977; 61:65–76.

44. Brown AG, Hamann WC, Martin HF. Descending influences on spinocervical tract cell discharge evoked by non-myelinated cutaneous afferent nerve fibers. *Brain Res* 1973a; 53:218–221.

45. Brown AG, Fyffe REW. Form and function of dorsal horn neurones with axons ascending the dorsal column in cat. *J Physiol* 1981; 321:31–47.

46. MacMahon SB, Wall PD. A system of rat spinal cord lamina 1 cells projecting through the contralateral dorsolateral funiculus. *J Comp Neurol* 1983; 214:217–223.

47. Basbaum AI. Conduction of the effects of noxious stimulation by short fiber systems in the spinal cord of rat. *Exp Neurol* 1973; 40:699–716.

48. Willis WD, Kenshalo DR Jr, Leonard RB. The cells of origin of the primate spinothalamic tract. *J Comp Neurol* 1973; 188:543–574.

49. Kevetter GA, Haber LH, Yezierski RP, Chung JM, Martin RF, Willis WD. Cells of origin of the spinoreticular tract in the monkey. *J Comp Neurol* 1982; 207:61–74.

50. Talbot JD, Marrett S, Evans AC, Meyer E, Bushnell MC, Duncan GH. Multiple representations of pain in cerebral cortex. *Science* March 15, 1991; 251(4999):1355–1358.

51. Reynolds DV. Surgery in the rat during electrical analgesia induced by focal brain stimulation. *Science* 1969; 164:444–445.

52. Fields HL, Basbaum AI. Brainstem control of spinal pain transmission neurons. *Ann Rev Physiol* 1978; 40:192–221.

53. Hosubuchi Y. Subcortical electrical stimulation for control of intractable pain in humans. *J Neurosurg* 1986; 64:543–553.

54. Kumar K, Wyant GM, Nath R. Deep brain stimulation for control of intractable pain in humans, present and future: a ten-year follow-up. *Neurosurgery* May 1990; 26(5):774–782.

55. Lovick TA, West DC, Wolstencroft JH. Responses of raphe spinal and other bulbar raphe neurones to stimulation of the periaquaductal grey in the cat. *Neurosci Lett* 1978; 8:45–49.

56. Willis WD, Haber LH, Martin RF. Inhibition of spinothalamic tract cells and interneurons by brain stem stimulation in the monkey. *J Neurophysiol* 1977; 40:968–981.

57. Morgan MM, Gold MS, Liebeskind JC, Stein C. Periaqueductal gray stimulation produces a spinally mediated, opioid antinociception for the inflamed hindpaw of the rat. *Brain Res* April 5, 1991; 545(1–2):17–23.

58. Dubuisson D, Wall PD. Descending influences on receptive fields and activity of single units recorded in laminae 1, 2 and 3 of cat spinal cord. *Brain Res* 1979a; 199:283–298.

59. Dubuisson D, Wall PD. Medullary raphe influences on units in laminae 1 and 2 of cat spinal cord. *J Physiol* 1979b; 300:33P.

60. Dubuisson D. Time course of descending excitation of single units recorded in laminae 1, 2 and 3 of cat spinal cord. *J Physiol* 1980; 307:56–57P.

61. Akil H, Mayer DJ. Antagonism of stimulation-produced analgesia by a serotonin synthesis inhibitor. *Brain Res* 1976; 44:692–697.

62. Eide PK, Hole K. Interactions between serotonin and substance P in the spinal regulation of nociception. *Brain Res* June 7, 1991; 550(2):225–230.

63. Basbaum AI, Marley NJE, O'Keefe J, Clanton CH. Reversal of morphine and stimulus-produced analgesia by subtotal spinal cord lesions. *Pain* 1977; 3:43–56.

64. King RB. Pain and tryptophan. *J Neurosurg* 1980; 53:44–52.

65. Terenius L. Families of opioid peptides and classes of opioid receptors. In: Fields HL, Dubner R, Cervero F, eds. *Advances in Pain Research and Therapy,* vol 9. New York: Raven Press; 1985:463–477.

66. Lord JAH, Waterfield AA, Hughes J, Kosterlitz HW. Endogenous opioid peptides: multiple agonists and receptors. *Nature* 1977; 267:495–499.

67. Wuster M, Rubini P, Schultz R. The preference of putative pro-enkephalins for different types of opiate receptors. *Life Sci* 1981; 29:1219–1227.

68. Hope PJ, Fleetwood-Walker SM, Mitchell R. Distinct antinociceptive actions mediated by different opioid receptors in the region of lamina I and laminae III-V of the dorsal horn of the rat. *Br J Pharmacol* October 1990; 101(2):477–483.

69. Tung S, Yaksh TL. In vivo evidence for multiple opiate receptors mediating analgesia in the rat spinal cord. *Brain Res* 1982; 247:75–83.

70. Moulin DE, Max M, Kaiko RF, et al. The analgesic efficacy of intrathecal D-Ala-D-Leu-enkephalin (DADL) in cancer patients with chronic pain. *Pain* 1985; 23:213.

71. Zorman G, Belcher G, Adams JE, Fields HL. Lumbar intrathecal naloxone blocks analgesia produced by microstimulation of the ventromedial medulla in the rat. *Brain Res* 1982; 236:77–84.

72. Levine JD, Lane SR, Gordon NC, Fields HL. A spinal opioid synapse mediates the interaction of spinal and brain stem sites in morphine analgesia. *Brain Res* 1981; 236:85–91.

73. Fields HL, Basbaum AI. Endogenous pain control mechanisms. In: Wall PD, Melzack R, eds. *Textbook of Pain.* London: Churchill-Livingstone; 1984:142–152.

74. Beitz AJ. The organization of afferent projections to the midbrain periaqueductal grey of the rat. *Neuroscience* 1982; 7:133–159.

75. Hosubuchi Y, Rossier J, Bloom FE, Guillemin R. Stimulation of human periaqueductal grey for pain relief increases immunoreactive β-endorphin in ventricular fluid. *Science* 1979; 203:278–281.

76. Jacob JJ, Tremblay EC, Colombel M-C. Facilitation des reactions nociceptives par la naloxone chez la souris et chez le rat. *Psychopharmacologia* 1974; 37:217–223.

77. Lewis JW, Cannon JT, Liebeskind JC. Opioid and non-opioid mechanism of stress analgesia. Science 1980; 208:623–625.

78. Simpson BA. Spinal cord stimulation in 60 cases of intractable pain. *J Neurol Neurosurg Psychiatry* March 1991; 54(3):196–199.

79. Spiegelmann R, Friedman WA. Spinal cord stimulation: a contemporary series. *Neurosurgery* January 1991; 28(1):65–70; discussion 70–71.

80. Woolf CJ, Mitchell D, Barret GD. Antinociceptive effect of peripheral segmental electrical stimulation in the rat. *Pain* 1980; 8:237–252.

81. Woolf CJ, Wall PD. Chronic peripheral nerve section diminishes the primary afferent A-fiber mediated inhibition of rat dorsal horn neurones. *Brain Res* 1982; 242:77–85.

82. Brown AG, Kirk EJ, Martin HF. Descending and segmental inhibition of transmission through the spinocervical tract. *J Physiol* 1973b; 230:689–705.

83. Melzack R. Acupuncture and related forms of folk medicine. In: Wall PD, Melzack R, eds. *Textbook of Pain* London: Churchill-Livingstone; 1984:691–700.

84. Le Bars D, Dickinson AH, Besson JM. Diffuse noxious inhibitory controls (DNIC). I. Effects on dorsal horn convergent neurones in the rat. *Pain* 1979; 6:283–304.

85. Mayer DJ, Price DD, Rafii A. Antagonism of acupuncture analgesia in man by the narcotic antagonist naloxone. *Brain Res* 1977; 121:368–372.

86. Sjolund BH, Ericksson MBE. Endorphins and analgesia produced by peripheral conditioning stimulation. In: Bonica JJ, Albe-Fessard D, Liebeskind JC, eds. *Advances in Pain Research and Therapy,* vol 3. New York: Raven Press; 1979:587–599.

87. Kayser V, Basbaum AI, Guilbaud G. Deafferentation in the rat increases mechanical nociceptive threshold in the innervated limbs. *Brain Res* February 5, 1990; 508(2):329–332.

88. Levitt M. The theory of chronic deafferentation dysesthesias. *J Neurosurg Sci* April–June 1990; 34(2):71–98.

89. Wall PD, Gutnick M. Properties of afferent nerve impulses originating from a neuroma. *Nature* 1974; 248:740–743.

90. Scadding JW. The production and prevention of experimental anesthesia dolorosa. *Pain* 1979; 6:175–182.

91. Scadding JW. Development of ongoing activity, mechanosensitivity, and adrenaline sensitivity in severed peripheral nerve axons. *Exp Neurol* 1981; 73:345–364.

92. Korenman EMD, Devor M. Ectopic adrenergic sensitivity in damaged peripheral nerve axons in the rat. *Exp Neurol* 1981; 72:63–81.

93. Devor M. Nerve pathophysiology and mechanism of pain in causalgia. *J Autonom Nerv Syst* 1983; 7:371–384.

94. Devor M, Govrin-Lippmann R, Raber P. Corticosteroids reduce neuroma hyperexcitability. In: Fields HL, Dubner R, Cervero F, eds. *Advances in Pain Research and Therapy,* vol. 9. New York: Raven Press; 1985:451–461.

95. Howe JF, Loeser JD, Calvin WH. Mechanosensitivity of dorsal root ganglia and chronically injured axons: a physi-

ological basis for radicular pain of nerve root compression. *Pain* 1977; 3:25–41.

96. Wall PD, Devor M. Sensory afferent impulses originate from dorsal root ganglia as well as from the periphery in normal and nerve-injured rats. *Pain* 1983; 17:321–339.

97. Ochoa H, Torebjork HE. Paraesthesia from ectopic impulse generation in human sensory nerves. *Brain* 1980; 103:835–854.

98. Nystrom B, Hagbarth KE. Microelectrode recordings from transected nerves in amputees with phantom limb pain. *Neurosci Lett* 1981; 27:211–216.

99. Loeser JD, Ward AA. Some effects of deafferentation on neurons of the cat spinal cord. *Arch Neurol* 1967; 17:629–636.

100. Rasminsky M. Ectopic excitation, ephaptic excitation, and autoexcitation in peripheral nerve fibers of mutant mice. In: Culp WJ, Ochoa J, eds. *Abnormal Nerves and Muscles as Impulse Generators*. New York: Oxford University Press; 1982:344–362.

101. Calvin WH, Devor M, Howe J. Can neuralgias arise from minor demyelination? Spontaneous firing, mechanosensitivity, and after-discharge from conducting axons. *Exp Neurol* 1982; 75:755–763.

102. Albe-Fessard D, Lombard MC. Use of an animal model to evaluate the origin of and protection against deafferentation pain. In: Bonica JJ, Lindblom U, Iggo A, eds. *Advances in Pain Research and Therapy,* vol. 5. New York: Raven Press; 1981:691–700.

103. Rinaldi PC, Young RF, Albe-Fessard D, Chodakiewitz J. Spontaneous neuronal hyperactivity in the medial and intralaminar thalamic nuclei of patients with deafferentation pain. *J Neurosurg* March 1991; 74(3):514–521.

104. Nashold B, Bullitt E. Dorsal root entry zone lesions to control central pain in paraplegics. *J Neurosurg* 1981; 55:414–419.

105. Smith KJ, MacDonald WI. Spontaneous and evoked electrical discharges from a central demyelinating lesion. *J Neurol Sci* 1982; 55:39–47.

CHAPTER 2

Pain Measurement

Peter White

Clinical pain is a persistent, unbearable personal experience that is often uncontrollable and accompanied by a level of stress or depression, often incapacitates physically and emotionally, and can totally disrupt and overwhelm the behavior of the sufferer. It prevents coherent thought and drives the patient to seek treatment or relief from the pain. Acute pain differs from chronic pain, not just in duration and intensity or the fact that acute pain is more closely linked to identifiable pathology, but because the noxious stimulus is more readily identifiable. In chronic pain particularly, there is no correlation between the amount of pathology and the degree of pain. Pain behavior lingers, often long after the pathologic process has healed.[35]

According to an accepted model, pain consists of four components, namely nociception, sensation, suffering, and behavior.[36] The term *pain* is a label that is loosely applied to all sorts of different unpleasant experiences. The actual perception of this state is based on a whole list of modifiers ranging from the memory of previous painful events to psychological influences including a state of stress,[31] an alteration in mood, and an expectation of treatment and recovery. Pain is not merely a sensory experience but rather a result of the processing that has gone on at a higher level.[97] The development of the signal detection theory recognized the complexity of neural processing of the pain signal by the brain.[16] It contends that the brain is not a passive receptacle for neural sensory or pain input but is rather a continually active processor of many sensory inputs that include nociception. The perception of pain sensation by the organism is determined by the resultant balance of all influences. Suffering is manifest in a physiologic or behavioural way. Malow has demonstrated that stress, in the form of induced anxiety, decreases pain sensitivity and reported pain experience when measured by verbal and physiologic indices.[89]

What do pain physicians themselves believe are appropriate, useful diagnostic tests? Physicians displayed substantial agreement about the differential utility of 18 common physical examination and diagnostic procedures such as plain radiography, CT scan, and electromyography.[128] However, there is little consensus and less empirical basis from which to choose the most appropriate instrument of pain measurement. Pain measurement is in evolution.

Categorization has changed as our methods of measurement and assessment have been developed and refined.[62]

When studying clinical pain, it is often impossible to examine the relationship between nociception and the pain response, since in certain chronic pain syndromes, such as phantom limb pain and trigeminal neuralgia, the original stimulus is absent. Consequently, to assess the pain experience, measurement instruments have traditionally relied upon subjective reporting, focusing on sensation, suffering, and behaviour rather than on nociception.

To categorize pain measurement, authors such as Frederickson[39] have recommended a subjective/objective approach. Pain variables such as intensity, frequency, and quality of pain are amenable to subjective (self-report) methods. Disability, expressed as a lack of mobility, an inability to work, or difficulty in interpersonal relationships, and pain behavior manifest as facial grimacing, vocalization, and posturing can be readily observed and measured. Similarly, the effects of therapy and other interventions can be quantified objectively.

An example of pure objective measurement is seen in the laboratory setting: The pain experience is artificially produced and potential variables can be controlled. These experiments are usually of short duration and involve healthy volunteers. Classically, a nociceptive stimulus can be standardized and inferences of the sensory experience are made by measuring the provoked response. No actual measurement of the pain experience has been made.

Another approach to pain measurement is based on the method of the assessment, for example, self-report, observed behavior, and physiologic approaches.[14,118,138] This is easily understood. Since pain is a personal experience, the only way we as physicians can judge a patient to be in pain is (1) to either rely on a description by the patient of the pain characteristics or effects, (2) to observe resultant behavior, or (3) to measure physiologic parameters that we believe to be characteristic of a patient in pain.

A comprehensive approach to chronic pain assessment is that recommended by Williams, who suggested that the information necessary to make the measurement could be grouped into six categories: physical, functional, behavioral/cognitive, emotional, economic, and sociocultural. He also reviewed the reliability and validity of each of the proposed measures.[154]

TYPES OF MEASUREMENT

Physical measures such as location of pain can be reliably assessed by self-report, whereas the spatial aspects of pain can be ascertained by the pain drawing. Physical symptoms can be assessed by self-report measures such as the Wisconsin Brief Pain Questionnaire.[22] Instruments such as the pressure algometer in myofascial trigger point studies[64,107] or the gnathodynamometer following dental extraction[55] allow objective pain measurement in specific pain syndromes. Measuring EMG activity of the frontal and temporal musculature has some usefulness in headache pain assessment.[7,113]

Functional measures include verbal or instrument quantification of uptime/downtime to assess 24-hour activity.[32,34,129] Physical, communicative, and social disabilities can be measured in several ways, including such valid and reliable self-report instruments as the Sickness Impact Profile,[3] the Health Assessment Questionnaire,[40] and the Pain Disability Index.[140] These measures are reliable and valid and provide considerable information on the ability of patients to care for themselves. As well, there are instruments such as the Activity Pattern Indicator,[36,126] a 64-item self-report measure, which provides information on the patient's actual functioning in terms of work and recreational activity, and the Chronic Illness Problem Inventory,[116] which can also assess the ability of patients to care for themselves. Another valid measure of function is to assess the ability of the patient to walk a standard distance.[23]

Information about the *behavioral/cognitive* aspects are measurable either observationally or by self-report measures. Behavior such as the amount of drugs needed,[70,87] the number of physician visits,[54] and assessment of nonverbal observable behavior such as posturing, limping, and guarding[72,73]; facial grimacing[29,63,68,83]; or sleep habits and ability to cope[11,127,143] are all appropriate measurable parameters. The Illness Behavior Questionnaire[114,150] is a reliable clinically useful instrument to test the neurotic symptoms of pain behavior such as denial, hypochondriasis, and somatic concern, although recent work has suggested the need to reconsider some of the items.[88]

Depression and anxiety are *emotional* factors which are often associated with the pain experience and are assessed by the administration of the Minnesota Multiphasic Personality Inventory and the Beck Depression Scale. The *sociocultural* factors on which information may be required include such areas as litigation, patient independence, quality of life,[140] family dynamics, and patient goals.

And what about the tests themselves? Do they reliably and sensitively measure what they are expected to measure? Unidimensional scales, such as the visual analog and the verbal category scales, are regularly used and are considered accurate measures of pain intensity. However, their use is limited because they do not reflect the complexity of the pain experience. Instruments such as the McGill Pain Questionnaire, because of their multidimensional approach, are believed to more truly reflect the many aspects of the pain experience.

The clinician expects a high correlation between the patient's report of behavior and observable behavior. There is often, however, marked disparity when comparing a patient's own assessment of acute pain with physician ratings of the same patient's pain experience.[37] Furthermore, the physician can strongly influence a patient's pain intensity ratings by antecedent reinforcement of pain talk or well talk.[152]

Why Measure Pain?

The initial measurement of the pain experience is valuable for several reasons. First, it produces a baseline on which to assess future therapeutic interventions. It is important to assess the degree of impairment or disability for therapeutic or compensation reasons. Many of the test instruments have discriminatory merit and may aid the clinician in diagnosing a specific condition. As well, certain test instruments have the specific ability to differentiate between the true sufferer and the malingerer[156] and to evaluate the influence of personality on the pain experience.[82,157]

What Are the Ideal Test Characteristics?

An ideal test should be reasonably simple to administer and directed at a level that most patients can understand. It should be accurate and reliable. As well, a test instrument must fulfill the criteria of validity and sensitivity and possess reliable scaling properties, free of random bias. Of these characteristics, reliability and validity are the two most important.[20]

An instrument is reliable if test scores provided by the same individual on two separate occasions are similar. The greater the consistency, the greater the reliability. There are three common types of reliability: internal consistency, test–retest reliability, and interrater reliability. For a questionnaire to be *internally consistent,* there should be a wide range of questions of single scale items. *Test–retest reliability* assesses the ability of the instrument to be repeated at intervals and to produce the same results over time. If two assessors of the same instrument produce the same results, then the measure has *interrater reliability.*

Validity is the extent to which a test measures what it is supposed to measure. There are many types of validity, including content, construct, and concurrent. A test has *content validity* if it assesses valid qualities that are reasonable and appropriate representatives of the particular entity that is being measured. For example, if a test assesses known characteristics of pain such as location, intensity, and interference with daily activities, it has content validity. The extent to which scores on the test behave as one would theoretically expect them to behave is *construct validity.*

A scale should also be as sensitive as is feasible. If intensity is the particular quality of pain that is to be measured, then the scale should cover the whole dimension of intensity. The more points within the scale, logically the more accurate the measurement should be. For example, a 7-point scale is an improvement over a 5-point scale.

SPECIFIC METHODS OF MEASUREMENT

Self-Reported Information

The personal nature of pain means a physician or pain therapist can only confirm the patient's report of pain by observing the resultant behavior and making an interpretation based on its consistency with known pain behavior.

The last 15 years have seen a proliferation of pain measurement instruments of varying complexity, which can collect and assess data of a subjective nature. The earliest and simplest self-report tests, such as the visual analog scale or simple descriptive scales continue to be used because of their ease of application and simplicity of understanding by both patient and clinician. This type of testing is limited because it tests only one dimension of pain at a time. More complex methods such as the McGill Pain Questionnaire, which analyzes the choice of word descriptions, can assess pain on several levels.

The self-report, verbal form of assessment is said to be limited because it relies heavily on the ability of the patient to recall pain. Studies have shown, however, that patients do retain accurate recall of specific pain experiences.[28,58,99,158]

On occasion, it may be necessary, because of language, intellectual, or functional difficulties such as ventilator dependence, to use next of kin or significant others to supply information about the patient's pain experience. O'Brien and Francis did confirm using the McGill instrument, that those individuals who lived with a patient with cancer pain and who professed a knowledge of the pain were able to closely match the patient's estimate of pain.[110]

There are inherent limitations in relying upon self-reporting measures. To accept self-reporting of pain behavior as a valid instrument, there must be consistency between what the patient says and what he or she does. There are often contradictions as exemplified by the work of Ready and associates, who reported on pain medication usage by pain patients in a hospital setting and found that there was a significant discrepancy between reported narcotic usage at home and that observed by hospital staff.[123] The patients tended to underreport their narcotic usage. Women, for reasons unknown, showed more tendency to underreport, than men. This contrasts with the work of Follick and associates who, in an outpatient setting, found a high correlation between self-report of activity, in the form of a pain diary, and that measured objectively by a electromechanical device.[32] The value of self-reporting can be influenced by compensation status;[8] use of drugs, in particular alcohol, benzodiazepines, and narcotics[53]; whether patients believe they are being observed[9]; and their treatment expectation.[61] Physicians' expectations can also introduce bias.[46] Nevertheless, the quality of information that can be derived from many self-report test instruments should not be underestimated.

SINGLE-DIMENSION SUBJECTIVE MEASURES

Visual Analog Scale (VAS):

This linear scale is the visual representation of a range of pain that a patient believes he or she might experience. It can take several forms, either as a pain scale or as a pain relief scale.[59,133] The range is represented by a line, usually 10 cm in length, with or without marks at each centimenter. The optimal length for measuring pain seems to be 10 cm.[135] Anchors at each end may be numerical or descriptive: One end represents "no pain" while the other represents "the worst pain the patient could possibly imagine." Other VAS variants include a numbered calibrated line 10 cm long, a series of adjoining boxes numbered 0 to 10, or a thermometer-like representation.

No pain at all ―――――――――――――. **The worst pain imaginable**

The scale is scored by the patient, who is asked to draw a mark on the line that represents the level of pain being experienced. The distance measured in millimeters from the lower anchor represents a measure of the particular modality which is being quantified. This can be readily reproduced over time. Visual motor errors, which are a measure of the patient's ability to accurately and reliably place the mark on the line, are minimal in young healthy patients.[60] There appears to be no difference between scores chosen whether the scale is presented vertically or horizontally.[25,134]

The VAS type of measurement has the advantage of simplicity. It is widely used and is independent of language. It is easily understood by most patients and can be readily reproduced on successive presentations.[124] Children from age 7 can understand it.[1] It is readily sensitive to a change in pain level when assessing the value of a specific treatment. It is far more accurate than a verbal category scale of pain relief which has insufficient words of ascending severity to critically grade pain relief.[111] The VAS can be used to scale pain at specific moments in time but is better limited to current rather than remembered pain experience.[85] Of the types of VAS, the absolute or unmarked line is less sensitive to bias.[12]

The disadvantage of this instrument is that it treats the pain experience as if it were monodimensional. It emphasizes intensity without due regard to other factors. There tends to be a grouping at the center numbers with greater reproducibility at the extremes of the line and at the midpoint.[60]

Another criticism is that the scale imposes limits by making the extremes absolute. Although "no pain" or "complete relief" is undisputably an absolute measure, the other anchor is not. The "worst pain one can imagine" leaves no room for even worse pain at a later time.

Not all patients can complete the VAS, there being a

quoted failure rate of 7 percent.[133] Responses to the VAS are influenced by several various biases affecting psychophysical responses.[43] It requires a certain amount of visual and motor coordination, which may be lacking in the postoperative period,[5] and measurements may be difficult to perform after anesthesia, when the patient may have trouble concentrating.[53,109]

A variant of the VAS is the *pain relief scale*, the anchors defining the degree of pain relief. The patient is asked to mark, on the line between the anchors, the amount of pain when compared to an earlier time.

No relief   **Complete relief**

0%————————————100%

Verbal Numerical Scale (VNS)

The VNS is a simple verbal pain rating scale with similarities to the VAS. It is linear and shows good correlation with the VAS over its full range.[108] The VNS is easily understood by the patient who merely chooses a number between zero and 10 to represent the level of pain.

No pain at all   **The worst pain imaginable**

0 1 2 3 4 5 6 7 8 9 10

The VNS eliminates the need for visual and motor coordination required to complete the VAS and is more likely to be completed.[108] It appears to be more useful than the VAS for pain measurement in the early phases of the postoperative period. Failure to complete the scale is of the order of 2 percent.[81] It may be easier to use than a VAS.[12]

Another *pain relief scale* is a variant of the visual numerical scale. The anchors define the degree of pain relief; zero indicates no relief while ten indicates complete relief.[59]

Other variants of the VAS include one that offers a series of facial expressions ranging from smiling through crying, often a helpful tool in children.

No relief   0 1 2 3 4 5 6 7 8 9 10   **Complete relief**

Verbal Rating Scale (VRS)

The verbal type of scale is the simplest and most likely to be completed because patients prefer verbal scales to the visual analog or numerical rating scales.[81] Scales defining pain intensity as mild, moderate, severe, or absent[74] or no pain, mild, discomforting, distressing, horrible, and excruciating as appears in the Present Pain Intensity Index of the McGill Pain Questionnaire are simple and easy to administer. Similarly, pain relief can be defined as none, slight, moderate,

or good. Distances between word descriptors on this scale are assumed to be equal.[86]

This scale has been shown to be sensitive to dosage and to sex and ethnic differences. The scale is superior to the visual analogue scale in assessing the effects of analgesics on acute pain.[111]

The verbal scale is limited because it offers a restricted choice of words that represent pain[24] and therefore does not allow for finer pain assessment.

MULTIDIMENSIONAL DESCRIPTIVE REPORTS

The Pain Diary

The pain diary is a personal, self-reported oral or written account of day-to-day experience and behavior. It is frequently used in the pain clinic context and has been used as an aid to diagnosis.[17] These reports are usually reliable and are a satisfactory method of monitoring day-to-day variation of the disease state and its response to therapy.[74,159] These measurements are dependent upon an accurate recording, by the patient, of common daily activities.

The patients are asked to make notes of pain intensity, particularly in relation to particular behavior such as:

Daily activities such as sitting, standing, and lying down
Sleep patterns
Sexual activity
Specific tasks
Pain medication taken
Meals eaten
Housekeeping activities performed
Recreational activities pursued

A pain diary has been included within the context of a larger instrument, for example, within the Pain Perception Profile[144] and the Dartmouth Pain Questionnaire.[19]

The information elicited from a pain diary has a use in clinical research. It is a more accurate record of actual drug ingestion than memory recall, considering that a patient relying on memory alone to recall drug use will tend to underestimate it, particularly if that drug is a narcotic.[123]

Pain Drawings

When pain drawings are used, patients are typically asked to shade in areas within a human figure outline or diagram corresponding to their area of pain sensation at specific times. Children from the age of 8 can reliably and validly complete this task.[131]

The drawing may be useful for assessing both the location and distribution of the pain and becomes a permanent record within the patient's chart.[90] Rating systems have been devised by Ransford and associates[117] and Margolis and associates.[92] The pain drawing may also be used to assess the changes of pain in response to therapy. It has been suggested that a visual representation may help the clinician in diagnosis and in selecting a rational form of therapy. This test, as a measure of percentage of body surface and location of pain, can be easily used by nonexpert assessors and has a high degree of test–retest reliability over time.[91]

There have been some differences of opinion about the psychological significance of these drawings.[42,112,117,131] It has been suggested that an analysis of the drawings could differentiate between the psychological and physical contributions to pain.[131,145] This view has been disputed.[42,56,149] Ransford and associates proposed that, when administered specifically to back pain patients, the pain drawing can identify those patients with a hysterical or hypochondriac psychological state as described by the MMPI.[11] Von Baeyer has disputed this specific proposition.[149]

This test instrument appears to have discriminatory ability. Patients, many of whom were involved in litigation stemming from their injury and disability, were given this test instrument.[132] Certain drawings were rated as inappropriate by an investigator who was blind to the patients' psychological and legal state. The patients whose drawings were so labeled were later identified as being involved in litigation and showed themselves to be more somatically preoccupied, obsessive, and hostile. They reported a higher level of general distress than patients whose pain drawings were rated as appropriate and who were not involved in litigation.

In summary, pain drawings are useful in assessing the site and distribution of pain, but they have certain limitations. They do not measure the actual intensity of pain. The instrument is inadequate for the measurement of pain in discrete areas, for example, headache. Certainly, there is a need for more objective criteria to assess the drawings, to avoid overinterpretation, and to determine the actual relationship between the significance of the pain drawing and psychological distress.

An alternative approach to the application of the pain drawing is its use in the assessment of pain in the pediatric population. The limited verbal ability of small children precludes the use of verbal self-reports of pain experience or pain behavior, hence the reliance on nonverbal or observed behavior techniques. One such technique described by Unruh and colleagues compared drawings made by a pediatric pain population of themselves in pain and categorized these drawings on the basis of color and content.[146] The result of their study confirmed the validity of color and content categorization. Their study also suggested that this method may have discriminative ability at least between children with musculoskeletal pain and headache.

The Faces Pain Scale

The measurement of pain in children is difficult but challenging. There is much more reliance on objective methods of data collection than occurs in adult pain assessment. An innovative nonverbal method is the use of a faces pain scale. These scales generally consist of sets of facial expression drawings that depict changes of severity of expressed pain (Fig. 2-1).

Several faces scales have been independently developed to overcome the cognitive complexity and metaphoric difficulty needed in many self-report, adult pain assessment instruments. Children do not have the verbal facility and conceptual understanding that adults possess, nor do they have the ability even to perform the visual analog scale until at least age 7.[1] Simply, children grade their pain by choosing the picture that represents their level of pain experience.

The Oucher, a well-known faces scale,[2,4] consists of a white cardboard poster with six photographs of a 3-year-old boy in increasing levels of pain on the right side, and a 0 to 100 scale on the left. The scaling is arbitrary, and children experience difficulty in establishing correspondence between two sets of two orders. Also, older children may not relate well to this very young face.[6]

The face scale of Frank and associates has a category scale that uses eight cartoon faces varying in expression from tears and misery to apparent laughter.[38] When this test was compared to an analog rating scale, there was good correlation with scores based on picture selection. Other face scales include those of McGrath and associates,[94] Maunuksela and associates,[93] and Whaley and Wong (see Fig. 2-1).[151] These tests, which include a smiling face at the no-pain end, have been criticized because its position assumes a continuous pleasure–pain dimension.[6]

More recently, Bieri and associates have introduced their own scale which contains a set of seven schematic faces that had been derived from several sets of drawings made by first- and third-grade children.[6] The subjects are simply told to point to the face that represents their level of pain. The response is scored by applying the scale number to the chosen face. These sets were found to be simple, easy to use, and nonverbal. They required minimal instruction. The pictures have been graded so that the facial differences are reasonably equidistant. They avoid the criticism of introducing the pleasure–pain dimension by ensuring that none of the faces on the presented cards are smiling. The scale ranges from no pain to the most pain possible. This

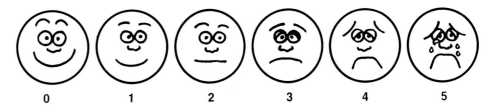

FIGURE 2-1. The Whaley and Wong faces pain rating scale. (Reproduced with permission from Whaley LF, Wong DL. *Nursing Care of Infants and Children.* 4th ed. St. Louis, MO: Mosby Year Book; 1991.)

test can be used in children from at least the age of 6 and possibly as early as the age of 2 years.

Wisconsin Brief Pain Questionnaire

Cancer pain often has an insidious onset, may involve many sites, and is frequently multicausal. Consequently, it is often difficult to assess with the better known pain test instruments.[24] The Wisconsin Brief Pain Questionnaire,[22] originally introduced to briefly assess pain in cancer, was designed to avoid some of the deficiencies of the McGill Pain Questionnaire (MPQ). The MPQ fails to assess such details as history of the pain and its interference with the patient's daily activities. It is time-consuming, and individual instruction may be needed to complete the test.

The Wisconsin Brief Pain Questionnaire contains 17 questions. It is self-administered and easily understood, and it can be easily completed unless the patient is most unwell. It uses simple instruments such as a pain drawing and verbal numerical scales to simplify the task. It assesses relevant pain data such as history, intensity, location, quality, and interference with everyday activities. It also examines the effects of pain upon the patient's mood and enjoyment of life.

Overall the test appears to have adequate reliability and validity. It is easy to administer either by an interviewer or by self-administration, and information is equally reliable. It does not address such issues as the emotional significance of pain or the situational influences of pain behavior. It has equal usage in noncancer forms of pain.

Self-Report: Use of Word Descriptors

The belief that language can provide a means of describing the pain experience was introduced by Dallenbach in 1939.[21] He created five groups of word descriptions which represented such characteristics of pain as its quality, time course, and emotional association.

In 1971 Melzack and Torgerson furthered this work on adjectival descriptors by using their own groups of words to represent several dimensions of pain.[101] In their original presentation, they included 102 words derived from the literature on clinical pain and grouped these words into classes and subclasses according to the similarity of their meaning. An independent panel further pruned the choice of words. The final selection of word descriptors were said to represent three interrelated but distinct components of the pain experience: affective, sensory, and evaluative dimensions. This three-dimensional idea of pain has been supported by factor analysis.[115] The groups of pain words were incorporated into a pain measurement instrument known as the Pain Rating Index which was incorporated into the McGill Pain Questionnaire.[96]

Using experimental psychophysical methods to substitute words that describe the sensory and unpleasant qualities of pain, it is possible to validate the use of word descriptors as representatives of the pain experience.[45] To independently confirm the discriminatory ability of words, Gracely and associates demonstrated that the use of a benzodiazepine anxiolytic, diazepam, resulted in changes of affective but not sensory word choices.[50] The same authors, using the narcotic agent fentanyl, applied the same method of cross-modality matching to induced dental pain and demonstrated a change in the choice of intensity but not sensory descriptors.[47]

Physicians have been found to agree on the use of word descriptors to discriminate between pain syndromes. The more involved they are in the care of pain patients, the more they value this mode of assessment. However, for reasons unclear, they rate word descriptors as being more useful for acute than chronic pain patients.[141] Chronic pain patients often have interrelated problems that are too complex to be reliably discriminated by simple word sets.[36]

There has been considerable examination of the appropriate word descriptors which could be incorporated into a pain questionnaire for use in a pediatric population.[1,41,67] Wilkie and associates recently published a list of 56 word descriptors that appear relatively free of gender, ethnic, and developmental bias for use in a pediatric population.[153] This list appears to have test–retest reliability and acceptable content and construct validity for potential use in the clinical situation.

The McGill Pain Questionnaire (MPQ)

In its final form, the MPQ instrument consists of four different parts.[96] The first part consists of a human figure drawing on which patients indicate their pain location (Fig. 2-2).

The second part, known as the Pain Rating Index, contains 78 adjective words divided into 20 groups. Each set contains up to 6 words in ascending order of quality. Ten of these groups describe sensory qualities in terms of temporal, spatial, thermal, and other properties and five are affective descriptors describing qualities such as tension, fear, or autonomic properties. A single set describes the evaluative dimension, while the remaining four groups are miscellaneous and contain words specific for certain conditions. Each word is assigned a value according to its position within its subclass. Patients are shown the word descriptors and requested to circle with a pen or pencil those words which most accurately describe their pain.

The third part supplements the measure by asking additional questions about prior pain experience and its location as well as information on current usage of pain medication.

The fourth part consists of the the Present Pain Intensity index (PPI). This scale is essentially a VRS of 0 to 5 with particular word descriptors such as "no pain," "mild," "discomforting," "distressing," "horrible," and "excruciating."

The test is administered in the following way. The particular words chosen are scored according to a predetermined rank, such that the word in each group implying the least severity is assigned a value of 1, the next least

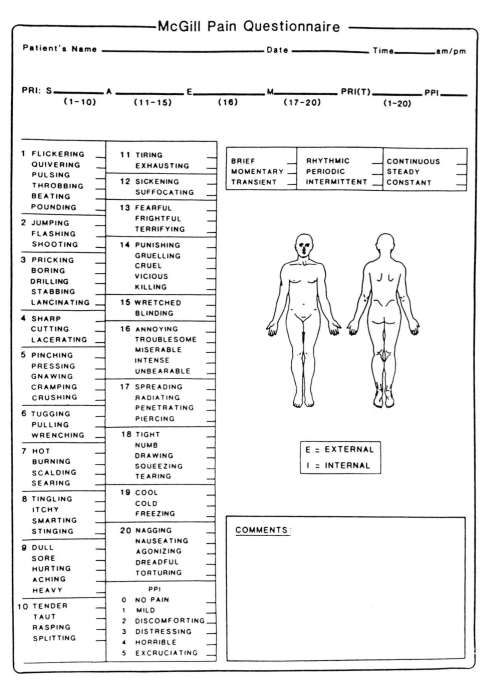

FIGURE 2-2. The McGill Pain Questionnaire. (Reproduced with permission from Wall PD, Melzack R, eds. *Textbook of Pain.* London: Churchil Livingston; 1984:199.)

severe a value of 2 and so on. It is assumed that the pain descriptors within a subclass are equidistant on an ordinal scale. The rank values are then added to obtain a score for each of the four classes of sensory, affective, evaluative, and miscellaneous, and the scales in turn are added to produce the Pain Rating Index Total (PRI-T). A second major scoring index is the number of words chosen (NWC). Combined with the PPI, the PRI-T and the NWC provide a quantitative assessment of the total pain experience.

There has been an enormous amount of critical examination of the way in which this test has been constructed, to assess its reliability, validity, and ability to discriminate between diagnostic groups.[79,80,81,95,96,115,121] The sensitiv-

ity of the MPQ to standardized stimuli has been documented.[78] All studies have found that the words of the Pain Rating Index (PRI) are appropriately grouped, although there is less consensus upon the scaling of the words within each group. Recent work suggests that the words within subsets are not equidistant.[122]

There is also an imbalance between the number of sensory, affective, and evaluative components of the PRI. The sensory dimension predominates over affective and evaluative dimensions in the number of subsets devoted to it. There is an inconsistency in the number of descriptor words within any one subset. Each word receives an absolute score, dependent upon its rank position within a subset. The possibility therefore exists that a word of particular potency in one subset might receive a lower rank score than a less potent word within another subset so that pain experiences of different intensities might have equal rating scores on the PRI-T. Charter and associates suggest that by converting the rank scores to a weighted score, reflecting more closely the position of the particular word within its subset, the potential for pain experience of differing intensities to produce equal rating scores will be much reduced.[15]

The three subscales do not display discriminant validity when subjected to factor analysis,[142] although the test–retest reliability of the PRI-T has been demonstrated.[51]

There is no mechanism within the test to determine which component truly reflects the patient's pain experience. Kremer and Atkinson have demonstrated that the affective scale can serve as an index of the overall affect of the chronic pain patient.[79] This outcome contrasts with the same authors' study of the affective scale in a cancer pain population.[80] Their patients reported a reliably higher affective emphasis when compared to a similar population with chronic pain not associated with cancer.

Attention has been directed to the correlation between the instruments measuring a particular quality of pain. A study by Reading reported a low correlation between the PPI and the VAS,[120] although Kremer and associates did not corroborate this finding.[81]

Does the type of format matter? Klepac and associates subjected patients to laboratory-inflicted pain and performed an MPQ in either the interview or self-administration formats. Word profile patterns were similar, although the mean levels were consistently higher on the interview format.[79]

Whatever the validity of these criticisms, this test does provide information about the qualitative and quantitative aspects of pain. It does treat pain as a multidimensional experience.

The questionnaire is widely applicable. It has been used to measure pain in patients with cancer[51,80] and chronic noncancer pain,[79] to discriminate between the different etiologies of facial pain,[100] to measure dental pain,[52,99] and to compare the pain experience in acute and chronic pain.[119] Also it has been used to measure laboratory-induced pain,[77] to assess those chronic pain patients involved in compensation,[98,102] and to study common postoperative complications.[18]

One such example of the discriminatory power of the test instrument is its ability to refute the belief that litigious patients have an exaggerated pain response.[102] For instance, in a study of 145 patients suffering from lower back pain to whom the MPQ had been administered, both compensation and noncompensation patients had identical pain scores and descriptor patterns.[102] Noncompensation patients, however, had significantly lower MPQ scores in affective and evaluative areas. This difference has been interpreted as indicating that compensation patients have less anxiety by virtue of their increased financial security. Furthermore, the patient is not "cured" by a favorable compensation settlement despite current belief.[103] There is no difference in sensory dimension and overall pain score that confirms the contention that compensation patients exaggerate their pain when compared to noncompensation patients.

If the MPQ has any limitations, it is the requirement that the patient possess an understanding of words used in the test. If the patient does not have the intellectual capacity or does not possess sufficient vocabulary, the value of this test is diminished. Similarly, particular word usage may not be understood by patients of differing culture or language. Consequently, the MPQ now forms the basis of similar pain questionnaires in other languages such as Finnish,[76] Dutch,[148] and Norwegian.[136]

The Dartmouth Pain Questionnaire (DPQ)

The Dartmouth Pain Questionnaire[19] is based upon the MPQ and is an adjunct to it. The DPQ is a five-part instrument incorporating features of the MPQ but adding four "objective" measures (pain complaints, somatic interventions, impaired functioning, and remaining positive aspects of function) and one subjective measure (change in self-esteem since the onset of pain).

Although the DPQ incorporates features of the MPQ by using a pain diary format, it also defines such pain characteristics as location, quality, emotional component, time course, and intensity. The DPQ assesses change in behavior, observed either by the clinician or a family member.

The test is easily self-administered or administered by an interviewer and can be completed within 20 minutes. Questions are given either a positive or negative score. The scoring is compiled by adding up the positive and negative values and producing a single score by dividing the total score by the total positive score.

This test can be used to differentiate between patients who have, and those who have not, benefited from pain therapy.[20]

The Short McGill Pain Questionnaire (SF-MPQ)

The short form McGill Pain Questionnaire[95] was developed because the long form MPQ is not readily applicable to research, in particular pharmacologic studies. The SF-MPQ contains 15 pain descriptor words, 11 sensory and 4 affective, that are commonly chosen in pain syndromes, as well as a visual analog scale and the Present Pain Intensity Scale. The sensory words used are throbbing, shooting, stabbing, sharp, cramping, gnawing, hot/burning, aching, heavy, and tender. The sensory word "splitting," which is discriminative for dental pain, was added. Other words used from the affective groups were tiring/exhausting, sickening, fearful, and cruel/punishing. These words were scaled on a VDS of none, mild, moderate, and severe.

To confirm the usefulness of the SF-MPQ in drug studies, the short and long form MPQ were administered to a group of postsurgical and postobstetric patients. Both tests were sensitive to the reduction in pain experiences produced by epidural blockade of labor pain and parenteral analgesic administered to postoperative pain patients.[98]

In summary, the test appears to be useful for rapid assimilation of data in specific studies and is sensitive to drug therapies.

Other MPQ Variants

The use of the MPQ to distinguish different patient pain experiences was analyzed by Dubuisson and Melzack.[26] They administered the MPQ to 95 patients suffering from one of eight specific pain syndromes. By using multiple discriminant analysis, they confirmed that each pain group was characterized by its own distinctive group of word descriptors. However, there was considerable overlap in the words chosen by particular diagnostic groups, suggesting that the diagnostic value of the MPQ varies with the etiology of the pain.

Subsequent application of the diagnostic value of the MPQ has led to the introduction of several word descriptor scales, for example the Back Pain Classification Scale,[72,73,80,82] the Headache Scale,[57] and the Facial Pain Scale.[100]

Memorial Pain Assessment Card

This self-administered test instrument was introduced to provide rapid evaluation of the subjective experience of pain intensity, pain relief, and psychological distress. This test is fast and easily administered to patients who are very ill and affected by sedatives and analgesics. Subjective measurements of pain, pain relief, and mood are made by the patient with reference to a visual analog scale. Furthermore they are asked to choose from a list of eight words that are graded descriptors of pain intensity. The instrument has been shown to correlate with other more complicated and longer test instruments.[30]

The West Haven–Yale Multidimensional Pain Inventory (WHYMPI)

The WHYMPI is a self-administered self-report of chronic pain behavior. It consists of a 52-item inventory divided into three sections, which in turn contain subscales. These three parts assess the impact of pain on the patient's life and the response of others to the patient's communication of pain. The text also measures the ability of the patient to conduct normal common daily activities.

Section 1 evaluates the perceived pain intensity in relation to several aspects of the patient's life. The six concepts measured on a seven-point scale are: pain severity, interference with life, dissatisfaction with level of functioning, appraisal of family support, perception of how much the patient has control over his or her own life, and affective distress.

Section 2 evaluates the patient's perceptions of response to and behavior toward the pain by close family members;

21 possible responses are scaled by the patient on a six-point scale.

Section 3 measures the patient's ability to conduct normal daily activities. There are four categories of activity ranging from domestic and social to recreational.

The test is scaled using the summed ratings procedure. It appears that the test has reliability and validity and is easy to complete.[75] The instrument does, however, have several limitations set by its self-reporting and nonobjectively gathered data. Also, the instrument does not quantify pain directly. The information gathered is specific only for that particular patient.

The Vanderbilt Pain Management Inventory (VPMI)

The Vanderbilt self-report questionnaire assesses the behavior of chronic pain patients by analyzing the frequency with which patients use active and passive coping mechanisms when their pain reaches a moderate or greater level of intensity.[11] This test instrument is based on 27 items that reflect both adaptive and maladaptive coping strategies. The patient rates each strategy on a five-point scale: 1 = never do, 2 = rarely do, 3 = occasionally do, 4 = frequently do, and 5 = very frequently do (when in pain).

When tested clinically, the instrument was found to be internally consistent and stable. It demonstrated that the more active coping the patient reported, the lower the depression, helplessness, pain, and functional impairment. The VPMI may have value in identifying patients who are likely to have adjustment difficulties.[11]

Psychophysical Measurement

To bridge the distance between laboratory and clinical approaches to pain measurement, cross-modality matching methods have been employed by several workers to measure the pain experience.[49,144] In this method a sensory experience, represented by a set of words that describe pain, is quantified by matching a stimulus in another sensory modality, such as handgrip force, time duration, line length, or loudness of sound. In this context these word descriptors can be response choices for subjects exposed to noxious stimuli. The concept of proportionality is central to the performance of the cross-modality matching procedure.[147] This procedure is likely to produce less biased and more consistent results than category scales measures. These techniques are able to scale pain on more than one dimension.

In the laboratory, the psychophysical technique has been used to test drugs.[47,50] Word descriptors are often used because the words chosen appear to produce objective scales of word meaning.[44] Several authors have demonstrated that when verbal descriptors are used, the two dimensions of stimulus intensity and unpleasantness appear to be independently scaled.[50,65,105]

Methods using word descriptor psychophysical techniques include the Pain Perception Profile,[144] the Descriptor Differential Scale,[48] and the multiple random staircase method.[49] All show potential for a broader clinical application in the future.

The Tursky *Pain Perception Profile* contains three sets of verbal descriptors, 12 words in each, which have been taken from the MPQ.[144] They are said to reflect the intensity, affective, and sensory qualities of pain. By psychophysical techniques each set is assigned a value, and each component is then given a ratio scale.

The intensity and affective, but not the sensory scales have been validated in patients with acute pain.[47] In chronic pain, only intensity was reliably scaled in studies by Urban[147] and Morley and Hassard.[106] Neither study demonstrated reliable scaling of the affective scales in this group of patients. These results are said to support the belief that intensity words chosen represent a single dimension construct whereas the affect words represent a multidimensional construct of affect.

The intensity, but not the affective or sensory, dimensions of the PPP has been validated by several authors.[44,106,144]

The *Descriptor Differential Scale* is currently used only experimentally. It employs the psychophysical principle of linear variance to scale word descriptors.[48] Twelve standard words, which represent each pain dimension to be assessed, printed in a random order, are each placed on a line representing the possible range of that word. Each word is scored, in turn, by the subjects, who place a mark on a line that is equivalent to their own pain experience when compared to that particular word. This method allows collection of multiple responses, reduces scaling error, and can assess both pain magnitude and scaling consistency.[48]

The reliability and objectivity of this instrument was confirmed by presenting it to a group of 91 patients undergoing dental extraction who completed the sensory, intensity, and unpleasantness forms. This test also can identify those subjects who performed inconsistently and who would not or could not, for uncertain reasons, assess their own pain experience.

MEASURING PHYSIOLOGICAL INDICATORS

An ideal assessment instrument could directly and objectively measure the pain experience and simplify what must be a complex neurophysiologic activity. If it were possible to measure the neuronal or cerebral activity manifestations of pain, the measurement would still be insufficient because strong components of the pain experience are the emotional or affective components. To date there have been few studies that have correlated the pain experience with physiologic parameters.

The usual physiologic manifestations of pain and suffering are often indistinguishable from the emotional dimension of anxiety, since anxiety often accompanies but is separate from the pain experience. Indices that are readily measurable include pulse rate, skin conductance, and temperature. These have been incorporated into the Autonomic Perception Questionnaire for use experimentally.[27]

Limited success has been demonstrated in the use of electromyographic measures in the study of muscle contraction in headache[7,113] and low back pain.[155] Correlation between muscle tension and perception of pain seems to be minimal.

The endogenous opioid beta-endorphin can be released during an acute pain experience, such as might follow severe burns; it can be quantified by immunoactivity techniques.[139] The release of this agent is associated with a reduction of the perceived pain intensity. It follows that beta-endorphin may be an objective marker of pain perception. Unfortunately, this substance is also released during stress.

The usefulness of laboratory and clinical measurements of evoked potentials in pain assessment has been reviewed by Chapman.[13] A relative but not absolute relationship has been found to exist between somatosensory event-related potentials and subjective pain reports.[104] It may be possible to monitor the effects of even weak analgesics using evoked cerebral potentials.[10] Evoked potentials have been used diagnostically to identify those patients suffering from trigeminal neuralgia who would benefit from posterior fossa decompression.[137]

In summary, although some areas appear promising for future clinical applicability, the usefulness of physiologic parameters, except perhaps in neonatal and infant pain assessment, is limited in current pain measurement.

OBJECTIVE MEASUREMENT OF PAIN

The experience of pain is currently impossible to measure directly. Therefore, the clinician must necessarily rely on the pain description (self-report) by the patient and substantiate this declaration by observing displays of appropriate physical behavior.

Manifest pain behavior can include pain complaints, the taking of medication or seeking of treatment, display of impaired physical or social function, and physical pain correlates such as facial grimacing, moaning, or rubbing the painful area.[33,69] Many of these activities can be objectively observed and quantified. To determine the accuracy of patient self-report, Sanders, for instance, compared the amount of uptime, using a patient activity diary, to that recorded by a mechanical instrument. Patients were found to consistently underreport uptime when compared to that shown by the clock.[129,130]

Objective measurement of pain behavior can be biased by many variables, including such areas as the observer influence on the patient's behavior, compensation status, and the role of spouses[9] or significant others. Such pain behavior can be reinforced and maintained by the act of observation despite the amelioration of pain sensation.[34] The knowledge that pain behavior which occurs for one set of reasons may persist for other reasons[33] adds to the difficulty of objectively measuring pain.

Alternatively, a strategy to take into account specific bias can be produced. Heaton and associates have developed the Psychosocial Pain Inventory, which can discriminate between exaggerated and nonexaggarated signs during physical examination.[54]

Is it worthwhile to make a distinction between objective and subjective measure of pain? We assume that objective clinical observations produce more reliable and valid measures than subjectively produced self-reporting. Yet even objective methods are not totally objective. These instruments do not directly measure the pain stimulus or the evoked psychological suffering. They rely on a method of quantification that by its very nature must have an inbuilt error.

Other limitations of the usage of observed behavior as a measure of pain are related to the environment in which the behavior is observed. Most observation occurs in a clinical setting, yet most of the patient's behavior happens at home. Alternatively, the use of a mechanical device to record uptime is limited to that behavior only.

Keefe and Block have developed a reliable observational method to objectively assess the pain experience of those with chronic low back pain.[72] Patients are asked to assume 10 different postural positions (static) or movements (dynamic) and their concomitant behavior is recorded on videotape. Trained observers review the film and rate the behavior according to the categories: guarding, bracing, rubbing, grimacing, and sighing. Interrater and test–retest reliability for this method have also been verified for a non-chronic back pain population.[66] More recently, Keefe and associates have simplified the method by having the behavior rated by an observer without reliance on videotaping.[71]

Other observational methods of pain measurement include those of Richards and associates, known as the UAB Pain Behavior Scale.[125] This instrument scales 10 specific behaviors on a daily basis: verbal and nonverbal complaints, downtime, facial grimacing, posture, mobility, body language, use of visible supportive equipment, stationary movement, and demands for either non-narcotic or narcotic analgesia. On the basis of predetermined criteria a member of the pain team scores each behavior as none (0), occasional (½) or frequent (1). The instrument can be rapidly scored. All behaviors are equally weighted. It appears to be a valid method for quantifying pain behavior.

Because of the difficulty of assessing pain in young children, it is often necessary to rely upon behavioral parameters such as facial activity.[63] One such method[84] is based upon the Facial Action Coding System,[29] in which facial activity is broken down into 44 separate action units. The modified version employs a limited number of rated facial expressions that are believed to be consistent with pain expression.[84]

CONCLUSION

In summary, the methods by which the clinician measures pain are imperfect. The personal nature of the pain experience does not lend itself easily to measurement and requires the gathering and assessment of both subjective and objective data. Many of the test instruments tend to measure only one dimension of pain. And how objective are so-called objective test methods which rely, at best, on measuring data with certain physical instruments that themselves have measurement error?

References

1. Abu-Saad H. Assessing children's response to pain. *Pain* 1984; 19:163–171.
2. Aradine CR, Beyer JE, Tompkins JM. Children's pain perception before and after analgesia: a study of instrument construct validity and related issues. *J Paediatr Nurs* 1980; 3:11–23.
3. Bergner M, Bobbit RA, Carter WB, Gilson BS. The sickness impact profile: development and final version of a health status measure, *Med Care* 1981; 19:787–805.
4. Beyer JE, Aradine CR. Content validity of an instrument to measure young children's perceptions of intensity of their pain, *J Paediatr Nurs* 1986; 1:386–395.
5. Bhachu HS, Kay B, Healy TEJ, Beatty P. Grading of pain and anxiety. *Anaesthesia* 1983; 38:875–878.
6. Bieri D, Reeve AR, Champion GD, Addicoat L, Ziegler JB. The Faces Scale for the assessment of the severity of pain experienced by children: development, initial validation and preliminary investigation for ratio scale properties. *Pain* 1990; 41:139–150.
7. Blanchard EB, Andrasik F, Ahles TA, Teders SJ, O'Keefe D. Migraine and tension headache: a meta-analytic review. *Behav Ther* 1980; 11:613–631.
8. Block AR, Kremer E, Gaylor M. Behavioural treatment of chronic pain: variables affecting treatment efficacy. *Pain* 1980; 8:367–375.
9. Block AR, Kremer E, Gaylor M. Behavioural treatment of chronic pain: the spouse as the discriminative cue for pain behaviour. *Pain* 1980; 9:243–252.
10. Bromm B. Assessment of analgesia by evoked cerebral potential measurement in humans. *Postgrad Med J* 1987; 63:9–13.
11. Brown GK, Nicassio PM. Development of a questionnaire for the assessment of active and passive coping strategies in chronic pain patients. *Pain* 1987; 31:53–64.
12. Carlsson AM. Assessment of chronic pain, 1: aspects of the reliability and validity of the visual analogue scale. *Pain* 1983; 16:87–101.
13. Chapman CR. Evoked potentials as correlates of pain and pain relief in man. *Agents Actions Suppl* 1986; 19:51–73.
14. Chapman, CR, Casey KL, Dubner R, Foley KM, Gracely RH, Reading AE. Pain measurement: an overview. *Pain* 1985; 22:1–31.
15. Charter RA, Nehemkis AM. The language of pain intensity and complexity: new methods of scoring the McGill Pain Questionnaire, *Percept Mot Skills* 1983; 56:519–537.
16. Clark WC, Pain sensitivity and the report of pain: an

introduction to Sensory Decision Theory. *Anesthesiology* 1974; 40:272–287.

17. Cohen MJ, McArthur DL. Classification of migraine and tension headache from a survey of 10,000 headache diaries. *Headache* 1981; 21:25–29.

18. Cohen MM, Tate RB. Using the McGill Pain Questionnaire to study common postoperative complications. *Pain* 1989; 39:275–279.

19. Corson JA, Schneider MJ. The Dartmouth Pain Questionnaire: an adjunct to the McGill Pain Questionnaire. *Pain* 1984; 19:59–69.

20. Cronbach LJ. Test validation. In: Thorndike RL, ed. *Educational Measurement*. Washington, DC: American Council on Education; 1971:462.

21. Dallenbach KM. Somesthesis. In: Boring EG, Langfield HS, Weld HP, eds. *Introduction to Psychology*. New York: Wiley; 1939:608–625.

22. Daut RL, Cleeland CS, Flanery RC. Development of the Wisconsin Brief Pain Questionnaire to assess pain in cancer and other diseases. *Pain* 1983; 17:197–210.

23. De Jong G, Hughes J. Independent living methodology for measuring long term outcome. *Arch Phys Med Rehabil* 1982; 63:221–229.

24. Deschamps M, Band PR, Coldman AJ. Assessment of adult cancer pain: shortcomings of current methods. *Pain* 1988; 32:133–139.

25. Dixon JS. Agreement between horizontal and vertical visual analogue scales. *Br J Rheumatol* 1986; 24:415–416. Letter.

26. Dubuisson D, Melzack R. Classification of clinical pain descriptions by multiple group discriminant analysis. *Exp Neurol* 1976; 51:480–487.

27. Dowling J. Autonomic measures and behavioural indices of pain sensitivity. *Pain* 1983; 16:193–200.

28. Eich E, Reeves JL, Jaeger B, Graff-Radford SB. Memory for pain: relation between past and present pain intensity. *Pain* 1985; 23:375–379.

29. Ekman P, Friesen WV. *Manual for the Facial Action Coding System*. Palo Alto: Consulting Psychologists; 1978.

30. Fishman B, Pasternak S, Wallenstein SL, Houde RW, Holland JC, Foley JM. The Memorial Pain Assessment Card: a valid instrument for evaluation of cancer pain. *Cancer* 1987; 60:1151–1158.

31. Follick MJ, Ahern DK. Outpatient behavioural management of chronic pain, *Behav Med Update* 1982; 3:7–10.

32. Follick MJ, Ahern DK, Laser-Wolston N. Evaluation of a daily activity diary for chronic pain patients. *Pain* 1984; 19:373–382.

33. Fordyce WE. *The Validity of Pain Behaviour Measurement*. St Louis, Mo: Mosby; 1976.

34. Fordyce WE, Lansky D, Calsyn DA, Shelton JL, Stolov WC, Rock DL. Pain measurement and pain behaviour. *Pain* 1984; 18:53–69.

35. Fordyce WE, Fowler RS, Lehman J, DeLateur B, Sand P, Trieschman R. Operant conditioning in the treatment of chronic pain. *Arch Phys Med* 1973; 54:399–408.

36. Fordyce WE, Brena SF, DeLateur BJ, Holcomb RJ, Loeser JD. Relationship of patient semantic pain descriptors to physician diagnostic judgements, activity level measures and MMPI. *Pain* 1978; 5:293–303.

37. Forrest M, Herman G, Andersen B. Assessment of pain: a comparison between patients and doctors. *Acta Anaesthesiol Scand* 1989; 33:255–256.

38. Frank AJM, Moll JMH, Hort JF. A comparison of three years of measuring pain. *Rheumatol Rehabil* 1982; 21:211–217.

39. Frederickson LW, Moll JMH, Hort JF. Methodology in the measurement of pain. *Behav Ther* 1978; 9:486–488.

40. Fries JF. The assessment of disability: from first to future principles. *Br J Rheumatol* 1983; 22:48–55.

41. Gaffney A. How children describe pain: a study of words and analogies used by 5–14 year olds. In: Dubner R, Gebhart GF, Bonds MR, eds. *Pain Research and Clinical Management*. Amsterdam: Elsevier; 1988:341–347.

42. Ginzburg BM, Merskey H, Lau CL. The relationship between pain drawings and the psychological state. *Pain* 1988; 35:141–146.

43. Gracely RH. Psychophysical assessment of human pain. In: Bonica JJ, Liebeskind JC, Albe-Fessard DG, eds. *Advances in Pain Research and Therapy*. New York: Raven Press; 1979.

44. Gracely RG, Dubner R. Reliability and validity of verbal descriptor scales of painfulness. *Pain* 1987; 29:175–185.

45. Gracely RH, McGrath P, Dubner R. Ratio scales of sensory and affective verbal pain descriptions. *Pain* 1978; 5:5–18.

46. Gracely RH, Dubner R, Deeter WR, Wolskee PJ. Clinician's expectations influence placebo analgesia. *Lancet* 1985; 1:43.

47. Gracely RH, Dubner R, McGrath P. Narcotic analgesia: fentanyl reduces the intensity but not the unpleasantness of painful tooth pulp sensations. *Science* 1979; 203:1261–1263.

48. Gracely RH, Kwilosz DM. The Descriptor Differential Scale: applying psychophysical principles to clinical pain assessment. *Pain* 1988; 35:279–288.

49. Gracely RH, Lota L, Walter DJ, Dubner R. A multiple random staircase method of psychophysical pain assessment. *Pain* 1988; 32:55–63.

50. Gracely RH, McGrath P, Dubner R. Validity and sensitivity of ratio scales of sensory and affective verbal pain descriptors: manipulation of affect by diazepam. *Pain* 1978; 5:19–29.

51. Graham C, Bond SS, Geekovich M, Cook MR. Use of the McGill Pain Questionnaire in the assessment of cancer pain: replicability and consistency. *Pain* 1980; 8:377–387.

52. Grushka M, Sessle BJ. Applicability of the McGill Pain Questionnaire to the differentiation of 'toothache' pain. *Pain* 1984; 19:49–57.

53. Hendler N, Cimi C, Ma T, Long D. A comparison of cognitive impairment due to benzodiazepines and to narcotics. *Am J Psychol* 1980; 137:828–830.

54. Heaton RK, Getto CJ, Lehman RA, Fordyce WE, Brauer E, Groban SE. A standardized evaluation of psychosocial factors in chronic pain. *Pain* 1982; 12:165–174.

55. High AS, Macgregor AJ, Tomlinson GE, Salkouskis PM. A gnathodynamometer as an objective means of pain assessment. *Br J Oral Maxillofac Surg* 1988; 26:284–291.

56. Hildebrandt J, Franz CE, Choroba-Mehnen B, Temme M. The use of pain drawings in screening for psychological involvement in complaints of low back pain. *Spine* 1988; 13:681–685.

57. Hunter M. The headache scale: a new approach to the

assessment of headache pain based on pain descriptors. *Pain* 1983; 16:361–373.

58. Hunter M, Philips C, Rachman S. Memory for pain. *Pain* 1979; 6:35–46.
59. Huskisson EC. Measurement of Pain. *Lancet* 1974; 2:1127–1131.
60. Huskisson EC. The visual analogue scale. In: Melzack R, ed. *Pain Measurement and Assessment*. New York: Raven Press; 1983.
61. Ignelzi RJ, Kremer EF, Atkinson JH. Patient pain intensity report to different health professionals. Paper presented at Assosciation for Advancement of Behaviour Therapy; November 25–27, 1980; New York, New York.
62. International Association for the Study of Pain, Subcommittee on Taxonomy. Classification of chronic pain: descriptions of chronic pain syndromes and definitions of pain terms. *Pain*. 1986; suppl 3:S1–S225.
63. Izard CE, Huebner RR, Risser D, McGinnes GC, Dougherty LM. The younger infant's ability to produce discrete emotion expressions. *Dev Psychol* 1980; 16:132–140.
64. Jaegger B, Reeves JL. Quantification of changes in myofascial trigger point severity with the pressure algometer following passive stretch. *Pain* 1986; 27:203–210.
65. Jamner LD, Tursky B. Discrimination between intensity and affective pain descriptors: a psychophysical evaluation. *Pain* 1987; 30:271–283.
66. Jensen IB, Bradley LA, Linton SJ. Validation of an observation method of pain assessment in non chronic back pain. *Pain* 1989; 39:267–274.
67. Jerrett M, Evans K. Children's pain vocabulary. *J Adv Nurs* 1986; 11:403–408.
68. Kahn EA. On facial expression. *Clin Neurosurg* 1966; 12:9–22.
69. Keefe FJ, Brantley A, Manuel GH, Crisson, JE. Behaviour assessment of head and neck cancer pain. *Pain* 1985; 23:327–336.
70. Keefe FJ, Block AR, Williams RB Jr, Surwit RS. Behavioural treatment of chronic low back pain: clinical outcome and individual differences in pain relief. *Pain* 1981; 11:221–231.
71. Keefe FJ, Wilkins RH, Cook WA. Direct observation of pain; behaviour in low back pain patients during physical examination. *Pain* 1984; 20:59–68.
72. Keefe FJ, Block AR. Development of an observation method for assessing pain behaviour in chronic low back pain patients. *Behav Ther* 1982; 13:363–375.
73. Keefe FJ, Hill RW. An objective approach to qualifying pain behaviour and gait patterns in low back pain patients. *Pain* 1985; 21:153–161.
74. Keele KD. The Pain Chart. *Lancet* 1948; 2:6–8.
75. Kerns RD, Turk DC, Rudy TE. The West Haven–Yale Multidimensional Pain Inventory (WHYMPI). *Pain* 1985; 23:345–356.
76. Ketovuori H, Pontinen PJ. A pain vocabulary in Finnish: the Finnish Pain Questionnaire. *Pain* 1981; 11:247–253.
77. Klepac RK, Dowling J, Rokke P, Dodge L, Schafter L. Interview v's paper and pencil administration of the McGill Pain Questionnaire. *Pain* 1981; 11:241–246.
78. Klepac RK, Dowling J, Hauge G. Sensitivity of the McGill Pain Questionnaire to intensity and quality of laboratory pain. *Pain* 1981; 10:199–207.

79. Kremer E, Atkinson JH. Pain measurement: construct validity of the affective dimension of the McGill Pain Questionnaire with chronic benign pain patients. *Pain* 1981; 11:93–100.
80. Kremer EF, Atkinson JH, Ignelzi RJ. Pain Measurement: the affective dimensional measure of the McGill Pain Questionnaire with a cancer pain population. *Pain* 1982; 12:153–163.
81. Kremer E, Atkinson J, Ignelzi RJ. Measurement of pain; patient preference does not confound pain measurement. *Pain* 1980; 10:241–248.
82. Leavitt F. Detecting psychological disturbance using verbal pain measurement; the back pain classification scale, In: Melzack R, ed. *Pain Measurement and Assessment*. New York: Raven Press; 1983.
83. LeResche L. Facial expression in pain: a study of candid photographs. *J NonVerbal Behav* 1982; 7:46–56.
84. LeResche L, Dworkin SF. Facial expression accompanying pain. *Soc Sci Med* 1984; 19:1325–1330.
85. Linton SJ, Gotestam KG. A clinical comparison of two pain scales: correlation, remembering chronic pain, and a measure of compliance. *Pain* 1983; 17:57–65.
86. Lodge M, Tursky B. Comparison between category and magnitude scaling of political opinion employing SRC/CPS items. Am *Polit Sci Rev* 1979; 73:50–66.
87. Lutz RW, Silbret M, Oldshan N. Treatment outcome and compliance with therapeutic regimens: long term follow-up of a multidisciplinary pain program. *Pain* 1983; 17:301–308.
88. Main CJ, Waddell G. Psychometric construction and validity of Pilowsky Illness Behaviour Questionnaire in British patients with chronic low back pain. *Pain* 1987; 28:13–25.
89. Malow RM. The effects of induced anxiety on pain perception; a signal detection analysis. *Pain* 1981; 11:397–405.
90. Margoles MS. The Pain Chart: spatial properties of pain. In: Mezack R, ed. *Pain Measurement and Assessment*. New York: Raven Press; 1983:309–321.
91. Margolis RB, Chibnall JT, Tait RC. Test-retest reliability of the pain drawing instrument. *Pain* 1988; 3:49–51.
92. Margolis RB, Tait RC, Krause SJ. A rating system for use with patient pain drawings. *Pain* 1986; 24:57–65.
93. Maunuksela EL, Olkkala KT, Korpela R. Measurement of pain in children with self reporting and behavioural assessment. *Clin Pharmacol Ther* 1987; 42:137–141.
94. McGrath PA, DeVeber LL, Hearn MT. Multidimensional pain assessment in children. *Adv Pain Res Ther* 1985; 9:387–393.
95. Melzack R. The short-form McGill Pain Questionnaire. *Pain* 1987; 30:191–197.
96. Melzack R. The McGill Pain Questionnaire: major properties and scoring methods. *Pain* 1975; 1:277–299.
97. Melzack R. *The Puzzle of Pain*. New York: Basic Books; 1973.
98. Melzack R, Katz J, Jeans ME. The role of compensation in chronic pain: analysis using a new method of scoring the McGill Pain Questionnaire. *Pain* 1985; 23:101–112.
99. Melzack R, Kent G. Memory of dental pain. *Pain* 1985; 21:187–194.
100. Melzack R, Terrence C, Fromm G, Amsel R. Trigeminal neuralgia and atypical face pain; use of the McGill Pain

Questionnaire for discrimination and diagnosis. *Pain* 1986; 27:297–302.

101. Melzack R, Torgerson WS. On the language of pain. *Anesthesiology* 1971; 34:50–59.

102. Mendelson G. Compensation, pain complaints and psychological disturbance. *Pain* 1984; 20:169–177.

103. Mendelson G. Not cured by a verdict: effect of legal settlement on compensation claimants. *Med J Aust* 1982; 2:132–134.

104. Miltner W, Johnson R Jr, Braun C, Larbig, W. Somatosensory event related potentials to painful and non-painful stimuli: effects of attention. *Pain* 1989; 38:303–312.

105. Morley S. The development of a self administered psychophysical scaling method: range effects. *Pain* 1988; 33:189–194.

106. Morley S, Hassard A. The development of a self administered psychophysical scaling method: internal consistency and temporal stability in chronic pain patients. *Pain* 1989; 37:33–37.

107. Mreskey H, Spear FG. The reliability of the pressure algometer, *Br J Soc Clin Psychol* 1964; 3:130–136.

108. Murphy DM, McDonald A, Power C, Unwin A, MacSullivan R. Measurement of pain: a comparison of the visual analogue with a nonvisual analogue scale. *Clin J Pain* 1988; 3:197–199.

109. Nayman J. Measurement and control of postoperative pain. *Ann R Coll Surg Engl* 1979; 61:419–426.

110. O'Brien J, Francis A. The use of next-of-kin to estimate pain in cancer patients. *Pain* 1988; 35:171–178.

111. Ohnhaus EE, Adler R. Methodological problems in the measurement of pain: a comparison between the verbal rating scale and the visual analogue scale. *Pain* 1975; 1:379–384.

112. Pawl RP. *Chronic Pain Primer*. Chicago: Yearbook; 1973:15.

113. Pearce S, Morley S. An experiemental investigation of pain production in headache patients. *Br J Clin Psychol* 1981; 20:275–281.

114. Pilowsky I, Spence ND. *Manual for the Illness Behaviour Questionnaire (IBQ)*. 2nd ed. University of Adelaide: Dept of Psychiatry; 1983.

115. Prieto EJ, Hopson L, Bradley LA, et al. The language of low back pain: factor structure of the McGill Pain Questionnaire. *Pain* 1980; 8:11–20.

116. Rames LO, Naliboff BD, Heinrich RL, Schag CL. The chronic illness problem inventory: problem oriented psychological assessment of patients with chronic illness. *Int J Psychiatry Med* 1984; 14:65–75.

117. Ransford AO, Cairns D, Mooney V. The pain drawing as an aid to the psychological evaluation of patients with lower back pain. *Pain* 1976; 2:127–134.

118. Reading AE. Testing pain mechanisms in person in pain. In: Wall PD, Melzack R, eds. *Textbook of Pain*. London: Churchill Livingston; 1984.

119. Reading AE. A comparison of the McGill Pain Questionnaire in chronic and acute pain. *Pain* 1982; 13:185–192.

120. Reading AE. A comparison of pain rating scales. *J Psychom Res* 1980; 24:119–126.

121. Reading AE. The internal structure of the McGill Pain Questionnaire in dysmenorrhoea patients. *Pain* 1979; 7:353–358.

122. Reading AE, Everitt BS, Sledmere CM. The McGill Pain Questionnaire: a replication of its construction. *Br J Clin Psychol* 1982; 21:339–349.

123. Ready LB, Sarkis E, Turner JA. Self-reported vs. actual use of medications in chronic pain patients. *Pain* 1982; 12:285–294.

124. Revill SI, Robinson JO, Rosen M, Hogg MIJ. The reliability of a linear analogue for evaluating pain. *Anaesthesia* 1976; 31:1191–1198.

125. Richards JS, Nepomuceno C, Riles M, Suer Z. Assessing pain behaviour: the UAB Pain Behavior Scale. *Pain* 1982; 14:393–398.

126. Rock DL, Fordyce WE, Brockway JA, Bergman JT, Spengler DM. Measuring functional impairment associated with pain: psychometric analysis of an exploratory scoring protocol for activity pattern indicators. *Arch Phys Med Rehabil* 1984; 65:295–300.

127. Rosentiel AK, Keefe FJ. The behavioural management of chronic pain: long term follow up with comparison groups. *Pain* 1980; 8:151–162.

128. Rudy TE, Turk DC, Brena SF. Differential utility of medical procedures in the assessment of chronic pain patients. *Pain* 1988; 34:53–60.

129. Sanders SH. Toward a practical instrument system for the automatic measurement of uptime in chronic pain patient. *Pain* 1980; 9:103–109.

130. Sanders SH. Automated versus self monitoring of uptime in chronic low back pain patients in a comparitive study. *Pain* 1983; 15:289–296.

131. Savedra MC, Tesler MD, Holzemer WL, Wilkie DJ, Ward JA. Pain location: validity and reliability of body outline markings by hospitalized children and adolescents. *Res Nurs Health* 1989; 12:307–314.

132. Schwartz DP, DeGood DE. Global appropriateness of Pain Drawings: blind ratings predict patterns of psychological distress litigation status. *Pain* 1984; 19:383–388.

133. Scott J, Huskisson EC. The graphic representation of pain. *Pain*, 1976; 2:75–84.

134. Scott J, Huskisson EC. Vertical or horizontal visual analogue scales. *Ann Rheum Dis* 1979; 38:560.

135. Seymour RA, Simpson JM, Charlton JE, Phillips ME. An evaluation of length and endphrase of the visual analogue scale in dental pain. *Pain* 1985; 21:177–185.

136. Strand LI, Wisnes AR. Development of a Norwegian pain questionnaire for pain measurement. *Tidsskr Nor Laegeforen* 1990; 110:45–49.

137. Stohr M, Petruch F, Scheglmann K. Somatosensory evoked potentials following trigeminal nerve stimulation to trigeminal neuralgia. *Ann Neurol* 1981; 9:63–66.

138. Syrjala KL, Chapman CR. Measurement of clinical pain: a review and integration of research findings. *Adv Pain Res Ther* 1984; 7:71–101.

139. Szyfelbum SK, Osgood PF, Carr DB. The assessment of pain and plasma beta-endorphin immunoactivity in burned children. *Pain* 1985; 22:173–182.

140. Tait RC, Chibnall JRT, Krause S. The Pain Disability Index: psychometric properties. *Pain* 1990; 40:171–182.

141. Tearnan BH, Dar R. Physician ratings of pain descriptors: potential diagnostic utility. *Pain* 1986; 26:45–51.

142. Turk DC, Rudy TE, Salovey P. The McGill Pain Question-

naire reconsidered: confirming the factor structure and examining appropriate uses. *Pain* 1985; 21:385–397.

143. Turner JA, Clancy S. Strategies for coping with chronic low back pain: relationship to pain and disability. *Pain* 1986; 25:355–364.

144. Tursky B, Jamner LD, Friedman R. The pain perception profile: a psychophysical approach to the assessment of pain report. *Behav Ther* 1982; 13:376–394.

145. Uden A, Astrom M, Bergenudd H. Pain drawings in chronic back pain. *Spine* 1988; 13:389–392.

146. Unruh A, McGrath P, Cunningham ST, Humphreys P. Childrens drawing of their pain. *Pain* 1983; 17:385–392.

147. Urban BJ, Keefe F, France RD. A study of psychophysical scaling in chronic pain patients. *Pain* 1984; 20:157–168.

148. Vanderiet K, Andriaensen H, Carton H, Vertommen H. The McGill Pain Questionnaire constructed for the Dutch language (MPQ-DV). Preliminary data concerning reliability and validity. *Pain* 1987; 30:395–408.

149. Von Baeyer CL, Bergstrom KJ, Brodwin MG, Brodwin SK. Invalid use of pain drawings in psychological screening of back pain patients. *Pain* 1983; 16:103–107.

150. Waddell G, Pilowsky I, Bond MR. Clinical assessment and interpretation of abnormal illness behaviour in low back pain. *Pain* 1989; 39:41–53.

151. Whaley L, Wong DL. *Nursing Care of Infants and Children*. St Louis, Mo: Mosby; 1987:1068–1070.

152. White B, Sanders SH. The influence on patient's pain intensity ratings of antecedent reinforcement of pain talk or well talk. *J Behav Ther Exp Psychiatry* 1986; 17:155–159.

153. Wilkie DJ, Holzemer WL, Tesler MD, Ward JA, Paul SM, Savedra MC. Measuring pain quality: validity and reliability of children's and adolescents' pain language. *Pain* 1990; 41:151–159.

154. Williams RCV. Toward a set of reliable and valid measures for chronic pain assessment and outcome research. *Pain* 1988; 35:239–251.

155. Wolf SL, Nacht M, Kelly JL. EMG feedback training during dynamic movement for the low back pain patients. *Behav Ther* 1982; 13:395–406.

156. Wolff BB. Laboratory Methods of Pain Measurement. In: Melzack R, ed. *Pain Measurement and Assessment*. New York: Raven Press; 1983.

157. Yang JC, Wagner JM, and Clark WC. Psychological distress and mood in chronic pain and surgical patients: a decision theory analysis. In: Bonica JJ, ed. *Advances in Pain Research and Therapy*. Florida: American Pain Society; 1983(5):901–906.

158. Strong MD, Roderick A, Chant D. Pain Intensity Measurement in Chronic Low Back Pain. *Clin J Pain* 1991; 7:209–218.

159. Jamison R, Brown G. Validation of hourly pain intensity profiles with chronic pain patients. *Pain* 1991; 45:123–128.

CHAPTER 3

Psychological Aspects of Pain

Dennis C. Turk, Thomas E. Rudy, and Charles D. Boucek

The quest to control pain has probably existed since the beginning of human history. Mention of pain treatment has been observed in Egyptian papyri dating back to 4000 B.C. Yet despite all this effort, no method that consistently and permanently ameliorates chronic pain for all individuals has yet been found. The development of potent narcotic analgesic medications has greatly improved our ability to alleviate acute pain, but adequate control of chronic pain remains elusive. As we will use the phrase, *chronic pain* refers to pain that persists beyond the time for healing of acute injury or pain associated with progressive diseases. This use can be contrasted with the commonly used and arbitrary classification of pain as chronic if it persists for a period of over 6 months.

The inability to identify a satisfactory method to control chronic pain has not been for lack of trying. The history of medicine is replete with strategies designed to provide relief. Cupping, trephining, leeching, bleeding, and purging are only a few of the procedures that have been tried. In addition, almost every organic and inorganic substance has been ingested in the pursuit of relief, frequently to no avail.

Systematic efforts to treat pain have been closely aligned with how pain is conceptualized. Historically, pain has been viewed as either the result of a psychological process *or* a sensory-physiologic event. Aristotle (cited in [1]) viewed pain as an emotion, and the Stoic philosophers taught that pain could be overcome by "rational repudiation," that is, through logic and reasoning. In marked contrast, the 17th-century French philosopher René Descartes conceptualized pain as a purely sensory phenomenon with its intensity determined exclusively by noxious sensory input. Descartes also proposed that a direct sensory transmission line existed from the periphery through the spinal cord to the brain where pain was registered. Thus, the Cartesian model of pain postulated that the amount of pain experienced was directly proportional to the amount of tissue damage. From this view, satisfactory treatment of pain should be achieved through blockage of the noxious sensory input by direct surgical means or pharmacologic agents.

The sensory-physiologic view espoused by Descartes gained increased acceptance and credibility in the late 1800s with advances in sensory physiology, neuroanatomy, and psychophysics. At that time, psychological factors, when considered at all, were relegated to positions of secondary interest. This "direct-connection" or unidimensional perspective continues to hold a position of prominence in current medical thinking. However, despite major advances in our understanding of the mechanics of the nervous system, the development of potent analgesic preparations, and increasingly sophisticated surgical procedures, permanent and consistent amelioration of pain has not been achieved.

The inadequacy of surgical and pharmacologic treatments has produced frustration because some patients continue to report pain despite the disruption or blockage of what are believed to be the pain pathways within the anterolateral spinothalamic tract and sensory registers within the brain. Many clinicians have observed that patients respond quite differently to ostensibly the same pain syndrome and report widely varying benefits from what would appear to be identical treatments. Frustrated by these apparent anomalies, physicians who adhere to a unidimensional sensory-physiologic view have suggested that the differences observed, if unrelated to known neuropathways, must be "psychogenic." In other words, if the pain pathways are severed or blocked and the patient continues to report pain, then the pain reported must ipso facto be *caused* by psychological mechanisms. Current usage of the term "psychogenic pain" is reminiscent of a long history in medicine of attributing diseases to psychological factors when the symptoms did not fit within the existing knowledge base (see Sontag's discussion[2] of the history of tuberculosis).

When pain is labeled psychogenic because "pain is reported in the absence of known or sufficient physical pathology," the assumption is that the true cause of all pain syndromes is known. This assumption is untenable; the physical bases for many pain syndromes are unclear.[3,4] Moreover, recent advances in diagnostic radiology have pinpointed some physical causes for syndromes that, before the availability of sophisticated technology, were thought to be of psychological origin. For example, before the development of computed tomography, reliable imaging of some lesions was difficult if not impossible. Developments in the area of nuclear magnetic resonance imaging may further advance our ability to identify pathologic factors that contribute to chronic pain. Thus, it must be remembered that "psychogenic pain" remains a diagnosis of exclusion and, consequently, the precision of this diagnosis is dependent on the our available knowledge and technology.[5,6]

BEYOND UNIDIMENSIONAL SENSORY-PHYSIOLOGIC MODELS OF PAIN

A major advance in conceptualizations about pain occurred as the result of the work of Henry Beecher, a pioneer in the field of anesthesiology. Beecher's observations during World War II led him to suggest[7] that the experience of pain has two components, namely, a sensory input component and a secondary emotional reaction to the sensory input. From this perspective, psychological factors (affect and cognition) were viewed as being capable of modulating the response to noxious sensory stimulation. It is important to note, however, that Beecher still tended to view the sensory input as primary and psychological factors as secondary components, or reactions to pain. Note, however, that Beecher did not refer to psychological factors as causal agents and consequently did not support a psychogenic view of pain. Rather, he was suggesting a linear model in which psychological factors were likely to influence the experience of pain after a physical cause.

Gate Control Model of Pain

The 1960s brought a resurgence of interest among investigators in pain and its treatment. Using published research and clinical observations, Melzack and his colleagues[8,9] proposed the gate-control model of pain, which was a radical departure from the predominant unidimensional model. The gate-control model emphasized the importance of both the central and the peripheral nervous systems in reports of pain. Unlike Beecher, who viewed psychological factors as reactions to pain, Melzack and his colleagues suggested that cognitive-evaluative and motivational-affective factors *interacted* with sensory phenomena to create the perception of pain. According to the gate-control model, it is the interaction among these factors that determines the experience of pain.

Although some of the physiologic bases of the gate-control model have been challenged,[10] its conceptual and multidimensional view along with its emphasis on pain as a perceptual and not solely a sensory phenomenon has received much support.[11] Current usage of the term *nociceptive stimuli* or *nociception* has evolved largely from the gate-control model and is employed to define the sensory phenomena, whereas the term *pain* is reserved for the *subjective perception* of pain.[12]

An Operant Conditioning Model of Pain

A second approach that has had a major impact on current therapeutic approaches to chronic pain is Fordyce's[13] operant conditioning model. According to Fordyce, pain is not directly observable but rather is based on verbal or nonverbal communications from the sufferer. These communications of pain are behavioral manifestations. As such, they can be observed by others and their expression reinforced. For example, expressions of pain (limping, moaning, grimacing, staying in bed) can lead to such positive outcomes as permission to avoid undesirable activities, financial compensation, solicitous attention from one's spouse, and so forth. These outcomes may serve to initiate or maintain the presence of these pain behaviors, which, according to the operant theory, can occur *even in the absence of nociceptive stimulation*. Thus, Fordyce's operant conditioning model emphasizes that these more objective pain behaviors rather than patients' subjective experiences of pain should be the targets of treatment interventions.

The history of pain appears to consist of a recycling of theoretical conceptualizations rather than a linear progression based on increased knowledge. The operant approach to pain is no exception. Early 20th-century authors addressed the importance of considering reinforcement of pain behaviors without using the terminology of operant conditioning.[14] The operant perspective departs from traditional sensory views in that nociception is viewed as neither a necessary nor a sufficient condition for the development of chronic pain. The operant conditioning model also departs from the gate-control model in that it ignores affective and cognitive components of the pain experience (see the debate on this topic by Rachlin[15] and the commentaries stimulated by this article).

A Cognitive-Behavioral Integration

Although the gate-control model[8] emphasized that cognitive, affective, and sensory factors are all components in pain perception, it is also important for the clinician to assess how psychological factors might influence the experience of pain over time. That is, patients' thoughts and appraisals may affect many aspects of their lives, including their level of physical activity. From the perspective of the gate-control theory, cognitive factors combine or interact with sensory factors to create the perception of pain per se: a cross-sectional or snapshot view. Cognitive-behavioral theory additionally focuses on the potential for psychological factors to influence the lives of patients who must live with unresolvable intractable pain: a longitudinal or motion picture view. Thus, this perspective places importance on how psychological processes can reciprocally determine and redefine the perceptual processes involved in reports of pain.

Even though the gate-control and the operant conditioning models offer quite different views of pain, they may be complimentary (see Ciccone & Grzesiak[16] and Sternbach[17] for an opposing view). Turk and his colleagues[11,18] have developed a cognitive-behavioral model that emphasizes the importance of sensory, cognitive, and affective, as well as behavioral, factors in the experience and treatment of pain. An important contribution of the cognitive-behavioral model is the increased attention given to the attitudes and beliefs of patients regarding their understanding of their condition, the health care system, appropriate behavioral responses to their disease, and their own resources and capabilities.

From a cognitive-behavioral view of pain, it is the patient's perspective that reciprocally interacts with emotional factors, sensory phenomena, and behavioral responses. Moreover, how the patient behaves will elicit responses from significant others that can reinforce both adaptive and maladaptive modes of thinking, feeling, and behaving. Thus, a synergistic model is proposed in place of the linear causation postulated by unidimensional models such as the sensory-physiological or operant concepts.

To summarize, from the cognitive-behavioral model, pain can best be described as a complex, multidimensional perceptual phenomena. Pain perception is not the end result of the passive transmission and registration of impulses from physically defined stimuli but a dynamic, interpretive process. To better understand and treat pain, consideration must be given to the role of thoughts, emotions, and behavior as well as sensory contributions to the processes involved in forming and maintaining pain perceptions.

PSYCHOLOGICAL FACTORS: DIRECT AND INDIRECT EFFECTS

One way to understand better the models of pain described above is to compare the direct and indirect interactions of physiologic, psychologic,[19] and behavioral factors. In Cartesian theory, pain is viewed as a direct reflection of nociceptive input; no credence is given to psychological or behavioral factors. From the gate-control perspective, psychological factors are believed to combine directly with nociceptive input; together, these factors define pain. From this perspective, sensory-nociceptive stimuli work in additive ways with cognitive and affective variables to determine whether pain is perceived. In this way psychological factors are believed to be directly related to an individual's perception of pain. However, the gate-control model does not address how these psychological factors in turn affect physical functioning.

In contrast, the operant-conditioning model pays little attention to nociceptive factors or the subjective experience of pain but rather views the reinforcement of pain behaviors as indirectly affecting the perception of pain and physiologic functioning. In other words, this model holds that reinforcement of pain behaviors may in fact lead to an increase in the expression of pain behaviors but that this increase does not necessarily have any direct impact on nociception. The increase in pain behaviors may then indirectly affect physical functioning and consequently nociception if these behaviors lead people to engage in fewer and fewer activities with consequent muscle atrophy and diminished physical capacity. Thus, the process outlined above would suggest that nociception is not necessary in the operant formulation of pain behaviors. Rather, reinforcement of maladaptive pain behaviors is sufficient to maintain these behaviors irrespective of any nociceptive stimulation experienced by the individual.

The cognitive-behavioral model explicitly considers how psychological and behavioral factors may both directly and indirectly affect the pain experience.[20] For example, psychological factors may induce muscular hyperreactivity in response to psychological stress. Research by Flor, Turk, and Birbaumer[21] examined the relationship of paraspinal lumbar EMG reactivity of chronic back pain patients, patients without back pain, and healthy controls. All subjects participated in a psychophysiological assessment that included four counterbalanced trials (discussion of personal stress, discussion of pain, performance of mental arithmetic, and recitation of the alphabet, a control condition). Bilateral paraspinal and frontalis EMG, heart rate, and skin conductance levels were recorded continuously. Psychological variables such as anxiety, depressed mood, and perceived control were also assessed.

The results of the Flor study indicated that back pain patients displayed EMG elevations and delayed recovery *only* in their paravertebral musculature and *only* when discussing personally relevant stress (the pain and stress trials) and not in the general stress (mental arithmetic) or control trials. Neither the non-back-pain nor the healthy control group displayed paravertebral hyperreactivity. Interestingly, the extent of abnormal muscular reactivity was best predicted by depressive mood and cognitive coping style (psychological variables) rather than by pain demographic variables such as number of surgeries or duration of pain. Similar results have been reported by Mercuri, Olson, and Laskin[22] and Dahlstrom, Carlsson, Gale, and Jansson,[23] who found that patients with temporomandibular joint disorders had a heightened EMG response to psychological stressors specifically at the site of their pain in comparison with the response of non-pain-related muscle groups.

Although increased muscle reactivity cannot be taken as a direct indication of pain,[24,25] muscular hyperreactivity to psychological stress may contribute to muscle spasm and thereby to increased nociception and exacerbation of pain. Flor and Turk[3] proposed that repeated and sustained muscular hypertension may produce ischemia and subsequently the release of pain-eliciting substances such as bradykinin. Stress-related sympathetic arousal may also lead directly to ischemia that may induce reflex muscle spasm and additional pain. Pain may subsequently act as a new stressor and increase the muscle tension and the formation of trigger points thereby perpetuating a pain–tension cycle. Furthermore, over time, fear of movement may develop (because movement increases pain in spastic muscles) leading to increasing immobility and greater tension and pain.

Additional support for the direct effect of psychological variables on pain comes from some of the preliminary work on endogenous opioids. Cognitive factors such as expectancy of relief have been shown to increase production of endorphins.[26] Moreover, psychological variables have been shown to potentiate the efficacy of known analgesic medications such as nitrous oxide[27] as well as other analgesic modalities such as audioanalgesia.[28]

Fear of movement, a psychological process, might also be considered to have an indirect effect on pain. Individuals suffering from chronic pain may reduce their levels of physical activity because they fear that physical activities may exacerbate their pain or cause additional physical damage. This reduction in physical activities can contribute to muscle atrophy with a concomitant reduction in strength and endurance. Further, engaging in fewer activities can lead to increased feelings of helplessness and dysphoric mood that subsequently increase the likelihood that individuals will still further reduce their involvement in reinforcing activities. As activity levels decline, there is frequently an increased self-focus and preoccupation with pain and consequently increased perceptions and reports of pain. Additionally, perceptions of helplessness and lack of control may interfere with the patient's compliance with physical therapy and other components of therapeutic regimens that require patients to make active efforts. An increase in pain behaviors then leads to an even greater attention to and reinforcement of these behaviors, as suggested by operant formulations. Finally, with increased complaints the opportunity for additional treatments and possible iatrogenic complications grows. In sum, a vicious cycle is created and perpetuated.

CLINICAL RESEARCH (See Chap. 34)

Psychologists involved in research and treatment of chronic pain have increasingly emphasized the importance of psychological factors in the individual's experience of pain. For example, cognitive variables have been implicated in the maintenance and exacerbation of chronic pain,[29] and have begun to be included as targets in treatments of chronic pain such as back pain,[30,31] headaches,[32] temporomandibular disorders,[33] and rheumatoid arthritis.[34] Psychological factors have also been suggested as a central mechanism in the reported efficacy of treatments such as biofeedback.[35,36] The utility of psychologically based interventions with diverse populations has been reviewed,[11,37,38] and the interested reader is encouraged to examine these papers for detailed presentations. Furthermore, neglect of psychological variables has been suggested as contributing to the failure of operant orientations.[39] Several studies illustrate some of the most recent relevant findings.

In a study examining the efficacy of biofeedback with rheumatology patients, Flor and associates[35] reported that a reduction in the duration, intensity, and quality of pain was associated with decreases in negative thoughts related to feelings of helplessness and lack of control. Thus, the main effects of the EMG biofeedback employed in this study appeared to be related to the psychological components of the pain experience and not, as would be predicted by sensory-physiologic models, the nociceptive stimulation of muscular tension. In another study employing biofeedback, this time with tension headache patients, Holroyd and Andrasik[40] interviewed patients after treatment with EMG

biofeedback and concluded on the basis of these interviews that the efficacy of biofeedback appeared to be unrelated to changes in muscular hyperreactivity. Rather, it seemed to the authors that the perceptions of self-control provided by biofeedback and the patients' attention to their own physiologic responses were the central active ingredients. These interview data are consistent with the results reported by Flor and colleagues.[35]

The post hoc explanation regarding the importance of cognitive variables in biofeedback treatment has subsequently been tested directly by Holroyd and colleagues.[36] Patients who suffered from tension headaches were provided with bogus feedback displays indicating that they were either highly successful in reducing their EMG activity or only moderately successful. Those patients who received the high success information demonstrated increased perceptions of self-efficacy and self-control as well as significant reductions in headache activity. The moderate success group, in contrast, showed minimal changes in perceived self-efficacy and no significant improvement in headaches. Since both groups received bogus feedback, it would appear that the cognitive factors of perceived self-efficacy and control were the sole determinants of symptom reduction (see also Courey and colleagues[25] and Neufeld and Thomas[41]).

Although many studies have reported on the efficacy of treatments that target psychological variables,[42,43] most of these studies have flaws that lead to difficulties in interpretation. Thus they must be viewed as suggestive rather than definitive. Moore and Chaney[44] reported a well-controlled study in which the efficacy of a brief outpatient group treatment program incorporating cognitive variables was described. This study is an important advance in that it included a treatment comparison group (often lacking from pain treatment outcome studies) as well as a waiting-list control group. Moreover, the authors included behavioral as well as self-report measures to evaluate treatment efficacy. The results of this study demonstrated quite convincingly that cognitive-behavioral treatment was successful not only in reducing self-reports of pain but also in reducing patients' use of the health care system, reducing pain behaviors (as observed by spouses), and improving physical indices of functioning such as ambulation, body control, and movement.

No single study is sufficient to demonstrate the importance of psychological factors, but taken as an aggregate these studies verify that self-appraisals, maladaptive thoughts, coping strategies, and other such variables affect the intensity and duration of pain. Most studies have not directly tested whether cognitive variables were actually altered by treatment. That is, modification of psychological variables is usually only inferred. When psychological variables have been examined directly, they have been assessed by measures that were not developed specifically for pain patients or for which appropriate psychometric properties have not been demonstrated. (Exceptions are the studies by Holroyd's group[36] and Neufeld and Thomas,[41] which directly manipulated expectancies).

MULTIAXIAL ASSESSMENT OF PAIN PATIENTS

Advances in the assessment of pain patients have not kept pace with theory and the development of therapeutic methods. Multidimensional conceptualizations of pain, as characterized by the gate-control and cognitive-behavioral models, have a good deal of face validity. There seems to be growing agreement among investigators[18,48,51] that adequate assessment of chronic pain requires measurement of three important dimensions, namely, medical–physical, psychosocial, and behavioral–functional. Such a multiaxial assessment of pain (MAP) incorporates these three dimensions to evaluate chronic pain patients, to improve clinical decision making, and to evaluate the efficacy of different treatments with diverse groups of patients and different pain syndromes.

Perhaps the earliest attempt to evaluate physical, cognitive, and affective contributors to the perception of pain was presented by Melzack[45] in the McGill Pain Questionnaire. Although this approach held great merit and served a heuristic function, subsequent research has suggested that the McGill questionnaire is not an adequate multidimensional measure of pain.[46] (See Chap. 2.)

Medical–Physical Axis

Until recently, assessment of chronic pain patients was characterized by several trends. First, evaluation of the medical–physical dimension relied on clinical judgment based on the practitioner's experience and some fairly standardized criteria.[47] Many of these approaches, however, have not been adequately normed. Some focus on a limited class of pain such as low back pain. For others, the adequacy of biometric properties (reliability, validity, utility) has not been established.

One early attempt to quantify and objectify assessment of the medical–physical dimension was reported by Brena and his colleagues[48–50] and is referred to as the Emory pain estimate model. It conceptualized chronic pain as consisting of two dimensions: The medical–physical and the psychological–behavioral. The latter was assessed using traditional psychological measures and ratings of some pain behaviors. The physical–medical dimension attempted to quantify traditional diagnostic and medical tests such as range of motion and trigger points. This early effort is laudatory, but the weighting system used to score its medical tests remains somewhat controversial and no adequate demonstration of the biometric properties of these ratings has been reported. Refinement of this type of quantification of medical–physical findings is sorely needed. The importance of such a system is evidenced by the fact that the Emory pain estimate model has been endorsed in the draft version of the American Medical Association Council on Scientific Affairs report on Benign Disease–Related Chronic Pain. Recent work by Waddell and his colleagues[47,51] in this area is most encouraging.

Behavioral–Functional Axis

The importance of behavioral factors in chronic pain has been emphasized for two decades,[52] but only recently have attempts begun to quantify specific behaviors so that the behavioral–functional dimension can be adequately assessed. The earliest studies focused on patients' reports of their activity level and use of medication. Patients were asked to estimate or to keep diaries of the number of hours or percentage of time during a day that they spent sitting, lying down, walking, standing, and so forth. Other behaviors recorded were physician visits specifically for pain and frequency of use of analgesic medication.

In addition to patient self-reports of functional activities attempts have been made to assess "pain behaviors objectively." As already noted, Fordyce's operant conceptualization[13] views pain behaviors as overt communications to others that patients have pain and that they are suffering. According to Fordyce, pain behaviors include (1) verbal complaints of pain and suffering, (2) nonlanguage sounds (e.g., moans, sighs), (3) body posturing and gesturing (e.g., limping, rubbing a painful body part or area), and (4) display of functional limitations or impairments (e.g., reclining for excessive periods of time, that is, "downtime").

In the first paper to report a quantifiable system to assess pain behaviors, Keefe and Block[53] videotaped patients assuming static postures and performing a range of dynamic movements (sitting, standing, walking, and reclining), each for a period of 2 minutes. Keefe and Block then rated five categories of pain behaviors: guarding, bracing, rubbing, grimacing, and sighing). Variations on this approach relying on the assessment of pain behaviors emitted during interviews and other observational periods have been reported.[54–56]

In a recent study, Turk, Wack, and Kerns[57] identified a group of 63 prototypic pain behaviors gleaned from the literature. Eight pain therapists rated these behaviors according to how typical they were of pain patients. Twenty specific behaviors were rated as very typical, for example, frequent shifting of position, clenching of teeth. These 20 behaviors were rated in terms of their similarity by 72 members of the International Association for the Study of Pain, 36 physicians and 36 psychologists. Two primary dimensions characterized the 20 pain behaviors, audible-visible and affective–behavioral. The pain behaviors also were classed within one of four clusters labeled (a) distorted ambulation or posture, (b) negative affective, (c) facial/audible expression of distress, and (d) avoidance of activity. There were no differences between the physicians and psychologists in these ratings. The results of this study support the conceptualization of pain behaviors originally outlined by Fordyce and provide an empirically derived basis for the assessment of pain behaviors.

These recent attempts to operationalize the construct of pain behaviors are quite promising, but, some approaches are quite cumbersome. They require videotape equipment and sophisticated behavioral sampling and scoring.[53] Other, simpler procedures have yet to establish the psychometric adequacy of these assessment methods.[55–57] These preliminary efforts do support the feasibility of developing procedures to operationalize the behavioral axis and serve as a starting point for inclusion within a MAP system.

Psychosocial Axis

If one adheres to the perspective that chronic pain is a complex, subjective phenomenon that is uniquely experienced by each patient, then knowledge about patients' idiosyncratic appraisals of their plight, their experience of pain, and their coping resources becomes critical for optimal treatment planning. For example, patients' subjective evaluations of the impact of pain on their lives are likely to be important in determining motivation for treatment and treatment adherence. Additionally, patients' perceptions of their life circumstances are likely to influence their communications with significant others and health care professionals. These sources of communication are likely to influence how others respond to them and potentially the therapeutic modalities to which people with pain are exposed.

A trend that has characterized assessment of the psychosocial dimension has been the reliance on instruments that were not specifically developed nor normed on chronic pain patients but rather were intended for use with psychiatric populations (e.g., Minnesota Multiphasic Personality Inventory, Beck Depression Inventory, Rorschach, Szondi). A detailed description of the use of these instruments with chronic pain patients is beyond the scope of this chapter, but the interested reader can consult Bradley and colleagues.[58]

More recently, comprehensive assessment instruments specifically to evaluate the psychosocial dimension of chronic pain have begun to appear: the Sickness Impact Profile,[59] the Illness Behavior Questionnaire,[60,61] the West Haven–Yale Multidimensional Pain Inventory.[62] Detailed description of each of these instruments is beyond the scope of this chapter. Such a discussion may be found in reference 18. One approach is described here to illustrate attempts to assess factors related to the psychosocial axis.

Kerns and associates[62] have developed a comprehensive assessment inventory, the West Haven–Yale Multidimensional Pain Inventory (WHYMPI). It is composed of three parts. The second part measures patients' perceptions of the range and frequency of responses by significant others to their displays of pain and suffering (i.e., pain behaviors) and part three comprises a daily activities checklist that is included as a component of the behavioral-functional axis. Part one is particularly relevant to the present discussion in that it was specifically designed to assess:

1. Chronic pain patients' reports of pain severity and suffering
2. Their perceptions of how pain interferes with their lives, including interference with family and marital functioning, work, and social-recreational activities
3. Dissatisfaction with their present level of functioning in each of the areas listed in 2
4. Appraisal of the support provided by spouses, family, and significant others
5. Perceived life control, incorporating the perceived ability to solve problems and feelings of personal mastery and competence
6. Affective distress, including ratings of depressed mood, irritability, and tension.

In addition to its comprehensive assessment of important psychosocial factors (i.e., content validity), the authors also demonstrated that the WHYMPI had good psychometric properties (internal consistency, temporal stability, and construct validity).

The development of psychometrically sound instruments such as the WHYMPI and procedures such as the pain behavior ratings described above hold great promise. Research is needed to confirm the utility of these procedures so that they can serve as assessment instruments to operationalize the psychosocial and behavioral axes within the more general MAP system. Once an acceptable system to assess each of the axes has been established, the MAP system outlined here can be directly tested. The development and testing of this type of system would permit the identification of sets or clusters of patients with specific characteristics that are based on a comprehensive consideration of physical, psychological, and behavioral findings. Once this taxonomy has been created and refined, it could be used prognostically, in clinical decision making, and in evaluating the efficacy of different treatments. The next section describes how this type of system might be developed and employed, using only the psychosocial and behavioral axes. In the more comprehensive approach that we have been suggesting, each of the assessment procedures comprising the three relevant axes would be incorporated within the analysis.

TOWARD A TAXONOMY OF CHRONIC PAIN PATIENTS

With increasing recognition that life with chronic pain can affect the patient in many ways (emotionally, socially, familially), investigators and clinicians frequently assess the chronic pain patient with a plethora of psychological measures, perhaps out of fear of missing an important psychosocial factor. For example, it is not uncommon for the patient coming to a pain clinic to answer over 500 questions that are related to psychological factors (an obvious parallel can be drawn to the medical–physical axis in that the chronic pain patient is frequently referred for numerous medical tests, examinations by specialists, x-rays, etc.). After this assessment battery, the difficult task is to "make sense" out of perhaps 20 to 30 derived scale scores. In other words, this kind of assessment may yield several measures of depression, anxiety, marital satisfaction, perceptions of control, health attitudes and behaviors, and so forth. An obvious solution to this dilemma is for the investigator to perform some type of data reduction strategy to achieve a general understanding of the psychosocial factors that are of special importance or unique to the chronic pain patient.

A frequently used data reduction procedure is to divide patients in terms of whether they scored above or below the mean average for a particular scale (eg, the Emory Pain Estimate model described above). Although simple enough, this method creates an insurmountable problem: It yields an enormous number of ways by which patients can be classified. For example, if one were to classify patients according to their scores on only eight measures, there would be 256 (28) unique categories to which patients could be assigned. Obviously, this approach is too broad and tells us very little about the typical psychosocial problems experienced by the chronic pain patient.

Although additional research is needed to advance our understanding of the basic psychosocial factors affected by living with chronic pain, all too often these approaches seem to us to provide little insight into understanding the individual pain patient or how living with chronic pain may differentially influence people's lives. In other words, more is learned about the performance of psychosocial assessment instruments than about the chronic pain patients for whom these instruments were developed.

We have begun to experiment with cluster analytic procedures as a method of discovering more about the similarities and differences among chronic pain patients on psychosocial measures by using the WHYMPI.[62] Instead of focusing on the similarities and differences among the psychosocial scales used to assess chronic pain patients, we used the reverse logic and looked at how subsets of patients fit together. The application of taxometric methods to the area of chronic pain may help the investigator identify and classify patients into categories that naturally exist. In other words, these methods help us discover subgroups or "homogeneous" samples of pain patients and guard against the investigator superimposing an a priori but potentially invalid structure on the data.

The general purpose of cluster analysis, which is a generic name for a wide variety of statistical procedures, is to (1) develop a typology or classification system, (2) investigate useful conceptual schemes for grouping entities, (3) generate hypotheses through data exploration, and (4) test hypotheses, or determine if types defined through other procedures are in fact present in a data set.[63] Specific to our particular application of cluster analysis, we wanted to determine whether primary subgroups of chronic pain

patients based on psychosocial and behavioral factors could be identified. To examine this question, we used patients' scores on nine scales of the WHYMPI. In other words, we wanted to determine whether there were unique response patterns or profiles on the nine WHYMPI psychosocial and behavioral scales that could be used to reliably classify patients into different groups that had theoretical or clinical implications.

K-means cluster analysis[64] was conducted on the WHYMPI scale scores of 121 heterogeneous chronic pain patients. This clustering technique was selected because it groups together *entities,* in this case chronic pain patients, with similar profiles across *attributes,* namely WHYMPI scale scores. Applying stringent criteria to the K-means clustering results indicated that a three-cluster solution was the most parsimonious solution to these data.

Although space does not permit a detailed discussion of the results of this cluster analysis, the primary findings of this statistical procedure are summarized in Table 3-1. Based on their mean scores on the WHYMPI scales, the first cluster appeared to reflect *inadequate social support.* That is, this cluster represented those pain patients who were experiencing an unusually high level of social distress at the time of their admission to a pain center. Specifically, these patients appeared to hold a common perception that their families and significant others were not very supportive of them, particularly as it related to their pain problem.

The second group of patients uncovered by the clustering procedure we labeled as *dysfunctional.* This cluster appeared to be composed of patients who perceived the severity of their pain to be at very high levels and who reported that it interfered to a great extent with many domains of their lives. Additionally, cluster 2 patients, when compared with cluster 1 patients, reported a higher degree of psychological distress due to pain, especially in terms of mood and their perceived ability to control their lives and solve their day-to-day problems. This group also reported low levels of daily activity.

Finally, the patients in cluster 3 appeared to have in common higher levels of social support, lower levels of pain severity and perceived interference, and higher daily activity levels. Thus, this group of pain patients appeared to be comprised of *adaptive copers.* In sum, this group of patients, perhaps because of more support from others or a less severe pain condition, appeared to be coping psychologically better with their pain in that they reported lower levels of dysphoric mood and, when compared with patients in clusters 1 and 2, believed that they had a better ability to control their lives.

If predictive validity can be established for these clusters, then developing this type of classification system for chronic pain patients may have important clinical implications. For example, patients presenting with a profile similar to the patients in cluster 1 may need more intensive family and marital interventions, whereas patients in cluster 2 may benefit from more intensive physical therapy and

Table 3-1
Interpretive Summary of K-Means Cluster Analysis of the WHYMPI Scales

Patient Cluster 1 (n = 34): Interpersonal Distress
Average levels of perceived interference and pain severity
Average levels of life control and negative mood
Average self-reported activity levels
Lower levels of perceived family and spousal support
Lower reported frequency of solicitous and distracting responses and higher reported frequency of
  punishing responses from spouse

Patient Cluster 2 (n = 51): Dysfunctional
Higher levels of perceived interference and pain severity
Lower levels of life control and higher levels of negative mood
Lower self-reported activity levels
Higher levels of perceived family and spousal support
Higher reported frequency of solicitous and distracting responses and lower reported frequency of
  punishing responses from spouse

Patient Cluster 3 (n = 36): Adaptive Copers
Lower levels of perceived interference and pain severity
Higher levels of life control and lower levels of negative mood
Higher self-reported activity levels
Higher levels of perceived family and spousal support
Higher reported frequency of solicitous and distracting responses and lower reported frequency of
  punishing responses from spouse

pain reduction treatment regimens and cluster 3 patients need a therapeutic approach designed to reinforce, enhance, and maintain their adaptive responding to their pain problem.

Although these preliminary results are promising, as with any study of this nature, these findings need to be replicated on additional populations and further validity needs to be established for these patient groups. Additionally, as we noted earlier, to create a more comprehensive patient classification system, information from the medical–physical axis also needs to be incorporated. This procedure may create further subdivisions of patient groups, establish more comprehensive profiles, and provide a more in-depth understanding of chronic pain patients' presenting problems and thereby enhance our ability to provide individual treatment approaches. We are currently conducting these studies. Some of our early findings support the validity and generalizability of the results reported above.

FUTURE DIRECTIONS

A growing body of empirical data support the inclusion of cognitive, affective, and behavioral factors in investigating, diagnosing, and treating chronic pain.[65–67] Currently there is much confusion in pain assessment because there is little agreement about how best to measure this complex and largely subjective phenomenon. We believe that the multiaxial assessment of pain (MAP) concept and the use of taxometrically based statistical procedures such as cluster analysis offer an advance over current assessment strategies. We are now attempting to refine this multiaxial system. Identifying clusters of patients according to physical, psychosocial, and behavioral data should enhance our understanding of pain, assist in the prescription of specific therapeutic interventions, and improve our ability to predict treatment outcome.

In the future, psychologists need to work more closely in interdisciplinary teams of health care professionals to provide the most appropriate treatment for patients with chronic pain. The single-modality approach to the treatment of chronic pain might seem a quaint anachronism, except that the word "anachronism" implies that such a concept was at one time useful. We are not sure this was ever the case. We believe that health care professionals abrogate their responsibilities when they try to treat chronic pain without considering all three of its dimensions: medical–physiological, psychosocial, and behavioral–functional.

References

1. Fulop-Miller, R. *Triumph over Pain*. New York: Literary Guild of America; 1938.
2. Sontag S. *Illness as Metaphor*. New York: Vintage Books. 1979.
3. Flor H, Turk DC. Etiological theories and treatments for chronic back pain, I: somatic factors. *Pain* 1984; *19*:105–121.
4. Loeser JD. Low back pain. *Research Publications of the Association for Research in Nervous and Mental Disease* 1980; 58:363–377.
5. Jenkins PL. Psychogenic abdominal pain. *Gen Hosp Psychiatry* January 1991; 13(1):27–30.
6. Feinmann C. Psychogenic regional pain. *Br J Hosp Med* February 1990; 43(2):123–124, 127.
7. Beecher, HK. *Measurement of Subjective Responses: Quantitative Effects of Drugs*. New York: Oxford University Press; 1959.

8. Melzack R, Casey KL. Sensory, motivational and central control determinants of pain: a new conceptual model. In: Kenshalo D, ed. *The Skin Senses*. Springfield, IL: Charles C Thomas; 1968:168–194.

9. Melzack R, Wall PD. Pain mechanisms: a new theory. *Science* 1965; 50:971–979.

10. Nathan PW. The gate control theory of pain: a critical review. *Brain* 1976; 99:123–158.

11. Turk DC, Meichenbaum D, Genest M. *Pain and Behavioral Medicine: A Cognitive-Behavioral Perspective*. New York: Guilford Press; 1983.

12. International Association for the Study of Pain. Pain terms: A list with definitions and notes on usage. *Pain* 1979; 6:249–252.

13. Fordyce WE. *Behavioral Methods for Chronic Pain and Illness*. St Louis, MO: Mosby; 1976.

14. Collie J. *Malingering and Feigned Sickness*. London: Edward Arnold; 1913.

15. Rachlin H. Pain and behavior. *Behav Brain Sci* 1985; 8:43–53.

16. Ciccone DS, Grzesiak RC. Cognitive dimensions of chronic pain. *Soc Sci Med* 1984; 19:1339–1346.

17. Sternbach RA. Behavior therapy. In: Wall PD, Melzack R, eds. *Textbook of Pain*. London: Churchill Livingstone; 1984:800–805.

18. Turk DC, Rudy TE. Assessment of cognitive factors in chronic pain: a worthwhile enterprise? *J Consult Clin Psychol* 1986; 54:760–768.

19. Rudy TE, Turk DC. Psychological aspects of pain. *Int Anesthesiol Clin* Winter 1991; 29(1):9–21.

20. Skinner JB, Erskine A, Pearce S, Rubenstein I, Taylor M, Foster C. The evaluation of a cognitive behavioral treatment programme in outpatients with chronic pain. *J Psychosom Res* 1990; 34(1):13–19.

21. Flor H, Turk DC, Birbaumer N. Assessment of stress-related psychophysiological reactions in chronic back pain patients. *J Consult Clin Psychol* 1985; 53:354–364.

22. Mercuri LG, Olson RE, Laskin DM. The specificity of response to experimental stress in patients with myofascial pain dysfunction syndrome. *J Dent Res* 1979; 58:1866–1871.

23. Dahlstrom L, Carlsson SG, Gale EN, Jansson TG. Stress-induced muscular activity in mandibular dysfunction: effects of biofeedback training. *J Behav Med* 1985; 8:191–200.

24. Bush C, Ditto B, Feuerstein M. A controlled evaluation of paraspinal EMG biofeedback in the treatment of chronic low back pain. *Health Psychol* 1985; 4:307–321.

25. Courey L, Feuerstein M, Bush C. Self-control and chronic headache. *J Psychosom Res* 1982; 26:519–526.

26. Pickar D, Cohen MR, Nabor D, Cohen RM. Clinical studies of the endogenous opioid system. *Biol Psychiatry* 1980; 17:1243–1276.

27. Dworkin SF, Chen ACN, Shubert MM, Clark DW. Cognitive modification of pain: information in combination with N_2O. *Pain* 1984; 19:339–351.

28. Melzack R, Weisz AZ, Sprague LT. Strategies for controlling pain: Contributions of auditory stimulation and suggestion. *Exp Neurol* 1963; 8:239–247.

29. Turk DC, Genest M. Regulation of pain: The application of cognitive and behavioral techniques for prevention and remediation. In: Kendall P, Hollon S, eds. *Cognitive-Behavioral Interventions: Theory, Research and Procedures*. New York: Academic Press; 1979:287–319.

30. Turner JA. Comparison of group progressive-relaxation training and cognitive-behavioral group therapy for chronic low back pain patients. *J Consult Clin Psychol* 1982; 50:757–765.

31. Nicholas MK, Wilson PH, Goyen J. Operant-behavioral and cognitive-behavioral treatment for chronic low back pain. *Behav Res Ther* 1991; 29(3):225–238.

32. Bakal DA, Demjen S, Kaganov JA. Cognitive behavioral treatment of chronic headache. *Headache* 1981; 21:81–86.

33. Stam HJ, McGrath P, Brooke RI. The effects of a cognitive-behavioral treatment program on temporomandibular pain and dysfunction syndrome. *Psychosom Med* 1984; 46:634–645.

34. Randich SR. Evaluation of a pain management program for rheumatoid arthritis patients. *Arthritis Rheum* 1984; 25 (suppl):11. Abstract.

35. Flor H, Haag G, Turk DC, Koehler G. Efficacy of EMG biofeedback, pseudotherapy, and convention medical treatments for chronic rheumatic pain. *Pain* 1983; 17:21–32.

36. Holroyd KA, Penzien DB, Hursey KG, et al. Change mechanisms in EMG biofeedback training: Cognitive changes underlying improvements in tension headache. *J Consult Clin Psychol* 1984; 52:1039–1053.

37. Turner JA, Chapman CR. Psychological interventions for chronic pain: a critical review, I: relaxation training and biofeedback. *Pain* 1982a; 12:1–22.

38. Turner JA, Chapman CR. Psychological interventions for chronic pain: a critical review, II: operant conditioning, hypnosis, and cognitive-behavioral therapy. *Pain* 1982b; 12:23–46.

39. Follick MJ, Ziter RE, Ahern DK. Failure in the operant treatment of chronic pain. In: Foe E, Emmelkamp P, eds. *Failures in Behavioral Therapy*. New York: Wiley; 1983:197–223.

40. Holroyd KA, Andrasik F. Coping and self-control of chronic pain. *J Consult Clin Psychol* 1978; 46:1036–1045.

41. Neufeld RWJ, Thomas P. Effects of perceived efficacy of a prophylactic controlling mechanism on self control under pain stimulation. *Can J Behav Sci* 1977; 9:224–232.

42. Murphy MA, Tosi DJ, Pariser RF. Psychological coping and the management of pain with cognitive restructuring and biofeedback: a case study and variation of cognitive experiential therapy. *Psychol Rep* June 1989; 64(3 pt 2):1343–1350.

43. Grunert BK, Devine CA, Sanger JR, Matloub HS, Green D. Thermal self-regulation for pain control in reflex sympathetic dystrophy syndrome. *J Hand Surg* Am July 1990; 15(4):615–618.

44. Moore JE, Chaney EF. Outpatient treatment of chronic pain: Effects of spouse involvement. *J Consult Clin Psychol* 1985; 53:326–334.

45. Melzack R. The McGill Pain Questionnaire: Major properties and scoring methods. *Pain* 1975; 1:277–299.

46. Turk DC, Rudy TE, Salovey P. The McGill Pain Questionnaire reconsidered: Confirming the factor structure and examining appropriate uses. *Pain* 1985; 21:385–397.

47. Waddell G, McCulloch JA, Kummel E, Venner RM. Nonorganic physical signs in low-back pain. *Spine* 1980; 5:117–125.

48. Brena SF, Chapman SL. Chronic pain: An algorithm for management. *Postgrad Medic* 1982; 72:111–117.

49. Brena SF, Koch DL. A "pain estimate" model for quantification and classification of chronic pain states. *Anesthesiology Review* 1975; 2:8–13.

50. Brena SF, Koch DL, Moss RM. Reliability of the "pain estimate" model. *Anesthes Rev* 1976; 3:28–29.

51. Waddell G, Main CJ. Assessment of severity in low-back disorders. *Spine* 1984; 9:204–208.

52. Fordyce WE, Fowler RS Jr, DeLateur B. An application of behavior modification technique to a problem of chronic pain. *Behav Res Ther* 1968; 6:105–107.

53. Keefe FJ, Block AR. Development of an observation method for assessing pain behavior in chronic low back pain. *Behav Ther* 1982; 13:363–375.

54. Cinciripini PM, Floreen A. An assessment of chronic pain behavior in a structured interview. *J Psychosom Res* 1983; 27:117–124.

55. Fordyce W, McMahon R, Rainwater G, et al. Pain complaints—exercise performance relationship in chronic pain. *Pain* 1981; 10:311–321.

56. Richards JS, Nepomuceno C, Riles M, Suer Z. Assessing pain behavior: The UAB Pain Behavior Scale. *Pain* 1982; 14:393–398.

57. Turk DC, Wack JT, Kerns RD. An empirical examination of the "pain behavior" construct. *J Behav Med* 1985; 8:119–130.

58. Bradley LA, Prokop CK, Gentry WD, Hopson L, Prieto EJ. Assessment of chronic pain. In: Prokop CK, Bradley LA, eds. *Medical Psychology: Contributions to Behavioral Medicine*. New York: Academic Press; 1981:35–52.

59. Bergner M, Bobbit RA, Carter WB, Gilson BS. The Sickness Impact Profile: validation of a health status measure. *Med Care* 1981; 19:787–805.

60. Pilowsky I, Spence ND. Pain and illness behavior: A comparative study. *J Psychosom Res* 1976a; 20:131–134.

61. Pilowsky I, Spence ND. Illness behavior syndromes associated with intractable pain. *Pain* 1976b; 4:61–71.

62. Kerns RS, Turk DC, Rudy TE. The West Haven-Yale Multidimensional Pain Inventory (WHYMPI). *Pain* 1985; 23:345–356.

63. Aldenderfer MS, Blashfield RK. *Cluster Analysis*. Beverly Hills, Calif: Sage Publications; 1984.

64. Everitt B. *Cluster Analysis*. London: Heinemann Educational Books; 1974.

65. Doody SB, Smith C, Webb J. Nonpharmacologic interventions for pain management. *Crit Care Nurs Clin North Am* March 1991; 3(1):69–75.

66. Benjamin S. Psychological treatment of chronic pain: a selective review. *J Psychosom Res* 1989; 33(2):121–131.

67. Harness DM, Rome HP. Psychological and behavioral aspects of chronic facial pain. *Otolaryngol Clin North Am* December 1989; 22(6):1073–1094.

CHAPTER 4

Diagnostic Measures

Ann-Marie E. Nehme and Carol A. Warfield

Pain is a noxious sensation elicited by stimuli that are capable of injuring tissue cells. As a totally subjective phenomenon, it cannot be precisely and objectively assessed. The patient's subjective description of his or her pain is often the physician's sole data base for diagnosis.

As the concept and reality of the pain clinic has evolved, the role of the anesthesiologist as a clinician in the field of diagnostic and therapeutic analgesia has developed.[1–7] Because the accurate evaluation of chronic pain problems can often be very difficult, diagnostic measures can play an important role in providing objective information about the mechanisms of pain in a particular patient.[8–12]

A clear understanding of the neuroanatomy and neurophysiology of pain pathways is necessary to understand the diagnostic procedures and is therefore briefly reviewed here. (See Chap. 1 for a more thorough discussion.)

Simplistically and more typically in acute somatosensory pain states, noxious stimuli from "injured" tissues are transmitted from peripheral receptors via specific pathways in the periphery to the central nervous system and sensory cortex. Unfortunately, our knowledge of the structure and physiology of the receptors and central pathways that mediate pain is not complete. Presumably, the peripheral receptors are fine branching nerve fibers that respond to different noxious stimuli. The pain fibers enter the spinal cord through the dorsal root and synapse with neurons in the posterior horn before advancing to the opposite lateral spinothalamic tract where they ascend to the thalamus and somesthetic area of the cortex. Generally the system is a relatively slow conducting system. It has many synapses and is integrated with the autonomic nervous system including reflex sympathetic activation. Pain fibers from the head and neck are carried in the trigeminal nerve (cranial nerve V) and its ganglion, as well as cranial nerves VII, IX, and X.

There are basically two types of pain: fast, sharp pain and slow, burning pain. The small, myelinated A-delta fibers are thought to convey sharp, fast pain as well as temperature, touch, and pressure sensations. The small, unmyelinated C-fibers are thought to transmit dull, burning pain and temperature sensation (Table 4-1).

Somatic nociceptive impulses are transmitted by peripheral somatic and somatosensory nerves and by sympathetic efferent nerves. Visceral pain is transmitted by afferent fibers closely associated with sympathetic nerve fibers.

Interpretation of these incoming nociceptive impulses as pain is a complex central process. Numerous factors play into both the interpretation and response including the circumstances under which the pain is occurring, the patient's cultural background, and the patient's perceptions and personality. Underlying psychological problems and secondary gains play a significant role here.

It is often useful to categorize pain, and certainly this is part of the approach to a diagnostic workup. Many of the diagnostic maneuvers will discern whether the pain is peripheral or central in origin. Because pain can be caused by

Table 4-1
Classification of Nerve Fibers

Type	Fiber Characteristics	Diameter, microns	Maximum Speed, m/s	Function	Anesthetic for Blocking % procaine
A	myelinated				
alpha		12–22	120	Large motor; sensory to muscle spindles and tendons	1.0
beta		5–13	70	Sensory to muscle spindles, touch, pressure, and vibration	1.0
gamma		3–8	40	Small motor to muscle spindles	1.0
delta		2–5	30	Touch, pressure, pain, and temperature	0.5
B	myelinated	3	15	Preganglionic autonomic fibers	.25
C	unmyelinated	1	2	Postganglionic autonomic fibers; pain and temperature	0.5

either organic or psychogenic factors, most tests will also address this issue. Finally, pain is categorized according to its onset and duration, that is, acute versus chronic pain. These categories represent very different situations. In almost all cases, the patient who would benefit from a diagnostic workup in the pain clinic setting is the one with a history of chronic pain resistant to both general diagnostic and therapeutic measures.

By the time the chronic pain patient reaches the pain clinic, he or she has typically undergone a thorough diagnostic workup and has been evaluated and treated by several doctors in different subspecialty areas. This in no way, however, obviates the need for the anesthesiologist as a clinician to approach the problem freshly, either to reconfirm the diagnosis and physical findings or to redefine the problem. The initial step, as in other areas of medicine, is a good history and physical examination.

HISTORY AND PHYSICAL EXAMINATION

The emphasis in the history, of course, is on the pain. The essential points include the circumstances at the onset of the pain and its initial presentation. Particularly important is the description of the present pain: Is it constant or intermittent, sharp, dull, gnawing, shooting, burning? Is it associated with diaphoresis, flushing, or temperature change in the affected area? Where exactly is the perceived distribution of the pain? What are the factors that worsen or improve it? Finally, what treatments has the patient tried and to what effect? Remember that in this patient group, it is not unusual for the history to be the major if not the sole source of data for the diagnostic workup.

It is well known that psychosocial factors affect both the perception of pain and the prognosis for recovery. Tests such as the Minnesota Multiphasic Personality Inventory (MMPI) are frequently part of the patient's diagnostic workup for identifying contributing emotional factors[9,13] (see Chap. 2). In addition, it is important to ascertain whether there is any secondary gain in the patient having pain. Whenever possible it is useful to know whether there is any litigation involved.

Regarding the physical examination itself, there are certain specific things for which one must look. The examination is concentrated primarily in the affected area. The clinician must evaluate any apparent deformity including asymmetry, scars, and changes in color or temperature. Examinations of joint mobility and of motor and sensory innervation are part of each evaluation. One must specifically look for areas of muscle spasm, trigger points (usually indicated by splinting and "ropiness"; see Chap. 19), and areas of allodynia, hyperalgesia, dyesthesia, hyperesthesia, paresthesia, or hypoesthesia.

Because the majority of patients in the typical pain clinic have chronic low back pain, a brief review of the basic examination of the back is worthwhile. With the patient standing, the back is examined for scoliosis or hyperlordo-

sis of the lumbar spine or excessive kyphosis of the thoracic spine. The patient is then instructed to walk, first normally, then on toes, and finally on heels, noting any weakness or onset of pain. With the patient sitting, tenderness over the spinous processes, facet joints, and sacroiliac joints is tested. Patellar (L3-4) and Achilles (L5-SI) deep tendon reflexes are elicited bilaterally. The patient is then instructed to lie supine on the examining table where motor strength of the lower extremities, particularly the ankle flexors (L5), and extensor (L5) and flexor (S1) hallucis longus muscles are tested. Response to light touch and pinprick is evaluated and any area of abnormal sensation noted. Tenderness of the quadriceps (L4), calf (S1) and anterior tibia (L5) is tested. Leg length is measured from the anterior superior iliac spines to the medial malleoli, and any discrepancy is noted. Finally, straight leg raising is done, noting the degree to which the patient can perform this, and what the limiting factor is, for example, back pain versus hamstring tightening.

By the end of this detailed history and physical examination, along with any previous study results, one should be ready to assess the situation and proceed with additional diagnostic maneuvers as indicated.

DIAGNOSTIC NERVE BLOCKADE: ANATOMIC APPROACH

The basis of diagnostic nerve blocks is the selective blockade of sympathetic and somatic nerve fibers of the affected painful area. This concept has been employed for several years, but recent advances in our understanding the complex nature of pain perception have challenged the basic premises on which these techniques rely. Differential neural blockade makes use of the known anatomic and/or physiologic differences in the sympathetic and somatic nerve pathways.[2,10,11,14–18] Psychogenic components of pain have been assessed with placebo injections, but this practice has been challenged because a placebo response may occur in about 30 percent of "normal" individuals; that is, a positive response to a placebo injection argues for but does not prove a psychogenic origin of pain. The specific procedure selected, of course, will be dependent on the site and type of pain (Table 4-2). Aside from differentiating between sympathetic and somatic pain, diagnostic blocks are also used to localize the source of pain. In the case of pain in the foot, for example, if a block at the ankle fails to relieve pain, the assumption has been made that the offending cause is more proximal and subsequent diagnostic measures can include sciatic block, paravertebral somatic block, and epidural block in an attempt to locate the source of nociception. If the pain remains after sciatic block and disappears with lumbar paravertebral somatic block, the assumption has been made that the offending cause is between the nerve root and sciatic notch. Recent understanding of the complexity of the central nervous system has, however, challenged these assumptions.

Table 4-2
Differential Nerve Blocks

Location of Pain	Somatic Block	Sympathetic Block
Head and neck	Cranial nerve V and branches; cervical roots and branches	Stellate ganglion
Upper extremity	Brachial plexus and branches	Stellate ganglion
Thorax	Intercostal	Thoracic epidural
Abdomen	Intercostal	Celiac plexus
Lower back	Lumbar paravertebral	Lumbar sympathetic
Lower extremity	Lumbar paravertebral blocks and branches or transsacral S1 blocks and branches	Lumbar sympathetic
Rectum and genitalia	Transsacral root blocks	Lumbar sympathetic

Head, Neck, and Upper Extremity

When the pain is of the head, neck, upper extremity, or upper chest a cervicothoracic (stellate ganglion) block may be useful. The stellate ganglion consists of the inferior cervical and first thoracic sympathetic ganglia, which are anatomically fused in about 80 percent of the population. As part of the cervical sympathetic trunk, it lies behind the carotid artery, medial to the vagus nerve, in the fascial plane between the carotid sheath anteriorly and prevertebral muscle fascia posteriorly. Specifically the stellate ganglion lies in the interval between the transverse process of the seventh cervical vertebra and the neck of the first rib, directly behind the vertebral artery. At its most inferior portion, the dome of the pleura may overlie the ganglion. Technically there are several methods of blockade, but the anterior approach first described by Leriche and Fontain[19] is the most commonly used. (See Appendix A, Section I.)

When a stellate ganglion block is used for differential diagnosis, normal saline is used for a placebo block. If the pain is relieved in this manner, one can assume a placebo effect. If there is no relief with a placebo injection, the block is done using 10 to 15 ml of local anesthetic, generally lidocaine or bupivacaine.

Signs of a successful block include Horner's syndrome (ptosis, miosis, anhydrosis, and enophthalmus), and a positive sympathogalvanic response or sweat test or temperature rise of the upper extremity. Once the examiner is assured that the block is successful, and if the patient still has no pain relief, a somatic block to the painful areas is performed. For the head and neck, for example, the block would include the trigeminal nerve and cervical plexus, whereas for the upper extremity the block would be at the brachial plexus.

Thorax

In the thoracic area, stellate ganglion block can confirm chest pain of sympathetic origin to the heart and lungs, whereas intercostal nerve blocks will ablate pain of chest wall origin. After giving off a short dorsal ramus to the paravertebral area, the ventral ramus or intercostal nerve courses laterally between the parietal pleura and around the internal intercostal membrane which is just deep to the external intercostal muscle. At about the angle of the rib, it gives off a collateral branch to the superior surface of the rib below. The main part of the nerve is in the groove on the undersurface of its rib with its associated artery and vein superior to it. It next gives off the lateral cutaneous branch, which supplies much of the skin of the chest and abdomen. It ends by turning anteriorly, piercing the external intercostal muscle and pectoralis major and the rectus abdominis in the abdomen to supply the skin of the breast, anterior thorax, and midabdomen. Only the third through sixth intercostal nerves are considered to be "typical." The first thoracic nerve has only a small intercostal branch with the rest joining the fibers of C8 in the brachial plexus. The second thoracic nerve, and occasionally the third, sends fibers in its lateral cutaneous branch to join the intercostobrachial nerve, which supplies sensation to the medial upper arm. The 7th to 11th intercostal nerves leave their grooves at about the point where the ribs turn superiorly to enter the abdominal wall musculature. The 12th nerve in the strictest sense is subcostal. (See Appendix A, Section IX for method.)

Most frequently this block is used to distinguish between chest wall or abdominal wall versus a deeper visceral source of pain.

Because of the high complication rate, particularly of pneumothorax, paravertebral thoracic sympathetic blocks are rarely employed. A differential epidural approach may be used instead and will be discussed shortly, under the section entitled "Differential Epidural Blockade."

Abdomen

In a patient with chronic upper abdominal pain of unknown etiology, a reasonable diagnostic approach would be to perform diagnostic intercostal blocks. If the pain is not relieved by these, despite effective block as evidenced by hypesthesia of the appropriate dermatomes, a celiac plexus block could be done to test for pain of sympathetic or visceral origin.

The celiac plexus is located anterolateral to the upper aspect of the body of the first lumbar vertebra overlying the celiac artery. It is primarily a sympathetic neural structure consisting mainly of two ganglia connected by a fiber network: preganglionic sympathetic fibers of the greater and lesser splanchnic nerves and postganglionic sympathetic branches which accompany the celiac artery. In addition, some parasympathetic vagal fibers pass through these ganglia.

Probably the best approach for this block is the percutaneous posterior approach performed under fluoroscopic guidance. (See Appendix A, Section III.)

Blockade of the celiac plexus with local anesthetic will affect the sympathetic and afferent pain fibers from the upper abdominal viscera. If a block of this structure relieves pain, one can conclude with a high degree of certainty that the pain is visceral in origin. A more permanent block with alcohol may then be considered for therapy. Note that unless a placebo injection was also done before the anesthetic block, a placebo response cannot be ruled out.

Lower Back, Lower Extremity

For pain of the lower back and lower extremity, differential nerve blocks can be achieved by following a placebo block with somatic blocks starting as distal in the extremity as the pain warrants, for example, blockade of the lateral femoral cutaneous nerve to diagnose meralgia paresthetica. If distal somatic blockade does not relieve the pain, more proximal blocks may be performed, eventually proceeding to a lumbar paravertebral somatic block. (See Appendix A, Section VII.) If pain persists, a lumbar sympathetic block may be performed. (See Appendix A, Section II.)

Each of the diagnostic procedures discussed so far falls under what is often referred to as the anatomic approach to pain diagnosis. As described, this employs the injection of placebo followed by sequential sympathetic and/or somatic neural blockade to nerves or ganglia that are anatomically discrete.

DIAGNOSTIC BLOCKADE: PHARMACOLOGIC APPROACH

An alternative approach, the pharmacologic approach, takes advantage of the neurophysiologic differences between the sympathetic and somatic nerve fibers and their differential sensitivity to the blocking effects of local anesthetic.[14] As far back as the late 1800s, the observation was made that certain nerve fibers were more susceptible to the anesthetizing effects of cocaine than others. Gasser and Erlanger's classic paper in 1929[20] reviewed this literature. Citing their experiment with cocaine, they concluded that ease of block-

ing was related mostly to fiber size. But because their results did not rigidly hold true, they believed another undetermined factor must also be in operation.

Subsequent studies[21–23] considered myelination in addition to fiber size, with small myelinated fibers being more susceptible to the action of local anesthetics than large ones. More recently studies by Gissen and associates[24] indicated that large, fast-conducting fibers are more susceptible to conduction blockade than smaller, slower-conducting fibers. These researchers believed that the discrepancies with previous studies are reconcilable if one considers conduction velocity as directly proportional to the distance between activation sites (nodes of Ranvier vs. myelinated nerves). Local anesthetic, by reducing the magnitude of sodium channel influx at the first activation site, should least affect the transmembrane potential at long distances from the initial site. Gissen's group concluded that conduction block, therefore, should occur in the largest fibers with the longest internodal distances, before the smaller fibers. They pointed out, however, that their studies were done in peripheral mixed nerves where small and large fibers are mixed at random in the neural bundle. This is in contrast to the dorsal spinal root where the small-diameter nerve fibers are more superficial and surround the deeper large-diameter fibers in the bundle. This would mean that local anesthetic would diffuse first to the smaller-diameter fibers. This phenomenon might explain their increased susceptibility compared to the larger-diameter fibers in this area and would be a feasible explanation of the discrepancies in these more recent studies. We must still state, as did Gasser and Erlanger in 1929, that "the problem can be considered to be only partly solved." Size of the fiber, whether or not it is myelinated, the concentration of anesthetic used as well as its lipid solubility, the length of the nerve fiber exposed to anesthetic, and the neuropathologic characteristics of the neural structure being blocked are all factors known to play a part in differential blockade.

Despite the unresolved issues, there are enough consistently reproducible results so that the differential pharmacologic blockade is a clinically useful method. It is generally observed and accepted that for blockade of spinal nerve roots, the B (3-micron diameter) myelinated, preganglionic autonomic fibers are blocked by the lowest concentration of anesthetic. (See Table 4-1.) Next the A-delta (2–5 microns) myelinated sensors for temperature and sharp pain are blocked, along with the C (0.5–1.0 micron) unmyelinated sensors for dull pain, temperature, and touch. At still higher concentrations of local anesthetics, one will get blockade of the A-alpha, beta, and gamma fibers (± 10–20 microns) which are responsible for motor function, touch, and pressure perception. It is because of this differential blockade that one can pharmacologically test sympathetic and somatic sources of pain in an area where there is no discrete anatomic separation of the sympathetic sensory and somatic nerves.

Differential Spinal Blockade

The differential spinal block is a time-consuming procedure that uses the foregoing knowledge to shed light on the etiology of the patient's pain.[14,25,26] Using standard sterile technique, the subarachnoid space is entered at the appropriate level. Four sequential injections are then performed until the patient reports relief of pain or all four injections are complete, whichever comes first (Fig. 4-1). The initial injection is of 5 to 10 ml of normal saline. If the patient reports relief, one can assume a placebo response and possibly pain of psychogenic origin. Approximately one fourth to one third of all patients will have a positive placebo response. In true psychogenic pain, the pain relief is usually long-lasting, whereas the more common placebo reaction is of short duration.

If the patient's pain is not relieved with normal saline, then one's goal is to block the nerve fibers requiring the weakest concentration of local anesthetic: the B sympathetic fibers. This is done by injecting 5 to 10 ml (*note:* the same volume is used for each injection) of 0.25% procaine. If these injections relieve the pain one can conclude it is of sympathetic origin, for example, reflex sympathetic dystrophy or causalgia. Of course, before arriving at this conclusion, one must confirm that there is sympathetic blockade but no sensory blockade.

Next a 0.5% concentration of procaine is used to extend the block to include the A-delta and C pain fibers. Once a sensory block is confirmed, relief of pain indicates a somatosensory source.

If there is no pain relief, the concentration of anesthetic is increased to 1% using the same volume as each of the previous injections to attain a motor block. If this fails to relieve the patient's pain despite complete sympathetic, sensory, and motor blockade, the etiology is most likely of central origin, although, again, psychogenic pain may also behave like this. At this point one might proceed with testing for centrally mediated pain as described in the section entitled "Intravenous Thiopental, Lidocaine, and Phentolamine Tests."

This technique of differential spinal blockade presents many practical problems. Generally, 10 to 20 min is required to evaluate the results of each of the four sequential blocks. It is often difficult, if not impossible, for the patient with severe chronic pain to lie still on his side for the prolonged time necessary for this testing. In addition to the lengthy procedure time, the patient must be observed for 1 to 2 h following the procedure until the block has entirely worn off. It may be impractical for the physician and staff in a busy pain clinic to devote the amount of time necessary for this procedure. There is some variability in the percentage concentration required for blockade at each level, and occasionally one must deviate from the guidelines until the proper level is achieved, again adding time.

FIGURE 4-1. Differential spinal blockade process.

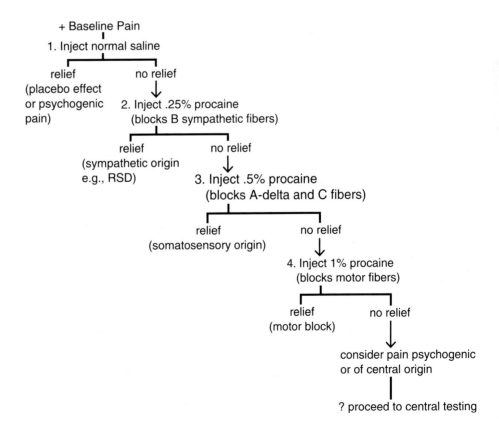

Modified Differential Spinal Blockade

Mainly for practical reasons, a modified differential spinal technique has been developed.[27] This approach is based on the knowledge that as a complete block wears off, it will do so in the order of motor first, then sensory, then sympathetic. In this modified technique, after subarachnoid tap, 2 ml of normal saline is injected to test for placebo effect and psychogenic pain as above. If the pain persists, one goes on to inject 2 ml of 5% procaine. The spinal needle is removed and patient placed supine. This concentration of procaine should induce a complete motor block. After confirmation of this complete blockade, pain is assessed. If there is no relief, then one may look to a central etiology. If there is pain relief, then one must continue to assess the level of blockade to identify the level at which the pain returns. If, for example, the pain recurs at the time the pinprick and temperature sensation returns, then one can conclude the source is the A-delta and C fibers. If the pain returns long after sensation has returned, one can conclude it is of sympathetic origin.

This modified method addresses three of the shortcomings of the original method: It requires considerably less time, the patient is not required to remain immobile, and the individual variability in concentration needed for specific levels of blockade are of no consequence secondary to the technique. It is certainly a more practical approach.

Differential Epidural Blockade

Another approach to diagnostic blockade of the spinal nerves is the differential epidural block.[28] In theory, the test is similar to the differential spinal blockade, the main difference being that the drugs are deposited in the epidural rather than the subarachnoid space. The technique is similar in that once the epidural catheter has been placed, a normal saline placebo test is followed sequentially by 0.5% lidocaine for testing sympathetic block, 1% for somatosensory block, and 2% for motor block. Results are determined as with the differential spinal. One disadvantage over the subarachnoid technique is that this adds more time to an already lengthy test, which in most cases makes it an impractical option.

A modified epidural technique could certainly be done using normal saline placebo followed by 10 to 20 ml of 2% lidocaine or 3% chloroprocaine and proceeding as with the modified spinal technique.

Another variation of the epidural method was described by Cherry and associates.[29] In their preliminary study, they placed an epidural catheter, then after a normal saline placebo injection, injected 1.0 μg/kg fentanyl and 20 minutes later gave 0.5 mg intravenous naloxone. Their purpose was to distinguish psychogenic pain from pain of organic origin. If the patient's pain was relieved by fentanyl, then worsened by naloxone, the pain was considered to be organic. No significant change after naloxone administration indicated an emotional or more central basis. This testing, of course, does not provide information regarding the specific pathway (e.g., sympathetic vs. sensory) but limits itself to the question of possible psychogenic versus somatic pain. One must also take into account the fact that intraspinal narcotics may be a more effective treatment for certain types of pain than others.

Intravenous Thiopental, Lidocaine, and Phentolamine Tests

If the results of a sequential, differential blockade is no pain relief at any level, the most likely explanation is an etiology proximal to the block, although psychogenic pain is not ruled out. Certain diagnostic maneuvers can test for pain of central origin. These tests are designed primarily to distinguish pain of central etiology from psychogenic pain or malingering. The two such tests most commonly used employ barbiturates and or lidocaine.

The barbiturate test is based on the assumption that if pain is of somatic origin then at light planes of barbiturate sleep the patient's response to the typical pain will be the same as when awake. If, however, the pain disappears completely, though the patient responds to other painful stimuli such as pressure over the anterior tibia, then pain of psychogenic origin is implicated. Basically, the test is done by slowly infusing thiopental until the patient falls into a light plane of sleep. The infusion is then stopped and the patient allowed to wake up slowly. At this point, the patient is periodically tested for response to pain other than his or her typical pain, for example, pressure over the anterior tibia or sternum. When patients respond to this stimulus they are tested for their typical pain using a stimulus known to elicit that pain. If the response is not positive then the pain is believed to be of psychogenic origin.

With the lidocaine test, the patient is given 1.2 to 2.0 mg/kg of lidocaine intravenously until he/she reports tingling or dizziness, which are signs of mild toxicity. Two minutes after this point, the patient's pain is reassessed. If intravenously administered lidocaine provides relief when other nerve blocking techniques have failed to do so, a central etiology is assumed. No relief argues against a central mechanism and for a psychogenic cause of the pain.

One certainly could argue that the interpretation of these results might be unreliable, or at least difficult, and conclusive studies proving the validity of these methods are lacking. In fact, there is a marked paucity of published reports or studies regarding these tests altogether.[30–32]

A third intravenous test useful in differential diagnosis is the phentolamine test for diagnostic and prognostic use in reflex sympathetic dystrophy (RSD). In his study of 48 patients, Arnér[33] showed that in those patients in whom pain was transiently relieved with intravenous phentolamine, intravenous regional guanethidine therapy was likely to provide effective pain relief. Although it has limited application, this test may be very useful in diagnosing and treating patients with RSD.

SUPPORTING DIAGNOSTIC STUDIES

A detailed discussion of the many supporting diagnostic studies available for the evaluation of a pain problem is beyond the scope of this chapter. However, several studies are worthy of mention because of the frequency of their use and their diagnostic helpfulness to the anesthesiologist in the pain clinic.

Electromyography and Nerve Conduction Studies

Not infrequently, the patient referred to the pain clinic will have previously undergone electromyography (EMG) studies in the evaluation of his or her pain. Briefly, EMG and nerve conduction studies are most useful in distinguishing between myopathic and neurogenic origin of peripheral neuromuscular pathology. Most important for the pain clinic, these studies assist in the diagnosis of a peripheral radiculopathy, with the distribution of abnormal findings helping to determine which nerve root is involved.

In general, low amplitude motor unit potentials of short duration suggest a muscular source of the pain, whereas large action potentials and fibrillation potentials come from a neurogenic pathologic process. Signs of disintegration of the integrity of the motor unit are associated with both. Fasciculations may be associated with nerve root irritation. Typically, in a patient with radiculopathy the EMG will demonstrate abnormal activity including fibrillations and large positive waves in the distribution of the affected nerve root. Unfortunately, the EMG may be falsely negative in a patient with known radiculopathy, and positive findings may not be obtained until long after the initial injury.

Radiologic Studies

X-rays, myelograms, computed axial tomographic (CT) scans, and magnetic resonance imaging (MRI) have often been previously been employed in diagnosis when the patient is referred to the pain clinic. Plain films have frequently been obtained at the initial evaluation and are useful in elucidating abnormal changes in bone, soft tissue, and air and fluid patterns. Unfortunately, as would be expected, there is a high false-negative rate in the patient who will ultimately come to the pain center for diagnosis. Even a positive finding does not necessarily lead to the etiology of a patient's pain.

For low back pain with or without radiculopathy, the myelogram was often used before CT and MRI were popularized.[34] Typically, metrizamide, a nonionic water soluble contrast material, is injected into the appropriate epidural space and the patient is then x-rayed. Extradural defects, as would be seen with a herniated disk, will show up clearly as a filling defect and can lead to the correct diagnosis (Fig. 4-2). It is important to realize that in the population without symptoms of back pain, there is an unknown percentage of people with disk protrusion.[35] Therefore, again, a posi-

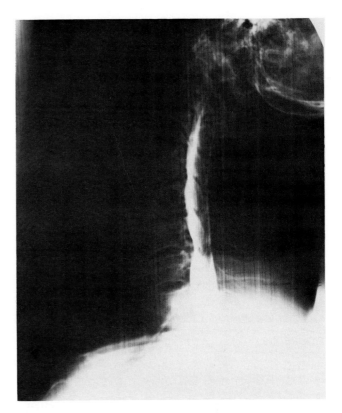

FIGURE 4-2. *Cervical myelogram showing filling defect at C5-6.*

tive finding does not absolutely lead to the true source of the pain.

More recently, CT scans and MRIs have been invaluable aids to diagnosis.[36,37] Each is a relatively noninvasive method of closely examining the spine, its bony structures and disk, and in the case of the MRI, the nerve root and soft tissue is well. Spinal stenosis, bony spurs, disk herniation, and nerve root compression each can potentially be seen by these scans, aiding in the diagnosis of low back pain and radiculopathy[38,39] (Fig. 4-3). Each method can be applied to virtually any part of the body in the diagnostic evaluation of pain of unknown etiology. Since CT scanning and MRIs are so noninvasive, many clinicians believe that their use is indicated to evaluate any pain that is disabling and accompanied by a neurologic deficit.

Thermography

Neuromuscular thermography is also used in the diagnosis of pain.[40,41] Changes in circulation regardless of the underlying cause will result in changes in temperature. Clinical thermographic equipment is based on the Stefan-Boltzmann law that a solid body heated to a temperature above absolute zero will radiate energy in the form of electromagnetic waves (in the infrared portion of the spectrum) at a rate proportional to the fourth power of the temperature. Fortunately skin, regardless of its pigmentation, is an excellent emitter of infrared rays. With the technology developed in

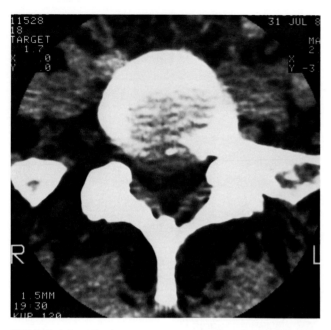

FIGURE 4-3. CT of lumbar spine showing central disk protrusion.

the 1960s of both liquid crystal and electronic infrared systems, the clinical usefulness of thermography was established.

It has been demonstrated that thermal symmetry exists in normal humans.[42] Asymmetry, defined as a difference of at least 1°C, or abnormal patterns can be correlated with certain disease states. For example, a patient with myofascial syndrome may exhibit a "trigger point" with a 1° to 2°F increase in temperature by thermogram. Likewise, areas of inflammation or acute pain generally exhibit an increase in temperature. Hypothermia, often associated with reflex sympathetic dystrophy, can be demonstrated with this method, as can the temperature decrease often associated with areas of chronic pain. Neuropathic pain has associated thermographic changes, at least in the animal model.[43] Chronic back pain exhibits certain findings.[44] Finally, nerve root irritation detected by thermography can be highly correlated (90%) with subsequent myelograms according to one study.[45] Another study,[46] however, concluded that thermography has little or no use as a diagnostic tool in lumbar radiculopathy.

CONCLUSIONS

As anyone who has worked with pain clinic patients knows, the underlying etiology of a chronic pain problem is often complex and elusive to the most scrupulous of diagnostic workups. With a clear understanding of neurophysiology, neuroanatomy, and the pharmacology of local anesthetics, the clinician is able to play a unique part in the diagnostic evaluation of the patient with a difficult problem. Although the exact details of our testing are still not clearly understood, we are able to employ certain principles in testing the underlying causes of pain. These, along with the many supplemental diagnostic tests, are often invaluable for subsequent care of these unfortunate patients.

References

1. Bonica JJ. *The Management of Pain*. Philadelphia: Lea & Febiger; 1953.
2. Bonica JJ. *Clinical Applications of Diagnostic and Therapeutic Nerve Blocks*. Springfield, IL: Charles C. Thomas; 1959.
3. Cousins MJ, Glynn CJ, Mather LE, Wilson PR, Graham JR. Selective spinal analgesia. *Lancet* 1979; 1:1141–1142.
4. Gross SG. Diagnosis anesthesia. Guidelines for the practitioner. *Dent Clin North Am* 1991; 35(1):141–153.
5. Ramamurthy S, Winnie AP. Diagnostic maneuvers in painful syndromes. *Int Anesthesiol Clin* 1983; 21:47–59.
6. Ramamurthy S, Winnie AP. Regional anesthetic techniques for pain relief. *Sem Anesth* 1985; IV(3):237–246.
7. Winnie AP, Collins VJ. The pain clinic: I. Differential neural blockade in pain syndromes of questionable etiology. *Med Clin North Am* 1968; 52:123–129.
8. Andrews DR, Warfield CA. Procedures used in the diagnosis of pain. *Hosp Pract* Off. 1986; 21(5A):108–121.
9. Aronoff GM, ed. *Evaluation and Treatment of Chronic Pain* Baltimore: Urban & Schwarzenberg; 1985.
10. Boas RA, Cousins MJ. Diagnostic neural blockade. In: Cousins MJ, Bridenbaugh PO, eds. *Neural Blockade in Clinical Anesthesia and Management of Pain*. 2nd ed. Philadelphia: Lippincott; 1988:885–898.
11. Bonica JJ. Diagnostic and therapeutic blocks: A reappraisal based on 15 years' experience. *Anesth Analg* 1958; 37:58–68.
12. Rudy TE, Turk DC, Brena SF. Different utility of medical procedures in the assessment of chronic pain patients. *Pain* 1988; 34(1):53–60.
13. Gentry WD, Newman MC, Goldner JL, Balyer C von. Relation between graduated spinal block technique and MMPI for diagnosis and prognosis of chronic low back pain. *Spine* 1977; 2:210–213.
14. Ahlgren EW, Stephen CR, Lloyd AAC, McCollum DE. Diagnosis of pain with a graduated spinal block technique. *JAMA* 1966; 195:813–819.
15. Bonica JJ. Current role of nerve blocks in diagnosis and therapy of pain. In: Bonica JJ, ed. *Advances in Neurology*. Vol. 4. New York: Raven Press; 1974:445–453.
16. Levy BA. Diagnostic, prognostic and therapeutic nerve blocks. *Arch Surg* 1977; 112:870–879.
17. Raj PP. Prognostic and therapeutic local anesthetic blockade. In: Cousins MJ, Bridenbaugh PO, eds. *Neural Blockade in Clinical Anesthetic and Management of Pain*. 2nd ed. Philadelphia: Lippincott; 1988:899–933.
18. Winnie AP, Ramamurthy S, Durrani Z. Diagnostic and therapeutic nerve blocks: Recent advances in techniques. *Adv Neurol.* 1974; 4:455–469.
19. Leriche R, Fontain R. L'anesthesie isoleé du ganglion étoile: Sa technique, ses indications ses resultatas. *Presse Med* 1934; 42:849.
20. Gasser HS, Erlanger J. Role of fiber size in establishment of

nerve block by pressure or cocaine. *Am J Physiol* 1929; 88:581–591.

21. Franz DN, Perry RS. Mechanisms for differential block among single myelinated and non-myelinated axons by procaine. *J Physiol* (Lond) 1974; 236:193–210.

22. Heavner JE, de Jong RH. Lidocaine blocking concentrations for B– and C– nerve fibers. *Anesthesiology* 1974; 40(3):228–233.

23. Nathan PW, Sears TA. Some factors concerned in differential nerve block by local anesthetics. *J Physiol* (Lond) 1961; 157:565–580.

24. Gissen AJ, Covino B, Gregus J. Differential sensitivities of mammalian nerve fibers to local anesthetic agents. *Anesthesiology* 1980; 53:467–474.

25. McCollum DE, Stephen CR. Use of graduated spinal anesthesia in the differential diagnosis of pain in the back and lower extremities. *South Med J* 1969; 57:410–416.

26. Sarnoff SJ, Arrowood JG. Differential spinal block. *Surgery* 1946; 20:150.

27. Akkineni SR, Ramamurthy S. Simplified differential spinal block. *Am Soc Anesth Annu Meeting* 1977:756–766.

28. Raj PP, McLennon JE, Phero JC. Assessment and management planning of chronic low back pain. In: Stanton-Hicks M, Boas R, eds. *Chronic Low Back Pain.* New York: Raven Press; 1982:71–99.

29. Cherry DA, Gourlay GK, McLachlan M, Cousins MJ. Diagnostic epidural opioid blockade and chronic pain: preliminary report. *Pain* 1985; 21:143–152.

30. Boas RA, Covino RB, Shahnarian A. Analgesic responses to I.V. lignocaine. *Br J Anaesth* 1982; 54:501–505.

31. Schwartz GR. Xylocaine viscous as an aid in the differential diagnosis of chest pain. *JACEP* 1976; 5(12):981–983.

32. Schoichet RP. Sodium amytal in the diagnosis of chronic pain. *Can Psychiatr Assoc J* 1978; 23(4):219–228.

33. Arnér S. Intravenous phentolamine test: diagnostic and prognostic use of reflex sympathetic dystrophy. *Pain* 1991; 46:17–22.

34. Hakelius A, Hindmarsh J. The significance of neurologic signs and myelographic findings in the diagnosis of lumbar root compression. *Acta Orthop Scand* 1972; 43:239–246.

35. McNab I. Negative disc explorations. *J Bone Joint Surg Am* 1971; 53A:891–896.

36. Glenn WV, Rhodes ML, Altschuler EM, Wiltse LL, Kostanek C, Yu Ming Kuo BA. Multiplanar display computerized body tomography applications in the lumbar spine. *Spine* 1979; 4(4):282–294.

37. Symposium. Computerized tomography of the lumbar spine. *Spine* 1979; 4:281–294.

38. Lindahl O, Rexed G. Histological changes in spinal nerve roots of operated cases of sciatica. *Acta Orthop Scand* 1951; 20:215–225.

39. Nachemson A. The lumbar spine—an orthopaedic challenge. *Spine* 1976; 1:59–68.

40. LeRoy PL, et al. Thermography as a diagnostic aid in the management of chronic pain. In: Aronoff GM, ed. *Evaluation and Treatment of Chronic Pain.* Baltimore: Urban & Schwarzenberg; 1985: 232–250.

41. Taylor H, Warfield CA. Thermography of pain: Instrumentation and uses. *Hosp Pract* Off. 1985; 20:164–169.

42. Uematsu S, et al. Thermography and electromyography in the differential diagnosis of chronic pain syndromes and reflex sympathetic dystrophy. *Electromygr Clin Neurophysiol* 1981; 21:165–182.

43. Bennet GJ, Ochoa JL. Thermographic observations on rats with experimental neuropathic pain. *Pain* 1991; 45(1):61–67.

44. Newman RI, Seres JL, Miller EB. Liquid crystal thermography in the evaluation of chronic back pain: a comparative study. *Pain* 1984; 20(3):293–305.

45. Wexler CE. An overview of liquid crystal and electronic lumbar, thoracic and cervical thermography. Tarzana, CA: Thermographic Services; 1983.

46. Harper CM, Low PA, Fealey RD, Chelimsky PC, Gillen DA. Utility of thermography in the diagnosis of lumbosacral radiculopathy. *Neurology* 1991; 41(7):1010–1014.

PART TWO

Pain by Anatomic Location

CHAPTER 5

Headache

John R. Graham and Dhirendra S. Bana

"When the head is not sound, the rest cannot be well."[1] Evolution has favored the brain as the nucleus of the human health care system. Physically, the brain receives the largest supply of blood, and generally, it is the last organ to be compromised when there is an impending blood shortage. As a control port for the nervous system and endocrine system, physical and psychological well-being depends highly on this vital organ. In short, the secret of humanity's success lies in the brain.

The natural association of head pain with a malfunction of the brain is the cause for great alarm. Any pain arising from the head leads to heightened response from the patient and fears of the worst consequences. Of the many pains felt by humans, pain in the head is perhaps the most distressing of all.

STRUCTURES IN THE HEAD SENSITIVE TO PAIN

Pain experienced in the head may arise in the head or may be referred from the neck or other organs. The pain-sensitive structures are distributed both intra- and extra-cranially.[2] It is convenient to divide pain arising in the head into these two catagories. This division helps to remind the physician that if a local cause of pain is not evident, there may be a more distant source.

Parts of the head that are pain sensitive include the following:

I. Extracranial structures
   A. Scalp and its integuments.
   B. Muscles.
   C. Fascia.
   D. Periosteum.
   E. Branches of the external carotid artery.
   F. Scalp veins.
   G. Eyes, ears, paranasal sinuses, and turbinates.
   H. Sensory nerves.
II. Intracranial structures
   A. Meninges lining the superior half of skull only in the vicinity of menigeal vessels and all of the meninges covering the brain at the base of the skull.
   B. Great venous sinuses.
   C. Tributory veins carrying blood to the great venous system.
   D. Meningeal blood vessels.
   E. Internal carotid artery, siphon, vessels constituting the circle of Willis, and extending 2 to 5 cm beyond the circle of Willis; anterior, middle, and posterior cerebral vessels; vertebral, basilar, cerebellar, and pontile arteries.
   F. Middle cerebral veins 3 to 4 cm nearest the sinuses.
   G. Tentorium.
   H. Sensory nerves and their ganglia.

In the supratentorial structure, pain is innervated by cranial nerve V, and it is felt in the anterior half of the head. Disorders below the tentorium register pain sensation through the upper cervical sensory roots, and the pain is felt in the posterior half of the head. One exception to this general rule is the nerve of Arnold, a branch of cranial nerve V that carries sensation from below the tentorium and is felt in the front of the head. Similarly, the upper two cervical roots are responsible for pain referred to the ipsilateral temporal area. Pain from the middle cranial fossa is carried over cranial nerves IX and X. It is felt in the ear and pharynx. Some sensory fibers exist in cranial nerve VII and are responsible for pain in the face and ear.

LOCATION OF PAIN

The location of the pain often can guide the physician to discover its likely source and possible responsible disorders. The potential sources of pain and some of their causes are shown in Figures 5-1 through 5-13. This list is not intended to be all inclusive, but it is a reminder of some of the common causes of pain at these locations.

MECHANISMS OF HEAD PAIN

Different ways in which pain can be produced in pain sensitive structures in the head include: (1) direct pressure on structures, (2) traction or distortion, (3) excessive generalized vasodilatation, (4) excessive localized vasodilatation, (5) prolonged muscle contraction, (6) inflammation, (7) neuralgia, (8) disorders of the nociceptive system and central endogenous control of pain, and (9) conversion or hysterical headache.

Sometimes more than one mechanism may be contributing to headache. For example, any movement during a migraine can intensify the throbbing. Consequently, patients tend to keep their neck muscles tight, an action that eventually may become another source of pain.

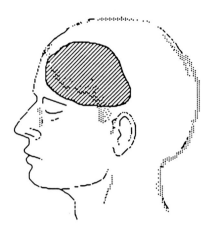

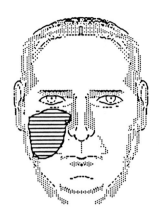

**Structures Potentially
Involved in Causing Pain**
Internal carotid artery
Middle cerebral artery
Superior sagittal sinus
Middle cerebral veins
Inferior cerebral veins
Maxillary sinus
Nasal middle turbinates
Nasofrontal ducts

Common Diseases
Migraine
Temporal arteritis
Temporomandibular joint
  syndrome
Diseases of the eye
Infections
Cluster headache
Trigeminal neuralgia
Herpes zoster
Cervical spine disorders

FIGURE 5-1. Temporal pain.

**Structures Potentially
Involved in Causing Pain**
Cranial nerve V root ganglion (V2)
Maxillary sinus antrum
Sphenopalatine ganglion
Vidian nerve
Cavernous sinus
Maxillary sinus
Teeth
Internal maxillary artery
Common carotid artery

Common Diseases
Acute sinusitis
Acoustic neuroma
Arachnoiditis
AV malformation
Osteoma of the foramen
  ovale
Sphenopalatine ganglion
  neuralgia
Vidian neuralgia
Cluster headache
Migraine headache
Tic douloureux
Dental diseases

FIGURE 5-3. Facial pain.

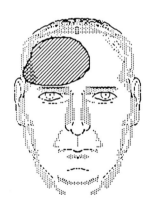

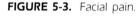

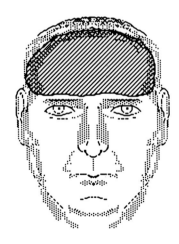

**Structures Potentially
Involved in Causing Pain**
Superior wall transverse sinus
Upper surface tentorium
  cerebelli
Frontal venous sinus
Superior sagittal sinus
Lateral ventricle
Tentorial nerves
Cranial nerve V nucleus (V1)
Pia–arachnoid near the arteries
  at the base of brain
Tentorium cerebelli (central portion)
Supraorbital artery
Anterior meningeal artery
Supraorbital nerve

Common Diseases
Migraine
Diseases of the eye
Frontal sinusitis
Ice cream headache
Cluster headache
Herpes zoster

FIGURE 5-2. Frontal pain.

**Structures Potentially
Involved in Causing Pain**
Temporal artery
Temporal muscle
Frontal muscle
Periosteum
Supraorbital artery
Supraorbital nerve
Frontal sinuses

Common Diseases
Tension (muscle contraction
  headache)
Hypertension
Traction headache
Combined headache
Cranial arteritis
Intracranial space-occupying
  lesions
Pseudotumor cerebri
Depression

FIGURE 5-4. Bifrontal headache.

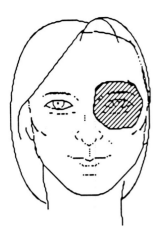

**Structures Potentially
Involved in Causing Pain**
Internal carotid artery
Anterior cerebral artery
Middle cerebral artery
Superior sagittal sinus
Sphenoid venous sinus
Cavernous sinus
Sphenoid sinus
Ethmoid sinus
Dural floor, anterior fossa
Diseases of the eye and
  surrounding structures

Common Diseases
Migraine
Cluster headache
Traction headache
Glaucoma
Keratitis–uveitis
Ruptured aneurysm
Inflammation

FIGURE 5-5. *Pain in and around the eye.*

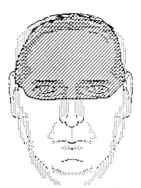
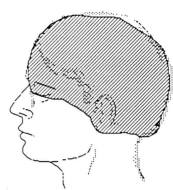

**Structures Potentially
Involved in Causing Pain**
Third ventricle
Cranial blood vessels
Cranial muscles and fascia
Periostium

Common Diseases
Anoxia
Hypercapnia
Fever
Nitroglycerine
Postseizure
Meningitis
Hemorrhage
Muscle contraction
Depression
Psychogenic headache
Excessive vasodilatation
Pseudotumor cerebri

FIGURE 5-7. *Generalized headache.*

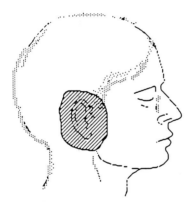

**Structures Potentially
Involved in Causing Pain**
Internal auditory artery
Pontile artery (up to 1.5 cm.
  from its origin)
Nasal septum (middle and
  lower turbinates)
Sigmoid sinus
Straight sinus (infratentorial)
Occipital sinus (near torcula)

Common Diseases
Inflammation of otologic
  structures
Blocked eustachian tube
Nasopharyngeal tumor
Tumors and diseases
  of cranial nerve IX
Tumors and diseases
  of cranial nerve X
Paget disease
Geniculate neuralgia
Glossopharyngeal neuralgia
Temporomandibular
  joint syndrome
Mastoiditis
Acoustic neuroma
Cerebellopontile angle tumor

FIGURE 5-6. *Pain in and around the ear.*

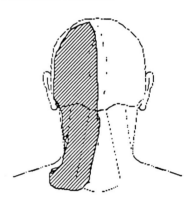

**Structures Potentially
Involved in Causing Pain**
Occipital artery
Greater occipital nerve
Annulus fibrosus (disc)
Periostium
Ligamentum flavum
Anterior longitudinal ligament
Posterior longitudinal ligament
Interspinous ligament
Posterior vertebral venous plexus
Anterior dura mater
Facet articulations
Paravertebral musculature
  and fascia
Vertebral arteries

Common Diseases
Compression of suboccipital
  artery
Greater occipital nerve
  compression
Cervical disc disease
Paget disease
Degenerative joint disease
Cluster headache
Muscle contraction
  headache
Vertebral artery aneurysm
  or tear
Basilar artery aneurysm
  or tear
Valsalva headache
  (cough headache)
Soft tissue and nerve
  injuries
Whiplash injury
Syringomyelia
Congenital anomalies
  (platybasia, etc.)

FIGURE 5-8. *Unilateral cervical headache.*

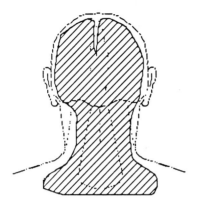

**Structures Potentially
Involved in Causing Pain**
Skull
Cervical vertebrae
Posterior fossa structures

Common Diseases
Platybasia
Occipitalization of C1
Posterior fossa tumors,
    abscess, cyst
Posttraumatic headache
Klippel–Feil syndrome
Prednisone withdrawal
Tension headache
Meningitis
Subarachnoid hemorrhage
Postlumbar puncture headache
Subluxation of odontoid
    (rheumatoid arthritis or
    prolonged cortisone use)
Lateral sinus thrombosis

FIGURE 5-9. Bilateral cervical headache.

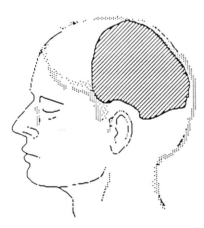

**Structures Potentially
Involved in Causing Pain**
Meninges
Meningeal arteries
Tributary veins
Skull
Mastoid

Common Diseases
Posttraumatic headache
Subdural hematoma
Arachnoid cyst
Vascular malformations
Migraine
Tumors
Cranial arteritis
Metastatic disease
Granulomas
Osteomyelitis

FIGURE 5-10. Parietal headache.

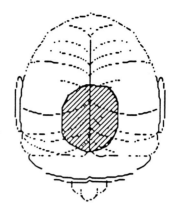

**Structures Potentially
Involved in Causing Pain**
Sphenoid sinus
Pituitary gland
Sagittal sinus
Skull

Common Diseases
Sphenoid sinusitis
Pituitary diseases
Sagittal sinus obstruction
Metastatic disease
Ice cream headache

FIGURE 5-11. Vertex headache.

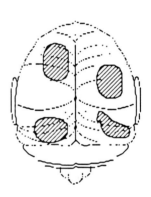

**Structures Potentially
Involved in Causing Pain**
Skull
Scalp vessels
Scalp sensory nerves

Common Diseases
Metastatic disease
Eosinophilic granuloma
Temporal arteritis
Cerebrovascular syphilis
Paget disease
Posttraumatic headache
Headache "jolts"
Localized inflammation
Sarcoidosis
Psychogenic headache

FIGURE 5-12. Multiple headache sites.

WORKUP OF A HEADACHE PATIENT

Headache History

The headache history is the most important part of the workup. In addition to determining the general medical condition, factual data about the headache and a description of its evolution over the years is important. A family history of headache is important. Migraine tends to run in families. Muscle contraction headache or the headache of a brain tumor rarely has such a tendency. If the patient has more

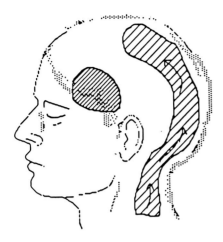

**Structures Potentially
Involved in Causing Pain**
Nerve root injury or
    compression
Occipital arteries

Common Diseases
Nerve entrapment syndromes
C2 syndrome
Cervical disc disease
Migraine
Cluster headache

FIGURE 5-13. *Cervical radiating pain.*

than one type of headache, it is best to determine the primary headache problem and then determine how other headaches differ from the main headache.

Headache Diary

The patient should be encouraged to keep a diary listing such details as the precipitating factors, accompaniments of the headache, duration of headache, and medication taken. It is also helpful to list the severity of headache (e.g., mild, moderate, severe, and excruciating) and the functional incapacity caused by the pain. The physician then can review the diary with the patient to see if there is any consistent pattern to the occurrence of the headaches that may aid the physician in making recommendations.

Life Profile

Often, major social and emotional trauma in the patient's life will trigger the onset of headaches or exacerbate an existing headache problem. Events such as the separation of parents, child abuse, depression, or head trauma are particularly important to explore. Information about the effect of menstrual periods and pregnancies on the headache also are valuable.

Headache Attack Diagram

A diagram showing the course of a headache attack is useful in advising patients about the importance of taking their medication on time. For example, Cafergot, taken at the onset of the headache, works more effectively than if it is taken when the headache is well established. The diagram

also gives the physician a good overview of the medications taken and details of how these were used during the headache attack.

Special Points in the Physical Examination

The workup should include a detailed neurologic examination to exclude any organic lesion. During the physical examination, we should examine and notice especially the following symptoms of endocrine disorders: acromegalic face, hypothyroid features, buffalo hump at the neck (as found in Cushing disease), or the dry eyes or mouth of Sjögren syndrome. In rheumatoid arthritis and after prolonged cortisone use, headache may arise from instability of the C1 odontoid process. We should check for tightness or pain in the trapezius muscle and look for any trigger points that may aggravate the existing headache or induce a headache. In temporal arteritis, there may be prominence of the artery with decreased pulsations and/or tenderness. The carotid artery also should be checked for tenderness or bruits and the heart, for mitral valve prolapse. In patients with neck pain, note whether a change in the headache occurs after the head is lifted passively off the neck. In cervicogenic headache and in some patients with posttraumatic headache, there may be a temporary relief in the headache using this maneuver. It is also important to check vision, the extremities for evidence of Raynaud disease, and the status of the peripheral vascular circulation.

Examination During Headache

If a patient is seen during a headache attack, the physician has the advantage of observing firsthand the characteristics of the headache. This may aid in making the headache diagnosis. For example, a patient during a migraine attack may look sick with pale, drawn face, dark circles around their eyes, and prominent temporal arteries. Occlusion of the temporal arteries by pressure may provide temporary relief in headache. A cluster headache may be diagnosed by the signs of unilateral tearing, redness of the eye and periorbital swelling, ptosis, miosis, and nasal stuffiness. These symptoms disappear within 1 to 2 h.

The behavior of the patient during a headache attack also can help to make the diagnosis. A migraine sufferer during an attack wants to be left alone and seeks the quietest, darkest place available. These patients prefer to lie still, whereas those with cluster headaches find no relief in any position and are apt to try different positions, including pacing the floor, sitting and changing position frequently, and even hitting their heads against the wall in desperation during the attack. Table 5-1 lists signs and symptoms that should prompt a physician to seek an underlying organic cause for the headaches.

Suggested Laboratory Tests for Headache Investigation

Each patient should be evaluated to determine the need for tests. Although laboratory investigation may not be neces-

Table 5-1
Warning of Organic Disease in Patient's History

Signs and Symptoms	Some Diseases to Consider
Headache accompanied by unconsciousness	Seizures, hemorrhage, posterior fossa lesions, and cervical spondylosis
No previous history of headache	Exclude bleed from aneurysm or AV malformation, sudden rise in blood pressure as in pheochromocytoma, embolic phenomenon, dissection of the carotid artery
Headache accompanied by neurologic abnormalities during and after the headache	Intracranial hemorrhage or thrombosis, tumors, ophthalmoplegic migraine, or hemiplegic migraine
Headache associated with fever or stiff neck	Exclude infection: bacterial, viral, or parasitic. Also check for emboli, thrombosis, hemorrhage, malignant disease, systemic lupus erythematosus, cranial arteritis
Headache first starting after the age 50 years[3,4]	Consider cervical spondylosis, disk disease, recent onset of hypertension, menopause, hormonal change such as hypothyroidism, cranial arteritis, metastatic disease, or depression
A change in character or response to treatment of previous headaches	Exclude tumor or other organic intracranial lesions, such as hemorrhage
Headache associated with alteration in personality or habits	Exclude tumor or infection
Headache associated with hypertension or endocrine disorders	Check for Cushing syndrome, parathyroid or pituitary tumors, hypothyroidism, and pheochromocytoma
Headache initiated by coughing, sneezing, straining, or coitus[5]	Look for posterior fossa or neck lesions, especially if Valsalva maneuver can initiate a headache rather than just aggravate an existing headache
Headaches that do not follow the course or pattern of well-established types of headache	Investigate for organicity of the headaches
Headache after injury	Ask for history of head and/or neck injury. Check for subdural hematoma, cervical disc, fractures. Also consider neck injury.
	Neck involvement may be caused by the soft tissues of the neck that are not visible on plain neck x-ray films. MRI may be more revealing. History of head injury may be remote, and patient may have forgotten about it. This should be explored especially in elderly patients where a subdural hematoma may remain asymptomatic for months before causing headache.

sary in all cases, Table 5-2 lists some of the conditions diagnosed by the tests commonly used for a headache workup. In general, the CT scan of the head is the most useful to exclude organic causes of headache. It is not useful, however, for diagnosing infections or small aneurysms. It is limited in the diagnosis of posterior fossa lesions. In this instance, MRI is a better test.

CLASSIFICATION OF HEADACHE

The classification of headache helps in planning the treatment strategy. Headaches cannot be classified using laboratory tests alone. A good history and physical examination is essential. Although there are many different classifications in vogue, the one recommended by the Ad Hoc Committee on Classification of Headaches[6] will be followed in this chapter. There are a few new types of headache that have been described since this classification was suggested, and these also will be discussed.

I. Vascular headache of migraine type.
   A. "Classic" migraine.
   B. "Common" migraine.
   C. "Cluster" headache.
   D. "Hemiplegic" and "ophthalmoplegic" migraine.
   E. "Lower half" headache.
II. Muscle-contraction headache.
III. Combined headache: vascular and muscle contraction.
IV. Headache of nasal vasomotor reaction.
V. Headache of delusional, conversion, or hypochondriacal states.
VI. Nonmigrainous vascular headaches.
VII. Traction headache.
VIII. Headache due to overt cranial inflammation.
IX–XIII. Headache due to disease of ocular, aural, nasal and sinusal, dental, or other cranial or neck structures.

Table 5-2
Tests Commonly Used in Headache Workup

Test	Conditions Checked
Temperature	Infection, cranial arteritis, autoimmune disease
Minnesota Multiphasic Personality Inventory, Zung scale	Emotional disorders
Cognitive testing	Organic cerebral dysfunction
Skull x-ray	Fracture, sinusitis, pituitary lesion, metastatic disease, bone destruction, Paget disease, calcified AV malformation, multiple myeloma, platybasia, sickle cell disease, pineal shift
Neck x-ray flexion and extension views	Fracture, disc disease, rheumatoid arthritis, congenital malformations, cervical spondylosis, tumors, dislocations
Doppler blood flow studies	Blood flow in major cerebral arteries
Technetium scan	Inflammation, granulomatous diseases, tumors, AV malformations, brain abscess
EEG	Seizure disorder, sleep disorder, space-occupying lesions
Beam EEG	Postraumatic damage, small foci of seizures, tumors, dysphasia, dyslexia, and other reading disabilities
CT Scan	Intracranial bleeding, space-occupying lesion, atrophy, AV malformations, large aneurysms (small and medium-size aneurysms may be missed)
MRI Scan	Intracranial bleeding, space occupying lesion, atrophy, AV malformations, aneurysms, multiple sclerosis, tuberous sclerosis. Soft tissue structures in the neck and scalp
Sleep studies	Sleep disorders including sleep apnea (obstructive and nonobstructive)
Thermogram	? Cluster headache (frontal "cold" spots)
Arteriogram	Complicated migraine, ophthalmoplegic migraine, tumors, aneurysms, AV malformations, intracerebral hemorrhage
Spinal tap	Infection, pseudotumor cerebri

XIV. Cranial neuritides.
XV. Cranial neuralgias.

Posttraumatic headache may arise from any one of several mechanisms.

Classic Migraine

Definition

"Recurrent attacks of headache, widely varied in intensity, frequency, and duration. The attacks are commonly unilateral in onset, are usually associated with anorexia and, sometimes, with nausea and vomiting. Headaches are preceded by sharply defined transient visual and other sensory or motor prodromes or both."[6] Occasionally, attacks consist only of the prodrome without a subsequent headache.

Cause

A familial disorder, for which the specific cause is unknown, characterized by an abnormal response to stress from the external, physiologic, and psychological environments.

Pathophysiologic Findings

The disturbed physiology in the migraine attack involves many bodily systems.[7] Chiefly affected are the brain, the central nervous system (CNS), the autonomic nervous system, and the cranial and systemic vasculature. Many other disturbances occur, such as fluid imbalance, hematopoietic changes, especially in platelet function, gastrointestinal disturbance, mood changes, and alteration in biochemical and enzyme functions. Fifty years ago, the original source of trouble was considered to be vasoconstriction in cranial blood vessels that caused ischemia and malfunction of brain cells, resulting in the neurologic symptoms of the prodrome.[8] More recently, evidence has been found that the initial aberration occurs in brain cells in the cortex and limbic system. This produces, or at least is accompanied by, ischemia similar to that seen in the "spreading depression of Leao" in the brain of experimental animals.[9] This latter phenomenon, caused by a stimulus to brain cells, results in a wave of nerve excitation that is followed by a longer wave of inhibition that spreads over the brain like ripples in a pool. The areas involved in the process show briefly increased blood flow that is followed by prolonged spreading ischemia.[10,11] Similar spreading depression, however, has not been observed directly in humans.[12] The factors that begin this sequence of events may vary from sludging (caused by platelet aggregation,[13] increased blood viscosity from high protein, lipoprotein[14] or fatty acid content[15]), disturbances of potassium metabolism, opening of arteriovenous (AV) shunts,[16] or even sudden physical trauma. During the period of the prodrome, changes occur in serotonin, dopamine, catecholamine receptors and transmitters, and the nociceptor system. These are influential in causing general symptoms of mood disturbance, pain, and gastrointestinal and peripheral vessel tone disturbances.

The painful or headache phase that follows the prodrome is associated with excessive painful pulsation of cranial vessels, especially the branches of the external carotid artery. At the site of the headache, substances that lower the pain threshold were found by Chapman and colleagues[17] in the vicinity of the dilated blood vessels. More recently, substance P was discovered to be an important putative agent in conveying sensory impulses from damaged or overstretched cranial vessel walls through the trigeminal nerve network to register in the brain as pain.[18] How much of the pain of migraine is caused by changes in the nociceptive centers of the CNS in the so-called central gray area and how much is caused directly by peripheral disturbances in intra- and extracranial vessel walls must be determined.

Age of Onset

The headache generally starts during childhood or teenage years, but many develop later, up to approximately age 40 years. At times, classic migraine recurs during the sixth or seventh decade of life, often in the form of a prodrome without a headache. It can be confused easily with transient ischemic attacks.

Attack Profile

Classic migraine can be conveniently divided into three phases including: (1) prodrome, (2) headache, and (3) post-headache phase.

Prodrome. Various types of prodromes reported by patients with classic migraine include: visual, sensory, motor, speech, cognitive function, and balance.[19] Visual prodromes are the most common. A classic visual phenomenon would be the gradual emergence of an incomplete oval scintillating shape with sharply angular zigzag lines that are of smaller magnitude at the ends and longer in the middle. The phenomenon starts as a small speck on one side of the visual field and progressively increases in size and shape (Fig. 5-14). As it evolves, it seems to move gradually upward and outward in the visual field. It may take 5 min to reach its full development, stay as a fully developed form for approximately 10 min, and then gradually fade. The disappearance does not follow a uniform pattern. Instead, a few lines fade and then more lines disappear until the whole visual field becomes clear. The whole process takes approximately 20 min. The phenomenon is hemianopic, is seen with the eyes open or closed, and is termed at *fortification spectrum* because of its crenelated formation. Other visual phenomena include wavy lines (as experienced while driving on a road on a hot summer day), silvery dots (which may have movement), dark areas in the visual field (reminiscent of the spots occurring after a camera flash light goes off), or there may be homonymous hemianopia.

Sensory prodromes may have positive features (such as tingling), followed by negative features (such as numbness creeping from one finger to another and up the hand and arm to the face). Motor prodromes are characterized by unilateral, or rarely bilateral, weakness involving the upper and/or lower extremeties in a gradual progression.

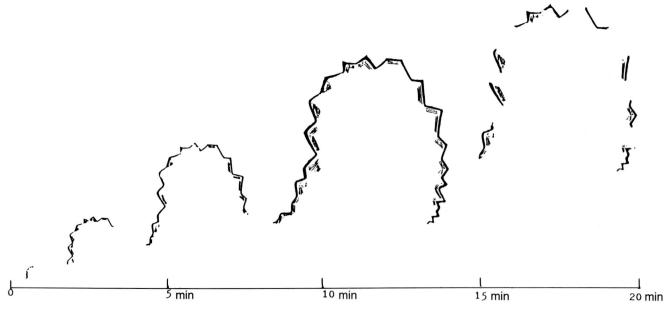

FIGURE 5-14. Progression of visual prodrome.

Headache Phase. The headache is usually, but not always unilateral. It is located commonly on the side opposite the prodrome. Occasionally, the headache is on the same side as the prodrome. In some patients, especially children, the headache may be bilateral. It is felt over the temporal area and may involve the frontal, parietal, and occipital areas, the eye, and the cheek. Its frequency is usually one to two times per month. Sometimes, however, attacks may come in flurries of several in a week followed by long headache-free periods. The headache may range from moderate and interfering with daily work to severe or incapacitating. Its duration is 6 to 10 h; in children, it often is much shorter. The quality of pain is throbbing. If the patient is resting, it may be a steady pain, but it starts to throb on exertion or by lying too flat. Its time of onset is any time; commonly, it may occur during relaxation after a stressful period, during sleep, or on waking. It is accompanied by nausea, vomiting, fatigue, and sensitivity to light, noise, or smells. Movements, such as bending over, coughing, or sneezing make the headache worse. The face looks pale or like "death warmed over." There is a painful expression on the face, often some blocking of the ipsilateral nostril, and slight watering of the eye. The patient usually answers questions in a slow low voice, using minimal words to converse; seeks a dark quiet place to lie down; and turns in bed, sits up, or moves around slowly to avoid increasing the exertion that causes more throbbing. The patient avoids reading, writing, watching television, listening to music, or making any decision that requires concentration. The factors that precipitate the attacks vary from patient to patient, although each patient has a fairly consistent list. Certain foods, such as cheese, chocolate, monosodium glutamate, alcoholic beverages (especially red wine), rapid changes in barometric pressure, humidity, or temperature; too much sleep or not enough sleep; being overtired; or relaxing after a stressful period frequently are reported.

Postheadache Phase. It may take almost 24 h for the patient to feel good after the headache. During this time, most patients feel exhausted, tired, as if they have been "through the mill." There is lingering mild soreness in the head. Occasionally, the patient feels elated or overenergetic during the postheadache period.

Relation of Headache to Significant Life Events

Patients who have headaches after stressful situations may learn to take prophylactic medications before such well-recognized situations (e.g., weddings, funerals, special events, or speeches).

Forerunners of the Main Headache

In childhood, car sickness, repeated episodes of bilious vomiting, and/or abdominal pain are common in patients who later in life get these headaches. These symptoms are regarded as childhood equivalents or forerunners of migraine.

Family History

This is commonly positive for headache in approximately 70 percent of patients, especially for those with "sick" headaches. Its mode of inheritance is probably multifactorial.[20]

Differential Diagnosis

This includes eye diseases, especially glaucoma. The halo seen around street lights is common in glaucoma but uncommon in classic migraine. Transient visual disturbances also can occur in transient ischemic attacks, cerebral emboli, other cerebrovascular accidents, carotid artery dissection, and hypoglycemia. Such disturbances rarely, if ever, have the clinical appearance and behavior of the migraine scintillating scotoma.

Treatment

Prophylactic Treatment. Because migraine is a disorder that is activated by stress in the patient's environment (external, physiologic, and emotional), it is important that physicians acquaint themselves, and the patient, with what those factors are and provide advice and guidance about eliminating as many of them as possible. This process takes time, some spent during each visit and usually over several visits, to establish an understanding of the relevance of this principle and make many life adjustments. Such changes often are hard to accomplish and may take weeks or months. Medication may be helpful in prophylaxis, but sometimes patients begin to depend on these drugs to solve their problems, many of which can be solved by alterations in their own behavior.

In general, the patient should avoid an overly busy schedule and, as a general rule, have 1 hour a day of free time to call their own and to unwind from a busy schedule. Similarly, it is wise to have 1 afternoon per week, 1 day per month, and 1 week every 6 months in which the patient can do whatever they please. If there is no known precipitating factor, make a list of events, stress factors, weather, foods, fasting, menses, or emotions the patient was experiencing before the headache that might be triggering the attacks.

For overly anxious patients, consider relaxation techniques, such as transcendental meditation, yoga, biofeedback, hypnotherapy, or books on relaxation. Some patients need psychotherapy when they have major problems or severe depression is present.[21]

During the prodromal phase, the patient may breathe into a plastic bag for 10 to 15 min (rationale: while vasoconstriction is occurring, this helps to open up the constricted vessels, thus avoiding later vasodilation). They then should hold their breath as long as possible and alternate with short periods of rapid breathing. Nitroglycerine 1/200 grains sublingually, if taken at the onset of the prodrome, may abort an attack. The timing of nitroglycerine use is crucial. Larger doses may make the headache worse.

A wide variety of drugs are available, some used specifically for migraine. Others may be used for other conditions. Common prophylactic drugs used and their modes of action are listed in Table 5-3.[22] Cyproheptadine and propranolol

Table 5-3
Prophylactic Agents

Drug	Constituents	Action	Dose	Comments
Anaprox	Naproxen	Anti-inflammatory, antiprostaglandin, analgesic, antiplatelet	275 mg twice a day	Gastric upset, renal failure, photoallergic reaction
Aspirin	Salicylates	Anti-inflammatory, analgesic, antiprostaglandin, antiplatelet	300 mg daily	Gastric irritation, bleeding tendency
Benadryl	Diphenhydramine	H_1 blocker, anticholinergic	25–50 mg	Drowsiness
Blocadren	Timolol	Nonselective β-blocker	20–40 mg	5–10 times more potent than Inderal
Butazolidin	Phenylbutazone	Anti-inflammatory, antiprostaglandin, analgesic, uricosuric	300–600 mg in divided doses	Hematologic, GI disturbances, avoid in children
Calan	Verapamil	Calcium-channel blocker, local anesthetic effect	80–320 mg in divides doses	Constipation, hypotension, cardiac conduction disturbance
Cardizem	Diltiazem	Calcium-channel blocker, local anesthetic effect	60–240 mg in divided doses	Cardiac conduction disturbance
Corgard	Nadolol	Nonselective β-blocker	40–160 mg	Long acting, other effects as above
Dilantin	Phenytoin sodium	Anticonvulsant	300 mg a day	Useful if EEG is abnormal, need blood Dilantin levels
Elavil	Amitriptyline	Interferes with reuptake of epinephrine and/or serotonin	25–150 mg a day	Once at night, dryness of mouth common
Inderal	Propranolol	Nonselective β-blocker	40–240 mg	Depression, bradycardia, asthma, hypotension
Indocin	Indomethacin	Anti-inflammatory, antiprostaglandin, analgesic, antiplatelet	25–150 mg a day in divided doses	Useful in neck pain, GI upset, fluid retention
Isoptin	Verapamil	Calcium-channel blocker, local anesthetic effect	80–320 mg in divided doses	Constipation, hypotension, cardiac conduction disturbance
Lisuride	Semisynthetic ergot alkaloid	Same as other ergot preparations		
Lopressor	Metoprolol	Selective β_1-adrenergic blocker	50–200 mg	Fatigue, hypotension
Marplan	Isocarboxazid	Monoamine oxidase inhibitor	30 mg a day, lower maintenance dose	Dietary precautions avoid sympathomimetic drugs*
Motrin	Ibuprofen	Anti-inflammatory, antiprostaglandin, analgesic, antiplatelet	300–1800 mg a day divided doses	GI upset, renal failure, photoallergic reaction
Mysoline	Primidone	Anticonvulsant	50–400 mg daily	Useful if EEG is abnormal, side effects: ataxia, vertigo†
Nalfon	Fenoprofen	Anti-inflammatory, antiprostaglandin, analgesic, antiplatelet	200–1800 mg divided doses	GI upset, renal failure, photoallergic reaction
Naprosyn	Naproxen	Anti-inflammatory, antiprostaglandin, analgesic, antiplatelet	250–1500 mg divided doses	GI upset, renal failure, photoallergic reaction
Nardil	Phenelzine	Monoamine oxidase inhibitor	15–60 mg, lower maintenance dose	Dietary precautions avoid sympathomimetic drugs, hypotension*
Periactin	Cyproheptadine	H_1 blocker, antiserotonin, anticholinergic, depressant	2–4 mg 2–3 times a day	Weight gain, drowsiness
Persantine	Dipyridamole	Prolongs platelet survival when combined with aspirin	50 mg 2–3 times a day	Hypotension
Procardia	Nifedipine	Calcium-channel blocker, local anesthetic effect	30–60 mg in divided doses	Edema, dizziness, flushing of the face, hypotension, headache
Sansert	Methysergide maleate	Antiserotonin, vasoconstrictor	2–6 mg	Pleuropulmonary fibrosis, edema, valvular fibrosis
Tegretol	Carbamazepine	Anticonvulsant	200–800 mg a day	Useful if EEG is abnormal, hematologic monitoring required
Trental	Pentoxifylline	Decreases blood viscosity and improves erythrocyte flexibility	400 mg 2–3 times a day	Avoid in caffeine sensitivity
Wytensin	Guanabenz	α_2-adrenergic agonist	4–24 mg daily	Useful in hypertensive headache patient

GI: gastrointestinal
*Increase the dose slowly over 1–2 months
†Read manufacturer's directions carefully before prescribing

are effective in the pediatric age group.[23,24] Other drugs commonly used for prophylaxis of migraine include: amitriptyline,[25] calcium-channel blockers,[26] and methysergide.[27] Physicians should consult the manufacturer's instructions before prescribing this[28] and other drugs discussed in this chapter. A drug soon to be released by the Food and Drug Administration (FDA) is sumatriptan, a serotonin-1 receptor (5-HT$_1$) agonist. In trial studies it has been shown to be effective by subcutaneous injection, oral, or intranasal route with minimal side effects.[28a–d]

Symptomatic Treatment. During the headache phase, antiemetics and analgesics may be needed. Common antiemetic medications include: trimethobenzamide, prochlorperazine, and metoclopramide. Analgesics include aspirin, acetaminophen, and ibuprofen. In severe headaches, we may need to resort to codeine-containing drugs and other narcotic analgesics. Commonly used drugs are listed in Table 5-4. The physician should watch for any addiction problem and dispense these drugs judiciously.

Ergot preparations are the mainstay of migraine therapy for patients in whom simple analgesics fail. They come in different forms. Table 5-5 lists some of their characteristics. The tolerance for ergot preparation varies widely from patient to patient. Women tend to be more sensitive than men and require smaller doses. In some patients, ergotamine may cause nausea, muscle and joint aches, and general malaise. It is wise, therefore, to prescribe a small dose the first time and repeat it in 1 hour if necessary. If the drug is well tolerated, a higher dose can be taken during the next attack. Each patient may need to find the best route and timing of ergotamine doses. Convenience and efficacy thus should be balanced, depending on the patient's daily life and occupation. Table 5-6 shows the routes by which the various drugs may be administered. Their efficacy and reliability of action are inversely proportional to convenience. Thus, a housewife may use a suppository early in an attack, but a secretary in a business meeting may prefer to take an oral or inhaled preparation. Ergotamine should not be used more than two or three times per week to avoid ergot dependency.

Common Migraine

Definition

"Vascular headache without striking prodromes and less often unilateral than classic migraine and cluster headache. Synonyms are: 'atypical migraine' or 'sick' headache. Calling attention to certain relationships of this type headache to environmental, occupational, menstrual, or other variables are such terms as: 'summer,' 'Monday,' 'weekend,' 'relaxation,' 'premenstrual,' and 'menstrual' headache."[6] Premonitory symptoms of mood disturbance, such as euphoria, depression, or irritability, or bouts of excessive yawning, sneezing, or hunger may be present several hours before the attack. The patient looks pale, sallow, in pain, and their eyes may lose their luster. There is a slight drooping of the eyelids. There may be prominence and tenderness of the temporal arteries.

Cause

See classic migraine section.

Pathophysiologic Findings

Same as classic migraine, although the oligemia phase before hyperemia may not be present as in classic migraine. Some contend these two conditions may be separate entities.

Attack Profile

The headache may start at any time. It commonly begins as a mild ache in the temporal areas or neck, gradually gaining in intensity, peaking in 3 to 4 h, and lasting for 8 to 10 h. Severe attacks may last 2 to 4 days. Lying down (with the head slightly raised) often improves the headache.

Age of Onset

This type of headache begins at points of increasing life stress from childhood to age 40 years, including beginning school, menarche, college, job, marriage, family, and business responsibilities.

Headache Phase

The frequency varies widely; commonly two to six attacks per month occur. Rare instances of daily occurrence lasting weeks or months exist, so-called migraine status. The quality of pain is a throbbing pain or a constant ache if the patient is lying still. The headache usually is unilateral, often shifting sides from one attack to another, and occasionally bilateral. Its location is temporal, parietal, or frontal, often with a suboccipital component. Its pattern of occurrence may be predictable, as in the so-called menstrual or weekend headache. It may involve a series of headaches for a few weeks, followed by headache-free periods of several weeks (as in cyclic migraine), or there may be no set pattern. Its severity is generally moderate to severe. The duration may last 8 to 10 h but may persist two to four days.

Frequently, nausea, or in severe headaches, vomiting, hypersensitivity to light, noise, and smell may occur during the headache phase. Polyuria, depression, irritability, and cold hands and feet also are seen. The patient shuns bright light, preferring to lie quietly in a dark room and avoiding conversation as much as possible because noise and speech can cause more pain. A cold wet cloth on the forehead or a tight band around the head may be helpful. The patient may try to induce vomiting because vomiting may bring relief occasionally.

Postheadache Phase

After the headache, the patient feels exhausted or tired and may require another day to regain full strength. Occasional patients feel exhilarated. After a common migraine attack,

Table 5-4
Symptomatic Treatment Agents

Drug	Constituents	Action	Dose	Comments
Advil	Ibuprofen (200 mg)	Nonsteroidal anti-inflammatory	1–2 at the onset, repeat every 3–4 h	GI upset, fluid retention, photo-allergic skin rash, bleeding
Aspirin	Salicylate	Analgesic, anti-inflammatory	300 mg 1–2 tab every 4 h as needed	GI upset, tinnitus, bleeding
Codeine	Codeine sulfate or phosphate	Analgesic	15–60 mg every 4 h	Drug dependence, constipation
Compazine	Prochlorperazine	Central antiemetic effect	5–10 mg 3–4 times a day, 25 mg suppository	Extrapyramidal symptoms, hepatotoxicity
Demerol	Meperidine	Analgesic	75–100 mg every 3 h as needed	Drug dependence
Ergot drugs	Ergotamine	See Table 5-5	See Table 5-5	See Table 5-5. Avoid in pregnancy; cardiovascular, hepatic, or renal diseases
Esgic	Butalbital 50 mg Acetaminophen 325 mg Caffeine 40 mg	Anxiolytic, muscle relaxant Analgesic	1 every 4–6 h	Barbiturate addiction
Fiorinal	Butalbital (50 mg) Aspirin (325 mg) Caffeine (40 mg)	Anxiolytic, muscle relaxant Analgesic	1 every 4–6 h	Barbiturate addiction
Fioricet	Butalbital (50 mg) Acetaminophen (325 mg) Caffeine (40 mg)	Anxiolytic, muscle relaxant Analgesic	1 every 4–6 h	Barbiturate addiction
Midrin	Isomethaptene mucate (65 mg) Dichloraphenazone (100 mg) Acetaminophen (325 mg)	Cranial and cerebral vasoconstrictor Mild sedative Analgesic	2 stat, repeat with 1 every h up to 5 doses	Avoid monoamine oxidase inhibitors, hypertension, glaucoma
Nuprin	Ibuprofen (200 mg)	Nonsteroidal anti-inflammatory	1–2 at the onset, repeat every 3–4 h	GI upset, fluid retention, photo-allergic skin rash
Percocet	Oxycodon hydrochloride (5 mg) Acetaminophen (325 mg)	Analgesic Analgesic	1–2 every 4 h as needed	Drug dependence, constipation
Percodan	Oxycodone hydrochloride (4.5 mg) Oxycodone terephthalate (0.38 mg) Aspirin (325 mg)	Analgesic Analgesic Analgesic, anti-inflammatory	1 for severe headache	Drug dependence, constipation
Phenergan	Promethazine	H_1 receptor blocker, antihistamine	25 mg every 6 h as needed	Sedation, dry mouth
Prednisone	Steroid	Anti-inflammatory, general well-being	5–20 mg (for resistant attacks)*	Carbohydrate metabolism, fluid retention, use for short course
Reglan	Metoclopramide	Increases tone and motility of gastric contractions	10 mg every 4–6 h tablet, syrup, suppository, or injection	Good for nausea, can cause extrapyramidal symptoms
Talwin	Pentazocine hydrochloride (12.5 mg)	Analgesic	30 mg every 6 h	Drug dependence
Tigan	Trimethobenzamide	Centrally acting antiemetic	100, 200 mg caps; 100, 200 mg suppositories, 100 mg injection	Extrapyramidal symptoms, hepatotoxicity, ? Reye syndrome in children
Tylenol	Acetaminophen	Analgesic	325 mg 1–2 tab every 4 h as needed	Hepatic and renal toxicity in prolonged use
Tylox	Oxycodone hydrochloride 4.5 mg Oxycodone terephthalate 0.38 mg Acetaminophen 500 mg	Analgesic Analgesic Analgesic	1 for severe headache	Drug dependence
Vistaril	Hydroxyzine pamoate	Potentiates action of opioids, muscle relaxant	25 mg intramuscular	Dry mouth, drowsiness

GI: gastrointestinal.

*Do not use more than 20 tablets (5 mg each) per month. 4 tablets at onset, 2 tablets 4 h later, one 4 h later and one 12 h later. For severe attacks, 60 mg can be used over 1-week period in reducing doses.

Table 5-5
Ergot Preparations

Trade Name	Contents and Route	Pharmacologic Action	Comments
Cafergot tab	Caffeine 100 mg Ergotamine 1 mg Bellafoline 30 mg	Cranial vasoconstrictor Serotonin antagonist Direct stimulation effect on peripheral and cranial vessel smooth muscles Depression of central autonomic reflexes, Closes A-V shunts. Anticholinergic, antiemetic	Nausea, leg cramps Daily use may lead to caffeine and ergot dependence
Cafergot PB tab	Caffeine 100 mg Ergotamine 1 mg Bellafoline 30 mg Pentobarbital 30 mg	Same as above Reduces nervous tension	Daily use can result in barbiturate and ergot dependence
Wigraine tab	Caffeine 100 mg oral Ergotamine 1 mg	Same as above Same as above	Nausea, leg cramps Daily use can cause ergot dependence
Wigrettes	Ergotamine 2 mg	Vasoconstrictor, uterine stimulant, α-adrenoreceptor antagonist	It is used when quick action is desired as in cluster headache
Bellergal tab	Phenobarbital 20 mg Ergotamine tartrate 0.3 mg Bellafoline 0.1 mg	Central sedative Sympathetic inhibitor Parasympathetic inhibitor	Same precaution as for Cafergot
Bellergal-S	Phenobarbital 40 mg Ergotamine tartrate 0.6 mg Bellafoline 0.2 mg	Same as above	Same precaution as for Cafergot
Ergomar Ergostat	Ergotamine 2 mg sublingual	Same as above	Used when quick action is needed, as in cluster headache or migraine, at the onset of headache
Medihaler ergotamine	Ergotamine 0.35 mg per whiff	Same as above	Same as above
Cafergot suppository	Ergotamine 2 mg Caffeine 100 mg	Same as above	Useful when nausea prevents oral use of Cafergot. Better absorption than tablets.
Cafergot PB Suppository	Ergotamine 2 mg Caffeine 100 mg Pentobarbital 60 mg Bellafoline 0.2 mg	Same as above	Better absorption than tablets. Precautions: Same as tablets.
Wigraine Suppository	Ergotamine 2 mg Caffeine 100 mg Tartaric acid 21.5 mg	Same as above	Same as above
Wigraine PB Suppository	Ergotamine tartrate 2 mg Caffeine 100 mg Belladona alkaloid 0.2 mg Pentobarbital 60 mg	Same as above	One case reported of reversible bilateral papillitis with ring scotoma in a patient who received five times the recommended dose over a 14-day period
DHE 45 Injection	Dihydroergotamine mesylate 1 mg	Central autonomic effects Peripheral vasocontriction	Low emetic potency
Sumatriptan	Oral 100 mg Subcutaneous 6 mg	5-HT$_1$ agonist	Minimal side effects. Not released by FDA yet.

Table 5-6
Drugs Used to Treat Headache Symptoms: Their Routes, Efficacy, and Convenience

Efficacy	Drug	Route	Convenience
* * * * *	DHE 45	Intramuscular injection	*
* * * *	Cafergot	Suppository	* *
* * * *	Cafergot PB	Suppository	* *
* * * *	Wigraine	Suppository	* *
* * * *	Wigraine PB	Suppository	* *
* * *	Ergomar	Sublingual	* * *
* * *	Ergostat	Sublingual	* * *
* * *	Wigrettes	Sublingual	* * *
* *	Medihaler Ergotamine	Inhaler	* * * *
*	Bellergal	Tablet	* * * * *
*	Bellergal S	Tablet	* * * * *
*	Cafergot	Tablet	* * * * *
*	Cafergot PB	Tablet	* * * * *
*	Wigraine	Tablet	* * * * *

* = least, ***** = most.

the patient may build up a temporary resistance against another attack, even though exposed to known precipitating factors.

Factors that Precipitate Attacks

The menstrual cycle, weather, or barometric pressure, a sudden change in altitude (for example, during air travel), fasting, prolonged sleep, a major change in pace of living, and emotional stress may lead to attack. Certain foods, such as cheese, chocolate, and monosodium glutamate, and drinks, such as red wine or any alcoholic beverage, also may cause an attack. Caffeine seems to induce headache in some patients, while others find it soothing. Excessive use of caffeine should be avoided.

Factors that Relieve Attacks

These include lying down in a dark quiet room, pressing on the temporal arteries, ice bags, freedom from stressful situations, and hydration.

Family History

This frequently is positive for common migraine or sick headaches. Recurrent so-called sinus headache in a parent often is migraine.

Differential Diagnosis

The main features that differentiate common migraine from tension headache are its unilaterality, throbbing quality, common accompaniment of nausea and vomiting, sensitivity to light and noise, and worsening of headaches with alcohol (the latter seems to relieve tension headaches). A family history of headache is less common in tension headache.

Prophylactic Treatment

See classic migraine section.

Symptomatic Treatment

See classic migraine section.

Cluster Headache

Definition

"Vascular headache, predominantly unilateral on the same side, usually associated with flushing, sweating, rhinorrhea, and increased lacrimation; brief in duration and usually occurring in closely packed groups separated by long remissions. Identical or closely allied are: erythroprosopalgia (Bing), ciliary or migrainous neuralgia (Harris), erythromelalgia of the head or histaminic cephalgia (Horton); and petrosal neuralgia (Gardner et al.)".[6]

The facial characteristics are so typical that a cluster headache diagnosis may be made from the patient's appearance during an attack. The patient generally has a leonine appearance with a thick-set jaw, accompanied by ipsilateral miosis, ptosis, conjuctival congestion, lacrimation, nasal stuffiness, or clear watery discharge. The autonomic symptoms disappear as the headache improves.

Cause

This is unknown.

Pathophysiologic Findings

There is considerable debate over whether cluster headache is a variant of migraine or a separate entity. Features of cluster headache that are migrainous are the following:

1. Visible unilateral dilatation of temporal artery during the attack.
2. Nasal blockage.
3. Ptosis.
4. Miosis (more marked in cluster headache).
5. Precipitation of headache by alcohol, nitroglycerine, naps,

rapid-eye-movement (REM) stage of sleep, and change of pace.

6. Definite response to ergotamine and steroids.[29]

Those who contend these two conditions are separate entities argue as follows:

1. Family history is strongly positive in migraine and less so in cluster headache.
2. Duration of attack is shorter in cluster headache.
3. Severity of attack is much greater in cluster headache.
4. Autonomic symptoms are increased markedly in cluster headache.
5. Multiple attacks in 24 h are more common in cluster headache.
6. Clustering of attacks in closely packed groups is typical of cluster headache. It occurs only occasionally in migraine.
7. Response to lithium is good in cluster headache but poor in migraine.
8. Sex ratio shows cluster headache is predominantly a male disease (male:female ratio, 4:1). In migraine, it is 3:1 in favor of women.
9. Corneal indentation pulse (CIP) is increased markedly in cluster headache but changed little, if any, in migraine.
10. Blood serotonin level drops during a migraine attack but not during a cluster headache.

The basic differences between cluster and migraine headaches seem to be in timing, intensity, duration of attack, and severity of headache.[30]

Cluster headache has developed after herpes simplex and other neurotropic viral infections, head and neck injuries, and major changes in emotional state. There is much to suggest an imbalance of the parasympathetic and sympathetic nervous systems in the cluster period and during attacks, probably of hypothalamic or limbic origin.

The exact source of pain is controversial.[31] Some investigators contend it results from parasympathetic activation in the fibers contained in the plexus and accompanying the internal carotid artery and its medium-size branches on to the pial arteries. Dilatation of these arteries causes severe pain.

Time of Onset

In some patients, the headaches tend to occur at approximately the same time each day, often at the end of the work day or 1 h after going to sleep. In others, there is no set time of onset. The patients may get more than one attack per day or night.

Attack Profile

The headache starts as a pressure sensation over and around the eye or temple area. Within minutes, it reaches its peak, remaining at that level for the next 30 to 60 min. Then it dissipates quickly (Fig. 5-15). The excruciating pain may be compounded by a sharp jabbing transient pain of higher intensity that repeats itself several times during the attack. Without medication, the headache usually subsides after approximately 45 min to 1 h. Occasionally attacks may last 3, 4, 6, or 8 h.

Patients generally know when they are in the cluster period because they may experience some low grade minor pressure sensations. Attacks generally are unilateral and usually, but not always, remain on the same side for the period of a given cluster of attacks.

Pattern of Occurrence

Cluster headache is classified based on its pattern of headache-free intervals into three catagories:

1. Episodic cluster headache commonly starts in the early spring or fall, and the cluster may last 4 to 6 weeks. The clusters may follow an almost carbon-copy pattern from 1 year to the next (Fig. 5-16).
2. Primary chronic cluster headache occurs in some patients where there is no distinct headache-free interval, although other characteristics of the headache are similar to episodic cluster headache (Fig. 5-17). If it continues steadily for 1 year or more, it is known as primary chronic cluster headache.
3. In the beginning, secondary chronic cluster headaches start as typical episodic cluster headaches. Over the years, the headache-free intervals become shorter and shorter until there is no such period, and secondary chronic cluster headache is diagnosed (Fig. 5-18).

Age of Onset

Attacks may begin at age 8 to 10 years. More often, they begin during the late teen-age years or 20s. Sometimes cluster headaches follow head or neck trauma or infections. More often, they occur after a change of pace or periods of stressful mental and emotional activity. Vacations are common times for cluster headache.

FIGURE 5-15. Cluster headache attack profile.

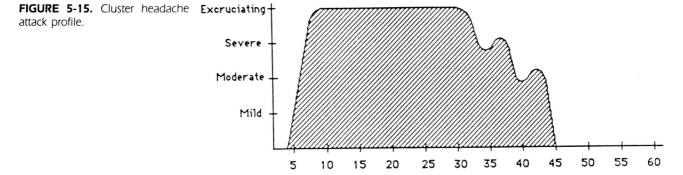

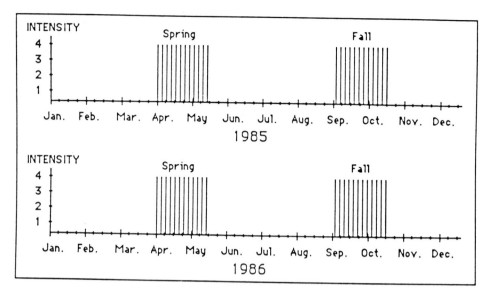

FIGURE 5-16. Episodic cluster headache.

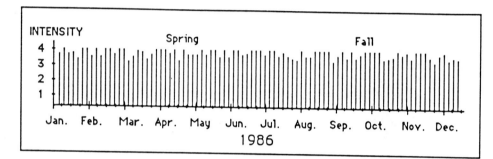

FIGURE 5-17. Primary chronic cluster headache.

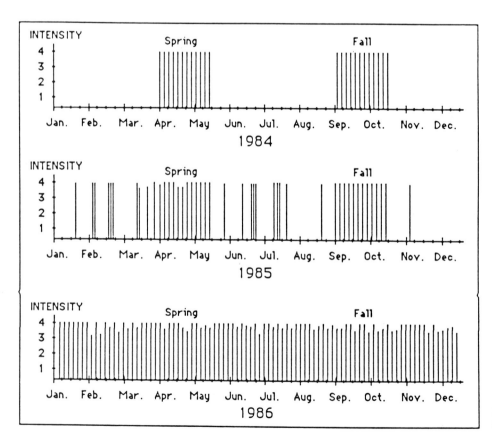

FIGURE 5-18. Secondary chronic cluster headache.

Headache Phase

The quality of pain is constant, boring and occasionally throbbing. The pain is located in and around the eye; over the temporal, maxillary, and frontal areas; and sometimes in the back of the neck in the suboccipital region. Pain in the upper teeth and gums is common and may lead to unnecessary tooth extraction. The pain is almost always severe to excruciating. There are no or occasional prodromal tightness, burning, or prickling in the neck or forehead. In rare instances, tearing, sweating, and nasal blockage may precede the onset of pain. Rarely, nausea, vomiting, photophobia, and sonophobia accompany the headache. These patients may try sitting or lying down but usually are found pacing the floor to relieve the intense pain. They press hard on the area over or around their eyes and on the back of their necks. They may try cold compresses in this area. Patients with cluster headache are known to become enraged and behave abnormally during an attack. Not infrequently, patients express the frustration of their inability to control the pain, by banging the wall, crying out, striking out, and rarely going into a trance.

Factors Precipitating Attacks

Precipitating factors include: smoking, certain foods (such as cheese, chocolate, or monosodium glutamate), and alcohol during the cluster period. These patients, however, can consume these items without any fear of getting a headache during the cluster-free period.

Factors Relieving Attacks

At the onset, counter stimulation with hot or cold application at the site may relieve an attack. Vigorous excersise for 5 to 10 min may be effective. Others cite inhalation of 100% oxygen at a rate of 8 liters/min for 5 to 10 min.[32] The use of ergotamine by inhalation, sublingually, orally, rectally or injection (see Table 5-5) may be effective.

Prophylactic Treatment

Steroid Therapy. Prednisone 40 to 60 mg daily for approximately 3 days is prescribed and then tapered. Do not use it for more than 4 to 6 weeks because long-term steroid administration can result in many complications, including, peptic ulcer, glaucoma, osteoporosis, fluid retention, and weight gain. If it is effective, we can taper the dose by 5 mg every 2 to 3 days. If headaches recur during the tapering period, we can administer the preceding next higher dose and, after a few days, resume tapering the dose. In the hospital setting, we can give 80 units of corticotropin intravenously or intramuscularly.

Lithium. Recently, lithium carbonate 300 mg three times a day after meals has been found to be effective. Lithium blood levels should be checked once a week. Thyroid function and hematopoietic and renal status also should be followed. On a long-term basis, this drug can cause hypothyroidism and interstitial nephritis. Lithium, however, can be used for longer periods than prednisone.[33] Tremors of the hands are a common side effect. After the cluster is under control, the lithium may be gradually tapered. In chronic cluster headache, it may be continued for months or years.

Calcium-Channel Blockers. Verapamil 80 mg three to six times a day may be effective. We should be careful if the patient is taking other cardiac medication when this drug is prescribed. Verapamil can cause conduction disturbances. Constipation is a common annoying side effect. Calcium-channel blockers should be given for at least 2 to 4 weeks as a trial.

Ergot Preparations. Used on a daily basis, these can be useful, especially in younger patients who have no cardiac or vascular problems. This is one of the few times when daily use of ergotamine is justified, provided attention is paid to vascular and other complications.[34] A dose on arising, before supper, and at bedtime may be indicated and tapered as improvement occurs.

Methysergide. Methysergide 2 mg three times a day can be effective. The patient should be monitored for cardiac murmur, pleuropulmonary fibrosis, or retroperitoneal fibrosis. These complications can be avoided if methysergide therapy is interrupted for 2 weeks after constant use for 3 months. Patients taking methysergide should be told these facts and urged to report any untoward symptoms while they are receiving this drug.

Cyproheptadine. Cyproheptadine 4 mg three to four times a day can be effective. Weight gain is a common side effect. Drowsiness may impair work function.

Other Treatments. In women with cluster headache during menopause, moderate doses of estrogen can be tried. Similarly, progesterone 250 mg can be given intramuscularly once a week. Progesterone intramuscularly also can be tried in men refractory to other therapies. There are no major side effects of progesterone therapy.

Occasionally, tricyclic antidepressants or monoamine oxidase inhibitors are helpful. A common side effect of tricyclic drugs is dry mouth. Dietary precautions are required when monoaminase oxidase inhibitors are used. A subcutaneous injection of 6 mg of sumatriptan, a 5-HT$_1$ agonist holds promise in the treatment of cluster headache.[34a]

Since the pain of cluster headache can be crippling, various surgical techniques have been tried where drug treatment failed. These include: (1) percutaneous radiofrequency thermocoagulation of trigeminal nerve rootlets,[35] (2) retrogasserian sensory rhizotomy with glycerol,[35] (3) resection of the greater superficial petrosal nerve,[36] (4) section of the nervus intermedius,[37] (5) sphenopalatine ganglionectomy,[38] (6) alcohol injection of the gasserian ganglion,[39] and (7) superficial temporal artery section.[40] Surgical procedures should be considered for patients who have not responded to medical therapy and are disabled by chronic cluster headache. Remissions are common after surgical procedures. In a 2-year follow-up of patients after sphenopalatine nerve crysurgical lesion, only 6 of 24 patients noticed improvement.[41]

Differential Diagnosis

Identical or closely allied are erythroprosopalgia (Bing),[41a] Ciliary or migrainous neuralgia (Harris),[41b] erythromelalgia of the head, histaminic cephalgia (Horton),[41c] and petrosal neuralgia (Gardner and associates).[36] Chronic paroxymal hemicrania is another diagnosis that also should be considered. In 1974, Sjaastad and associate[42] described a new headache entity seen in women who had headaches resembling cluster headache but more frequently. Pain occurred in and around the eye, forehead, and face (always unilaterally) and was accompanied by secretions from the ipsilateral eye and nostril. The frequency of attacks varied between 6 and 18 per day. Each headache lasted 15 to 45 min. Aspirin was helpful somewhat, but indomethcin 100 to 200 mg daily eradicated the headaches completely within 1 day. A trial of indomethacin for 2 to 3 days is indicated especially in women who have five or more headache attacks per day.

In one case, an AV malformation in the occipital lobe presented as a cluster headache.[43] In this patient, although there was the typical periodicity of cluster headache associated with lacrimation, nasal congestion, and rhinorrhea, the pain was located ipsilaterally in the temporoparietal area rather than periorbitally as is typical in cluster headache.

Hemiplegic Migraine

Definition

"Vascular headache featured by motor phenomena which persists during and after the headache."[6]

Cause

The cause is unknown.

Pathophysiologic Findings

Prolonged vasoconstriction and/or ischemia and hypercoagulable state accompanied by increased platelet aggregability are seen.

Description

The patient commonly has a history of classic or common migraine. The headache, when accompanied by hemiplegia, is usually a more severe headache. Motor or sensory prodromes persist through the headache phase and may continue for several days afterward. Visual field defects are also common. There may be numbness of the face, arm, or leg; paresthesia, aphasia, and confusion are also common. Headache usually is unilateral. The phenomena may switch sides from one attack to another.

The frequency of hemiplegic migraine is 0.3% of patients with migraine.[44] The hemiplegia usually reverses after the first attack, but it can become permanent after repeated attacks. It is likely to occur in women receiving oral contraceptives or heavy users of ergotamine and/or tobacco before hemiplegia. The mortality rate is 5%.[45]

Age of Onset

It is more common in women in their 20s to 30s.

Headache Phase

The headache is generally unilateral. A constellation of neurologic signs and symptoms may accompany complicated migraine. These include nausea and vomiting, motor aphasia, confusion, hemiparesis, hemiplegia, ataxia, and rarely, Jacksonian jerks, amnesia, or fugue-like state.

Investigations

It is mandatory to exclude organic lesions in these patients. An electroencephalogram (EEG) during and after a headache attack is helpful. A CT scan of the head, MRI scan, radionucleide scan, and cerebral arteriogram are indicated in patients who have persistence of prodromes after or beyond the onset of headache. An arteriogram, however, should not be done during the attack. Wait until all the symptoms have cleared before doing this test; otherwise, there is danger of causing a permanent deficit. Lumbar puncture done after the attack to exclude bleeding also may be indicated.

Family History

This frequently is positive for classic or common migraine. In some families, other members of the family may have strikingly similar hemiplegic migraine.

Variants of Hemiplegic Migraine

Basilar artery migraine includes, along with the headache, dysarthria, aphasia, ataxia, severe visual loss, tinnitus, and vertigo. Sometimes global amnesia can occur with the migraine. Locked-in syndrome is characterized by a conscious patient who is paralyzed totally except for the movement of their eyes. The patient is aware of their surroundings but is unable to speak or show emotion. This locked-in state is a transient occurrence in migraine; if it is caused by an organic lesion of the pons, it may be fatal.[46] These attacks require constant medical supervision and emergency room admission where practical. Lateral medullary syndrome is migraine that rarely may be complicated by permanent occlusion of the posterior inferior cerebellar artery resulting in lateral medullary syndrome.[47] Other types of strokes also have been reported after a complicated migraine.[48,49]

Prophylactic Treatment

If attacks occur frequently, papaverine hydrochloride and aspirin 325 mg three to four times daily, used either singly or in combination, may prevent hemiplegic migraine. If these are ineffective, propranolol prophylaxis and/or calcium-channel blockers should be tried. Also, consider drugs that inhibit platelet formation, such as aspirin and dipyridamole. Avoiding oral contraceptives and smoking is recommended. If hypertension is present, it should be treated. The role of anticoagulants in complicated migraine currently is not established.

Symptomatic Treatment

During these severe episodes, the patient should be attended by another person. Rest, sedation, and analgesic medications are indicated. At the onset, attempts to increase cerebral vasodilatation by carbon dioxide inhalation, breathing in a bag, or vigorous exercise (if possible) helps in some patients. Breathing oxygen or inhalation of small doses of amyl nitrite at the onset of the prodrome can be tried. Prednisone 15mg orally repeated in 4 h is another therapy that sometimes is effective. Ergot preparations should be avoided because they increase vasoconstriction and ischemia. The use of calcium-channel blockers at the onset of such an attack has been tried and appears promising.

Ophthalmoplegic Migraine

Definition

"Vascular headache featured by ocular phenomena which occur during and after the headache. It may lead to permanent neurologic deficit."[6]

Cause

The cause is unknown.

Pathophysiologic Findings

This type of headache most likely results from mechanical compression of the affected nerve from dilated edematous adjacent arteries. The artery undergoes changes during migraine headache, and the nerve is probably not involved.

Attack Profile

Temporary paralysis of cranial nerve III is most common. Other nerves also can be involved, including IV, VI, or portions of V. These deficits usually begin during the headache and often continue after the headache is over. The pupil is dilated ipsilaterally in contrast to diabetic oculomotor paralysis where the pupil is normal in size. The deficits may last days or weeks. Occasionally, after repeated attacks, there may be permanent impairment of the affected eye muscles.

Age of Onset

Generally, this disorder begins in childhood, sometimes as early as 2 to 3 years of age.

Headache Phase

Visual prodromes (usually diplopia) develop together with the headache and persist after it for days, weeks, and occasionally, permanently. The frequency varies; a few attacks per year are most common. The quality of pain is usually throbbing. The headache is unilateral, on the same side as ophthalmoplegia. Its location is behind and over the eye. If the headache is severe, it may involve the whole head. There is no predictable pattern of occurrence. Its severity is usually moderate to severe in intensity. Its duration is 8 to 10 h, but the eye weakness may last several days to weeks. After repeated attacks, there may be permanent eye weakness, including permanent pupillary dilatation. Nausea, vomiting, and with severe attacks, vertigo occur frequently as in common migraine.

Factors Precipitating Attacks

These are unknown but may be the same factors that cause classic and common migraine.

Family History

This usually is positive for migraine and, sometimes, for ophthalmoplegic migraine.

Differential Diagnosis

Attacks of ophthalmoplegic migraine closely resemble episodes of leaking aneurysms of the internal carotid artery or posterior or anterior communicating arteries. It is important to exclude a bleeding aneurysm in every case of ophthalmoplegic migraine. Other differential diagnoses include fibrochondroma of cranial nerve III, neurofibroma of cranial nerve III, thrombosis of the central retinal artery, and diabetic oculomotor paralysis.

Investigations

A CT scan of the head, an arteriogram, and lumbar puncture are indicated in ophthalmoplegic migraine to exclude a bleeding aneurysm. A thorough eye examination by an ophthalmologist is also part of the workup.

Treatment

Ergotamine preparations prescribed as in classic migraine are useful in ophthalmoplegic migraine. In severe cases, a short course of corticosteroids for 4 to 6 days may reduce the duration of the attack and prevent permanent damage from frequent attacks. Prophylactic measures are the same as those used for common migraine.

Lower Half Headache

Definition

"Headache of possibly vascular mechanism, centered primarily in the lower face. In this group, there may be some instances of 'atypical facial' neuralgia, sphenopalatine ganglion neuralgia (Sluder) and vidian neuralgia (Vail)."[2] This is termed *atypical* to differentiate it from trigeminal or typical facial neuralgia.

Cause

The cause is unknown.

Pathophysiologic Findings

Headaches are probably of vascular origin. Often, at first, the headaches are intermittent, as in common migraine. Then, gradually, they become more frequent and last longer. In an established case, the vascular features of the headache are lacking, and headache is felt constantly for months or years.

Attack Profile

This disorder affects predominantly women. The attacks, at first, may occur around menstrual periods. Later, they occur more often and last longer, eventually becoming a daily headache. At times, there may be a constant daily headache from the start.

Age of Onset

This disorder generally starts in the 20s to 30s, but occasionally, it begins after a head or neck injury or a dental or surgical procedure.

Headache Phase

Although more commonly patients feel throbbing pain, constant deep-seated aching, pulling, or boring pain also is found. Generally, the headache is located in the maxillary and periorbital areas, but it may involve the temple, ear, jaw, and mandible. Occasionally, it spreads, causing aching in the neck and shoulders.[50] It is usually unilateral but can be bilateral. At first its pattern of occurrence is episodic, around menstrual periods. Later, the headaches are more frequent, last longer, and eventually become constant. It may, however, be a constant ache from the start. Its severity is mild to moderate. Its duration is 8 to 10 h, but as mentioned, these headaches can be constant. There is no prodrome. Depression is a prominent accompaniment during the headache.

Factors Precipitating Attacks

Menstrual periods, an exacerbation of depression, and digestive system disturbances can precipitate attacks.

Differential Diagnosis

Underlying local disease related to the sinuses, ear, nose, throat, teeth, gums, or temporomandibular joint should be excluded.

Treatment

Patients can be refractory to any mode of therapy. Treatment requires a strong commitment on the physician's part to be understanding, patient, and not feel disappointed if the headaches cannot be "cured" in a few visits. Psychiatric intervention is recommended in patients who are depressed or have other emotional problems.

In the episodic variety, ergot preparations are administered as used in migraine headaches (see Table 5-5). In the constant variety, tricyclic antidepressants, such as amitriptyline 25 to 150 mg at bedtime, may be beneficial. Monoamine oxidase inhibitors also may be helpful. β-Blockers (propranolol 40 mg three or four times a day) can be tried. A trial of methysergide and calcium-channel blockers also may be used in the same way as in migraine prophylaxis.

There is a great tendency for patients to seek a surgical "cure." Physicians should resist the temptation to refer the patient for some form of surgery. In intractable cases, a neurosurgical opinion may be sought but should be handled by a neurosurgeon well acquainted with this syndrome. The advice of an experienced psychiatrist also should be obtained before neurosurgical treatment is done.

Muscle-Contraction Headache

Definition

"Ache or sensations of tightness, pressure, or constriction widely varied in intensity, frequency, and duration. Sometimes long lasting and commonly suboccipital. It is associated with sustained contraction of the skeletal muscles in the absence of permanent structural change, usually as part of the individual's reaction during life stress. The ambiguous and unsatisfactory terms 'tension,' 'psychogenic,' and 'nervous' headache refer largely to this group."[6]

Cause

The cause is a response to stressful situations[51] or mechanical irritation of muscles, tendons, or fascia. In migraine headache, if movement makes the head hurt more, the patient may keep their head still. This constantly contracts the neck muscles, which in turn, eventually become another cause of pain. Conversely, in some cases, migraine headache can be precipitated by prolonged neck and scalp muscle contraction.

Pathophysiologic Findings

Muscle contraction of the scalp and cervical region or muscle ischemia from sustained muscle contraction are found. Such increased muscle contraction is shown readily in many patients, but it is not always present. Other unknown factors also may be important.

Age of Onset

These headaches may start at any age. Frequently, this headache is a response to stresses in life. The cause of stress may be different at different ages. For example, in childhood, it may be abusive (physically and emotionally) behavior of the parent or parents. In school-aged children, added pressure of studies, teachers, or teasing from classmates may occur. In adulthood, lack of communication or respect for each other among spouses is a common cause of stress. Depression commonly surfaces when we realize that the time to fulfill dreams of the future gradually is slipping away. This is likely to cause stress and muscle contraction headache ("the train of life's happiness is beginning to pull out of the station, all aboard??").

Headache Phase

The quality of pain is a tight band, pressure, vice-like pressure, or a tight cap around the head. The neck muscles feel as if they are in a knot. The location of the headache is in the forehead, neck, shoulders, and all around the head; it usually is bilateral. Its pattern of occurrence is during the period of stress or anticipation of stress. Migraines, however, occur during the relaxation phase after the stressful period. Its severity varies in intensity from mild to severe. Its duration is from a few hours to 1 day to several days. In some cases, these headaches persist for months or years. Their time of onset is before or during a stressful time. It is rare for the patient to wake up from a sound sleep as a result of a tension headache unless there is some abnormality of the cervical vertebrae that, during sleep, may put the neck in a position that causes the neck muscles to tighten up. There is no prodrome. The patient appears anxious, tense, and at times, depressed. There may be soreness in tight shoulder and neck muscles. Nausea, vomiting, photophobia, or sonophobia are uncommon. The patient may continue to function through the headache.

Factors Precipitating Attacks

Anticipation of impending stress generally alerts the patient of a coming headache. In addition to emotional stress, mechanical stress, such as having the neck in a position that eventually causes muscle tension (for example, assembly-line work where the neck is kept in a fixed position for long periods) may produce a headache.

Relation of Headache to Significant Life Events

Muscle contraction headaches are likely to occur in domestic or office situations where feelings are suppressed or during stressful situations, such as job interviews, weddings, or family gatherings. The patient is often a tense or anxious person, described as a worrier or a type A personality.

Family History

Other family members also may be tense or nervous. A family history of headache is not as common as in migraine, but it may be present.

Differential Diagnosis

Migraine headaches usually surface after a stressful period and tension headache, before or during the stress. Alcoholic beverages may precipitate migraine headaches. A tension headache usually is relieved by alcohol. Exercise during a headache makes a vascular headache of the migraine type throb and hurt more, but it has no effect or may have some

beneficial effect in tension headache. Headache that wakes the patient out of a deep sleep generally is not a tension headache. Sensitivity to light or noise is uncommon in tension headache. The response to ergot is good in migraine but poor in tension headache.

Headache of delusional, conversional, or hypochondric states (so-called psychogenic headaches) may mimic tension headache. Headaches caused by disorders of the cervical vertebrae, such as bony spurs or impingement of the greater occipital nerve, can be detected by physical examination and cervical spine x-rays. Depression commonly can present as tension headache. Organic causes, such as cervical abnormalities, posterior fossa tumors, or metabolic abnormalities, can cause neck muscles to tighten and resemble muscle contraction headache.

Symptomatic Treatment

If the physician can identify the underlying cause of tension, the treatment may be obvious. If the patient is a nervous worrier, regardless of the level of exogenous stress, methods aimed at learning to relax may help. Biofeedback is useful in this situation. Most patients find massage of the neck or shoulder muscles soothing. Psychotherapy may help deal with unresolved issues that are causing anxiety. Behavior modification is combined frequently with biofeedback. Autogenic phrases and progressive relaxation exercises also are used commonly with biofeedback. The patient can learn to relax by following techniques in self-help books that are available in most bookstores. Transcutaneous nerve electrical stimulation and acupuncture sometimes help but often only temporarily. An understanding physician is an integral part of the treatment.

Over-the-counter analgesics, such as aspirin and acetaminophen, are helpful and commonly used by patients, sometimes in excessive amounts. Each patient has their own favorite brand that "does the trick" for them. Most drugs except ergot preparations and corticosteroids listed in migraine therapy also have been used in tension headache.

Analgesic abuse can occur readily in these patients. They should be discouraged from excessive use of over-the-counter analgesics, which can cause gastric, hepatic, or renal damage. Drugs containing caffeine may perpetuate the headache by caffeine withdrawal. Barbiturate dependence is another danger in patients taking drugs containing this compound.

Prophylactic Treatment

Aspirin or acetaminophen in combination with caffeine[52] and butalbital may be used in tension headache in limited amounts but only for short-term protection during special events. If depression is a major factor in perpetuating tension headache, tricyclic antidepressants (amitriptyline 25 to 150 mg or doxepin 25 to 150 mg) at bedtime can be tried. In patients with prolonged tension headache, tricyclics may be useful even though depression is not overt.

Muscle relaxants, such as diazepam or methocarbamol

with aspirin may be useful for specific periods. Supervision regarding the duration and quantity of therapy is needed to avoid dependence on these agents. Special attention in this regard needs to be paid to combinations of caffeine, analgesics, and sedatives before these drugs, when used in excess, may lead to prolongation of the problem and dependency requiring detoxification. Short courses of anxiolytic drugs like clorazepate, chlordiazepoxide, diazepam, and alprazolam, alone or in combination with antidepressants also may be helpful.

Combined Headache: Vascular and Muscle Contraction

Definition

"Combinations of vascular headache of the migraine type and muscle-contraction headache *prominently co-existing in an attack*."[6]

Headache Phase

These headaches may start in teen-age years or later in life. They have the quality of migraine (throbbing pain) and a feeling of a tight band around the head (tension headache). Occasionally, pain is felt all over. Nausea and occasionally vomiting are fairly common. Menses may be a precipitating factor in some patients.

The headache is moderate to severe in intensity, lasting 8 to 10 h. Sometimes, it continues for 1 to 3 days. The headache may awaken the patient from sleep or may start during the morning hours.

There are no prodromes; if the headache is severe, nausea, vomiting, photophobia, or sonophobia may accompany it. The face looks pale. The patient may be depressed.

Treatment

Biofeedback, behavior modification, general relaxation, and psychotherapy are useful in combined headache. Drugs used in the symptomatic and prophylactic treatment of migraine are also useful in combined headache. Propranolol is especially effective. Drug abuse frequently is seen in these patients. Tricyclic antidepressants in full doses up to 150 mg daily may be valuable.

Nasal Vasomotor Reaction

Definition

"Headaches and nasal discomfort (nasal obstruction, rhinorrhea, tightness or burning), recurrent and resulting from congestion and edema of nasal and paranasal mucous membranes, and not proven to be due to allergens, infectious agents, or local gross anatomic defects. The headache is predominantly anterior in location and mild or moderate in intensity. The illness is usually part of the individual's reaction during stress. This is often called 'vasomotor rhinitis.' "[6]

Cause

Although unknown, these headaches can occur in hypothyroidism. More commonly, patients have deep-seated emotional stress from chronic hidden resentment and anger.

Pathophysiologic Findings

There is blockage of the nasal passages.

Age of Onset

This disease usually begins in the teen-age years or adulthood.

Headache Phase

The quality of pain is constant. The location is the nose, cheeks, frontal sinuses, eyes, and behind the eyes. Its pattern of occurrence is not set. Its severity is usually mild to moderate in intensity. Its duration is continuous. The headache usually starts in the early morning. There is no prodrome or accompaniments during headache. The patient manages to continue to function, although he/she may try various forms of nose drops and over-the-counter analgesics (often in excess).

Factors Precipitating Attacks

The pain usually gets worse whenever the cause of suppressed resentment becomes active.

Differential Diagnosis

Allergic or infectious diseases of the nasal sinuses, retention cysts, deviated septum, and excessive use of nasal decongestants should be excluded.

Treatment

Hypothyroidism should be treated if that condition exists. Tricyclic antidepressants, such as amitriptyline or monoamine oxidase inhibitors, such as phenelzine, may be helpful. Psychotherapy in a patient who recognizes an unresolved underlying emotional stress can be useful. The physician should be supportive of the patient's suffering and be willing to listen to the patient's explanations for why they are not able to make changes that they know will improve the headache. The mere process of being a patient listener is a form of therapy any physician can provide and does not require special training in psychotherapy. Sometimes, the patient needs the help of specialists in psychotherapy, behavior modification, relaxation, hypnosis, and family counseling. Surgery on the nose or sinuses solely to improve headaches should be avoided.

Headache of Delusional, Conversional, or Hypochondriacal States

Definition

"Headaches of illnesses in which the prevailing clinical disorder is a delusional or a conversion reaction and a peripheral pain mechanism is nonexistent. Closely allied are the hypochondriacal reactions in which the peripheral disturbances relevant to the headache are minimal. These also have been called 'psychogenic' headaches."

Cause

The cause is unknown.

Pathophysiologic Findings

These are unknown.

Age of Onset

The headaches frequently start in the teen-age years.

Headache Phase

The quality of pain can be described variously as pressure, exploding, fullness, or weight on the head and neck. There is no localized area, but the whole head is involved. Sometimes the patient may experience pain in one particular area, such as in the temporal area or occipital region. The pain is described as moderate to severe in intensity, and it interferes in activities of daily living. These patients commonly complain that the pain never leaves them during their waking hours. There are no prodromes. These patients usually have blurring vision, concentric narrowing of the visual field, light-headedness, faint feeling, and difficulty in concentration.

Family History

This generally is not present.

Differential Diagnosis

If the patient describes localized headache, it may mimic migraine headache. The patient's manner of describing the severity of the headaches, with indifference, may be a clue to the correct diagnosis. Often, organic causes should be excluded for the patient's vague and multiple complaints, but multiple somatic complaints easily can sway the physician to do an unnecessarily extensive workup. This should be avoided as much as possible.

Treatment

The role of the physician as a patient listener and as a general guardian advising about daily activities, eating habits, vacation, and exercise is helpful and may make a difference between the patient becoming a drug abuser or maintaining a reasonable life without overuse of medication. These patients can associate the onset of the headache with some stressful situation in their life, such as action in combat during the war or sexual abuse. The patient generally is hard to reach emotionally and tends to avoid situations with close emotional ties. They may be refractory to all forms of therapy.

If the headache starts in childhood, referral to a psychiatrist may be beneficial to uncover any underlying unresolved issues. Sometimes after several interviews, psy-

chotherapy may be needed or hypnosis or an analytic interview may be required to uncover the major issues. If there is secondary gain in having a headache, it may be impossible to get rid of headache and may be an unrealistic goal to achieve. If the symptoms are not controlled, the physician still may be valuable in the patient's care by avoiding unnecessary treatments and planning achievable reasonable goals. This is an example where less is better.

Drug therapy with tricyclic antidepressants, such as amitriptyline or doxepin may be helpful.

Nonmigrainous Vascular Headaches

Definition

"Nonmigranous vascular headaches associated with generally nonrecurrent dilatation of cranial arteries. Causes include:
   A. Systemic infections, usually with fever[53]
   B. Miscellaneous disorders, including hypoxic states, carbon monoxide poisoning, effects of nitrites, nitrates, and other chemical agents with vasodilator properties; caffeine-withdrawal reactions, circulating insufficiency in the brain (in certain circumstances); postconcussion reactions, post convulsive states, 'hang over' reactions,[54] foreign protein reactions, hypoglycemia, hypercapnia, acute pressor reactions (abrupt elevation of blood pressure, as with paraplegia or pheochromocytoma), and certain instances of essential arterial hypertension (eg. those with early morning headaches)."[6]

Cause

The headache is secondary to the underlying metabolic, physiologic, or mechanical disturbance.

Pathophysiologic Findings

Vasodilatation of extracranial vessels can cause headache. Vasodilatation and stretching of pain-sensitive intracranial arteries, venous sinuses, and their tributaries are also painful.

Different Types of Headache

There are many infectious diseases associated with headaches. The clue is fever and/or other constitutional symptoms, which should prompt investigation for infectious or inflammatory causes.

Intracranial vasodilatation is the source of headache in hypoxic states and carbon monoxide poisoning. Nitrite ingestion is the cause of headache from eating hot dogs, salami, and occupational hazards (such as, gun powder factories). Nitrates (such as, nitroglycerine, isosorbide dinitrate, amyl nitrate, erythrityl tetranitrate, and pentaerythritol tetranitrate) all can cause headache, especially in a headache-prone patient. Some of the other vasodilator chemicals that can lead to headache include: hydralazine, minoxidil, calcium-channel blockers (especially, nifedipine), sodium nitroprusside, diazoxide, and theophylline-like drugs.

Caffeine, a vasoconstrictor, when withdrawn after prolonged continued use, causes rebound vasodilatation of the cranial vessels, resulting in vascular headache. Daily use of ergotamine can cause similar rebound headache after sudden withdrawal.

Headache is common in cerebrovascular disease (such as, transient ischemic attacks and stroke). It usually occurs on the side of ischemia. In the vertebrobasilar system, gradual narrowing of the vessels may cause occipital headache and other symptoms (such as, visual disturbance, vertigo, sensory loss, dysarthria, numbness of one side of the face or extremities, and motor weakness). Although generally mild, not throbbing, and lasting for a few minutes to a few hours, it can be a severe throbbing headache as described in 1664 in association with asymptomatic occlusion of the carotid artery. The headache probably is multifactorial rather than caused solely by dilatation of anastomotic arteries.[55] The return of migraine-like headache in an older person may represent a change in their arteries and their behavior.

Some patients who had migraine headache in the past notice aggravation of their symptoms after an injury causing concussion. The headache may have vascular features. Similarly, in the postconvulsive period, a patient may have headaches from vasodilatation of the cerebral vessels.

Headache felt the morning after heavily drinking is multifactorial. It may be the result of loss of sleep, overtiredness, hypoglycemia after alcohol ingestion, or overindulgence in substances known to cause headaches, such as cheese, nitrites, monosodium glutamate, and cigarette smoking. Remorse is also a prominent feature. The headache has vascular throbbing qualities.

A foreign-protein reaction (for example, to a vaccine) causes headache and other reactions (such as, fever and malaise). Prolonged fasting in a migraine sufferer can precipitate an attack. Other causes of hypoglycemia are drug induced (insulin or oral hypoglycemic agents, salicylates, propranolol, alcohol, disopyramide, sulfamethoxazole, and trimethoprim in a patient with impaired renal function).

Chronic hypercapnia, as occurs in a patient with chronic obstructive pulmonary disease, is a potent cerebrovasodilator. These patients commonly complain of throbbing headaches. In acute carbon dioxide retention, there is a mixture of vascular responses, including vasoconstriction, vasodilatation, and local CO_2 accumulation. The neurologic symptoms vary depending on which is the predominant factor.

Abrupt elevation in blood pressure (for example, in pheochromocytoma or paraplegia) causes a generalized throbbing headache of short duration from cranial arterial dilatation. The headache directly is correlated with the level of the blood pressure. The headache in essential hypertension, however, as in migraine, is caused largely by dilatation of branches of the external carotid artery. Only one half of the patients with essential hypertension complain of headaches. The intensity of the headache correlates with the severity of the hypertension, but there is no direct correlation between the level of blood pressure at the time and the presence or absence of headache. It is not uncommon in essential hypertension for headache to occur when the blood pressure is falling or low. It is thought that vasoconstriction in hypertension stimulates vasodilatation. As the vasoconstrictive stimuli diminish, vasodilatation occurs, resulting in headache. This might explain early-morning headache in essential hypertension when the blood pressure is generally low or falling.

With renal insufficiency, even without hypertension, some patients develop headache. This is a vascular headache akin to migraine, even though they may have no history of migraine.

Patients who undergo chronic hemodialysis also have chronic headaches. This is related temporally to the process of hemodialysis and occurs near the end of dialysis. Patients who have a history of migraine headache are particularly prone to getting dialysis-induced headaches. The pain is throbbing in nature and worsened by straining. It is more likely to occur when there is a significant drop in blood pressure or a decrease in serum sodium and osmolality. The headaches can be improved by increasing the sodium in the dialysate. These headaches, unlike dialysis dysequilibrium syndrome, do not disappear with continued long-term dialysis. Studies have shown that those who have dialysis-induced headaches have lower renin and aldosterone levels than those who do not get headaches. These headaches disappear when the patient gets a renal transplant, but they reappear if the kidney shows signs of rejection.

Traction Headache

Definition

"Headaches resulting from traction on intracranial structures, mainly vascular, by masses.

A. Primary or metastatic tumors of meninges, vessels, or brain.

B. Hemotomas (epidural, subdural, or parenchymal).

C. Abscesses (epidural, subdural, or parenchymal).

D. Post-lumbar puncture headache ('leakage' headache).

E. Pseudotumor cerebri and various causes of brain swelling."[6]

Pathophysiologic Findings

Pain is caused by distortion or stretching of pain-sensitive structures (such as, portions of the tributary veins, venous sinuses, meningeal vessels, carotid, vertebrobasilar, cerebellar, and cerebral arteries and tentorium) or by sudden or subacute overall or local changes in intracranial compartmental volume.

Primary or Metastatic Tumors

Description. Primary tumors constitute 70 percent to 75 percent of all brain tumors. Secondary metastatic tumors can occur when any primary tumor metastasizes to the brain, but bronchogenic and breast tumors are the most common. Seventy percent of all intracranial tumors in children are located infratentorially. In adults, 70 percent are located supratentorially. Headache generally occurs during the early part of the day. There may be localized tenderness of the skull at the site of a meningioma or at the mastoid area in a cerebellopontine angle tumor. Pain in the back of the head is present in almost all patients with infratentorial tumors. These also can cause unilateral muscle contraction in the neck and occipital region with characteristic tilting of the head. Frontal headache is more common with supratentorial tumors, although it also can occur with infratentorial tumors. Sudden rotation of the head, inducing frontal and temporal headache, may be diagnostic of a tumor. The headache may be aggravated by the onset of minor infections. Increased intracranial pressure is not necessary to produce a headache.

Headache Phase. The headache is intermittent. If there is no traction involved, there may be no headache. Its quality of pain is generally deep, aching, steady, or dull. Its severity is usually severe but not as severe as migraine. It rarely interferes with sleep. Nausea is common, and the patient may have vomiting when intracranial compression is made worse by coughing, Valsalva maneuver, or displacement of the medulla. In approximately one third of cases, during the early stages, the headache overlies the tumor. Later, after distortion of intracranial barriers, it may become bilateral. Posterior fossa tumors most commonly present with headache as their first symptom, except in cerebellopontine angle tumor. Supratentorial tumors present with other symptoms first, such as visual disturbances, paresthesias, convulsions, and personality changes before headaches. Headache in the postauricular area is almost specific for cerebellopontine angle tumors. Posterior fossa tumors may cause frontal pain by the nerve of Arnold, a branch of cranial nerve V.

Treatment. Prognosis depends on the treatment of the tumor. Headache may be relieved by aspirin.

Hematomas

Cause. In epidural hematoma, there is a collection of blood between the skull and dura mater, usually the result of a tear in the middle meningeal artery or more rarely in the vein. This process may progress rapidly. In subdural hematoma, there is a collection of blood between the dura and arachnoid. Subdural hematoma is of two types: (1) acute where bleeding occurs from a tear of a bridging vein between the venous sinus and cortex or from torn vessels in the underlying CNS, and (2) chronic where the site of bleeding is a bridging vein between the dura and meninges or between the middle meningeal artery and its branches. A related condition, subdural hygroma is a subdural collection of cerebrospinal fluid (CSF), sometimes blood tinged. It is thought to result from a tear in the arachnoid membrane.

Clinical Description. One percent to 3 percent of all head injuries include epidural hematoma. An overlying skull fracture is almost always present. The patient initially is unconscious, later regains consciousness, and then finally loses consciousness. The blood clot does not resolve or organize. It is a medical emergency and should be drained. Otherwise, it leads to increased intracranial pressure and herniation of temporal lobes with midbrain and medullary compression. If the patient is conscious, headache is a prominent early symptom. Later on, restlessness and combativeness is predominant and should alert the physician to an expanding intracranial lesion.

Skull fracture is uncommon in subdural hematoma. More commonly, these are located on the convexity of the cerebral hemispheres. There are five clinical subtypes of subdural hematoma.

1. Acute subdural hematoma that is common with more severe injury and loss of consciousness; it becomes clinically significant within 48 h of injury. There is a fluctuating level of consciousness.
2. Subacute subdural hematoma becomes clinically significant 2 to 14 days after the injury, and surgical therapy is different than for acute subdural hematoma.
3. Chronic subdural hematoma that is seen more than 14 days after the injury with headache as the most common complaint; later, apathy, inappropriate behavior, and confusion may occur. Intracranial pressure may be normal, but papilledema is uncommon. Sudden head movement or tapping the head can induce a headache.
4. Subdural hematoma of the elderly presents as mental deterioration without headache. When present, the headache may be bilateral. The original head injury may be relatively trivial, and the patient may not even remember the incident.
5. Infantile subdural hematoma can occur, but expansion of the infantile skull minimizes the increase in intracranial pressure. The child is usually restless and irritable.

Intracerebral hematoma is commonly associated with contusion or laceration of the brain. A contusion is an area of hemorrhagic necrosis that results when a blunt force crushes or bruises cell tissue. The most common site of contusion is the surface of the brain, frequently in the subfrontal, anterior temporal, and occipital regions. It may occur at the site of injury, a so-called coup lesion, or at a distance from the site of injury, usually on the opposite side of the brain, a contrecoup lesion. Headache is produced if the blood leaks into the subarachnoid space or if there is traction on pain-sensitive structures. The headache is dull and poorly localized; later, it may become more severe.

Treatment. This depends on the type, extent, and accessibility of the hematoma to surgery.

Abscesses

The source of infection can be (1) direct implantation by trauma or surgery, (2) extension from nearby foci of infection (especially mastoiditis, frontal, or ethmoid sinusitis), or (3) hematogenous spread where the primary source is usually the lung, heart, or bones. This is common with cyanotic congenital heart diseases.

Clinical Presentation. It takes approximately 2 months for a brain abscess to become of significant size to cause traction. An abscess from mastoiditis may first show signs of cerebritis. The disease then gradually grows, destroying and compressing the tissue. An infection in a sinus can spread to the extradural space, subdural space, meninges, or brain tissue and may rupture into the ventricles.

The patient has general complaints of increased intracranial pressure that occur early in cerebellar abscesses and later in frontal or temporal abscesses. A clinical deficit always is present. A source usually can be found in the mastoid, paranasal sinuses, lungs, heart, or skull. Rupture of the abscess into the brain ventricles may lead to ventriculitis or meningitis. Involvement of venous sinuses can cause sinus thrombosis. CSF is under increased pressure, with leukocytosis and high protein levels but a normal glucose content.

Gram-positive organisms are common with frontal or ethmoid sinusitis. Anaerobic bacteroides infection also can occur. Gram-negative organisms are common with middle ear disease.

Early signs of temporal lobe abscess are headaches, dysphasia (where the dominant temporal lobe is involved), upper quadrant homonymous hemianopia, papilledema, and muscle weakness. Patients with cerebellar abscess give a history of headache, vomiting, nystagmus (slower toward the side of the lesion), and ataxia. Subdural abscesses present with high fever and seizures. There may be frontal tenderness and redness and swelling of the eyelids.

Diagnosis. A CT scan should be done. The physician should avoid lumbar puncture and seek neurosurgical consultation.

Treatment. Proper culture and antibiotic treatment is essential. Dexamethasone, dehydration therapy, and anticonvulsants are indicated. Patients are best managed by an experienced neurosurgeon. In general, superficial supratentorial abscesses can be aspirated unless there is evidence of coning. In the latter case, they should be excised. Cerebellar abscesses should be excised immediately. When otitis media has caused the abscess, surgery of the infected ear must be done immediately after treatment of the abscess. The mortality rate is approximately 10 percent. Misdiagnosis and resistant bacteria are the main causes of mortality. Residual effects include epilepsy.

Postlumbar Puncture Headache

Definition. This is a headache that appears a few hours to several days after lumbar puncture and lasts a variable period of days or rarely weeks.

Cause. There is constant leakage of the spinal fluid from the hole in the dural membrane. It usually occurs when the fluid volume is less than 90 percent of its usual amount.

Pathophysiologic Findings. Traction on sensitive vascular structures in the head can occur because of low CSF volume and pressure.

Headache Phase. The headache shows a predictable response to position. It starts and progressively gets worse in the vertical position. It improves or totally disappears within minutes on lying down. The quality of the pain is a dull ache or throbbing. Its location, commonly, is bifrontal and occipital. Nausea, dizziness, and photophobia are common. It occurs in approximately 15 percent of spinal taps but is proportional to the size of the needle used. Headache occurs every time there is a change in position.

Treatment. Generally, the headaches improve with bed rest, increased fluid intake, and analgesics. If they continue, an autologous blood patch, applied in the epidural space at the same site as the original lumbar puncture is helpful and gives almost immediate relief. Occasionally, the patient may require a repeat blood patch.[56] Some patients need up to five blood patches. In rare cases, the hole must be sealed by surgically placing a suture in the dura.

Prophylaxis. A small needle should be used (20 gauge if a manometric reading is required or 25 to 26 gauge if a pressure reading is not necessary). A lateral approach, 2 to 3 cm from the midline, prevents overlapping of holes in the dura and arachnoid and may prevent the spinal fluid leak.[57] The subject should remain immobile during the procedure.

Spinal fluid leakage also can occur in posttraumatic situations. This may be secondary to skull fracture, congenital abnormalities in the floor of the skull, or pituitary fossa tumor. It also may occur postoperatively after yttrium implantation or transsphenoidal hypophysectomy. Diagnosis of this condition can be suspected by a dry tap or spontaneous rhinorrhea. The fluid has a higher sugar content than normal nasal secretions. On lateral skull x-ray, a fluid level may be seen in the sphenoid sinuses.

Pseudotumor Cerebri

Definition. There are features of raised intracranial pressure without any evidence of intracranial mass or obstructive hydrocephalus.

Cause. Causes include: (1) lateral sinus thrombosis after infections of the middle ear, (2) diminished absorption of CSF, (3) lead encephalopathy, (4) accelerated arterial hypertension, (5) chronic pulmonary disease with CO_2 retention, (6) polycythemia vera, (7) hypoparathyroidism, (8) excessive vitamin A intake, (9) treatment with nalidixic acid, tetracycline in infants, amitriptyline, or some hormone preparations, (10) corticosteroid therapy, and (11) adrenal insufficiency.

Headache Phase. This headache is most common in late teen-age years and menopausal overweight women. The headache is generalized. Its intensity varies but usually is mild to moderate. Its frequency is daily. Papilledema usually is present and may be marked despite a minimal amount of symptoms. Visual impairment and diplopia (from partial or complete cranial nerve VI palsy) may occur; vision may become gray or black for a few seconds on any change of posture of the head. There is risk of loss of vision as a result of optic atrophy.

Differential Diagnosis. Papilledema without intraocular mass can be seen in Guillian Barré syndrome and tumors of cauda equina. In both cases, CSF protein is elevated; in pseudotumor cerebri, it is normal. Ischemic papillitis from temporal arteritis and optic neuritis can cause optic disc swelling. Pseudopapilledema caused by drusens (hyaloid bodies) around the disc may be confused with papilledema.

Laboratory Data. CT scan shows normal or small ventricles with no midline shift. Spinal fluid is under increased pressure, varying between 220 and 600 mmH$_2$O. The fluid is clear with a normal chemical analysis and cell count.

Treatment. Weight loss is recommended in obese patients. Thiazide diuretics and corticosteroids are useful, and repeated lumbar puncture may provide headache relief. We should search for any underlying treatable factor.

Prognosis. Some patients recover within a few weeks; others require diuretic therapy for long periods. Relapse occurs in 10 percent of the patients.

Headache Due to Overt Cranial Inflammation

Definition

"Headaches due to readily recognized inflammation of cranial structures, resulting from usually nonrecurrent inflammation, sterile or infectious.

A. Intracranial disorders: infectious, chemical, or allergic meningitis, subarachroid hemorrhage, post-pneumoencephalographic reaction, arteritis, and phlebitis.

B. Extracranial disorders: arteritis and cellulitis."[6]

Intracranial Infections and Chemical or Allergic Meningitis

There are numerous infections and chemical agents responsible for headache. Infections from bacteria, fungi, parasites, spirochetes, and viruses can involve the head. Cryptococcal infection can cause headache without fever or other neurologic symptoms.

Acute meningitis after a diagnostic lumbar puncture or spinal anesthesia could be a result of chemical contamination of instruments or anesthetic agents. Such a headache is not worse on standing nor relieved by lying down. Chemical meningitis also can result from leakage into the subarachoid space of material from an epidermoid tumor or a craniopharyngioma.

Generalized severe angioedema is reported to produce headache, epilepsy, hemiplegia, and coma. Allergy to parabens (a chemical stabilizer in injectable medications) can cause cerebral edema, headache, and semicoma.

Intracranial hemorrhage can be caused by a subarachnoid hemorrhage, intracerebral hemorrhage, or a combination of subarachnoid and intracerebral hemorrhage. Subarachnoid hemorrhage results from the arteries on the surface of the brain, and it is limited to the area between the pial and arachnoid membranes that contains the CSF. Intracerebral hemorrhage is caused by rupture of vessels in the substance of the brain. Causes of intracerebral hemorrhage include: (1) arterial aneurysm, (2) cerebrovascular malformations, (3) hypertensive–atherosclerotic hemorrhage, (4) hemorrhage into brain tumor, (5) bleeding disorders, (6) intracranial vasculitis, or (7) intracranial venous infarction.

Cause. This includes bleeding from aneurysms and bleeding from arterioles in hypertension or arteriosclerosis.

Pathogenic Findings. A sudden change in intracranial pressure and chemical irritation of meninges may be seen.

Headache Phase. Unruptured aneurysms are asymptomatic except in enlarging lesions pressing on painful structures.[58] The location of the bleeding is the main determinant of the clinical presentation. Posterior communicating and basilar artery aneurysms cause cranial nerve III palsy. Rupture causes the sudden onset of violent headache that is felt in the neck and occipital area and spreads to involve the whole head, neck, and even the lower spine. There may be previous episodes of warning leaks of minor neurologic signs or occipital or cervical headache of short duration. At the onset of a major leak, there may be dizziness, brief loss of consciousness, or seizure. Vomiting and neck rigidity are common. There may be early development of papilledema.

Acute pulmonary edema and the syndrome of inappropriate antidiuretic hormone also can develop. Intracerebral bleeding is more common with AV malformations.

Laboratory Tests. Immediate CT scan without contrast (and then with contrast if indicated) should be done. This will establish the diagnosis in 95 percent of cases. If the scan is delayed more than 4 days after the hemorrhage, it will be positive in only 3 percent of cases. Aneurysms larger than 5 mm in diameter can be visualized on the scan, but those smaller than 5 mm might be missed.

Lumbar puncture should not be done as the first test because the pressure may be elevated and cause herniation. If there is no evidence of papilledema, and the scan is negative, a spinal tap must be done to exclude a small subarachnoid hemorrhage. These cases then are managed by a neurologist and neurosurgeon.

Prognosis. The prognosis for AV malformation is better than for an aneurysm; the prognosis in the latter is grave. The risk of dying in the first 8 weeks after the rupture is 40 percent.

Treatment. The treatment is surgical for aneurysms. The aim of therapy is to prevent further ruptures of the aneurysm while maintaining normal cerebral perfusion. A large AV malformation should not be removed if it has not bled, especially if its removal would cause damage to vital neurologic functions. Those located in frontal or occipital poles sometimes can be removed. The treatment of other causes of intracranial hemorrhage is to treat the underlying pathologic condition.

Pneumoencephalographic Reaction

The headache is caused in part by a decrease in the buoyant support of the brain, causing traction on pain-sensitive structures in the brain. The availability of CT scan has practically replaced the need for pneumoencephalography. The latter rarely is positive, if the scan is negative.

Arteritis

Polyarteritis nodosa can cause aneurysmal dilatation or intracerebral hemorrhage by necrosis of the artery. Amyloidosis also can cause intracerebral hemorrhage, is six times more common in women, and is not associated with systemic amyloidosis. Drug abuse, particularly with amphetamines, can cause vasculitis and result in intracerebral hemorrhage.

Intracranial Phlebitis

The large dural sinuses may become thrombosed spontaneously when they are infected or when there is infection in the adjacent epidural or subdural spaces. The lateral, cavernous, and petrosal sinuses are involved most often. This may result in increased intracranial pressure, multifocal brain ischema, or cerebral infarction.

Lateral Sinus Thrombosis

This is a complication of acute or chronic otitis media or mastoiditis. Infants and children most commonly are affected. Symptoms include fever, headache, nausea and vomiting, drowsiness, and eventually coma and seizures. There is papilledema, which may be unilateral.

Cavernous Sinus Thrombosis

This usually is caused by infection in the orbit, nasal sinuses, or upper half of the face. It causes high fever, headache, malaise, nausea, vomiting, convulsions, tachycardia, chemosis, edema, and cyanosis of the upper face, particularly the eyelids and the base of the nose. Distension of superficial veins over the forehead may occur. Cerebral venous thrombosis of pregnancy also can lead to headaches and seizures.

Extracranial Disorders

Arteritis. Temporal arteritis is a type of giant cell arteritis. It may involve other large arteries. The smaller arterioles are not involved. It is seen chiefly in patients older than 55 years of age. It causes narrowing of the lumen,

leading to complete occlusion. If the ophthalmic artery is involved, it leads to sudden blindness, the most feared complication of the temporal arteritis. Pain on chewing food is caused by facial artery ischemia; mandibular artery occlusion may cause jaw and tooth pain. The headache can be fleeting in nature, involving different parts of the head. The involved artery usually is swollen, tender, and less pulsatile, compared with the prominent tender arteries of migraine that have increased pulsations, which subside after the headache. Systemic symptoms include malaise, poor appetite, low grade fever, anemia, weight loss, and often polymyalgia rheumatica. The diagnosis is made by an elevated erythrocyte sedimentation rate and biopsy of the involved artery.

Treatment consists of high-dose steroids (prednisone 40 to 60 mg daily initially and continued for 4 weeks followed by gradual tapering). The reduction in dose should be monitored by the clinical response to corticosteroids rather than the sedimentation rate. The latter may remain elevated long after clinical improvement. It is prudent to add H_2-blocker drugs to prevent the possibility of gastric ulcer or bleeding complications from corticosteroids. Therapy may have to continue for months or years. Eye examination by an ophthalmologist is mandatory to exclude retinal artery ischemia and glaucoma, which can be worsened by steroid therapy. Steroids should be started without waiting for confirmation of the diagnosis because sudden irreversible blindness can occur without any warning. Biopsy should be obtained as soon as practical and should involve examination of 3 to 4 cm of artery cut longitudinally because skipped lesions are common and the diagnosis can be missed if a normal portion of the artery is examined.

Other causes of extracranial vasculitis that can cause headache include: periarteritis nodosa, Takayasu vasculitus, Wegener vasculitis, systemic lupus erythematosus, and disorders of collagen.

Headache Due to Diseases of Ocular, Aural, Nasal, and Sinusal, Dental, Cranial, and Neck Structures

Headaches from Ocular Structures

Headaches may be caused by spreading of pain from noxious stimulation of ocular structures (such as, increased intraocular pressure, excessive contraction of ocular muscles, trauma, new growth, or inflammation). If pain occurs on moving the ocular globe or if there is a change in visual acuity, ocular diseases should be excluded by an ophthalmologist.

Headaches from Aural Structures

Herpes zoster in the ear should be obvious because the lesions can be seen in the external ear canal or ear drum. Tumors in the pharynx and fossa of Rosenmuller in the middle ear cause referred pain to the ear. An ear, nose, and throat consultation is indicated if the patient's earache is unexplainable.

Headache of Nasal and Sinusal Structures

Although acutely infected sinuses may be a source of the headache, incidental findings in the sinuses (such as, retention cysts or a deviated septum) may be repaired surgically without improvement of headache. These disorders should be corrected only when the indications are appropriate and not with a hope to cure a long-standing headache problem.

Dental Structures

As with deviated septum, many innocent impacted teeth get pulled without relieving the headache.

Headaches from Other Structures of the Cranium and Neck (Such As Periostium, Joint, Ligaments, Muscles, or Cervical Roots)

Periosteal involvement caused by infection, inflammation, or separation from the bone can induce pain. The common joints implicated in headache include the temporomandibular joint, atlantoaxial joint, cervical apophyseal joints, and uncovertebral joints (joints of von Luschka).

Pain-sensitive structures in the neck include the outer fibers of anulus fibrosus, the vertebral periosteum, the ligamentum flavum, the anterior and posterior longitudinal ligaments, the interspinous ligaments, the posterior vertebral venous plexus, the anterior dura mater, the facet articulations, the paravertebral muscles and their fascia, and the vertebral arteries. These structures can be affected by traumatic, degenerative, and inflammatory processes in the neck.[59] (See Chap. 17.)

The posterior ramus of C1 (suboccipital nerve) often has no sensory distribution. The dorsal ramus of the second cervical (greater occipital nerve) has sensory fibers and is vulnerable to pressure and trauma as it exits between the bony surfaces and muscles in the suboccipital area.

The pain arising from the lower cervical region may be felt as orbital or facial pain through complex synapses between the cervical afferent fibers and lower cervical fibers of cranial nerve V. A small area overlying the mandibular angle and parotid gland is supplied by cranial nerves II and III.

Occipital Neuralgia. Entrapment of the sensory roots of the C2 or C3 nerves causes tenderness over the greater occipital nerve. Pain is exaggerated by hyperextension and rotation of the head to the painful side. Injections of local anesthetic and corticosteroid (see Appendix A, Section XI) at the painful site or rarely enlarging the opening for the greater occipital nerve can relieve the headache. This headache starts in the occipital region and radiates to the vertex, temporal area, periorbital area, and/or face. The attacks frequently occur at night, often associated with tearing, flushing of the face, alteration of sweating, at times occlusion of the nasal passage ipsilaterally, and dizziness.[60]

Referred Pain of Muscular Origin. Constant contraction of cervical muscles can lead to pain felt in a distant area. There is pain at the local site with tenderness to pressure at a few spots in the muscle, so-called trigger points (fibrocystic nodules) (see Chap. 19). When the trigger point is pressed, it may induce or worsen the pain at the referred site. Injection of local anesthetic, such as procaine at the trigger point, can relieve the pain at the referred site. The physician should explore the cause of the muscle spasm (physical or emotional), and treat the underlying condition. This is likely to give lasting relief in muscle tightness.

Temporomandibular Joint Syndrome (See Chap. 6). Diseases of the temporomandibular joint (TMJ) or its cartilage can cause pain in this area. There is usually muscle tenderness, crepitus in the joint, limitation of motion, and pain. An x-ray of the joint may show erosion or subluxation. These patients tend to grind their teeth. The pain usually is present in the morning over the joint area and ipsilateral temporal muscle. Patients tend to be anxious and tense. A systematic approach by an oral surgeon experienced in treatment of this condition is necessary. Correcting a bad bite does not correct a tense personality.

Cranial Neuritides Caused by Trauma, New Growth, or Inflammation

Description

Direct trauma to sensory nerves may cause injury, impaired function, and pain. The trauma may occur from an orbital or jaw fracture that may result in damage, entrapment, or neuroma formation of the sensory nerve. Infection and inflammation, such as lymphadenitis, may cause tic-like sharp jabs of pain if it is near a sensory nerve. Inflammation in the ear may cause pressure on the facial nerve resulting in Bell's palsy. This may respond to corticosteroids if they are given early in the illness. Injury to the sensory and sympathetic fibers in accompanying vessels can result in causalgic pain that may respond to sympathetic blocks with local anesthetics. In resistant cases, an ablation procedure may be necessary.

Postherpetic Neuralgia (See Chap. 21)

Herpes zoster may involve any dermatome and is more likely to occur in patients whose immune system is deranged, in the aged, and in those taking immunosuppressive drugs, including corticosteroids. Growing evidence suggests that a short course of acyclovir at the onset of this condition may be helpful in shortening the duration of eruption, severity of the disease, and its painful sequelae.

Narcotics may be necessary to control the worst phase of postherpetic neuralgia but should be reduced as soon as possible. Local treatment, such as the use of calamine lotion or calamine combined with diphenyldramine lotion and ointments that contain pain-reducing substances, may produce some benefit. Covering the area to prevent stimulation from garments and other objects may also reduce pain.

Cranial Neuralgias (See Chap. 6)

Definition

> "Trigeminal (tic douloureux) and glossopharyngeal. The pains are lancinating ('jabbing'), usually in rapid succession for several minutes or longer; are limited to a portion or all of the domain of the affected nerve; and are often triggered by end-organ stimulation. Trigeminal neuralgia must be distinguished, in particular, from cluster headache, with which it is often confused."[6]

Tic Douloureux

Cause. Trigeminal neuralgia can be caused by compression of the trigeminal nerve by arteries or veins of the posterior fossa. It also may be associated with multiple sclerosis, gasserian ganglion tumor, or brain stem infarction involving the descending root of the trigeminal nerve. In some cases, no cause may be found.

Pathophysiologic Findings. There is sudden and excessive discharge from the involved nerve.

Description. Sudden lightning-like jabs occur in the distribution of the involved nerve. Each episode lasts 1 to 2 seconds; shocks are repeated every few seconds for periods of minutes or hours. The pain is triggered by touching or moving the face, eating hot soup, chewing, or swallowing. It frequently involves the second and third division of cranial nerve V and rarely occurs at night. Generally, the physical examination is otherwise normal. If there are abnormal sensory findings in the distribution of the nerve, an underlying organic cause should be sought. Multiple sclerosis should be considered if tic douloureux occurs in a patient younger than 55 years of age.

Treatment. Carbamezapine is the treatment of choice; if there is no response, adding phenytoin or phenytoin alone can be tried. Baclofen or chlorphenesin carbamate may be helpful.[61]

Often, if medical therapy has failed, surgical intervention is successful. Radiofrequency lesions of the gasserian gangion are most popular, but recurrences are common. Trigeminal nerve decompression in the posterior fossa also is helpful. Other procedures include injection of glycerol into Meckel's cave, surgical section of sensory rootlets, and bulbar tractomy. (See Chap. 35.)

Differential Diagnosis. Cluster headache should be excluded because the treatment for the two conditions is different. During a pain attack, the patient with cluster headaches often presses the area around the eye or temple hard to relieve the pain; in tic douloureux, the patient keeps their hands off their face because the slightest touch can trigger another attack. Autonomic signs and symptoms,

with Horner syndrome on the affected side along with nasal stuffiness ipsilaterally, are common in cluster headache but not tic douloureux. If questioned closely, the duration of pain is constant, lasting 35 to 40 min in cluster headache; several quick jabs each lasting 1 s but coming in repeated succession for 30 to 45 min occur in tic douloureux. There are no trigger points in the face in cluster headache, which frequently occurs at night and wakes the patient up from a sound sleep. Tic douloureux rarely occurs during sleep. Cluster headache usually starts in the late teen-age years or early 20s and is predominantly a disease of men. Trigeminal neuralgia is common in older people.

Glossopharyngeal Neuralgia

This is a rare condition. The quality of pain is a sharp jabbing lightning-like pain as in tic douloureux, but triggering factors are chewing, swallowing, and factors stimulating the tonsils and pharynx. The pain spreads toward the angle of the jaw and ear. Organic causes of glossopharyngeal neuralgia include tonsillar tumor. A thorough ear, nose, and throat evaluation is necessary in glossopharyneal neuralgia. Treatment with carbamazephine usually is effective. Jabbing jolts in the ear also may occur in the rare condition of trifacial neuralgia related to the occasional sensory nerve found in the seventh nerve. Treatment is the same as for the other neuralgias. Occasionally, surgical treatment is successful if medications fail.

Posttraumatic Headache Syndrome

Definition

> "So-called chronic posttraumatic headache may arise from one of several mechanisms. Such headache may represent sustained muscle contraction, recurrent vascular dilatation, or rarely, local scalp or nuchal injury. In some patients, the posttraumatic pain is part of a clinical disorder characterized by delusional, conversion, or hypochondriacal reactions."[6]

Description

There are three varieties of posttraumatic headache[62,63]: (1) severe pain or tenderness in a scar or site of impact with local tenderness, (2) a steady pressure sensation or aching pain in a circumscribed area, often in a band-like distribution, that is thought to be related to muscle contraction, and (3) throbbing and aching pain occurring in attacks, usually unilateral and in the temporal, occipital, and frontal regions. This is a result of arterial vasodilation and responds to ergotamine.

In the acute form, the headache may be related to accumulation of blood in the epidural, subdural, or subarachnoid space. Sustained headache after the injury may be related to adhesions involving pain-sensitive structures in the arachnoid. There is no correlation between the duration of coma, disorientation, or amnesia and the incidence of posttraumatic headache. In whiplash injury, there is sudden hyperextension followed by hyperflexion. Most patients complain of diffuse muscular soreness followed by head and neck pain shortly after the accident. The cervical discomfort spreads upward from the neck to the occiput and over the vertex to the frontal region. It localizes in the area behind the eyes. It may be a dull ache, but sometimes, it is throbbing without nausea or vomiting. It may last for several days to weeks. There may be unilateral or bilateral localized painful areas in the suboccipital and neck region. If the neck was laterally rotated at the time of whiplash, the neck injury may be more severe than if the neck was in the resting position. Neck injuries in lateral rotation can cause damage to the vertebral–basilar arteries with subsequent subarachoid hemorrhage, leading to coma and even death soon after the injury.

Because the headaches start to interfere in the patient's daily routine, other psychological changes come into play. Depression should be recognized early and treated. The emotional responses seem to be more prominent if the accident was someone else's fault rather than the patient's. These include anger at the assailant and anxiety about courts, lawyers, and the patient's family. As time passes, there is lack of self-esteem and ego strength. On psychological testing, patients with posttraumatic headache syndrome score higher on hysterical, depressive, and hypochondriacal scales.

Posttraumatic pain syndrome may present as chronic subdural hematoma especially in elderly patients, who may have suffered a trivial head injury and might have forgotten about the incident. Sometimes during the posttraumatic period, other problems appear such as seizures, accentuation of previous vascular headache, causalgia from injured blood vessels and nerves, neuromas, and the onset of cluster headache or muscle contraction headache syndromes. Conversion headache syndrome arises out of post concussion dreams, phobias, and fear of repetition of the injury. Analgesic abuse can be common.

Treatment

This consists of active rehabilitation and treatment of depression, anger, tension, and frustrations. Use of antidepressant drugs and avoidance of analgesics and tranquilizers is helpful. Trials of physical therapy, heat, ultrasound, and transcutaneous nerve stimulation also can be helpful. In selected cases, cervical collars and neck traction can be useful. Surgical treatment of definite demonstrable lesions believed to cause the headache (such as, cervical disc disease, nerve trauma, and soft tissue damage) should be done only when clearly indicated. A sympathetic physician who is willing to understand the patient's pretrauma personality and family background and who will take the time to explain to the patient the underlying cause of their complaints (such as, dizziness and pain) will have better results. Many patients improve in group therapy and nondrug therapies in pain clinics. Early settlement of the ongoing suit might help the patient to return to work sooner and improve self-esteem.

SUMMARY

When a person experiences headache for the first time, especially when it is preceded or accompanied by neurologic symptoms, it can be alarming. It raises the worst fear.

A detailed history, complete physical examination, and appropriate tests and x-rays help to establish a diagnosis. The various forms of headache span a broad range. There is the occasional nuisance headache, the predictable headache after stressful periods or the more severe and frustrating recurrent headache that tends to rule the patient's life. The patients in this latter headache group find it difficult to make plans because previous engagements often had to be changed as a result of a headache. Also, they often find little sympathy from loved ones or colleagues who are tired of listening to the same complaints. These patients seek help in various places hoping someone finally will find something "wrong" with their head and "fix it."

Patients facing relentless headaches generally will find medicines that work for them by trial and error. Often, however, this use eventually leads to abuse. Some patients realize this problem; others underestimate their use and may need to have this pointed out to them. A detailed history of drug use will be beneficial in these cases.

For some patients, the reassurance of knowing that there is nothing seriously wrong with them is all that is needed, and they can tolerate the headache without requiring medication. Most patients seek a remedy to their problem, but there are others who "need" their headache to help cope with a stressful situation. For them, knowing that the physician is available if needed is a form of therapy. In many instances, it is important to tell patients with headache that the symptom usually is a result of the overactivity of a good central nervous system—a signal of overuse of a good instrument rather than a deficiency.

Treatment of analgesic abuse requires patience, perseverance, and the patient's trust in the physician. Our late colleague, Dr. Hiro Iida, used to remind us of a Japanese saying, "To catch a running horse, you have to run with the horse for some time." Similarly, the physician may have to prescribe analgesics and preventive medicines temporarily until the patient is "reined in" and gradually taught to change their life.

The physician frequently has to deal with headache on different levels. Often, psychological factors have to be addressed. In such cases, unless the patient has gained confidence in the physician and agrees to participate in psychotherapy, referral to a psychotherapist or psychiatrist will not be helpful.

Treatment of headache usually requires active participation by both the doctor and patient. The physician should seek and understand the patient's expectations and be able to outline goals for each patient. The patient should be made aware of his/her role in achieving these goals and conscientiously complete the therapy and maintain a relationship with the physician over a considerable period of time.

We hope these patients often-asked question of why they get a headache will stimulate cooperative research between the basic sciences and clinicians interested in this important field of medicine that plays such a vital role in the quality of human life.

References

1. DuBartas S; Bartlett J, ed. *Divine Weeks and Works, Familiar Quotations.* 15th ed. Boston: Little, Brown; 1980:169.

2. Coodley EL. Headache as an initial manifestation of systemic disease. *Funct Neurol* October–December 1990; 5(4):371–373.

3. Silberstein SD, Merriam GR. Estrogens, progestins and headache. *Neurology* June 1991; 41(6):786–793.

4. Baumel B, Eisner LS. Diagnosis and treatment of headache in the elderly. *Med Clin North Am* May 1991; 75(3):661–675.

5. Sands GH, Newman L, Lipton R. Cough, exertional, and other miscellaneous headaches. *Med Clin North Am* May 1991; 75(3):733–747.

6. Ad Hoc Committee on Classification of Headache. (Friedman AP, Finley KH, Graham JR, et al.) Classification of headache. *JAMA* 1962; 179:717–718.

7. Moskowitz MA. Basic mechanisms in vascular headache. *Neurol Clin* November 1990; 8(4):801–815.

8. Graham JR, Wolff HG. Mechanism of migraine headache and action of ergotamine tartarate. *Arch Neurol Psychiatry* 1938; 39:737–763.

9. Leao AAP. Spreading depression of activity in the cerebral cortex. *J Neurophysiol* 1944; 7:359–390.

10. Skinhoj E. Hemodynamic studies within the brain during migraine. *Arch Neurol* 1973; 29:95–98.

11. O'Brien MD. Cerebral blood changes in migraine. *Headache* 1971; 10:139–143.

12. Gloor P. Migraine and regional cerebral blood flow. *Trends Neurosci* 1986; 9:21.

13. Deshmukh V, Meyer JS. Cyclic changes in platelet dynamics and the pathogenesis and prophylaxis of migraine. *Headache* 1977; 17:101–108.

14. Leviton A. Migraine associated with hyper pre-beta hyperlipidemia. *Neurology* 1969; 19:963–965.

15. Anthony M. Role of individual free fatty acids in migraine. *Res Clin Stud Headache* 1978; 6:110–116.

16. Heyck H. Pathogenesis of migraine. *Res Clin Stud Headache* 1969; 2:1–28.

17. Chapman LF, Ramos AO, Goodell H, Silverman G, Wolff HG. A humoral agent implicated in vascular headache of the migraine type. *Arch Neurol* 1960; 3:223–229.

18. Moskowitz MA. The neurobiology of vascular head pain. *Ann Neurol* 1984; 16:157–168.

19. Pederson DM, Wilson WM, White GL Jr, Murdock RT, Digre KB. Migraine aura without headache. *J Fam Pract* May 1991; 32(5):520–523.

20. Refsum S. Genetic aspects of migraine. In: Vinken PS, Bruyn GW, eds. *Handbook of Neurology: Headache and cranial neuralgias.* Vol. 5. Amsterdam: North Holland Pub Co; 1968:258–269.

21. Holroyd KA, Penzien DB. Pharmacological versus nonpharmacological prophylaxis of recurrent migraine headache: a meta-analytic review of clinical trials. *Pain* July 1990; 42(1):1–13.

22. Solomon GD. Pharmacology and use of headache medications. *Cleve Clin J Med* October 1990; 57(7):627–635.

23. Ludvigsson J. Propranolol in treatment of migraine in children. *Lancet* 1973; 2:799.

24. Rothner AD. Headaches in children: a review. *Headache* 1979; 19:156–162.

25. Couch JR, Ziegler DK, Hassanein R. Amitriptyline in the prophylaxis of migraine. *Neurology* 1976; 26:121–127.

26. Meyer JS, Hardenberg J. Clinical effectiveness of calcium entry blockers in prophylactic treatment of migraine and cluster headache. *Headache* 1983; 23:266–277.

27. Graham JR. Methysergide for the prevention of headache. Experience in 500 patients over 3 years. *N Engl J Med* 1964; 270:67–72.

28. Graham JR, Selby HI, LeCompte PM, et al. Fibrotic disorders with methysergide therapy for headaches. *N Engl J Med* 1966; 274:359–368.

28a. Goadsby PJ, Zagami AS, Donnan GA, et al. Oral sumatriptan in acute migraine. *Lancet* 1991; 338:782–783.

28b. Sumatriptan International Study Group. Subcutaneous sumatriptan in the acute treatment of migraine. *J Neurol* 1991; 238(Suppl 1):S66–S69.

28c. Subcutaneous Sumatriptan International Study Group. Treatment of migraine attacks with sumatriptan. *N Engl J Med* 1991; 325:316–321.

28d. The Finnish Sumatriptan Group and the Cardiovascular Clinical Research Group. A placebo-controlled study of intranasal sumatriptan for the acute treatment of migraine. *Eur Neurol* 1991; 31:332–338.

29. Graham JR. The relation of cluster headache to migraine. In: Mathew NT, Ed. *Cluster Headache.* Jamaica, NY: Spectrum Publications; 1984:79–87.

30. Kudrow L. Diagnosis and treatment of cluster headache. *Med Clin North Am* May 1991; 75(3):579–594.

31. Sicuteri F, Fanciullacci M, Nicolodi M, et al. Substance P theory: a unique focus on the painful and painless phenomena of cluster headache. *Headache* January 1990; 30(2):69–79.

32. Kudrow L: Symptomatic treatment of cluster headache, oxygen inhalation. In: Kudrow L, ed. *Cluster Headache: Mechanisms and Management.* New York: Oxford University Press; 1980:142–145.

33. Ekbom K. Lithium for cluster headache: review of the literature and preliminary results of long term treatment. *Headache* 1981; 12:132–139.

34. Mathew NT. Prophylactic pharmacotherapy of cluster headache. In: Mathew NT, ed. *Cluster Headache.* Jamaica, NY: Spectrum Publications; 1984:97–109.

34a. The Sumatriptan Cluster Headache Study Group. Treatment of acute cluster headache with sumatriptan. [Comment in: *N Engl J Med* 1991; 325(5):353–354.] *N Engl J Med* 1991; 325(5):322–326.

35. Onofrio BM, Campbell JK. Surgical treatment of chronic cluster headache. *Mayo Clin Proc* 1986; 61:537–544.

36. Gardner WJ, Stowell A, Dutlinger R. Resection of the greater superficial petrosal nerve in the treatment of unilateral headache. *J Neurosurg* 1947; 4:105–114.

37. Sachs E Jr. The role of nervus intermedius in facial neuralgia; report of four cases with observations on the pathways

for taste, lacrimation and pain in the face. *J Neurosurg* 1968; 28:54–60.

38. Meyer JS, Binns PM, Ericsson AD, Valpe M. Sphenopalatine ganglionectomy for cluster headache. *Arch Otolaryngol* 1970; 92:475–484.

39. Harris W. Alcohol injection of the gasserian ganglion for migrainous neuralgia. *Lancet* 1940; 2:481–482.

40. Watson CP, Morley TP, Richardson JC, Schultz H, Tasker RR. The surgical treatment of chronic cluster headache. *Headache* 1983; 23:289–295.

41. Kudrow L. The management of cluster headache. In: Kudrow L, ed. *Cluster Headache: Mechanisms and Management.* New York: Oxford University Press; 1980:146–148.

41a. Bing R. *Lehrbuch der Nervenkrankheiten.* 1st ed. Berlin: Ukban and Schwarzenberg; 1913.

41b. Harris W. Ciliary (migrainous) neuralgia and its treatment. *Br Med J* 1936; 1:457–460.

41c. Horton BT. Histaminic cephalgia: differential diagnosis and treatment. *Mayo Clin Proc* 1956; 31:325–333.

42. Sjaastad O, Dale I. Evidence of a new (?) treatable headache entity. *Headache* 1974; 14:105–108.

43. Mani S, Deeter J. Arterio venous malformation of the brain presenting as a cluster headache—a case report. *Headache* 1982; 22:184–185.

44. Bradwhaw P, Parsons M. Hemiplegic migraine, a clinical study. *Aust J Med* 1965; 34:65.

45. Featherstone HJ. Clinical features of stroke in migraine: a review. *Headache* 1986; 26:128–133.

46. Sulkava R, Kovanen J. Locked-in-syndrome with rapid recovery: a manifestation of basilar artery migraine. *Headache* 1983; 23:238–239.

47. Solomon GD, Spaccavento LJ. Lateral medullary syndrome after basilar migraine. *Headache* 1982; 22:171–172.

48. Spaccavento LJ, Solomon GD. Migraine as an etiology of stroke in young adults. *Headache* 1984; 24:12–22.

49. Welch KM, Levine SR. Migraine-related stroke in the con-text of the International Headache Society classification of head pain. *Arch Neurol* April 1990; 47(4):458–462.

50. Lovshin L. Carotodynia. *Headache* 1977; 17:192–195.

51. De Benedittis G, Lorenzetti A, Pieri A. The role of a stressful life events in the onset of chronic primary headache. *Pain* January 1990; 40(1):65–75.

52. Ward N, Whitney C, Avery D, Dunner D. The analgesic effects of caffeine in headache. *Pain* February 1991; 44(2):151–155.

53. Goldstein J. Headache and acquired immunodeficiency syndrome. *Neurol Clin* November 1990; 8(4):947–960.

54. Mathew NT. Drug-induced headache. *Neurol Clin* November 1990; 8(4):903–912.

55. Edmeads S. The mechanism of ischemic cerebrovascular disease. *Headache* 1979; 19:345–349.

56. Casement BA, Danielson DR. The epidural blood patch: are more than two ever necessary? *Anesth Analg* 1984; 63:1033–1035.

57. Hatfalvi BI. The dynamics of post spinal headache. *Headache* 1977; 17:64–66.

58. Ostergaard JR. Headache as a warning symptom of impending aneurysmal subarachnoid haemorrhage. *Cephalalgia* February 1991; 11(1):53–55.

59. Besson JM. Arthritis and headache. *Can J Physiol Pharmocol* May 1991; 69(5):635–636.

60. Hunter CR, Mayfield FH. Role of the upper cervical nerve roots in the production of pain in the head. *Am J Surg* 1949; 78:743–749.

61. Fromm GH. Clinical pharmacology of drugs used to treat head and face pain. *Neurol Clin* February 1990; 8(1):143–151.

62. Delessio DJ; Dalessio DJ, ed. *Post Traumatic Headache in Wolf's Headache and Other Head Pain.* 4th ed. New York: Oxford University Press; 1980:324–338.

63. Goldstein J. Posttraumatic headache and the postconcussion syndrome. *Med Clin North Am* May 1991; 75(3):641–651.

CHAPTER 6

Orofacial Pain

David A. Keith

Pain in the oral and facial structures is a common symptom. Although in most cases, the cause can be determined readily,[1,2] the anatomy of the area is so complex that the diagnosis may be difficult.

Pain originating in the mouth and face is mediated mainly by the 5th (trigeminal) cranial nerve. This has three branches: ophthalmic, maxillary, and mandibular. In addition, the facial (nervus intermedius root), glossopharyngeal, vagus, and cervical nerves also innervate parts of this region. These nerves have a tortuous anatomic course and distribution and do not follow an orderly pattern. All pain fibers from this region (with the exception of those from the cervical nerves) travel to the spinal nucleus of the cranial nerve V. From there, they are connected to higher centers.[3]

The emotional significance of pain in this region may be heightened for several reasons. The mouth and face are innervated highly by sensory fibers. (This area is represented on the sensory homunculus as much larger than its actual size.) The trigeminal nervous system develops early, and reflex suckling activity has been observed in utero. Furthermore, in most western civilizations, the face is one of the few parts of the body exposed to view. It is through the face that we communicate and express our feelings toward our fellow human beings.

THE PAIN HISTORY

It is imperative that a thorough history be obtained before the patient is examined or special tests are ordered. In most cases, the diagnosis may be made with this information alone.

It also is important to obtain the patient's description of the pain. Primary neuralgias frequently are described as sharp and lancinating, vascular headaches as throbbing, and muscle pain as a continuous and dull ache. The intensity of the pain should be measured against the patient's own experience of pain, need for medication, and effect on life style, for example, sleep, work, and social activities. The origin of the pain should be ascertained by asking the patient to indicate this with one finger. Its distribution pattern should be traced accurately in terms of the local anatomy. The patient should be urged to remember the events surrounding the original onset of the pain, even though this may have occurred several years previously.

Any other instances of similar pain should be determined, although the patient may not associate these with the current problem. The time relationship of the pain should be clarified in terms of its duration, frequency of attacks, and possible remissions of pain. In many instances, aggravating factors (e.g., lying down, chewing, the sight or smell of food, alcohol, or stress) and relieving factors (e.g., heat and cold) are important clues. The effect of past treatment should be elucidated carefully (which medications helped, did surgery alter the nature of the pain, did endodontic treatment or extractions affect the pain). Finally, the presence or absence of associated factors, such as swelling, flushing, tearing, and nasal congestion, must be ascertained. The patient may not be able to answer all questions during the first interview. Collaborating information may be required from relatives and friends to obtain a general picture of the pain and its effect on and perception by the patient. This information usually will lead to a diagnosis.

A complete physical examination and appropriate tests, including blood and urine analyses, radiographs, and where indicated, referral to other specialists or more sophisticated tests, for example, MRI or CAT scan, will help to confirm the clinical diagnosis and exclude other underlying conditions.[4]

CLASSIFICATION OF ORAL AND FACIAL PAIN

There are various classifications of oral and facial pain, but none[5-13] are entirely satisfactory. From a clinical point of view, pain in the mouth or face may be divided into the following groups:

I. Pain due to local disease
   A. Teeth and jaws
   B. Temporomandibular joint and muscles of mastication
   C. Salivary glands
   D. Nose and paranasal sinuses
   E. Blood vessels
II. Pain arising from nerve trunks and central pathways
   A. Group A: no abnormal central nervous system signs (e.g., idiopathic paroxysmal trigeminal and glossopharyngeal neuralgia)
   B. Group B: abnormal central nervous system signs (e.g., nerve involved by pressure, infiltration, or degenerative disease at an intra- or extracranial location)

III. Pain from outside the face (e.g., ears, eyes, heart, cervical spine)

IV. Chronic atypical facial pain

Characteristic Features of Oral and Facial Pain

Pain Due to Local Disease

This category includes the greatest number of oral and facial pains encountered in clinical practice. By means of a careful history and appropriate tests, the etiology can be determined.

Teeth and Jaws. Pain arising from the teeth, supporting structures, and jaws usually is diagnosed accurately by the patient. Hypersensitivity of a tooth as a result of an exposed root surface or a recent deep restoration is described as sharp, usually transient, and well localized. It is aggravated by hot, cold, or sweet foods. A cracked tooth also may cause transient sharp pain on biting. This may be difficult to identify and lead to an erroneous diagnosis. If the pulp is involved in an inflammatory reaction resulting from dental caries, the pain is spontaneous, severe, and less well localized. Heat aggravates and cold relieves the pain; it may persist for minutes or hours. In time, the pain suddenly stops, indicating complete necrosis of the pulpal tissue. This may progress to a periapical abscess in which signs of infection are present, and the tooth is tender to bite on and to percussion. Endodontic treatment will save the tooth and eliminate the infection.

The infection, however, may progress to cellulitis and abscess formation. Incision and drainage sometimes can be done under local anesthesia, but occasionally, a general anesthetic is required. In the most extreme situation, Ludwig angina may develop. The infection spreads to the sublingual, submental, submandibular, and pterygomandibular spaces bilaterally and then through the retropharyngeal, pretracheal, and carotid sheath to the mediastinum. In these cases, the airway may be compromised severely. These infections were invariably fatal before antibiotics were discovered. Even today with aggressive antibiotic therapy, surgical drainage, and supportive care, fatalities can occur.

A particularly painful condition occasionally arises after tooth extraction, usually of a mandibular molar. This is termed *localized osteitis* (frequently called, *dry socket*). The pain is severe and constant, starting 2 to 3 days after the extraction and lasting for 10 to 14 days thereafter. The socket should be irrigated and dressed on a regular basis until granulation occurs. Osteomyelitis of the jaw (usually the mandible) is rare today, but it may present as an intense deep-seated pain, accompanied by appropriate physical and radiographic signs. The chronic sclerotic variety is more insidious and less readily diagnosed. Treatment is surgical debridement with vigorous antibiotic therapy. Osteoradionecrosis is a relentless extremely painful condition characterized by postirradiation bone necrosis, predominantly of the mandible, with exposure of the bone into the mouth or externally. In most cases, the condition can be controlled only by radical surgical excision of the affected bone.

Referred pain occasionally is encountered. The patient complains of pain in the mandible, but a maxillary tooth is found to be the cause or vice versa. More common is the complaint of earache accompanying an unidentifiable toothache. Referred pain to the ear indicates mandibular tooth disease. The perception of the anatomic site apparently is mistaken in the branches of the trigeminal nerve.

Temporomandibular Joint Disorders and Diseases. Masticatory pain can arise from the muscles of mastication[14] or the temporomandibular joint itself.[15–17] Although it is a common cause of facial pain, a thorough history and examination must be done to exclude other potentially more serious diagnoses.

Masticatory system disorders have been classified in many different ways. Because of the difficulty encountered in establishing a precise cause, these disorders often are defined on the basis of symptoms and signs. However, broad categories of masticatory problems include: masticatory muscle spasm, internal derangement of the temporomandibular joint, chronic hypomobility, trauma, degenerative joint disease, growth disorders, infections, tumors, and congenital abnormalities.

It is imperative to take a detailed history and do a thorough clinical examination. In addition, the patient's family, social, and medical history should be ascertained. Clinical examination should include: (1) palpation of the muscles of mastication (temporalis, masseter, and medial and lateral pterygoids); (2) observation of mandibular motion: opening, closing, lateral excursion, and protrusion; (3) palpation and/or auscultation of joint noises; (4) examination of the dentition and occlusion; and (5) brief neurologic examination of the trigeminal system.

Masticatory muscle spasm (temporomandibular joint or myofascial pain dysfunction) is the most common of all masticatory system disorders. Epidemiologic studies from many countries show that signs and symptoms of such disorders are widespread, and that 28 percent to 88 percent of people have detectable clinical signs of dysfunction. Fewer individuals (12 percent to 19 percent) are aware of symptoms. A smaller group (5 percent or more) may require treatment.

It is generally agreed that patients with temporomandibular joint dysfunction will exhibit one or more of the following signs: (1) decreased range of mandibular motion, (2) impaired function (e.g., deviation, sounds, or sticking), and (3) pain on palpation of the masticatory muscles or joint or after movement of the joint. One or more of the following symptoms also may occur: (1) temporomandibular joint sounds, (2) fatigue or stiffness of the jaws, (3) pain in the face or jaws, (4) pain on opening the mouth wide, and (5) locking. Radiographic studies of the temporomandibular joint show no evidence of disease.

The cause of this clinical complex is multifactorial. Among those most commonly cited are functional, psychological, and structural factors. It is important to understand that, for a particular patient, a single clear etiologic factor rarely is apparent. More often, several possible factors are identified. Likewise, treatment goals should be formulated that address the several likely causes.

Most patients respond to simple noninvasive treatment plans. These should include, but are not necessarily limited to, the following.

1. *Reassurance.* It is important that patients realize they are not alone with their symptoms, that the symptoms are essentially self-limited, and that no disease exists. The role of muscle spasm and its benign nature should be explained carefully.
2. *Rest.* Although it is not prudent to immobilize the mandible, patients should be instructed to have a mechanically soft diet for 2 weeks and avoid yawning and laughing with the mouth open. Such habits as chewing gum and biting fingernails should be discouraged.
3. *Heat.* The application of heat to the sides of the face by heating pad, hot towel, or hot water bottle will be comforting and relieve the muscle spasms. More vigorous treatment can be achieved with ultrasound or short-wave diathermy heat treatments. These are available in physical therapy departments.
4. *Medications.* Nonsteroidal anti-inflammatory analgesics are valuable in the acute stage. The drugs ibuprofen, naproxen, and indomethocin at a low dose for 2 weeks are used most widely. Anxiolytic agents, such as the benzodiazepines, also are used commonly. Several regimens exist, and doses should be individualized. The usual regimen consists of diazepam 2.5 to 10 mg two to four times daily, with an increased bedtime dose as necessary to ensure restful sleep. It is important that this treatment be limited to approximately 2 weeks because there is a potential for dependency. Narcotic analgesics should be avoided.

   Antidepressants have a long history of effectiveness in the treatment of chronic pain. In view of the strong association between temporomandibular joint dysfunction and psychological factors, their use often is justified especially when this disorder is a part of a more global complex of muscle pains and other signs and symptoms of depression are evident. The tricyclic antidepressants are used most widely. A bedtime-only schedule of 25 to 100 mg of amitriptyline or doxepin often can relieve the symptoms in 1 or 2 weeks. Treatment is maintained for 2 to 4 months; then it is tapered to a low maintenance dose or discontinued.
5. *Occlusal therapy.* There are many interocclusal appliances, and their multiplicity suggests that the optimal design has not been found. These devices usually are made of processed acrylic and serve the following functions: (1) improve the function of the temporomandibular joint, (2) improve the function of the masticatory motor system and reduce abnormal muscle function, and (3) protect teeth from attrition and abnormal occlusal loading. In essence, a full-arch occlusal stabilizing appliance (Fig. 6-1) is the type that has been most effective. Partial-coverage appliances tend to produce significant and irreversible changes in dentition. An

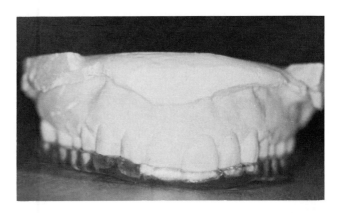

FIGURE 6-1. *Full-arch occlusal stabilizing appliance. (Reproduced with permission from Guralnick WC, Keith DA. Osteoarthritis of the temporomandibular joint. In: Moskowitz, et al, eds.* Osteoarthritis: Diagnosis and Management. *Philadelphia: Saunders; 1984:530.)*

appropriate appliance is effective in most patients (70 percent to 90 percent). They are most successful in reducing masticatory muscle pain and controlling attrition and adverse tooth loading.

There have been numerous claims that occlusal interferences of various types are the chief cause of masticatory muscle pain and that their elimination by occlusal adjustments will result in improvement. Because masticatory dysfunction is a multifactorial problem, this is unlikely to be true. The negative influence of malocclusion, loss of teeth, and occlusal interferences on masticatory dysfunction is not well supported. On general principles, however, occlusal disharmony (including premature contacts) should be eliminated and missing teeth replaced. The long-term efficacy of repositioning adult nongrowing jaws with occlusal splints or functional appliances has not been proved satisfactorily.

6. *Behavioral modification.* Bearing in mind the psychological effect in this disorder, attempts to lower patient stress are important. Relaxation techniques, conditioning, and biofeedback all have been advantageous approaches. The most important factor, however, is undoubtedly the therapeutic interaction of the practitioner with the patient.

Internal derangement is another cause of masticatory system disorders. Despite the fact that temporomandibular joint arthrography was developed in the 1940s by Norgaard,[18] the dental profession was reluctant to recognize the potential contribution of internal derangement of the meniscus to the spectrum of temporomandibular joint disorders. In recent years, this lack of interest has been replaced by too much interest; no doubt, a balance will be found in future. The meniscus can, either temporarily or permanently, be displaced and cause the symptoms.[19]

The main categories of internal derangement are, first, anterior displacement with reduction. This occurs when the meniscus is displaced in the closed-mouth position and reduces, with a click, to a normal relationship at some time during opening. In these circumstances, the patient complains of the click and a variable amount of pain. On opening, the jaw deviates toward the affected side until the click occurs and then returns to the midline. Preventing the mouth from closing fully by using a splint, tongue blades, or dental-mirror handle eliminates the click. An arthrogram will show a displaced meniscus that is reduced on opening. This situation may include an intermittent locking and may progress to the second category, anterior displacement without reduction (closed lock). Patients again have a variable amount of pain, and if muscle spasm has been relieved adequately, may be pain free. They feel, however, that something in the joint is stopping it from opening. There is usually a history of clicking with intermittent locking. Opening may be limited to 25 to 30 mm, with restriction of motion to the contralateral side. An arthrogram or MRI shows displacement without reduction (closed lock) and also may demonstrate perforation and degenerative changes. In such cases, the signs and symptoms of degenerative joint disease also may be present.

Initial treatment for internal derangements consists of the noninvasive therapies used for temporomandibular joint syndrome (as discussed previously). In patients with anterior displacement with reduction (intermittent locking), these strategies often are successful. In patients with a closed lock, especially those in which the condition is long standing, these treatments may reduce muscle spasm and pain and restore some motion, but the underlying displacement will remain. When noninvasive treatment has been attempted for several months and the patient remains restricted, arthroscopy or surgical repair should be considered.

Chronic hypomobility is a rare but important cause of masticatory system disorders. Ankylosis is the persistent inability to open the jaws. It may result from pathologic involvement of the joint structures (true ankylosis) or limitation produced by extraarticular causes (false ankylosis). Infection and trauma (including previous surgery) are the prime causes of true ankylosis. The findings are severe limitation of opening, possibly with mandibular retrognathism if mandibular growth has been restricted. Radiographs show destruction of the joint surfaces, loss of joint space, and in extreme cases, ossification across the joint. False ankylosis may be caused by various disorders that can be categorized as: myogenic (such as, masticatory muscle contracture), neurogenic (tetanus), psychogenic (conversion reaction), bone impingement (enlarged coronoid process), fibrous adhesions (after temporomandibular joint surgery, temporal flap, or trauma), and tumors.

Many patients require surgery. In those with true ankylosis, even under general anesthesia it will not be possible to open their mouths. A careful awake fiber-optic–assisted intubation is required.

The key to successful therapy is to identify, as far as possible, the cause of the ankylosis and treat it as aggressively as possible. It should be recognized, however, that true ankylosis with fibrosis and calcification can be extremely recalcitrant to treatment.

Trauma is the fourth cause of masticatory system disorders. A blow to the jaw can sprain the temporomandibular joint, cause a joint effusion, or fracture the neck of the mandibular condyle. In an acute sprain, the joint is painful, and there is severe limitation of motion caused by muscle spasm. Heat, rest, and nonsteroidal anti-inflammatory medications will resolve the acute symptoms, but other forms of treatment may be required to alleviate residual muscle spasm and pain. In the case of a joint effusion, in addition to pain and limitation, the patient will be unable to close their teeth together on that side. In a more severe injury, a hemarthrosis may develop, with damage to the meniscus. Active physical therapy is required to restore range of motion and prevent the development of ankylosis. A fracture of the neck of the condyle is a common maxillofacial injury, and if undisplaced, it requires analgesics and a soft diet for a few days. In the unilateral displacement or dislocated variety, the patient will have a premature bite on the affected side and deviation to that side on opening. Intermaxillary fixation for 10 days may be required with active physical therapy thereafter to restore function. The patient with bilateral fractures will have an anterior open bite and posterior displacement of the mandible. More aggressive treatment will be required to restore the bite and function. Depending on the position of the displaced fragment, it may interfere with mandibular motion.

Degenerative joint disease (osteoarthritis, osteoarthrosis) of the temporomandibular joint is the fifth cause of masticatory system disorders, and it may be the result of several different insults to the joint structure that exceed its capacity to remodel and repair. These insults may be traumatic (acute or chronic), chemical, infectious, or metabolic. The patient complains of pain on jaw movement and limitation of movement, with deviation to the affected side. There may be acute tenderness over the joint itself. Joint sounds are described as grating, grinding, or crunching (but not clicking or popping). Initially, radiographs may be normal, but marked degenerative and remodeling changes will be seen later, possibly at a time when the symptoms have subsided. The natural course of the disease suggests that the pain and limitation will disappear after several months.

The features of degenerative temporomandibular joint disease are different from those of most other joints in the body. There is a strong predeliction for women to be affected. A significant number of patients are in their third or fourth decade of life. Few have generalized osteoarthritis.

Most patients can be kept comfortable until remission using the noninvasive techniques outlined earlier. Some require injections of corticosteroids into the joint. This treatment generally is reserved for older patients and is limited to two or three injections. In those who are refractory to these techniques, surgery may be indicated to remove loose fragments of bone (so-called joint mice) and to reshape the condyle. Attention should also be directed toward the meniscus because its displacement may be a primary reason for the degenerative changes.

Rheumatoid arthritis also can afflict the temoromandibular joint and reports of its incidence range widely. The disease may attack any elderly person. In young patients, an association with micrognathia may be found. In advanced cases, ankylosis may be the presenting complaint. Radiographic findings show joint destruction, possibly involving both the condyle and the articular eminence. Other stigmas of the disease will be evident, and if medical management is ineffective, alternative treatment of the degenerative joint disease or ankylosis may be necessary.

Postnatal growth abnormalities are the sixth cause of masticatory system disorders. Studies of facial growth show the major contribution made by the mandibular condyle to the adaptive growth of the mandible in the functional soft tissue matrix. Several conditions may reduce growth, including hypothyroidism, hypopituitarism, and nutritional deficiency, such as, vitamin D deficiency. In gigantism, all skeletal structures are enlarged; in acromegaly, a marked prognathism is produced. Several local conditions such as trauma, infection, rheumatoid arthritis, exposure to radiation, and scarring from burns or surgery are other causes of reduced growth.

Infections are the seventh cause of masticatory system disorders. Temporomandibular joint infections are uncommon today. When seen, the preauricular area is swollen, hot, and tender. Patients have difficulty opening and closing their mouths. Radiographs may show increased joint space, bony destruction, and sclerosis in the chronic stage. Treatment includes drainage, debridement, and appropriate antibiotic therapy.

Tumors are the eighth cause of masticatory system disorders. Temporomandibular joint tumors are rare, but several varieties of primary and metastatic tumors have been reported. The most common are benign cartilaginous or bony tumors. These may cause limitation of motion or malocclusion, but they are not always painful.

Congenital abnormalities constitute the final cause of masticatory system disorders. Complex coordinated growth of the facial structures is necessary to achieve normal form and function. On occasion, the developmental process is altered, and malformations occur. It is beyond the scope of this chapter to review all the possible anomalies encountered in clinical practice, but many abnormalities of the temporomandibular joint occur in conjunction with recognized syndromes, for example, lateral facial dysplasia or Treacher Collins syndrome. A full clinical and radiologic workup is necessary to evaluate the defect fully. Treatment usually is undertaken by a multidisciplinary team.

Salivary Glands. The parotid and submandibular salivary glands are occasionally the site of infection or disease. In the more common condition of submandibular sialolithiasis, Wharton's duct becomes blocked by a stone or nonopaque "sludge." Characteristically, the gland swells, and pain is felt by the patient at the sight, smell, or thought of food. The swelling and pain may decrease after the meal, but they recur at the next meal. If the stone is in the duct, a sialolithotomy often can be done to relieve the problem. Surgical excision of the submandibular gland, however, frequently is necessary because the gland structure is damaged considerably by repeated infections.

Nose and Paranasal Sinuses. Experimental stimulation of various areas in the nose and paranasal sinuses refers pain to well-defined regions of the mouth, face, and cranium. Therefore, in any diagnosis of pain, rhinologic causes should be sought. The most common diagnostic dilemma is differentiating maxillary toothache from maxillary sinusitis, especially because periapical infection from a maxillary premolar or molar occasionally may cause sinusitis.

Blood Vessels. The many names ascribed to facial migrainous neuralgias have confused clinicians, as shown by the considerable length of time between onset of symptoms and appropriate diagnosis and treatment of this condition. The Subcommittee on Taxonomy of the International Association for the Study of Pain has provided a provisional summary description for pain of vascular origin.[20]

Cluster headache (see Chap. 5) usually is unilateral in the ocular, frontal, and temporal areas, but it also may be situated in the infraorbital region and maxilla. The condition afflicts men predominantly and usually starts between 18 and 40 years of age. Attacks are grouped in bouts of several weeks to months with pain-free intervals of several months duration. Bouts often last from 4 to 8 weeks with 1 to 3 attacks every 24-h period and a maximum of 8 attacks daily. The pain is excruciating. It is described as constant, stabbing, burning, and throbbing. Associated features include ipsilateral ptosis/miosis, tearing, rhinorrhea, and blocked nose. Treatment includes ergot preparations, prednisone, and methysergide. Chronic cluster headache is similar to cluster headache, but it is rarer. The diagnosis requires at least two or more attacks per week over a period of more than a year. Treatment is the same as that for cluster headache, but lithium carbonate tends to work better in chronic cluster headache.

Chronic paroxysmal hemicrania (see Chap. 5) involves the ocular, frontal, and temporal areas and occasionally the occipital, infraorbital, aural, mastoid, and nuchal areas (invariably on the same side). It occurs predominantly in women. Patients have attacks every day, usually for 15 to 30 min in a 24-h period. Characteristically, the attacks fluctuate in frequency and severity. Attacks may last 5 to 45 min; at their maximum, they are excruciating. Ipsilateral conjunctival injection, lacrimation, nasal stuffiness, and rhinorrhea occur in most patients. Attacks occur at regular intervals through the day and night, and patients may be awakened by a nocturnal attack. Indomethacin provides immediate and absolute relief. Although these vascular pains usually are situated in the cranium, they can occur in the infraorbital region of the maxilla and lead to confusion with sinus or dental disease. Such patients frequently undergo extensive dental treatment before the correct diagnosis is made.

Temporal giant cell arteritis (see Chap. 5) afflicts patients older than 60 years of age. There is a dull persistent pain in the temple after chewing. The temporal artery is nonpulsatile, tortuous, and tender. Referral to an ophthalmologist is essential to exclude ophthalmic artery involvement and the possibility of permanent blindness. Corticosteroids will ameliorate this condition.

Pain Arising from Nerve Trunks and Central Pathways

Group A: No Abnormal Central Nervous System Signs.

Facial neuralgias include the primary idiopathic neuralgias.[21] These have been recognized for many centuries and are among the most severe pains felt by humans. The features of trigeminal neuralgia are well defined and diagnosed.[22] Characteristically, there is a trigger zone in the area of the nasolabial fold or upper or lower lip. When stimulated by washing, shaving, talking, or any slight movement, pain will occur which is severe, lancinating, and lasts only a few seconds. There is no objective sensory loss. An untreated patient initially may present in an unkempt state, drooling from the mouth and unwilling to move or touch the trigger area. Injection of a local anesthetic into the area will abolish the trigger for the duration of the anesthesia. Remission for months or years commonly occurs.

Although this description is classic and usually well recognized, patients who have undergone various treatments in the past may give different descriptions that may confuse the diagnosis. Furthermore, several less typical features may be reported, such as continuous or long-lasting aching or burning between paroxysms and spontaneous changes in sensation.

Although no cause has been found, some patients describe a previous traumatic event. Pathologic examination of resected nerve tissue has shown evidence of hypomyelination or demyelination in the region of the trigeminal ganglion. Some neurosurgeons believe that impingement of blood vessels on the nerve in the region of the ganglion is the cause of this disease. It is important to recognize that, in some patients, especially those younger than 40 years of age, symptoms of trigeminal neuralgia may indicate an underlying disease, such as multiple sclerosis or a space-occupying lesion at the cerebellopontine angle.[23]

A similar condition, glossopharyngeal neuralgia, has the same characteristics except that the trigger zones are in the tonsil, lateral pharyngeal wall, or base of the tongue. This condition should not be confused with Eagle syndrome[24] in which an elongated styloid process may impinge on the soft tissue of the throat during neck movement or swallowing or Trotter syndrome[25] in which a tumor of the nasopharynx may cause pain in the lower jaw, tongue, and side of the head. In these cases, however, other signs such as deafness (from occlusion of the eustachian tube) and asymmetry in mobility of the soft palate (from tumor invasion of the levator palati muscle) should be sought.

Treatment of the primary neuralgias initially is medical. Carbamazepine or phenytoin are effective in many cases.[22]

Some patients, however, are allergic to these medications or develop bone marrow depression as an adverse effect. Traditionally, peripheral neurectomy of the maxillary or mandibular division of cranial nerve V or phenol or alcohol blocks have been used to denervate the area permanently. With the introduction of the radiofrequency lesion, the pain fibers specifically supplying the trigger zone may be destroyed selectively without necessarily interfering with sensory function. This is a relatively benign procedure with excellent long-term results.[26] Other neurosurgeons prefer intracranial surgery in which vascular structures are dissected off the trigeminal ganglion; good results can be obtained despite the greater risks of this major surgical intervention.[27,28] Glycerol injection and other surgical procedures also have been used successfully (see Chap. 35).

Another Group A disorder is postherpetic neuralgia[29,30] (see Chap. 21). A significant number of patients (approximately 25 percent) develop chronic pain after acute herpes zoster, and its incidence increases with age. Although the mechanism is poorly understood, it appears that the initial acute inflammation results in fibrosis of the nerve sheath and dorsal root ganglion with loss of large myelinated axons.

Herpes zoster also may occur in the distribution of the trigeminal nerve. The first division especially is affected, and the possibility of corneal ulceration and scarring should be remembered. The pain is described as a constant burning sensation, with a stabbing component. Hyper- or hypesthesia may be present.

Treatment is not entirely satisfactory. Various medications may reduce the pain of acute herpes zoster, such as topical idoxuridine, oral amantadine, intramuscular interferon, intravenous acyclovir, and intravenous vidarabine. Steroids also have been advocated, and sympathetic block can be useful.

In chronic postherpetic neuralgia, few approaches provide significant relief. Anticonvulsants, antidepressants, and antipsychotic agents all have been used. Occasionally, neurosurgical procedures are indicated.

Group B: Abnormal Central Nervous System Signs.

The cause in these syndromes may be extracranial or intracranial. It includes trauma, osteomyelitis, Paget disease, primary or metastatic tumors[31] or space-occupying lesions at the cerebellopontine angle[17] or the middle cranial fossa, disseminated sclerosis, cerebrovascular disease, syphilis, and syringobulbia.

Pain Arising from Outside the Face

Pain perceived in the face may be a result of irritation of pain receptors in tissues that are related embryologically to the segmental innervation of the face. This pain may originate in the eyes, ears, heart, or cervical spine. Common ocular causes of pain[32] include: refractive error, convergence insufficiency, extraocular muscle imbalance, trauma (e.g., abrasion, contact lens damage, or foreign body), otitis, angle-closure glaucoma, and so-called dry eye syndrome. Common causes of ear pain are outlined in Table 6-1.

Coronary artery disease classically is described as left substernal pain referred to the arm and side of the neck that is brought on by physical exertion, emotional upset, or ingestion of food. It is relieved rapidly by rest or sublingual nitroglycerine. On occasion, the pain sweeps up the neck and into the angle of the jaw. If the pain occurs in the jaw without other related symptoms, the diagnosis may be missed.

The dorsal root of cervical nerve III supplies the skin overlying the angle of the mandible. A cervical strain injury, cervical osteoarthritis, or spondylitis may irritate these nerves and cause pain in their distribution. Pressure on the occipital nerve (cervical nerve II) can cause occipital neuralgia with a sharp lancinating quality that shoots forward over the head. Local anesthetic and steroid injections may be necessary (see Chap. 5).

Chronic Atypical Facial and Oral Pain[5,9,33–36]

Many patients have intractable facial pain that may have been termed *atypical facial pain* or *psychogenic facial pain*. In these patients, the pain is a multifactorial problem characterized by equivocal physical findings, diffuse descriptions, and ill-defined psychiatric symptoms. In addition, malingerers, drug abusers, and patients with Munchausen syndrome may be encountered.

In an effort to diagnose and treat patients with chronic joint pain, we established a Chronic Facial Pain Group (consisting of an oral and maxillofacial surgeon, psychopharmacologist, neurologist, and neurosurgeon). We in-

Table 6-1
Common Causes of Ear Pain

Types	Examples
Intrinsic	
Infection	Acute otitis media
	Acute otitis externa
	Malignant otitis externa
	Infected cyst of ear canal
Trauma	Barotrauma
	Foreign body
	Direct trauma
Tumor	Carcinoma of the ear
Extrinsic	
Infection	Pharyngitis or tonsillitis
	Sinusitis
	Any cause of cervical adenopathy
	Ramsey Hunt syndrome
Tumor	Carcinoma of the oropharynx, nasopharynx, hypopharnyx, or larynx
Other	Temporomandibular joint syndrome
	Dental problems
	Glossopharyngeal neuralgia
	Atypical facial neuralgias

terview and examine patients at the same time. The pain is classified using the McGill–Melzack scale,[37] the International Association for the Study of Pain axes, the *Diagnostic and Statistical Manual III* [R] psychiatric classification, and the *International Classification of Disease*. In a study[38] of 107 patients, 88 patients were women, and 19 were men (mean age, 44.6 years; range, 17 to 87 years). These patients had experienced pain for a mean of 7.8 years (range, 0.5 to 46 years) and had consulted a mean of 5.8 physicians. They typically described their pain as continuous and fluctuating in intensity. All patients had used some medications (mean, 5.7); 58 percent had used narcotic analgesics, and 34 percent had used antidepressant medications.

Fifty-one percent of these patients had undergone some previous surgical intervention, and 14 percent had undergone temporomandibular joint surgery (15 patients and 23 operations). Forty percent of the patients had been treated with physical therapy, and 33 percent of the patients had used occlusal splints of one type or another. In addition to the facial pain (42 percent bilateral, 30 percent left, and 28 percent right), 58 percent of the patients had cranial pain, 36 percent had neck pain, and 46 percent had pain in other areas.

Most of these patients had more than one diagnosis. According to the classification systems, 65 percent of the patients had definable psychiatric problems, chiefly depression (38 percent); 36 percent had symptoms attributable to the masticatory system (temporomandibular joint and muscles); 29 percent had neuralgias of the trigeminal nerve; and 15 percent had pain of vascular origin. The rest were classified as atypical facial pain of unknown or mixed cause.

A variant of atypical facial pain is phantom-tooth pain or atypical odontalgia[39] in which pain is reported in a tooth or its supporting structures. Fillings, endodontic treatment, extractions, and bone currettage often are done without relief. The same sequence is followed in a neighboring tooth until a whole region of the mouth is rendered edentulous.

Burning mouth and burning tongue (glossodynia) is a troublesome condition with several different causes.[40] On first presentation, a complete oral examination should be done and a comprehensive history taken. Laboratory tests are necessary to exclude diabetes mellitus, pernicious anemia, and vitamin B_{12} and folate deficiency. Other causes include xerostomia, geographic tongue, median rhomboid glossitis, trauma, candidiasis, and psychogenic factors. In all cases of atypical pain, a thorough physical and radiographic examination is necessary, and a psychiatric workup is indicated.

As indicated, depression frequently is associated with chronic pain either as a premorbid (before the onset of pain) or reactive condition. In both instances, the patient will benefit greatly from treatment. Antidepressant medications have a long history of effectiveness and safety. They can reduce anxiety, reverse both mood and vegetative signs and symptoms of depression, and improve sleep patterns. The tricyclic antidepressants (amitriptyline and doxepin) are used most widely, and a bedtime-only schedule of 25 to 100 mg often will achieve improvement in 1 to 2 weeks.[41] The treatment can be continued for several months and then tapered to a low maintenance dose. Monoamine oxidase inhibitors and lithium salts also may be prescribed on occasion.

Anxiety sometimes is associated with chronic facial pain, and it may or may not be associated with a specific major life change, for example, illness, death, or acute stress. A careful history usually uncovers many symptoms, including tachycardia, dizzy spells, headaches, unsteadiness, paresthesias, breathing difficulties, trembling, excessive perspiration, a choking sensation, or hyperventilation. Relaxation techniques (such as meditation, hypnotherapy, behavior therapy, and biofeedback) are useful, and the minor tranquilizers (chlordiazepoxide and diazepam) are prescribed widely.[42]

Other psychiatric conditions also may present with pain, for example, hysteria, schizophrenia, and hypochondriasis. Even when these diagnoses have been excluded, there remain many patients with various emotional problems that may contribute to or cause pain. Hackett[43] developed the Madison scale to describe the characteristics that correlate with the psychogenicity of pain and are helpful in evaluating such patients.

Treatment for patients with chronic facial pain depends on its cause and may consist of multiple concurrent approaches.[44,45] A multidisciplinary approach has been found to be helpful in the diagnosis and treatment of these patients, but it is evident that, despite the best efforts of physicians and the use of sophisticated imaging techniques and tests, the needs of many of these patients are not met. They continue to seek medical consultations and undergo surgical intervention with no relief of their pain. A pain management program may ultimately be helpful for these individuals.

References

1. Austin DG, Cubillos L. Special considerations in orofacial pain. *Dent Clin North Am* January 1991; 35(1):227–244.
2. Mandel S. Facial pain. "Why does my face hurt, doctor?" *Postgrad Med* January 1990; 87(1):77–80.
3. Wyke B. The neurology of facial pain. *Br J Hosp Med* October 1968:46–65.
4. McDonald JS, Pensak ML, Phero JC. Differential diagnosis of chronic facial, head, and neck pain conditions. *Am J Otol* July 1990; 11(4):299–303.
5. Bell WE. *Orofacial Pains: Classification, Diagnosis, Management.* 3rd ed. Chicago: Yearbook Medical Publishers Inc; 1985.
6. Guernsey LH. Facial pain. In: Irby W, ed. *Current Advances in Oral Surgery, 2.* St Louis, MO: Mosby; 1977.
7. Gregg J. Neurological disorders of the maxillofacial region. In: Kruger GO, ed. *Textbook of Oral Surgery.* 4th ed. St Louis, MO: Mosby; 1974:620–660.
8. Young RR. Basic principles underlying craniofacial pain. In: Shaw JH, Sweeney EA, Cappuccino CC, et al., eds. *Textbook of Oral Biology.* Philadelphia: Saunders; 1978.
9. Alling CC III, Mahan PE. *Facial Pain.* 2nd ed. Philadelphia: Lea & Febiger; 1977.
10. Mumford JM. *Orofacial Pain—Aetiology, Diagnosis and Treatment.* 3rd ed. Edinburgh: Churchill Livingstone; 1982.
11. Sharar Y: Orofacial pain. In: Wall PD, Melzack R, eds. *Textbook of Pain.* Edinburgh: Churchill Livingstone; 1984:338–349.
12. Loeser JD: Tic douloureux and atypical facial pain. In: Wall PD, Melzack R, eds. *Textbook of Pain.* Edinburgh: Churchill Livingstone; 1984.
13. Pertes RA, Heir GM. Chronic orofacial pain. A practical approach to differential diagnosis. *Dent Clin North Am* January 1991; 35(1):123–140.
14. Dayal PK, Desai KI, Shah TN. Orofacial manifestations of myofascial pain dysfunction syndrome amongst dental patients. *Indian J Dent Res* January–March 1990; 2(1):145–152.
15. Laskin DM, Greenfield W, Gale E, et al. The President's Conference on the examination, diagnosis and management of temporomandibular joint disorders. Chicago: American Dental Association; 1989.
16. Zarb GA, Carlsson GE. *Temporomandibular Joint Function and Dysfunction.* Copenhagen: Munksgaard; 1979.
17. Sarnat BG, Laskin DM. *The Temporomandibular Joint: A Biological Basis for Clinical Practice.* 3rd ed. Springfield, IL: Charles C. Thomas; 1979.
18. Norgaard F. *Temporomandibular Arthrography.* Copenhagen: Munksgaard; 1947 Thesis.
19. Helms CA, Katzberg RW, Dolwick MF. Internal derangement of the temporomandibular joint. San Francisco, CA: Radiology Research and Education Foundation; 1983.
20. Merskey H. Development of a universal language of pain syndromes. *Adv Pain Res Ther* 1983; 5:37–52.
21. Donlon WC, Jacobson AL, Truta MP. Neuralgias. *Otolaryngol Clin North Am* December 1989; 22(6):1145–1158.
22. Sweet WH. The treatment of trigeminal neuralgias (tic douloureux). *N Eng J Med* 1986; 315:174–177.
23. Nguyen M, Maciewicz R, Bouckoms A, Poletti C, Ojemann R. Facial pain symptoms in patients with cerebellopontine angle tumors. A report of 44 cases or cerebellopontine angle meningioma and a review of the literature. *Clin J Pain* 1986; 2:3–9.
24. Eagle WW. Elongated styloid process. Further observations and a new syndrome. *Arch Otolaryngol Head Neck Surg* 1948; 47:630.
25. Trotter W. On clinically obscure malignant tumours of the nasopharyngeal wall. *Br Med J* 1911; 2:1057–1059.
26. Sweet WH, Wepsic JG. Controlled thermocoagulation of trigeminal ganglion and rootlets for differential destruction of pain fibers. *J Neurosurg* 1974; 40:143–146.
27. Janetta PJ: Trigeminal neuralgia: treatment of microvascular decompression. In: Wilkins RH, Rengachary SS, eds. *Neurosurgery 3.* New York: McGraw-Hill; 1985:2357–2363.
28. Zakrzewska JM. Surgical management of trigeminal neuralgia. *Br Dent J* January 19 1991; 170(2):61–62.

29. Hope-Simpson RE. Postherpetic neuralgia. *J R Coll Gen Pract* 1975; 25:571–575.

30. Taub A. Relief of post herpetic neuralgia with psychotropic drugs. *J Neurosurg* 1973; 39:235.

31. Marbach JJ. Current concepts in the management of pain in the head and neck cancer patient. *Dent Clin North Am* April 1990; 34(2):251–263.

32. Hitching R: Eye pain. In: Wall PD, Melzack R, eds. *Textbook of Pain*. Edinburgh: Churchill Livingstone; 1984:331–337.

33. Feinman C, Harris M. Psychogenic facial pain, I: the clinical presentation; II: management and prognosis. *Br Dent J* 1984; 156:165–168, 205–208.

34. Feinman C, Harris M, Cowley R. Psychogenic facial pain: presentation and treatment. *Br Med J* 1984; 288:436–438.

35. Friction JR. Behavioral and psychosocial factors in chronic craniofacial pain. *Anesth Prog* January–February 1985; 32(1):7–12.

36. Marbach JJ, Lipton JA. Aspects of illness behavior in patients with facial pain. *J Am Dent Assoc* 1978; 96:630–638.

37. Melzack R. The McGill Pain Questionnaire: major properties and scoring methods. *Pain* 1975; 1:275–279.

38. Keith DA. Chronic facial pain: a review of 107 patients. Paper presented at the Ninth International Conference on Oral and Maxillofacial Surgery, May 1986; Vancouver, Canada.

39. Marbach JJ, Hulbrock J, Hohn C, Segal AG. Incidence of phantom tooth pain. An atypical facial neuralgia. *Oral Surg* 1982; 53:190–193.

40. Zegarello DJ. Burning mouth. An analysis of 57 patients. *Oral Surg* 1984; 58:34–38.

41. Brown RS, Bottomly WK. Utilization and mechanism of action of tricyclic antidepressants in the treatment of chronic facial pain: a review of the literature. *Anesth Prog* September–October 1990; 37(5):223–229.

42. Keefe FJ, Beckman JC. Behavioral assessment of chronic orofacial pain. *Anesth Prog* March–June 1990; 37(2–3):76–81.

43. Hackett TP: The pain patient: Evaluation and treatment. In: Hackett TP, Cassem NH eds. *Handbook of General Hospital Psychiatry*. St Louis, MO: Mosby; 1978:41–63.

44. Hutchison I, Nally F. Management of orofacial pain. *Practitioner* January 1991; 235(1498):72–77.

45. McDonald JS, Pensak ML, Phero JC. Thoughts on the management of chronic facial, head, and neck pain. *Am J Otol* September 1990; 11(5):378–382.

CHAPTER 7

Neck Pain

Richard L. Gilbert and Carol A. Warfield

Neck pain is a common complaint. The neck is composed of many pain-sensitive tissues in a small area. The cervical spine is mobile and situated between an immobile thorax and a relatively weighty head; therefore, it is subject to varying degrees of trauma. The patient with minor self-limited neck pain might not consult a physician. Those who see a primary-care physician with a complaint of neck pain often can be helped by conservative management. A patient with severe chronic neck pain might be helped by therapies offered by a clinician in a pain management clinic setting. However, a knowledge of the many causes of neck pain is required.

The cause of a patient's neck pain is determined by a careful history, physical examination, and appropriate radiologic and laboratory tests.[1] It is necessary to be aware of the more serious disorders that can cause neck pain and require referral to an orthopedist or neurosurgeon. Table 7-1 lists many causes of neck pain, and it can be used as an extended reference (reference modified from DeGowin and DeGowin).[9]

DIAGNOSIS

A careful history, physical examination, appropriate laboratory studies, and an understanding of the mechanism of pain production will aid the clinician in the diagnosis and treatment of the patient's neck pain. In addition, a more serious disorder can be excluded.

History

Some of the more salient aspects of the history that the clinician should focus on include:

1. Precipitating and associated events (trauma, infection, emotional stress, or use of medications)
2. Duration (acute or chronic)
3. Aggravating and alleviating factors
4. Areas of maximal pain
5. Point of origin, and if present, points of radicular pain
6. Character of pain (sharp, dull, burning, or throbbing)
7. Associated neurologic symptoms (weakness, numbness, clumsiness, or long tract signs)
8. Associated medical symptoms (dyspnea, fever, chest tightness, or weight loss)
9. Other bony or muscular pains
10. Previous treatment
11. Other medical and surgical history
12. Pending litigation

Acute trauma requires careful neurologic and radiologic investigation. A history of significant or progressive upper extremity weakness or long track signs indicates neurosurgical or orthopedic referral. The presence of meningeal signs in the appropriate setting requires hospitalization. The patient's emotional state often can aggravate and perpetuate chronic neck pain.

Physical Examination[10]

Inspection should begin by watching the unaware patient enter the examination room and during history taking. The patient's normal posture and attitude of the head and neck might reveal an underlying disorder. The neck region should be inspected for normal characteristics and disease, including masses, muscular asymmetries, scars, discolorations, and cutaneous lesions. Palpation of the anterior neck can be done best on a patient in the supine position. The bony structures, including the hyoid bone, thyroid cartilage, cricoid cartilage, and first cricoid ring should be examined for normal contour and motion. The thyroid gland should be assessed for enlargement, tenderness, nodules, and bruits. The carotid artery is examined for bruits, tenderness, and tumor. Abnormal lymphadenopathy may indicate infection or malignancy. Cervical adenitis also may cause torticollis. Parotiditis must be excluded. The sternocleidomastoid muscle should be palpated for trigger points (myofascial pain or disease), hypertrophy and size discrepancy (torticollis, tenderness and swelling, or hematoma). The supraclavicular fossa must be assessed for masses (tumor, subclavian artery aneurysm, or pathologic lymphadenopathy) and fullness (superior vena cava syndrome).

The posterior bony palpation can be done best with the examiner's hands cupped underneath the neck of the supine patient because tense muscles inhibit assessment of the bony prominences. Palpation of the occiput may reveal occipital neuralgia. The mastoid process and superior nuchal line are examined. Each cervical vertebral spinous process is palpated, beginning with C2, and tenderness, irregularity, malalignment, and step-offs are investigated. The facet joints can be assessed by moving each hand

Table 7-1
Classification of Neck Pain

<table>
<tr><td colspan="2" align="center">**Neck Pain without Stiffness**</td></tr>
<tr>
<td valign="top">

Enhanced by swallowing
  Carotid artery (carotidynia,[2] carotid body tumor, or inflamed thyroglossal duct)
  Esophagus (inflamed diverticulum, peptic esophagitis, or radiation esophagitis)
  Mediastinum (spontaneous pneumomediastinum)[3]
  Pharynx (pharyngitis or Ludwig angina)
  Salivary gland (mumps or suppurative parotiditis)
  Thyroid gland (acute suppurative thyroiditis, subacute thyroiditis with pain radiating to the ear, hemorrhage, or thyroid cystadenoma)
  Tongue (ulcers or neoplasm)
  Tonsils (tonsillitis or neoplasm)
Neck pain enhanced by chewing
  Mandible (fracture, osteomyelitis, or periodontitis)
  Salivary gland (mumps or suppurative parotiditis)
  Temporomandibular joint (associated with myofascial pain syndrome in neck)
Neck pain enhanced by head movement
  Cervical spine (whiplash, acute or subacute fracture, dislocation, ligamentous damage, herniated intervertebral disk, rheumatoid neck,[4] facet joint syndrome,[5] or occipital neuralgia with C1 to C2 arthrosis syndrome[6]
  Nuchal muscles or trapezius muscles (viral myalgia or myofascial pain syndrome)
  Sternocleidomastoid (torticollis, hematoma, or myofascial pain)

</td>
<td valign="top">

Neck pain enhanced by shoulder movement
  Cervical rib
  Costoclavicular syndrome
  Scalenus anticus syndrome
  Pectoralis minor syndrome
Neck pain not enhanced by movement
  Branchial cleft remnant (inflamed pharyngeal cyst)
  Lymph node, acute (adenitis) or chronic (Hodgkin disease, scrofula, gummas, actinomycosis, or carcinomatous metastasis)
  Nervous system (cervical herpes zoster, spinal cord neoplasm, Arnold-Chiari malformation, syringomyelia, epidural abscess or hematoma, or poliomyelitis)
  Salivary gland (calculus in duct)
  Skin and subcutaneous tissue (furuncle, carbuncle, or erysipelas)
  Soft tissue calcium deposit at first and second cervical vertebrae[7]
  Spinal vertebrae (primary metastatic neoplasm, infectious osteomyelitis, tuberculosis, or herniated intervertebral disk)
  Subclavian artery (aneurysm)
Referred pain to the neck
  Angina
  Bronchus (broncial tumor)[8]
  Pain from sixth cervical dermatomal band
  Pancoast tumor

</td>
</tr>
<tr><td colspan="2" align="center">**Stiff Neck: Neck Pain and Limitation of Motion**</td></tr>
<tr>
<td valign="top">

Acquired (spasmodic torticollis)
Acute infections
  Fibrositis (transient stiff neck)
  Reflex spasms (meningitis or adenitis from acute pharyngitis)
  Torticollis
Acute traumatic
  Cervical spine strain
  Dislocations
  Facet dislocation
  Fractures
  Herniated disk
  Ligamentous rupture
  Subluxation

</td>
<td valign="top">

Chronic infection
  Infectious arthritis
  Intramuscular gummas
  TB spondylitis
Chronic posttraumatic
  Contracture from burns
  Nerve injury
  Untreated acute injuries
Congenital (congenital torticollis)
Degenerative (cervical spondylosis with fibrositis)
Inflammatory bone lesions
  Calcific tendinitis of the longus colli
  Subluxation of atlas

</td>
</tr>
</table>

laterally about 1 in from the spinous process. Facet tenderness and increased pain with neck extension and rotation should be observed (facet joint syndrome or osteoarthritis). Soft tissues of the posterior neck can be examined with the patient sitting in front of the examiner. The trapezius muscle is palpated for spasm, trigger points, and tenderness. If there is no evidence of an unstable cervical spine, full range of motion and cervical muscle strength should be tested. The presence of atrophy or hypertrophy and the reproduction of pain symptoms are assessed. The upper extremities and hands are observed for signs of atrophy, cyanosis, and differences in skin temperature (reflex sympathetic dystrophy). Maneuvering the upper extremities to elicit compression syndromes is done.

The neurologic examination is critical in evaluating the patient with neck pain because radicular symptoms and neurologic deficits localize the area of disease. (Table 7-2 and Fig. 7-1.)

Table 7-2
Motor and Reflex Distribution of Cervical Roots

Disk	Reflex	Muscles
C4, C5, and root C5	Biceps	Deltoid or biceps
C5, C6, and root C6	Brachioradialis	Wrist extensors or biceps
C6, C7, and root C7	Triceps	Wrist flexor, finger extensory, or triceps
C7, T1, and root C8	—	Finger flexors or hand intrinsic muscles
T1, T2, and root T1	—	Hand intrinsic muscles

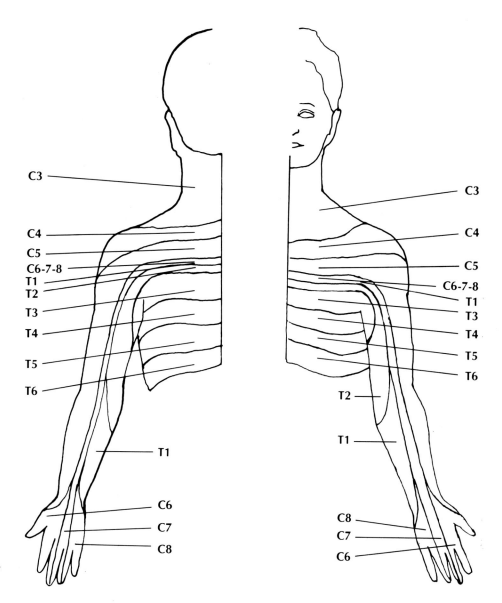

FIGURE 7-1. Dermatomes of the chest and upper extremity.

Other useful tests of the cervical spine include:

1. *The distraction test.*[10] In this test, manual and in-line traction done by the examiner simulates effective traction on the cervical spine and can relieve pain from nerve root compression and facet joint irritation.
2. *The compression test.*[10] The examiner presses down on the seated patient's head to reproduce the nerve impinged by the neural foramina or facets.
3. *The Valsalva test.*[10] This test can increase intrathecal pressure, exacerbating nerve root impingement by a tumor or disk in the cervical canal.
4. *Tests for the compression syndromes.* These include the scalenus anticus syndrome test (the Adson test)[10] and tests for costoclavicular syndrome and pectoralis minor syndrome. Where the history and physical examination warrant, x-rays and additional laboratory studies may be indicated.

NEUROANATOMY AND FUNCTIONAL ANATOMY[11]

There are eight cervical nerves. Each exit above the cervical vertebrae except C8; this exits below the C7 cervical vertebra. The spinal nerves divide into anterior and posterior primary rami, after giving off a meningeal branch that supplies the local vertebral structures. The posterior primary rami of C1 is entirely motor and runs over the posterior arch of the atlas to the suboccipital triangle where it supplies the capital movers and neck extensors. The C2 posterior ramus emerges between the axis and the atlas and divides, forming the greater occipital nerve. It is joined by the branches of C3 and supplies cutaneous sensation of the occipital regions. The lateral branch is motor and supplies the posterior cervical muscles. The medial branch of C3 supplies the skin of the lower occiput. The lateral branch supplies the posterior cervical muscles. The posterior rami of C4 through C8 supply the posterior cervical muscles. The medial branches of C4 and C5 supply the overlying skin. The anterior primary rami of the cervical spinal nerves supply the motor and sensory innervation to the front and side of the neck.

The cervical plexus is composed of the anterior divisions of C1 through C4. It supplies: (1) the superficial cutaneous branches (lesser occipital nerve (C2), greater auricular nerve (C2 and C3), anterior cutaneous nerve (C2 and C3), and supraclavicular nerve (C3 and C4); (2) deep branches that innervate the anterior vertebral muscles (recti capitus, longus capitus, scalenus medius, and branches of the levator scapular) and contribute to the sternomastoid (C2 and C3) and trapezius (C3 and C4); (3) the phrenic nerve (C3, C4, and C5); and (4) the communicating branches to the vagus and sympathetic chain.

The brachial plexus is formed by the anterior primary rami of C5 through T1 and provides motor and sensory innervation to the upper extremity. The plexus runs from roots, trunks, divisions, cords, and branches. The pattern of radicular symptoms and motor, sensory, and reflex deficits localize nerve root involvement as discogenic or other. Table 7-2 and Figure 7-1 summarize the neuroanatomy of the brachial plexus (see Chap. 14).

There are various pain-sensitive tissues in the neck, and there are areas considered to be pain insensitive.[12] The musculoskeletal anatomy will be considered. The cervical disk, including the nucleus pulposus, has no nervous tissue. The vertebral body, excluding the periosteum, is considered to be insensitive to pain. The posterior longitudinal ligament is pain sensitive and subjected to pressure from a herniated disk. The anterior ligament also is pain sensitive. The nerve root is a site of pain production from its origin to the dural sleeve and throughout its course in the cervical area. Ischemia secondary to stretching may be the mechanism of pain production. The facet joint is a source of pain; this can be elicited by extension and rotation toward the involved side. Cervical muscular pain may be caused by sustained contracture with resultant ischemia, myofascial pain syndrome, tearing or traction of muscles from the periosteum, and muscular hematoma.

The healing of torn ligaments and joint capsules may result in hyperplasia, fibrosis, and scarring with resultant nerve root irritation and compression and characteristic radiculopathy along the distribution of the involved nerve root.[13] Skeletal fractures with degenerative changes can occur. Articular cartilage injury from acute deforming forces, although initially painless because cartilage has no nerves, later results in joint wear and tear. Trauma to the sympathetic chain and fascial structures of the neck can result in a reflex sympathetic dystrophy with abnormal sympathetic response. This often is amenable to stellate ganglion or cervical sympathetic blockade.

CERVICAL TRAUMA: SOFT TISSUE INJURIES OF THE NECK

Neck pain from a traumatic origin includes many injuries from self-limited acute cervical strain to cervical fracture with paralysis. This section will consider soft tissue injuries without spinal cord paralysis.

The anatomic characteristics of the cervical spine predispose it to injury by direct and indirect forces. The neck is situated between the inflexible thoracic spine and the head, a relatively heavy structure that it must support. Reports indicate that 85 percent of neck disorders result from acute or repetitive neck injuries or chronic stresses and strain.[13]

Minor trauma resulting in acute cervical pain often is secondary to musculoskeletal injury and most frequently is self-limited using conservative treatment. One study[14] examined patients with acute cervical pain without neurologic symptoms in their arms. These patients were divided into three treatment groups: (1) neck collar and analgesics; (2) neck collar, analgesics, and TENS three times a week; and (3) neck collar, analgesics, and physical therapy. All patients also were encouraged to rest. Most patients markedly improved after 1 week. By 6 weeks, 95 percent of the patients in all groups were pain free. The TENS improved early cervical mobility.

The Whiplash Syndrome

Neck injuries often result from automobile accidents. One study[15] showed that 60 percent of patients who were injured in a car accident and presented to a hospital had neck pain. After 1 year, 26 percent of the original group had persistent neck pain. The term *whiplash* describes a resultant injury caused by an abrupt hyperextension of the neck from an indirect force.

When forward flexion of the neck is produced by acceleration or deceleration, the forward flexion of the head is limited by the chin touching the chest.[16] Lateral flexion movement stops when the ear hits the shoulder. These movements are within the physiologic range of motion of the cervical spine. No strain is placed on the intervertebral joints. By contrast, backward extension of the head stops when the occiput hits the posterior chest wall. This is beyond the physiologic range of motion. In a rear-end collision,[17] the body is propelled in a linear horizontal direction. The head abruptly moves backward, necessitating acute hyperextension of the cervical spine. This is followed by a recoil of the head with severe cervical neck flexion and finally a return to the neutral position. The opposite sequence occurs in head-on collisions.

The Symptom Complex

Because muscular hemorrhage and edema are involved, patients often do not have symptoms for 12 to 24 h after a whiplash injury. The cervical flexor muscles, specifically the sternocleidomastoid, the scalenus, and the longus colli undergo an acute stretch reflex.[18] Some fibers are torn. Hohl[19] reported characteristic symptoms of patients after a motor-vehicle accident. This author followed 146 walk-in patients for 5 years after motor-vehicle accidents that caused soft tissue neck injury without fractures or dislocations. Seventy percent of these accidents were rear-end collisions. Almost all patients complained of neck pain and stiffness. Two-thirds of patients had headaches, and one-third had shoulder or intrascapular pain. Ten percent had arm and hand pain or arm and hand numbness. There was loss of consciousness in 10 percent. Only 3 percent had a neurologic deficit.

Characteristically, the pain is localized to the neck and later may radiate from the neck to the shoulders, arms, or back of the head. Persistent suboccipital pain does not necessarily involve a local lesion at the atlantoaxial region but may be referred pain from a damaged cervical segment.[16] Injection of the occipital nerve with a local anesthetic and corticosteroid may be useful in this setting. Similarly, pain and numbness radiating down the arm (although a poor prognosticator in terms of the chronicity of the pain) may not necessarily indicate nerve root pressure but may be referred pain.[19] Nonneurogenic radiation of pain and numbness may be caused by chronic irritation of the musculoligamentous joint and intervertebral disk rather than by organic nerve pressure. These radicular symptoms are nonneurogenic, and therefore, they follow no specific nerve pathway. They are not well defined by the patient in contradistinction to well-defined neurogenic symptoms. Subjective numbness in the ulnar distribution may represent anterior scalenus spasm and entrapment of the brachial plexus; this is amenable to injection of the muscle with a local anesthetic and corticosteroid. Although reportedly rare in a whiplash injury, tearing of the longitudinal ligament and intervertebral disk herniation may cause discogenic pain. Radicular symptoms may be present in the posterior scapular muscles, across the back and shoulder, and into the arms.[17] Neurogenic pain is characterized by a clearly defined pattern of sensory, motor, and reflex findings. Persistent radicular pain after cervical trauma requires additional investigation to exclude nerve root involvement.

Severe hyperextension injury may stretch the esophagus with resulting edema or retropharyngeal hematoma; this may cause dysphagia. Hoarseness can occur, and bilateral vocal cord paralysis has been reported after severe flexion–extension injuries.[17] Damage to the cervical sympathetic chain may occur with the resultant symptoms of nausea, dizziness, Horner syndrome, and tinnitus. Vertebral artery spasm may be responsible for some of these symptoms.[16] The long-term complications of trauma to the sympathetic chain include reflex sympathetic dystrophy; this may be amenable to stellate ganglion blockade.

Injury to the brain itself from abrupt flexion and extension can cause concussion and cerebral contusion, with symptoms of loss of consciousness, dizziness, and headache.

Psychosomatic reactions after soft tissue neck injuries are the result of several factors. The chronicity of symptoms, associated emotional reaction to the accident, and secondary gain are all factors. One study showed that, in those patients with persistent symptoms after a motor-vehicle accident, if litigation claims were settled within 6 months, 83 percent were symptom free at 5 years. If litigation settlement occurred 18 months after the accident, then follow-up at 5 years revealed that only 38 percent were symptom free.[19]

In the patient with neck trauma, a plain-film x-ray study may be useful. Two views are necessary, the anteroposterior (AP) and lateral. If we consider the less severely injured patient (who is conscious, with radiculopathy, but without a neurologic deficit), x-ray studies should include: (1) AP of the atlantoaxial articulation (open mouth), (2) AP of the lower cervical spine, (3) lateral view, and (4) each oblique view.[20] These should be obtained and examined before additional studies. After excluding an unstable cervical spine, lateral flexion–extension views have been suggested for those with flexion–extension injuries, such as whiplash. Some suggest obtaining a pillar view, especially if there is a suspicion of an articular mass. X-rays should be assessed, not only for bony damage, but also for soft tissue injury. Persistent symptoms and neurologic findings may warrant additional investigations, including possibly CT scan, magnetic resonance imaging, myelography, or EMG.

Treatment

The initial treatment is conservative. Most authors recommend a soft cervical collar, analgesics, and bed rest with gradual increase in activity for the first 1 to 2 weeks. Some suggest physical therapy, Greenfield isometric neck exercises, heat, and traction if the symptoms respond.[16] TENS has been found to be useful for acute cervical strain; it hastens pain relief and the return of neck range of motion.[14] Mealy and associates[15] found that patients with acute whiplash injuries who were treated with early mobilization (ice for the first 24 h and then repetitive and passive movement within the patient's tolerance) had a lower pain score at 4 and 8 weeks and increased cervical movement at 8 weeks compared with those treated conservatively.

Despite improvement in most patients' symptoms, a substantial number of patients with whiplash have chronic symptoms. Hohl's study[19] of 150 walk-in patients who were assessed 5 years after an automobile accident that caused soft tissue injuries to the neck reported 43 percent with persistent symptoms. Poor prognostic indicators for chronic pain included: (1) numbness and pain in the upper extremity, (2) use of a cervical collar for more than 12 weeks, (3) requirement of home traction, and (4) physical therapy restarted more than once. Although a sharp reversal of the cervical curve on x-ray after the injury predicted degenerative changes, it was not associated with persistent symptoms. MacNab[16] found 45 percent of 266 patients had persistent symptoms despite court settlements. Gotten's survey[21] of 100 cases of whiplash injury found 12 percent of patients with persistent symptoms after litigation settlements.

These patients with chronic pain often are referred to a pain management center. A detailed history, physical examination, and a review of radiologic information will identify patients requiring neurosurgical or orthopedic referral. The patient with chronic neck pain after a soft tissue injury of the neck often can be helped by administering a nerve block with a local anesthetic with or without corticosteroids. These include patients with: (1) reflex sympathetic dystrophy amenable to stellate ganglion block, (2) occipital neuralgia amenable to occipital nerve block, (3) traumatic torticollis amenable to accessory nerve block or injection into the muscle belly, (4) myofascial pain syndrome after trauma amenable to trigger-point injections and stretch-and-spray therapy, and (5) suprascapular pain amenable to injection of the suprascapular nerve. In addition, patients with radicular and nonradicular neck pain often derive benefit from cervical epidural corticosteroids.

Neck Pain of Myofascial Origin (See Chap. 19)

One of the most common and frequently overlooked causes of neck pain is the myofascial pain syndrome. This syndrome is characterized by pain and/or autonomic phenomena referred from active trigger points. A myofascial trigger point is a hyperirritable locus that is palpable as an exquisitely tender taut band or knot in a skeletal muscle. Digital compression causes a characteristic reproducible pattern of referred pain and autonomic phenomena (sweating, vasoconstriction, and pilomotor activity) that is remote from the location of the trigger point.[22] The pain pattern is not limited to a specific dermatome or peripheral nerve segment. Moreover, an active trigger point is tender, prevents full lengthening of the muscle, weakens the muscle, and can mediate a local twitch response if stimulated adequately.

On a cellular level, the myofascial trigger point seems to originate after an acute muscle stress or strain, causing tissue damage and impairment of calcium regulation. A state of localized sustained muscle contraction is initiated with increased metabolites and decreased blood flow to the area. Multiple afferent fibers of varying types emanating from the trigger point to the spinal cord are stimulated and initiate the characteristic referred pain and/or autonomic phenomena.[22]

The myofascial pain syndrome is essentially a diagnosis of exclusion because the character of the pain may mimic other cervical disorders; these must be excluded. Myofascial pain is often abrupt in onset, and patients may remember a specific precipitating event, often traumatic, for example, a whiplash injury. However, the pain may be more gradual in onset from a chronically overused muscle. Myofascial pain may develop after, or be worsened by, psychogenic stress, viral illness, visceral disease, exposure to cold or damp weather, and strenuous exercise or prolonged tensing of the involved muscle.[22] The patient often will describe pain that is steady, deep, and aching in quality.[22] Although the pain may follow a dermatomal–myotomal pattern, it does not follow a characteristic nerve root pattern nor is there usually dysesthesia or paresthesia, which often is present with nerve root irritation.

In neck pain of myofascial origin, the muscles of the shoulder and neck are often tense. Palpation of a taut band-like trigger point reproduces the patient's pain. There may be associated weakness but not atrophy of the involved muscles.[22] Trigger points commonly responsible for pain referred to the cervical area are located in several muscles (Table 7-3).

Nerve entrapment by myofascial taut bands has been

Table 7-3
Cervical Myofascial Trigger Points

Muscle	Area of Referred Pain
Trapezius	Neck, shoulder, or temporal region[22]
Splenius capitus and cervicis	Head, occiput, shoulder, or neck (there may be blurred vision)[22]
Posterior neck muscles (semispinalis capitis, cervicis, or multifidi)	Suboccipital area, neck, or shoulders[22]
Levator scapulae	The angle of the neck or along vertebral border of the scapula[22]
Scalenus	Chest, upper central border of scapula, or along arm[22]
Infraspinatus	Posterior neck, suboccipital area, deltoid, deep in shoulder joint, or front and lateral aspects of arm and forearm[22]

described. Brachial plexus entrapment by the scalenus and/or pectoralis minor can occur. Greater occipital nerve entrapment by the semispinalis capitus also can occur.[22–24]

Management

Treatment of the myofascial pain syndrome and eradication of acute myofascial trigger points may be achieved primarily by spraying the involved muscle with vapocoolant coupled with passive stretching of the muscle. A stream of fluorimethane or ethyl chloride is sprayed in parallel sweeps in the direction of the referred pain over the skin of the involved muscle. The muscle then is stretched passively and slowly to the normal full muscle length in an effort to inactivate the trigger point. Hot packs then are applied.[22] The spray facilitates stretching by inhibiting pain and spinal stretch reflexes and, in essence, acting as a distraction.[22] When a smaller number of well-defined trigger points are not eliminated fully by the stretch-and-spray technique, they may be injected with a local anesthetic and corticosteroid and then stretched. It is important to identify the trigger point accurately at its point of maximal intensity and inject directly into the taut band. Needling of the trigger point should reproduce the patient's referred pain pattern. Bupivacaine 0.25% or 0.5% or lidocaine 1% often are used. These local anesthetics sometimes are mixed with local corticosteroids, for example, triamcinolone approximately 1 ml (40 mg of the steroid can be mixed with 10 ml of the anesthetic). Hot packs are applied after injection and stretching. Injections in proximity to the thorax, great vessels, and nerve chains warrant monitoring for complications. Travell and Simons'[22] manual on trigger points shows appropriate stretch-and-spray positions for those trigger points resulting in cervical pain.

Nonsteroidal anti-inflammatory agents are useful as adjuvant therapy for decreasing musculoskeletal inflammation in patients with myofascial pain syndrome. A tricyclic antidepressant agent prescribed at bedtime also is useful because it alleviates some of the depression element in chronic pain of myofascial origin and acts directly as an analgesic and bedtime sedative.

Because many conditions of daily living contribute to the formation and exacerbation of myofascial trigger points, therapy must incorporate a multifaceted approach. Self-hypnosis and biofeedback are useful in diminishing the psychogenic stress that can cause and exacerbate pain from myofascial trigger points. Driving, typing, heavy shoulder bags, exposure to cold drafts, and improper sleeping are a few conditions that contribute to and exacerbate myofascial trigger points and result in cervical pain. Practices and activities that lead to prolonged overutilization, strain, or tensing of the shoulder and neck muscles should be avoided. In addition, a formal physical therapy program often is beneficial. A program that encompasses stretch-and-spray techniques, strengthening exercises, and utilization of moist heat, ultrasound, and electrical stimulation is useful.[25] The patient also can institute a program of passive stretching while taking a hot shower or with application of moist hot packs.

Torticollis

Torticollis is a severe state of neck muscle contracture. Contracture, sometimes spasmodic, usually is unilateral, and the head often is twisted painfully to one side with the chin, to the opposite side. Torticollis results from disease or injury to the central nervous system or musculoskeletal tissues of the neck.[26] It can be congenital or acquired.

The congenital types of torticollis of musculoskeletal origin include:

1. Congenital muscular and postural torticollis (muscle trauma, tumor, and inflammation)
2. Congenital C1 to C2 articulations (atlantoaxial dislocation)
3. Congenital anomalies of the cervical vertebrae (Klippel-Feil syndrome)
4. Congenital absence of cervical muscles.[27]

Congenital neurogenic torticollis may be caused by Arnold-Chiari malformations, spina bifida, hydrocephalus, syringomyelia, or syringobulbia.[27]

Acquired types of torticollis associated with musculoskeletal conditions include:

1. Traumatic, such as neck muscle injuries; fracture; subluxation of the odontoid, C1, C2, and C3; atlantoaxial instability; and trauma to the clavicle, scapula, or cervical ligaments
2. Infectious, such as nasopharyngeal torticollis associated with upper respiratory tract infection; cervical adenitis associated with viral, bacterial, and tubercular organisms; cervical abscess; osteomyelitis; and fascitis
3. Postinfectious, such as influenza, diphtheria, or scarlet fever
4. Neoplastic, such as neoplasm of the bones, muscle, lymphatics, or vascular structures of the neck
5. Scar formation
6. Vascular abnormalities
7. Anterior scalenus syndrome
8. Pharmacologic, such as drugs resulting in dystonic reactions, for example, phenothiazines.

Acquired types of torticollis associated with neurologic conditions include:

1. Syringomyelia
2. Dystonic syndrome
3. Posterior fossae disease (tumors)
4. Herniated cervical disk
5. Hydrocephalus
6. Postencephalitis.[27]

Spasmodic Torticollis

The cause of this disorder is unclear, although it is considered to be a type of torsion dystonia.[28] The disorder begins in the fourth and fifth decades of life and presents with jerky movements of the head and painful neck spasms.[29] There is an association with writer's cramp, general torsion dystonias, essential tremor, parkinsonism, familial cases,[28] and hyperthyroidism.[30] The course is progressive deterioration during the first 5 years, static for the next 5 years, and a final relapse. A small number of patients have a hysterical conversion symptom. Psychological factors can aggravate the problem.

Long-standing torticollis can produce permanent contracture of the cervical muscles, fibrotic changes in the tissue, and degeneration of the cervical spine. There may be variable degrees of pain associated with the course of the disease.[31] Evaluation of a patient with torticollis should include the history (e.g., trauma, drugs, familial tendencies, and infection), physical findings (including careful neurologic examination and evaluation of the cervical spine), and x-ray findings (including cervical spine films of the odontoid and AP, lateral, and oblique views of the neck). This enables the clinician to classify torticollis as acquired or congenital, of traumatic origin, or involving musculoskeletal or neurologic structures. When torticollis is associated with a neurologic deficit, additional radiographic investigations are warranted, including CT scan with contrast and/or myelography.[26]

Treatment

Pharmacologic therapy of spasmodic torticollis has been somewhat effective. Therapies manipulating the dopaminergic, cholinergic, adrenergic, and serotonergic systems, and the use of γ-aminobutyric acid agonists have had varying degrees of success. Lee[32] suggests anticholinergics for mild symptoms of torticollis, including trihexyphenidyl (2 to 4 mg per day) or benztropine (1 to 3 mg per day), diazepam (5 to 15 mg per day), or amantadine (100 to 300 mg per day). For moderate to severe symptoms, he recommends haloperidol (1 to 8 mg per day). Psychological approaches, such as psychotherapy, hypnosis, behavior modification, and biofeedback also have been advocated.[31]

Blocking the accessory nerve with a local anesthetic can relax the trapezius and sternocleidomastoid muscles in torticollis. Alternatively, the local anesthetic may be injected diffusely into the muscle belly. Because other neck muscles frequently are involved, blocking the cervical plexus with a local anesthetic may be required to relieve the muscle spasm. If blocking the cervical plexus and accessory nerve improve the symptoms, repeated blocks, coupled with physical therapy to strengthen opposing muscles, can be used. Neurolytic blockade of the accessory muscles with phenol may be considered. More recently, injection of botulinum toxin has been advocated.[33]

Surgical options for neurogenic torticollis, including Arnold-Chiari malformation, syringomyelia, and colloid cysts, have been described. The patient may be considered for surgical management if medical management and other conservative measures have not provided symptomatic relief. Cervical approaches include cervical rhizotomy, selective excision of the hyperkinetic cervical muscles, stereotactic ablative procedures directed to the thalamus, and neuroaugmentative procedures such as thalamic and cervical dorsal column stimulation. These surgical approaches have had varied degrees of success.[26]

CERVICAL SPONDYLOSIS

Disk degeneration and cervical spondylosis is a common cause of neck pain. Approximately 50 percent of people older than age 50 years and 75 percent of those older than 65 years of age have radiologic evidence of cervical spondylosis.[34] Not all of them have associated symptoms.

Pathophysiologic Findings

As a consequence of aging the vascular supply to the disk is diminished resulting in disk degeneration. The anulus dehydrates, leading to approximation of the vertebrae. This leads to disk bulging and fibrosis, ultimately resulting in calcification and osteophyte formation. The bone formation can lead to narrowing of the spinal canal with subsequent cord compression or narrowing of the intervertebral foramina, resulting in nerve root compression. In addition, the ligaments and facet joints hypertrophy.[12,34]

The nerve roots most often involved in spondyloradiculopathy are C5 and C6 because of the increased mobility, angulation, and degeneration that can occur in the mid-cervical region.[12]

Symptoms

Presenting symptoms were reported in 100 patients with radiographic evidence of cervical spondylosis.[35] Approximately 30 percent of patients had symptoms of headaches or brachial radiculopathy. Fifteen percent of patients had vertigo, myelopathy, or neck pain. Vertebral basilar ischemic symptoms, loss of consciousness, or drop attacks were seen in 5 percent of patients.

Neck Pain

Neck pain from a cervical root is caused by acute intermittent nerve irritation, generally a result of nerve impingement in a narrowed intervertebral foramen. The pain may occur insidiously, as in cervical spondylosis, and be precipitated by minor trauma. Alternatively, more acute severe neck pain may occur with a herniated cervical intervertebral disk in the setting of a degenerated spondylitic spine. The pain in the neck often is poorly localized and worsens with movement. Muscular spasm often is present.[34] Cailliet[12] described ill-defined intrascapular pain with muscle spasm and tenderness as a result of anterior disk disease rather than nerve root irritation. This can occur months before evidence of root entrapment. Plain-film x-rays and a CT scan of the neck are helpful in excluding other causes of neck pain, including primary osteomyelitis, tuberculous osteitis, malignancy, and retropharyngeal abscess.[34]

Brachial Radiculopathy

The symptom of brachial plexus nerve root impingement at the level of the intervertebral foramen usually is shooting or burning pain, originating in the posterior neck with radiation across the shoulder and down the outer arm to the elbow or hand.[34] Persistent nerve root impingement leads to a characteristic sensory loss (hypesthesia or anesthesia), motor loss (weakness or atrophy), and diminished reflexes.

An acute protruded disk is associated with more severe pain, occurring acutely after trauma or violent movement, with symptoms radiating down the arm. Neurologic deficits soon appear. Other conditions that may produce symptoms similar to brachial radiculopathy include myofascial pain syndrome, apical tumors, and shoulder disorders (including capsulitis, rotator cuff injuries, bursitis, and thoracic outlet compression of the brachial plexus nerves and/or subclavian artery.

Suboccipital Neuralgia

Headache may result from occipital neuralgia. The occipital nerve rises from the posterior primary ramus of C2 and supplies the skin overlying the occiput and scalp. Typically, a nagging pain begins in the occipital region with radiation to the ipsilateral forehead. Paroxysmal pain may become continuous. Atlantooccipital disorders must be excluded radiographically.

Cervical Myelopathy

Cervical myelopathy can be a result of compression of the spinal cord by ligaments or protruded disks, trauma, or compromise of the blood supply. If compression originates anteriorly, for example, by an osteophyte or central disk protrusion, the resulting deficit is mostly motor. However, posterior compression, for example, from a hypertrophied ligament, causes dorsal column loss. The limited mobility of the spinal cord in the cervical area associated with cervical spondylosis magnifies the effect of movement because it contributes to spinal cord compression. Spinal cord compression often is painless, although in the early stages the patient may complain of foot numbness and an unsteady gait.[34] It is essential to examine the patient carefully for neurologic deficits that typically include lower motor deficits of the upper extremities and associated long tract signs affecting the lower extremities.

Other disorders that may mimic cervical spondylitic myelopathy and must be excluded including dorsal column loss from subacute combined degenerative disease (e.g., vitamin B_{12} deficiency), multiple sclerosis (although often other evidence of central nervous system plaques and deficits are present), motor neuron disease (e.g., amyotrophic lateral sclerosis), and syringomyelia.[34] Other causes of cord compression (including spinal cord tumors, metastatic disease, infectious processes, and Arnold-Chiari syndrome) may be excluded by more specific radiographic investigations.

Patients with neck pain and cervical radicular symptoms should undergo plain-film x-rays of the cervical spine, including: AP and lateral views, flexion–extension views, atlantooccipital views, and oblique-plane x-rays. A cervical CT scan may demonstrate disk herniation and nerve root impingement. However, because most elderly patients have some degree of spondylosis, these findings are not necessarily the cause of the symptoms. A chest x-ray is warranted to exclude apical thoracic disease, for example, Pancoast tumor. Progressive neurologic deficit or signs of cord compression are indications for the patient to undergo spinal myelography, nuclear magnetic resonance imaging[36] or CT scanning, and evaluation by an orthopedist or neurosurgeon.

Treatment

A patient who has neck pain and/or cervical radicular symptoms, with a normal neurologic examination and radiographic investigations that exclude diseases other than cervical spondylosis, may be treated conservatively. Treatments include a soft collar, analgesics, and possibly traction. Some authors do not recommend traction because they find this to be an irritant.[37] Myofascial trigger points or local areas of tender muscle nodules can be injected with a local anesthetic and corticosteroids. After other disorders have been excluded, cervical spondylosis involving occipital neuralgia can be managed by injecting the occipital nerve with local anesthetics and corticosteroids. Jeffries[34] suggests that, in children, suboccipital neuralgia must be investigated by a pediatric neurologist or neurosurgeon. Other aspects of conservative management include cervical isometric exercises recommended to increase cervical muscle strength.[34,37] In addition, anti-inflammatory medications, TENS, and local heat can be used. Surgery usually is reserved for progressive neurologic deficits or signs of cord compression. Minor neurologic deficits that do not seem to interfere with function can be managed nonsurgically. Neurologic deficits that do interfere with important functions should be managed surgically.[34,37] Surgery for pain alone is controversial. Some authors recommend it for unremitting pain, recurrent neck pain, and radicular symptoms.[37] Cervical epidural corticosteroids for chronic neck pain and cervical radiculitis have been reported to be effective. Schulman[38] reported a 41 percent incidence of substantial pain relief in approximately 100 patients undergoing cervical epidural steroid injection. Indications for injection included spondylosis, spinal stenosis, cervical arthritis, radiculopathy, and cervical disk syndrome. There were no major complications in this study. In addition, Warfield and colleagues[39] reported on 16 patients with complaints of severe neck and arm pain and numbness in the radicular distribution for at least 3 months with negative CT and myelographic studies. Conservative therapy, including rest, cervical collars, traction, and nonsteroidal anti-inflammatory agents was ineffective in these patients. Eleven of them had substantial improvement in their pain. Six patients who had abnormal neurologic signs before the injection had improvement in these signs. There were no complications in this study.

COMPRESSION SYNDROMES

Compression of the neurovascular bundle in the area of the cervical thoracic dorsal outlet can produce symptoms that mimic the neck pain and extremity dysesthesia and numbness found in cervical radiculopathy. The brachial plexus is formed by the anterior primary rami of C5, C6, C7, C8, and T1.[11] These roots emerge from the intervertebral foramina and become sandwiched between the scalenus anticus and medius. At this point, the roots unite to form three trunks: an upper trunk (C5 and C6), a middle trunk (C7), and a lower trunk (C8 to T1). The three trunks are grouped closely and emerge laterally and between the scalenus, across the posterior triangle of the neck, and across the first rib. At the lateral portion of the first rib and posterior to the clavicle, each trunk separates into an anterior and posterior division. These six divisions descend into the axilla. In the apex of the axilla, the divisions join to form three cords. Grouped around the axillary artery are (1) the lateral cord, composed of the anterior division of the upper (C5 to C6) and middle (C7) trunk; (2) the medial cord, a continuation of the anterior division of the lower trunk (C8 to T1); and (3) the posterior cord, the posterior division of all three trunks (upper, middle, and lower). Behind the pectoralis minor, the cords orient around the axillary artery according to their names. They continue and form the peripheral nerves and branches of the upper extremity. The lateral and medial cords comprise the median nerve, the medial cord gives rise to the ulnar nerve, and the posterior cord becomes the radial nerve. The subclavian artery arches over the first rib and joins the brachial plexus immediately behind where the anterior scalenus inserts into the first rib. The subclavian vein runs over the first rib, but usually it is anterior to the anterior scalenus muscle.[12,40]

The compression syndromes include the following:

1. Anterior scalene syndrome,[12] in which the neurovascular bundle (the nerve, artery, and sometimes a vein) is compressed in the triangle formed by scalenus anticus and medius and the first rib
2. The clavicular costal syndrome,[12] in which the neurovascular bundle (nerve, artery, and vein) is compressed between the clavicle and first rib
3. The pectoralis minor or hyperabduction syndrome,[12] in which the neurovascular bundle (nerve, artery, and vein) is compressed between the pectoralis minor and the rib cage.

Anterior Scalene Syndrome

Neurovascular entrapment at the level of the anterior scalene may involve the nerve and artery and possibly the vein or lymphatic vessels. Hand edema and finger stiffness may be present[22] because the subclavian vein is compressed between the first rib and clavicle secondary to a taut scalenus. Most often, brachial plexus compression occurs with symptoms of numbness, tingling, and hypesthesia in the arms and hands, chiefly in the ulnar distribution. The pain is often dull and aching in quality and may include the neck, shoulders, arm, or hand. Symptoms may occur during the early morning and awaken the patient from sleep or after prolonged activity using the hands.

These patients may have mild hypesthesia to light touch and pinprick, although other findings often are absent. The Addson test (tensing the scalenus and elevating the first rib) reproduces the patient's symptoms. This test is done with the examiner abducting and extending the involved arm while monitoring the radial pulse. The patient faces the involved side, extends their neck, and takes a deep breath. Reproduction of the symptoms and obliteration of the pulse constitute a positive result. Normal subjects may have obliteration of the radial pulse with this maneuver, but they do not have the characteristic symptoms. Spasm of the scalenus (myofascial syndrome) generally is believed to be the most likely cause. It may result from cervical nerve root irritation from cervical spondylosis or facet syndrome; trauma or stress and strain of the scalenus also may be causes. Uncommonly, the presence of a cervical rib with an associated fibrous band attached may predispose to neurovascular entrapment.[12] However, most patients with cervical ribs have no symptoms, most patients with symptoms have no cervical ribs, and removal of the rib often does not afford relief. Surgery rarely is indicated. Treatment involves conservative measures including: a soft collar and strengthening, stretching, and posture exercises to decrease the cervical lordosis and increase shoulder girdle strength. The anterior scalenus and associated trigger points may be injected with a local anesthetic and corticosteroid to diminish spasms and relax trigger points.

Clavicular Costal Syndrome[12]

As described, the neurovascular bundle courses between the first rib and the clavicle. Its compression leads to the clavicular costal syndrome. Poor posture, fatigue, and trauma may predispose to this syndrome. Pain, paresthesia, and numbness in the arms and hands occur chiefly at night or in the early morning. The diagnosis is made by eliciting symptoms and obliterating the radial pulse by bringing the shoulders back and down (chest elevation and shoulder retraction).

The treatment involves increasing neck flexibility and improving posture by strengthening exercises for the shoulder girdle. Poor posture secondary to psychogenic factors should be addressed.

Pectoralis Minor Syndrome (Hyperabduction Syndrome)

As described, the neurovascular bundle may be compressed between the pectoralis minor and the rib cage. The symptoms are similar to the costoclavicular syndrome.[12]

Entrapment often may involve the ulnar and medial distribution. The symptoms usually are transient and without objective physical findings. They frequently occur at night or in the early morning. The diagnosis is made by reproducing the symptoms and obliterating the radial pulse by placing the arms abducted over the head, externally rotated and backward. This stretches the pectoralis minor and compresses the underlying neurovascular bundle.

In addition, hyperirritability and tautness of the pectoralis minor (myofascial syndrome) that cause shortening of the muscle may be responsible for this syndrome. A poor slumped posture may contribute. Treatment includes improvement in posture and spraying or injection and stretching the pectoralis minor trigger points.

The compression syndromes should be suspected in the patient who has cervical pain and associated extremity symptoms, which may be reproduced by appropriate positioning of the arms and neck. However, it is necessary to exclude other causes, including cervical disk disease, degenerative joint disease, carpal tunnel syndrome,[41] pericapsulitis,[12] and shoulder–hand syndrome.[12] Moreover, disorders of the apical thorax, including a Pancoast tumor, subclavian artery aneurysm, or other supraclavicular fossa or axillary disease, must be excluded.

CERVICAL FACET JOINT SYNDROME

Cervical facet joint syndrome can cause both local and radicular symptoms often indistinguishable from cervical disk disease.[42] Often cervical facet and disk disorders, leading to cervical pain, occur together.

Each posterior facet joint has a dual nerve supply, with one branch arising from the posterior primary ramus at the same level and the other from the posterior primary ramus from above. Therefore, to block the C4 to C5 facet joint, for example, the nerves from C4 and C5 must be blocked. Acute facet joint irritation may occur from local trauma or excessive movement. More commonly, facet joint irritation arises from chronic changes of facet joint thickening and hypertrophy initiated by disk degeneration and spondylosis, trauma, or excessive load-bearing stress.[43]

Upper cervical facet joint irritation may be responsible for symptoms of upper neck pain, with radiation to the occipital region and ipsilateral frontal area. Associated are occipital and vascular headaches.[5] Lower cervical discogenic nerve root irritation resulting in muscular spasms also may lead to secondary upper facet joint irritation. The findings include facet joint tenderness (located 3 to 4 cm from the midline), a normal motor and sensory examination, and x-ray findings, which, in addition to degenerative changes, reveal facet disease (hypertrophy and thickening).

Low cervical pain characterized by neck pain with radicular symptoms to the shoulder and arms more often is caused by discogenic nerve root irritation. However, concomitant or secondary facet joint irritation often contributes. Facet joint tenderness may be present.

Management

The initial therapy is conservative. Similar to facet syndrome in the lumbar sacral region, patients often respond to injection of the facet joint with corticosteroids and local anesthetics. Dory[44] reported his findings on cervical facet injections for cervical syndrome. Arthrography was done during facet joint injections on 14 patients undergoing a total of 22 joint injections. He selected the level to be injected by the localization of the symptoms from the history or palpation on physical examination and by the site of the referred pain. All patients in this study had not responded to conservative therapy. Disk disease was excluded by plane x-rays, and nerve root compression was excluded by EMG studies.

The patients were placed prone, and a 22-gauge spinal needle was inserted into the facet joint under fluoroscopic guidance. Placement was confirmed by contrast material injected into the joint space. He injected 1 ml of corticosteroid in the joint because he believed this was the limit of the cervical facet joint volume. Nine patients had pain relief lasting 3 days to 13 months. Improvement was more likely if the typical pain was reproduced on distension of the facet joint during the injection.

Blockade of the facet joint also may be achieved by blocking the posterior primary ramus that supplies the facet joint and the posterior primary ramus above the involved facet joint. A needle is inserted at the junction of the superior facet joint and the transverse process. The nerve curves around the superior facet and innervates the joint. A local anesthetic and corticosteroid are injected in this area.[31] If the injection relieves the symptoms, permanent blockade can be accomplished with a cryoprobe or phenol.

Sluijter and Koetsveld-Baart[5] described percutaneous facet denervation in patients with cervical syndrome emanating from the facet joint who did not respond to conservative therapy (not including facet injections) and were not surgical candidates (disk surgery, foraminotomy, or spinal fusion).

A preliminary block of the posterior primary ramus was done to evaluate the contribution of the facet joint to cervical pain. This alleviated the pain. A percutaneous facet denervation, with a 12-gauge thermal electrode (60 s and 80°C) was used. They found 70 percent to 100 percent improvement in pain symptoms in 40 percent of patients with upper cervical syndrome or lower cervical syndrome. The follow-up was no less than 18 months. Complications consisting of localized neck pain occurred in 20 percent of patients and lasted 3 to 12 weeks.

CERVICAL EPIDURAL STEROIDS

The following section reviews studies in which epidural corticosteroids were administered for the treatment of cervical pain. Rowlingson[45] reported a retrospective study of 25 patients with cervical radiculopathy symptomatic for an average duration of 15 months (range, 1 to 60 months). These patients did not respond to conservative treatment. Using a 17-gauge Weiss winged epidural needle and a hanging-drop technique, they injected 50 mg of triamcinolone and lidocaine 1% (total volume, 4 ml) into the cervical epidural space. They entered midline at C6 to C7 or C7 to T1 and 30° caudad to the perpendicular line of the skin. The patients were seated with their necks flexed. There were no complications.

Sixty-five percent of the patients had either complete resolution of symptoms or an overall improvement of 75 percent in symptoms that lasted an average of 6 months. All patients in the group had a history of cervical radiculopathy characterized by neck pain with radicular symptoms to the extremities. Eighty percent had an appropriate sensory loss. Sixty percent had appropriate motor loss. In general, a history, physical examination, and appropriate radicular findings consistent with cervical radiculopathy increased the likelihood of successful amelioration of symptoms.

Schulman[38] retrospectively examined 96 patients with chronic neck pain. Of these, 66 had spondylosis, 2 had spinal stenosis; 5 had cervical arthritis; 21 had radiculopathy of nonspecific origin; and 5 had cervical disk syndrome. In this group, 75 percent of patients received a single injection, and 20 percent received two injections. Most injections were done at the C5 to C6 or C6 to C7 level. A 17-gauge Weiss needle was inserted into the epidural space by loss of resistance. They injected 80 to 160 mg of methylprednisolone with either lidocaine 1% (25 to 200 mg) or bupivacaine 0.5% (20 to 75 mg). Forty percent of patients had either complete pain relief or 50 percent to 75 percent pain relief for 1 month to 1 year. Fair pain relief (25 percent to 50 percent) was reported in approximately one-third of patients. No particular pattern of success could be based on a diagnostic group. Minor complaints occurred, such as nausea in 8 percent, shortness of breath in 3 percent, and abdominal bloating in 3 percent of patients.

Warfield and associates,[39] at our institution, reported on 16 patients with severe radicular neck and arm pain and numbness of at least 3 months' duration (range, 3 to 72 months). Twelve patients had neurologic signs before treatment (12 percent with diminished deep tendon reflexes, 60 percent with sensory loss, 80 percent with motor loss, and 88 percent with decreased range of motion of the neck). In all patients, CT scan and/or myelography were negative. All patients had not responded to conservative therapy, including rest, cervical collar, traction, and nonsteroidal anti-inflammatory medications. These authors injected 80 mg of methylprednisolone in 5 ml of normal saline into the epidural space at C6 to C7 or C7 to T1 using a 17-gauge Touhy needle by a loss-of-resistance technique. The patients were seated. Eleven patients had improvement of their pain in 1 week that lasted for at least 3 months. The only factor predicting a positive response was decreased cervical range of motion before the injection. EMG findings did not predict improvement. Fifty percent of the patients with neurologic findings had objective improvement in their signs. There were no complications.

Pawl and colleagues[46] studied whether injecting cervical epidural corticosteroids would diminish the need for surgical intervention for discogenic spondylosis. This study included approximately 100 patients with cervical syndrome who underwent epidural steroid injection. One-third of these patients ultimately underwent surgical intervention. One-third of the initial patients had radicular symptoms (upper extremity pain with weakness or paresthesia in a dermatomal pattern). In this group, 80 percent had more than 50 percent relief after treatment. The remaining one-third of patients in the study were characterized as having neck pain without radicular symptoms. In this group of patients who underwent epidural steroid injection, 50 percent noted a 50 percent improvement in their symptoms. However, if the patients who were in litigation were eliminated, 70 percent in this group noted improvement in their pain relief of 50 percent or more. It was concluded that cervical epidural steroid injections diminished the requirement for cervical surgery by 40 percent.

We may conclude, from a review of the preceding studies, that cervical epidural corticosteroid injection is a safe technique. In patients with chronic neck pain and symptoms that are radicular in nature, a response rate of approximately 70 percent can be expected. In patients with chronic neck pain that is not radicular in nature, a 50 percent response rate can be expected. After careful evaluation, in patients with chronic neck pain, cervical epidural steroids may be used to treat chronic pain before surgical intervention. They may diminish the requirement for surgical intervention.

SUMMARY

The causes of neck pain are many and varied. They may be self-limited and require little intervention or life-threatening and require immediate invasive action. A knowledge of the anatomy of the neck and a thorough history and physical examination are invaluable to the clinician who diagnoses and treats painful cervical conditions.

References

1. Pawl RP. Chronic neck syndromes. *Compr Ther* April 1990; 16(4):43–51.
2. Roseman DM. Carotidynia a distinct syndrome. *Arch Otolarygol* 1967; 85(1):81–84.
3. Rose VP, Veach JS, Tehranzdeh J. Spontaenous pneumomediastinum as a cause of neck pain, dysphagia, and chest pain. *Arch Intern Med* 1984; 144(2):392–393.
4. March JS. Rheumatoid neck. *Br J. Hosp Med* 1985; 33(2):96–100.
5. Sluijter ME, Koetsveld-Baart CC. Interruption of pain pathways in the treatment of the cervical syndrome. *Anaesthesia* 1980; 35:302–307.
6. Ehni G, Benner B. Occipital neuralgia and the C$_{1-2}$ arthrosis syndrome. *J Neurosurg* 1984; 61(5):961–965.

7. Bernstein SA. Acute cervical pain associated with soft tissue calcium deposition anterior to the interspace of the first and second cervical vertebrae. *J Bone Joint Surg* 1975; 57(3):426–428.

8. Wilson DS. Pain in the neck and arm. *Rheum Rehab* 1979; 18(3):177–180.

9. DeGowin E, DeGowin R. *Bedside Diagnostic Examination*. New York: MacMillan; 1981:206–210, 717–720.

10. Hoppenfeld S. Physical examination of the cervical spine and temporomandibular joint. In: Hoppenfeld S, ed. *Physical Examination of the Spine and Extremities*. New York: Crofts; 1976:106–127.

11. Ellis H, Feldman S. *Anatomy for the Anaesthetist*. Boston: Blackwell Scientific Publications; 1983:164–170.

12. Cailliet R. *Neck and Arm Pain*. Philadelphia: FA Davis Co; 1981.

13. Jackson R. Cervical trauma: Not just another pain in the neck. *Geriatrics* 1982; 37(4):123–126.

14. Nordemar R, Thorner C. Treatment of acute cervical pain—comparative group study. *Pain* 1981; 10:93–101.

15. Mealy K, Brennan H, Fenelon GCC. Early mobilization of acute whiplash injuries. *Br Med J* 1986; 292:656–657.

16. MacNab I. The whiplash syndrome in symposium on disease of the intervertebral disk. *Orthop Clin North Am* 1971; 2(2):389–403.

17. Cloward R. Acute cervical spine injuries. *Clin Symp* 1980; 32(1):4.

18. Silverman JL, Rodrigues AA, Agre JC. Quantitative cervical flexor strength in healthy subjects and in subjects with mechanical neck pain. *Arch Phys Med Rehabil* August 1991; 72(9)679–681.

19. Hohl M. Soft tissue injuries of the neck in automobile accidents. *J Bone Joint Surg* 1974; 56a(8):1675–1681.

20. Harris JH, Jr. Radiographic evaluation of spinal trauma. *Orthop Clin North Am* 1986; 17(1):75–86.

21. Gotten N. Survey of 100 cases of whiplash injury after settlement of litigation. *JAMA* 1956; 162:865.

22. Travell JG, Simons DG. *Myofascial Pain and Dysfunction. The Trigger Point Manual*. Baltimore: Williams & Wilkins; 1983.

23. Grosshandler S. Chronic neck and shoulder pain focusing on myofascial origins. *Postgrad Med* 1985; 77(3):149.

24. Byrn C, Borenstein P, Linder LE. Treatment of neck and shoulder pain in whip-lash syndrome patients with intracutaneous sterile water injections. *Acta Anesthesiol Scand* January 1991; 35(1):52–53.

25. Foley-Nolan D, Barry C, Coughlan RJ, O'Conner P, Roden D. Pulsed high frequency (27MJz) electromagnetic therapy for persistent neck pain. A double blind, placebo-controlled study of 20 patients. *Orthopedics* April 1990; 13(4):445–451.

26. Maxwell R. Surgical management of torticollis. *Postgrad Med* 1984; 75(7):147–155.

27. Kiwak K. Establishing an etiology for torticollis. *Postgrad Med* 1984; 75(7):129–138.

28. Spasmodic torticollis. *Br Med J* 1978; 2:786. Editorial.

29. Spasmodic torticollis. *Lancet* 1978; 2:301–302. Editorial.

30. Gilbert G. The medical treatment of spasmodic torticollis. *Arch Neurol* 1972; 27:503.

31. Ramamurthy S. Cervical pain. In: Raj P, ed. *Practical Management of Pain*. Chicago: Year Book Pub; 1986:426–428.

32. Lee C. Spasmodic torticollis and other idiopathic torsion dystonias. Medical management. *Postgrad Med* 1984; 7:139.

33. Jedynak CP, de Saint Victor JF. Treatment of spasmodic torticollis by local injections of botulinum toxin. *Rev Neurol* (Paris) 1990; 146(67):440–443.

34. Jeffries RV. Cervical spondylosis in persistent pain. In: Lipton S, ed. *Modern Methods of Treatment, 2*. New York: Grune & Stratton; 1980:115.

35. Brain L. Some unsolved problems of cervical spondylosis. *Br Med J* 1963; 1:771–777.

36. Nagata K, Kiyonaga K, Ohashi T, Sagara M, Miyazaki S, Inoue A. Clinical value of magnetic resonance imaging for cervical myelopathy. *Spine* November 1990; 15(11):1088–1096.

37. Rothman R. The acute cervical disc. *Clin Orthop* 1975; 109:59–68.

38. Schulman M. Treatment of neck pain with cervical epidural steroid injections. *Reg Anaesth* 1986; 2(2):92–94.

39. Warfield C, Biber M, Crews D, Nath DGK. Epidural steroid injection as a treatment for cervical radiculitis. *Clin J Pain* 1987; 3(1):13–15.

40. Ellis H, Feldman S. *Anatomy for the Anaesthetist*. Boston: Blackwell Scientific Publications; 1983:325, fig. 194.

41. Strandness DE, Jr. (1980) Vascular diseases of the extremities. In: Isselbacher AJ, Adams RD, Petersdorf RJ, Wilson JD, eds. *Harrison's Principles of Internal Medicine*. New York: McGraw-Hill; 1980:1185.

42. Aprill C, Dwyer A, Bogduk N. Cervical zygapophyseal joint pain patterns, II: a clinical evaluation, *Spine* June 1990; 15(6):458–461.

43. Boas R. Facet joint injections. In: Stanton-Hick M, Boas R, eds. *Chronic Low Back Pain*. New York: Raven Press; 1982.

44. Dory MA. Arthrography of the cervical facet joints. *Radiology* 1983; 149:379–382.

45. Rowlingson JC. Epidural analgesic technique in the management of cervical pain. *Anesth Analg* September 1986; 65(9):938–942.

46. Pawl RP, Anderson W, Shulman M. The effect of epidural steroids in the cervical and lumbar region on surgical intervention for discogenic spondylosis. In: Fields HL, ed. *Advances in Pain Research and Therapy, 9* New York: Raven Press; 1985:791–798.

CHAPTER 8

Chest Pain

Anthony M. Lin

Chest pain is a common chief complaint; its differential diagnosis remains challenging.[1] The importance of correctly diagnosing potentially lethal causes of chest pain, such as myocardial ischemia, is obvious. This chapter will review the more common causes of chest pain. Attention to detail in history taking and physical examination and a selective use of laboratory tests usually will guide the clinician to the correct diagnosis.[2,3]

Understanding the pathophysiology of chest pain is useful in its differential diagnosis. Pain is a warning that signals potential or actual damage to tissue. It usually is secondary to noxious stimuli that affect a specific organ system and transmit impulses to the brain by the peripheral nervous system.

Visceral pain (e.g., angina) is carried mostly by unmyelinated C fibers; somatic pain is transmitted by the much larger, myelinated, rapidly conducting A fibers. Thus, there is a qualitative difference between visceral and somatic pain. The latter tends to be sharp and well circumscribed, whereas the former often is dull, aching, and diffuse.

The sensory fibers of the heart are conducted by the superior, middle, and inferior cardiac nerve to the cervical and upper thoracic ganglia of the sympathetic chain (Fig. 8-1). In turn, these fibers enter the posterior roots at the T1 to T5 levels of the spinal cord. Other thoracic structures, such as the esophagus, aorta, mediastinum, and portions of the chest wall, have sensory nerves with the same general afferent distribution. The intercostal and phrenic nerves supply the pain fibers for the parietal pleura and the diaphragmatic surface of the parietal pericardium.

Visceral pain usually is referred to the dermatomes that send sensory fibers to the spinal roots that innervate the diseased organ (Fig. 8-2). The distribution of pain is thus segmental, in part, but it may affect only a portion of the segment or overflow into adjacent levels. For example, angina most often is felt in the T1 to T5 dermatomes, but it can radiate to the left arm in areas innervated by C8.

When a patient has chest pain, a complete history is mandatory. The following characteristics of chest pain always should be discussed in detail: location, quality, duration, frequency, radiation, aggravating or alleviating factors, depth and intensity, and associated symptoms and findings.[4]

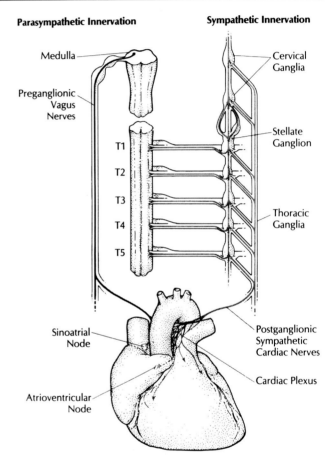

FIGURE 8-1. Pathways of sympathetic and parasympathetic innervation of the heart are traced. The heart's afferent sensory fibers pass through the sympathetic chain and enter the spinal cord in the upper thoracic posterior roots (T1 to T5). (Reproduced with permission from *Hosp Pract* 1989; 24(4):44. Illustration by Susan Tilberry.)

If the history and physical examination are equivocal, examination of the patient during an episode of chest pain may be diagnostic. For example, ECG changes seen during an episode of angina may be absent when the patient is pain free.

The clinician also may try to reproduce the pain. For example, pain from costochondritis usually is elicited by deep pressure over the affected area. A patient's response to medications also can be helpful in the differential diagnosis,

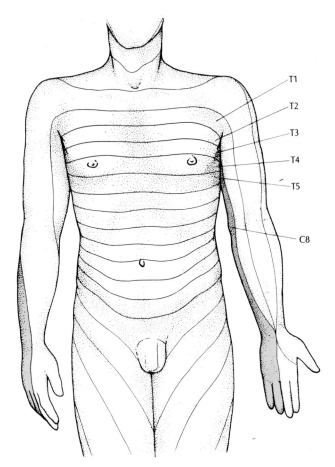

FIGURE 8-2. Segmental distribution of anginal pain is referred in a dermatomal pattern corresponding to the distribution of sensory fibers to the spinal roots that innervate the heart. Pain usually is felt in the T1 to T5 dermatomes but can radiate to the left arm in areas innervated by C8. (Reproduced with permission from *Hosp Pract* 1989; 24(4):47. Illustration by Susan Tilberry.)

for example, when pain from a peptic ulcer is relieved by antacids.

CARDIOVASCULAR CAUSES

Myocardial Ischemia

Angina occurs when the oxygen demand of the heart exceeds the supply, usually in the setting of coronary artery disease. Angina usually is felt retrosternally and may radiate to either arm or both, especially the ulnar aspect of the left arm (Fig. 8-3). It also can radiate to the anterior part of the neck or lower jaw. It rarely extends beyond the area between the epigastrium and lower jaw (C3 to T6). Atypical angina may be localized to the jaw and arm and mistaken for a dental or orthopedic problem. Angina rarely is so localized that it can be isolated using a finger to follow the pain course. Patients may use a clenched fist (Levine sign) to describe the quality of the pain.

Chest pain that radiates to the left arm is not specific for

angina. Nerve impulses from visceral and somatic structures converge in the spinal cord. Their origin could be confused by the brain. Thus, any disorder that stimulates the afferent fibers of the left upper thoracic region could cause pain in the left arm, chest, or both.

Angina often is described as a heavy pressure in the chest. The pain usually is deep and accompanied by diaphoresis, dyspnea, nausea, and vomiting when infarction has occurred. Precipitating factors include physical exertion, excitement, cold, and a postprandial state. Pain that is worsened by respiration or can be reproduced by direct pressure usually is not angina.

Angina generally lasts 1 to 30 min. Transient pain (less than 30 s) that resolves despite continued physical activity is unlikely to be angina. Pain that lasts longer than 30 min may suggest myocardial infarction or unstable angina. Relief within 1 to 3 min after administration of sublingual nitroglycerin is highly suggestive of angina, although cer-

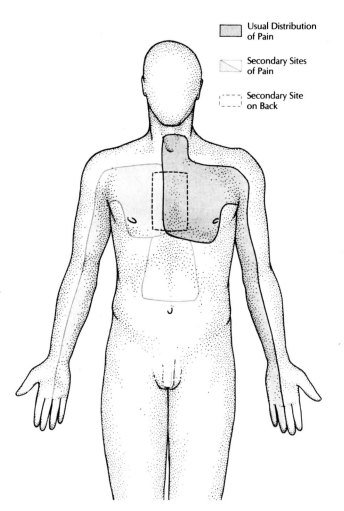

Usual Distribution of Pain

Secondary Sites of Pain

Secondary Site on Back

FIGURE 8-3. Myocardial ischemia produces anginal pain commonly felt in all or part of the sternal region, in the left side of the chest, in the neck, and down the ulnar side of the left arm. Other sites are sometimes involved, as shown. (Reproduced with permission from *Hosp Practr* 1989; 24(4):48. Illustration by Susan Tilberry.)

tain gastrointestinal disorders (e.g., esophageal spasm) also may respond to nitrates. During an angina attack, the ECG will show ST-segment depression but may revert completely within seconds after the resolution of pain.

Coronary artery spasm also can cause chest pain (Prinzmetal angina), with or without concomitant coronary artery disease. Such episodes are not necessarily related to physical exertion or increased myocardial oxygen demand. Nitroglycerin or calcium-channel blockers can produce prompt relief. ST elevation is seen on the ECG during the acute episode because a spasm may cause transmural myocardial ischemia. Provocative tests with ergonovine or cold pressors can be used to confirm the diagnosis of coronary artery spasm.

Pericarditis

The visceral pericardium is insensitive to pain. The parietal pericardium has no pain fibers except in the portion adjacent to the diaphragm. Pericardial pain usually is described as sharp, burning, and precordial. It may radiate from the diaphragmatic parietal pericardium, through the phrenic nerves, to the left shoulder. The pain typically is relieved when the patient sits and leans forward. Causes of pericarditis include infection, myocardial infarction, cardiotomy, trauma, collagen vascular disease, irradiation, uremia, and metastatic cancer. Physical examination may reveal a friction rub. The ECG typically shows ST elevation. A pericardial effusion may be present.

Aortic Dissection

Patients with dissecting aortic aneurysms often have chest pain. Anterior chest pain with radiation to the interscapular area is the typical pattern of presentation. Ascending aortic dissection frequently is associated with anterior chest pain; dissection of the descending thoracic aorta usually causes posterior chest pain. Patients with a history of hypertension, Marfan syndrome, cystic medial necrosis, and blunt chest trauma are at risk for aortic dissection. Physical examination may reveal a murmur of aortic regurgitation. Chest x-ray may show a widened mediastinum. Definitive diagnosis is made by aortography. Proximal dissections require emergency surgery. Dissections distal to the left subclavian artery may be managed with vasodilators and β-adrenergic blockers; surgery may be necessary if there is aortic rupture or compromise of vital organs.

Other Cardiovascular Causes

Idiopathic hypertrophic subaortic stenosis, mitral valve prolapse,[5,6] myocarditis, and aortic stenosis all can cause chest pain. More recently, cardiac-induced chest pain has been described after cocaine use.[7]

PULMONARY CAUSES

Chest pain may be present in various pleuropulmonary diseases. Most parenchymal lung disorders cause pain by involving the pleura (inflammation) and mediastinum. Obstructive lung diseases can cause chest pressure by overworking the accessory muscles of respiration. Pain of pleural origin usually is exacerbated by respiration as is pericardial and chest-wall pain. It is not surprising that certain cardiac and pleuropulmonary disorders are mistaken for each other.

Pleurisy

Inflammation of the pleura is a common cause of chest pain. The visceral pleura has no sensory innervation; pain arises from the parietal pleura. Intercostal nerves innervate the costal part of the parietal pleura and the lateral portion of the diaphragmatic pleura. The phrenic nerves innervate the central part of the diaphragm. Therefore, radiation to the ipsilateral shoulder may occur in pain caused by diaphragmatic pleurisy.

Pleural pain usually is unilateral and restricted in distribution. It tends to be located along intercostal nerve zones. It is usually severe, sharp, and burning and is exacerbated by deep breathing. Movement of the torso may aggravate the pain. Pleurisy may result from pulmonary infarction, pneumonia, cancer, asbestos exposure, and pneumothorax.[8] A rapid onset of pain at rest suggests a pneumothorax; a slower onset implies infectious causes. The development of pleurisy over weeks that is accompanied by constitutional symptoms suggests malignancy, tuberculosis, or connective tissue disease. A pleural rub may be found during the physical examination. Chest x-ray may reveal an associated pleural effusion.

Embolism

Massive pulmonary embolism can cause acute pulmonary hypertension, with substernal chest pain similar to angina. The mechanism of chest pain is unclear. It may result from the acute distension of the pulmonary artery or from right ventricular ischemia secondary to the acute rise in afterload. A smaller embolism usually causes pleuritic pain, probably as a result of pulmonary infarction and subsequent pleural inflammation. Dyspnea and tachycardia usually are present with pulmonary emboli. Chest pain may resolve quickly with anticoagulation therapy, but sometimes it persists for days. In the latter case, a chest x-ray may show an elevated hemidiaphragm and pleural effusion. ECG, ventilation–perfusion scans, and pulmonary angiography may be useful in the diagnosis of pulmonary emboli.

Mediastinal Disease

Mediastinitis and mediastinal tumors can result in dull poorly localized chest pain. Alcohol ingestion often can cause acute chest pain in patients with mediastinal Hodgkin lymphoma. Chest x-rays will help confirm the presence of mediastinal disease.

Pneumomediastinum can be caused by pneumothorax, acute airway obstruction, or a Valsalva maneuver during labor. The resultant pain is substernal or precordial and can radiate to the jaw, neck, and arm. Dyspnea usually occurs. A Hamman sign (a crunching sound over the precordium) may be present. Chest x-ray may show air in the subcutaneous tissue and the mediastinum.

GASTROINTESTINAL CAUSES

Pain arising from the gastrointestinal tract, especially from the esophagus, can be confused with angina.[9,10]

Esophagus

Substernal chest pain often is esophageal in origin, and it is caused by reflux, motility disorders, infection, cancer, or connective tissue disease (especially the syndrome of calcinosis, Raynaud phenomenon, esophageal dysmotility, sclerodactyly, and telangiectasia associated with scleroderma).[11] Esophageal pain usually is felt in areas innervated by C7 to T12.

Heartburn is the result of esophageal reflux of gastric acid. It is a burning retrosternal pain that can be severe especially after meals and when the patient is recumbent. It typically is relieved by antacids. Pain may occur because of the direct toxic actions of the gastric acid on nerve endings in the esophageal mucosa and secondary esophageal spasm. Endoscopy may show reflux esophagitis. Upper intestinal studies may reveal a hiatal hernia and associated reflux. Provocative testing also may be useful.[12,13]

Heavy chest pressure with meals or physical exertion also can be caused by esophageal spasm. It can mimic angina so closely that nitroglycerin or calcium-channel blockers may relieve the pain. Useful studies include barium radiography and esophageal manometry. The former may show disorganized contractions if recorded cinegraphically. Manometry may show repeated and abnormal contractions of high amplitude; it is diagnostic if the pain occurs during the study. Esophageal spasm may be the result of a number of disorders, including achalasia.[14]

Gallbladder

Biliary colic usually is caused by passage of a stone or biliary dilation secondary to obstruction from a stone or cancer. It often is felt over the right upper quadrant or epigastrium, but sometimes it can be retrosternal or radiate to the right shoulder. After an acute attack, residual soreness may persist for days. Fever and jaundice may help in the differential diagnosis.

Pancreas

The pain of pancreatitis usually is epigastric, with radiation to the back, but it sometimes can be substernal in location. The pain frequently is intermittent but may become constant with time. It often decreases when the patient sits leaning forward with the trunk flexed and knees drawn up. ST and T-wave changes may be present on the ECG and confuse the clinical diagnosis. A history of alcohol abuse or gallstones may be helpful in differentiating pancreatic pain from other causes of chest pain.

Peptic Ulcer

Peptic ulcer pain also can mimic angina. It may be a burning gnawing ache or just a vague discomfort in the epigastrium or the lower chest. Typically, it is postprandial, usually starting 1 to 2 h after meals. It can be differentiated from angina by a response to antacids, no response to nitrates, and the absence of ECG changes during an acute episode. Endoscopy and an upper gastrointestinal series are useful in confirming the diagnosis.

Liver or Spleen

Inflammation of the liver or spleen can cause subcapsular swelling and pain that radiates to the diaphragmatic pleura. The splenic flexure syndrome is marked by left upper quadrant discomfort; this may radiate to the left shoulder. The pain is the result of gaseous distension of the descending colon with secondary diaphragmatic irritation.

SKELETAL CAUSES

Disorders of the thoracic skeleton are common causes of chest pain. Pain caused by diseases of the ribs and costal cartilage usually occurs anterolaterally. Pain that involves the spine usually is posterior, but it also can radiate anteriorly.

Rib Fracture

Trauma and metastatic cancer are common causes of rib fracture. The more exposed fourth to eighth ribs especially are prone to fracture from an impact with a steering wheel. Pneumothorax, hemothorax, and cardiac tamponade are potential complications. Chest pain caused by a rib fracture frequently is aggravated by breathing, coughing, or bending. The diagnosis can be made by physical examination (point tenderness, swelling, or crepitus) and chest x-rays. Splinting after a fractured rib can compromise respiration. TENS, intercostal nerve blocks, epidural anesthesia, and parenteral analgesics are used to decrease splinting in patients at high risk for respiratory insufficiency.

Costochondritis

Pain and tenderness of the costochondral junction are common. This pain usually is described as dull and gnawing. The most common sites of involvement are the second, third, and fourth cartilages. Costochondritis should not be confused with Tietze syndrome; the latter is marked by painful noninflammatory swelling of one or more costochondral junctions. Single joints often are affected, and multiple joint involvement tends to be unilateral. The syndrome typically develops gradually, but its onset sometimes may be acute. Point tenderness usually can be elicited.

Injection with local anesthetics and corticosteroids may provide pain relief. Excision rarely is necessary. Analgesics and physical therapy are sometimes useful.

Xiphoiditis

Chest pain that can be reproduced by palpation of the xiphoid process is called xiphoiditis or xiphodynia. It is uncommon and may be related to costochondritis. The pain usually is felt as a deep retrosternal ache that may radiate to the epigastrium or precordium. Overlapping of cardiac afferents and xiphoid nerves explains the clinical resemblance to angina pectoris. In xiphoiditis, however, the pain can be elicited easily with pressure over the xiphoid process. Nonsteroidal anti-inflammatory drugs and TENS have been used. Surgery rarely is necessary.

Osteoarthritis

Cervical and thoracic osteoarthritis can be confused with angina pectoris. The pain arises as a result of nerve root compression from narrowed neural foramina and is referred to dermatomes innervated by the affected nerves. It usually is bilateral and extends in a dermatomal distribution across the back. Some patients may feel a substernal component (so-called cervicoprecordial angina) with radiation to the arms, neck, or jaw.

The pain may have the pressure-like quality that typifies angina. Cervical symptoms usually are present but may be minimal. Activities involving the upper torso and arms and prolonged sitting or lying can precipitate the pain. It often can be reproduced by palpation of posterior trigger points. Radiographic studies show osteoarthritis. Treatment includes traction and anti-inflammatory medication. If conservative treatment fails, laminectomy may be necessary.

Other skeletal causes of chest pain include primary rib tumors, infections of the chest wall, and osteoporosis (which may result in fracture or collapse of the thoracic vertebrae).

MUSCULAR CAUSES

Strain of the accessory thoracic muscles can result in chest pain that may radiate to the shoulder and arm. It can be confused with angina. Contractile muscle tissues are subject to daily use and can develop trigger points. Pain from a myofascial trigger point is aching, constant, and deep.[15] Affected muscles often have a decreased range of motion. Palpation of the trigger point can elicit the painful symptoms and muscle spasm. Treatment includes muscle relaxation, stretch-and-spray therapy, injections with local anesthetics with or without corticosteroids, TENS, and the use of nonsteroidal anti-inflammatory drugs.

NEUROLOGIC CAUSES

Intercostal Neuralgia

There are many causes of intercostal neuralgia. This is associated with a superficial tenderness or ache along an intercostal nerve. Herpes zoster and postherpetic neuralgia are the most common. In addition, metastatic and spreading tumors of the thoracic cavity and postthoracotomy scars can entrap intercostal nerves and result in severe pain in the distribution of the nerve. Intercostal nerve blocks with local anesthetics, alone or in combination with corticosteroids, may be helpful in entrapment syndromes. Trauma to the chest wall is another cause of intercostal neuralgia.

Herpes Zoster (See Chap. 21)

Herpes zoster occurs when dormant varicella viruses become activated in the dorsal root ganglion. Unilateral pain spreads and intensifies along one or more thoracic dermatomes for several days after onset. After the rash appears, the diagnosis can be made easily. A band of hyperesthesia and the dermatomal distribution are helpful in the differential diagnosis before the appearance of the telltale rash. The pain usually will disappear in weeks, but it may persist in some patients (especially those who are elderly or immunocompromised) as postherpetic neuralgia. In this disorder, the pain persists in a dermatomal pattern long after the vesicular eruption has healed. Postherpetic neuralgia occurs in approximately 10 percent of patients with herpes zoster.

Treatment of herpes zoster is directed toward early resolution of the infection and prevention of postherpetic neuralgia. Management includes drug therapy (antiviral agents and analgesics), sympathetic nerve blocks (for prevention), and psychosocial and physical therapy. Postherpetic neuralgia is difficult to treat. Tricyclic antidepressants, anticonvulsants, and phenothiazines have been tried with inconsistent results. Infiltration of the painful region with corticosteroids and local anesthetics has been beneficial in some patients. TENS and sympathetic or somatic nerve blocks with local anesthetics also have been tried. Neurosurgery is a possibility when the patient is disabled by the pain; dorsal root entry zone lesions are advocated by some physicians.

OTHER CAUSES

Painful scars can occur after thoracic surgery. They cause a characteristic pain syndrome that usually persists for at least 2 months after the procedure. There is a continuous aching or burning sensation, often extending beyond the scar. In addition, there is sensory loss and absence or sweating along the scar. Temperature, touch, pressure, and emotional factors can aggravate the pain. The appearance of the scar is not significant. Smooth scars can be painful, and indurated scars can be painless. Histologic examination shows a chaotic formation of neural elements; neuromas may be present. The pain has been attributed to imperfect nerve regeneration. TENS, analgesics, antidepressants, anticonvulsants, local infiltration of anesthetics and corticosteroids, and nerve blocks have been used with varying success. Many patients have undergone scar resection with no pain relief. Delayed chest pain also may occur as a result of sternal wire sutures.[16,17]

Chest pain may be felt after extensive breast surgery, such as radical mastectomy. Patients usually have a burning pain in the axilla and upper chest; this may radiate to the medial part of the arm. The pain probably is secondary to the transection of the intercostobrachial nerve. Postmastectomy pain rarely lasts longer than 3 months after surgery. Some patients may have chronic pain after mastectomy. This pain frequently is in a nonanatomic area on the anterior chest wall and is extremely sensitive to touch.

Panic disorder, depression, and other psychiatric maladies also may be manifested as chest pain.[18-22]

References

1. Ott DJ, Abernethy WB, Chen MY, Wu WC, Gelfand DW. Radiologic evaluation of esophageal motility: results in 170 patients with chest pain. *AJR Am J Roentgenol* November 1990; 155(5):983–985.

2. McCroskery JH, Schell RE, Sprafkin RP, Lantinga LJ, Warner RA, Hill N. Differentiating anginal patients with coronary artery disease from those with normal coronary arteries using psychological measures. *Am J Cardiol* March 15, 1991; 67(7):645–646.

3. Amin M, Gabelman G, Karpel J, Buttrick P. Acute myocardial infarction and chest pain syndromes after cocaine use. *Am J Cardiol* December 15, 1990; 66(20):1434–1437.

4. Carney RM, Freedland KE, Sapira JD, Jaffe AS. Panic disorder and depression in patients with chest pain not due to coronary artery disease. *Am J Cardiol* April 15, 1990; 65(15):1048. Letter.

5. Cattau EL Jr. Noncardiac chest pain evaluation: clearing the air or more smoke? *Am Gastroenterol* July 1991; 86(7):920–921.

6. Cheng TO. Etiology of chest pain in mitral valve prolapse. *Am J Med* July 1991; 91(1):103. Letter.

7. Carney RM, Freedland KE, Ludbrook PA, Saunders RD, Jaffe AS. Major depression, panic disorder, and mitral valve prolapse in patients who complain of chest pain. *Am J Med* December 1990; 89(6):757–760.

8. Cannon RO III, Cattau El Jr, Yakshe PN, et al. Coronary flow reserve, esophageal motility, and chest pain in patients with angiographically normal coronary arteries. *Am J Med* March 1990; 88(3):217–222.

9. Bassotti G, Pelli MA, Morelli A. Clinical and manometric aspects of diffuse esophageal spasm in a cohort of subjects evaluated for dysphagia and/or chest pain. *Am J Med Sci* September 1990; 300(3):148–51.

10. Eastridge CE, Mahfood SS, Walker WA, Cole FH Jr. Delayed chest wall pain due to sternal wire sutures. *Ann Thorac Surg* January 1991; 51(1):56–59.

11. Fine PG, Karwande SV. Sternal wire-induced persistent chest pain: a possible hypersensitivity reaction. *Ann Thorac Surg* January 1991; 49(1):135–136.

12. Bensard DD, St. Cyr JA, Johnston MR. Acute pleuritic chest pain and lung mass in an elderly woman. *Chest* June 1990; 97(6):1473–1474.

13. Dalton CB, Hewson EG, Castell DO, Richter JE. Edrophonium provocative test in noncardiac chest pain. Evaluation of testing techniques. *Dig Dis Sci* December 1990; 35(12):1445–1451.

14. Browning TH. Diagnosis of chest pain of esophageal origin. A guideline of the Patient Care Committee of the American Gastroenterological Association. *Dig Dis Sci* March 1990; 35(3):289–293.

15. Katon WJ. Chest pain, cardiac disease, and panic disorder. *J Clin Psychiatry* May 1990; 51(suppl):27–30; discussion 50–53.

16. Roll M, Kollind M, Theorell T. Clinical symptoms in young adults with atypical chest pain attending the emergency department. *J Intern Med* September 1991; 230(3):271–277.

17. Richter JE. Practical approach to the diagnosis of unexplained chest pain. *Med Clin North Am* September 1991; 75(5):1203–1208.

18. Brand DL, Beck JG, Wielgosz AT. Unexplained chest pain. Future directions for research. *Med Clin North Am* September 1991; 75(5):1209–1218.

19. Bradley LA, Scarinci IC, Richter JE. Pain threshold levels and coping strategies among patients who have chest pain and normal coronary arteries. *Med Clin North Am* September 1991; 75(5):1189–1202.

20. Eagle KA. Medical decision making in patient with chest pain. *N Eng J Med* May 2, 1991; 324(18):1282–1283. Editorial.

21. Pearce MJ, Mayou RA, Klimes I. The management of atypical non-cardiac chest pain. *Q J Med* September 1990; 76(281):991–996.

22. Pellegrino MJ. Atypical chest pain as an initial presentation of primary fibromyalgia. *Arch Phys Med Rehabil* June 1990; 71(7):526–528.

CHAPTER 9

Low Back Pain

John C. Rowlingson

Low back pain is a common malady, but effective treatment is not always available. The practitioner must have a holistic attitude when evaluating patients with complaints of low back pain because musculoskeletal structures of the back rarely operate alone in producing the pain. The evaluation protocol must be thorough and systematic because the differential diagnoses are numerous and no laboratory test is available that can quantify the patient's pain.[1] A diagnosis that encompasses both the physical qualities of the pain and its impact on the patient's self-perception, lifestyle, social relationships, and ability to work must be made. Appropriate treatment will follow only after this has been achieved. The distinction between acute and chronic pain will guide the choice of treatment options. In general, the pain can be decreased with medications, surgery, nerve blocks, and/or counterstimulation techniques. As the pain's frequency and intensity are reduced, recommendations can be made for corrective or restorative physical therapy. Additional lifestyle and vocational restoration may require psychotherapeutic interventions to aid the patient in coping with the residual pain and interacting with the compensation–disability systems. The patient must become active in the treatment program and acknowledge that, when the pain is chronic in nature, simply removing the pain will not be the answer to all pain-related problems.

The facts and figures that document the prevalence of low back pain are impressive.[2–10] Data show that 80 percent of the American population has had a back injury at some time during their lives, low back pain is second only to the common cold as a cause of disability from work in people younger than 55 years of age, and low back pain is second only to headaches as a chronic pain problem. In general, low back pain complaints are common and, by implication, extremely costly because of the health-care funds used, days lost from work, money spent per injury, and percentage of disability and workmen's compensation funds required.[11] For example, although only 7.4 percent of patients with low back pain in the Quebec Task Force on Spinal Disorders study did not improve, this group accounted for 75 percent of the money spent on back pain.[12]

Pain is so pervasive in life; however, low back pain remains difficult to treat effectively. Because pain specialists are becoming increasingly involved in the management of patients with acute and chronic pain, it is extremely likely that patients with complaints of low back pain will be referred to them. These specialists should understand the anatomy of the low back, the rationale for the thorough evaluation scheme for patients with low back pain, and the reputable treatments available. To help decrease the disproportionate share of health-care costs that low back pain demands, more effective intervention must be provided earlier in the course of the disease. Most low back episodes will end in less than 2 months.[13,14] Anesthesiologists can contribute abundantly to pain management, not only because of their ability to provide temporary decreases in pain by regional anesthetic procedures, but equally because of their familiarity with the pharmacology of analgesic and adjunctive drugs, the neuroanatomy of pain pathways, and the high quality patient interaction skills that reflect a sensitivity to both the physical and nonphysical aspects of the patient's being.

EVALUATION OF THE PATIENT WITH LOW BACK PAIN

Low back pain is a classic pain problem because the differential diagnosis for such complaints is lengthy and definitive proof of every complaint is not feasible. Complaints of low back pain often reflect changes in the musculoskeletal structures of the lumbosacral area, but other causes must be excluded by the patient's workup.[15] As Keim and Kirkaldy-Willis[16] succinctly note in their monograph, other causes of low back pain include congenital disorders, tumors (benign and malignant), heavy metal poisoning, metabolic disorders, inflammatory disease, degenerative disease, infectious disease, circulatory disorders, intrinsic and extrinsic mechanical disorders, and psychoneurotic problems. There also can be referred pain; trauma; genitourinary, gastrointestinal, or gynecologic pain; and postsurgical scarring.[3,17–19]

Pain specialists most frequently play a consultant role when dealing with the patient who has low back pain. The primary physician frequently does the preliminary workup of the patient, and a reasonable diagnosis will have been established. It is important that the patient's relevant records be reviewed before the clinical evaluation of the patient actually occurs. This provides the physician with an evolutionary outline of the patient's complaint and allows for a more structured and less random interview. Because of the many differential diagnoses for low back pain, the evaluation scheme must be thorough and systematic.[20] Although pain specialists may not have the time or office capability to assure this, they must be satisfied that the workup is proceeding in a logical progressive way. Record review will help to document this and validate the patient's history, indicate past physical changes, detail the results of diagnostic laboratory testing, and recount past treatments.

In any patient with a complaint of pain, the specific history of the onset, site, character, and quality of the pain; the factors that make it better or worse; and the degree of activity interference must be elicited.[21] Also the history of response to past therapies, whether medical, surgical, rest, or whatever, should be obtained. The general medical history of the patient will be critical also, not only in light of the many differential diagnoses of low back pain, but also because other medical conditions may influence the patient's complaints.

As the duration of the pain increases, the important differences between acute and chronic pain become significant.[22,23] The clinician must be concerned enough to investigate the psychosocial aspects and other consequences of the patient's complaints of chronic pain.[24,25] There can be significant nonphysical factors that influence the patient's descriptions of and reactions to pain.[26] Unless a complete diagnosis is made, including all physical and nonphysical components of the pain, appropriate comprehensive therapy is not as likely to be recommended. The practitioner is advised to follow the example of pain centers by using standardized questionnaires and forms to elicit the historic information in an organized consistent manner.

A physical examination of the patient is mandatory.[25] This will correlate the pain complaints with anatomic possibilities; help identify nerve, muscle, bone, and vessel disorders; and contribute to making the proper diagnosis. In patients whose complaints are more chronic in nature, the examination will substantiate earlier findings or reveal progression or regression of the disease. These patients can have physical changes over time, especially given the likelihood of cumulative trauma to the low back secondary to a stressful posture. Physical examinations done serially can be useful in documenting improvement, or lack thereof, with treatment.

The standardized neurologic examination will elicit changes in vascular, sensory, motor, and reflex activity in the lower extremities. A musculoskeletal examination will assess the range of motion of the low back (flexion and extension and straight leg raising supine and seated) and hip or leg joints, shortening of and/or spasm in muscles, muscular trigger points, and postural changes, such as those associated with scoliosis or changes in lumbar lordosis. Physical assessment also must include a functional review, that is, the patient's ability to walk, stand, sit, and bend. As in history taking, standardized forms that guide the accumulation of these data are beneficial. We must be aware that the contemporary physical workup of patients

with chronic pain includes sophisticated functional assessment of the patient's aerobic capacity, trunk strength, lifting power, mobility, elasticity, and endurance.[27]

Laboratory tests may or may not supplement the information gained from history taking and physical examination.[28] The results of these investigations will be significant to the anesthesiologist because nerve block intervention frequently can be applied when there is a focal disorder, but we must know where the problem is located to achieve the best results. All practitioners should acknowledge that there are no diagnostic laboratory tests for every cause of low back pain.[15,27] Thus, we must avoid the temptation to conclude that negative laboratory test results imply there is no pain. As will be discussed later, many common causes of musculoskeletal low back pain involve structures that are not tested by the routine of x-rays, EMG, myelogram, and CT scan.

Plain posteroanterior and lateral x-rays of the lumbosacral spine will reveal anatomic changes, such as transitional vertebrae (found in 5 percent to 7 percent of the population), bony tumors, compression fractures, scoliosis, and disk space narrowing.[16,29,30] Oblique x-rays are needed to reveal spondylosis and spondylolisthesis. Myelography can detail disk herniation and nerve root compression, although false-positive and -negative results are possible.[15] CT scans may replace the need for this. They provide a versatile noninvasive method for assessing the relationship of lumbosacral structures to the neural elements.[31] Magnetic resonance imaging probably will continue to improve the accuracy of diagnosis in the future.[32] EMG studies complete the thorough neurologic examination and help differentiate acute from chronic changes.[33,34] Thermography is a diagnostic imaging technique whose specific place in pain evaluation currently is not clarified[35,36] (see Chap. 4). There are many criteria that contribute to the validity of this test. At least the technique is not invasive, has only a 5 percent to 8 percent false-negative rate, and could be used as a screening test.

Even with this high technology, all pain cannot be documented by laboratory testing. In addition, positive results on these tests do not necessarily explain the patient's pain complaints. Given the increasing financial constraints on reimbursement, all physicians must be sensitive to the cost of medical care. No one should duplicate diagnostic tests needlessly, expecting that laboratory studies can prove the presence of pain. Only those tests that would change the course of referral or treatment should be ordered, especially in patients with chronic pain. Patients who have had surgery in the lumbar area present a greater challenge because any findings must be interpreted in light of postsurgical alterations in anatomy.[37]

In patients with persistent (chronic) complaints of low back pain, an additional realm of assessment must be the nonphysical or psychosocial one.[10,24,26,38] Some patients have the tendency to manifest psychological conflict through physical complaints. Physical pain can disrupt more than just the patient's physical capabilities. It markedly can affect the quality of the patient's life, and this has an impact on the whole family socially and economically.[3] Relationships between employers and workers deteriorate as a result of absences from work and uncertainty about returning to work.[39] Strang[10] showed that patients with chronic low back pain who are receiving compensation are more likely to have had work-related events causing their pain, litigation pending, vague diagnostic and objective findings, more resistance to conservative therapy, greater medical and compensation costs, and lower likelihood of returning to work. Thus, the presence or absence of these nonphysical factors must be identified in the workup of the patient.

ANATOMIC CONSIDERATIONS

A brief review of the functional musculoskeletal anatomy of the low back area will help the practitioner understand more readily the common causes of low back pain for which consultation is sought. In normal posture, the anterior vertebral column is the main weight-bearing structure of the low back.[40] The disks that are interposed between the vertebral bodies allow for shock absorption, flexibility, and motion. In the lumbar spine, the disks account for one-third of the total height of the spine; in the other vertebral column sections, they account for only one-fifth of the total height.[7] The disk is composed of a viscous liquid center surrounded by a tough fibrous anulus. This is thinnest in its posterior portion, and this finding may explain the likelihood of posterior herniation of the disk when forces are applied unevenly or suddenly to the spinal column. Also the posterior longitudinal ligament thins in the L2–L5 area, also allowing posterior herniation. As people age, the disks lose some of their resiliency and become less capable of evenly distributing the mechanical forces applied with activity.[40] Eighty-five percent of herniated disks occur at the L4–5 and L5–S1 levels.[7]

The posterior elements of the spine include the lamina, pedicles, and facet joints. They form the protective circular arch for the spinal cord and emerging nerve roots. These structures impose restrictions on the range of the motion of the spine and serve as anchors for muscles, ligaments, and tendons. The intervertebral foramina formed by the pedicles and the apposition of the facets allow for the exit of the spinal nerves. Usually the nerve root fills 35 percent to 50 percent of the foraminal volume.[40] The paraspinal muscles (semispinalis, multifidus, and quadratus lumborum) act on the spine to provide posture, motion, and support. Disruptions in the coordination of musculoskeletal activity can prevent the spine from being in an optimal position for lifting, bending, or twisting, and an injury can result.

Only 1 percent to 2 percent of patients with low back pain have disk herniation. Far more common (80 percent to 90 percent of patients) is postural low back pain. This suggests that disturbed posture contributes to the patient's complaints. As outlined by Cailliet,[40] the following changes occur: the lumbar lordotic curve is increased secondary to pain and reflex muscle spasm, the weight-bearing function is transferred from the anterior spine (vertebral bodies) to the posterior elements, the facet joints are stressed, the sheer forces on the disks (especially in the posterior axis) are increased, the intervertebral foramina may be compromised, and the nerve roots may be impinged. The main sites of origin of low back pain are listed as the posterior longitudinal ligament, the interspinal ligaments, the nerve roots and their dural coverings, the facet joints, and the deep muscles. We must keep these structures in mind when considering the positive and negative results of routine laboratory tests that are obtained with the hope of identifying the cause of the patient's pain complaint.

CHARACTERISTICS OF COMMONLY REFERRED CASES

Most patients with low back pain have postural back pain. These strains and sprains of the low back area are a direct result of injury to the supporting muscles and ligaments. Frequently, the patient will have diffuse low back pain limited to the lumbosacral area and describe the pain as dull and aching. There are no complaints of radiating pain, although some pain into the buttocks or toward the hip can occur. The physical examination is unrevealing except for possible tenderness over the sacroiliac joints and paraspinal muscle spasm associated with subsequent stiffness on range-of-motion testing. Laboratory assessment usually does not reveal the cause of the pain. Patients with degenerative joint disease may have similar symptoms although their diagnosis suggests some baseline disorder of the facet joints in addition to the postural changes.

Patients with acute disk syndromes frequently have a positive history for a specific event (lifting in a bent and twisted stance) that started their low back pain. Often the pain is sharp and shooting in character. The pain follows dermatomal pathways into the lower extremity and is decreased when the patient lies down. The patient may have typical changes on neurologic examination, and straight leg raising (and even sitting) will reproduce complaints of radicular pain. Those with the combination of positive straight leg raising, crossed straight leg raising, and bowstring sign have the three signs most indicative of radicular low back pain.[15] Paraspinal muscle spasm may be marked and range of motion limited. Maneuvers that increase intraabdominal pressure (straining during bowel movement or coughing) may exacerbate the pain. Laboratory studies may show nerve root compression. Patients with metastatic disease may have acute radicular pain related to tumor infiltration of nerve roots[41] or bony invasion that causes structural faults such as compression fractures that allow the nerve root impingement. Hypertrophic changes of the vertebral margins and facet joints (associated with osteoarthritis of the spine) also may result in radicular pain. Spinal stenosis is said to be present when there is fibrous and bony proliferation of the disk and the protective bony arch of the spine on a chronic basis.[42]

After lumbar laminectomy with or without fusion procedures, a certain percentage of patients will continue to have complaints of low back pain. Often these patients with postlaminectomy syndrome have diffuse ill-defined residual low back pain that is dull and aching in character. Occasionally, episodes of sharper pain occur. The pain is not localized in the low back area but commonly involves the hips, buttocks, or upper posterior thighs. Their physical examination findings will be confused by residual neurologic changes from the earlier surgery, but frequently they reveal various sensory changes, loss of reflex, and muscle weakness. Flexibility of the lumbar spine usually is diminished, as is hip motion and straight leg raising, secondary to muscle spasm. Laboratory studies are problematic because positive findings must be discriminated from residual effects from earlier studies and surgery.

TREATMENT CONCEPTS

With a bout of acute low back pain, the patient's expectation is that the onset of pain symptoms will result in evaluation and then treatment that, at least, reduces, but more likely eliminates, the pain. The fundamental treatment options in the management of acute pain are medications (narcotics, non-narcotics, and adjuncts), surgery, nerve blocks, and stimulation techniques. The goal is rapid elimination of the pain symptoms and restoration of normal function. When the patient's complaints of pain are chronic (arbitrarily defined as pain of longer than 6 months' duration in the past, but now the time frame is 7 weeks), the realistic goals of treatment are different from those for acute pain. There may be valid structural reasons why the pain cannot be eliminated totally (e.g., soft tissue scarring, nerve root fibrosis, or bony derangement). Furthermore, chronic pain, by its very nature, implies the probable presence of numerous nonphysical factors that can modify the description of the pain, the patient's tolerance for it, or ability to cope with it. Thus, the treatment program for chronic pain first aims to decrease the frequency and intensity of the patient's pain. When this begins to occur, less consideration should be given to surgical solutions for the pain, less potent medications will be required, and the patient can be encouraged to participate in a physical rehabilitative program plus therapy that helps to provide insight into the intense interaction of the physical and nonphysical components.

Many patients with low back pain complaints will benefit from conservative therapy. A review of the literature, looking at the components of conservative therapy, did not demonstrate conclusively the efficacy of these treatments.[43] However, Nachemson[44] reported that 70 percent of patients with discogenic low back pain and sciatica obtained relief of symptoms in 3 weeks with conservative therapy and that 90 percent of such patients had relief in 2 months. Conservative therapy is a generic term that includes many treatments but excludes the surgical therapy. Initially, such a program aims to rest the low back. Bed rest or at least diminished activity (time off from work or temporary discontinuation of strenuous physical activities) will be recommended. The inclination for rest may be reinforced by the use of potent analgesic drugs and indirect muscle relaxants, many of which have mild-to-moderate sedative qualities, depending on the dose prescribed. Physical therapy (ultrasound, diathermy, whirlpools, TENS, or massage) may be included as additional components of the program when the patient is comfortable enough to travel to the treatment or arrangements are made for their application at home. Eventually, a progressive return to activity is allowed as the pain subsides. Deyo and Diehl[43] reported that the patient's satisfaction with the care they received for back pain was related directly to the quality of the explanation they were given.

The pain specialist may be asked to evaluate patients with low back pain at any time during their illnesses. Patients may be referred with acute symptoms related to disk herniation or strain or sprain injuries of longer duration. The patient's recovery may not be progressing with conservative therapy, and consultation may be sought before surgical options are explored. Alternatively, the patient may progress to chronic low back pain syndrome, in which the physical disease is magnified by the patient's psychological, social, and occupational considerations.

Depending on the time, interest, and knowledge of the pain specialist, many options for pain management can be offered to the patient. In general, we try to decrease the pain with judicious medication programs, various regional analgesic procedures, and counterstimulation techniques. When pain reduction begins, specific recommendations are made about physical rehabilitation. In all patients, encouragement and verbal support will enhance their progress and compliance. Some, especially those with chronic pain syndrome, may need frequent supportive therapy and even formal psychotherapy. The ultimate goal of treatment is rehabilitation to a functional life style that includes normal levels of social interaction and occupational pursuits. Many patients will require a program of treatment that is based on a coordination of therapies that each provides an additive effect in achieving the overall desired result. The Quebec Task Force on Spinal Disorders suggests that, after 3 months of conservative therapy or accumulated time lost from work as a result of low back pain, the patient should be referred to a multidisciplinary pain center.[12]

TREATMENT OPTIONS

Medications

Much has been written about the use of medications in the management of pain.[45–51] When we consider the ready availability, the ease of use, the variety, and simplicity of medications, it is easy to understand why their prescription is so prevalent. The problem with medication use is that, for this approach to be most effective, we must know what the cause of the pain complaint is. For instance, aspirin and the other nonsteroidal anti-inflammatory drugs (NSAIDs) have potent anti-inflammatory properties. If the patient's complaints of low back pain probably are based on inflammatory changes in musculoskeletal structures, an anti-inflammatory drug (such as aspirin) should be prescribed. Furthermore, the patient must be compliant with the recommended therapy to guarantee an adequate clinical trial. There are many NSAIDs to try. When patients cannot tolerate aspirin or other NSAIDs because of gastrointestinal upset, fluid retention, or renal insufficiency, acetaminophen is an alternate drug choice. However, we must recognize that this drug lacks the potent anti-inflammatory action of the NSAIDs and, therefore, may not be as effective in reducing the pain. Tables with equianalgesic doses of drugs commonly prescribed are published elsewhere[47,50] (see Chap. 26). Most nonnarcotic analgesics offer the advantages of low cost, lack of synergistic physiologic depressive effects, ready availability, and nonaddictiveness.

Because reflex muscle spasm may complicate low back pain, many patients will receive indirect muscle relaxants. Familiar drugs include cyclobenzaprine, methocarbamol, and combinations. Baclofen is a neuronal depressant reported recently to be safe and effective in 30 to 80 mg/day doses.[52] Many of these drugs have sedative side effects. Thus, caution must be taken when prescribing them for ambulatory patients who are working and driving or in patients already receiving other sedative drugs.

In patients with the acute onset of severe musculoskeletal low back pain or those with chronic pain who have a flare-up of pain above their usual baseline, the need for narcotic medications may arise. The tendency to underprescribe these medications secondary to exaggerated fears about the side effects has been well documented.[47,53,54] The physician prescribing these drugs must ensure that they are given in doses that achieve the desired effect and that the doses are not constrained by arbitrarily set limits. When the medications are so used for periods of 7 to 21 days, either the patient will begin to improve (and the medications can and should be reduced and eliminated) or the pain will persist and additional workup is recommended to identify the cause of the severe pain for which the drug trial has not been effective.

It is common practice to attempt to augment the analgesics with adjunctive drugs so that the overall dose can be reduced and the side effects minimized or eliminated (see Chap. 26). Such drugs as hydroxyzine, promethazine, doxepin, amitriptyline, and trazodone are common choices.[55–57] These drugs can be used, not only in combination with the narcotic analgesics, but also frequently, they are recommended as adjuncts to nonnarcotic drugs. The prolonged use of sedative–hypnotic drugs such as the benzodiazepines in patients with chronic pain is not desirable because of the potential for physical dependence and the antalgesic effect associated with central nervous system serotonin depletion.

If potent medications are prescribed in effective doses for short periods of time (days), the expectation is that prolonged use will not be necessary because the episode of pain will be terminated or at least the pain reduced to such a level that potent medications no longer are indicated. Some of the rationale for using adjunctive medications is based on manipulating endogenous analgesic systems. For instance, anatomic, physiologic, and pharmacologic studies have shown that serotonin is important in the ascending and descending pathways of neural transmission involved with pain.[57,58] The tricyclic antidepressants act pharmacologically by blocking the reuptake of norepinephrine and serotonin, and they can enhance analgesia at doses not associated with an antidepressant effect and faster than such an effect would occur.[59]

As the complaints of pain become more chronic in nature, there is a diminishing likelihood that a simple pharmacologic solution to the problem will be found. In chronic conditions, all problems secondary to pain cannot be treated satisfactorily by drug use. As the medications that may be effective in managing acute pain continue to be used, patients can develop tolerance (narcotics) or achieve a ceiling effect (NSAIDs). The doses of such medications then may be increased with the hope of reestablishing effectiveness, but most commonly, the patient suffers drug-related side effects. Thus, medications to treat the side effects are added, and the patient is at risk of having symptoms secondary to ill-advised (e.g., sedative drugs used with other sedative drugs) or illogical (narcotics with narcotic agonist–antagonist drugs) drug combinations. Many times, patients with complaints of chronic pain will benefit by detoxification from most of the drugs they are using. This is reasonable because a careful history will reveal long trials of drug use (weeks to months) with no decrease in pain and only drug-related effects as a result of drug use.

Surgery

The pain specialist may be consulted about patients who have surgically accessible lesions but who choose to try all nonsurgical methods of pain management before undergoing an operation. Alternatively, the patients referred may have had a surgical procedure, but the pain persists or returns. Operative intervention in the management of low back pain is certainly an option in these patients. Because surgery is an invasive technique, a specific diagnosis is necessary, and both the patient and the surgeon must have a realistic expectation of such an approach. Before surgical intervention, the workup must identify the structural and mechanical cause of the pain (e.g., herniated disk, spondylolisthesis, foraminal encroachment on nerve roots, or pseudoarthrosis).

Given the limitations of even the most sophisticated diagnostic laboratory techniques,[27] we still cannot be certain which herniated disk needs surgery and which does not.[60] Lumbar laminectomy frequently is used in patients who do not respond to full conservative therapy, in those with foraminal encroachment on nerve roots, and in those with progressive neurologic deficits. Waddell and associates[61] studied surgical outcomes in patients with low back pain after industrial injuries. They showed that 97 percent of patients receiving compensation after laminectomy had some persistent complaints of pain and 72 percent reported some continued impairment of function. As the complaints become more chronic and factors other than tissue damage contributed to the pain, surgical solutions become inadequate. Plasticity and neuron recruitment are compensatory mechanisms of the nervous system that attempt to overcome pain system interruption; they may cause more pain ultimately.[19]

Chymopapain injection of disks has been resurrected in recent years as an alternative method to surgery (*not* to conservative therapy) for relieving nerve root compression by herniated disk material.[3,60,62] Most workups do not indicate reliably in a routine manner those patients for whom this is the treatment of choice. This is not a benign treatment because life-threatening anaphylactoid reactions and other complications have been reported.[63] There may be irregular distribution of the chymopapain in the disk after injection; therefore, successful results range between 59 percent and 90 percent.[3]

Nerve Blocks

Anesthesiologists have the unique skills to provide regional analgesic procedures. These techniques can be used in a diagnostic fashion (for instance, in differential neural blockade) to help identify the cause of the patient's pain,[64,65] (see Chap. 4) or more commonly, they are used therapeutically. At all times, the absolute contraindications to regional anesthesia must be remembered so that these techniques are not used in patients who are inappropriate to receive such therapy. The anesthesiologist must decide whether the relative contraindications (such as doing nerve blocks on patients with active neurologic disease, for example, acute herniated disk or in those receiving drugs with anticoagulant properties, such as NSAIDs) preclude intervention with invasive regional analgesic techniques. We must not compromise the potential advantages of therapeutic nerve blocks by basing their use on an incomplete data base, using faulty technique, or showing a lack of discretion in applying regional procedures. Being technically capable of doing a nerve block *is not* an indication for its use.

There are many procedures to choose, and the specific type of nerve block is determined by the diagnosis.[66] One of the most common techniques advocated for use in selective patients with complaints of low back pain is that of epidural corticosteroid injection (see Chap. 29). There is a long evolutionary history of the development of this technique. Briefly, irritation of primarily neural structures (but perhaps other structures such as musculoskeletal) in the lumbar spine suggests the presence of inflammation.[67–69] Thus, corticosteroids, as potent anti-inflammatory drugs, can play a beneficial role in the management of pain secondary to these inflammatory changes.[70]

Additional mechanisms for low back pain, especially those occurring after surgery, have been suggested recently. Loeser[19] proposed that some of the persistent low back pain may result from injury to the peripheral nerves or nerve roots. Damage in the nervous system can trigger changes in neuronal activity and central modulation of afferent input and efferent output; it can encourage neuroma formation. Experimental evidence indicates that corticosteroids may suppress abnormal discharges in neuromas. Therefore, the pain relief after epidural injections thought secondary to reduction of inflammatory conditions may be too simplistic a conclusion.[71] The concept of using intraspinal narcotics in patients with complaints of low back pain is too new to have its proper place and efficacy documented at this time.[72–74]

Although the subarachnoid injection of depot corticosteroids has been advocated in the past for treating radiculopathy,[75,76] the technique is less popular now. Mechanically, the compression and irritation of nerve roots occur in the epidural space and not in the subarachnoid space; therefore, the placement of the drug is more exact when epidural injection is used. Few patients with the diagnosis of arachnoiditis really have inflammatory changes in the arachnoid membrane; instead, they have scarring. Abram[77] showed a poor response rate in patients given subarachnoid triamcinolone diacetate, and recent reviews provide additional discouragement of such use of these drugs.[78–80]

Other less commonly used regional anesthetic techniques are paravertebral,[81,82] lumbosacral fascia,[83] and transsacral blocks.[84] These procedures are most useful when the pain is away from the midline or the midline–paramedian approach for the injection of the drug bolus is precluded by earlier surgery or traumatic changes. These techniques place the drug distal to the intervertebral foramen and count on retrograde diffusion to produce a clinical result.[85–87]

A final form of nerve block therapy is related to treating trigger points[88,89] (see Chap. 19). These are discrete areas in muscles or their connective tissue that are exquisitely painful to palpation and seem to initiate some of the patient's pain. Biochemically, they are areas of focal ischemia that result when pain causes reflex muscle and vascular spasm. They may be the primary source of the patient's complaints, but more commonly, they occur in patients with chronic low back pain from prolonged imbalances in posture. Abnormal posture occurs in such patients secondary to the pain causing the muscle spasm and fatigue; over time, this results in a transfer of mechanical stress to areas of the muscle not capable of handling it.

Trigger points may be identified in the paraspinal muscles in the thoracolumbar area. Pain over the sacroiliac joints may be treated as a trigger point as can pain in the sciatic notch that is associated with the piriformis syndrome.[90,91] Patients with piriformis syndrome may have peripheral complaints consistent with sciatica because the piriformis muscle directly overlies the sciatic nerve in its course through the pelvis. However, these patients usually do not have concurrent complaints of low back pain. Careful history taking usually will elicit that the patient's pain seems to originate in a consistent area, and then, as the day progresses and muscles fatigue from persistent spasm, the pain begins to spread. Physical examination usually will identify the trigger areas. Infiltration injection with local anesthetic, Sarapin (High Chemical, Philadelphia, PA), and occasionally, corticosteroids may be beneficial, especially when used in conjunction with active physical therapy.

Stimulation Procedures

We all have used the stimulation concept in treating pain. When we suck our thumbs after hitting them with hammers or rub our shins after getting kicked, there is an augmentation of sensory input beyond that initiated by the hammer strike or kick. Melzack and Wall[92] proposed the gate-control theory in 1965.[92] Basically, this hypothesis states that small pain fibers (C or A-delta) bring in sensory information from the periphery to the central nervous system and that this input can be modified if larger faster transmitting fibers (A-alpha or A-beta) are excited.

Methods to stimulate the nervous system, such as dorsal column stimulation and epidural stimulation, have been advocated.[93] However, they are invasive and lack the simplicity and practicality of TENS. If we were to list the positive features of a pain treatment, our list would be similar to these characteristics of TENS: noninvasive, simple enough for home use and without a formal therapist (after an orientation session), basically without age restrictions, not interfering with other treatments, having no systemic side effects, being patient controlled, and using the body's own endogenous mechanisms (at least in part) for handling pain.

TENS units readily are available by prescription from medical-supply houses, physical-therapy departments, and commercial health-care outfits. The patient must be instructed in the proper use of the machine. The pain may not be reduced but the pain-induced reflex muscle spasm may be interrupted. If the patient has less muscle fatigue and improved range of motion from TENS, they are more likely to cooperate with the recommendations about improving muscle tone and strength and overall function.

Physical Rehabilitation

Relief from back pain is a primary goal of treatment. A secondary objective that is the need to keep the patient comfortable enough to cooperate with recommendations made about rehabilitative physical therapy and exercise prescription. Even during episodes of low back pain when the patient is bedridden for just a few weeks (and certainly when the period of disability is longer), there are physical and emotional changes in the patient. The enforced inactivity and disruption of the patient's routine may provoke anxiety, despair, anger, agitation, frustration, or depression. In addition, the patient can lose muscular tone and strength, have joint range-of-motion compromises, develop inflexible postures, and gain weight. These consequences of chronic pain also must be reversed because attention is directed at the patient's ultimate rehabilitation. Unfortunately, the brief time spent with the patient during most follow-up visits is dominated by descriptions of pain and primary treatment of it. Little consideration may be given to the patient's functional status. Thus, the patient's faulty physical condition persists, and the emotional ravages linger.

It is routine to recommend exercise to improve the patient's overall fitness.[2,3,6,7,9,16–18,34,94] There have been long battles not yet won as to which exercises are best for a given patient, although pelvic tilt and knee-to-chest maneuvers have been traditional. A generic prescription is not likely to be the answer. A formal physical therapy assessment, especially in more chronic cases, is recommended strongly. In addition to providing a proper assessment, the patient will receive instruction when the exercises are demonstrated and cannot pretend ignorance of what to do.[95] Follow-up by the physical or exercise therapist will provide an indication of the patient's motivation for and compliance with the therapeutic program.

The fundamental principle is that all patients with musculoskeletal low back pain need regular daily exercise that restores muscular tone, strength, coordination, and endurance to the groups that are operative in the mechanical function of the lumbar spine.[96] Thus, not only muscles in the paraspinal group (semispinalis, multifidus, or quadratus lumnorum), but also the anterior abdominal wall, gluteal, hamstring, iliopsoas, and rectus femoris muscles must be considered. If the patient's workup has revealed that the ongoing pain does not imply ongoing tissue damage, then pain is not necessarily a reason to stop or avoid activity. When the patient begins to stretch and use muscles long rested, generally, the pain will increase. However, in most cases, this muscle soreness subsides in a few weeks. Gradually, the patient finds that more activity is possible with less pain or at least with no major increase above the baseline. Patients must be cautioned not to assume that the activities of daily living substitute for exercise.

A method of encouraging the patient's rehabilitation that has become popular in recent years is the concept of back school programs.[34,97] In general, these involve educational components that teach the patient about the anatomy and function of the low back; demonstrations that highlight proper body mechanics for lifting, bending, and sitting; practice sessions that emphasize correct performance of exercise; and encouragement and support from the group nature of the program. Basically, the patients are encouraged to adopt an active self-care philosophy rather than act as passive recipients of treatment. Research must document that back school programs can decrease the cost of back injuries and/or decrease the incidence of back injuries before industry fully will support such programs.

Regardless of the formal program provided for a patient, the most important component is the patient's doing the exercises at home and gradually increasing their number, frequency, and difficulty. In terms of behavior modification, having the patient exercise to a given quota of repetitions rather than to the point of pain is crucial. On a temporary basis, selective patients may benefit from back braces or other orthotic devices. As Wilensky[34] observed, orthotics can decrease pain and provide protection against additional injury, aid in early rehabilitation when muscles are weak, and correct deformities. However, prolonged reliance on a back brace or cane can result in muscle atrophy, posture abnormality, continued weakness in muscles, loss of motivation for complete rehabilitation, and soft tissue contracture.

Psychological Strategies

All pain, whether it is acute or chronic, provokes a concurrent emotional response. In the evaluation, the exact emotional reaction must be identified and considered during treatment. Pain can occur without positive laboratory confirmation of its cause, and the absence of an obvious physical cause for pain does not necessarily imply the presence of a psychological one.[98] The extraphysical aspects of a patient's pain problem will be handled according to the doctor's interest, knowledge of the options for management, and the local professional resources.

In acute low back pain, in which anxiety is likely to dominate the patient's physical presence, antianxiety agents such as the benzodiazepines play a definite role. Their main function is as sedatives rather than true muscle relaxants, but this quality is beneficial to reinforce bed rest and reduce muscle spasm. On a prolonged basis, the benzodiazepines are not beneficial because the anxiety does not linger, the drugs are associated with physical dependence and undesirable side effects, an antalgesic effect mediated by decreasing serotonin may arise, and they impair the patient's ability to cooperate fully with rehabilitative efforts.

The use of versatile psychotherapeutic techniques in low back pain management can be beneficial. In selected patients, nonmedication approaches, such as biofeedback, self-regulation techniques, or hypnosis, can be used to control anxiety, muscle tension, and spasm. Many acute episodes of low back pain are over before these techniques can be learned and applied. However, patients with chronic low back pain who have a flare-up above their baseline may be helped. In patients with chronic low back pain and failed low back syndrome, psychotherapeutic interventions more likely are offered as coping strategies.[99,100] That is, when the patient acknowledges that some part of their chronic low back pain will not disappear no matter what treatment is provided, reality dictates that the residual pain must be tolerated. Psychotherapeutic techniques give the patient the perception of having some degree of control over the pain and encourage daily functions despite residual pain.[101]

Rehabilitation

The ultimate goal of treatment in patients with low back pain is to return them to their full productive lives.[102] In general, the sooner their complaints of pain are handled effectively, the greater will be the likelihood that this lofty objective can be achieved.[103] Unfortunately, as the pain becomes more chronic and more unmeasurable influences modify the perception of pain, there are impediments for many patients to achieve a functional return to their social contacts with family and community life, let alone their occupational pursuits.[5,10,24,104]

By and large, the pain specialist will not be involved in this aspect of the patient's care, but rather will recommend a therapeutic plan to the patient's primary physician. Many professionals have difficulty in determining exactly who is disabled and to what degree, what the patient can do and should be expected and allowed to do, and what compensation they should receive. Carron and associates[105] showed that having a less fulfilling compensation system (as in New Zealand), resulted in patients with low back pain using the compensation and disability system less and for shorter periods of time and suffering less life-style disruptions than similar patients in the United States.[105] Catchlove and colleagues[106] showed that workmen's compensation patients who participated in directed return-to-work programs were more successful in returning to work, used fewer compensation benefits, and required less additional treatment for pain.[106]

The implications are clear. Improvements must be made in the disability–compensation system to make it more equitable, productive, and successful.[5,12–14] The pain specialist's major role in this issue is to be available to evaluate and treat patients with low back pain, hoping that early intervention can have positive results and minimize disability–compensation issues.

References

1. Borenstein D. Low back pain: epidemiology, etiology, diagnostic evaluation, and therapy. *Curr Opin Rheumatol* April 1991; 3(2):207–217.
2. Addison RG. Chronic low back pain (CLO-BAP). *Clin J Pain* 1985; 1:50–59.
3. Belkin S. Back pain. In: Aronoff GM, ed. *Evaluation and Treatment of Chronic Pain.* Baltimore-Munich: Urban & Schwarzenberg; 1985:333–350.
4. Bonica JJ. The nature of the problem. In: Carron H,

McLaughlin RE, eds. *Management of Low Back Pain.* Littleton, MA: John Wright-PGS Inc; 1982:1–15.

5. Carron H. Compensation aspects of low back claims. In: Carron H, McLaughlin RE, eds. *Management of Low Back Pain.* Littleton, MA: John Wright-PSG Inc; 1982:17–26.

6. Deyo RA. Conservative therapy for low back pain. *JAMA* 1983; 250:1057–1062.

7. Finneson BE. *Low Back Pain.* 2nd ed. Philadelphia: Lippincott; 1981.

8. Grazier KL, Holbrook TL, Kelsey JL, Stauffer RN. *The Frequency of Occurrence, Impact, and Cost of Musculoskeletal Conditions in the United States.* Chicago: American Academy of Orthopaedic Surgeons; 1984.

9. MacNab I. *Backache.* Baltimore: Williams & Wilkins; 1977.

10. Strang JP. The chronic disability syndrome. In: Aronoff GM, ed. *Evaluation and Treatment of Chronic Pain.* Baltimore-Munich: Urban & Schwarzenberg; 1985:603–623.

11. Frymoyer JW, Cats-Baril WL. An overview of the incidences and costs of low back pain. *Orthop Clin North Am* April 1991; 22(2):263–271.

12. Quebec Task Force on Spinal Disorders. Scientific approach to the assessment and management of activity-related spinal disorders. *Spine* 1987; 12(7S):S16.

13. National Institute for Disability and Rehabilitation Research on Acute Low Back Pain. Report on workshop on low back pain. September 1989; Charlottesville, VA.

14. Roland M, Morris R. A study of the natural history of back pain. *Spine* 1983; 2:145–150.

15. McCulloch JA. Differential diagnosis of low back pain. In: Tollison CD, ed. *Handbook of Chronic Pain Management.* Baltimore: Williams & Wilkins; 1989:335–336.

16. Keim HA, Kirkaldy-Willis WH. Low back pain. *Clin Symp* 1980; 32(6):6–28.

17. Flor H, Turk DC. Etiological theories and treatments for chronic back pain, I: somatic models and interventions. *Pain* 1984; 19:105–121.

18. Gross D. Multifactorial diagnosis and treatment for low back pain. In: Bonica JJ, Liebeskind JC, Albe-Fessard DG, eds. *Advances in Pain Research and Therapy, 3.* New York: Raven Press; 1979:671–724.

19. Loeser JD. Pain due to nerve injury. *Spine* 1985; 10:232–235.

20. Rowlingson JC, Tooney TC. Multidisciplinary approaches to the management of chronic pain. In: Ghia JN, ed. *The Multidisciplinary Pain Center.* Boston: Kluwer Academic Publishers; 1988:45–73.

21. Vukmir RB. Low back pain: review of diagnosis and therapy. *Am J Emerg* July 1991; 9(4):328–335.

22. Hobbs WR, Yazel JJ. Psychological aspects. In: Carron H, McLaughlin RE, eds. *Management of Low Back Pain.* Littleton, MA: John Wright-PSG Inc; 1982:69–89.

23. Rowlingson JC, Stehling L. Anesthesia update #10. The evaluation and treatment of the patient with chronic pain. *Orthop Rev* 1982; 11:79–85.

24. Follick MJ, Smith TW, Ahern DK. The Sickness Impact Profile: a global measure of disability in chronic low back pain. *Pain* 1985; 21:67–76.

25. Naliboff BD, Cohen MJ, Swanson GA, Bonebakker AD, McArthur DL. Comprehensive assessment of chronic low back pain patients and controls: physical abilities, level of activity, psychological adjustment and pain perception. *Pain* 1985; 23:121–134.

26. Abram SE, Anderson RA, Maitra-D'Cruze AM. Factors predicting short-term outcome of nerve blocks in the management of chronic pain. *Pain* 1981; 10:323–330.

27. Frymoyer JW. Back pain and sciatica. *N Eng J Med* 1988; 318:291–299.

28. McCowin PR, Borenstein D, Wiesel SW. The current approach to the medical diagnosis of low back pain. *Orthop Clin North Am* April 1991; 22(2):315–325.

29. Frymoyer JW, Newberg A, Pope MH, et al. Spine radiographs in patients with low-back pain. *J Bone Joint Surg Am* 1984; 66–A(7):1048–1055.

30. Morris JL. Radiologic evaluation. In: Carron H, McLaughlin RE, eds. *Management of Low Back Pain.* Littleton, MA: John Wright-PSG, Inc; 1982:107–147.

31. Kieffer SA, Cacayorin ED, Sherry RG. The radiologic diagnosis of herniated lumbar intervertebral disk. *JAMA* 1984; 251(9):1192–1195.

32. Modic MT, Ross JS. Magnetic resonance imaging in the evaluation of low back pain. *Orthop Clin North Am* April 1991; 22(2):283–301.

33. Sanders DB. Electromyography in diagnosis. In: Carron H, McLaughlin RE, eds. *Management of Low Back Pain.* Littleton, MA: John Wright-PSG Inc; 1982:91–99.

34. Wilensky J. Physiatric approach to chronic pain. In: Aronoff GM, ed. *Evaluation and Treatment of Chronic Pain.* Baltimore-Munich: Urban & Schwarzenberg; 1985:199–230.

35. LeRoy PL, Christian CR, Filasky R. Diagnostic thermography in low back syndromes. *Clin J Pain* 1985; 1:4–13.

36. Newman RI, Seres JL, Miller EB. Liquid crystal thermography in the evaluation of chronic back pain: a comparative study. *Pain* 1984; 20:293–305.

37. Byrd SE, Cohn ML, Biggers SL, et al. The radiographic evaluation of the symptomatic postoperative lumbar spine patient. *Spine* 1985; 10(7):652–660.

38. Turk DC, Herta F. Etiological theories and treatments for chronic back pain, II: psychological models and interventions. *Pain* 1984; 19:209–233.

39. Feuerstein M, Sult S, Houle M. Environmental stressors and chronic low back pain: life events, family and work environment. *Pain* 1985; 22:295–307.

40. Cailliet R. Low back pain. In: Cailliet R, ed. *Soft Tissue Pain and Disability.* Philadelphia: FA Davis Co; 1977:41–106.

41. Mehta M. The nature of cancer pain. In: Mehta M, ed. *Intractable Pain.* London: Saunders; 1973:129–130.

42. Haglund MM, Schumacher JM, Loeser JD. Spinal stenosis: an annotated bibliography. *Pain* 1988; 35:1–37.

43. Deyo RA, Diehl AK. Patient satisfaction with medical care in low-back pain. *Spine* 1986; 11:28–30.

44. Nachemson AL. The lumbar spine. An orthopedic challenge. *Spine* 1976; 1:59–71.

45. Amadio P Jr. Peripherally acting analgesics. *Am J Med* 1984; 77(3A):17–26.

46. Huskisson EC. Non-narcotic analgesics. In: Wall PD, Melzack R, eds. *Textbook of Pain.* New York: Churchill Livingstone; 1985:505–513.

47. Inturissi CE. Role of opioid analgesics. *Am J Med* 1984; 77(3A):27–37.

48. Khoury GF. Therapeutic use of pain relieving drugs in chronic pain patients. *Semin Anesth* 1985; 4(4):300–304.

49. Monks R, Merskey H. Psychotropic drugs. In: Wall PD, Melzack R, eds. *Textbook of Pain.* New York: Churchill Livingstone; 1985:526–537.

50. Stimmel B. Pain, analgesia and addiction: an approach to the pharmacologic management of pain. *Clin J Pain* 1985; 1(1):14–22.

51. Twycross RG. Narcotics. In: Wall PD, Melzack R, eds. *Textbook of Pain.* New York: Churchill Livingstone; 1985:514–525.

52. Dapas F, Hartman SF, Martinez L, et al. Baclofen for the treatment of acute low-back syndrome. *Spine* 1985; 10(4):345–349.

53. Marks RM, Sachar EJ. Undertreatment of medical inpatients with narcotic analgesics. *Ann Intern Med* 1973; 78:173–181.

54. Porter J, Jick H. Addiction rare in patients treated with narcotics. *N Engl J Med* 1980; 302:123.

55. Atkinson JH, Kremer EF, Garfin SR. Psychopharmacological agents in the treatment of pain. *J Bone Joint Surg Am* 1985; 67–A:337–342.

56. Feinmann C. Pain relief by antidepressants: possible modes of action. *Pain* 1985; 23:1–8.

57. Kanner R: Psychotropic drugs in the management of pain. *Curr Concepts Pain* 1983; 1(2):11–15.

58. Rosenblatt RM, Reich J, Dehring D. Tricyclic antidepressants in treatment of depression and chronic pain: analysis of the supporting evidence. *Anesth Analg* 1984; 63:1025–1032.

59. Clifford DB. Treatment of pain with antidepressants. *Am Fam Physician* 1985; 31:181–185.

60. Watts C. Spinal surgery. In: Tollison CD, ed. *Handbook of Chronic Pain Management.* Baltimore: Williams & Wilkins; 1989:317–319.

61. Waddell G, Kummel EG, Lotto WN, et al. Failed lumbar disk surgery following industrial injuries. *J Bone Joint Surg Am* 1979; 61:201–207.

62. Javid MJ, Nordby EJ, Ford LT, et al. Safety and efficacy of chymopapain (Chymodiactin) in herniated nucleus pulposus with sciatica. *JAMA* 1983; 249:2489–2494.

63. Moss J, Roizen MF, Nordby EJ, et al. Decreased incidence and mortality of anaphylaxis to chymopapain. *Anesth Analg* 1985; 64:1197–1201.

64. Ghia JN, Toomey TC, Mao W, et al. Towards an understanding of chronic pain mechanisms: the use of psychological tests and a refined differential spinal block. *Anesthesiology* 1979; 50:20–25.

65. Ramamurthy S, Winnie AP. Regional anesthetic techniques for pain relief. *Semin Anesth* 1985; 4(3):237–246.

66. Rowlingson JC. Appropriate use of therapeutic nerve blocks. In: Tollison CD, Kriegel ML, ed. *Interdisciplinary Rehabilitation of Low Back Pain.* Baltimore: Williams & Wilkins; 1989:63–73.

67. Benzon HT. Epidural steroid injections in low back pain and lumbosacral radiculopathy. *Pain* 1986; 24:277–295.

68. McCarron RF, Wimpee MW, Hudkins PG, et al. The inflammatory effect of nucleus pulposus. A possible element in the pathogenesis of low-back pain. *Spine* 1987; 12:760–764.

69. Hakelius A. Prognosis in sciatica: a clinical follow-up of surgical and non-surgical treatment. *Acta Orthop Scand Suppl* 1970; 129:1–73.

70. El-Khoury GY, Renfrew DL. Percutaneous procedures for the diagnosis and treatment of lower back pain: diskography, facet-joint injection, and epidural injection. *Am J Roentgenol* October 1991; 157(4):685–691.

71. Devor M, Govrin-Lippman R, Raber P. Corticosteroids suppress ectopic neural discharge originating in experimental neuromas. *Pain* 1985;22:127–137.

72. Dallas TL, Lin RL, Wu WH, Wolskee P. Epidural morphine and methylprednisolone for low back pain. *Anesthesiology* 1987; 67:408–411.

73. Rocco AG, Frank E, Kaul AF, Lipson SJ, Gallo JP. Epidural steroids, epidural morphine and epidural steroids combined with morphine in the treatment of post-laminectomy syndrome. *Pain* 1989; 36(3):297–303.

74. Auld AW, Maki-Jokela A, Murdoch M. Intraspinal narcotic analgesic in the treatment of chronic pain. *Spine* 1985; 10(8):777–781.

75. Winnie AP, Hartmann JT, Meyers HL Jr, et al. Pain Clinic, II: intradural and extradural corticosteroids for sciatica. *Anesth Analg* 1972; 51:990–1002.

76. Sehgal AD, Tweed DC, Gardner WJ, et al. Laboratory studies after intrathecal corticosteroids. *Arch Neurol* 1963; 9:64–68.

77. Abram SE. Subarachnoid corticosteroid injection following inadequate response to epidural steroids for sciatica. *Anesth Analg* 1978; 57:313–315.

78. Bernat JL. Intraspinal steroid therapy. *Neurology* 1981; 31:168–171.

79. Kepes ER, Duncalf D. Treatment of backache with spinal injections of local anesthetics, spinal and systemic steroids. A review. *Pain* 1985; 22:33–47.

80. Nelson DA. Danger from methylprednisolone acetate therapy by intraspinal injection. *Arch Neurol* 1988; 45:804–806.

81. Carron H, Korbon GA, Rowlingson JC. *Regional Anesthesia: Techniques and Clinical Application.* New York: Grune & Stratton, Inc; 1984:28–29.

82. Moore DC. *Regional Block.* Springfield, IL: Charles C. Thomas; 1975:206–210.

83. Cailliet R: Low back pain. In: Cailliet R, ed. *Soft Tissue Pain and Disability.* Philadelphia: FA Davis Co; 1979:83.

84. Carron H, Korbon GA, Rowlingson JC. *Regional anesthesia: techniques and clinical applications.* New York, Grune & Stratton, Inc; 1984:64–66.

85. Carron H, Korbon GA, Rowlingson JC. *Regional Anesthesia: Techniques and Clinical Applications.* New York: Grune & Stratton, Inc; 1984:142–144.

86. Cailliet R. Low back pain. In: Cailliet R, ed. *Soft Tissue Pain and Disability.* Philadelphia: FA Davis Co; 1979:95–97.

87. Destouet JM, Murphy WA. Lumbar facet block indications and technique. *Orthop Rev* 1985; 5:280–288.

88. Goldenberg DL. Fibromyalgia syndrome: an emerging but controversial condition. *JAMA* 1987; 257:2782–2787.

89. Graff-Radford SB. Myofascial pain: an overview. *Semin Anesth* 1985; 4(4):281–286.

90. Cailliet R. Low back pain. In: Cailliet R, ed. *Soft Tissue Pain and Disability*. Philadelphia: FA Davis Co; 1979:99–100.

91. Wyant GM. Chronic pain syndromes and their treatment, III: the piriformis syndrome. *Can Anaesth Soc J* 1979; 26:305–308.

92. Melzack R, Wall PD. Pain mechanisms: a new theory. *Science* 1965; 150:971–979.

93. North RB. Neural stimulation techniques. In: Tollison CS, ed. *Handbook of Chronic Pain Management* Baltimore: Williams & Wilkins; 1989:136–146.

94. Sikorski JM. A rationalized approach to physiotherapy for low-back pain. *Spine* 1985; 10(6):571–579.

95. Linton SJ, Bradley LA, Jensen J, et al. The secondary prevention of low back pain: a controlled study with follow-up. *Pain* 1989; 36:197–207.

96. Koes BW, Bouter LM, Beckerman H, Van der Heijden GJ, Knipschild PG. Physiotherapy exercises and back pain: a blinded review. *BMJ* June 29 1991; 302(6792):1572–1576.

97. Grimes D, Bennion D, Blush K, Duncan ME. Back school—teaching patients to love their backs. *Residents Staff Phys* May 1980:60–68.

98. Giddon DB, Rabinovitz SL. The psychological aspects of treatment of chronic pain patients. *Reg Anesth* 1980; 5(3):16–23.

99. Hobbs WR, Yazel JJ. Psychological management. In: Carron H, McLaughlin RE, eds. *Management of Low Back Pain*. Littleton, MA: John Wright-PSG Inc; 1982:181–187.

100. Krishnan KRR, France RD, Pelton S, McCann UD, Davidson J, Urban BJ. Chronic pain and depression, II: symptoms of anxiety in chronic low back pain patients and their relationship to subtypes of depression. *Pain* 1985; 22:289–294.

101. Beekman CE, Axtell L, Noland SK, West JY: Self-concept: an outcome of a program for spinal pain. *Pain* 1985; 22:59–66.

102. Oland G, Tveitan G. A trial of modern rehabilitation for chronic low-back pain and disability. Vocational outcome and effect of pain modulation. *Spine* April 1991; 16(4):457–459.

103. Wigley RD, Carter N, Woods J, Ahuja M, Couchman KG. Rehabilitation in chronic pain: employment status after four years. *N Z Med J* January 24 1990; 103:9–10.

104. Cats-Baril WL, Frymoyer JW. Identifying patients at risk of becoming disabled because of low back pain. The Vermont Rehabilitation Engineering Center predictive model. *Spine* June 1991; 61(6):605–607.

105. Carron H, DeGood DE, Tait R. A comparison of low back pain patients in the United States and New Zealand: psychosocial and economic factors affecting severity of disability. *Pain* 1985; 21:77–89.

106. Catchlove R, Cohen K: Effects of a directive return to work approach in the treatment of workmen's compensation patients with chronic pain. *Pain* 1982; 14:181–191.

CHAPTER 10

Abdominal Pain

Yvona Trnka

Despite recent technologic advances, the diagnosis and treatment of chronic recurrent abdominal pain remains a challenge. Pain is a subjective sensation that patients often find difficult to describe. By contrast with other areas of the body, the abdominal organs have relatively poorly developed sensory systems that also may contribute to the patient's difficulty when trying to describe and localize the pain. The purpose of pain is to protect the organ and the patient from injury. After the source of the pain is found, every effort should be made to control the pain. In chronic pancreatitis or diffuse malignancy, for example, pain control may become as much a challenge as in instances where no underlying cause can be found.

For a patient to perceive pain, the autonomic nervous system must be intact; the anatomy and physiology of pain have been described in detail in previous chapters. Abdominal organs are relatively insensitive to many stimuli compared with a sensitive organ such as the skin. In addition to the relative paucity of sensory nerve endings, several viscera may be innervated by the same group of nerves. Therefore, pain patterns are not well differentiated, either as to the location of the pain or the cause of the pain. Nevertheless, there are some recognizable pain patterns, and a careful history often can lead to the correct diagnosis.

Abdominal pain can be classified as visceral,[1] somatic, or referred pain. The latter can be explained easily by our knowledge of the segmental distribution of the spinal nerves. The pain can be referred to remote areas of the body if they are supplied by branches of the same spinal nerve. In addition, the pain may spread cranially to adjacent segments. Lower lobe pneumonia may be associated with severe upper abdominal pain and even some associated guarding; this is the most frequently used example of referred pain.

DIAGNOSIS

Superficial abdominal pain can be differentiated easily by the patient; it usually is caused by a local process in the abdominal wall.[2] Pain over the xiphoid or costal margins that is exacerbated by movement or touch often is attributable to costochondritis, a form of arthritis that usually responds to appropriate therapy with anti-inflamatory agents or intraarticular injections. Sharp burning pain near a recently healed incision may indicate nerve irritation from surgical transection, entrapment in the healing tissue, or regeneration with neuroma formation. Pain originating in the abdominal wall frequently can be obliterated (and thus diagnosed) by blocking the appropriate intercostal or paravertebral nerves. Block of the celiac plexus can be helpful in differentiating abdominal wall or genitourinary pain from intraabdominal visceral pain because the plexus supplies all abdominal viscera except the rectum, sigmoid, bladder, and reproductive organs.

The more common deep abdominal pain is, by definition, either of visceral or somatic origin. Visceral pain is described most often as dull, aching, or diffuse mid-abdominal discomfort. The pain from the stomach, pancreas, and hepatobiliary tree localizes to the epigastrium. Periumbilical localization occurs from the small bowel and right colon; the rest of the colon and the genitourinary organs cause pain that localizes to the hypogastrium. The common midline pain location is a result of the bilateral innervation of the abdominal organs from both sides of the spinal cord. When it is severe, visceral pain may generate a secondary physiologic reaction mediated by the autonomic nervous system and manifested by nausea, vomiting, sweating, lightheadedness, and salivation.

Somatic pain that originates in the parietal peritoneum and the root of the mesentery is more intense, better circumscribed, and in closer proximity to the area of origin.

To determine the source of the pain, it is important to assess, not only its intensity, location, and character, but also its onset, whether acute or insidious, and its temporal profile.[3] The circumstances that intensify or alleviate the pain are significant. Relief with eating or antacids suggests ulcer disease or gastroesophageal reflux. Postprandial pain, depending on its location, character, and timing, could be biliary, ischemic, or associated with a more benign condition, such as lactose intolerance or irritable bowel syndrome. Seasonal patterns frequently are seen in ulcer disease and occasionally with regional enteritis. The pain of inflammatory bowel disease and irritable bowel syndrome may be relieved by defecation, whereas heat usually relieves pain of musculoskeletal origin. Posture, sudden movement, coughing, straining, and sneezing may worsen the pain from peritoneal irritation or spinal origin. The abdomen is not exempt from psychogenic pain. This may be manifested as a component of irritable bowel syndrome. Although common, psychogenic pain should and does remain a diagnosis of exclusion.

CLASSIFICATION OF PAIN PATTERNS

Esophagus

Heartburn is the most common symptom referable to the esophagus.[4] It is a burning or hot substernal discomfort frequently moving up toward the neck, but it may be localized only to the epigastrium. Eating, bending down, lying down after eating, and occasionally vigorous exercise may precipitate it. Whether it is caused by discomfort from chemical irritation by acid or bile or secondary muscle spasm plays a role is not entirely clear. Occasionally, the pain is described more as a heaviness or tightness in the chest with secondary restricted respiration and subsequent shortness of breath, simulating myocardial ischemia. The shortness of breath may be caused by an intercostal muscle spasm mediated by spinal reflex arcs. Usually the pain from the esophagus is felt at the level of the lesion. In some patients, however, pain caused by a lesion in the lower third of the esophagus is felt in the throat or in the high retrosternal area. The opposite is uncommon. When it is severe, such as that associated with an ulcerating or infiltrating process, esophageal pain can radiate into the back, between the shoulder blades.

Stomach and Duodenum

The character of pain from ulcer disease varies widely. Typically, it is located in the epigastrium.[5] It may be a sharply localized burning or gnawing pain or just a vague discomfort occurring from 0.5 to 2 h after eating. Occasionally, it occurs shortly before meals or on an empty stomach; it may wake the patient up in the early hours of the morning. It is relieved by food or antacids. The pain may, at times, be more localized to the right or left upper quadrant. When the pain bores through into the back, it usually indicates a posterior duodenal-wall ulcer with secondary irritation of, or penetration into, the pancreas. This pain usually is deep, persistent, poorly localized, and does not respond well to treatment. Unlike heartburn, ulcer pain frequently occurs in clusters; several weeks of daily pain may be followed by variably long pain-free intervals. There may be seasonal variation with the symptoms; they may be worse during the spring and fall.

Pain from gastritis tends to be more persistent and may be more difficult to abolish. The associated nausea and vomiting may be particularly troublesome. As in heartburn, it is not known whether the pain is produced by acid irritation of the nerve endings in the ulcer bed or whether it is secondary to a spasm of antral or duodenal smooth muscle.

Epigastric pain occurring soon after eating, unrelieved by antacids, and with lack of periodicity does not necessarily exclude ulcer disease. Pyloric channel ulcers may present in such a manner, and unless there is associated postprandial vomiting, the diagnosis may not be made until frank gastric outlet obstruction occurs.

Small Intestine

As a rule, pain originating in the small intestine is periumbilical in location and crampy or colicky in nature. Jejunal lesions tend to be associated with pain in the left upper quadrant. Ileal pain tends to localize in the right lower quadrant, and it may result from abnormal bowel motility patterns. It also can be caused by a lowered threshold to the pain of bowel distension or contraction. A lesion obstructing the lumen of the bowel, such as regional enteritis or a malignant process, may be the precipitating factor.

The pain of irritable bowel syndrome frequently is chronic, and at times, it can be incapacitating. It is unusual, however, for it to wake the patient from sleep. The pain usually is in the lower abdomen, in either the right or left lower quadrants. Its description ranges from burning, sharp, and stabbing to dull. Most commonly, it is intermittent, but it may be constant with superimposed acute attacks. The pain may remain localized or may migrate with time. Eating usually precipitates it; defecation or fasting tends to relieve it. Nausea, bloating, and dyspepsia frequently occur and may simulate peptic ulcer or biliary tract disease. A change in bowel habits is not universal finding, but classically, diarrhea alternates with constipation. Predominant diarrhea or constipation, however, can be part of the syndrome.

Pain from partial small bowel obstruction also occurs after meals. The closer the lesion is to the stomach, the earlier the pain occurs. Moreover, nausea and vomiting are more likely to occur when the lesion is close to the stomach. The pain frequently is described as crampy and comes in waves. Regional enteritis is suggested by localization of the discomfort to the right lower quadrant and associated diarrhea, fever, weight loss, or extraintestinal manifestations, such as arthritis and mouth ulcers. Significant weight loss and cachexia may suggest an underlying lymphoma or metastatic disease to the bowel. It may be several months before complete obstruction occurs. At this time, the diagnosis is more obvious. As in appendicitis, the initial pain may be a nonspecific discomfort, but as the underlying process develops and eventually involves the overlying peritoneum, the pain localizes and approximates the site of the underlying disease.

Postoperative adhesions frequently are blamed for chronic or recurrent abdominal pain. Before exploration is considered, definitive evidence of bowel obstruction using plain abdominal x-rays or angulation and proximal dilatation of the bowel using a barium study should be documented.

Colon

Pain from the colon usually is poorly localized to the lower midabdomen. However, adenocarcinoma of the colon or diverticulae[6] of the colon with secondary microperforation and abscess formation may have localized symptoms overlying the area of disease. Pain from the rectosigmoid area, in addition to being in the left lower quadrant, also may be located in the sacral area.

Pancreas, Liver, and Biliary Tract

Because the pancreas, liver, biliary tract, stomach, and duodenum share some of the same afferent neuropathways, it is easy to understand some of the difficulties involved in the differential diagnosis of chronic epigastric pain. Diseases of the pancreas, particularly pancreatic cancer, are the most difficult to diagnose. Pain resulting from pancreatic cancer usually signifies infiltration of the retroperitoneal area or celiac axis with its neural plexus or spreading to surrounding organs. Some of the pain may be a result of pancreatic duct obstruction and surrounding pancreatitis. Tumors in the head of the pancreas cause pain that is more localized to the epigastrium or right upper quadrant. Those in the tail tend to cause pain in the left upper quadrant. Lesions in the body of the pancreas can cause the pain to radiate into the back. Back pain alone also can be a presenting symptom. Because pancreatic cancer is rarely resectable, the physician often is able only to treat the sometimes severe pain. The retroperitoneal celiac plexus often is involved by the tumor, and the anesthesiologist frequently will be asked to guide and help manage the pain (see Chap. 28)

The pain of chronic pancreatitis, mainly a result of alcohol abuse, can be constant, debilitating, and frequently lead to drug abuse. The persistent inflammation of the pancreas causes some of the pain as does the ductal dilatation secondary to ductal obstruction by concretions or strictures. The pain is dull or sharp, burning, and steady. It commonly radiates into the back. Superimposed more acute attacks last from days to several weeks.[7] Eating, moving, or lying down may aggravate the pain; sitting up or leaning forward may relieve it. In patients who are not surgical candidates, the anesthesiologist may be asked to intervene. Neurolytic celiac plexus blocks have been used to treat patients who have not responded to conservative or surgical therapies. It often is used as a last resort because rendering the abdomen insensitive may allow future abdominal disease to be missed.

Placement of stents during endoscopic retrograde cholangiopancreatography was used initially to decompress a dilated biliary tree. Only recently, however, this technique also has been used to decompress the pancreatic duct. Relief may occur if the dilated biliary (or pancreatic) duct was the cause of the pain. Both benign and malignant lesions are amenable to this technique.[8]

Biliary pain usually is caused by passing a stone or biliary tree dilatation secondary to an obstruction. Contrary to the commonly used term *biliary colic,* the pain tends to be of gradual onset. After it peaks, it tends to reach a plateau until again, hours later, it diminishes. An attack may last from several hours to a day. The pain characteristically is localized to the right upper quadrant and may radiate into the right shoulder and shoulder blade, but it also is felt commonly in the epigastrium with radiation into the back. Vomiting occurs in most patients and may provide some relief. After an acute attack subsides, residual soreness may persist for several days. Commonly, these symptoms occur after eating, but they may become constant if the common bile duct is impacted by a stone or infiltrated by a malignant process. Associated dyspepsia is common. In approximately one-quarter of patients, it responds to antacids, further confusing its cause. The appearance of complicating cholangitis (with its symptoms of fever and jaundice) usually leads quickly to the correct diagnosis.

The liver parenchyma is insensitive to pain, but relatively rapid distension of the liver capsule will initiate well-localized right upper quadrant pain. Acute processes like viral hepatitis, alcoholic hepatitis, and cardiac decompensation with secondary liver congestion rarely may appear as right upper quadrant pain, but this does not evolve into a chronic complaint. Chronic active hepatitis may, however, follow a course of recurrent attacks of right upper quadrant pain. The pain usually is well localized and accompanied by worsening liver function tests.

Benign focal nodular hyperplasia or adenomas associated with the use of birth-control pills may cause recurrent right upper quadrant discomfort or, occasionally, a dramatic crisis of severe abdominal pain and hypotension from a hemorrhage into the capsule or peritoneum. The recurrent warning pains probably are caused by small bleeding episodes into the lesions. Bleeding into or necrosis of malignant lesions in the liver will cause a similar pain, but they usually are accompanied by fever and jaundice. The pain may be well localized, sharp, and steady. It may be exacerbated by any movement producing friction between the liver surface and the ribs. When sought, a bruit over the lesion may be identified in approximately 25 percent of patients.

Vascular Diseases of the Bowel

Although mainly asymptomatic, occlusive vascular disease may be associated with chronic recurrent dull periumbilical or epigastric pain. The pain of intestinal angina presents approximately 0.5 h after eating and lasts while digestion and absorption of the ingested meal is occurring. Usually at least two of the three major splanchnic vessels are affected by significant obstruction from atherosclerotic changes. It is, therefore, postulated that the collateral supply is insufficient to meet the increased need during digestion and that a state of relative ischemia and subsequent pain is created. Classically, this recurrent pain may create fear of eating and secondary severe weight loss. When patients with acute ischemia are questioned closely, retrospectively, they often will report postprandial abdominal discomfort preceding the acute event by weeks to months.

Superior mesenteric artery syndrome and celiac compression syndrome frequently are mentioned in the differential diagnosis of chronic abdominal pain, but their validity is controversial. Superior mesenteric artery syndrome is described as occurring in so-called asthenic patients or patients with significant weight loss. The postprandial epigastric pain, vomiting, and distension are believed to be caused by compression of the duodenum by the superior mesenteric artery. The pain of celiac compression syndrome is not necessarily related to meals. The celiac axis frequently has a high take off and may be compressed by the median arcuate ligament of the diaphragm or by the tissue of the celiac ganglion. Whether bowel ischemia is the cause of the pain or whether the pain originates from the celiac ganglion also is unclear.

Abdominal aortic aneurysm usually presents more acutely, but a slowly expanding or leaking aneurysm may be associated with recurrent dull midepigastric or back pain over several months. This pain, like pancreatic pain, occasionally may be relieved by sitting up or leaning forward. The pulsating, sometimes tender, mass can be palpated, and a bruit may be heard.

Peritoneum

The parietal peritoneum is well innervated by the branches of the spinal nerves, and consequently, the pain perceived is well localized. Such pain frequently is associated with secondary muscle spasm of the overlying abdominal wall. The visceral peritoneum, however, has no pain receptors, and any pain that is generated is poorly defined. Chronic pain originating in the peritoneal cavity is mostly caused by a malignant process. Metastatic bowel or ovarian tumors and lymphoma are common. Mesothelioma is the most common primary tumor; teratoma, carcinoid, or sarcoma are less common. The abdominal discomfort often is compounded by the presence of ascites, which distends the peritoneum further and causes more pain.

In young patients of Mediterranean descent who have chronic recurrent attacks of sudden diffuse or localized peritoneal pain, familial Mediterranean fever should be considered. Abdominal tenderness, fever, and arthritis are common. Despite feeling very ill, the patient recovers in several days and is well until the next attack.

Mesentery and Omentum

Recurrent localized or generalized abdominal pain in an older patient, associated with displacement of the stomach or bowel on x-ray studies, should suggest a mesenteric or omental lesion. Fever, weight loss, nausea, vomiting, and a palpable tender mass may be associated with mesenteric paniculitis or retractile mesenteritis. Metastatic tumors to the mesentery are more common than primary lesions. The latter usually are fibromas, myomas, or histiocytic or lipomatous tumors. Leiomyomas and leiomyosarcomas tend to involve the omentum.

Genitourinary

The acute pain of renal colic or pyelonephritis is classic and easy to diagnose. The triad of hematuria, flank pain, and a palpable mass suggests renal cell carcinoma, but it occurs infrequently. The tumor often is diagnosed from systemic complaints (dull upper abdominal or flank pain may be included). Perinephric abscess, although uncommon, should be considered in a patient with a history of urinary tract infections or pyelonephritis. Typically, dull upper quadrant or flank discomfort is present and accompanied by malaise and low grade fevers.

Gynecologic problems usually cause acute pain. Depending on the patient's age, chronic lower abdominal pain, usually more localized to one of the lower quadrants, could be a presenting symptom of chronic pelvic inflammatory disease or uterine or ovarian cancer. The pain can be dull, steady, or crampy. The local irritation by the mass or inflammatory process can cause changes in the urine or bowel pattern (see Chap. 11).

Metabolic Causes of Abdominal Pain

Metabolic causes of chronic abdominal pain are rare but should always be sought, particularly when the usual diagnostic avenues have been exhausted. The hepatic porphyrias have many features in common, including their clinical presentation. Abdominal pain is the most prominent symptom. It is thought to result from autonomic neuropathy that causes disturbances in gastrointestinal motility. Spasm and dilatation of the bowel can cause severe pain. The frequent association of fever and leukocytosis mimics an inflammatory process. Although vomiting and constipation frequently are present, the abdomen is soft, without marked tenderness. These attacks may last from days to weeks. Fasting, infections, the menstrual cycle, and drugs whose metabolism involves the hemoproteins of cytochrome P_{450} are often the precipitating factors. Such drugs include alcohol, barbituates, anticonvulsants, estrogens, and contraceptives. A knowledge of so-called safe or probably safe drugs may be useful to the clinician treating the pain. Drugs that are considered safe include morphine and related opiates, which may be required to treat the pain in an acute attack.

In our society, lead poisoning mainly is encountered in children. Although anemia, peripheral neuritis, and encephalopathy complete the picture, the young patient may have only lead colic, sometimes called *painter's cramps*.

Severe, migrating, poorly localized, crampy abdominal pain may be accompanied by guarding and rigidity of the abdominal wall, raising the suspicion of an acute intraabdominal event.

When in a hemolytic crisis, a patient with paroxysmal nocturnal hemoglobinuria may have substernal, lumbar, or abdominal pain in addition to generalized weakness. The pain may be colicky and last for several days. The abdomen may be tender with some guarding and even a rebound phenomenon. Venous thrombosis occurs with increased frequency in these patients. It always should be considered if a sudden increase of liver size accompanies these attacks, suggesting thrombosis involving the portal system.

Hyperparathyroidism has been called the syndrome of bones, stones, and groans. The abdominal pain usually is caused by associated peptic ulcer disease or pancreatitis.

The lightening-sharp abdominal pain of tabes mainly is associated with syphilis, but it also may occur with diabetes and meningeal tumors. This is a radicular syndrome resulting from damage to the large posterior lumbosacral roots.

The diagnosis of chronic recurrent abdominal pain often can be a challenge to both the therapeutic and diagnostic abilities of the involved physician. Unfortunately, many of these patients undergo multiple surgical procedures without any significant findings. Good knowledge of the underlying anatomy and pain patterns should make the diagnosis and subsequent treatment easier.

TREATMENT

Most of this chapter has dealt with the diagnosis of abdominal pain syndromes. When a treatable disorder is identified, appropriate therapy should be instituted. Unfortunately, many patients have chronic abdominal pain without a specific diagnosis despite an extensive workup. Others have a condition diagnosed, but conventional methods have failed to treat their pain. Nerve blocks rarely are helpful in treating chronic benign abdominal pain. Nonspecific methods, such as antidepressants, stress reduction techniques, and behavioral approaches often are useful in treating these difficult problems.

References

1. Ness TJ, Gebhart GF. Visceral pain: a review of experimental studies. *Pain* May 1990; 41(2):167–234.
2. Gallegos NC, Hobsley M. Abdominal wall pain: an alternative diagnosis. *Br J Surg* October 1990; 77(10):1167–1170.
3. Avorn J, Everitt DE, Baker MW. The neglected medical history and therapeutic choices for abdominal pain. A nationwide study of 799 physicians and nurses. *Arch Intern Med* April 1991; 151(4):694–698.
4. Trnka Y, Warfield CA. Chronic abdominal pain. *Hosp Pract Off.* 1984; 19:201–209.
5. Currie DJ. Abdominal pain. 5th ed. New York: McGraw-Hill; 1970.
6. Cheskin LJ, Bohlman M, Schuster MM. Diverticular disease in the elderly. *Gastroenterol Clin North Am* June 1990; 19(2):391–403.
7. Karanjia ND, Reber HA. The cause and management of the pain of chronic pancreatitis. *Gastroenterol Clin North Am* December 1990; 19(4):895–904.
8. Zimmerman D. Stenosis and dilatation of the biliary and pancreatic ducts. In: Sivak MV, ed. *Gastroenterologic Endoscopy.* Philadelphia: Saunders; 1987.

CHAPTER 11

Pelvic Pain

Eric D. Lichter and Scott P. Laff

The physician treating a woman with pelvic pain may need to play many roles: gynecologist, internist, surgeon, and psychiatrist. Understanding the varied causes and symptoms of pelvic pain is essential for selecting the proper diagnostic workup, thereby avoiding ineffective therapeutic interventions that may complicate the patient's condition further and obscure a correct diagnosis.

The cyclic course of many types of pelvic pain is the reason for much misdiagnosis and mistreatment. When the diagnosis is uncertain, the patient most commonly is thought to have pelvic inflammatory disease (PID) and treated with antibiotics. In reality, many of these patients actually have endometriosis, a functional ovarian cyst, mittelschmerz, or pelvic pain of nongynecologic origin. The pain from many of these noninfectious entities resolves spontaneously (at least temporarily) without treatment. The assumption that the antibiotics have alleviated the pain only confirms the misdiagnosis and delays proper evaluation. The next time the patient has a similar complaint, proper evaluation will be bypassed, and again she will be treated with an unnecessary course of antibiotics. The symptoms also will subside, and thus she will begin a cycle of misdiagnosis and mistreatment. To break this pattern, the physician must understand, not only the clinical signs that characterize pelvic pain, but also the specific neuropathways involved.

NEUROANATOMY

Although the parenchyma of internal organs do not contain pain receptors, both the arterial walls and peritoneum are innervated richly. Pain from visceral organs therefore is apt to be poorly localized by the patient and often is perceived at a surface site far removed from its actual source (that is, referred pain). The visceral sensory fibers are believed to be discharged into the same pool of neurons in the spinal cord as the impulses arising in the somatic nerve fibers in the skin. This results in an overflow of impulses and a subjective misinterpretation of the true origin of the pain at the level of the sensory cortex. Pain from the fundus of the uterus most commonly is referred to the hypogastrium and

elicits a complaint of midline lower abdominal pain. Pain from the cervix is felt as pain over the lower back and sacral area, although it also may be transmitted to the hypogastrium. Pain from the area of the ovaries is the most difficult to interpret because of the intercommunication of the ovarian and pelvic nerve plexuses and the variability of ovarian location (e.g., freely mobile, adherent in the cul-de-sac, or at the pelvic side wall). As a rule, the ovarian parenchyma is insensitive to pain. Pain from pathologic conditions of the ovaries is a late manifestation, arising from stretching of the surrounding peritoneum or vascular structures.

HISTORY

A proper history may be the most important factor in the diagnosis of pelvic pain. In many instances, the physician may be able to make a preliminary diagnosis before examining the patient.

It is important to ascertain all qualities of the pain. How did the pain begin? Was it sudden or gradual? A gradual onset more likely would be associated with infection compared with a sudden onset that may indicate rupture or torsion of an ovarian cyst. Did the pain awaken the patient from sleep? What was she doing when the pain began? Many patients report the rupture of a cyst occurring during physical activity (such as sexual intercourse), although it may occur at any time. What was the relation of pain onset to the menstrual cycle? Recurrences of PID tend to occur during or after menstrual periods. The pain of endometriosis usually begins with menstrual flow, peaks with onset of maximum flow, and then gradually decreases.

Has the patient had pain of this type before and, if so, how often? This may indicate whether the patient has a chronic or acute condition. What is the character of the pain? Is it sharp, dull, or colicky? Is it constant or intermittent? Is it localized or does it radiate? Pain associated with dysmenorrhea often is described as crampy; pain from PID is dull; and pain from a twisting ovarian cyst may be sharp and intermittent. Free fluid in the peritoneal cavity may cause pain that radiates to the left shoulder. Masses in the cul-de-sac may be felt as rectal pressure.

Are there accompanying symptoms, such as nausea, vomiting, diarrhea, or urinary complaints? This may make us consider a gastrointestinal or genitourinary cause.

Portions of this chapter taken from Lichter ED, et al. The pain clinic: pelvic pain syndrome. Reprinted with permission from *Hosp Pract* 1985; 20(3):32e.

Has the patient been under increased stress lately? Has there been a recent death in the family? Are there recent marital problems? This may indicate underlying psychologic factors that should be addressed.

Abdominal, vaginal, and rectal examination should be done gently to minimize the patient's discomfort. The rectal examination, although underestimated and poorly used, can provide significant clinical information. For example, in a woman with significant cervical motion tenderness that seems inconsistent with other findings, rectal manipulation of the cervix can help evaluate her pain. A rectal examination can disclose masses in the cul-de-sac that may indicate early carcinoma, nodularity in the rectovaginal septum (suggesting endometriosis), or evidence of gastrointestinal disease (e.g., diverticulitis or inflammatory bowel disease).

SPECIFIC PAIN SYNDROMES

Dysmenorrhea

Pain associated with the menstrual period usually is described as lower midabdominal cramping that radiates to the back. It may be associated with premenstrual molimina and can include nausea, vomiting, diarrhea, anxiety, breast tenderness, and headache. The pain generally begins 2 to 12 h before the menstrual flow. Its peak intensity coincides with full flow, and it gradually subsides before the flow ends.

There are two categories of dysmenorrhea: primary and secondary. The primary type usually occurs at or a short time after menarche and has no identifiable pelvic disease. It is estimated that 50 percent of postpubescent women have dysmenorrhea, and 10 percent are incapacitated for 1 to 3 days each month.[1]

Currently, primary dysmenorrhea is thought to be caused by increased endometrial prostaglandin production and release. This leads to myometrial contractility. If excessive, this leads to uterine ischemia and pain.[2,3] Penetration of excess prostaglandin into the general circulation may cause the systemic symptoms (e.g., nausea, bloating, and breast tenderness) of dysmenorrhea.[3] This hypothesis has led to the use of antiprostaglandin agents for treatment. The nonsteroidal anti-inflammatory agents with prostaglandin synthetase inhibitory properties frequently are used (e.g., naproxen, indomethacin, and ibuprofen).[4] A good response also has been claimed with oral contraceptives; these decrease endometrial prostaglandins by inhibiting endometrial growth and development.[1]

Secondary dysmenorrhea occurs later in life, usually after age 30 years. It is caused by acquired pathologic conditions. These include endometriosis, adenomyosis, leiomyomas, cervical stenosis, and salpingitis. The pain of secondary dysmenorrhea may be similar to that of primary dysmenorrhea. In extensive disease, it may precede or extend beyond the menstrual period. It may progress to continuous pain that is exacerbated only during menses.

The diagnostic workup of these patients should include a complete blood count, urinalysis, erythrocyte sedimentation rate, and pelvic ultrasonography. A trial of antiprostaglandins often is worthwhile. If the patient needs birth control and there is no contraindication, oral contraceptives may be a good choice. If the patient remains symptomatic, laparoscopy is the next logical step.

Endometriosis

Endometriosis is the presence of endometrial tissue outside the endometrial cavity. The most common location is on or within the ovaries. In descending order of frequency, the rest of these lesions are found in the pouch of Douglas, uterine ligaments, pelvic peritoneum, rectovaginal septum, and rectosigmoid.[5] Distant spread also is possible to the appendix, vagina, vulva, bladder, umbilicus, lymph nodes, lungs, brain, and scar tissue after previous surgery.

Although the exact cause is unknown, three theories should be mentioned. The most popular is the transtubal regurgitation theory that attributes the spread to retrograde reflux of menstrual blood into the pelvic cavity. A second theory attributes the development of ectopic endometrium to activation and differentiation of coelomic rests in various parts of the peritoneum. Distant spread has been explained by metastasis of endometrial tissue through lymphatic and hematologic channels.

Most patients with endometriosis are 25 to 45 years of age. Because the endometriosis responds to the cyclic rise and fall of ovarian hormones, pregnancy (with its persistent high hormone levels and natural suppression of the cyclic nature of hormone production) is thought to be protective. This has led to the stereotypical characterization of the patient with endometriosis as a white woman who delayed marriage and child bearing while pursuing a career. However, endometriosis may be encountered in very young women and in nonwhites. A positive family history for endometriosis is found in 15 percent to 20 percent of patients.[6]

It is estimated that 30 percent to 40 percent of women with endometriosis are infertile.[7] A combination of peritubal adhesions, distortion of pelvic architecture, scarring, and the possibility of increased levels of prostaglandin causing decreased tubal motility makes endometriosis a major cause of infertility and a common presenting complaint.

The diagnosis is hampered by the lack of a uniform symptom complex and a poor correlation between disease progression and severity of symptoms.[8,9] Minimal disease can cause great discomfort; extensive pelvic involvement may be associated with only mild symptoms.

Endometrial implants on peritoneal surfaces appear as multiple bluish-red nodules, patches, or cysts. Although the lesions usually are small, foci in the ovary and uterosacral ligaments may attain sufficient size to be palpated easily.

Microscopic examination of these lesions shows endometrial glands and stroma that may reflect the cyclic changes of proliferative and secretory endometrium. It is this activity that causes the symptoms and pathologic findings of this disease. Menstruation in these ectopic locations provokes a connective tissue reaction to contain the shed material. This leads to adhesions, scarring, tissue distortion, and pain. Because endometrial tissue contains prostaglandins, the role of these chemicals in disturbances of fertility and pain also has been stressed.[10]

Menstrual disturbances are common, as is dysmenorrhea. Dyspareunia may be the presenting symptom, especially when there is involvement of the uterosacral ligaments. Gastrointestinal complaints may predominate in the presence of rectal lesions, and urinary tract symptoms may prevail if the bladder is affected. A small portion of patients have an acute abdomen, resulting from rupture of an endometrioma.

During the physical examination, the uterus may be found to be fixed in the cul-de-sac, and the ovaries may be enlarged. Nodularity of the uterosacral ligaments is considered pathognomonic. In some instances, the examination may be completely normal. Because of the great variation in presenting clinical patterns, laparoscopy should be used liberally whenever the diagnosis is considered seriously and before any long-term therapy is begun.

The treatment varies depending on the extent of disease and the patient's desire to have a child. Hormonal therapy to induce a pseudopregnancy state commonly is prescribed, usually by administering continuous high-dose oral contraceptives. However, weight gain, initial exacerbation of pain, and the possibility of thromboembolism limit the use of these drugs.[11] More recently, induction of pseudomenopause using danazol therapy has been introduced as an alternative method of treatment. This drug appears to have a direct effect on hypothalamic–pituitary function by preventing the midcycle surge of luteinizing hormone and acting on numerous other sites to inhibit several enzymes involved in steroidogenesis.[12] Its most common side effects (weight gain and edema) are reversible.[11] Surgery is recommended for patients with moderate-to-severe disease, those who have not responded to medical therapy, or those with no desire for pregnancy.[13]

Adenomyosis

Adenomyosis is a benign invasion of the wall of the uterus by endometrial tissue. Most patients are 35 to 50 years of age and have had children. Presenting complaints usually are dysmenorrhea and menorrhagia.

Although a definitive diagnosis requires direct pathologic examination of uterine tissue, a presumptive determination can be made in a symptomatic woman who, on examination, has a moderately and diffusely enlarged uterus with one or more small nodules palpated in the uterine wall. These nodules are adenomyomas, tumors composed of stroma and endometrium, as distinct from leiomyomas (which contain no glandular components).

Adenomyosis has been found in association with leiomyomas, endometrial hyperplasia, endometrial carcinoma, and endometriosis.[14,15] All these conditions may have a similar symptom complex. Therefore, an appropriate workup should be done before therapy is begun.

The severity of the menorrhagia and dysmenorrhea and the patient's desire for a future pregnancy will determine the choice of therapy in confirmed adenomyosis. Temporizing is preferred for the woman who wishes to continue child bearing; she can be treated with analgesics and hematinics. Simple hysterectomy is curative.

Leiomyomas

Leiomyomas (commonly called fibroids) are benign tumors arising from smooth muscle. Although their cause is unknown, estrogen, growth hormone, and progesterone may play a role in their genesis.[16] These tumors (single or multiple) can appear at various locations in the uterus. They may occur in the submucosa (extending into the uterine cavity), intramurally (confined in the uterine wall), or in the subserosa (projecting into the abdominal cavity).

Various symptoms are attributed to fibroids, including menorrhagia, infertility, fetal wastage, polycythemia, and ascites.[16] Although occasionally present, pain is not a common characteristic symptom of leiomyomas. Associated conditions (such as salpingitis, endometriosis, and diverticulosis) should be excluded before attributing the pain to fibroids. When present, the pain usually is described as a sensation of lower abdominal heaviness and pressure (described as bearing down). Urinary or intestinal symptoms may occur if the leiomyoma impinges on the bladder or rectum.

Pain and tenderness in a patient with a previously asymptomatic myoma generally indicates rapid growth with associated vascular compromise and infarction. This event occurs most commonly during pregnancy; the hyperestrogenic state favors growth of the myoma. In the absence of pregnancy, rapid growth may represent sarcomatous change. Although this complication is uncommon (estimated to occur in 0.1 percent or less of women with myomas[16]), it is potentially fatal.

In rare instances, torsion of a pedunculated fibroid will cause acute pain that may suggest an acute surgical abdomen. Large growths can become impacted in the pelvis, and pressure on the back and legs or urinary retention may occur.

Not all myomas require surgery. Treatment depends on symptoms and the patient's desire to have children. For the woman still planning to conceive, myomectomy with conservation of the uterus often is possible. In the patient not wishing to bear children who is symptomatic or has a rapidly enlarging myoma, hysterectomy is recommended. Many patients who are asymptomatic can be watched closely with follow-up evaluations every 6 months.

Ultrasonographic examination of the pelvis will aid in

differentiating uterine from ovarian enlargement. Myomas tend to shrink during the perimenopausal period as a result of decreasing estrogen production.

Functional Ovarian Cysts

During the reproductive period, functional ovarian cysts may occur. These cysts are called functional because they are related to normal cyclic ovarian function. Follicle cysts may occur during the follicular phase as the time for ovulation approaches. After ovulation, the normal corpus luteum may enlarge and form a corpus luteum cyst. In most patients, these cysts resolve spontaneously over the next menstrual cycle and cause no problems. Occasionally, they may create symptoms by rupturing or becoming twisted. Pain from a ruptured cyst usually is described as sharp and sudden in onset. It may occur during physical activity, such as sexual intercourse. The clinical presentation varies from a quick onset and resolution of pain within hours to an acute abdomen requiring laparotomy. The corpus luteum cyst poses a vexing diagnostic problem because it may mimic the same symptom complex as that of an ectopic pregnancy (that is, unilateral pain, delayed period, and a palpable mass). When time permits, pregnancy testing in association with ultrasonography will help make the diagnosis.

Torsion of an ovarian cyst usually presents as episodic unilateral pain that eventually becomes constant and localized. The diagnosis is made by palpating a tender mass; it may be confirmed by ultrasonography. After torsion has occurred, laparotomy for oophorectomy usually becomes necessary.

PID

Although all pelvic organs can be affected in PID, the fallopian tubes usually are the most extensively involved and sustain the most damage. Offending organisms include *Neisseria gonorrhoeae, Chlamydia trachomatis,* and *Mycoplasma hominis* in the acute phase, and a host of gramnegative and anaerobic organisms in the chronic and recurrent stages. Risk factors for PID include previous episodes of gonococcal PID, sexual activity with multiple partners, and use of an intrauterine device.

During the acute stage, pain is the prominent symptom. It is usually bilateral and associated with increased vaginal discharge, fever, and chills. Irregular bleeding may occur, but this is uncommon. Symptoms typically begin during or shortly after menses. Physical examination shows a purulent cervical discharge, with tenderness on cervical motion and palpation of the adnexa. Direct or rebound abdominal tenderness may be found. In severe cases, upper adominal tenderness also may be present. Fever, leukocytosis, and an increased erythrocyte sedimentation rate will be present. The acute phase either resolves completely with appropriate therapy or progresses to a chronic state with exacerbations of infection and pain often at the time of menstruation.

Laparoscopy should be used liberally to confirm the diagnosis of PID because the differential diagnosis is extensive.[17] Other gynecologic disorders include ectopic pregnancy, ruptured ovarian cyst, and septic abortion. Gastrointestinal disorders include appendicitis and inflammatory bowel disease. Urologic conditions include pyelonephritis and renal calculi.

Appropriate therapy involves intravenous or oral antibiotics, depending on the clinical situation. Surgery is done in patients with intractable disease or abscesses.

CONFOUNDING FACTORS

Adhesions

Whether adhesions cause pelvic pain is controversial.[18] How to treat them is even more controversial.[19] If surgery is considered, the surgeon must be wary. Lysis of adhesions for pain relief may fail and cause additional adhesions.

Tipped Womb

The retroverted uterus once was considered a cause of chronic pelvic pain. This condition is mentioned merely to be dismissed. A retroverted uterus with no other associated pathologic condition is not a cause of pelvic pain and is not an indication for surgery.

Nongynecologic Pain

In the evaluation of pelvic pain, nongynecologic sources should be considered.[20] It is not within the scope of this article to examine the long list of possibilities; we merely remind clinicians that they exist. Possible nongynecologic causes of pelvic pain include appendicitis, inflammatory bowel disease, diverticulitis, and diseases of the urinary tract, such as interstitial cystitis.[21]

Psychogenic Pain

With the workup complete and the diagnosis still a mystery, psychogenic pain becomes a possible diagnosis.[22] Patients and physicians seem uncomfortable with the notion that emotional suffering may be experienced as bodily pain.[23] Although physicians may acknowledge the existence of ordinary tension headaches (which have no definable somatic cause), they are less likely to accept a chronic complaint of abdominal or lower back pain in the absence of demonstrable disease.

Beard[24] examined the psychological characteristics of women with complaints of pelvic pain and no apparent disease. He compared this group with a group of women who had pelvic disease and a normal control group. He found that women who had pelvic pain in the absence of organic disease were different psychologically from the other two groups and tended to have abnormal attitudes about their own sexuality and that of their partners.

The basic problem appeared to be a difficulty in externalizing feelings of stress. Because the area of conflict centered around their difficulties in personal relationships, their stress was converted into pelvic pain. This was a symptom that was used to avoid physical contact. In such patients, psychiatric treatment can help, not only to relieve the pain, but also to avoid unnecessary surgery.[25] Depression also has been associated with a high incidence of pelvic pain.[26]

Chronic pelvic pain can be a perplexing diagnostic dilemma. Fortunately, many options are available for patients with intractable pelvic pain, including presacral neurectomy, recently reinvestigated as a therapeutic option for the treatment of this problem.[27,28] With any type of pelvic pain, a systematic and understanding multidisciplinary approach to diagnosis and treatment can provide the patient with prompt and effective therapy.[29,30]

References

1. Dawood MY. Dysmenorrhea and prostaglandins: pharmacological and therapeutic considerations. *Drugs* 1981; 22:42.
2. Akerland M. Pathophysiology of dysmenorrhea. *Acta Obstet Gynecol Scand Suppl* 1979; 87:27.
3. Csapo AI. A rationale for the treatment of dysmenorrhea. *J Reprod Med* 1980; 25(suppl): 213.
4. Furniss LD. Nonsteroidal anti-inflammatory agents in the treatment of primary dysmenorrhea. *Clin Pharm* 1982; 1:327.
5. Fox H, Buckley CH. Current concepts of endometriosis. *Clin Obstet Gynecol* 1984; 11:279.
6. Runney B. Endometriosis, IV: hereditary tendency. *Obstet Gynecol* 1971; 137:735.
7. Kistner R. (1979) Management of endometriosis in the infertile patient. In: Wallach EE, Kempers DD, eds. *Modern Trends in Infertility and Conception*. Baltimore: Williams & Wilkins; 1979.
8. Stout AL, Steege JF, Dodson WC, Hughes CL. Relationship of laparoscopic findings to self-report of pelvic pain. *Am J Obstet Gynecol* January 1991; 164(1 pt 1):73–79.
9. Al-Suleiman, SA. Laparoscopy in the management of women with chronic pelvic pain. *Aust N Z J Obstet Gynaecol* February 1991; 31(1):63–65.
10. Young S, Moon DV, Lenny PS. Prostaglandin F in human endometrial tissue. *Am J Obstet Gynecol* 1981; 141:344.
11. Raible MD. Pathophysiology and treatment of endometriosis. *Am J Pharm* 1981; 38:1696.
12. Barbieri RL, Ryan KJ. Danazol: endocrine pharmacology and therapeutic applications. *Am J Obstet Gynecol* 1981; 141(4):453.
13. Luciano AA, Pitkin RM. Endometriosis: approaches to diagnosis and treatment. *Surg Ann* 1984; 16:297.
14. Owolabi TO, Strickler RC. Adenomyosis: a neglected diagnosis. *Obstet Gynecol* 1977; 50:424.
15. Fukamatsu Y, Tsukahara Y, Fukuta T. A clinicopathologic study on adenomyosis uteri. *Hippou Sauka Fujinka Gakkal Zasshi* 1984; 36:431.
16. Buttram VC, Reiter RC. Uterine leiomyomata: etiology, symptomatology and management. *Fertil Steril* 1981; 36:433.
17. Faro S, Maccato M. Pelvic pain and infections. *Obstet Gynecol Clin North Am* June 1990; 17(2):441–455.
18. Stovall TG, Elder RF, Ling FW. Predictors of pelvic adhesions. *J Reprod Med* May 1989; 34(5):345–348.
19. Steege JF, Stout AL. Resolution of chronic pelvic pain after laparoscopic lysis of adhesions. *Am J Obstet Gynecol* August 1991; 165(2):278–281. Discussion of 281–283.
20. Reiter RC, Gambone HC. Nongynecologic somatic pathology in women with chronic pelvis pain and negative laparoscopy. *J Reprod Med* April 1991; 36(4):253–259.
21. Levine DZ. Interstitial cystitis. An overlooked cause of pelvic pain. *Postgrad Med* July 1990; 88(1):101–102, 107–109.
22. Wood DP, Wiesner MG, Reiter RC. Psychogenic chronic pelvic pain: diagnosis and management. *Clin Obstet Gynecol* March 1990; 33(1):179–195.
23. Reiter RC, Shakerin LR, Gambone JC, Milburn AK. Correlation between sexual abuse and somatization in women with somatic and nonsomatic chronic pelvic pain. *Am J Obstet Gynecol* July 1991; 165(1):104–109.
24. Beard RW. Pelvic pain in women. *Am J Obstet Gynecol* 1977; 128:566.
25. Peters AA, Van Dorst E, Jellis B, Van Zuuren E, Hermans J, Trimbos JB. A randomized clinical trial to compare two different approaches in women with chronic pelvic pain. *Obstet Gynecol* May 1991; 77(5):740–744.
26. Hahn MB, Jones MM, Carron H. Idiographic pelvic pain. The relationship to depression. *Postgrad Med* March 1989; 85(4):263–266, 268, 270.
27. Vercellini P, Fedele L, Bianchi S, Candiani GB. Pelvic denervation for chronic pain associated with endometriosis: fact or fancy? *Am J Obstet Gynecol* September 1991; 165(3):745–749.
28. Fliegner JR, Umstad MP. Presacral neurectomy—a reappraisal. *Aust N Z J Obstet Gynaecol* February 1991; 31(1):76–79.
29. Gambone JC, Reiter RC. Nonsurgical management of chronic pelvic pain: a multidisciplinary approach. *Clin Obstet Gynecol* March 1990; 33(1):205–211.
30. Kames LD, Rapkin AH, Naliboff BD, Afifi S, Ferrer-Brechner T. Effectiveness of an interdisciplinary pain management program for the treatment of chronic pelvic pain. *Pain* April 1990; 41(1):41–46.

CHAPTER 12

Perineal Pain

Jeffrey Uppington and Carol A. Warfield

Generally speaking, patients with chronic perineal pain are difficult to treat. This also is true of pain felt in nearby parts of the body. Thus, the following discussion will cover, not only pain in the perineum, but also pain in the groin, genitalia, urethra, anus, and coccyx. In clinical practice, there is much overlap in these anatomic locations because pain commonly is referred from one area to another as a result of the relationship in the nerve supply. Usually pain in one region will predominate, and therefore, a classification into anatomic region becomes valid.

ANATOMIC CONSIDERATIONS

The somatic nerve supply to this area comes from L1 to L2 and S2 to S5. The parasympathetic supply is from the sacral segments; the sympathetic supply arises from T10 to L2.[1]

The skin over the inguinal region is served by the ilioinguinal and the iliohypogastric nerves (L1 to L2). Leaving the anterior rami of the lumbar roots, these nerves course laterally and inferiorly through the psoas muscle, then between the quadriceps lumborum muscle and the parietal peritoneum, until they reach the region medial to the iliac crest (Fig. 12-1). There they pierce the transversus abdominis and travel between the transversus and the internal oblique muscles (Fig. 12-2). The iliohypogastric nerve provides sensation to the suprapubic region. The ilioinguinal nerve pierces the internal oblique muscle, enters the inguinal canal, joins the spermatic cord, and leaves by the external inguinal ring. It provides sensory innervation to the skin over the inguinal ligament and perhaps part of the base of the scrotum or labia.

The skin of the penis is supplied by the two dorsal nerves of the penis, lying deep to the Buck fascia and lateral to the dorsal artery. These are end branches of the pudendal nerve (S2 to S4). Additional cutaneous innervation from the base of the penis is supplied by branches of the ilioinguinal nerve. The erectile bodies are innervated by the autonomic nervous system. The sensation from the skin of the scrotum, especially the posterior two-thirds, is relayed by the posterior scrotal nerves (S2 to S4). The anus and anal sphincters derive their nerve supply from the inferior rectal and perineal nerves, both branches of the pudendal nerve. The perineal skin is innervated by the sacral roots (S2 to S4), and the skin between the anus and the coccyx derives its innervation from the lower sacral and coccygeal plexus.

The genitofemoral nerve derives from L1 to L2 and is formed in the substance of the psoas major (see Fig. 12-1). It descends along the medial border of the psoas onto the common and then external iliac artery. It divides into two branches as it approaches the inguinal ligament. The genital

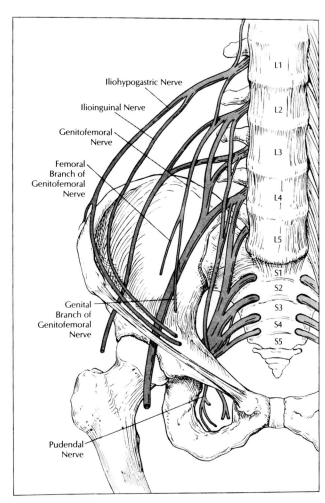

FIGURE 12-1. *Somatic nerve supply to the genital region comes predominantly from the lumbar (L1 to L2) and sacral (S2 to S4) segments. In general, the parasympathetic nerves arrive from the sacral segments, whereas the sympathetic nerves arrive from the lumbar segments (and from more distant thoracic segments, not shown here). The end branches of the pudendal nerve (S2 to S4) supply the skin of the penis (or the lowest part of the vagina). (Reproduced with permission from* Hosp Pract *1988; 23(7):39. Illustration by Pauline Thomas.)*

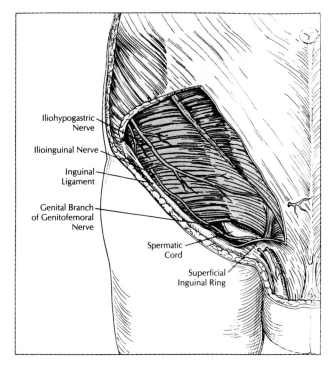

FIGURE 12-2. *The skin over the inguinal region is served by three nerves from the lumbar plexus: the iliohypogastric, the ilioinguinal, and the genital branch of the genitofemoral. The iliohypogastric nerve provides sensation to the suprapubic region. The ilioinguinal nerve supplies the skin over the inguinal ligament and possibly also part of the base of the scrotum (or labia). The genital branch of the genitofemoral nerve serves the lateral part of the scrotum (or vulva). (Reproduced with permission from* Hosp Pract *1988; 23(7):38. Illustration by Pauline Thomas.)*

branch enters the deep inguinal ring and passes down the inguinal canal. It emerges at the superficial inguinal ring (see Fig. 12-2), supplies the lateral side of the scrotum or vulva, and innervates the cremaster muscle. The femoral branch follows the external iliac artery beneath the inguinal ligament, below which it is contained in the femoral sheath. It supplies the skin on the upper part of the femoral triangle. The afferent nerve supply of the upper vagina and cervix is through the pelvic splanchnic (parasympathetic) nerves (S2 to S4), but the lowest part of the vagina is supplied by the pudendal nerve.

The details of the nervous connections of the testis and scrotum are mentioned later as part of the discussion of scrotal pain.

PERINEAL PAIN

Perineal pain may have a local cause or be referred from the urinary tract, lumbosacral nerve roots, or pelvic organs. All possibilities must be investigated. However, even with vigorous investigation, an organic cause of perineal pain often is difficult to find. Woodhouse and Riggs,[2] for example, report a ratio of 1:12 of chronic prostatitis (known

cause) to prostatodynia (unknown cause). One scheme of investigation is outlined in Figure 12-3.

Bladder Pain

Pain from the bladder may be referred to the perineum. True bacterial cystitis includes acute symptoms of dysuria and frequency and usually responds promptly to the appropriate antibiotic regimen. Recurrent cystitis in men frequently is associated with chronic prostatitis. In women, it may present a difficult therapeutic challenge. Flat carcinoma in situ of the bladder mucosa often is called malignant cystitis. The diagnosis may be missed without urine cytologic examination or biopsy of the affected bladder mucosa. Bladder neck dyssynergia usually includes problems of voiding, but its symptoms may overlap prostatodynia; urodynamic studies are useful in some patients. The dyssynergia may respond to small doses of phenoxybenzamine or other α-adrenergic blocking drug.

Prostatic Pain

In men, perineal pain often is ascribed to the prostate. Direct pain from the prostate is unusual.[3] Carcinoma from the prostate or rectum involving the prostatic capsule may cause local pain. This is an uncommon cause of perineal pain and is diagnosed by a rectal examination. Pain or fullness in the perineum may be felt when the prostate is inflamed. The classification and nomenclature of prostatitis is now defined[4] (Table 12-1). Prostatodynia is the preferred term to prostatosis.

Acute bacterial prostatitis, in rare instances, can cause a prostatic abscess. It can be diagnosed readily by culturing the prostatic fluid and urine. It is treated with the appropriate antibiotic and drainage of any abscess cavity. Chronic prostatitis describes acute relapsing episodes of bacterial cystitis with intervening periods when the same organism is found in the prostatic secretion. Between the acute attacks, there may be perineal or pelvic discomfort; the patient may not volunteer this information because of the severity of the acute episodes.

A diagnosis of chronic prostatitis depends on bacterial localization studies.[5] Voided urine and expressed prostatic secretion are collected in aliquots. The first 10 ml of voided urine (VB1), a conventional midstream urine (VB2), prostatic secretions after prostatic massage (EPS), and the first 10 ml of urine after prostatic massage (VB3) are collected. Prostatic massage is considered by some to be contraindicated in acute bacterial prostatitis because of the risk of inducing bacteremia. For the same reason, a prostatic biopsy should not be attempted for chronic prostatitis. In addition, irrelevant inflammatory changes are common in the adult prostate.[6] In chronic prostatitis, between the acute attacks, bacteria can be grown from EPS and VB3 specimens only. During an acute attack, growth occurs in all specimens, although to a greater degree in the prostatic

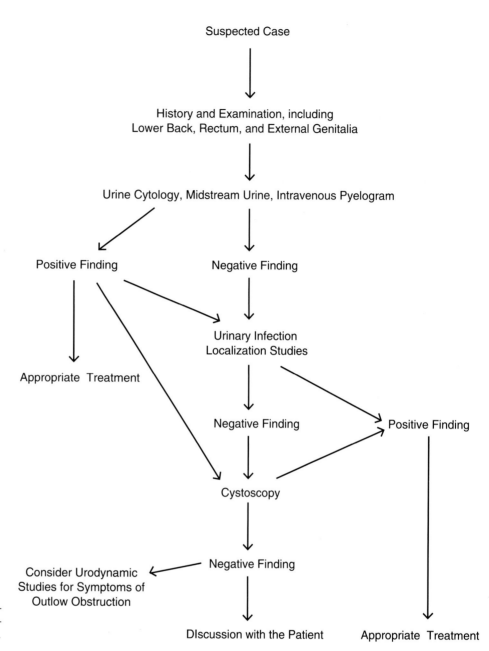

Suspected Case

History and Examination, including
Lower Back, Rectum, and External Genitalia

Urine Cytology, Midstream Urine, Intravenous Pyelogram

Positive Finding   Negative Finding

Appropriate Treatment

Urinary Infection
Localization Studies

Negative Finding   Positive Finding

Cystoscopy

Consider Urodynamic
Studies for Symptoms of
Outlow Obstruction   Negative Finding

DIscussion with the Patient   Appropriate Treatment

FIGURE 12-3. Scheme of investigation of perineal pain (modified from Woodhouse and Riggs[2]).

Table 12-1
Classification of Prostatitis

Condition	Prostate Examination	Prostatic Fluid		Bladder and Urine	Systemic Symptoms
		Microscopy	*Culture*		
Acute bacterial prostatitis	Hot, tender, swollen	Purulent	Positive	Culture positive	Pyrexia, myalgia, malaise
Chronic bacterial prostatitis	Normal	Purulent	Positive	Culture positive in acute exacerbations	Mild; severe with exacerbations
Nonbacterial prostatitis	Normal	Purulent	Negative	Negative	Mild or none
Prostatodynia	Normal	Normal	Negative	Negative	Marked polysymptoms

secretions (EPS and VB3). If the prostatic secretion is purulent (a leukocyte count greater than 10 to 20 cells per high-power field), but no organisms are grown, then the diagnosis is chronic nonbacterial prostatitis. Organisms difficult to culture, such as *Trichomonas, Chlamydia,* or *Mycoplasma* rarely are found in prostatitis. If there is no clinical response to a trial of antimicrobial agents, such as tetracycline, it is reasonable to abandon an infective diagnosis. Most men, as indicated earlier, will have prostatodynia, a diagnosis of exclusion.

Pelvic Floor Tension Myalgia

It should not be assumed that patients with a diagnosis of prostatodynia have pain that originates in the prostate, despite this implication in the terminology. Some (or many) of them may have pelvic floor tension myalgia, a problem that causes pain in the pelvic floor muscles and their areas of attachment, such as the sacrum, pubic rami, ischial tuberosity, and coccyx.[7] Symptoms include perineal pain or discomfort that may be associated with aching discomfort in the rectum, pelvis, testes, or lower back. It often is made worse by sitting. Variable urinary symptoms may occur. A vicious cycle of tension, leading to pain, leading to increasing tension develops. This syndrome is equally or even more common in women than men and may be associated with dyspareunia. The only abnormal finding is pain or tenderness of the pelvic floor musculature during the rectal examination. Usually involved are the piriformis, coccygeus, levator ani, sacrococcygeal ligaments, muscular attachment areas to the sacrum or coccyx, or a combination of any of these. In particular, the prostate is not tender, and the external genitalia are normal. The muscle tension may have originated from some local inflammatory process, such as proctitis, cervicitis, urethritis, anal fissure, or hemorrhoids (which have since subsided), poor posture, gynaecologic surgery, or psychological stress. Habit contraction can develop. This may be accentuated further by hypochondriac or hysteriac neurosis and anxiety, thus producing the symptom complex.

The treatment tries to induce temporary relief of pain by deep heat (rectal diathermy or external application of heat such as warm baths), muscle relaxation by massage of the pelvic floor muscles, and reeducation of the pelvic floor musculature. Relaxation of the pelvic floor muscles can be induced by asking the patient to expel an examining finger in the rectum without straining. Successful relaxation of the levator ani, in particular, can be demonstrated by placing a hand over the anal crease and feeling a widening of the crease. Contraction of the muscles is felt by a deepening of the anal crease. The patient may use this technique at home to achieve sensory feedback of pelvic relaxation to help reestablish habitual relaxation of the pelvic floor. Precipitating factors (such as poor posture or prolonged sitting without a pillow or other support) should be identified and avoided.

Tumor

Cancer may cause perineal pain, either directly or as a pain referred to the perineum. The most common primary tumor is colorectal, but prostatic, bladder, cervical, and uterine cancers also may be involved. A tumor of the sacral roots always should be considered as part of the differential diagnosis.

Trauma

Trauma may result in chronic perineal pain. The most common trauma that causes chronic pain is surgical, particularly abdominoperineal resection of the rectum and anus. The pain is essentially a phantom rectal pain, and often it is localized to the rectum. It can extend to or be confused with the perineum, however. Pain after an episiotomy often is slow to resolve after delivery.[8] Occasionally, it may persist for years. Care should be taken to ensure the pain is caused by and not coincidental with the episiotomy scar. Repeated infiltration of the scar with local analgesics or caudal blocks may be beneficial.

Inflamed Cowper Glands

Chronic perineal and urethral pain in men has been ascribed to inflammation of one or both of the bulbourethral (or Cowper) glands.[9] Inflamed, but not normal, glands can be palpated with the index finger in the rectum, using the thumb of the same hand to palpate the perineal structures anteriorly beside the bulbous urethra. Ideally, the patient is placed in the knee–chest position. Local excision of the inflamed glands successfully relieved the pain in the patient reported by Casey.[9]

Psychological Factors

There are a proportion (perhaps the majority) of patients with perineal pain where no diagnosis can be made. In men, the condition is called prostatodynia. In women, the term *perineal neuritis* has been applied.[10] If all organic causes have been eliminated, the pain may be psychosomatic.[11] Psychological factors that have been found in these patients include depression,[12] anxiety,[13] hypochondriasis,[2] and neuroticism.[14] The patients have a variation of what Addison[15] termed *chronic pain syndrome.* Treatment is difficult and requires a multidisciplinary approach, including initial recognition of the psychological and psychosocial factors involved. Drug therapy should be as simple as possible. Peripherally acting analgesics and nonsteroidal anti-inflammatory agents are preferred. Antidepressants may act as analgesics in addition to their antidepressant action.[16] Behavior modification, biofeedback, progressive relaxation therapy, or hypnotherapy all may be valuable in individual patients[17] (see Chaps. 3, 32, and 34).

Nerve Blocks

Nerve blocks may be valuable in patients with organic pain that has a reasonably defined nerve or root distribution. This applies particularly to cancer pain.[18] If caudal blockade with small amounts (e.g., 6 to 8 ml) of local anesthetics is effective, then caudal cryoanalgesia should be considered. The technique has been well described[10] and is useful to treat for cancer pain or coccydynia localized to the lower sacral or coccygeal nerves. Generally, it is disappointing for pain with a large functional component. Neurolytic blocks for perineal (and rectal) pain present a problem primarily because of the serious risk of bladder or anal sphincter involvement when neurolytic agents or ablation are applied to the lower lumbar and sacral segments.[19] A unilateral block sometimes will produce good relief without complications. If successful, the other side can be done later. Transsacral neurolytic nerve block using aqueous phenol through the S4 sacral foramen has been used for rectal cancer and perineal pain.[20] The block may not last long, but it can be repeated easily with little bladder dysfunction. Sacrococcygeal rhizotomy has produced good results in patients with neoplastic disease and well-localized pain.[21] The results have not been as successful for noncancer pain, and the technique cannot be recommended for pain of nonmalignant origin because postoperative numbness and dysfunction are common complications.

COCCYGEAL PAIN

Coccygeal pain is termed *coccydynia* or *coccygodynia*. The main symptom is pain in the area of the coccyx that is worsened by coccygeal pressure from sitting and eased when standing. Thin patients with flat buttocks probably should carry a foam cushion to sit on. Obese patients might avoid soft chairs. Other symptoms may be associated with the pain, such as rectal fullness, rectal pain, and pain on defecation.

Coccydynia implies chronicity. Pain from acute trauma settles progressively and is over in 4 to 8 weeks. This term should be restricted to pain that persists beyond this time.

Many cases of coccygeal pain follow some kind of trauma.[22] This is usually a direct blow from a projecting object, but it may follow vaginal delivery. Rarely, it may occur in association with lumbar disc syndrome[23] or lumbosacral strains. Thiele[17] found a high percentage of patients with coccygeal pain to have spasms of the levator ani and coccygeus muscles. He believed the pain originated in these muscles or the medial fibers of the gluteus maximus and was referred to the coccygeal area.[24] These patients have a variant of pelvic floor tension myalgia.

The coccyx can be examined best using the finger of one hand inserted into the rectum with the other hand over the coccyx. Any coccygeal tenderness, mobility of the coccyx, or any tenderness of the surrounding viscera, levator ani, and coccygeus muscles should be noted. If movement of the coccyx simulates the patient's pain, relief may be achieved by injecting the sacrococcygeal joint with a local analgesic and corticosteroid (40 mg of methylprednisolone).[25,26] If tenderness and pain can be elicited from the pelvic floor muscles, treatment can follow similar guidelines as used in tension myalgia of the pelvic floor. Repeated contraction and relaxation of the gluteal muscles also may be helpful.

If a definite coccygeal trauma has occurred that can be related directly to the patient's pain, then occasionally, coccygectomy is helpful. However, this operation frequently is ineffective, and it may make subsequent treatment more difficult. In most patients, the pain does not originate from the coccyx itself but from surrounding structures, such as ligaments, joints, and muscle.

Repeated sacral blocks may be beneficial. Cryoanalgesia of the caudal canal (which may require repetition) has been helpful in many cases.[10] Neurolytic blocks with aqueous phenol (again repetition may be required) bilaterally into the fifth sacral and coccygeal nerves have been described as giving long-lasting pain relief.[27] If neurolytic blocks are used for benign pain, great care should be taken in patient selection. Sacrococcygeal rhizotomy has not been beneficial in patients with coccygeal pain.[21]

PAIN IN THE GROIN

Pain in the groin can be caused either by a local cause or a distant lesion with pain radiating to the groin. The main local causes are the entrapment neuropathies or hernias, either femoral or inguinal.

Entrapment Neuropathies

Perhaps the most common nerves entrapped are the ilioinguinal and iliohypogastric. The usual cause of damage is surgery. Because of the oblique course of the nerve, various incisions may be involved. The most common are inguinal or femoral hernia repair, a low McBurney muscle-splitting incision (for appendicitis), pelvic laparotomy with a transverse incision, incision for a lumbar sympathectomy, and a low renal incision. Direct blunt trauma may involve these nerves, and spasms of the abdominal muscles also may stretch or compress them. The pain ranges from a mild ache to lancinating pain, continuous or intermittent, within the cutaneous innervation of these nerves. Standing tends to worsen the pain, and lying down may help. Hip flexion on the affected side also may be beneficial. Occasionally, a pain in this region occurs spontaneously without trauma. This type of inguinal neuritis may have psychosomatic elements.

Damage to the genitofemoral nerve may occur during groin surgery or injury. A psoas abscess or a compressing abdominal mass also may involve the nerve. The pain is similar to ilioinguinal pain, but it also may occur on the inside of the upper thigh.

The obturator nerve (L2 to L4) leaves the pelvis through

the obturator foramen. Obturator neuritis may occur here, either from an obturator hernia or from osteitis pubis.[25] Obturator neuralgia may follow childbirth. The pain characteristically radiates from the groin along the inner aspect of the thigh. In the case of an obturator hernia, coughing or sneezing raises the intraabdominal pressure and worsens the pain. The association with osteitis pubis presumably is a result of surrounding tissue edema and nerve compression. In addition to pain, a dysesthesia or paresthesia may be present, and there may be some loss of sensation. There also may be associated weakness of thigh adduction. Patients with severe obturator neuritis have a distinctive gait, with an increased outward swing of the involved leg because of the partially unopposed action of the thigh abductors.

Hernia

A common cause of groin pain is an inguinal or femoral hernia. Most patients with obvious hernias are referred to a surgeon, not a pain clinic. Hernias, however, may be present despite negative physical findings, and thought must be given to this cause in any patient with obscure groin pain. There are two investigations that may show these occult hernias. One, ultrasonography, is reliable in the femoral, but not the inguinal region.[28] The second, herniography, with or without femoral phlebography, has been useful for demonstrating both types of hernias. In one series of 250 patients,[29] herniography revealed nonpalpable but symptomatic hernias in 51 percent of men and 21 percent of women. Direct inguinal hernia was the most common finding, with twice as many right-sided as left-sided cases. Femoral hernia was less common; an obturator hernia was found in only one patient. Some had combined hernias. Of the surgically treated patients, 87 percent were free of groin pain postoperatively (follow-up, 1 to 66 months; mean, 31 months).

However, the presence of a hernia, even an occult one, does not necessarily explain the cause of the pain. In 13.4 percent of patients with a demonstrable hernia by herniography, the pain was not relieved by surgery. Many patients who complain of pain after herniorrhaphy will, on careful questioning, say that their pain was present before the surgery and was the same afterward. Thus not all patients postherniorrhaphy with groin pain may have surgical nerve damage that explains their pain. Other causes should be sought.

Referred Groin Pain

The origin of referred groin pain may be discovered by careful questioning and examination of the organs known to refer pain to the inguinal area. Pain referred to the groin also may be felt in other areas, such as the testes and scrotum. The urinary tract and testes are well known to refer pain to the groin, but the lumbar plexus as an origin must not be forgotten. Pelvic fracture or retraction of the pelvis against the psoas may cause nerve damage involving the L1 distribution. The plexus also may be involved in tumor spread from pelvic organs. Unilateral motor and sensory changes usually are present. Root pain felt in the groin may arise from arachnoiditis, intervertebral disc prolapse, or spinal stenosis. Back symptoms and/or sciatica may be present in addition to the groin pain.

Pain in the groin also may be referred from facet joints in the vertebral column. Experiments on humans have shown that noxious stimulation of upper and lower lumbar facet joints gives pain that can be felt in the groin; stimulation of the lower lumbar facet joints (L4 to L5) also may refer pain to the anterior and lateral aspects of the upper thigh. In one study, referred pain arose with both intra- and pericapsular stimulation.[30] Thus the back should be examined carefully and evidence for the facet syndrome sought,[31] particularly if the symptom of back pain is worse on extension and on straightening the back from flexion. Injections of local analgesics and corticosteroids and application of the cryoprobe to the facet joints has helped some patients with groin pain (Uppington J. In preparation.).

Diseases of the retroperitoneal structures, such as malignant tumors may evoke pain in the dorsal or lumbar spine with radiation to the groin, lower abdomen, and anterior thighs. Spinal tumors also may radiate pain to the inguinal region.

Pain from arthritis of the hip may be associated with significant groin pain. Gluteal fibrosis and pelvic lipomatosis may refer pain to the groin and testicles.

The treatment depends on the cause. Pain from nerve entrapment or neuritis may be helped by selective blocks of the ilioinguinal and iliohypogastric, genitofemoral, or obturator nerves. Repeated local analgesics and corticosteroid injections may be enough to break the cycle of pain and cause long-term relief. Freezing of the ilioinguinal nerve (which must be done with surgical exposure of the nerve because it is difficult to locate with sufficient accuracy by the cryoprobe percutaneously) has not produced long enough relief to justify this surgical operation to our knowledge.

Drug therapy is necessary for resistant cases. Simple analgesics including nonsteroidal anti-inflammatory agents may be useful. Combination analgesics, carefully selected, also have a place.[32] If there is an element of deafferentation pain (that is, pain occurring in an area of diminished or abnormal sensation[33]), conventional analgesics may not be effective. Tricyclic and other antidepressants may be tried[34] because there is evidence they relieve deafferentation pains, such as postherpetic neuralgia.[16] Anticonvulsant drugs also have been used for this type of pain.[35] TENS has been helpful for some patients.[36]

There will be some patients in whom the diagnosis is unknown and who do not respond to therapy. In these patients, psychological or psychiatric factors should be explored.[37] Being aware of the psychodynamics of pain behavior and developing an understanding of the stress response to continuing pain (a vicious cycle of denial, anger, and depression) can help the physician approach these patients.[38] The proper use of listening and educational techniques may help the patient understand and tolerate pain. A multidisciplinary approach to these patients should be adopted.[15]

PAIN IN THE MALE GENITALIA

Penis

Pain in the penis can be caused by inflammatory lesions of the glans and foreskin; the patient may be predisposed if phimosis is present. Phimosis also may cause discomfort as a result of irritation of the glans from adhesions. In paraphimosis, the retracted foreskin cannot be drawn forward from behind the corona. This is a medical emergency causing severe pain, but it can be diagnosed easily. The foreskin should be replaced manually under sufficient analgesia or anesthesia. If this is impossible, a dorsal slit in the foreskin may be necessary. If neglected, gangrene may ensue.

Priapism is another painful condition that requires urgent attention. This is persistent penile erection without sexual desire caused by lack of venous outflow from the corpora cavernosa. The corpus spongiosum and the glans are relatively flaccid, and although painful, the penis is not tender to palpation. Ischemic changes will occur with time. The cause usually is idiopathic, but it may be secondary to sickle cell disease, polycythemia, leukemia, prostatic disease, drugs, or central nervous system infections.[3] Conservative therapy consists of sedation, ice packs, or administration of heparin or estrogen. If severe, nerve block, aspiration of the corpora, or vascular surgery may be necessary. The prognosis depends on the severity of the problem and the rapidity of treatment. Thrombosis, fibrosis, and permanent impotence may result.

Peyronie disease, the cause of which is obscure, frequently involves curvature of the penis and pain during sexual intercourse. A plaque-like lesion may be found on the dorsum of the penis. The inflammatory process seems to start in the areolar layer deep to the tunica albuginea, and it can progress to a dense fibrous plaque near the glans penis. The pain may occur during erection. Treatment has included oral potassium, para-aminobenzolaid, vitamin E, and steroid injections into the plaque. Surgical removal of the plaque with dermal grafts has been successful. In addition, division of the plaque and a penile prosthesis have been used.[39]

After bilateral vasectomy, some patients have severe pain on ejaculation. In these cases, small tender nodules are palpable along the course of the vas deferens, and the discomfort probably is caused by a congested epididymis. Excision of these sperm granulomas or opening the testicular end of the cut vas may cure this condition.

Severe penile pain can occur many months or years after the insertion of a penile prosthesis. Apart from the presence of the prosthesis, there are no other physical findings. The pain may be relieved after injection of a local anaesthetic into the corpora cavernosum or by removing the prosthesis.[3]

Scrotum and Testes

The nerve supply to the scrotum and its contents is complex and somewhat controversial. Essentially, it consists of an organ with a distant splanchnic supply (T10 to T12) surrounded by structures supplied by somatic nerves of widely separate segments (L1 to L2 and S2 to S3) that also supply other viscera with autonomic nerves. The potential for referred pain in both directions is obvious. One generally accepted view[40] is as follows. The testes are supplied by sympathetic nerves from T10 to T12. The vas and epididymis are supplied by sympathetic fibers from T10 to L1. The cremaster, cord structures, and tunica vaginalis are supplied by somatic fibers from L1 to L2 (genital branch of the genitofemoral nerve). Essentially, the entire skin of the scrotum (not just the posterior aspect) is innervated by S2 to S3 (posterior scrotal nerves). It is difficult to combine these findings with the mechanism of localization of testicular pain, but it would seem that gentle compression of the testis actually stimulates superficial tissues supplied by S2 to S3 (scrotal pain), greater compression stimulates the tunica vaginalis and L1 to L2 (groin pain), and only severe compression stimulates the testis itself to produce pain in the T10 to T12 region (lower abdominal pain). In other words, splanchnic nerves normally require heavy stimulation to produce pain that is poorly localized. Pain localized accurately in the scrotum is transmitted by somatic nerves, even if the primary lesion is in the testis or epididymis.

Pain in the scrotum can be classified in three ways. First, pain can be produced and felt in the scrotum. Second, pain can be produced in the scrotum but felt elsewhere. Third, the pain can be produced elsewhere but felt in the scrotum.

Acute Pain

Acute pain can be caused by cellulitis of the skin of the scrotum. Rarely, a mixed infection can lead to intense necrosis with massive sloughing of the skin of the scrotum and even the penis (Fournier gangrene). The treatment is surgical drainage and antibiotics.

Acute epididymoorchitis, by stimulating the surrounding somatic nerves, involves fever, scrotal pain, swelling, induration, and nodularity. It may be associated with urinary tract infection, urethritis with meatal discharge positive for gonococci or *Chlamydia,* or tuberculosis. A long course of appropriate antibiotic therapy usually is sufficient therapy.

An important differential diagnosis is torsion of the spermatic cord. This usually occurs in teen-agers, but the age range can be 9 months to 40 years.[41] Torsion involves sudden scrotal pain that, in severe cases, may be referred to the groin or lower abdomen and associated with nausea and vomiting. The testis is swollen and tender. Urgent surgical exploration is necessary to prevent vascular compromise and ischemia with loss of the testis. The diagnosis may be confirmed by technetium pertechnetate blood flow scans. Intermittent torsion may cause intermittent scrotal pain. Late torsion of a testicular appendage may present similarly to early torsion of the spermatic cord. Sometimes, however, the purplish infarcted appendage may be seen through the scrotal skin, and transillumination will show it as a black area.

Viral orchitis may occur in 15 percent to 40 percent of adult men with mumps, but testicular inflammation occurs rarely with other viral infections, such as infectious mononucleosis.

Chronic Pain

Chronic pain from local lesions is more difficult to diagnose. Large testicular tumors may include scrotal or testicular discomfort more commonly than generally thought,[42] presumably from dragging on the cord. Prompt surgical exploration by an inguinal approach is indicated if a tumor is suspected. Pain from advanced inoperable cancer may be helped by radiotherapy, chemotherapy, or a combination of both.[43] Testicular discomfort also may occur as a result of large hydroceles and inguinal hernias, especially those in which the hernial sac approaches the scrotum.

Varicoceles are common. They may be found in 8 percent to 22 percent of the general population and usually are left-sided because the left internal spermatic vein inserts into the left renal vein at a right angle. A right-sided varicocele is unusual and should lead the physician to suspect possible retroperitoneal disease causing increased pressure on the right internal spermatic vein. This enters the vena cava at an oblique angle and is thus less prone to varicocele formation. Small varicoceles[44] may be found only with the patient standing and doing a Valsalva maneuver. The incidence of pain from a varicocele is debatable. Nocks[3] claims it frequently is painful; Yeats[40] questions whether an uncomplicated varicocele is a genuine cause of scrotal pain. Pain can occur from a thrombotic varicocele when, incidentally, the cough impulse is no longer present. High ligation of the internal spermatic vein in patients presumed to have a painful varicocele only has an approximately 30 percent success rate.[40] Many patients who are thought to have a painful varicocele have associated latent inflammatory conditions of the prostate and epididymis.[45,46]

Cremasteric spasm causes pain when the testis forcibly is drawn up to the external inguinal ring. This may occur at times of mental stress or for no apparent reason. Division (or circumcision) of the cremaster, which also divides the genital branch of the genitofemoral nerve, has been described as being curative.[40]

Other rarer causes of local testicular pain are polyarteritis nodosa, Henoch-Schönlein purpura, and thrombosis of testicular arteries in cases of repeated trauma.

Referred Scrotal Pain

The most common cause of referred pain to the scrotum is a stone in the lower part of the ureter. The pain probably is referred from splanchnic ureteric stimulation (L1) to the same somatic segment as the genitofemoral nerve. An aching pain in the groin and testis may be caused by degenerative lesions of the lower thoracic and lumbar spines. An intervertebral disc protrusion may cause scrotal pain.[47] An iliac artery aneurysm has caused scrotal pain,[48] and testicular pain has been the first manifestation of epilepsy.[49]

Gluteal fibrosis (consisting of a definite, often large, fibrotic nodule in the gluteal fascia just lateral to the posterior superior iliac spine) may cause an ache in the testes or groin. Pressure on the nodule produces the pain, and infiltration of it with local anesthetic temporarily removes it. The genital pelvic viscera (prostate, seminal vesicles, and proximal part of the vas) theoretically can refer pain both in the distribution of the genitofemoral nerve (L1) and posterior sacral nerves (S2 to S3). How often this happens is not known.

Retroperitoneal lesions, particularly tumors, can cause pain in the scrotum. The most common tumors are those from the bladder, prostate, and bowel, but lymphomas also are possible, although rarer. There frequently are other complaints, such as gastrointestinal or genitourinary problems and scrotal pain. A retroperitoneal bleed (as may occur in a patient receiving anticoagulants) can do the same. Retroperitoneal fibrosis may be felt first as referred pain. The diagnosis requires an intravenous pyelogram, retrograde pyelogram, or CT scan. Pelvic lipomatosis is a disease of unknown origin involving the proliferation of the retroperitoneal fat. Most patients are overweight men with groin and testicular discomfort. The ureter can be compressed, causing hydronephrosis. The diagnosis is made on plain x-ray film of the abdomen when radiolucent areas of lipomatous tissues can be seen. Surgery may be necessary in those with progressive urinary obstruction.

After orchidectomy, some patients have phantom testicular pain. Repeated blocks of the genitofemoral nerve may provide some relief.

There are many cases of scrotal pain in which no diagnosis can be made. Some patients relate worsening of the pain with mental stress; most will not. The physical examination and investigations will be unremarkable. Some may be helped by blockade of T10 to T12, L1 to L2 or S2 to S4 roots by epidural or caudal blocks, ilioinguinal or genitofemoral nerve blocks, or TENS. In many cases, the attending doctor will be tempted to use destructive procedures, such as division of the ilioinguinal or genitofemoral nerves, or even recommend surgical removal of the testis. Great care should be taken in selecting patients for destructive nerve procedures. Most patients with benign conditions, especially those of unknown cause, may not improve, and they risk permanent side effects. Therefore, we are left with a patient with pain in a denervated area that may be extremely difficult to treat. Patients with pain without demonstrable organic cause may receive a trial of antidepressants, but a multidisciplinary approach using psychological and/or psychiatric input may be the preferred therapeutic route.[15,37,38]

PAIN IN THE FEMALE GENITALIA

Chronic Vulval Pain

Pain in the vulva is termed vulvodynia and has several causes. One of these is idiopathic vulvodynia (that is, pain for which investigations have not found a cause). It has been suggested that this pain now be called *burning vulva syndrome*.[50] Some authorities, however, still use vulvodynia.[51] This pain should be differentiated from itching, the main complaint in pruritus vulvae.

The most likely causes of chronic vulval pain are vestibulitis, chronic candidiasis, postherpetic neuralgia, subclinical papillomavirus infection, Sjögren disease, and psychophysiologic problems.[51] Vestibulitis[52] is suggested by the presence of one or more minute trigger points; when stimulated by pressure, they cause the patient's pain. Biopsy will confirm the diagnosis if there are inflammatory cells clustered around the ostia of the minor vestibular glands. Chronic candidiasis may or may not have the classic thick white potassium hydroxide-positive discharge. This diagnosis should be considered in those whose pain started during a proven acute episode of candidiasis, or who have recurrent documented candidal vulvovaginitis. Postherpetic neuralgia usually is unilateral with a history of acute herpes zoster infection. Confirmation may be difficult without a good history. Identification of subclinical papillomavirus infection requires the use of vulval colposcopy to investigate typical lesions and biopsy to confirm the cause. In some cases of prolonged vulval pain, a viral explanation may be found for symptoms previously considered psychosomatic.[53] Sjögren disease may cause dryness and irritability of the vulval mucosa without visible changes. A Schirmer test for ocular tearing and the demonstration of Ro(SSA) and La(SSB) antibodies may be helpful in evaluating this possibility. If redness is found on examination, a biopsy may be necessary to exclude systemic lupus erythematosus, lichen planus, lichen sclerosis, plasma cell vulvitis, and similar conditions.

In those patients in whom an organic cause cannot be found, there may be a psychological basis for their pain. However, it is not that simple. We never can be absolutely sure we have excluded all organic causes of pain. Even if we find a physical explanation, this does not exclude a psychological element superimposed on the organic problem. Women with chronic vulval pain have similar personality characteristics as some men with chronic pain of the penis, scrotum, or anus.[54] They also resemble patients with idiopathic pelvic pain.[55] They share many of the psychological features of patients with psychosomatic vulvovaginitis,[56] with whom their symptoms overlap. They may have generalized symptoms of a nonspecific nature such as fatigue, gastrointestinal and sleep disturbances, evidence of depression, dependancy, hostility, and anger. Their involvement in a relationship often is regarded as less than satisfactory, although they are unwilling to sever the relationship. They have decreased libido and sexual activity. However, they do have pain, requiring our assistance. This might be done either by professional counseling or treatment strategies devised by their own physician.

Pruritus Vulvae

Pruritus vulvae is the sensation of itching in the vulva. This may be severe enough to be interpreted as pain. The sensation of itch is received by free nerve endings lying at the epidermal junction, and like pain, it is conducted along small slowly conducting sensory neurons to the lateral spinothalamic tracts. It has been suggested that itch is mediated by histamine, to which the tissue may be sensitized by prostaglandins[57] and other pharmacologically active substances such as kallikreins, kinins, complement components, and cathepsins. There may be other mechanisms of pruritus that do not rely on histamine release.

The most common cause of vulval itching is infection; candida and *Trichomonas* are the most frequent causes.[58] The differential diagnosis is shown in Table 12-2. Treatment is directed at the cause. Most cases of pruritus vulvae are treated in gynecologic clinics, but a few chronic severe cases not been helped by conventional means may reach pain clinics. Those patients without a physical cause are a variation of those with psychosomatic vulvovaginitis.

Dyspareunia

Dyspareunia is pain during sexual intercourse. Etiologic clues are present in the clinical classification[59]. Primary dyspareunia is present during the first coital experience and is likely to be psychogenic. Secondary dyspareunia has a later onset and is more likely to be organic in origin.[60] In introital dyspareunia, pain occurs at the entrance of the penis into the vagina. Deep-thrust dyspareunia relates to pain on deep penetration into the vagina.[61] Functional dyspareunia is that without a physical basis, and it is not accompanied by other psychiatric illnesses. Dyspareunia is differentiated from vaginismus (the latter is defined as failure to allow penetration caused by an involuntary muscle spasm and the patient may complain of pain at the same time). Vaginismus usually is psychological in origin, except for that caused by local vulvovaginal lesions.

Primary introital dyspareunia may be caused by a fibrotic hymenal ring or vaginal agenesis. Anxiety, which may be generated by feelings about the sexual act, can inhibit sexual arousal, and any discomfort during early intercourse can be accentuated by a lack of lubrication. If this continues

Table 12-2
Causes of Pruritus Vulvae

Local Causes

Infection

Fungal	Candidiasis
	Dermatophytosis
Viral	Herpes genitalis
	Genital warts
	Molluscum contagiosum
	Condyloma lata
Parasitic	Scabies
	Pediculosis pubis
	Threadworm
Protozoan	Trichomoniasis
Bacterial	Gonorrhea
	Syphilis, condyloma lata, chancroid, lymphogranuloma venereum

Inflammation   Contact dermatitis (allergic or irritant)
Lichen simplex
Seborrheic dermatitis
Acrodermatitis enteropathica
Psoriasis
Juvenile dermatitis herpetiformis

Atrophic dermatoses of the vulva
Lichen sclerosis
Primary atrophy of the vulva
Senile genital atrophy
Lichen planus

Tumor   Benign (Fox-Fordyce disease)
Malignant (extramammary Paget disease, Bowen disease, squamous cell carcinoma)

Fixed drug eruption

Miscellaneous   Retained foreign bodies
Poor hygiene

General Causes

Part of a generalized dermatosis

Part of generalized pruritus associated with internal disease
Hepatic disease (jaundice)
Endocrine (thyroid disease)
Renal (chronic renal failure)
Blood disorders (polycythemia)
Gastrointestinal (Crohn disease)
Tropical (filariasis or onchocerciasis)
Neurologic (thalamic tumor)
Drugs (opiates, cocaine, or chloroquine)

Psychogenic

and is not overcome, then a vicious cycle may occur with increasing discomfort and pain. These patients have developed primary dyspareunia. In a more severe cycle, this can lead to vaginismus.

Secondary introital dyspareunia may be caused by obstetric scarring,[62] postepisiotomy pain, or acute vulvovaginal infection. Psychological problems also may occur, such as situational rejection, lack of adequate arousal, and occasionally fear of pregnancy.

Primary deep-thrust dyspareunia is less likely to have an organic cause than secondary deep-thrust dyspareunia, but one must be sought. The cause of the latter may be endometriosis, chronic pelvic inflammatory disease (especially with adnexal fixation), previous pelvic surgery if an ovary becomes fixed to the cul-de-sac, and cervical or forniceal lacerations with scarring. Another cause of deep-thrust dyspareunia and postcoital ache is the so-called pelvic congestion syndrome.[63] Synonyms are pelvic relaxation, pelvic congestion, and broad ligament laceration.[64] In addition to deep-thrust dyspareunia, the symptoms include pelvic heaviness, low back pain, chronic lower abdominal ache, and vague pelvic pain. They usually are worse after standing for long periods. The pathologic process seems to be pelvic and uterine venous congestion, probably from the sex steroids and accentuated by gravitational effects during pregnancy and broad ligament scarring after childbirth. There is probably an autonomic nervous system component related to psychic stress. The overall process is similar to the parasympathetically and sympathetically mediated physiologic changes associated with sexual arousal. Most patients are multiparous. There is no specific diagnostic test, but pelvic examination may detect changes from the morning to the afternoon. A paracervical block may help the symptoms temporarily. Management is directed mainly at excluding other serious lesions, explaining the benign nature of the disease to the patient, and exploring any underlying psychological manifestations. Diuretics, hormones, or psychoactive drugs may be beneficial. If severe symptoms persist, hysterectomy will offer a 95 percent reduction of the problem,[62] but it does nothing for (or even worsens) the psychological problems. Pelvic congestion must be differentiated from psoas muscle spasm (this also can cause low back and pelvic pain) and deep-thrust dyspareunia. It is caused by poor abdominal tone and posture and is more likely to occur after pregnancies and in midlife as a result of decreased physical activity and decreased concentration on maintenance of the abdominal musculature. A program of exercises to strengthen the paraspinal muscles and increase abdominal muscle tone will help. Pelvic floor tension myalgia also may cause dyspareunia. A hysterectomy will not help these muscle pains.

In any patient with dyspareunia, organic and psychological problems may coexist. Most of the organic lesions are treated on gynecologic principles. Counseling for the functional aspects may be done either by the primary physician or a specialist. Functional dyspareunia may be helped by either psychotherapy or behavioral therapy.[65]

URETHRAL PAIN

Urethral pain may be a result of urethral strictures or infections in the bladder, urethra, or seminal vesicles in men. Pain with voiding (which accompanies acute bladder infection) often is felt in the glandular urethra, an area innervated by S2 to S3. There may be tenderness along the course of the urethra. A clear, purulent, or bloody discharge may be seen at the urethral meatus. Urethral diverticulitis may be an obscure cause of pain. In women, the pain can be felt in the pelvis. During examination of the urethra, gentle pressure may express urine or pus and confirm the diagnosis. Urethral polyps also may be found.

Some women complain of persistent or recurrent frequency and dysuria. Such symptoms have been termed the urethral syndrome.[66] Bacteria may or may not be present (some regard the urethral syndrome as being abacteriuric).[67] The diagnosis depends on the absence of significant urologic disease. In some postmenopausal patients, it is thought that the urethral mucosa atrophies after the reduction in estrogen levels, similar to atrophic vaginitis. A caruncle may develop. Estrogen replacement may reactivate the urethral epithelium and abolish the inflammation. Urethral caruncles also are thought to disappear with estrogen therapy.[68] Some women with the urethral syndrome have a urethra that is high in the vagina. This may be traumatized more readily during sexual intercourse. Advice on changing sexual positioning may be helpful.

Investigating urethral pain initially consists of urinalysis, wet smear, and Gram staining. A smear of the discharge or swabbing the urethral mucosa should be cultured for *Chlamydia*. Subsequent investigations may include cystourethrography, retrograde urethrography, and cystourethroscopy.

Treatment of bacterial infection with appropriate antibiotics and surgically correctable lesions should be referred to a urologist. The urethral syndrome itself is more difficult to treat. After relieving any bacterial contamination, the pain may be relieved by fluids, bicarbonate, and introital hygiene. Estrogen therapy, when appropriate, may be beneficial. If these fail, a wide urethral dilatation has been helpful. Urethroplasty and urethrolysis play a role in selected patients, particularly where postcoital symptoms predominate.[66] Many of these women have a marked functional overlay that must not be ignored. A simple explanation coupled with supportive counseling will benefit most of them.

PAIN IN THE ANUS AND LOWER RECTUM

Pain in the anus may be acute or chronic. Table 12-3 lists the common causes. These acute pains usually are treated primarily by surgeons, and details of their treatment can be found in a surgical text. Anal ulcers, however, may be difficult to manage, especially those associated with radiotherapy. Caudal blocks may be helpful, and if the ulcer is low enough, caudal cryoanalgesia[10] may be effective for long-term pain relief.

Proctalgia fugax is a disorder of undetermined origin consisting of a fleeting rectal pain, occurring episodically, without demonstrable organic cause.[69] The symptoms are rare before puberty and usually disappear by age 70 years. Men and women are affected, and the patient may seem in otherwise good health. The pain occurs just above the anus, is severe, and lasts a few minutes to less than 0.5 h. The

Table 12-3
Pain in the Anus

Acute
Hemorrhoids
Anorectal abscess
Fissure-in-ano
Fistula-in-ano
Anal ulcers (postradiotherapy)
Chronic
Proctalgia fugax
Rectal neuralgia
Rectal tabetic crisis
Pruritus ani

duration and location of the pain is constant for each individual patient. The pain may occur at night or during the day, and it is not associated with bowel disturbance. The onset in men is sometimes related to ejaculation and, in both sexes, to straining at stool. Proctalgia is a relatively common phenomenon and has been reported in 14 percent of 301 subjects studied.[70] Physical examination is normal. Although the pathogenesis is obscure, it may be related to muscle spasm of the pelvic floor musculature, especially the pubococcygeus, transverse perineal muscles, bulbocavernosus, ischiocavernosus, and puborectalis. These are innervated by S3 to S4 (which controls their tonic and clonic contractions during ejaculation). The personality characteristics of these patients have been described variously as irritable, perfectionist, meticulous, obsessional, tense, and anxious. One study showed that many sufferers were perfectionist, most tense, or anxious; approximately one-third had severe or persistent neurotic symptoms in childhood.[71] Proctalgia fugax was believed to be of psychogenic origin, but this was not proved. Each attack may be attenuated with upward pressure on the anus or by a hot sitz bath. Amyl nitrite and nitroglycerine have no effect. Quinine has been recommended for night attacks, but this drug was not proved to be efficacious. Reassurance is important, and psychotherapy may help adjust these patients to their illness. Currently, we believe proctalgia fugax is harmless, unpleasant, and incurable.[72]

Rectal neuralgia consists of burning pain radiating from the rectum to the perineum, sacral region, and genitalia that is accompanied by paresthesia and hyperesthesia. As a deafferentation pain, it is difficult to treat and may require antidepressants or anticonvulsants.

Rectal tabetic crisis may mimic proctalgia fugax, but it can be differentiated by the abnormal neurologic findings and positive serologic results. Tabes dorsalis responds less to penicillin than other late manifestations of syphilis[73] because the neurologic damage already has occurred.

Pruritus ani may be severe enough to be interpreted as pain. Its relationship to anal pain is similar to the relationship of pruritus vulvae to vulvodynia. Hyperesthesia may be present. Symptoms are intermittent rather than continuous and are more common at night rather than during the day. Constipation is common. The main known causes[74] are listed in Table 12-4. No cause can be discovered in more than one-half of patients. Although no specific personality traits have been described in these patients, it is often assumed that there are psychogenic problems.

If a secondary cause can be found, it should be treated appropriately. Idiopathic cases require an explanation of the diagnosis, should be instructed to avoid scratching if possible to reduce the cycle, to practice anal hygiene (using sitz baths and cleansing), and to avoid dietary factors (such as seasoned food, pickles, or others, that may be associated with the pruritus). Cotton may be substituted for toilet paper, and medicated soaps should be avoided. Talcum powder may be useful in hot weather or for obese patients. Diphenhydramine may be helpful in severe cases. X-ray therapy in the past had some success,[75] but there are significant unacceptable irradiation hazards. Surgical therapy (undercutting and denervation of the perianal skin or excision of the skin) is reserved for the most severe cases, has no guarantee of success, and may be the basis for later denervation pain. Continued support for the patient is necessary; psychotherapy may play a role in extreme situations.

CONCLUSION

On the whole, acute pain in this region has well-defined causes and therapy. Chronic pain, however, is another story. In many cases, the physician is unable to find an organic treatable cause. This is one reason why pain in this area can depress the clinician, who feels helpless when presented with a patient with long-standing pain of no apparant cause and in whom no specific therapy is known. However, careful history taking, coupled with a thorough examination and appropriate laboratory tests, can detect treatable lesions in many patients. Other patients, even with apparent psychogenic elements, often are helped by various combinations of nerve blocks, caudal blocks, cryotherapy, and careful use of simple and nonsteroidal anti-inflammatory analgesics, antidepressants, and even anti-convulsants. They need continued psychological support; behavioral or psychotherapy may be required in selected cases.

Table 12-4
Causes of Pruritus Ani

Primary or Idiopathic

Secondary

Skin disease	Neurodermatitis
	Lichen planus
	Psoriasis
	Eczema
	Lichen sclerosis
	Contact dermatitis
	Bowen disease
Infections	Candidiasis
	Fungal infection
	Intestinal parasites (especially thread-worms)
	Anal warts
Gastrointestinal disease	Rectal disorders causing discharge
	Hemorrhoids
	Fissures
	Fistulas
	Proctitis
	Polyps
	Rectal neoplasm
	Irritable bowel syndrome
	Ulcerative colitis
	Malabsorption disorder
Miscellaneous	Drugs
	Quinidine
	Antibiotics (especially tetracycline)
	Obesity

References

1. Blacklock NJ. Surgical anatomy. In: Williams DI and Chisolm GD, eds. *Scientific Foundations of Urology.* 2nd ed. London: Heinemann; 1982:473–485.
2. Woodhouse CRJ, Riggs AJ. Chronic perineal pain. *Br J Hosp Med* 1984; 32:302–304.
3. Nocks BN. Pain in the male genitalia. In: Aronoff GM, ed. *Evaluation and Treatment of Chronic Pain.* Baltimore: Urban & Schwarzenberg; 1985:393–405.
4. Drach GW, Meares EW, Fair WR, Starey TA. Classification of benign disease associated with prostrate pain: prostatitis or prostatodynia. *J Urol* 1978; 120:266.
5. Meares EM, Starey TA. Bacteriologic localization patterns in bacterial prostatitis and urethritis. *Invest Urol* 1986; 5:492–518.
6. Cameron KM. Pathology of the prostate. *Br J Hosp Med* 1974; 11:348–355.
7. Smaki M, Merrit JL, Stillwell GK. Tension myalgia of the pelvic floor. *Mayo Clin Proc* 1977; 52:717–722.
8. Kitzinger S. Episiotomy pain. In: Wall PD, Melzack R, eds. *Textbook of Pain.* Edinburg: Churchill Livingstone; 1984:293–303.
9. Casey WC. Recurrent perineal and urethral pain. *JAMA* 1983; 249:3174.
10. Evans PJD, Lloyd JW, Jack TM. (1981) Cryoanalgesia for intractable perineal pain. *J R Soc Med* 1981; 74:804–809.
11. Schover LR: Psychological factors in men with genital pain. *Cleve Clin J Med* November–December 1990; 57(8):697–700.
12. Magui G, deBertolini C, Dodi G, Infantino A. Treatment for the chronic pain patient. *Ala J Med Sci* 1982; 19:121–122.

13. Osborn DE. Prostatodynia—physiological characteristics and rational management with muscle relaxants. *Br J Urol* 1981; 53:621–623.

14. Smart CJ, Jenkins JD, Lloyd RS. The painful prostate. *Br J Urol* 1975; 47:861–869.

15. Addison RG. Chronic pain syndrome. *Am J Med* September 10 1984; 77(3A) (suppl):54–58.

16. Watson CF, Evans RJ, Reed K, Merskey H, Goldsmith L, Warch J. Amitriptyline versus placebo in postherpetic neuralgia. *Neurology* 1982; 32:671–673.

17. Thiele GH. Coccygodynia and pain in the superior gluteal region and down the back of the thigh, causation by tonic spasm of the levator ani, coccygeus and piriformis muscles and relief by massage of these muscles. *JAMA* 1937; 109:1271–1275.

18. Patt R, Jain S. Long-term management of a patient with perineal pain secondary to rectal cancer. *J Pain Symptom Manage* April 1990; 5(2):127–128.

19. Swerdlow M. Intrathecal and extradural block in pain relief. In: Swerdlow M, ed. *Relief of Intractable Pain*. Amsterdam, New York, Oxford: Elsevier; 1983:175–214.

20. Robertson DH. Transsacral neurolytic nerve block: an alternative approach to intractable perineal pain. *Br J Anaesth 1983;* 55:873–874.

21. Saris SC, Silver JM, Vieira JFS, Nashold BS Jr. Sacrococcygeal rhizotomy for perineal pain. *Neurosurgery* 1986; 19:789–792.

22. Wray CC, Easom S, Hoskinson J. Coccydynia. Aetiology and treatment. *J Bone Joint Surg* Br March 1991; 73(2):335–338.

23. Nelson DA. Coccydynia and lumbar disk disease—historical correlations and clinical cautions. *Perspect Biol Med* Winter 1991; 34(2):229–238.

24. Thiele GH. Coccygodynia: cause and treatment. *Dis Colon Rectum* 1963; 6:422–436.

25. Finneson BE. *Low Back Pain*. 2nd ed. Philadelphia: Lippincott; 1980:533–555.

26. Hodge J. Clinical management of coccydynia. *Med Trial Tech Q* Winter 1979; 25(3):277–284.

27. Churcher M. Peripheral nerve blocks in relief of intractable pain. In: Swerdlow M, ed. *Relief of Intractable Pain*. Amsterdam, New York, Oxford: Elsevier; 1983:147–174.

28. Deitch EA, Soncrant MC. Ultrasonic diagnosis of surgical disease of the inguinal–femoral region. *Surg Gyn Obstet* 1981; 152:319–322.

29. Sneedberg SGC, Brooré AEA, Elmé O, Gullaro A. Herniography in the diagnosis of obscure groin pain. *Acta Chir Scand* 1985; 151:663–667.

30. McCall IW, Park WM, O'Brien JP. Induced pain referral from posterior lumbar elements in normal subjects. *Spine* 1979; 4:441–446.

31. Mooney V, Robertson J. The facet syndrome. *Clin Orthop* 1976; 115:149–156.

32. Beaver WT. Combination analgesics. *Am J Med* September 1984; 77(3A):38–52.

33. Tasker RR. Deafferentation. In: Wall PD, Melzack R, eds. *Textbook of Pain*. Edinburgh: Churchill Livingstone; 1986:119–132.

34. Rosenblatt RM, Reich J, Dehring D. Tricyclic antidepressants in the treatment of depression and chronic pain. *Anesth Analg* 1984; 63:1025–1032.

35. Swerdlow M. Anticonvulsant drugs and chronic pain. *Clin Neuropharmacal* 1984; 1:51–82.

36. Hameroff SR, Carlson GL, Brown BR. Ilioinguinal pain syndrome. *Pain* 1981; 10:253–257.

37. Blumer D. Psychiatric consideration in pain. In: Rothman RH, Simeone FA, eds. *The Spine*. Vol. II. Philadelphia: Saunders; 1975:871–906.

38. Posner RB. Physician–patient communication. *Am J Med* September 1984; 77(suppl):59–64.

39. Devine CJ Jr, Horton CE. Surgical treatment of Peyronie's disease with a dermal graft. *J Urol* 1974; 111:44–49.

40. Yeats KW. Pain in the scrotum. *Br J Hosp Med* 1985; 33:101–104.

41. Ransler CW III, Allen TD. Torsion of the spermatic cord. *Urol Clin North Am* 1982; 9:245–250.

42. Prout GR Jr, Griffin PP. Testicular tumors: delay in diagnosis and influence on survival. *Am Fam Physician* 1984; 29:205–209.

43. Jackson SM. (1983) Radiotherapy, anticancer drugs and hormones in the relief of pain. In: Swerdlow M, ed. *Relief of Intractable Pain*. Amsterdam, New York, Oxford: Elsevier; 1983:347–379.

44. Demas BE, Hricak H, McClure RD. Varicoceles. Radiologic diagnosis and treatment. *Radiol Clin North Am* May 1991; 29(3):619–627.

45. Biggers RD, Soderdahl DW. The painful varicocele. *Milit Med* 1981; 146:440–441.

46. Takihara H, Sakatoku J, Cockett AT. The pathophysiology of varicocele in male infertility. *Fertil Steril* May 1991; 55(5):861–868.

47. White SH, Leslie IJ. Pain in scrotum due to intervertebral disc protrusion. *Lancet* 1986; 1:504.

48. Ali MS. Testicular pain in a patient with aneurysm of the common iliac surgery. *Br J Urol* 1983; 44:447–448.

49. York GR, Gabor AJ, Dreyfus PM. Paroxysmal genital pain: an unusual manifestation of epilepsy. *Neurology* 1979; 29:516–519.

50. McKay M. Burning vulva syndrome. Report of the ISSVD task force. *J Reprod Med* 1984; 29:457.

51. Lynch PJ. Vulvodynia: a syndrome of unexplained vulval pain, psychological disability and sexual dysfunction. *J Reprod Med* 1986; 31:773–780.

52. Friedrich EG Jr. The vulvar vestibule. *J Reprod Med* 1983; 28:773–777.

53. DiPaulo GR, Rueda NG. Deceptive vulvar papillomavirus infection: a possible explanation for certain cases of vulvodynia. *J Reprod Med* 1986; 31:966–970.

54. Cotterill JA. Dermatological non-disease: a common and potentially fatal disturbance of cutaneous body image. *Br J Dermatol* 1981; 104:611–619.

55. Pearson JW. Chronic pelvic pain: its evaluation and therapy. In: Symonds EM, Zuspan FP, eds. *Clinical and Diagnostic Procedures in Obstetrics and Gynecology*. New York: Marcel Dekker; 1984:381–395.

56. Dodson MG, Friedrich EG. Psychosomatic vulvovaginitis. *Obstet Gynecol* 1978; 51(suppl):23s–25s.

57. Greaves MW, McDonald-Gibson W. Itch: Role of prostaglandins. *Br Med J* 1973; III:608–609.

58. Goolamali SK. Pruritis vulvae, In: Fisher AM, Gordon H, eds. *Clinics in Obstetrics and Gynaecology. Gynaecological Enigmas, 8*. No. 1. London: Saunders; 1981:227–240.

59. DeWitt DE. Dyspareunia. Tracing the cause. *Postgrad Med* April 1991; 89(5):67–68, 70, 73.

60. Lackritz RM, Weinberg PC. Dysmenorrhea, premenstrual syndrome, dyspareunia. In: Pauerstein CJ, ed. *Gynecologic Disorders. Differential Diagnosis and Therapy*. New York: Grune & Stratton; 1982:51–66.

61. Oates JK. Focal vulvitis and localized dyspareunia. *Genitourin Med* February 1990; 66(1):28–30.

62. Perineal pain after childbirth. *Med J Aust* April 2 1990; 152(7):386–387. Letter.

63. Bolling DR, Jr. Pelvic floor dysfunction: genital prolapse, pelvic relaxation and urinary incontinence. In: Pauerstein CJ, ed. *Gynecologic Disorders. Differential Diagnosis and Therapy*. New York: Grune & Stratton; 1982:265–290.

64. Allen WM, Masters WH. Traumatic laceration of uterine support. The clinical syndrome and the operative treatment. *Am J Obstet Gynecol* 1955; 70:500–513.

65. Masters WH, Johnson VE. *Human Sexual Inadequacy*. London: Churchill Livingstone; 1970.

66. Smith P. The urethral syndrome. In: Fisher AM, Gordon H, eds. *Clinics in Obstetrics and Gynaecology. Gynaecological Enigmas, 8* No. 1. London: Saunders; 1981:161–172.

67. O'Grady FW. Urinary tract infection in women. *J R Coll Physicians Lond* 1979; 13(2):70–73.

68. Parsons L, Sommers SC. *Gynecology*. 2nd ed. Philadelphia: Saunders; 1978:352.

69. Schuster MM. Constipation and anorectal disorders. In: Almy TP, Fielding JF, eds. *The GI Tract in Stress and Psychological Disorders*. Clinics in Gastroenterology, 6(3):643–658.

70. Thompson WG, Heaton KW. Proctalgia fugax. *J R Coll Physicians Lond* 1980; 14:247–248.

71. Pilling LF, Swenson WM, Hill JR. The psychologic aspects of proctalgia fugax. *Dis Colon Rectum* 1965; 8:372–376.

72. Douthwaite AH. Proctalgia fugax. *Br Med J* 1962; III:164–165.

73. Holmes KK. Syphilis. In: Isselbacker KJ, Adams RD, Braunwald E, Petersdorf RG, Wilson JD, eds. *Harrison's Principles of Internal Medicine*. 9th ed. New York: McGraw-Hill; 1980:716–726.

74. Shearman DJC, Finlayson NDC. *Diseases of the Gastrointestinal Tract and Liver*. Edinburgh: Churchill Livingstone; 1982:934.

75. Shapiro AI, Rothman S. Pruritis ani: a clinical study. *Gastroenterology* 1945; 5:155–167.

CHAPTER 13

Joint Pain

Tobin Gerhart and Lena E. Dohlman

This chapter provides the pain specialist with a background for treating the many conditions that cause joint pain. A detailed discussion of all the rheumatologic, neurologic, and orthopedic aspects of this topic is not intended. Instead, the clinical presentation and treatment of those conditions most likely to be referred for pain management will be emphasized. Although, typically, patient referrals are sent with a diagnosis and a previous treatment history, there may be pitfalls for the unwary physician. The diagnosis may have changed and be in error. The duration or kind of medical treatment may have been inadequate. An example of this sort of problem is a patient referred with an undiagnosed low grade chronic joint infection or tumor. Proper pain management for patients with joint symptoms requires a knowledge of the clinical presentation, pathologic condition, and therapy of joint disease.[1]

Patients with joint pain are a common clinical challenge to the practicing physician. Large public health surveys group together many joint conditions under the term *arthritis,* an affliction affecting 23 million Americans with symptoms severe enough to restrict activities and require medical attention.[2] Approximately 55 percent of patients with arthritis report that it bothers them all the time, and 60 percent report that it bothers them a great deal.[1] Because only a small fraction of the patients with arthritis actually are referred to a pain management unit, these patients may have special problems.

Not all of the conditions causing pain described by these patients as originating from the region of the joint involve intraarticular disease. Acute and chronic periarticular inflammatory conditions, such as tendinitis, bursitis, and adhesive capsulitis occur commonly. Much less frequent, but more important to remember, are tumors and indolent infections, both intraarticular and those in the adjacent bone and soft tissues. Pain also can be referred to the joint from either nerve root irritation (such as that caused by cervical disc disease) or from intraabdominal or intrathoracic disease. A correct understanding of the cause of joint pain can be difficult at times, but it is crucial for proper management.[3] We must not attribute joint symptoms caused by some treatable serious underlying medical condition to a nonspecific pain syndrome.

An organized and systematic approach to joint pain is important to provide the best possible treatment (Table 13-1). One simple way to evaluate joint pain is to determine whether the cause of the pain is a result of an intrinsic or extrinsic disorder. Intrinsic disorders involve the joint itself and characteristically have three features: (1) the patient gives a history of pain that is aggravated when the joint is stressed (e.g., sitting typically aggravates sciatica, and walking is painful with hip joint arthritis), (2) physical examination reveals tenderness to palpation that can be either localized or diffuse, and (3) the pain can be elicited by active or passive range of motion of the joint. Extrinsic disorders are those originating outside the joint area. They do not fulfill these three criteria. Usually the distinction is easy to make, but the boundaries occasionally can be blurred, particularly with neurologic causes. Extrinsic causes of pain in the joints are covered elsewhere in this book. This chapter will focus on intrinsic causes of joint pain.

CATEGORIZATION OF INTRINSIC CAUSES OF JOINT PAIN

A first step in approaching intrinsic joint pain is to determine from which of three anatomic locations the condition originates: intraarticular, periarticular soft tissues, or the adjacent bone (see Table 13-1). Although occasionally

Table 13-1
Organization of Conditions Causing Joint Pain

Intrinsic Disorders
Intraarticular
  Inflammatory
    Immunologic
    Crystal-induced
    Infections
  Intraarticular derangement
  Osteoarthritis
Periarticular soft tissues
  Bursitis and tendinitis
  Mechanical instability (dislocations)
  Adhesive capsulitis
Adjacent bone
  Fractures
  Metabolic disease
  Heterotopic bone formation
  Neoplasms
Extrinsic Disorders

there is some overlap between these anatomic regions, a distinct localization usually can be made by physical examination and radiographic studies. Intraarticular disease causes joint effusions and synovial or joint-line tenderness. Periarticular conditions also may cause tenderness around the joint, but they lack joint effusions. Lesions in the adjacent bone can be identified either by plain radiographs or with a bone scan.

Conditions in each anatomic region of the joint can be organized by their causes into broad categories. Intraarticular causes of joint pain may be divided into three categories: inflammatory, intraarticular derangement, and osteoarthritis. These three categories usually can be distinguished by taking a careful history.

Inflammatory Joint Disease

Inflammatory conditions of the joint often have an insidious or nontraumatic pattern of onset. The patient typically complains of pain and stiffness that is more severe in the morning. This usually improves somewhat with a little activity or joint motion. The joints themselves usually are tender, but weight-bearing activities do not necessarily worsen the symptoms. The symptoms frequently can be relieved by administering anti-inflammatory agents. The patients may have characteristic systemic signs, such as rashes, fever, and other organ system pathologic findings. The involvement can be monoarticular or polyarticular. Three causes of inflammatory joint conditions include: immunologic, crystal-induced, and infectious.

Immunologic Arthropathies

Rheumatoid arthritis is the most important example of an immune-mediated joint disease, with an estimated 5 million Americans afflicted in the United States currently.[4] It is usually polyarticular and pursues a slow relentless course. Although periods of remission can be obtained with therapy, these patients have recurrent painful rheumatoid flares[5] until all the articular cartilage has been destroyed leaving a so-called burned-out joint. Women more frequently are affected than men. The diagnosis of rheumatoid arthritis is made based on the clinical picture, analysis of the joint fluid, and serum tests for rheumatoid factor, an immunoglobulin M.[6] Approximately 85 percent of patients with rheumatoid arthritis test positive for rheumatoid factor compared with less than 5 percent of normal subjects and 20 percent to 40 percent of patients with other collagen diseases or chronic inflamatory conditions.

Mild to moderately symptomatic rheumatoid arthritis usually responds well to nonsteroidal anti-inflammatory drugs (NSAIDs) such as aspirin, ibuprofen, indomethacin, and naproxen (Table 13-2).[7] These drugs have immediate analgesic and anti-inflammatory effects, and their efficacy, therefore, can be assessed quickly. There is no convincing evidence that one NSAID is better than another, but often a patient who has not responded to one NSAID will respond to another. Therefore, trials on several of these agents should be attempted before the patient's pain is considered refractory to NSAIDs. All these drugs can cause gastrointestinal irritation, although many believe that some of the newer (and more expensive) NSAIDs cause fewer gastrointestinal side effects than aspirin. The nonacetylated salicylates seem to have the least gastrointestinal effects. All NSAIDs also affect platelet functions and cause an increase in bleeding time with the exceptions of some of the nonacetylated salicylates (such as salsalate). Apparently, salsalate and magnesium salicylate may be among the few NSAIDs that can be used in patients who have had an asthmatic reaction to aspirin. All NSAIDs can have adverse central nervous system effects (such as confusion). Indomethacin can have more severe effects than some of the other NSAIDs, especially in elderly patients. There are several slower acting drugs used to treat rheumatoid arthritis that have no immediate analgesic effects, but they are used to control symptoms over a longer period. They also may delay progression of the disease, but most have severe adverse side effects. They include hydroxychloroquine, gold compounds, penicillamine, and the cytotoxic drugs azathioprine, methotrexate, and cyclophosphamide.

Corticosteroids are anti-inflammatory and immunosuppressive. Occasionally, they are used for symptomatic treatment of patients with severe rheumatoid arthritis. Their use is controversial, however, because of serious side effects, including osteoporosis, gastrointestinal bleeding, and cataracts. Corticosteroids also can be injected locally for temporary control of symptoms in an acute episode where one or two joints are especially painful. Triamcinolone diacetate and methylprednisolone acetate appear to suppress inflammation for the longest time. The injection of the joint should be done using careful aseptic technique. A 20- or 22-gauge needle is inserted on the extensor surface of the joint that is furthest from the nerves, arteries, and veins and closest to the joint cavity. Synovial fluid is aspirated first for analysis and to decrease joint distension. After assurance that no joint infection is present, the corticosteroid is injected at a dose appropriate to the joint size. This use of corticosteroids also is controversial because there is no evidence that any long-term benefit is obtained with this form of treatment. Repeated and long-term use of corticosteroids may be damaging to the joint, and injections should not be done more frequently than two to three times a year. Total joint replacement surgery is an option for suitable candidates with uncontrolled pain and functional impairment.

Psoriatic arthritis and systemic lupus erythematosus are other examples of immunologically mediated conditions causing polyarthritis.

Crystal-Induced Arthropathies

Crystal-induced arthropathy includes gout and pseudogout.[8] Uric acid and calcium pyrophosphate crystals, respectively, precipitate in the joints of these patients, causing a dramatic

Table 13-2
Nonsteroidal Anti-Inflammatory Drugs for Treatment of Rheumatoid Arthritis

Drug	Usual Dosage Range	Side Effects	Special
Aspirin	3.6–5.4 g/day	*	Inexpensive, GI effects more severe, probably best choice for early pregnancy
Fenoprofen	300–600 mg tid–qid	*	GI effects less severe than with aspirin
Ibuprofen	400–600 mg tid–qid	*	GI effects less severe than with aspirin
Naproxen	250–500 mg bid	*	GI effects less severe than with aspirin, long half-life
Indomethacin	25 mg tid–50 mg bid	*	High incidence of adverse effects, especially CNS, but effective
Sulindac	150–200 mg bid	*	High incidence of adverse effects
Meclofenamate sodium	200–400 mg in 3–4 doses	*	High incidence of diarrhea, allergic reactions more common
Naproxen sodium	275 mg bid–tid	*	
Piroxicam	20 mg qd	*	Allergic reactions more common
Tolmetin	200–600 mg tid	*	GI side effects common
Nonacetylated salicylates			
Magnesium salicylate	2 tablets tid–qid	GI, CNS, otic	No platelet dysfunction, bronchospasm less likely than with aspirin, avoid use in renal failure
Choline salicylate	4.8–7.2 g/day	GI, otic, respiratory	No platelet dysfunction
Choline magnesium salicylate	3 g/day	GI, otic	No platelet dysfunction, GI effects mild
Diflunisal	250–500 mg bid	GI, liver, CNS, renal, hypertensive	No platelet dysfunction at low doses
Salsalate	3–4 g/day	GI, otic	No platelet dysfunction, asthmatic reaction less likely than with aspirin, less effective

*GI, platelet dysfunction, hypersensitivity reactions, CNS, hepatic, otic, hematopoietic, renal, and cardiac.

GI includes dyspepsia, heartburn, nausea, vomiting, GI bleeding, and constipation.

CNS includes drowsiness, headache, and dizziness, sweating, depression, tinnitus, confusion, and anorexia.

Hepatic includes abnormal liver function tests and hepatitis.

Otic includes tinnitus and temporary hearing loss.

Hematopoietic includes neutropenia, thrombocytopenia, and rarely aplastic anemia.

Renal includes decreased renal blood flow, causing renal failure in patients with compromised renal function.

Cardiac includes congestive heart failure, palpitations, hypertension, and edema.

Respiratory includes bronchospasm.

inflammatory response. The patients often have severe symptoms of acute joint pain and swelling. Acute flare-ups of gout usually are monoarticular (with a predilection for the lower extremity). A diagnosis of gout is made by identifying (in a sample of joint fluid) the needle-shaped uric acid crystals; these are brightly birefringent when seen through a polarizing microscope. Colchicine is the drug of choice for initial treatment, and the response usually is dramatic. Nonsteroidal anti-inflammatory drugs (such as indomethacin) also can be useful in treating an acute attack. After resolution of the acute attack, treatment should begin with allopurinol to decrease the production of urates and probenecid to increase excretion of uric acid.

Pseudogout, also known as chondrocalcinosis, usually does not appear until the third or fourth decade of life. Typically, attacks are less severe than gout. Radiographs show punctate or linear calcifications in the fibrocartilage of the menisci and articular cartilage, especially in the wrist and knee. The diagnosis is confirmed by identifying the rectangular dimly birefringent crystals of calcium pyrophosphate found in the joint fluid. Treatment includes NSAIDs; these usually provide relief of symptoms.

Joint Infections

Joint infections can occur either hematogenously or through direct contact. The possibility of a septic joint always must be considered in a patient who previously has received a corticosteroid injection. The clinical course of the disease depends on the infectious agent. Gonorrhea and pyogenic infections of staphylococci or streptococci characteristically are fulminant, with a dramatically swollen painful joint, systemic signs of fever, and an elevated leukocyte count. More indolent and easier to overlook are joint infections from tuberculosis and fungi. Fluid aspirated from infected joints is turbid, has a low glucose level, and has a leukocyte count above 50,000/dl with a predominance of polymorphonuclear leukocytes (polys). Gram staining may identify an organism tentatively; antibiotics can be started pending the results of cultures. Pyogenic joint infections constitute a medical emergency because the lysozomal enzymes released by the polys can destroy articular cartilage permanently within 24 hours. Lavage of the joint using repeated aspirations or surgical means removes these damaging enzymes. The inflamed synovium offers no barrier to antibiotics; high concentrations can be achieved in the joint fluid. Intraarticular antibiotic injection should be avoided because this can cause an intense chemical reaction.

Intraarticular Derangement

Mechanical blocking of the joint, commonly called intraarticular derangement, occurs when some damaged or abnormal structure in the joint prevents normal motion of the joint surfaces. The joint most frequently involved is the knee, but intraarticular derangement occasionally occurs in other joints. Patients have three characteristic symptoms: locking, giving way, and swelling of the joint as a result of effusions. Typically, the extremity is functioning normally when, during some activity, the joint suddenly becomes locked painfully. The patient is unable to either flex or extend the joint fully until, with a fortuitous movement, something seems to slide out of place, and the joint regains mobility. After one of these episodes, the joint remains painful for a few days and may develop an effusion. Trauma may result in mechanical blocking when structures such as the meniscus are torn, and its fragments lodge abnormally between the joint surfaces. Loose bodies or so-called joint mice are produced when small pieces of the articular surface break off, usually after repetitive trauma. The cartilage cells, nourished by the synovial fluid, grow in size while drifting around inside the joint. When the free fragment drifts between the joint surfaces and is large enough to cause impingement, the patient experiences a sudden locking episode. Large loose bodies also can be formed when a piece of the articular surface that has been damaged by osteochondritis dissecans falls out into the joint. A much rarer cause of intraarticular impingement is a tumor (such as a pigmented villonodular synovitis and synovial chondromatosis). A history of episodic locking, giving way, and joint effusions is a primary indication for arthroscopy. Not only can an accurate diagnosis be made, but frequently the problem can be corrected by removing the abnormality arthroscopicly.[9,10]

Osteoarthritis (Degenerative Joint Disease)

Osteoarthritis (or degenerative joint disease) is the most common form of arthritis. It is characterized by a progressive loss of articular cartilage, subchondral bony sclerosis, and cartilage and bone proliferation at the joint margins, eventually leading to osteophyte formation.[4] The resulting joint deformities produce progressive pain and limitation of the movement of the joint. The cause of osteoarthritis is not clear, but it occurs when cartilage repair does not match with cartilage degeneration. Osteoarthritis, therefore, often develops in patients whose joints previously have been injured by inflammatory conditions or intraarticular derangements. It also occurs more commonly in those who have been exposed to frequent joint injury (such as sports professionals) and in those who have stressed their joints (obese patients). Osteoarthritis is more common in middle to late age; this is consistent with the greater incidence of disease in joints they are used more. It disproportionately involves weight-bearing joints (hips and knees), and there is a direct relationship between the amount of activity or loading a joint undergoes and the extent of the patient's symptoms. By contrast with inflammatory arthritis, the pain usually is less intense in the morning and steadily worsens throughout the day. The symptoms are relieved by unloading the affected extremity, such as lying down when a leg joint is involved or using a sling for the arm. On physical examination, the tenderness is localized to the joint-line itself and is not as severe as in inflammatory conditions. Intermittent effusions occur; the joint fluid essentially is normal when analyzed. Four diagnostic radiographic findings include: a narrowed joint space, presence of osteophytes, subchondral sclerosis, and some cyst formation. Radiographs of the hips and knees must be taken with the patient standing and bearing weight to assess the extent of joint space narrowing and malalignment.

Osteoarthritis is the most common indication for which nonsteroidal anti-inflammatory drugs are prescribed. They can be effective in controlling the pain and reducing inflammation in the early stages of the disease. As in rheumatoid arthritis, it is important to try several different NSAIDs because patients who do not respond to one frequently have a good result with another. Lower doses of NSAIDs generally should be used to treat osteoarthritis compared with those in rheumatoid arthritis. Unfortunately, these drugs have not been shown to retard the disease process itself, and often, more radical treatments are required when the symptoms worsen. Tricyclic anti-depressants and TENS can be helpful adjuncts to NSAID therapy in controlling the pain. They may help to delay the need for surgical joint replacement and improve the comfort of patients who are poor surgical candidates. The use of intraarticular corticosteroid injections is controversial. Temporary relief of symptoms may be produced at the expense of accelerating joint destruction through interference with normal articular healing mechanisms. A neurotrophic arthropathy also may result from decreased antalgic joint feedback. Recent experimental evidence suggests that repeated intraarticular injections of glucocorticoids in patients with osteoarthritis can induce or accelerate the deposition of hydroxyapatite in the articular cartilage.[11]

Prosthetic joint replacement surgery is an option for patients with severe disabling disease who do not respond to medical management. The primary indication is pain relief, although sometimes improved range of motion is a secondary consideration. Current clinical studies of patients with hip and knee replacements report 90 percent to 95 percent good-to-excellent results at 10 years' follow-up. The major unsolved problem in prosthetic joint replacement is loosening of the components at the interface between the cement and the patient's bone. Loose components are painful and predispose the patient to secondary hematogenous infection. Loosening occurs because the polymethylmethacrylate cement is inert and stabilizes itself in the bone solely by mechanical interlock. Repetitive stresses lead to accumulation of material-fatigue damage in the cement, causing component failure. Excessive weight and high activity levels, therefore, will accelerate the loosening process. Younger patients are much poorer candidates for prosthetic joint replacement because they can be expected to live longer and have higher activity levels.

Revision of a failed prosthetic joint is more difficult than a primary procedure as a consequence of scarring and deficient bone stock. The infection rate has been reported to be from 2- to 10-fold that for primary arthroplasties. Revision surgery in the United States now constitutes an estimated 10 percent to 15 percent of all prosthetic arthroplasties. A new approach to the loosening problem is cementless arthroplasty. In this procedure, a special porous coating is placed on the components that allows direct ingrowth of the patient's bone, thereby creating a living bone that theoretically is not subject to fatigue failure. Clinical studies show that results are comparable with conventional cemented arthroplasty, but follow-up studies with appreciable numbers of patients extend only to 5 years or less. Conventional arthroplasty has such an excellent record (even at 10 to 15 years) that proving the superiority of another approach will take many years.

Surgical treatment for younger or heavier patients may include an osteotomy. In this procedure, the bone is cut near the joint to realign it. The correction of bowleg (genu varus) deformities by making a proximal tibial osteotomy is an important example of this procedure. The abnormal mechanical forces across the medial part of the joint are relieved by the osteotomy, slow the progression of osteoarthritis, and provide pain relief. Osteotomy around the hip is used similarly to rotate areas of the femoral head damaged by avascular necrosis or osteoarthritis out of the weight-bearing region. Osteotomy has been viewed more favorably in Europe than in the United States. The pain relief is not as satisfactory as after prosthetic arthroplasty, but these patients can return to activities (such as farming) without restrictions because loosening of components is not an issue.

Another surgical alternative is fusion; this provides a completely pain-free joint. The main disadvantage is lack of motion. For some joints (such as the ankle and nondominant shoulder), this procedure causes little disability because adjacent joints (subtalar and scapulothoracic) provide compensating motion. Hip and knee fusions cause more functional restrictions and are contraindicated if there is a possibility that more than one joint requires fusion. The young patient with end-stage joint disease who is not a suitable candidate for prosthetic replacement or the alternatives of osteotomy or fusion remains a frustrating unsolved problem.

PERIARTICULAR SOFT TISSUE DISORDERS
Bursitis and Tendinitis

Acute inflammatory conditions (such as bursitis and tendinitis) are the most common causes of joint pain. The classic presentation involves a history of overuse, with excessive or unusual activity followed by symptoms of pain 6 to 24 h later when inflammation has occurred. During the physical examination, patients have well-localized areas of tenderness corresponding to the specific anatomic site affected. The joint itself is not involved, and no effusion is present. Certain maneuvers can cause the pain to be referred to the affected area. For instance, asking the patient to dorsiflex a clenched fist and then resist efforts to straighten the wrist will cause pain at the lateral epicondyle of patients with tennis elbow or lateral epicondylitis.

Most patients are relieved to hear a simple medical explanation of their problem. For example, repetitive excessive motion of any structural material causes the accumulation of fatigue damage similar to that when a paper clip is bent repetitively until it breaks. In living animals, this damage can be repaired in most instances by the normal healing response. However, if the injury is excessive, an inflammatory response may occur, resulting in swelling, redness, and tenderness, usually many hours after the activity that caused it. Structures, such as tendons and bursas, that permit motion around the joints are affected by this problem because of repetitive high loading forces involved as a result of the leverage exerted by the extremities.

Therapy for tendinitis, bursitis, and similar conditions consists of rest and anti-inflammatory medication. Most patients respond to oral NSAIDs in a few days. If the symptoms are persistent or are severe, then glucocorticoid injections can provide dramatic relief. The patients who respond best to injection therapy have a well-localized area of moderate-to-severe tenderness that can be touched with a single finger during the physical examination. Water-insoluble forms of glucocorticoids (such as methylprednisolone acetate) are preferable because they have less systemic uptake and a prolonged local duration of action. Mixing 1 to 2 ml of lidocaine with the glucocorticoid also is desirable. The patient should feel immediate relief, and the physician will have the advantage of knowing before the patient leaves whether the medication was injected into the correct location. Common suitable anatomic locations include the supraspinatus bursa at the shoulder, the pes anserinus bursa and the ileotibial band at the knee, the greater trochanteric bursa at the hip, and the lateral epicondyle at the elbow. Because injection at these sites is extraarticular, there is no detrimental effect to the articular cartilage. Considerable restraint should be exercised in injections administered for inflammation of certain tendons, particularly the Achilles and quadriceps. Glucocorticoids will impair collagen metabolism and can lead to weakening and rupture after multiple injections. A poor response to rest and anti-inflammatory therapy is a worrisome sign and indicates the need for reevaluation of the diagnosis.

Mechanical Instability (Dislocations)

Pain associated with chronic joint instability can pose perplexing management problems. Acute subluxations and dislocations after joint trauma usually heal well with standard orthopedic treatment. Sometimes, however, the instability goes unrecognized initially or persists for other reasons, resulting in a difficult chronic pain problem. Proper management of these patients depends on an understanding of the underlying instability. Recognition usually is easy, but in some patients, the diagnosis can be overlooked if careful attention is not paid to the history. The shoulder and knee joints are afflicted most frequently by chronic laxity because they depend on capsular soft tissues for stability.

The shoulder frequently is dislocated because the glenohumeral articulation is shallow, with little inherent bony constraint. The initial dislocation usually requires high energy trauma to stretch or tear the capsule and supporting ligaments, but subsequent episodes can occur under milder conditions (such as during sleep). Anterior dislocations predominate. For these, the most vulnerable position is an elevated arm that is rotated externally. When the shoulder is dislocated, patients feel acute pain and are unable to move their arms. Although reduction usually requires medical assistance, some patients (after many dislocations) are able to reduce their own shoulders. Recurrent trauma causes the ligamentous stabilizers to become lax. Treatment of recurrent anterior dislocations surgically is recommended after several episodes have occurred because future recurrent dislocations are likely and, eventually, may result in degenerative joint changes. Surgical procedures have a 90 percent to 95 percent success rate in preventing later dislocations.

Voluntary dislocators, many of whom have psychological problems, can both dislocate and relocate their shoulders at will. Experience has shown that they respond poorly to surgical procedures, and operative treatment is not recommended for these patients. Eventually, many have chronic pain as a result of the degenerative changes. They should be managed using (1) physical therapy to attempt to improve stability by strengthening the stabilizing musculature and (2) psychiatric counseling.

Posterior dislocation of the shoulder is easier to miss during the physical examination because of the concealing muscle mass. Furthermore, posterior dislocations frequently occur in patients who are seizing, an event not always associated with major skeletal trauma. For these reasons, patients with posterior dislocations can go unrecognized and present as chronic shoulder pain. Absence of a full range of motion is an important clue. Anteroposterior radiographs can give the false impression of a normal shoulder because of the fortuitous superposition of the humeral head near the glenoid. The diagnosis can be confirmed by an axillary view laterally; this shows that the true position of the humeral head is posterior to the glenoid.

Even anterior dislocations sometimes are overlooked, especially in elderly patients. They have pain and limited shoulder motion. If the joint has been dislocated more than several weeks, then the usual gentle closed reduction maneuvers usually are unsuccessful; more aggressive closed or open surgical procedures, however, are hazardous. Such patients consequently are left dislocated and treated symptomatically. The range of motion remains limited, but the pain eventually improves.

True dislocations of the knee are major limb-threatening injuries associated with high energy trauma. Chronic recurrent dislocations do not occur. Transient subluxation of the knee from a tear or laxity of the anterior cruciate ligament, however, is one of the most frequent causes of chronic disability and pain in the lower extremity. Patients with anterior cruciate laxity give a characteristic history. They can participate in many sports activities, but when they try to turn on a weight-bearing slightly flexed knee, a sudden giving way occurs. Afterward, pain and joint effusion can result. Most patients can be rehabilitated with muscle-strengthening exercises. Frequently, they can return to their previous sports, especially if they are willing to wear a properly designed derotational-type brace. Serious athletes and certain laborers who require reliable performance from their knee may be candidates for reconstructive surgery.

Adhesive Capsulitis

Loss of normal joint motion also can lead to chronic pain secondary to adhesive capsulitis. Although this condition can affect any joint, the shoulder is afflicted most commonly. Understanding the course of a simple limited case of adhesive capsulitis helps put into perspective these difficult patients who may be referred for pain management. The history usually includes some form of trauma, such as a fracture or acute episode of bursitis or tendinitis. These patients tend to keep their arms immobilized at their sides because motion of their shoulders is painful. This immobilization allows the inflamed synovial folds to contract and scar together. This scarring worsens the initial problem of pain with shoulder motion, and the arm is kept immobilized by the patient. Inability to elevate the arm more than 90° during physical examination is worrisome. This test should be done with the patient supine so that the difficulty of lifting the arm against gravity is obviated. The primary aim of treatment should be prevention. Immobilization of the injured shoulder or arm with a sling should not be prolonged beyond 1 to 2 weeks without instituting daily range-of-motion exercises, especially in elderly patients. These should include pendulum exercises, in which the patient bends forward and lets the hanging arm swing in widening arcs. As motion improves, the patient should lie supine and slowly raise the involved arm fully overhead using their contralateral hand. The importance of persistence with the exercises, despite initial discomfort, must be stressed to the patient. After adhesive capsulitis occurs, treatment can be difficult and prolonged. A physical therapist can be helpful in severe cases in assisting the patient with range-of-motion exercises. A suprascapular nerve block done in a pain clinic just before the physical therapy session sometimes can allow the patient to make more rapid progress. The suprascapular nerve is a fairly superficial nerve, and it can be blocked easily using a 22-gauge needle and 2 to 4 ml of a local anesthetic, such as lidocaine 1% or bupivacaine 0.5%. The injection is made by locating the scapula notch with the needle tip using a posterior approach and injecting at a depth of approximately 1.5 cm. This will block sensory fibers to the shoulder joint and surrounding structures and allow the shoulder to be moved with minimal pain during the physical therapy session. Oral anti-inflammatory medication and analgesics also can be used to allow the patient to do the arm exercises in greater comfort.

ADJACENT BONE

Fractures

Most acute fractures are obvious because they are associated with a history of trauma and diagnostic x-ray findings. Because stress fractures and pathologic fractures are atypical in this regard, they are easy to overlook. Stress fractures occur most frequently in the lower extremities, and the patient typically has pain associated with weight bearing or active motion of the limb. The cause is excessive repetitive loading that produces microfractures in the bone. The body's initial reaction is to resorb bone in preparation for a secondary bone-forming phase to heal the microfractures. If the patient ignores the pain signals during this stage and continues heavy activity, then the damage accelerates because the bone temporarily is weaker. Eventually, a fracture results. Bone scans show increased uptake early and help to make the diagnosis. X-ray findings may be normal initially and often are just subtle radiolucent lines when they do occur. The treatment is protection from weight bearing and sometimes cast immobilization.

Pathologic fractures also occur without a convincing history of trauma. In a sense, they are stress fractures through areas of bone weakened by metabolic bone disease or tumor. The importance of a pathologic fracture, therefore, is to recognize the underlying disease process. Treat-

ment of the underlying medical condition should always be considered first, for instance, correction of hyperparathyroidism or irradiation or chemotherapy to treat a metastatic lesion. Often, surgical stabilization of the affected bone by prophylactic internal fixation is necessary for pain relief and prevention of a true displaced fracture.

Metabolic Disease

Paget disease is a focal bony disorder of bone of unknown cause. It is rare before the age of 40 years, but autopsy incidence figures show that it occurs in 3 percent to 4 percent of the population. It is more common in England and northern Europe and less common in Scandinavia and the Mediterranean countries. The histopathologic findings consist of three phases: an initial osteolytic phase, a mixed phase, and generally a late osteoblastic phase. The problem is abnormally high bone turnover, with excessive resorption, followed by subsequent formation of new bone. Radiographic diagnosis is made using four criteria: (1) enlargement of the bones, (2) a coarsened trabecular pattern, (3) alternating lytic and sclerotic areas, and (4) thickening of the bone cortex. These patients have an elevated alkaline phosphatase level, and their bone scans are positive early. Most patients with Paget disease are asymptomatic. Others have minimal pain readily controlled by analgesics. The hip usually is the most symptomatic joint. Salicylates in high doses suppress Paget activity and should be considered first. Currently, several agents are being evaluated for therapy, including plicamycin, diphosphonates, and calcitonin.

Heterotopic Bone Formation

Myositis ossificans, or heterotopic bone formation, constitutes an abnormal bone response to injury. Typically, these patients have a history of blunt trauma, surgery, or joint dislocation. They complain of pain and a tender swelling located most often near a joint. After the process begins, the cycle takes 3 to 6 months to run its course, and little can be done to alter this. It is important not to mistake myositis ossificans for a sarcomatous lesion. Even with a biopsy, they are easily confused. With myositis ossificans, the most mature tissue is in the periphery of the lesion; in a sarcoma, the reverse is true. Initially, a hot area appears on the bone scan. Then on radiographs, a hazy enlarging mass forms; this eventually will differentiate into mature bone.

Myositis ossificans progressiva is a rare condition of unknown cause affecting interstitial tissue, muscle, ligament, and fascia. Associated anomalies are common, especially underdeveloped thumbs and great toes. As the name implies, these patients essentially have multiple progressive areas of involvement with myositis ossificans. Some patients undergo many operations for excision of the heterotopic bone, but only temporary relief is provided because recurrence is the rule.

Neoplasms

Primary malignant bone tumors are rare. Less than 3000 new cases occur annually in the United States. Benign bone tumors (such as osteoid osteoma, osteoblastoma, enchondroma, fibrous dysplasia, fibrous cortical defects, nonossifying chondroma, and bone cysts) are more common. Even more frequent are metastatic lesions. Often a bony metastasis will be the first manifestation of an occult primary lesion. Because malignant lesions tend to metastasize more centrally, the proximal limb more often is affected than the distal. Patients typically complain of pain at night in addition to that associated with weight-bearing activities. The radiographic appearance of a malignant lesion is characteristic. The lesions are large and show destruction of the adjacent cortex. Their outlines are irregular, without a well-defined sclerotic border. Solid tumors may include a soft-tissue mass. A bone scan is indicated if a neoplastic lesion is suspected.

SUMMARY

This chapter provided the pain management physician specialist with a background knowledge of the clinical presentation and treatment of common diseases causing joint pain. The importance of reevaluating a patient's referral diagnosis before treatment was emphasized to facilitate proper management. Only joint pain from intrinsic disorders of the joint was discussed because pain caused by extrinsic disorders is covered in other chapters of this book. A discussion of intrinsic joint pain was approached by determining from which of three anatomic areas the pain originates: intraarticular, periarticular soft tissue, or adjacent bone. Conditions occurring in each anatomic region were organized further by their causes into categories for more detailed discussion.

References

1. Buckelew SP, Parker JC. Coping with arthritis pain. A review of the literature. *Arthritis Care Res* December 1989; 2(4):136–145.
2. Grazier KL, Holbrook TL, Kelsey JL, Stoufer RN. *The Frequency of Occurrence, Impact and Cost of Musculoskeletal Conditions in the United States.* Chicago: American Academy of Orthopedic Surgeons; 1984.
3. Guilbaud G. Central neurophysiological processing of joint pain on the basis of studies performed in normal animals and in models of experimental arthritis. *Can J Physiol* May 1991; 69(5):637–646.
4. Altman RD. Osteoarthritis. Differentiation from rheumatoid arthritis, causes of pain treatment. *Postgrad Med* February 15, 1990; 87(3):66–72, 77–78.
5. Lovell DJ, Walco GA. Pain associated with juvenile rheumatoid arthritis. *Pediatr Clin North Am* August 1989; 36(4):1015–1027.
6. Rigby AS, Wood PH. A review of assignment criteria for rheumatoid arthritis. *Scand J Rheumatoid* 1990; 1:27–41.
7. Bradley LA. Adherence with treatment regimens among adult rheumatoid arthritis patients: current status and future directions. *Arthritis Care Res* September 1989; 2(3):33S–39S.
8. Zuckerman JD, Mirabello SC, Newman D, Gallagher M, Cuomo F. The painful shoulder: part II. Intrinsic disorders and impingement syndrome. *Am Fam Physician* February 1991; 43(2):497–512.
9. Jacobson KE, Flandry FC. Diagnosis of anterior knee pain. *Clin Sports Med* April 1989; 8(2):179–195.
10. Mrose HE, Rosenthal DI. Arthrography of the hand and wrist. *Hand Clin* February 1991; 7(1):201–217.
11. Ohira T, Ishikawa K. Hydroxyapatite deposition in articular cartilage by intra-articular injections of methylprednisolone. *J Bone Joint Surg* 1986; 68A:509–519.

CHAPTER 14

Pain in the Extremities

Michael J. Stabile and Carol A. Warfield

The causes of extremity pain are many and varied. This chapter will attempt to provide a comprehensive differential diagnosis of pain in these areas. After the specific diagnosis is established, the reader can consult the chapter dealing with the particular pain syndrome to find treatment options.

VASCULAR DISORDERS

Acute Arterial Insufficiency (See Chap. 23)

The important distinguishing feature of the pain of acute arterial insufficiency is its sudden onset. Emboli lodge at points where arteries branch. Branch points also are more likely to be affected by atherosclerosis. Emboli may occlude more than one vessel at a branch point and thereby limit collateral flow. Muscle necrosis and irreversible changes may occur if blood flow is not reestablished within 4 to 6 h.[1]

The five cardinal features of arterial insufficiency (the five "P's") are well known: pain, pallor, paresthesias, paralysis, and pulselessness. The pain is well localized to an extremity and severe. It may be attenuated by good collateral circulation, that is, occlusion of a brachial artery may not produce as dramatic a clinical picture as occlusion of a common femoral artery or popliteal artery. Nerve endings and muscle tissue are extremely sensitive to hypoxia, and acute obstruction soon leads to anesthesia and paralysis in an affected extremity.[2]

As a rule, pulses will be absent distal to the site of obstruction. However, there may be manifestations of acute arterial occlusion with detectable distal pulses. Therefore, pain and associated signs and symptoms of ischemia in the presence of detectable pulses warrants further investigation.[3] Conversely, pulses may be unusually strong proximal to the site of the occlusion.

Acute ischemia in an extremity also will be accompanied by a change in the skin temperature distal to the site of occlusion. The extremity will appear pale, and the veins may seem to be empty. Palpation along the course of the artery may reveal tenderness over the site of occlusion. The muscles will begin to feel hard and inelastic as the ischemia progresses.[4] Muscular fatigue and weakness will be apparent.

Chronic Arterial Insufficiency

Chronic arterial insufficiency can produce a wide variety of painful symptoms. Affected patients can have numbness, coldness, tingling, or total paresis. The type of pain in the lower extremity (intermittent claudication or rest pain) is determined by the degree of insufficiency. Atherosclerosis is the most common cause of chronic lower limb ischemia. The incidence of this disease and its progression in individual patients is increased in the presence of hypertension, diabetes mellitus, hypercholesterolemia, and cigarette smoking.[5] Buerger disease or thromboangiitis obliterans is a less common cause of chronic arterial insufficiency. Popliteal artery entrapment and cystic adventitial disease are rare causes of lower limb ischemia; both generally occur in young active people.

The pathophysiology of atherosclerosis begins with a fatty intimal streak caused by either increased permeability of damaged intima to low density lipoprotein or a thrombus of platelet and fibrin encountering collagen through an intimal tear and forming a seal. The thrombus accumulates, and this leads to plaque formation and progressive luminal occlusion.[6,7]

Claudication is cramping pain that occurs when the blood flow cannot be increased to a muscle mass in response to the increased metabolic demands of exercise. Blood flow is adequate in the extremity at rest. Claudication has several diagnostic features: (1) it is always relieved by rest after exercise, (2) it is produced by a consistent amount of exercise, and (3) it is always experienced in a functional muscle group.[8]

Ischemic rest pain occurs when blood flow in the extremity falls below resting tissue requirements. It is a manifestation of severe chronic arterial insufficiency. The pain occurs in the toes and metatarsal joints and is not confined to functional muscle groups. These patients may experience relief by hanging the affected limb over the side of the bed. The pain is constant and aggravated by limb elevation and exposure to cold.[9] Differentiating between intermittent claudication and ischemic rest pain is important even though the two groups can be considered different points in the continuum of chronic arterial insufficiency. Nondiabetic patients with claudication rarely require extremity amputation, although many patients with ischemic rest pain do.[10,11]

The diagnosis of both acute and chronic arterial insufficiency of the lower limbs is facilitated by measuring systolic blood pressure at the ankle. The cuff encircles the ankle, and a Doppler probe is placed over the dorsalis pedis or posterior tibial arteries. The pressure obtained in the ankle then is compared with the pressure in the arm. This is known as the ankle pressure index. As the pulse travels to the lower extremities, there is some systolic augmentation, and the ankle pressure should exceed the arm pressure by 15 to 20 mmHg in the absence of a proximal occlusion.[12] Therefore, a normal ankle pressure index would be 1.10 to 1.20. An ankle pressure index less than 1.0 suggests some degree of arterial insufficiency. These indexes also correlate with angiographic evidence of occlusive disease.[13–15] The diagnosis also is aided by doing arterial angiography of the lower extremities.

Popliteal Artery Entrapment

Popliteal artery entrapment results in unilateral claudication in young patients.[16,17] The popliteal artery, instead of coursing downward between the two heads of the gastrocnemius muscle, passes medially to the muscle. Its compression by muscle or fiber spans results in calf and foot claudication. The symptoms may mimic chronic arterial insufficiency. The patient has numbness, paresthesias, and cramping associated with exercise. The unilateral nature of the symptoms and the young age of the patient should suggest the diagnosis. Physical examination may reveal either present or absent popliteal and dorsalis pedis pulses. Alternatively, the dorsalis pedis artery may disappear with exercise. Palpation may show increased collateral blood flow (palpable geniculate arteries) near the knee. This distinguishes this entity from chronic arterial insufficiency. Active plantar flexion or passive dorsiflexion may obliterate the pedal pulses and aid the diagnosis. A bruit also may be heard over the popliteal artery.

Arteriography is essential for diagnosis and should be done bilaterally (25 percent of cases will be bilateral even in asymptomatic patients).[18] Angiographic confirmation relies on medial deviation of the popliteal artery and segmental occlusion of the popliteal artery.

Adventitial Cystic Disease of the Popliteal Artery

Adventitial cystic disease of the popliteal artery is a rare cause of claudication in young patients.[19] The symptoms are produced by a cyst within the adventitial layer of the popliteal artery leading to gradual occlusion. These patients are men who describe a short onset of severe claudication. The diagnosis is aided by a murmur in the popliteal fossa and the absence of pedal pulses. If pedal pulses are present, they can be eliminated by acute knee flexion. The cysts contain mucoproteins and mucopolysaccharides; their exact cause is unclear. Radiographic evidence for the diagnosis includes an "hourglass" appearance using angiography.[20]

Buerger Disease or Thromboangiitis Obliterans

Buerger disease involves the entire neurovascular bundle of the small vessels of the hands and feet. It appears as an intermittent claudication of the arch of the foot and can progress to ischemic digital pain at rest and frank gangrene. These patients are men younger than 40 years of age and heavy smokers.[21,22] The disease involves more than one limb. Unlike atherosclerosis, Buerger disease can cause ischemic lesions of the fingers, and there may be recurrent episodes of superficial thrombophlebitis. Angiography shows many small artery occlusions with tapering proximal to the occlusion and the absence of plaques.[23] Its pathologic features include a panangiitis that preserves vessel architecture and infiltration of the vessel walls by giant cells and lymphocytes.

Raynaud Syndrome

Raynaud syndrome is defined as episodic digital vasospasm precipitated by cold or stress that affects mostly the fingers and hands. It also may affect the feet and toes. The classically described attack has three components: (1) initial blanching with relative numbness secondary to arterial vasoconstriction, (2) cyanosis resulting from the saturation that occurs because of the small quantity of blood entering the capillaries and small veins, and (3) reactive hyperemia.[24] Usually, neither pallor nor cyanosis predominates. Seventy percent to ninety percent of patients with Raynaud syndrome are women.[25] The pain, which initially may be mild, becomes more severe and constant as the condition progresses.

The underlying pathophysiology in an attack is digital artery closure.[26] This may occur secondary to a vasoconstrictive mechanism (generally in younger women with connective tissue disease) or an obstructive mechanism (usually in older patients with atherosclerosis). The former may be caused by abnormal arterial adrenoreceptors or adrenoreceptor–immune complex interactions. In the latter group of patients, there are baseline proximal luminal obstructions.

Raynaud syndrome is associated with various other diseases (Table 14-1).[27] It also is associated with occupational hazards, such as operating a chain saw or pneumatic drill. The vibration frequency of these tools (110 to 140 Hz) supposedly causes severe sheer stresses in the arteries of the hands and fingers.[28] Pathologic studies show subintimal fibrosis after long-term exposure to these tools.

The diagnosis is confirmed by the ice-water immersion test. Using a thermistor probe, a baseline digital tip pulp temperature is determined (which must be greater than 32°C even if external warming must be used). The patient's

Table 14-1
Diseases that May Be Associated with Raynaud's Syndrome

Immunologic and Connective Tissue Disorders
  Scleroderma
  Mixed connective tissue disease
  Systemic lupus erythematosus
  Rheumatoid arthritis
  Dermatomyositis
  Polymyositis
  Hepatitis B antigen-induced vasculitis
  Drug-induced vasculitis
  Sjögren syndrome
  Undifferentiated connective tissue disease
Obstructive Arterial Diseases without Immunologic Disturbance
  Arteriosclerosis
  Thromboangiitis obliterans
  Thoracic outlet syndrome
Occupational Raynaud Syndrome
  Vibration injury
  Direct arterial trauma
  Cold injury
Drug-Induced Raynaud Sydrome without Arteritis
  Ergo
  β-Adrenergic blocking drugs
  Cytotoxic drugs
  Oral contraceptives
Miscellaneous
  Vinyl chloride disease
  Chronic renal failure
  Cold agglutinins
  Cryoglobulinemia
  Neoplasia
  Neurologic disorders
    Central nervous system
    Peripheral nervous system
  Endocrinologic disorder

fingers then are submerged in ice water for 30 s. The temperatures are recorded every 5 min for up to 45 min.[29] A normal patient's digital temperature returns to baseline within 10 min. Patients with Raynaud syndrome have a prolonged return to baseline temperature.

Other laboratory diagnostic tests include an erythrocyte sedimentation rate, complete blood count, antinuclear antibody, and rheumatoid factor. Hand radiographs are useful for detecting subcutaneous calcinosis typical of scleroderma or CRST syndrome (that is, calcinosis cutis, Raynaud phenomena, sclerodactyly, and telangiectasia).

Sympathetic Dystrophies (See Chap. 16)

The term *sympathetic dystrophy* includes a range of syndromes,[30] such as: (1) causalgia, (2) mimocausalgia states, (3) postfracture, (4) shoulder–hand, and (5) minor trauma.

The cause of reflex sympathetic dystrophy after trauma seems to involve increased sympathetic activity plus abnormal reflexes that allow sympathetic stimulation to per-

petuate itself. Normally, trauma produces a stimulant through efferent sensory fibers that travels to the posterior root ganglion and synapses in the posterior horn. The impulse is relayed to the lateral horn where the sympathetic nerve body sends efferent sympathetic impulses from the anterior root. These impulses then synapse in the sympathetic ganglion and mediate vasoconstriction in the affected extremity. Healing attenuates the sympathetic response. However, affected patients have an abnormal sympathetic response with continuing vasoconstriction and resultant ischemia.[31]

The hallmarks of this disorder are pain, swelling, discoloration, and stiffness. Pain is the most important symptom. It is constant and may be of several types (burning, cramping, or cutting). It is aggravated by active or passive motion of the extremity. Hyperpathia is a characteristic symptom. Tenderness may be elicited over the joints also. Swelling is the most common physical sign. The soft swelling of Stage I progresses to the harder edema of Stage II with resultant thickening about the joints. The swelling, which also may begin at the point of initial trauma, generally will involve the whole extremity. Discoloration can occur. Patients may have early capillary vasodilation with redness, especially over the joints. The vasoconstriction of the latter stages of the syndrome results in a whitish pallor. The fourth characteristic feature is stiffness.[32] This results from the intense pain of motion combined with the increased swelling. As the disease progresses, fibrosis of ligamentous structures and adhesion formation further limit joint motion. Forearm and shoulder motion are limited to a much greater extent than elbow motion.

Affected patients also have other signs and symptoms, such as positive responses to cold and the ice-water emersion test, and there is decreased skin temperature in the affected extremity. Trophic skin changes may be seen as tight shiny skin; these are a later feature caused by atrophy of subcutaneous tissue. There may be tapering of the pulp area of the fingers (the so-called pencil-pointing sign).

Causalgia

Major causalgia can be distinguished from minor causalgias by the site of nerve injury. Major causalgia (described first in 1864 among Union soldiers after gunshot wounds to nerves) involves injury to proximal major mixed nerves with resultant pain in the entire extremity.[33,34] Minor causalgia involves injury to distal sensory nerves; generally, it is confined to one or several fingers.[35]

The Shoulder–Hand Syndrome

The shoulder–hand syndrome is seen after trauma to the neck, chest, or shoulder. However, it also may occur after ulcers, strokes, lung tumors, and myocardial infarctions. The symptoms begin in the shoulder with pain and stiffness and then spread to the entire extremity. Soon, trophic changes appear, such as muscle atrophy, thickening of the palmar fascia, demineralization, and nail atrophy.[36,37]

In summary, the diagnosis of reflex sympathetic dystrophy depends on the findings of (1) pain, (2) swelling, (3) discoloration, (4) stiffness, and (5) temperature changes. The diagnosis also can be confirmed if sympathetic blockade provides pain relief and vasodilatation.

Thrombophlebitis

Thrombophlebitis of the superficial venous system can occur either in the upper or lower extremities. The factors responsible for both thrombosis of the superficial venous system and deep vein thrombosis (DVT) are defined in the Virchow triad: stasis, abnormalities of the vessel wall, and hypercoagulability. Thrombophlebitis occurs after an injury to a limb or secondary to intravenous cannulation. Other causes include varicose veins and carcinoma. Patients may have pain and redness along the course of a superficial vein. Hardness along the vein or a small knot also may be found. The diagnosis may be aided by Doppler studies that show diminished or absent flow through the vein. Treatment is directed toward the underlying disease process and should involve bed rest, elevation of the extremity, and application of moist compresses.

DVT

DVT can develop near valves in the lower extremity. Initial platelet aggregation is followed soon by a fibrin thrombus. Both platelets and fibrin contribute to the growing thrombus; there are various presentations. Calf vein thrombosis usually presents with calf tenderness and minimal swelling. The skin temperature may be increased in the extremity secondary to diversion of blood flow from the deep veins to the superficial veins. Increased tenderness with dorsiflexion (Homan sign) is notoriously unreliable in the diagnosis of DVT.[38] Femoral vein thrombosis usually is associated with calf tenderness, popliteal fossa tenderness, and leg swelling. Ileofemoral vein thrombosis will be accompanied by sudden severe pain, edema, and discoloration. Patients also may feel tingling, numbness, and weakness. The pain begins in the area of the femoral triangle or in the calf, but soon it involves the entire leg. This acute venous outflow obstruction can progress to venous gangrene with interference of arterial inflow and limb cyanosis (phlegmasia cerulea dolens).[39]

The conditions that predispose to DVT include obesity, the postpartum state, pelvic surgery, lower extremity fractures, prolonged bed rest, estrogen use, and carcinoma. Detection depends on several noninvasive tests as follows.[39–42]

1. Doppler ultrasonography recognizes the distorted flow patterns
2. Impedance plethysmography quantifies venous obstruction by measuring the rate at which a vein empties when a pneumatic cuff at the thigh is released
3. Radioactive fibrinogen uptake tests include the use of labeled fibrinogen that is taken up by newly formed thrombi. This is the most sensitive test to detect below-the-knee thrombi.

Ascending contrast phlebography also can be used to diagnose DVT, but it is invasive, often painful, and difficult to interpret.

Cellulitis in an extremity, although it does not have a vascular cause, must be differentiated from both superficial and deep venous thrombi. These infections occur after trauma to the skin and subcutaneous tissue. Inflammation is accompanied by edema, hyperemia, and leukocytic infiltration. The hallmarks of infection (swelling, tenderness, heat, and redness) will be apparent. Lymphangitis may be evident with reddish painful streaks and regional node tenderness and enlargement. These patients generally have more systemic symptoms than those with superficial thrombophlebitis. Gram staining of needle aspirates is helpful in diagnosing this disorder and crucial for further therapy.

Compartment Syndrome

Compartment syndrome is defined as a condition in which increased tissue pressure in a confined space compromises the circulation, resulting in muscle necrosis and neurologic injury.[43] Of the compartment syndromes described (acute, subacute, and chronic Volkman contracture), only the acute compartment syndromes are painful. Acute compartment syndromes are seen after tibial fractures, supracondylar fractures, brachial arteriograms, gunshot wounds, circumferential burns, snake bites, reflow after limb reattachment, and crush injuries. The pathophysiology involves raised tissue pressure in a compartment leading to altered microcirculation in the compartment.[44–46] Early investigators believed the increased tissue pressure led to arterial spasm and subsequent compromised tissue perfusion. However, newer hypotheses describe increasing tissue pressure that compromises transmural pressure across the walls of the arterioles. At a critical transmural pressure, the vessels close. Small arterioles close at a lower transmural pressure than larger arteries. This explains the clinical finding of obvious tissue ischemia in the presence of palpable pulses. Another hypothesis involves a rise in venous pressure in a compartment in response to the rise in tissue pressure. The venous pressure increase allows blood flow to continue. However, this venous hypertension in the compartment soon disturbs the normal capillary AV gradient. This, in turn, compromises tissue perfusion and capillary blood flow. The Starling gradients also are disrupted, leading to decreased extracellular fluid absorption and increased extracellular fluid transudation, and causing a further increase in tissue pressure in the compartment.

Acute compartment syndromes usually are intensely painful. The pain is well localized to the involved muscle groups. A distinguishing feature is that passive stretching of the involved muscle groups greatly aggravates the pain. For example, passive finger extension in a patient who has flexor forearm compartment syndrome leads to excruciating pain. The second typical finding is a firm induration over the involved muscle groups. Less importantly, patients may have weakness of the involved muscles and paresthesias in the distribution of the involved nerves. Palpable pulses are an unreliable clinical sign.

Measuring the tissue pressure in the compartment can aid in the diagnosis. The normal tissue pressure is between 0 and 10 mmHg. Permanent nerve dysfunction can occur with tissue pressures as low as 30 mmHg for 6 to 8 h. The tissue pressure may be measured by the injection method of Whitesides and associates,[47] the wick catheter method of Owen and colleagues,[48] or the continuous infusion method of Matsen and colleagues.[49,50]

Arterial Thrombosis in the Drug Abuser

Extremity pain after drug injection can result from a number of complications (Table 14-2).[51] Intraarterial injection of many agents can result in extremity pain and gangrene. The theoretic mechanisms cited include: (1) vasospasm, (2) norepinephrine release, (3) intimal damage, (4) necrotizing arteriitis, and (5) particulate embolism. However, the final common pathway is arterial thrombosis. Diluants used in street drugs (lactose, quinine, starch, and talcum powder) compound the vascular insult.[52]

The history is essential to establish the diagnosis. With an intraarterial injection, patients may describe a so-called *hand trip* that begins with a burning from the point of insertion of the needle to the tip of the fingers.[53,54] This

Table 14-2
Complications of Drugs-Induced Vascular Insufficiency

Infections
 Cellulitis
 Abscesses
 Osteomyelitis
 Septic arthritis
Lymphatic Complications
 So-called puffy hand
Vascular Complications
 Volkmann ischemic contracture
 Crush syndrome
 Rhabdomyolysis
 Necrotizing angiitis
 Direct arterial injury
  Thrombosis
  Embolism
  Mycotic aneurysm
 Skin ulcers
 Thrombophlebitis
Neurologic Complications
 Direct injury to nerve
 Polyneuritis
 Ischemic neuritis
 Acute transverse myelitis

Reprinted with permission from Ritland D, Butterfield W. Extremity complications of drug abuse. *Am J Surg* 1973; 126:639.

burning is followed immediately by blanching, severe pain, and cyanosis. Addicts also use belts or vigorous tourniquets for injections; these inadvertently may be left on during the postinjection stupor and further compromise the vascular supply. Finally, pressure necrosis from an abnormal posture after sedation may lead to muscle breakdown and ischemia. The needle itself, which causes perivascular hematomas, production of an intimal flap, or a false aneurysm, also can lead to thrombosis.[55]

The so-called puffy hand syndrome results from widespread destruction of lymphatic vessels and veins in an extremity used for injections.[56,57] Extremity drainage will depend on the deep venous system after the superficial lymphatic vessels and veins are destroyed. When perivascular injection or hematomas compromise the deep venous system, swelling and venous hypertension can lead to gangrene. The diagnosis of extremity pain in drug abusers depends on the history and signs of acute ischemia. Identification of the drug used is also helpful. Adjuvant tests include Doppler ultrasonography, digital temperature readings, and plethysmography. Angiography also may be useful.

Mycotic Aneurysm[58,59]

Mycotic aneurysms in the extremities can arise through several recognized mechanisms as follows.[60,61]

1. Septic embolization in the arterial lumen causes a gradual weakening of the arterial wall, subsequent aneurysm formation, and enlargement of the artery. This occurs during bacterial endocarditis and accounted for most mycotic aneurysms in the past.[62]
2. Local spread from an abscess or area of cellulitis destroys the arterial wall with resulting aneurysm formation.[63]
3. Trauma to an artery and subsequent contamination can cause the formation of a mycotic aneurysm. This commonly occurs after penetrating trauma, radiologic procedures, or inadvertent arterial injection by drug abusers.[64]

Most mycotic aneurysms are arterial because the low pressure in the venous system prevents dilatation. An exception to this rule are the aneurysms that result from repeated punctures of AV dialysis fistulas. The venous punctures coupled with the high venous pressure seen in these fistulas can cause aneurysm formation.

Mycotic aneurysms are found in patients with a history of rheumatic fever, intravenous drug abuse, immunosuppression, prolonged illness, penetrating trauma, and invasive radiologic procedures. A warm tender pulsatile mass will be palpated in an extremity. A systolic bruit will be heard over the mass; this distinguishes aneurysms from AV fistulas. The latter have both a systolic and dystolic component to their bruits.[65] Signs and symptoms of generalized sepsis also may be present. Occasionally, septic arthritis or petechial skin lesions can develop from emboli originating in the aneurysms.

An arteriogram is a useful aid to confirm the diagnosis. Needle aspiration also may be warranted.

Traumatic Aneurysms[66,67]

Traumatic aneurysms actually are false aneurysms from arterial penetration. These perivascular hematomas follow laceration of all layers of the arterial wall. They may be classified as: (1) acute traumatic hematomas in which through-and-through disruption of the arterial wall leads to a gradual enlarging hematoma contained by surrounding tissue or (2) chronic traumatic aneurysms in which the perivascular hematoma is absorbed, and a tissue sac and surrounding fibrosis provide boundaries.

Traumatic aneurysms result from penetrating trauma, invasive radiologic procedures, placement of intraaortic balloon pumps, vascular procedures, orthopedic reconstructive procedures, and internal fixation of bones.[68]

The interval from initial insult to aneurysm detection is longer than 1 month in more than 50% of cases. Affected patients have a tender pulsatile mass near the course of the artery. Like mycotic aneurysms, a systolic bruit will be present. Occasionally, compression by the expanding aneurysm will lead to a secondary peripheral neuropathy or venous occlusion. Suspected traumatic aneurysms in the extremity can be evaluated using percutaneous angiography.

NEUROGENIC SYNDROMES

Brachial Plexus Lesions

Several anatomic relationships become important when referring to brachial plexus disorders. The plexus is superficial in the supraclavicular fossa and protected by skin, subcutaneous tissues, and fascia. Also, the brachial plexus is in close proximity to the subclavian artery in the fossa, and both structures lie near the apex of the lung. More distally, the plexus lies close to the first and second parts of the axillary artery, and both are surrounded by a thick pad of fat and connective tissue. Therefore, many causes can lead to brachial plexus neuropathies (Table 14-3). For example, traction on the upper cervical roots when the shoulder is depressed forcibly and the head turned to the opposite side can lead to neuropathy. Apical lesions of the lung also may depress both the plexus and the vessels that run close to it.

Generally, all lesions of the brachial plexus cause paralysis or muscle weakness at the shoulder. Any lesion involving the T1 root or sympathetic trunk will be accompanied by Horner syndrome. Sensory deficits will be combined with disturbances of sweating. Most plexus lesions also have long-term complications (Table 14-4).[69]

It is instructive to divide plexus lesions anatomically regardless of the cause. First, superior plexus lesions (Duchenne-Erb) result from damage to the fifth and sixth

Table 14-3
Brachial Plexus Neuropathies[69]

Traumatic
  Birth injuries
  Stab and gunshot wounds
  Motorcycle accidents
  Football injuries
  Backpack injuries
  Electric shock
  Laborers carrying heavy loads
Iatrogenic
  Axillary artery injuries during cardiac catheterizations
  Radiotherapy
  Plexus neuropathies from general anesthesia
Vascular
  Emboli
  Generalized vasculopathies
  Heroin injection
Tumors
  Primary
  Secondary infiltration from lung (Pancoast tumor)
  Metastases (e.g., breast cancer or Hodgkin disease)
Cryptogenic
  Neuralgic amyotrophy
  Serum sickness
Anatomic
  Thoracic outlet syndrome

cervical roots. The deltoid, biceps, brachioradialis, and brachialis muscles are affected. There is an inability to abduct and externally rotate the shoulder and an inability to flex the elbow or pronate the forearm. The arm hangs loose, internally rotated, and the palm is visible from behind (so-called porter's-tip position). Sensory loss may be apparent over the deltoid and radial side of the forearm. An isolated middle brachial plexus lesion (C7) is unusual. It is manifested by sensory deficits on the back of the forearm or the radial aspect of the dorsum of the hand. Inferior plexus lesions (C8 to T1) include paralysis of small hand muscles and finger flexors with preservation of finger and wrist extensors. These lesions, therefore, result in hyperextension at the metacarpophalangeal joints and flexion at the interphalangeal joints. Horner syndrome may be seen. These inferior plexus lesions may result from sudden upward pulling on the shoulder. *Lower plexus lesions* are divided anatomically into three types. First, posterior lesions cause sensory deficits along the distribution of the axillary and radial nerves and weakness of abduction of the arm and

Table 14-4
Long-Term Complications of Plexus Lesions

Skin blisters

Ulceration and secondary infection

Joint contractures

Reflex sympathetic dystrophy

Osteoporosis

inability to extend the wrist or fingers. Second, medial cord lesions cause weakness of the muscles innervated by the ulnar nerve and medial head of the median nerve, thereby leading to severe hand disability. Sensory deficits produce dysfunction of the medial cutaneous nerve of the upper arm and forearm. Isolated medial cord lesions are rare except after radiotherapy. Third, lateral cord lesions involve the lateral part of the median nerve and musculocutaneous nerve, causing weakness of flexion and pronation of the forearm, wrist, and fingers. Sensory loss is limited to the radial aspect of the forearm (Table 14-5).

Because of its superficial position in the supraclavicular fossa, the brachial plexus can be susceptible to traction and exogenous compression. Upper brachial plexus injuries have been reported in laborers that carry heavy loads on their shoulders. Paralysis from the heavy backpacks carried by soldiers (so-called rucksack paralysis) has been recognized since World War II.[70–72] The whole plexus (usually on the nondominant side) is affected initially. However, soon only the upper plexus lesions remain, and it is common to see involvement of the nerve to the serratus anterior with winging of the scapula. Upper plexus injuries also have been reported in American football players.

Hematomas after anticoagulation or percutaneous axillary artery cannulation may lead to plexus injuries.[73,74] Of special concern to physicians are brachial plexus injuries occurring during general anesthesia. There are three causes.

First, shoulder braces may be placed too far medially near the posterior triangle and injure the plexus before it descends behind the clavicle. Second, if the arm is abducted to 90° or more, the head of the humerus descends into the axilla and presses into the plexus as it descends from the supraclavicular area to the axilla. Third, excessive depression of the shoulder girdle with the patient in the Trendelenburg position can stretch the upper roots of the brachial plexus.[75,76]

Vascular insufficiency is a rare cause of brachial plexus lesions, but this may occur after acute axillary artery occlusions secondary to emboli. Intravenous injection of contaminated heroin can lead to a painless paresis of muscles supplied by the posterior and medial cord.[77]

Radiotherapy to the clavicular region or axilla has been reported increasingly as a source of plexus lesions. Although occasionally it is difficult to determine whether the lesion is caused by the radiation per se or by local tumor infiltration and/or metastases, certain features characterize each. Postradiation intervals shorter than 3 months or longer than 5 years favor metastases. Intense pain, lower plexus lesions, and Horner syndrome all favor metastases. Skin changes, lymphedema of the extremity, induration over the supraclavicular fossa, and upper plexus lesions favor radiotherapy as the source of the neuropathy. Paresthesias frequently can be elicited by tapping the supraclavicular fossa after radiation-induced lesions (Table 14-6).[78,79]

Table 14-5
Physical Findings in Brachial Plexus Injuries

Vertebral Level	Motor Deficit	Sensory Deficit	Reflex Affected
C5	Shoulder abduction, deltoids, biceps	Radial aspect of arm	Biceps
C6	Wrist extension	Lateral forearm	Brachioradialis
C7	Wrist flexion, finger extension	Middle finger	Triceps
C8	Finger flexion	Medial forearm	—
T1	Finger abduction	Medial aspect of arm	—

Modified from Sola A. Upper extremity pain. In: Melzack R, Wall PD, eds. *Textbook of Pain*. New York: Churchill-Livingston, 1984:252–262.

Table 14-6
Characteristics of Brachial Plexus Injuries Caused by Radiation Versus Tumor[78,79]

Characteristics	Radiation	Tumor
Site	Upper plexus	Lower plexus
Pain	<50%	>75%
Lymphedema	Usually present	Usually absent
Time of onset to 1 year	Between 3 months and 5 years	3 months
Horner	Usually absent	Usually present
Skin changes	Usually present	Usually absent

Primary tumors of the brachial plexus are rare. They usually are benign and are painful without motor or sensory deficits.[80,81] Pancoast tumors are the most frequent tumors of the brachial plexus. Excruciating pain extending down the ulnar side of the hand may be the presenting symptom, followed by motor and sensory loss. Anatomically, it is easy to see why the lower brachial plexus is involved initially. A Horner syndrome usually occurs. Breast tumors are the most common source for metastases to the brachial plexus. Hodgkin disease and lymphosarcoma are the other common sources for metastases.

Inherited Brachial Plexus Neuropathy

There is a familial occurrence of recurrent episodes of brachial plexus neuropathy.[82–86] Clinically, this familial brachial plexus neuropathy is similar to neuralgic amyotrophy except for several distinguishing features. Unlike neuralgic amyotrophy, the familial form is characterized by recurrent episodes over several years separated by intervals of full recovery. Both diseases occur most commonly during the third and fourth decade of life, but in the familial form, affected patients may have their first attacks during the first decade of life. The familial form does not seem to be precipitated as commonly by infections as neuralgic amyotrophy. However, several authors reported a dramatic onset of attacks in women several hours after childbirth.[84,87] There may be minor dysmorphic features (e.g., hypotelorism, epicanthic folds, and cleft palate) associated with the familial form of the disease.[84] Finally, there is nerve involvement outside the brachial plexus with such diverse manifestations as Horner syndrome, Bell palsy, and lumbosacral weakness in the familial form of the disease.[86]

Pain is the initial manifestation of a familial attack. It is described as sharp and burning, particularly in the shoulder. The pain is aggravated by movement; therefore, affected patients keep their shoulders immobile. Weakness soon follows, and although any muscle in the plexus may be involved, those innervated by the upper trunk of the plexus generally are affected. Sensory dysfunction is not a prominent feature. Affected patients usually have an excellent recovery of strength, but they may accumulate deficits after multiple attacks.[85]

Guillain-Barré Syndrome

Guillain-Barré syndrome occurs worldwide; there is an incidence of 1 to 1.5 cases per 100,000 persons annually. There is no age or gender preference; 60 percent to 70 percent of cases are preceded by an upper respiratory or gastrointestinal illness 1 to 3 weeks before the onset of the syndrome.[88]

An ascending weakness involving both proximal and distal muscles is the distinguishing feature of Guillain-Barré syndrome. The weakness generally begins in the lower extremities and then can progress to upper extremity muscles, intercostals, and neck muscles. Affected patients also have decreased sensation and possibly transient autonomic dysfunction.

Pain occurs in one-third of the cases of Guillain-Barré syndrome as a result of involvement of the posterior roots. There may be tenderness after deep pressure on the muscles. Paresthesias are common. Affected patients also describe a burning radiating pain.

The clinical diagnosis is aided by examining the cerebrospinal fluid. Normal pressures, increased protein, and acellular fluid will be found. Nerve conduction studies show slowing after the paralysis begins.[89] A syndrome identical to Guillain-Barré syndrome can occur after infectious mononucleosis.

Fabry Disease (Angiokeratoma Corporis Diffusum)

Fabry disease refers to an X-linked recessive disorder characterized by accumulation of a lipid, ceramide trihexoside, in many organs. These patients are young boys or men with intense burning pain in their feet and lower legs.[90]

The enzymatic defect in Fabry disease is a deficiency of the enzyme ceramide trihexosidase; the terminal molecule of galactose is missing from this enzyme.[91] Stored glycolipid accumulates in different organ systems. Renal involvement initially is characterized by albuminuria and inability to concentrate urine; then it progresses to uremia. Glycolipid accumulates in the endothelial cells of the glomeruli and distal tubular cells. Angiokeratomas are found over the perineum, upper thighs, and buttocks; these are the first manifestations of this disease. Less commonly, they may be seen on the lip and oral mucosa.[92]

The vascular elements that supply the ganglions of the peripheral nervous system accumulate the lipid. The ganglion cells themselves and the perineural cells may contain the storage material, possibly causing the anhidrosis and pain that are features of this disease.[93]

Other systems that accumulate glycolipid include the eye, liver, and reticuloendothelial system. The diagnosis can be confirmed by enzyme assays done on biopsy specimens of small intestinal mucosa.[91] Tissue α-galactosidase activity is decreased in patients with Fabry disease; there are commercially available kits that assay this substance. Urine sediment also can be examined for glycolipids, but this is time consuming.

Compression Neuropathies

Compression neuropathies are caused by pressure damage to peripheral nerves.[94] The pressure may be external (a brace or cast), or the nerves may be compressed by adjacent body tissues (tumors, muscle, or synovial thickening). Entrapment neuropathies occur at sites where the nerves normally would be somewhat confined (Table 14-7). It is

Table 14-7
Common Compression Neuropathies

Nerve	Site of Entrapment
Anterior interosseous nerve	Between the two heads of the pronator teres
Median nerve	Carpal tunnel
Ulnar nerve	Condylar groove, cubital tunnel at the elbow, palmar fascia–pisiform bone at the wrist
Radial nerve (radial tunnel syndrome)	Radial tunnel between the superficial and deep heads of the supinator
Suprascapular nerve	Spinofenoid notch on upper border of scapula
Lateral femoral cutaneous nerve (meralgia paresthetica)	Inguinal ligament
Obturator nerve	Obturator canal
Deep peroneal nerve (anterior tibial syndrome)	Muscle swelling in the anterior compartment
Posterior tibial nerve (tarsal tunnel syndrome)	Tarsal tunnel, medial malleolus–flexor retinaculum
Sural nerve	External pressure over posterior lower calf
Phantom nerve or interdigital nerve (Morton neuroma)	Adjacent metatarsal heads of third and fourth toes, phantom fascia

Modified from Adams RD, Victor M, eds. *Principles of Neurology.* 3rd ed. New York: McGraw-Hill; 1985:166.

important to note that individual peripheral nerves are more sensitive to compression involving disease states associated with generalized peripheral neuropathies (e.g., diabetes mellitus, renal failure, or alcoholism).[95,96]

Affected patients have symptoms of sensory nerve dysfunction. Paresthesias and numbness usually are confined to the cutaneous distribution of the nerve. The pain is localized, can occur at rest, but may be referred to other sites.

There are several diagnostic aids that are useful to localize and assess these neuropathies.[97] Nerve conduction studies may reveal: (1) slowing of conduction secondary to focal demyelination, (2) reduced amplitudes of both sensory action potentials and compound muscle potentials secondary to axonal damage, and (3) the presence of a generalized polyneuropathy. Electromyography is another useful tool in evaluating compression neuropathies. These studies may show: (1) denervation potentials in the muscle secondary to anterior horn cell loss and (2) motor unit potential variation secondary to reinnervation of the muscle by axons. CT scans and radiography may reveal bone or joint abnormalities responsible for compression.[98]

Ulnar Nerve Syndromes

The ulnar nerve is formed from the C7, C8, and T1 roots. It courses medially in the upper arm and gives off no branches. At the elbow, it lies behind the medial epicondyle in the ulnar groove. It then descends under a roof formed by the aponeurosis of the flexor carpi ulnaris muscle in the cubital tunnel. Motor branches arise in the cubital tunnel and supply the flexor carpi ulnaris. The nerve then gives off branches to the flexor digitorum profundus of the fourth and fifth digits. The palmar cutaneous branch arises and supplies the hypothenar region. More distally, the dorsal cutaneous branch arises and innervates the medial half of the back of the hand and half of the fourth and fifth digits. The nerve enters the hand superficial to the flexor retin-aculum and runs between the hook of the hamate and pisiform bone into the Guyon canal where it bifurcates and gives rise to a superficial terminal branch and deep motor branch that supplies the hypothenar muscles, third and fourth lumbricales, the adductor pollicis, and all the interossei.

Compression above the Elbow and at the Elbow

The elbow is the most common site of ulnar nerve entrapment, particularly in the condylar groove and cubital tunnel. The nerve lies superficially in the groove and is susceptible to compression by leaning on the elbow or improper arm position during general anesthesia. Deformities from injuries to the elbow can cause the ulnar nerve to stretch, and palsy may occur, with a neuropathy appearing long after the actual time of injury (so-called tardy ulnar palsy).[99] The ulnar nerve also may be compressed in the cubital tunnel (so-called idiopathic cubital tunnel syndrome); this may be caused by prolonged flexion tightening the aponeurosis at the proximal end of the tunnel.[100,101]

Ulnar nerve injuries during anesthesia may result when the patient's arm is adducted along the side of the body and the hand supinated. The patient's elbow may slip out of the restraints, and with the ulnar groove located posteromedially, the edge of the table may compress the nerve. Pronating the forearm will rotate the ulnar groove more posteriorly and laterally and prevent compression by the table or equipment rail.[102]

Patients with entrapment neuropathies at or above the elbows may have pain at the elbow or spreading to other parts of the arm. Tingling and numbness along the medial portion of the palm and the fourth and fifth digits also occurs. Muscle wasting is prominent in the hypothenar eminence, and affected patients have weakness of the interossei. Severe ulnar neuropathy at the elbow results in a so-called claw-hand deformity. Proximal ulnar entrapment is characterized by weakness of the flexor carpi ulnaris and flexor digitorum profundus muscles; this distinguishes it from more distal entrapments.

Ulnar Nerve Compression in the Wrist or Hand

Ulnar nerve compression in the wrist or hand may result in intermittent paresthesias along the volar aspect of the fifth digit and half or all the volar aspect of the ring finger.[103] The sensory branch of the ulnar nerve to the hand is in the Guyon canal and encased by fibrous tissue. Repetitive trauma to the area (e.g., striking a stapler) can lead to compression. Other causes include pressure from a wrist watch band or overuse of the flexor carpi ulnaris. Finally, space-occupying lesions (e.g., ganglions or lipomas), thrombosis of the ulnar artery, or a rapid weight gain may cause nerve compression at the edge of the Guyon canal.

Radial Nerve Syndromes

The radial nerve receives contributions from the C5 to T1 roots. It spirals around the shaft of the humerus in the spiral groove and descends along the lateral aspect of the humerus superficially. It passes distally in front of the lateral epicondyle and divides into the deep motor nerve (posterior interosseous nerve) and superficial radial nerves variably 4 to 5 cm above or below the lateral epicondyle. The deep motor branch (posterior interosseous nerve) passes into the supinator muscle through the arcade of Frohse and finally supplies the extensor muscles of the digits. The superficial radial nerve passes over the supinator and pronator teres muscles along the lateral forearm and supplies sensation to the dorsal aspect of the hand, the thumb, and adjacent fingers.

The radial nerve may be compressed in the axilla secondary to the misuse of crutches. Along with the signs and symptoms described subsequently for more distal radial neuropathies, these patients characteristically have triceps weakness.

Most radial nerve compressions occur between the mid to upper arm and elbow where the nerve courses laterally around the spinal groove and then passes superficially along the humerus. Improper positioning of the arm during sleep or intoxication (so-called Saturday-night palsy) results in involvement of the extensors of the wrist and fingers and the brachioradialis muscles with resultant wrist drop and associated variable sensory disturbances.[104] Misuse of tourniquets, external pressure from ether screens and Mayo stands, and failure to pad the dependent arm when a patient is in the lateral decubitus position can produce a radial nerve palsy during anesthesia. Fractures of the shaft of the humerus with callus formation compress the nerve and may cause radial neuropathy.

The posterior interosseous nerve (deep motor branch) can be compressed in the radial tunnel between the superficial and deep heads of the supinator. Radial tunnel syndrome is characterized by deep aching pain of the extensor–supinator muscles in the dorsal forearm. Affected patients are unable to extend their thumbs and fingers at the metacarpophalangeal joints and cannot deviate their hands in the ulnar direction. Superficial radial nerve compressions can be caused by wearing handcuffs or watch bands or by fractures of the radius. Affected patients feel pain and paresthesias on the dorsum of the thumb and index finger.

Median Nerve Syndromes

The median nerve receives contributions from the C5 to T1 roots. It courses medially in the upper arm where it gives off no branches. The nerve crosses the elbow anteriorly and passes between the two heads of the pronator teres. It then passes deep to the tendon (so-called subliminis bridge) and runs distally between the flexor digitorum profundus muscles and flexor digitorum superficialis muscles. Motor nerves branch off before the median nerve passes between the pronator teres, the muscles responsible for wrist and finger flexion. A purely motor branch, the anterior interosseous nerve, is given off just after the median nerve emerges from the pronator teres. It innervates the flexor digitorum profundus to the second and third digits. The median nerve passes under the flexor retinaculum at the wrist and innervates the first two lumbrical muscles and the adductor pollicis brevis. The digital nerves then provide sensory innervation to the distal palm and palmar surfaces of the first through fourth digits.

Compression in the Carpal Tunnel

Compression of the median nerve in the carpal tunnel is the most common compression neuropathy of the upper extremity.[105] Women between the ages of 40 and 60 years are affected predominantly. Any condition that reduces the capacity of the carpal tunnel can precipitate the symptoms.[106] These include: (1) fractures, (2) ganglions, (3) xanthomas, and (4) synovial disorders. Systemic conditions associated with an increased incidence include: (1) obesity, (2) pregnancy, (3) hypothyroidism, (4) acromegaly, (5) myeloma, (6) amyloidosis, (7) Raynaud disease, (8) chronic renal failure, and (9) diabetes mellitus.

The syndrome is characterized by paresthesias and pain occurring during sleep. The paresthesias usually are localized to the palmar aspects of the fingers and hands. These patients, however, may complain of wrist and forearm pain. The paresthesias and pain are aggravated by repeated wrist and finger flexion. Affected patients also may feel clumsy and have hand weakness. The symptoms usually begin in the dominant hand, although in more than one-half of cases, the disorder is bilateral.[107]

Physical examination reveals decreased sensation over the palmar aspect of the thumb through the ring finger. A late sign of median neuropathy is atrophy of the thenar muscles. The diagnosis is aided by both the Tinel sign and Phalen test. The Tinel sign refers to distal paresthesias elicited by percussion of the median nerve either proximal to the flexor retinaculum in the wrist or distally at the base of the palm. The Phalen test is done by applying a tourniquet to the arm at 60 mmHg pressure.[108] The venous congestion will elicit paresthesias in patients with carpal tunnel syndrome. Alternately, acute flexion of the wrist for 60 s will accomplish the same goal.

Median Nerve Compression Proximal to the Carpal Tunnel

The median nerve may be compressed proximally in the axilla as a result of the misuse of crutches. The pronator syndrome results from median nerve entrapment between the two heads of the pronator teres; this may appear spontaneously or be caused by excessive forearm pronation (e.g., in tennis players).[109] These patients have unlocalized forearm pain combined with numbness in the fingers innervated by the median nerve.[110] Anterior interosseous syndrome is caused by damage to this purely motor branch from fractures or fibrous band compression. Affected patients have proximal forearm pain that increases with exercise.[111]

Diagnostically, these proximal nerve compressions can be distinguished from carpal tunnel syndrome by the characteristic weakness of the flexor digitorum muscles and flexor pollicis longus. These patients are asked to oppose the tip of the thumb to the second digit and are unable to flex both distal phalanges (so-called circle test). Weakness of pronation also is characteristic of proximal median nerve entrapment.[111,112]

Digital Nerve Compression of the Thumb and Fingers

So-called bowler's thumb is caused by constant irritation of the digital nerve at the thumb. There is perineural fibrosis, and a painful nodule results. So-called harp player's thumb is caused by strumming musical instruments; painful nodules or hypersensitivity to touch may occur.

Suprascapular Nerve

The suprascapular nerve is a purely motor nerve arising from the upper branch of the brachial plexus. It runs under the trapezius muscle through a notch on the upper border of the scapula and supplies the supraspinatus and infraspinatus muscles.

Injury to the nerve occurs after damage to the scapula or brachial plexus injuries. The syndrome is characterized by no sensory loss and weakness confined to spinatus muscles. Affected patients have pain after shoulder abduction.[113,114] Tenderness may be elicited by palpating the suprascapular notch. Needle EMG shows denervation of the spinatus muscles.

Femoral Nerve Entrapment Syndrome

The femoral nerve is formed from the posterior branches of L2 to L4 behind the psoas muscle. Then it courses around the lateral wall of the psoas muscle into the iliacus compartment located between the psoas and iliacus muscles and covered by the iliacus fascia. The femoral nerve then di-

vides into branches that supply the quadriceps and sensory branches to the anterior thigh. The nerve terminates as the saphenous nerve; this supplies sensation to the skin on the medial aspect of the leg.

Femoral neuropathy is characterized by wasting of the quadriceps muscles and sensory disturbances over the anteromedial aspect of the thigh and medial aspect of the lower leg. The patellar reflex also will be diminished or absent.

Femoral neuropathy may result from various causes. Diabetes is the most common cause.[115] Others include: injury of the nerve beneath the inguinal ligament as a result of scar tissue or prolonged lithotomy position[116] and compression of the nerve in the iliacus compartment from hematomas secondary to trauma or anticoagulants.[117]

Femoral neuropathy must be differentiated from L3 to L4 radiculopathy. EMGs are helpful in determining whether motor dysfunction is confined to the femoral nerve distribution. CT scans and radiographs of the lumbar and sacral spine are useful for excluding disk disease.

Meralgia Paresthetica or Lateral Femoral Cutaneous Nerve Entrapment (Roth Disease or Bernhardt Disease)

The lateral cutaneous nerve of the thigh is a purely sensory nerve formed from the posterior division of L2 and L3 roots; these supply the anterolateral aspect of the thigh. The nerve emerges along the lateral border of the psoas muscle and courses peripherally around the pelvis between the iliac muscle and its overlying fascia (Fig. 14-1). The nerve then descends under the lateral aspect of the inguinal ligament to the anterior–superior iliac spine; finally, it runs beneath the deep fascia and subcutaneous tissue of the upper thigh.[118] The nerve divides into anterior and posterior branches; these supply the anterolateral aspect of the thigh and posterior aspect of the thigh, respectively. Affected patients with this syndrome have burning pain and dysesthesias along the lateral aspect of the thigh. These symptoms are exacerbated by prolonged walking or standing.

The most common site of lateral femoral cutaneous nerve entrapment appears to be as the nerve passes from the pelvis into the thigh.[119] Thus, pressure from belts, girdles, and tight pants is cited as a precipitating cause. Also, direct trauma to the area of the anterior–superior iliac spine can lead to increased tension on the nerve. The diagnosis can be confirmed by blocking the nerve with a local anesthetic. A wheal is raised medially and inferiorly to the anterior–superior iliac spine. After the fascia above the inguinal ligament is pierced, 10 to 12 ml of a local anesthetic is injected in a fan-like distribution. (See Appendix A.X.)

Sciatic Nerve Syndromes

The sciatic nerve is composed of two distinct nerves, the tibial nerve and the common peroneal nerve. The common peroneal nerve arises from the posterior divisions of L4, L5, S1, and S2. The tibial nerve arises from the anterior divisions of L4 and L5, and S1 to S3. The sciatic nerve leaves the pelvis through the sciatic notch below the piriformis muscle where it may be compressed by masses. Then it courses between the greater trochanter and ischial tuberosity covered by the gluteus maximus muscle and hamstrings.

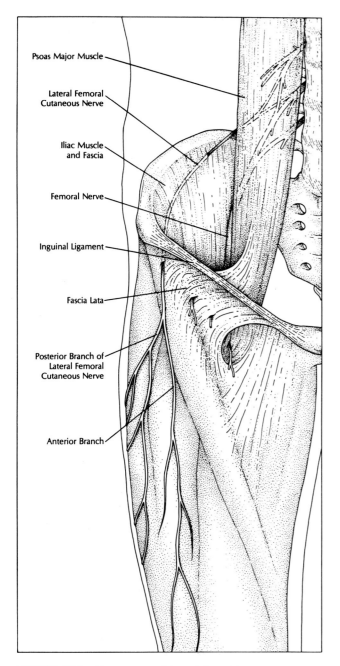

FIGURE 14-1. Entrapment of lateral femoral cutaneous nerve commonly occurs when nerve passes through inguinal ligament. Entrapment also may occur in fascia of iliac muscle. Tension, mechanical friction, and neural irritation may arise along entire anatomic course, with eventual formation of pseudoganglions and consequent meralgia. (Reproduced with permission from Warfield CA. Meralgia paresthetica: causes and cures. *Hosp Pract Off* 1986; 21(2):40c.)

The superior and inferior gluteal nerves and posterior cutaneous nerve of the thigh pass with the sciatic nerve through the notch. This is useful for localizing sites of sciatic compression.

Aside from penetrating trauma, most injuries to the sciatic nerve occur as a result of fracture dislocations of the hip joint and hip replacement. Deep injections in the buttock may cause muscle fibrosis that compresses the nerve or direct injury to the nerve.[120] Masses, such as endometriomas, may compress the nerve at the sciatic notch.[121] In addition to the buttock pain and paresthesias along the back of the leg, a sciatic nerve injury can cause foot drop, impaired hip extension, and decreased sensation over the lateral leg and foot.

The piriformis syndrome is caused by spasm or scarring of the piriformis muscle. Affected patients have symptoms similar to "sciatica," such as buttock pain and burning dysesthesias down the back of the leg.[122,123]

The common peroneal nerve syndrome involves the common peroneal nerve, a branch of the sciatic, that diverges from the tibial nerve in the upper popliteal fossa and passes laterally to the head of the fibula close to the median margin of the tendon of the biceps femoris. Then it passes superficially to the neck of the fibula. Distal to this, it divides into the superficial peroneal nerve (musculocutaneous nerve) and the deep peroneal nerve. The superficial peroneal nerve courses along the shaft of the fibula with the peroneal muscles that it supplies. Its cutaneous nerve innervates the skin of the lateral and distal portion of the lower leg and dorsal aspect of the foot. The deep peroneal nerve descends in the anterior compartment of the leg and supplies the tibialis anterior, extensor hallucis longus, and extensor digitorum brevis muscles in the foot.

The common peroneal nerve may be compressed near the neck of the fibula during general anesthesia or coma. Rarer causes include prolonged squatting[124] or crossing of the legs.[125] The nerve also may be compressed by ganglions or cysts in the knee joint. Affected patients have foot drop and sensory deficits over the anterolateral aspect of the lower leg and dorsum of the foot (Fig. 14-2).

Anterior tibial syndrome involves compression of the deep peroneal nerve. This is caused by muscle swelling in the anterior compartment. These patients have exquisite anterior lower leg pain and motor dysfunction. The syndrome may occur after trauma, reperfusion after arterial occlusion, or excessive exercise.

Tibial nerve syndromes involve the tibial nerve that branches from the sciatic nerve, descends through the popliteal fossa, and passes deep between the heads of the gastrocnemius muscle, which it supplies. The nerve becomes superficial along the medial aspect of the ankle and passes under the flexor retinaculum into the foot. The flexor retinaculum forms the roof of the tarsal tunnel. Distal to this site, the tibial nerve divides into plantar nerves and sensory branches that supply the sole of the heel. The plantar nerve innervates motor and sensory elements of the anterior two-

The image labels read:
Psoas Major Muscle
Lateral Femoral Cutaneous Nerve
Iliac Muscle and Fascia
Femoral Nerve
Inguinal Ligament
Fascia Lata
Posterior Branch of Lateral Femoral Cutaneous Nerve
Anterior Branch

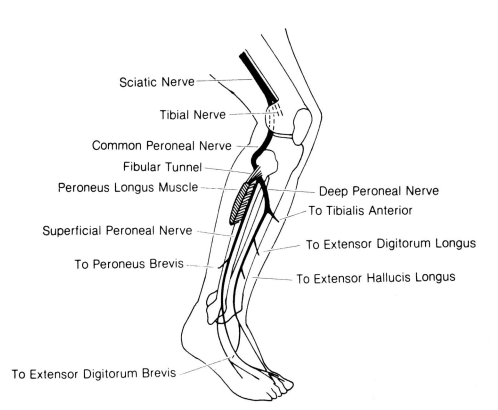

FIGURE 14-2. Common peroneal nerve (anterolateral aspect of the right leg). Schematic representation of its course, clinically relevant anatomic relations, and major branches. (Reproduced with permission from Dyke PJ, Thomas PK, Lambert EH, Bunge R, eds. *Peripheral Neuropathy.* 2nd ed. Philadelphia: Saunders; 1984:1448.)

thirds of the sole. The sural nerve leaves the tibial nerve in the popliteal fossa and descends in the middle of the calf to supply the skin over the lateral aspect of the ankle.

Compression of the distal part of the tibial nerve or two plantar nerves can cause diffuse foot pain and paresthesias in the sole of the foot. Weakness of foot muscles may be noticed, and physical examination shows plantar nerve sensory abnormalities. Compression or palpation over the medial aspect of the Achilles tendon may elicit pain and paresthesias. This syndrome is called the *tarsal tunnel syndrome,* and it can result from ill-fitting foot wear or compression by tendon sheaths.[126,127]

Morton neuroma or Morton neuralgia is caused by compression of the interdigital nerves by adjacent metatarsal heads (generally between the third and fourth toes). The pain radiates from the site of the neuroma into the toes. Initially, the pain occurs while walking, but eventually it becomes continuous.

Sural neuropathy causes paresthesias and pain over the lateral aspect of the ankle and foot. This results from prolonged pressure over the posterior lower calf.[128]

Hypothyroid Neuropathy

The peripheral nervous system manifestations of myxedema are well described. Affected patients may have either mononeuropathy or polyneuropathy.

The most common mononeuropathy involves compression of the median nerve as it passes through the carpal tunnel at the wrist. With myxedema, the extracellular tissue in the perineurium, endoneurium, and tendons acquires increased amounts of acid mucopolysaccharides. These attract fluid and diminish the available space for nerve in the carpal tunnel.[129]

The extremity pain associated with the polyneuropathy of hypothyroidism has two distinct origins: (1) skeletal muscle and (2) peripheral nerve. Affected patients may have myoedema of the skeletal muscle that is manifested as cramping.[130] Movement is slowed, and there is prolonged relaxation and contraction. The relaxed muscles feel firmer and larger. Proximal weakness is another feature. Neuropathy (e.g., slowed conduction velocity, decreased tendon reflexes, dysesthesias, and sensory deficits) is the other source of distal extremity pain in hypothyroid patients.

A distinct type of muscle cramping has been noticed in both patients with hypo- and hyperthyroidism. These patients experience an undulatory muscular twitching, the so-called myokymia. This may be caused by repetitive discharges from many single motor nerve fibers. The cramping is accompanied by excessive sweating.[131]

Neuropathy in Acromegaly

Patients with acromegaly may have intense pain and tingling in their extremities as a result of hypertrophic neuropathy.[132] In addition, bilateral carpal tunnel syndrome has been reported frequently in association with acromegaly.[133] Growth hormone, released by the active pituitary tumor, causes proliferation of the connective tissue and synovium. This diminishes the available space in the carpal tunnel. Hypertrophic connective tissue also may compress axons, resulting in sensorimotor disturbances.

Thoracic Outlet Syndrome

The thoracic outlet syndrome is a result of compression or irritation of the brachial plexus and subclavian vessels as they pass through the costoclavicular space and thoracic outlet.[134,135] Actual compression of the brachial plexus (compared with subclavian venous or arterial compression) is responsible for the symptoms in most patients. Therefore, the disease probably should be viewed as a neuropathy (Fig. 14-3).[136] The syndrome primarily affects young and middle-aged women. The history is essential to separate thoracic outlet syndrome from other causes of upper extremity pain, such as carpal tunnel syndrome and cervical disc disease (Table 14-8).[137] The symptoms may occur spontaneously or after trauma[138] to the shoulder and neck, resulting in chronic muscle spasms.[138,139] The pain initially is intermittent, but it increases in severity and frequency with time and is unilateral. It begins over the anterior and posterior shoulder region and radiates down the lateral arm to the hand. The pain also may radiate up the back of the neck to the mastoid and occipital region of the skull and cause severe headaches. Paresthesias accompany the pain, and because the compression typically involves C8 to T1 of the plexus, affected patients localize their numbness and tingling to the ulnar nerve distribution.

A striking feature of the history is that elevating the arm and increased arm activity can initiate or aggravate the symptoms. Muscle cramping per se is not a feature of the syndrome. The hands may or may not show increased sensitivity to cold.

As mentioned previously, the signs and symptoms of arterial occlusion are rare with thoracic outlet syndrome. An unusual form of the syndrome is caused by subclavian vein thrombosis[140] after exertion, resulting in cyanosis and edema of the extremity (the so-called effort thrombotic syndrome of Paget and Schroetter).

The physical examination should include blood pressure measurement in both arms to identify any differences. Muscle atrophy of ulnar-innervated interosseous muscles can be assessed by an interphalangeal card test or spreading the digits against resistance. Triceps strength may be diminished. Bruits may be heard over the supraclavicular fossa. Moderate pressure over the supraclavicular fossa for 15 s may reproduce the symptoms. The reflexes generally are normal. Pinprick sensation may be diminished over the C8 to T1 dermatome.

Several maneuvers that have questionable diagnostic value should be mentioned.[141] The Adson maneuver consists of monitoring the radial pulse while patients take deep breaths, extend their necks, and then turn their chin toward the affected side. A decrease or disappearance of the pulse is a positive test result. A bruit may be heard over the supraclavicular area using this maneuver. The deep breath elevates the first rib and turning the neck narrows the interscalene triangle. The costoclavicular compressive maneuver consists of monitoring the radial pulse while the patient throws back their shoulders and presses them down-

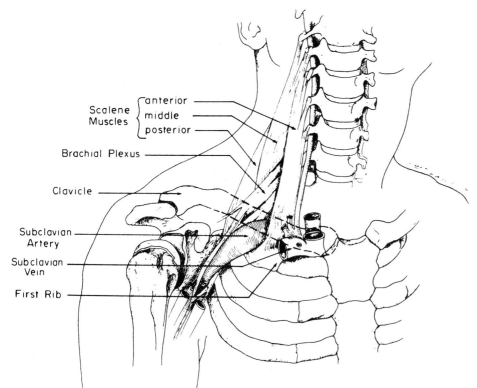

FIGURE 14-3. Course of the brachial plexus and subclavian artery between the anterior scalene and middle scalene muscles. Dilatation of the subclavian artery just distal to the anterior scalene muscle is illustrated. Immediately distal to the anterior and middle scalene muscles is another potential area of constriction, between the clavicle and the first rib. With extension of the neck and turning of the chin to the affected side (Adson maneuver), the tension on the anterior scalene muscle is increased and the subclavian artery compressed, resulting in a supraclavicular bruit and obliteration of the radial pulse. (Reproduced with permission from Adams RD, Victor M. Polymyositis and other acute and subacute myopathic paralyses. In: Adams RD, Victor M, eds. *Principles of Neurology.* 3rd ed. New York: McGraw-Hill; 1965.)

Scalene Muscles ⎰anterior ⎱middle ⎱posterior

Brachial Plexus

Clavicle

Subclavian Artery

Subclavian Vein

First Rib

Table 14-8
Thoracic Outlet, Carpal Tunnel, and Cervical Disk Syndromes

	Thoracic Outlet	*Carpal Tunnel*	*Cervical Disk*
Symptoms			
Pain	Neck, shoulder and arm (intermittent)	Wrist, volar forearm, fingers 1, 2, and 3 (intermittent)	Neck and shoulder (constant)
Numbness	Ulnar nerve or whole hand or arm asleep	Median nerve, fingers 2, 3, and 4	Radial nerve (dorsal web between fingers 1 and 2)
Awkwardness	All fingers or digits 4 and 5	Fingers 1, 2, and 3	Thumb
Aggravation	Arm elevation	Sustained grasp, pinch	Neck turn or arm stretch
Color	Normal, pallid, cyanotic, or splotchy	Normal, red, or splotchy	Normal or splotchy
Edema	±	±	0
Signs			
Percussion	+ Brachial plexus	+ Tinel volar wrist	+ Neck at disc level
Compression	+ Brachial plexus	+ Phalen (wrist flexion)	+ Neck and brachial plexus
Symptoms reproduced	Arm elevation and brachial plexus compression	Wrist flexion	Head turn and tilt, cranial compression
Nerve conduction	± (Unreliable if negative)	± (Unreliable if negative)	
X-rays	Normal, long C7 process, anomalies (venoarteriogram)	Normal, arthritis or old trauma	Degenerative arthritis, narrowed disc myelogram + 85 per cent
Treatment			
Conservative	Shoulder shrug, physical therapy, exercises, avoid arm elevation	Wrist splint, avoid grasp, steroid injection	Cervical traction and collar
Indications for operation	Treatment failure, severe pain, loss of hand function	Return of symptoms, severe pain, loss of function; thenar atrophy	Severe pain unrelieved by treatment
Operation	Resection of first rib and congenital band	Resection of carpal ligament	Discectomy with fusion

Reprinted with permission from Rutherford RD. *Vascular Surgery.* 2nd ed. Philadelphia: Saunders; 1984:710.

ward. A positive test result is a decrease or disappearance of the radial pulse with or without a bruit. This maneuver compresses the subclavian artery between the clavicle and the first rib.

By contrast, the elevated-arm stress test described by Roos[139] seems to have some diagnostic value. This test involves a 90° abduction and external rotation of the arms. The patient then is instructed to open and close their hands for 3 min. A reproduction of symptoms of the thoracic outlet syndrome constitutes a positive test result.

In addition to the history and physical examination, some other tests should be discussed when diagnosing thoracic outlet syndrome. Although thoracic outlet syndrome can be considered an ulnar neuropathy, the actual irritation of the plexus is intermittent and rarely results in neuropathic changes. Hence, nerve conduction studies generally are not useful.[142,143] Also, because the C8 to T1 part of the plexus is both inferior and deep, stimulation would be difficult technically. Only a small minority of patients with thoracic outlet syndrome have disease that involves subclavian arterial compression, therefore, angiograms generally are not indicated. There are two exceptions to this general rule as follows: (1) there is a large differential blood pressure between the arms or (2) there is interest in excluding a subclavian artery aneurysm. Cervical spine films generally are valuable in patients with thoracic outlet syndrome to exclude any coexisting cervical disc disease.

Cervical Disk Disease (See Chap. 7)

Cervical disk disease is another common cause of neck, shoulder, and arm pain. The root or cord compression may result from ruptured disk material or a degenerative osteophytic lesion. The radiculopathy usually involves, in descending order: C7, C6, C5, and C8. The symptoms may occur after trauma or sudden hyperextension.[144,145]

The syndrome involving lateral disk lesions between the fifth and sixth cervical vertebrae includes pain felt at the trapezium ridge, tip of the shoulder, radial forearm, and thumb. Affected patients have sensory loss and paresthesias in the same distribution. Unilateral paracervical muscle spasm will be present. The patient may feel tenderness in the biceps and supraclavicular regions. A motor deficit in the biceps may be noticed with absence of the biceps reflex. The patient has a secondary weakness after forearm flexion.

The other common syndrome is caused by lateral protrusion between the sixth and seventh cervical vertebrae with involvement of the seventh cervical root. The pain occurs in the shoulder and radiates down the elbow and dorsal forearm to the index and middle fingers. There is tenderness over the third and fourth thoracic spinous processes and the triceps region. The patient has sensory deficits and paresthesias in the second and third fingers. The physical examination shows an absent triceps reflex with weakness in forearm extension, wrist extension, and hand grip.

Regardless of the cervical root involved, affected patients relate a history of chronic sharp pain. Events such as coughing or sneezing tend to exaggerate the pain. Most changes in head position (particularly hyperextension) intensify the pain. On examination, turning the head to one side and hyperextending the neck will produce neck pain and characteristic radicular paresthesias (Table 14-9).

Neuralgic Amyotrophy

Neuralgic amyotrophy is a syndrome characterized by an acute onset of shoulder pain. The pain can be severe or aching. Although it frequently affects the shoulder alone, it also may involve the arm, neck, and back. The pain is worse at night and intensifies with movement.[146] The syndrome involves mostly the right side, and almost 25 percent of cases are bilateral.

At varying intervals, the pain is followed by proximal motor weakness in the shoulder and arms, particularly affecting the muscle innervated by the axillary and suprascapular nerves.[147] Complete limb paralysis is rare. Pain relief often occurs after resting the limb with the elbow flexed and the shoulder adducted. This may aggravate the weakness. Sensory involvement is not a characteristic feature of this syndrome.

The cause is unknown. However, a brachial neuritis similar to neuralgic amyotrophy may appear after serum inoculations or infections caused by influenza, typhus, or vareola viruses.

The diagnosis depends on obtaining a history consistent with neuralgic amyotrophy. The physical diagnosis is aided by eliciting pain after arm abduction, externally rotation at the shoulder, and then extension of the elbow (the so-called flexion–adduction sign described by Waxman).[148] EMG studies show a peripheral plexus lesion with normal spinal roots.[149]

Neuropathy of Serum Sickness

Before the age of antibiotics, bacterial infections often were treated with large volumes of horse or rabbit antisera. The serum sickness that patients had occasionally was accompanied by neuropathy, usually brachial neuropathy.[150]

Heterologous serum rarely is used today, but neuropathies still may occur as a sequela of typhoid or paratyphoid vaccinations or drugs that form complexes with serum proteins.[151]

The usual clinical features of serum sickness (e.g., lymph node swelling, joint pain, myalgias, and albuminuria) generally are present when the neuropathy appears. There is no relationship between the amount of serum given, the severity of systemic manifestations, and the development of neuropathy.

The onset of pain is sudden. It generally occurs in the shoulder girdle or upper arm. The pain should be distinguished from more typical myalgic or arthritic types seen during serum sickness in other joints and muscles. Physical examination may find tenderness over the brachial plexus. Weakness involving the shoulder muscles soon follows the onset of pain, and affected patients may be paralyzed totally and have striking atrophy. The reflexes also are decreased or absent, and vasomotor changes may appear. Sensory signs are not prominent, a feature that is found in other brachial neuropathies. The radial nerve is a less common site of involvement.

The pathologic basis of the neuropathy of serum sickness seems to be that immune-complex deposition causes vasculitis and perivascular edema. This, in turn, leads to edema of the nerves. This swelling impinges on the nerves as they exit from the foramina. If the swelling progresses, it may compromise flow further and lead to frank necrosis of the nerves. This explains why severe lancinating pain is such a prominent feature of the neuropathy of serum sickness.[150,152]

Neuropathy in Connective Tissue Diseases

Peripheral neuropathy may occur in conjunction with various connective tissue diseases. The clinical manifestations and histopathologic findings are similar regardless of the disease. The pathogenic lesion is arteritis involving the small nutrient arteries of the nerves. Thus it is described as an angiopathic neuropathy that will occur with varying frequencies in rheumatoid arthritis, polyarteritis nodosa, Churg-Strauss vasculitis, systemic lupus erythematosus, and giant cell arteritis.[153]

Patients with rheumatoid arthritis and peripheral neu-

Table 14-9
Most Frequent Clinical Findings with Cervical Disk Disease[145]

Cervical Root Involved	Clinical Findings		
	Motor Deficit	*Sensory Change*	*Reflex Loss*
C5	Deltoid	Proximal shoulder	None
C6	Biceps	Thumb	Biceps
C7	Triceps	Long finger	Triceps
C8	Intrinsic hand muscles	Ring and little fingers	None

ropathy have certain distinguishing features. First, usually, they have had rheumatoid arthritis for an average of 10 years before the onset of neuropathy. Second, rheumatoid nodules and destructive joint changes are present. Third, elevated titers of rheumatoid factor are common.[154] Fourth, these patients have other complications of arteritis (such as nail-bed infarctions, skin ulcers, and Raynaud phenomenon). Finally, these patients often describe a change in their clinical status involving fever, anorexia, or weight loss. It previously was believed that patients receiving corticosteroids were at risk for an increased incidence of neuropathy. However, these are patients with severe disease, and it is thought currently that corticosteroids may help to check the progression of the arteritis. Thus, rapid tapering of these drugs may exacerbate the arteritis and precipitate the onset of the neuropathy.

The latter usually includes a gradual onset of numbness and tingling confined to the lower extremities. The sensory deficits are symmetric and not accompanied by motor deficits. Patients with rheumatoid arthritis and other connective tissue diseases also may have mononeuritis multiplex or a sudden onset of pain and paresthesias along the course of a peripheral nerve followed by wrist or foot drop.

Although only a small percentage of patients with rheumatoid arthritis have symptomatic neuropathy, a large percentage have histologic evidence of disease involving the peripheral nerves at autopsy.[154] The range of arterial pathologic changes in the peripheral nerves includes: perivascular infiltration with mononuclear cells, fibrinoid necrosis of the media with infiltration of eosinophils and mononuclear cells, intimal proliferation and reduplication of the internal elastic lamina, and hemorrhage around the vessel walls. The damage to nutrient vessels results in both segmental demyelination and wallerian degeneration in the affected nerves.[155]

The diagnosis of rheumatoid arthritis generally is well established before the neuropathy appears. However, patients with neuropathy have an elevated erythrocyte sedimentation rate, mild normochromic normocytic anemia, and significantly elevated titers of rheumatoid factor.

Polyarteritis nodosa is a multisystem disease characterized by a vasculitis of small and medium-sized muscular arteries with particular involvement of the kidneys and gastrointestinal tract. Clinical neuropathy is a common manifestation of this disease. The clinical presentation may be similar to that of rheumatoid arthritis. One important distinguishing feature is that the neuropathy of polyarteritis nodosa will involve the upper extremities as frequently as the lower extremities. The neuropathy may occur in conjunction with other manifestations of this disease, such as fever, weight loss, renal insufficiency, and skin lesions.[156] Patients with both polyarteritis nodosa and rheumatoid arthritis also may have an accompanying arthritis. The arthritis of polyarteritis nodosa is mild and of short duration. It does not involve the extensive joint destruction and nodule formation seen with rheumatoid arthritis.

The pathologic changes noticed in the peripheral nerves involve an arteritis of nutrient arteries that is similar to that described in rheumatoid arthritis. The diagnosis depends on a histologic demonstration of vasculitis in the involved organs.

Peripheral neuropathy may be associated with Churg-Strauss vasculitis (eosinophilic granulomatosus). It is considered a variant of polyarteritis nodosa that is characterized by peripheral eosinophila and a strong association with severe asthma.[157] Both systemic lupus erythematosus and giant cell arteritis (involving the temporal arteries) may include secondary neuropathy.

Porphyric Neuropathy

The porphyrias are a group of metabolic disorders characterized biochemically by an overproduction of porphyrins and porphyrin precursors. Recurrent attacks are common. They often are precipitated by drugs (such as barbiturates, phenytoin, sulfonamides, and estrogens). The neuropathy and extremity pain is a feature only of one subgroup, the so-called hereditary hepatic porphyrias, that includes: (1) acute intermittent porphyria, (2) variegate porphyria, and (3) hereditary coproporphyria.[158]

Acute intermittent porphyria, inherited as an autosomal dominant trait, is most common in women of English and Scandinavian origin.[159] Attacks are rare before puberty and are distinguished temporally by three phases: (1) abdominal pain, (2) psychologic disturbances, and (3) polyneuropathy. Abdominal pain initiates the attack. The pain is described as colicky and may be diffuse or confined to one region of the abdominal wall. It often radiates to the back but is not accompanied by abdominal wall guarding or tenderness. Tachycardia is a constant physical sign during attacks.[160] Radiographic studies show distended loops of bowel. Psychologic manifestations follow the acute abdominal attacks. This phase is characterized by restlessness, insomnia, hallucinations, and/or confusion.[161] Neuropathy is the final phase of the attack. It is symmetric, progressive, and initially involves mostly motor nerves. The upper extremities are affected more than lower extremities and the proximal, more so than the distal muscles. Tendon reflexes are diminished or absent.[162,163] The extremity pain that occurs can result from various factors. Proximal muscle aching and cramps are common. Paresthesias and dysesthesias also occur in half the cases.

The diagnosis depends on the characteristic history and is confirmed by demonstrations of increased levels of porphobilinogen and δ-aminolevulinic acid in the urine. Variegate porphyria is most common among European descendants in South Africa. The acute attacks are similar to those of acute intermittent porphyria, but in addition, they are accompanied by cutaneous photosensitivity. Hereditary coproporphyria is a rare cause of neuropathy and is distinguished by a predominantly fecal excretion of porphyrins.

Hepatic Neuropathy

Several types of peripheral neuropathy may accompany hepatic dysfunction. These are distinct from alcoholic neuropathy or illnesses that affect both the liver and peripheral nervous system concomitantly.[164] Specifically, the conditions are (1) a painless demyelinating neuropathy that accompanies hepatic dysfunction, regardless of the cause;[165,166] (2) an acute polyneuritis identical to that seen with Guillian-Barré syndrome occurring late in the course of viral hepatitis as jaundice is regressing;[167,168] and (3) a rare but painful neuropathy that occurs with biliary infections.[169]

Patients with biliary cirrhosis and neuropathy have the other common manifestations of this disease: hepatomegaly, pruritus, jaundice, and cutaneous xanthomatosis. Hypersensitivity and paresthesias have been recognized for a long time as a feature of biliary cirrhosis. However, Thomas and Walker[169] also documented the presence of sensory deficits. Xanthomatous involvement of the connective tissue sheaths of the cutaneous nerves is the cause of the painful dyesthesias.

The So-Called Burning-Feet Syndrome

The burning-feet syndrome described among prisoners of war after World War II initially was believed to be a distinct deficiency syndrome. Currently, experts agree that it is one manifestation of vitamin B deficiency and can be found in patients with (1) alcoholic neuropathy, (2) beriberi, (3) pellagra, and (4) Strachon syndrome. The symptom of burning feet or acrodysesthesia begins as a persistent burning pain over the metatarsal on the soles of the feet. This may be accompanied by various other dysesthesias, tingling, electric shocks, or coldness. Soon, the entire soles and dorsal surface of the feet are involved symmetrically. The pain worsens at night. Affected patients try a number of methods to relieve the burning: immersing their feet in ice water, constant massage, or walking (despite pain caused by contact stimuli). Many authors believed the syndrome had a causalgic basis as a result of findings such as cyanosis and hyperhidrosis. Other features of peripheral neuropathy (e.g., absent reflexes, impairment of sensation, and muscle wasting) may or may not be present. Occasionally, the patient's hands may be involved.

Isoniazid or Hydralazine-Induced Neuropathy

The occurrence of isoniazid-induced neuropathy was discovered shortly after the drug was first used to treat tuberculosis. The neuropathy generally was confined to the lower extremities and involved motor functions, sensation, and reflexes. The initial symptoms consisted of numbness and tingling. These began in the toes and feet, followed by calf tenderness, and finally continuous burning paresthesias and painful dysesthesias caused by contact stimuli. The progression of symptoms was coupled with proximal spreading of the neuropathy to the knees. Also, patients had weakness during toe movements and dorsiflexion and loss of the Achilles reflex.[170] The incidence of the neuropathy varies with the dose of drug administered. It ranges from less than 10 percent with a dose of 4 to 9 mg/kg/day to 40 percent with doses of 20 mg/kg/day in other series.[171] The cause of the neuropathy is vitamin B_6 deficiency. Isoniazid produces marked excretion of pyridoxine. Adding supplemental doses of this vitamin can prevent the occurrence of the neuropathy.[172]

Pyridoxine deficiency presumably is the basis for the neuropathy that complicates therapy with hydralazine also. This drug is related chemically to isoniazid.[173]

Pellagra

Pellagra was described first in 1730 among peasants in northwestern Spain whose diet consisted almost entirely of corn. The role of sunlight, the seasonal variation (highest in the spring), and the rash that appeared on exposed areas (so-called Casd collar) were noticed. The first reports of pellagra in the United States were made in the late 1800s, and the disease soon attained epidemic proportions among alcoholic populations in northern and southern farmers. The disease rarely is seen in the continental United States currently (except among faddists), but it occurs commonly among poorer vegetarian populations and the black population of South Africa.

Initially, it was believed that pellagra was caused solely by a niacin-deficient diet. Subsequently, it was shown that (1) administration of tryptophan to humans resulted in increased urinary excretion of niacin metabolites and (2) the dermal and gastrointestinal manifestations of pellagra responded to large doses of tryptophan. Thus, currently, it is believed that pellagra is the result of a deficiency of niacin and its amino acid precursor, tryptophan.

Pellagra is manifested by a clinical triad of dermal, gastrointestinal, and neurologic lesions. The skin lesions first appear to be erythematous; then they become brown and hyperkeratotic. They are seen on the face, neck, sternum, and dorsum of the hands and feet. Affected patients have anorexia, diarrhea, weight loss, and dysphagia. The neurologic involvement is varied. It consists of depression, insomnia, and irritability. There also may be signs of spinal cord involvement. The neuropathy, which is identical to that observed with beriberi, is the most common neurologic manifestation. Affected patients have exquisite tenderness to palpation of the muscles of their calves and feet. Many also feel an intense burning pain in a so-called glove-and-stocking distribution. This is accompanied by a loss of vibratory sensation and decreased deep tendon reflexes.

The Syndrome of Amblyopia, Painful Neuropathy, and Orogenital Dermatitis (Strachan Syndrome)

Strachan (in 1888) and Scott (in 1918) both described a deficiency syndrome among Jamaicans consisting of amblyopia, painful neuropathy, and orogenital lesions that was distinct from beriberi and pellagra. These manifestations since have been described among World War II prisoners in Johore and Singapore, survivors of German concentration camps, and natives in Trinidad and Senegal. Currently, the syndrome has not been related to a specific vitamin deficiency, although a riboflavin deficiency has been suggested. The few neuropathologic studies done reveal spinal cord posterior column demyelination, particularly in the cervical region.

These patients classically have numbness and tingling in their hands and feet. The dysesthesias consist of severe burning in their soles and palms, which often is worse at night. The numbness extends progressively to the knees or hips, and the patient's gait may be impaired. Often the symptoms are confined to the lower extremities, or alternatively, they may begin in the fingertips and involve the hands and arms symmetrically. Muscle wasting is progressive, and extremity cramps are common.

Amblyopia is the other constant feature of this syndrome. Visual impairment is accompanied by central and centrocecal scotomas that progress to complete blindness. Ophthalmologic evaluation shows little, except occasionally disk hyperemia is found.

The dermatitis involves the corners of the mouth and eyes, prepuce, anus, and vulva. Deafness and vertigo (so-called camp dizziness) were a common feature of some outbreaks of the syndrome.

Alcoholic Neuropathy

In a consecutive series of 1030 alcoholic patients admitted to Boston City Hospital,[173a] a 9 percent incidence of peripheral neuropathy was observed with a disproportionately higher incidence in women. The cause of alcoholic neuropathy is a nutritional deficiency that accompanies alcoholism and a toxic effect of the alcohol per se. Alcoholic patients with neuropathy subsist on a diet of carbohydrates. They also have an impaired capacity to absorb folate and thiamine and to digest fats. The characteristic pathologic feature is axonal degeneration with destruction of both myelin and axons. The changes are seen predominantly in the longest and largest myelinated fibers. As the neuropathy advances, anterior and posterior nerve root involvement occurs.

Alcoholic neuropathy is a progressive symmetric disorder of the extremities that generally spares both the cranial and truncal nerves. The lower extremities (particularly the feet and ankles) are affected more than the upper ex-

tremities; 70 percent of patients had lower extremity involvement alone. Motor disability and sensory deficits occur concomitantly. These signs can range from mild asymptomatic depression of the Achilles reflex to gross motor deficits (wrist and foot drop). All sensory modalities, both superficial and deep, may be affected with a characteristic distribution (so-called glove and stocking).

The pain that accompanies alcoholic neuropathy is located in several areas. Affected patients have a highly characteristic tenderness when pressure is applied to the muscles of their feet and calves. The dysesthesias may be a dull constant ache in their distal lower extremities or a sharp lancinating tabes-like pain. These patients also describe a burning-feet syndrome that consists of severe paresthesias of the soles aggravated by contact stimuli. Another annoying sensory disturbance is excessive sweating on the volar surfaces of the feet and hands; presumably this is related to involvement of postganglionic sympathetic efferent fibers. The neuropathy may be accompanied by many other signs (e.g., stasis edema, glossiness of the skin, pigmentation changes, and dystrophic changes in the feet).

Herpes Zoster (See Chap. 21)

Herpes zoster or shingles is an infection by the DNA virus varicella-zoster that occurs with an incidence of approximately 125 cases per 100,000 annually in the general population. The varicella-zoster virus also causes chicken pox in children, and herpes zoster is thought to be a reactivation and multiplication of a virus that has remained in the dorsal root ganglia of nerves for many years.

Varicella or chicken pox occurs after the introduction of the virus from an outside source into a patient with no immunity. It is believed that the virus then passes from the sensory ending to the sensory ganglia. It remains there during the latent phase. With the declining antibody titers to the virus in elderly or immunocompromised patients, the reactivated virus begins to replicate. This can lead to damage in the sensory ganglia and secondary neuralgia. The virus then spreads peripherally to the sensory nerve endings in the skin, causing a vesicular eruption. Herpes zoster is more common and its course is more severe in immunosuppressed patients. However, most affected patients are healthy (Table 14-10).

Table 14-10
Patients at Increased Risk for Herpes Zoster

Hodgkin lymphoma
Lupus erythematosus
Non-Hodgkin lymphoma
Status-post bone marrow transplantation
Status-post radiochemotherapy
Malignancies
Syphilis
Malaria

Zoster usually is limited to the dermatome of a single spinal or cranial sensory nerve. Affected patients have pain and dysesthesia along a dermatomal distribution. The pain is variable; at first, it usually is mild. It then can increase in intensity over the succeeding days. Occasionally, patients have accompanying systemic symptoms: fever, malaise, adenopathy, or headache. After 4 to 5 days, the typical lesions appear. They begin with swelling and erythema; then red papules appear that progress to clear vesicles, blebs, and pustules that crust over in 2 to 3 weeks. The lesions are unilateral in a dermatomal distribution. The thoracic dermatomes most commonly are involved, followed by the cranial dermatomes, the lumbosacral, and the cervical.

During the acute phase, patients feel continuous dysesthesias that are aggravated by movement or pressure on the skin. As the blebs begin to dry and scale, the intense pain subsides, but many still have hyperesthesia and, only gradually, become asymptomatic.

Paresis may accompany the rash. This is seen more commonly in elderly patients. It follows the appearance of the rash and usually occurs with cervical and lumbosacral eruptions rather than thoracic. Involvement of the facial nerves is common (Ramsay Hunt syndrome).

The virus may be recovered from early vesicles, cerebrospinal fluid, and blood. The base of the skin lesions contain multinucleated giant cells and eosinophilic intranuclear inclusions.

From 10 percent to 50 percent of patients with acute herpes zoster have postherpetic neuralgia. This is defined as pain persisting 4 to 6 weeks after the skin lesions have disappeared. The incidence of postherpetic neuralgia increases with advancing age. These patients generally describe burning pain with associated hyperesthesia.

INTRODUCTION TO PERIPHERAL NEUROPATHIES (See Chap. 22)

Peripheral neuropathies are a common source of extremity pain. Such diverse entities as diabetic neuropathy, carpal tunnel syndrome, lumbar and cervical disc disease, and herpes zoster are examples of neuropathic syndromes. The peripheral nervous system has several unique features that make it particularly susceptible to trauma or metabolic derangements. First, the peripheral nervous system (which includes all neural structures outside the pial membrane of the brainstem and spinal cord) is composed of long axons (1 to 2 m). Second, the spinal roots pass through narrow foramina centrally and many ligaments and tendon sheaths peripherally, making them susceptible to compression. Third, the axons depend on a complex longitudinal network of nutrient arteries that run in the epineurium and perineurium.

Not all peripheral neuropathies are painful. Those neuropathies involving smaller afferent fibers are painful. Those affecting large diameter afferent fibers and Schwann cells generally are painless. The pain associated with a peripheral neuropathy usually is not a distinguishing feature of the neuropathy. Therefore, diagnosis depends first on establishing whether the patient has a peripheral neuropathy and second on determining the cause of the neuropathy.

Peripheral neuropathies, regardless of their cause, have several characteristic signs and symptoms: (1) paresthesias and dysesthesias, (2) sensory loss, (3) loss or diminution of tendon reflexes, and (4) impaired motor function. Paresthesias and dysesthesias are a common feature of certain types of neuropathies (e.g., diabetic and alcoholic neuropathy). The paresthesias can manifest as tingling, lancinating pain, or numbness. Perversion of sensation also occurs (e.g., a tactile stimulus may cause a burning pain or tingling). Another unusual feature is that the pain persists after the stimulus is withdrawn. With a neuropathy, the sensory threshold is raised, but the experience or response is intensified (hyperpathia). The mechanism of paresthesias is not understood. One hypothesis cites the loss of large touch–pressure fibers no longer inhibiting pain-receiving cells in the posterior horn. Another states that ectopic discharges may result from regenerated nociceptive fibers. Most neuropathies are accompanied by some type of sensory loss. All the sensory types (touch–pressure, vibratory, joint position, pain, and temperature) may be affected, or one may be affected more than the rest. Loss or diminution of tendon reflexes is another characteristic sign of peripheral neuropathy. Depression or loss of the Achilles reflex is a particularly sensitive index of polyneuropathy. Reflexes will be diminished as a result of sensory impairment combined with loss of muscle strength.

Other signs and symptoms, such as tremors and disorders of autonomic function, also may be seen with peripheral neuropathies. Laboratory tests (e.g., nerve conduction studies, nerve biopsies, and cerebrospinal fluid examination) may be useful when diagnosing neuropathies.[174,175]

Diabetic Neuropathy

Diabetic neuropathy includes a wide range of clinical manifestations. Traditionally, it has been categorized anatomically (Table 14-11). For our purposes, the diabetic neuropathies can be classified into separate pain syndromes:

Table 14-11
The Diabetic Neuropathies

Symmetric Polyneuropathies
    Sensory polyneuropathy
    Acute motor neuropathy
    Autonomic neuropathy
Focal and Multifocal Neuropathies
    Cranial neuropathy
    Limb mononeuropathy
    Diabetic amyotrophy

Table 14-12
Features of the Diabetic Neuropathies

Syndrome	Features
Polyneuropathy	Numbness, painful paresthesias, hyperesthesia, Charcot joints, loss of distal reflexes, edema
Radiculopathy	Lancinating pain in root distribution with segmental sensory and reflex loss
Mononeuropathy	Sudden or gradual loss of cranial nerves (3rd, 4th, 6th, 7th, or 10th) or peripheral nerves (ulnar, median, radial, or femoral)
Amyotrophy	Proximal asymmetric weakness and pain in thighs, or lumbar region with muscle wasting, absence of sensory loss

polyneuropathy, mononeuropathy, radiculopathy, and amyotrophy (Table 14-12).[176,177]

The incidence of diabetic neuropathy varies from a low of 5 percent to 6 percent to a high of 60 percent in different series, depending on the criteria used to establish the diagnosis. Pirart[178] noticed the prevalence of neuropathy increased from 7.5 percent at the time of discovery of diabetes mellitus to almost 50 percent after 25 years; neuropathy rarely occurs in young patients.[179] Neuropathy is found both in Type I or insulin-dependent diabetes mellitus, and in Type II or noninsulin-dependent diabetes mellitus. It also may occur in diabetes after pancreatectomy and hemochromatosis. Several authors cited the triad of neuropathy, nephropathy, and retinopathy (diabetic triopathy).[180] From this list, we can see there is a close association between sensory neuropathy and autonomic neuropathy.

Symmetric Sensory Polyneuropathy

A symmetric sensory polyneuropathy is the most frequent form of peripheral nerve disorder in diabetic patients. It may occur acutely after a diabetic coma or as a result of poor control.[181] Others found that it occurred after initiation of therapy with insulin or oral hypoglycemic agents and periods of emotional stress.

In most instances, the physical signs are minimal, and the neuropathy is diagnosed by a loss of ankle jerks and vibratory sense in the feet. The symptoms generally are confined to the lower extremities, and they consist of burning paresthesias with tingling and numbness. A deep aching pain (described by patients as "arising from the bones") that intensifies at night can affect the feet and legs. Symmetric distal sensory impairment occurs in a glove-and-stocking distribution.

Some authors believe that diabetic sensory neuropathy occurs along a continuum. At one extreme, are patients with loss of position sense, decreased reflexes, and no pain. At the other end, are those with cutaneous hyperesthesia, distal burning pain, and autonomic dysfunction but preserved reflexes and large fiber sensory function. This latter type shows involvement of small myelinated and unmyelinated nerve fibers using sural nerve biopsy samples.[182]

Others describe less common variants of symmetric sensory polyneuropathy. Archer and associates[183] documented severe distal burning pain in men without sensory loss and no autonomic features after rapid weight loss. The neuropathy subsided after these patients gained weight and had improved diabetic control.

The term *diabetic pseudotabes* refers to a variant that includes symmetric distal loss of cutaneous sensibility, joint position, and vibration, all leading to gait abnormalities and foot ulcers. Autonomic signs and symptoms, including atonic bladder and Argyll Robertson pupils, also may occur.

Neuropathy arthropathy, seen in established cases of sensory polyneuropathy, affects mainly the joints of the feet and, less commonly, the ankle points. The interphalangeal and metatarsophalangeal joints are affected.[184]

Autonomic dysfunction is almost a constant companion of sensory polyneuropathy and has a wide range of clinical manifestations (see Table 14-13). Diabetic autonomic neuropathy seems to affect the longer fibers first, like its sensory counterpart. The earliest changes involve vascular and sudomotor innervation of the legs. Anhidrosis, a result of postganglionic lesions of the sudomotor fibers, initially is detectable in the feet, but it may extend over other areas in a symmetric fashion. It is associated with an absence of piloerection. Peripheral edema of unknown origin also frequently occurs with diabetic neuropathy.[185]

Table 14-13
Manifestations of Diabetic Autonomic Dysfunction

Cardiac	Orthostatic hypotension Diminished beat-to-beat variation Peripheral edema
Genitourinary	Neurogenic bladder Retrograde ejaculation Erectile impotence
Gastrointestinal	Nocturnal diarrhea Constipation Decreased gastric motility
Others	Anhidrosis Abnormal pupil reaction

Focal and Multifocal Neuropathies

The peripheral nerves most commonly affected by diabetic neuropathy are the following: ulnar, median, radial, femoral, lateral cutaneous of the thigh, and peroneal nerves. The onset may be abrupt or insidious. These isolated peripheral nerve lesions often occur at sites common for external pressure palsies (e.g., carpal tunnel).

Diabetic Amyotrophy/Proximal Motor Neuropathy

Diabetic amyotrophy is a syndrome usually encountered in older diabetic patients that consists of asymmetric proximal muscle wasting in the lower limbs. The muscles commonly affected include the iliopsoas, quadriceps, and adductor muscles but not the hamstrings.[186,187] Pain, both in the thigh muscles and lumbar region, is a common feature of the syndrome. It generally is most severe at night. The patellar reflex may be depressed, but loss of sensory function is not a typical feature.

Uremic Neuropathy

The incidence of neuropathy is 60 percent to 70 percent in patients about to begin dialysis for chronic renal failure.[188,189] The progression of the neuropathy depends solely on the duration and severity of renal failure and has no relationship to the underlying cause. Men seem to have a several-fold higher incidence than women.

Uremic neuropathy is invariably distal, symmetric, and combines motor and sensory dysfunction.[190] The legs are affected before and more often than the upper extremities. This correlates with histopathologic studies that show a distal axonal degeneration with shrinkage and nerve fiber loss predominantly involving larger fibers.

The exact cause of the neuropathy is unknown, although the accumulation of toxic substances with molecular weights of 300 to 2000 Daltons (the so-called middle-molecule hypothesis) that are not removed during hemodialysis is considered the most likely explanation.[191] This is supported by the appearance of increased signs and symptoms of neuropathy with normal blood levels of creatinine and urea during hemodialysis and the improvement of the neuropathy with increased number of hours of dialysis beyond that needed for chemical control. Two other observations support the middle-molecule hypothesis as the source of neuropathy are: (1) the striking remission of neuropathy after successful renal transplantation and (2) the fact that peritoneal dialysis, which presumably passes toxic molecules more selectively than hemodialysis, is not associated with neuropathy despite having higher blood levels of urea and creatinine.

Uremic patients can have extremity pain from various causes. Nielsen[192] noticed muscular cramps and the restless-leg syndrome in two-thirds of patients in his series. The cramps, which also can occur during acute uremia, probably reflect muscular irritability in the presence of uremic toxins. They are not necessarily associated with any other signs and symptoms of neuropathy (e.g., slowing of conduction velocity). The restless-leg syndrome of Ekbom[193] characterized by night pain relieved by movement is associated with clinical neuropathy. Dysesthesias can occur with a variety of manifestations. They range from the burning-feet type identical to that seen in alcoholic patients to painful tingling, electric shocks, or constrictive feelings around the ankles and feet. The diagnosis depends on demonstrating a neuropathy with symptomatic uremia and excluding other causes of neuropathy, such as toxins.

Gold Neuropathy

Gold has been used traditionally to treat rheumatoid arthritis. Common side effects of this drug include fever and rashes. The incidence of patients who have peripheral neuropathy after gold therapy is less than 1 percent. Affected patients have painful paresthesias, followed by sudden onset of asymmetric weakness. They may have fever and rashes before the onset of the neuropathy.[194]

There is some controversy as to whether the neuropathy is a result of the direct toxic effect of the drug or a hypersensitivity reaction.[195]

Perhexiline Neuropathy

Perhexiline maleate was introduced for the treatment of angina in the early 1970s. Peripheral neuropathy was seen in some patients who were treated with doses of 300 to 400 mg/day for 4 months to 1 year. These patients had pain and distal paresthesias, followed by severe distal and proximal muscle weakness. They also had a high incidence of bilateral papilledema, abnormal liver function tests, and weight loss. Perhexiline apparently causes cellular accumulation of abnormal gangliosides, particularly in Schwann cells and liver cells.[196]

Vincristine Neuropathy

Casey and associates[197] demonstrated that vincristine, a chemotherapeutic agent, predictably produced peripheral neuropathy. Paresthesias beginning in the fingers were the most common initial symptom. Affected patients also had painful cramping and weakness in the extensor muscles of their hands and wrists. Most lost their ankle reflexes. The neuropathy improved somewhat after decreasing or discontinuing the drug. Vincristine has been shown to produce a breakdown of neurotubules and proliferation of neurofilaments in both human and animal nerve cells.[198]

Nitrofurantoin Neuropathy

Nitrofurantoin may cause peripheral neuropathy characterized by distal weakness and sensory loss. Pain and paresthesias are the common presenting symptoms.[199] The onset of neuropathy may occur as early as several weeks after drug therapy begins; most commonly, it is seen in patients with impaired renal function who have higher blood levels of the drug.[200]

Disulfiram Neuropathy

Neuropathy is a rare complication of disulfiram therapy for alcohol abuse.[201] Affected patients generally have taken 1.0 or 1.5 g daily of this drug. They have paresthesias beginning in the lower extremities. The mechanism is unclear; however, carbon disulfide, a by-product of disulfiram, is a known neurotoxin.[202]

Carcinomatous Neuropathy

An association between malignant disease and peripheral neuropathy independent of metastases has been recognized for a long time. In 1948, Denny-Brown[203] described two patients with carcinoma of the lung and sensory neuropathy from degeneration of dorsal root ganglion cells.

Studies among different groups of workers revealed an incidence of clinical peripheral neuropathy in the range of 1.7 percent to 5 percent of patients with cancer.[204,205] The highest incidence occurs among those with carcinoma of the lung, followed by those of the stomach, colon, and breast.

A sensorimotor type of neuropathy is the most common type, followed by a sensory type.[205] The predominantly sensory neuropathy is characterized by painful dysesthesias that begin distally and then spread proximally. Aching pains also are common. Tendon reflexes are depressed, and the position and vibratory sense may be impaired. The neuropathy often precedes other symptoms of the neoplasm by 1 year. This type of neuropathy seems to have a predilection for women. The course of the neuropathy is unaffected by the underlying disease state.

Pathologic changes associated with sensory neuropathy include severe degeneration of the posterior columns secondary to degeneration of dorsal nerve roots.[203] Axonal degeneration and segmental demyelination occur with sensorimotor neuropathy.[206] The actual cause of the neuropathies is unclear.

RHEUMATOLOGIC DISORDERS (See Chap. 13)

Polymyalgia Rheumatica

Polymyalgia rheumatica is a clinical syndrome characterized by morning stiffness in the proximal portion of the extremities or torso.[207] It is relatively common in those older than 50 years of age. One study documented an annual incidence of 53.7 cases per 100,000 persons aged 50 years or older with a prevalence of 500 per 100,000.[208] There is also a close relationship between polymyalgia rheumatica and giant cell arteritis; polymyalgia rheumatica occurs in 40 percent to 60 percent of patients with giant cell arteritis.[209]

Some authors suggest that polymyalgia rheumatica may be an expression of an underlying arteritis.

The diagnosis is made by the presence of symptoms in two of the three commonly affected areas (neck, hip, or shoulder) for at least 1 month plus other evidence of a systemic reaction, such as an increased erythrocyte sedimentation rate to more than 40 mm/h using the Westergren method.[210] Some definitions also include a rapid response to small doses of corticosteroids. The presence of other diseases, such as rheumatoid arthritis, polymyositis, malignancy, or chronic infection excludes the diagnosis.

The cause is unknown. The increased incidence of the disease in those older than 50 years of age suggests some relationship to aging. Reports of familial aggregation and the finding that the disease appears almost exclusively in whites suggest a genetic predisposition. Several results show a humoral or cellular immune basis: (1) the granulomatous histopathologic features of giant cell arteritis, (2) the presence of immunoglobulins and complement deposits adjacent to the elastic lamina in some involved temporal arteries, and (3) the finding that sera from patients with polymyalgia rheumatica contains increased levels of circulating immune complexes during active disease.[211]

These patients are generally in good health before polymyalgia rheumatica develops. Arthralgias and myalgias may occur either slowly or abruptly; they generally begin in one shoulder girdle. However, the disease soon becomes bilateral and eventually involves most of the tendinous attachments, and there is proximal muscle pain with movement (versus the joint pain in rheumatoid arthritis).[212,213] Muscular strength is normal. An associated finding may be synovitis in the knees or sternoclavicular joints. More than half the patients have systemic symptoms (such as weight loss or a low grade fever before the onset of muscle pain).[212,213]

Laboratory findings during its active phase include: (1) a markedly elevated erythrocyte sedimentation rate (more than 100 mm/h using the Westergren method), (2) a mild-to-moderate normochromic anemia, and (3) an increase in α-2-globulin and fibrinogen.[214] Significant normal laboratory values include serum creatine kinase, muscle biopsies, and electromyograms.

The differential diagnosis of polymyalgia rheumatica includes rheumatoid arthritis, polymyositis, and systemic processes (such as bacterial endocarditis). The absence of swelling and peripheral joint pain should distinguish polymyalgia rheumatica from arthritis. Polymyositis is characterized by muscle weakness, elevated muscle enzyme studies, and abnormal electromyograms.

Psoriatic Arthritis

Psoriatic arthritis is an inflammatory asymmetric polyarthritis found in patients with psoriasis. The cause is unknown, but up to 30 percent of patients are positive for HLA-B27 antigen.[215] The onset of the arthritis generally follows the psoriasis by months or years. The course of arthritis may or may not parallel that of the skin lesions. The pattern of the arthritis is that of a typical inflammatory arthritis that affects predominantly the upper extremities. The proximal joints of the hands and feet are tender and swollen. The arthritis is limited to several joints and is asymmetric. There are no rheumatoid nodules. Laboratory tests do not show rheumatoid factor. Affected patients may have an increased erythrocyte sedimentation rate and anemia.[216]

The radiologic features of psoriatic arthritis include erosions of the articular surfaces and the so-called pencil-in-cup deformity observed in joints of the fingers and toes. The diagnosis depends on findings consistent with psoriasis and an accompanying inflammatory arthritis without rheumatoid factor or nodules.

Reiter Syndrome

Reiter syndrome is an asymmetric inflammatory arthritis coupled with urethritis or cervicitis. Classically, the syndrome also included conjunctivitis. The syndrome has two clinical forms. The postvenereal form occurs predominantly in young men; the postdysenteric form affects both sexes in all age groups. The actual pathogenesis of the disease involves infection of the urogenital tract or gut with one of several organisms in genetically susceptible patients. Sufferers generally have the HLA-B27 alloantigen.[217]

Clinically, the syndrome begins with an asymptomatic serous urethral discharge. This is followed by conjunctivitis in some cases.[218] Finally, the patient has an acute onset of inflammatory arthritis of the lower extremities. Keratoderma blennorrhagia frequently appear on the palms or soles. Painless mucocutaneous lesions may appear in the mouth, on the palms and soles, or on the glans penis.[218]

Synovial fluid analysis reveals an increased leukocyte count and inflammatory arthritis. The diagnosis, therefore, relies on documenting nonspecific urethritis or cervicitis without rheumatoid factor.

Gout

Gout is a painful disorder of the joints secondary to deposition of crystals of monosodium urate monohydrate. Urate values greater than 7.0 mg/dl in the plasma cause saturation; chronically elevated uric acid leads to gouty attacks. Hyperuricemia per se is not synonymous with gout, and most hyperuricemic patients are asymptomatic. Men tend to have higher values for uric acid, and more than 95 percent of cases occur in adult men. Hyperuricemic patients also are prone to acute nephrolithiasis, and approximately 20 percent of gout sufferers have attacks of renal colic before gouty attacks.[219]

The pathogenesis of an acute gouty attack after years of chronically elevated uric acid levels probably involves crystal deposition and resultant phagocytosis by leukocytes, leading to activation of Hageman factor, coating of crystals with gamma globulins, and complement activation.[220] Lowering the local tissue pH then results in additional precipitation of urate crystals.

The initial attack of gouty arthritis is exquisitely painful and usually monoarticular. Affected patients may describe prior mild attacks (twinges). The attacks generally are confined to the distal lower extremities, particularly the great toe (podagra). The following are involved in order of decreasing frequency: instep, ankle, heel, knee, and upper extremities. The attacks may be triggered by trauma, alcohol, surgery, or dietary excesses. Affected patients may have accompanying systemic signs: fever, increased erythrocyte sedimentation rate, and leukocytosis. The attacks abate spontaneously and are separated by periods when the patient is completely asymptomatic.[221]

In untreated patients, the hyperuricemia causes deposits of monosodium urate (tophi) in tendons, membranes, and soft tissues. However, these tophi rarely occur before the onset of acute gouty attacks.

The diagnosis is confirmed by finding monosodium urate crystals in the leukocytes from synovial aspirates using polarized-light microscopy. These crystals appear needle shaped and negatively birefringent. The leukocyte count of the synovial fluid during attacks may vary from 1000 to 70,000/dl. Extracellular crystals may be found in the synovial fluid during asymptomatic periods. In the absence of microscopic confirmation, the diagnosis can be presumed by the combination of: (1) the presence of hyperuricemia, (2) a history typical of gout, and (3) response to colchicine.

Pseudogout

Pseudogout is a crystalline arthritis seen in elderly patients that is characterized by calcium deposits in articular cartilage and caused by release of calcium pyrophosphate crystals into the joint space. There is a definite association with hyperparathyroidism, osteoarthritis, and hemochromatosis. Pseudogout also is seen in the following metabolic disorders: Wilson disease, hypothyroidism, gout, and ochronosis.[222]

Patients with pseudogout have elevated fluid levels of inorganic pyrophosphate. Crystals then form in articular cartilage (chondrocalcinosis). The crystals found in synovial fluid are released from the cartilage, possibly after trauma that disrupts the cartilage or as a result of lowering the Ca^{2+} levels in the synovium. Regardless, the presence of calcium pyrophosphate crystals then causes a classic inflammatory response, and polymorphonuclear leukocytes enter the joint.[223]

The acute arthritic attacks of pseudogout are usually monoarticular. The knee is the most common site. The joint is warm, swollen, and painful. The attacks may be preceded by surgery or trauma.

The diagnosis is based on showing calcium pyrophosphate dihydrate crystals in the synovial fluid during acute attacks. Under a polarized-light microscope, the crystals appear as positive birefringent blunt rods. They may be intra- or extracellular. Radiologically, these patients have calcium deposits in their articular cartilage.[224]

Osteoarthritis

Osteoarthritis affects elderly patients, and stress on the joints appears to be a factor. Articular cartilage in the joints absorbs the bulk of the stress from use. Because the cartilage is subjected to increased pressure, there is an increased number of chondrocytes and increased production of synovial fluid. The cartilage soon shows focal erosions, and the water content and proteoglycan content is reduced. Eventually, joint margins reveal new bone and thickened synovium. The end point of this process is a progressive loss of chrondrocytes, development of fissures, osteophyte formation, and replacement of cartilage with bone.[225]

The pain of osteoarthritis usually is limited to one or several joints. It is described as diffuse and aching. Rest relieves the pain, and activity aggravates it. Affected patients may describe an increase in symptoms with changes in weather. Stiffness generally is not a symptom.[226]

Heberden nodes, which are prominent knobs along the medial and lateral aspect of distal interphalangeal joints, are a common finding during the physical examination. These are painless as are the Bouchard nodes found on the proximal interphalangeal joints. Occasionally, the joints may appear swollen and warm as a result of the inflammatory synovitis that accompanies an exacerbation of symptoms. The pattern of joint involvement (proximal interphalangeal and distal interphalangeal involvement with sparing of the wrist joint) distinguishes osteoarthritis from rheumatoid arthritis.[227]

The radiologic findings typical of osteoarthritis include: loss of joint space, presence of osteophytes, and subchondral sclerosis. Synovial fluid contains a low leukocyte count with predominantly mononuclear cells.

Rheumatoid Arthritis

Rheumatoid arthritis is distinguished by inflammatory synovitis, resulting in eventual cartilage and bone destruction. The cause is unknown; however, a genetic influence has been established by its association with HLA-DR4.[228] Women are affected threefold more than men. The onset of symptoms is most frequent between the ages of 35 and 50 years.

The joint pain of rheumatoid arthritis generally is preceded by systemic symptoms: fatigue, generalized weakness, and anorexia. The pain affects joints in a symmetric distribution and is aggravated by passive or active motion.[229] Morning stiffness is a universal feature and is an important criterion for the diagnosis. Physical examination reveals synovitis with accompanying swelling, tenderness, and increased warmth in the joints. The pain is secondary to

joint swelling; this stretches the joint capsule. The wrist joints, proximal interphalangeal joints, and metacarpophalangeal joints usually are involved; it rarely involves the distal interphalangeal joints. Hand involvement with destruction of cartilage, tendons, and ligaments can cause a number of typical deformities: (1) boutonnière deformity (which results from flexion deformity of the proximal interphalangeal joints and extension of the distal interphalangeal joints), (2) swan-neck deformity (which results from hyperextension of proximal joint and flexion of distal interphalangeal joints), and (3) radial deviation at the wrist with ulnar deviation at the digits.

The diagnosis depends on the presence of criteria listed by the American Rheumatism Association (Table 14-14). There are no specific diagnostic tests for rheumatoid arthritis. Affected patients may have rheumatoid factor (autoantibodies to immunoglobulin G) in their serum. In addition, there may be a normochromic normocytic anemia. Most patients also have increased erythrocyte sedimentation rates. Evaluation of the synovial fluid shows increased leukocytes with polymorphonuclear leukocytes, suggesting an inflammatory process.

MUSCULAR DISORDERS

Most skeletal muscle pain is associated with exercise or trauma.[230] The pain is related temporally to exercise and is of limited duration. Muscle pain is transmitted by the thin myelinated fibers (Group III or A delta) and unmyelinated fibers (Group IV or C). These afferent fibers have unencapsulated branching endings throughout the muscle with increasing density in the region of fascia, tendons, and aponeuroses. There are two types of muscle pain receptors: chemoreceptors and mechanoreceptors. The former respond to chemical changes in the environment; the latter are affected by mechanical changes. These receptors can be

Table 14-14
American Rheumatism Association Criteria for the Diagnosis of Rheumatoid Arthritis*

1. Morning stiffness
2. Pain on motion or tenderness in at least one joint
3. Swelling (soft tissue thickening or fluid) in at least one joint
4. Swelling of at least one other joint
5. Symmetric joint swelling
6. Subcutaneous nodules
7. Typical radiologic changes
8. Demonstration of rheumatoid factor in serum
9. Poor mucin precipitate from synovial fluid
10. Characteristic histologic changes in synovium
11. Characteristic histologic changes in nodules

*Criteria 1 to 5 must be continuous for at least 6 weeks. Criteria 2 to 6 must be observed by a physician. The presence of seven or more criteria indicates classic disease; five to six criteria indicate definite disease; three to four criteria indicate probably disease.
From Martin JB. *Harrison's Principles of Internal Medicine.* New York: McGraw-Hill; 1987:1950.

stimulated by potassium ions, hydrogen ions, histamine, serotonin, or bradykinin.[231–234]

Muscle pain or myalgia most often is described as dull or aching in quality. The term *cramp*[235] refers to an acute onset of a painful contraction, and although they can be intensely painful, the quality of pain is described as dull. A muscle *contracture* is similar to a cramp, but of a longer duration; it is seen in disorders of muscle metabolism. Muscle *spasms* are reflex contractions of muscles surrounding injured tissues or structures (e.g., abdominal muscle spasm associated with an inflamed appendix). *Myotonia* is tonic spasm of a muscle after voluntary contraction caused by a high frequency firing of muscle fibers. *Tetany* refers to involuntary cramp-like spasms associated with reductions in ionizable calcium or magnesium and attributed to repetitive firing in motor axons. *Dystonia* is an involuntary contraction of muscle that involves both agonist and antagonist activities.

Myalgias can be difficult to distinguish from pain arising from other sites. Pain from the joints is well localized and exacerbated by movement. Bone pain is poorly localized but tends to have a deep boring quality that generally worsens at night. It is important to determine whether the muscle pain is accompanied by weakness (failure to achieve strength) or fatigue (failure to maintain strength). As a rule, proximal muscle weakness suggests primary muscle disease; peripheral and localized pain and weakness tends to occur with nerve entrapments. Excessive fatiguability is seen in disorders of muscle metabolism, myotonic disorders, and mitochondrial myopathies.

The relationship of diet, alcohol intake, and fasting to muscle pain should be determined. Drinking bouts may precipitate myopathy and myoglobinuria in alcoholic patients. Fasting or prolonged exercise with fasting may precipitate pain and weakness in patients with carnitine palmityl transferase deficiency. A diet lacking in vitamin D may lead to osteomalacic myopathy with bone and muscle pain.

Signs of muscle pain are confined to weakness, fatiguability, tenderness, and swelling. Muscle swelling per se is rare, but it may be occur in the polymyositis–dermatomyositis complex, acute alcoholic myopathy, phosphofructokinase deficiency, and myophosphorylase.

Useful clinical tests to evaluate muscle pain and disease include: (1) presence of myoglobinemia and myoglobinuria, (2) serum creatine kinase levels, (3) erythrocyte sedimentation rate, (4) EMG, (5) quantitation of muscle force generation, (6) exercise testing, (7) ischemic forearm tests, and (8) muscle biopsy.

Myoglobin is a muscle protein involved in oxygen storage. Muscle breakdown or rhabdomyolysis can release the myoglobin molecules, which may pass into the urine as a result of their small size (molecular weight, 17,500 Daltons) and precipitate oliguric renal failure. Myoglobinemia and myoglobinuria may arise from various causes.[236]

Creatine kinase is a muscle enzyme that catalyzes the breakdown and synthesis of phosphoryl creatine. Abnormal increases in serum levels of creatine kinase may indicate muscle damage; however, exercise and intramuscular injections also may cause elevated serum levels.[237] This enzyme is elevated in muscular dystrophies, acute rhabdomyolysis, McArdle disease, and polymyositis–dermatomyositis complex.

EMG is helpful in distinguishing myopathies from neurogenic diseases. Denervation from entrapment is characterized by fibrillation and giant action potentials; myopathies are associated with brief small amplitude motor unit potentials. EMG also can provide information about which nerve roots are involved.

Quantitation[238] of muscle force generation can be done using a hand-held dynamometer or muscle-testing chair. The latter involves electrical activation of the quadriceps with large surface electrodes and provides data concerning muscle fatiguability and frequency characteristics. These tools can track the progression of the disease or the distribution of muscle weakness.

Exercise testing uses submaximal effort at approximately 70 percent of previously determined maximal rate while simultaneously measuring heart rate and blood pressure and levels of blood lactate and pyruvate. Exercise testing can elicit symptoms in patients with muscle disorders, and it is a particularly useful tool in those with suspected metabolic disorders.

The simplicity and advantages of muscle biopsy, particularly in the diagnosis of inflammatory myopathies and mitochondrial myopathies, have been well described. Percutaneous needle biopsy is atraumatic and appears to be as reliable clinically as an open biopsy of muscle.

Muscle Pain and Exercise

Normally, muscle pain and exercise can occur under two situations. First, pain can occur with exercise and increase in intensity until the muscle relaxes. When the voluntary contraction stops, the pain disappears immediately. This type of concentric contraction or positive work has a high metabolic cost.[239] The mechanism for this type of ischemic pain appears to be an accumulation of metabolites that occludes blood vessels and stops the blood supply to the muscle. Second, vigorous exercise leads to delayed muscle pain. This results from eccentric muscle contractions or negative work where the muscle is lengthened during a contraction.[240] The mechanism of this delayed soreness after eccentric contraction is unknown; however, the muscles show evidence of damage, both biochemically and morphologically.[241]

Cramps are painful involuntary contractions of acute onset that occur more often at night. Stretching of voluntary muscle produces an involuntary contraction that cannot be relaxed. The cramping results from spontaneous firing of groups of anterior horn cells with motor unit contractions.

Cramps in the calf muscles generally are considered benign. More generalized cramps may be a sign of muscle disease.[235] Cramps that are recurrent and confined to one specific muscle group may indicate nerve root entrapment. They also occur with increasing frequency during pregnancy, with electrolyte imbalances, and in patients undergoing hemodialysis. Physical examination during muscle cramping shows a taut contracted muscle. This can be a distinguishing feature of the cramps caused by intermittent claudication where patients have cramp-like pain without muscle contraction. The cause of the pain is not understood completely, but it may involve an accumulation of metabolites or a relative ischemia of the muscle. There is a benign form of muscle cramping (idiopathic cramp syndrome) where no neuromuscular disorder is apparent.

The stiff-man syndrome refers to a progressive form of painful muscle spasm.[242,243] These patients have a board-like stiffness of their muscles, paroxysms of cramping, and a normal sensory examination. The muscle stiffness resolves during sleep or after the administration of large doses of diazepam. Isaac syndrome is manifested by excessive sweating, widespread fasciculations, generalized stiffness, and continuous motor unit activity that persists during sleep and anesthesia.[244]

Tetany results from a reduction in ionizable calcium and magnesium. This leads to increased neuromuscular irritability and involuntary cramp-like spasms. The actual level of ionizable calcium needed to produce tetany varies individually and is related to the concentration of other electrolytes in the extracellular fluid. Hyperventilation and ischemia increase the tendency for spasm to occur. The full clinical spectrum of tetany is manifested by perioral and peripheral paresthesias, carpal spasm, pedal spasm, laryngospasm, Chvostek and Trousseau signs, and Q-T prolongation on an ECG. Hypocalcemia causes unstable depolarization of the nerve fiber axons. Thus, there is increased sensitivity of the facial nerve to percussion (Chvostek sign) and spasm with ischemia (Trousseau sign).

Drugs also may be a source of muscle pain. Focal myopathy may occur after intramuscular injections from local irritation (e.g., paraldehyde) or after histamine release (opiates).

Painful proximal myopathy with tenderness and weakness can occur after administration of clofibrate, aminocaproic acid, and emetine, particularly after prolonged treatment and elevated serum blood levels. Serum levels of muscle enzymes are elevated, and myoglobinuria may occur. Muscle biopsy reveals multifocal muscle-fiber necrosis. A painful necrotizing proximal myopathy with an associated peripheral neuropathy has been reported in patients treated with vincristine.[245] Chronic hypokalemia from drug use generally results in painless weakness and hypotonia. However, painful quadriparesis and myoglobinuria has been reported after administration of amphotericin B and chlorthalidone.[245] Finally, some drugs may cause myalgias and cramps from unknown mechanisms. These

include lithium carbonate, danazol, isoetherine, cimetidine, and the diuretics, metolazone and bumetanide.[245]

The glycogen storage diseases are a group of diseases in which there is an inborn error of glycogen metabolism. When the energy supply for muscle contractions is compromised, muscle fatigue and pain may result.

McArdle disease or Type V occurs during adolescence with cramps, weakness, and contractions induced by vigorous exercise. The cramps and pain are relieved by rest, but the contractions may persist for hours. Moderate exercise may be well tolerated. This disorder is caused by a deficiency of the enzyme myophosphorylase. Tarui disease or Type VII is a rarer enzyme deficiency that begins during early childhood and is characterized by exercise-induced pain without muscle contractions.

Idiopathic Polymyositis and Dermatomyositis

Idiopathic polymyositis and dermatomyositis refer to a category of relatively common diseases that may affect striated muscle only (polymyositis) or skin and muscle (dermatomyositis). They also may occur associated with arthritis, connective tissue diseases, or malignancy. Pain may be a prominent feature.[246]

The cause of polymyositis–dermatomyositis is unknown. Theories include autoimmune processes or a possible viral mechanism.[247] Polymyositis–dermatomyositis may have several different clinical presentations. Polymyositis, confined to striated muscles, begins with an insidious onset over 3 to 6 months of a symmetric weakness of the proximal limb and trunk muscles. In a minority of patients, this subacute muscle weakness is preceded by a febrile illness. Women outnumber men 2:1, and the age range is generally 30 to 60 years.[248] Rarely, severe muscle weakness occurs acutely with associated myoglobinuria.

Affected patients first notice weakness of the proximal limb muscles when climbing steps, rising from chairs, or combing their hair. The muscle pain that occurs in a minority of patients is of a constant aching quality and follows the same distribution as the weakness.[249]

Physical examination shows a symmetric weakness of the muscles of the hips, shoulders, and thighs. Weakness of the facial and pharyngeal muscles also is common. The muscles are not tender to examination, and atrophy is not a prominent feature.

Dermatomyositis is characterized by skin lesions that may precede, accompany, or follow the muscle involvement. The rash may take one of several forms: localized erythema, maculopapular eruption, or exfoliative dermatitis. The areas most predisposed are the eyelids, the bridge of the nose, and the cheeks. The extensor surfaces of elbows, knees, and knuckles may develop flat plaques known as Gottron papules.[250] The myositis that accompanies these skin changes is indistinguishable from polymyositis.

Polymyositis or dermatomyositis may occur associated

with an underlying neoplasm (Group 3) (Table 14-15). The muscle and skin manifestations may antedate the discovery of a carcinoma by 1 to 2 years. This generally occurs with bronchogenic carcinoma.[251] The actual incidence of underlying carcinomas with polymyositis is 2 percent to 3 percent; it rises to 15 percent to 20 percent with dermatomyositis.

Idiopathic polymyositis and dermatomyositis occurs less frequently in childhood than in adults. The childhood form constitutes 8 percent to 22 percent of cases in most large series. The clinical features of the disease in children are similar to those in adults; however, children have a high incidence of vasculitis.[252]

Finally, polymyositis or dermatomyositis may occur in collagen vascular disease. Mixed connective tissue diseases also may have an accompanying arthritis that limits joint motion and further diminishes strength.

Laboratory findings common to all the clinical subsets of dermatomyositis–polymyositis include: (1) elevated serum levels of skeletal muscle enzymes, particularly creatine kinase (which may be elevated 10 to 80-fold normal), (2) sometimes positive tests for circulating rheumatoid factor and antinuclear antibody, (3) myoglobinuria, (4) EMG showing an increase in the insertional activity of the muscle with numerous fibrillation potentials and positive sharp waves at rest,[253] and (5) resultant muscle biopsy consisting of inflammatory infiltrates (lymphocytes and histiocytes) between the muscle fibers and around the small blood vessels in the muscle.[254]

Other Forms of Polymyositis

Trichinosis in humans is contracted by ingesting meat (usually pork) containing the larvae of *Trichinella spiralis*. There are no intermediate hosts. The larvae are freed from their cysts by gastric digestion and migrate into the intestinal mucosa where copulation occurs. The offspring (up to 1500 larvae per female) enter the circulation and are distributed to muscles throughout the body. When the larvae enter the muscle, they grow and become encysted; eventually, the cysts become calcified. The life cycle then

Table 14-15
Classification of the Dermatomyositis–Polymyositis Complex

Group 1. Primary idiopathic polymyositis

Group 2. Primary idiopathic dermatomyositis

Group 3. Dermatomyositis (or polymyositis) associated with neoplasia

Group 4. Childhood dermatomyositis (or polymyositis) associated with vasculitis

Group 5. Polymyositis or dermatomyositis associated with collagen vascular disease (overlap group)

Proposed by Bohan and Peter.[246]

ends. The muscles most affected include the eye muscles, diaphragm, deltoid, pectorals, and gastrocnemius.[255]

The clinical severity of the symptoms correlates well with the number of larvae disseminated to the tissues. Patients with less than 10 larvae per gram of muscle are asymptomatic; those with greater than 50 larvae per gram of muscle are symptomatic. Gastrointestinal symptoms (e.g., diarrhea and abdominal pain) appear 1 to 2 days after the infected meat is eaten. This brief period is followed by a stage of muscular invasion that may last up to 6 weeks. Affected patients have muscle pain and tenderness with accompanying weakness. They also may have fever, periorbital edema, conjunctivitis, and a maculopapular rash. Severe cases may have various central nervous system manifestations. Finally, myocarditis may occur with resultant congestive heart failure and ECG changes.

Laboratory findings include an eosinophilic leukocytosis (>500 eosinophils/μl) within the first few weeks. Serologic tests are available that become positive within the first month and remain positive for years. A definitive diagnosis is made after muscle biopsy. A gram portion of muscle is excised from the gastrocnemius or deltoid and examined microscopically for the presence of larvae or calcified cysts.[256]

Eosinophilic Myositis

Eosinophilic myositis consists of three separate clinical entities: (1) eosinophilic fasciitis, (2) eosinophilic monomyositis, and (3) eosinophilic polymyositis.[257] Eosinophilic fasciitis involves tenosynovitis with local pain and stiffness of unknown cause. The disease progresses from one muscle to another, but generally it is confined to an extremity. These patients have no systemic manifestations. The muscle per se is not involved, and the biopsy of fascia and tendon sheaths reveals an inflammatory process with eosinophilic leukocytes. Eosinophilic monomyositis includes muscle pain confined to one calf muscle. A tender mass is found in the muscle. A muscle biopsy shows an inflammatory necrosis and edema of interstitial tissues. Eosinophilic polymyositis as described by Layzer and colleagues[258] is the third form of eosinophilic myositis. This is characterized by multiple systemic problems (congestive heart failure, anemia, and pulmonary infiltrates) plus painful proximal muscle weakness. The muscles themselves are swollen and exquisitely tender.[259]

References

1. Malan E, Tattoni G. Physio- and anatopathology of acute ischemia of the extremities. *J Cardiovasc Surg* (Torino) 1963; 4:2.

2. Perry MO. Acute arterial insufficiency. In: Rutherford RB, ed. *Vascular Surgery*. 2nd ed. Philadelphia: Saunders; 1984.

3. Perry MO. Acute arterial insufficiency. In: Rutherford RB,

ed. *Vascular Surgery*. 2nd ed. Philadelphia: Saunders; 1984.

4. Perry MO. Acute arterial insufficiency. In: Rutherford RB, ed. *Vascular Surgery*. 2nd ed. Philadelphia: Saunders; 1984.

5. Kempczinski RF. The management of chronic ischemia of the lower extremities. In: Rutherford RB, ed. *Vascular Surgery*. 2nd ed. Philadelphia: Saunders; 1984.

6. Walton KW. Pathogenic mechanisms in atherosclerosis. *Am J Cardiol* 1975; 35:542.

7. Haust MD, More RH. Development of modern theories on the pathogenesis of atherosclerosis. In: Wissler RW, Gees JC, eds. *The Pathogenesis of Atherosclerosis*. Baltimore: Williams & Wilkins; 1972:1–9.

8. Kempczinski RF. Peripheral arterial atheroembolism. In: Miller DC, Roon AJ, eds. *Diagnosis and Management of Peripheral Vascular Disease*. Menlo Park: Addison-Wesley; 1982.

9. Kempczinski RF. The differential diagnoses of intermittent claudication. *Pract Cardiol* 1981; 7:53.

10. Boyd AM. Natural course of atherosclerosis of lower extremities. *Proc R Soc Med* 1962; 53:591.

11. Imparato AM, Kim GE, Davidson T, Crowley JG. Intermittent claudication: its natural course. *Surgery* 1975; 78:795.

12. Sumner DS. Measurement of segmental arterial pressure. In: Rutherford RB, ed. *Vascular Surgery*. 2nd ed. Philadelphia: Saunders; 1984.

13. Carter SA. Indirect systolic pressure and pulse waves in arterial occlusive disease of the lower extremities. *Circulation* 1968; 37:624.

14. Carter SR. Clinical measurement of systolic pressures in limbs with arterial occlusive disease. *JAMA* 1969; 207:1869.

15. Cutajar CL, Marston A, Newcombe JF. Value of cuff occlusion pressures in assessment of peripheral vascular disease. *Br Med J* 1973; 2:392.

16. Love JW, Whelan TJ. Popliteal artery entrapment syndrome. *Am J Surg* 1965; 109:620.

17. Insua JA, Young JR, Humphries AW. Popliteal artery entrapment syndrome. *Arch Surg* 1970; 101:771.

18. Ezzet F, Yettra M. Bilateral popliteal artery entrapment: case report and observations. *J Cardiovasc Surg* 1971; 12:71.

19. Bergan JJ. Adventitial cystic disease of the popliteal artery. In: Rutherford RB, ed. *Vascular Surgery*. 2nd ed. Philadelphia: Saunders; 1984.

20. Bergan JJ. Adventitial cystic disease of the popliteal artery. In: Rutherford RB, ed. *Vascular Surgery*. 2nd ed. Philadelphia: Saunders; 1984.

21. McPherson JR, Juergens JL, Gifford RW Jr. Thromboangiitis obliterans and arteriosclerosis obliterans: clinical and prognostic differences. *Ann Intern Med* 1963; 59:288.

22. Juergens JL. Thromboangiitis obliterans. In: Rutherford RB, ed. *Vascular Surgery*. 2nd ed. Philadelphia: Saunders; 1984.

23. Rivera R. Roentgenographic diagnosis of Buerger's disease. *J Cardiovasc Surg (Torino)* 1973; 14:40.

24. Allen EV, Brown GE. Raynaud's disease: a critical review of minimal requisites for diagnosis. *Am J Med Sci* 1932; 183:187.

25. VeLayos EE, Robinson H, Porciuncula FV, Masi AT. Clinical correlation analysis of 137 patients with Raynaud's phenomenon. *Am J Med Sci* 1971; 262:347.

26. Blunt RJ, Porter JM. Raynaud's syndrome. *Semin Arthritis Rheum* 1981; 11:282.

27. Porter JM. Raynaud's syndrome and associated vasospastic conditions of the extremities. In: Rutherford RB, ed. *Vascular Surgery*. 2nd ed. Philadelphia: Saunders; 1984.

28. Taylor W, Pelmar PL. Raynaud's phenomenon of occupational origin: an epidemiological survey. *Acta Chir Scand Suppl* 1976; 465:27.

29. Porter JM. Raynaud's syndrome and associated vasospastic conditions of the extremities. In: Rutherford RB, ed. *Vascular Surgery*. 2nd ed. Philadelphia: Saunders; 1984.

30. Patman RD. Post-traumatic pain syndromes: recognition and management. In: Rutherford RB, ed. *Vascular Surgery*. 2nd ed. Philadelphia: Saunders; 1984.

31. Patman RD. Post-traumatic pain syndromes: recognition and management. In: Rutherford RB, ed. *Vascular Surgery*. 2nd ed. Philadelphia: Saunders; 1984.

32. Lankford LL. Reflex sympathetic dystrophy. In: Evarts CM, ed. *Surgery of the Musculoskeletal System*. New York: Churchill Livingstone; 1983.

33. Mitchell SW, Morehouse GR, Keen W. *Gunshot Wounds and Other Injuries of Nerves*. Philadelphia: Lippincott; 1864.

34. Lankford LL, Thompson JE. Reflex sympathetic dystrophy, upper and lower extremity: diagnosis and management. In: *AAOS Instructional Course Lectures*. Vol. 26. St. Louis: Mosley; 1977.

35. Lankford LL, Thompson JE. Reflex sympathetic dystrophy, upper and lower extremity: diagnosis and management. In: *AAOS Instructional Course Lectures*. Vol. 26. St. Louis: Mosley; 1977.

36. Steinbrocker O. The shoulder–hand syndrome: associated painful homolateral disability of the shoulder and hand with swelling and atrophy of the hand. *Am J Med* 1947; 3:402–407.

37. Steinbrocker O, Spitzer M, Friedman HH. The shoulder–hand syndrome in reflex dystrophy of the upper extremity. *Ann Intern Med* 1948; 29:22–52.

38. Bernstein EF. Operative management of acute venous thromboembolism. In: Rutherford RB, ed. *Vascular Surgery*. 2nd ed. Philadelphia: Saunders; 1984.

39. Sumner DS. Hemodynamics and pathophysiology of venous disease. In: Rutherford RB, ed. *Vascular Surgery*. 2nd ed. Philadelphia: Saunders; 1984.

40. Sumner DS. Evaluation of venous circulation with the ultrasonic Doppler velocity detector. In: Rutherford RB, ed. *Vascular Surgery*. 2nd ed. Philadelphia: Saunders; 1984.

41. Wheeler HB. Plethysmographic diagnosis of deep venous thrombosis. In: Rutherford RB, ed. *Vascular Surgery*. 2nd ed. Philadelphia: Saunders; 1984.

42. Baxter BT, Blackburn D, Payne K, Pearce WH, Yao JS. Noninvasive evaluation of the upper extremity. *Surg Clin North Am* February 1990; 70(1):87–97.

43. Matsen FA III. Compartmental syndromes: a unified concept. *Clin Orthop* 1975; 113:8.

44. Rorabeck CH, Clark KM. The pathophysiology of the anterior tibial compartment syndrome: an experimental investigation. *J Trauma* 1978; 18:299.

45. Rorabeck CH, Macnab I. The pathophysiology of the anterior tibial compartmental syndrome. *Clin Orthop* 1975; 113:52.

46. Sheridan GW, Matsen FA III, Krugmire RB Jr. Further investigations on the pathophysiology of the compartmental syndrome. *Clin Orthop* 1977; 123:266.

47. Whitesides TE, Haney TC, Morimoto K, et al. Tissue pressure measurements as a determinant for the need of fasciotomy. *Clin Orthop* 1975; 113:43.

48. Owen CA, Mubarak SJ, Hargens AR, et al. Intramuscular pressure with limb compression. Clarification of the pathogenesis of the drug-induced compartment syndrome/crush syndrome. *N Engl J Med* 1979; 300:1169.

49. Matsen FA III, Winguist RA, Krugmire RB Jr. Diagnosis and management of compartmental syndrome. *J Bone Joint Surg Am* 1980; 62A:286.

50. Hargens AR, Mubarak SJ. Laboratory diagnosis of acute compartment syndromes. In: Mubarak SJ, Hargens AR, eds. *Compartment Syndromes and Volkmann's Contracture. Monographs in Clinical Orthopaedics, III*. Philadelphia: Saunders; 1981.

51. Ritland D, Butterfield W. Extremity complications of drug abuse. *Am J Surg* 1973; 126:639.

52. Wright CB, Geelhoed G, Hobson R, et al. Acute vascular insufficiency due to drugs of abuse. In: Rutherford RB, ed. *Vascular Surgery,* 2nd ed. Philadelphia: Saunders; 1984.

53. Gay GR. Intra-arterial injection of secobarbital sodium into the brachial artery: sequelae of a "hand trip." *Anesth Analg (Cleve)* 1971; 50:979.

54. Maxwell TM, Olcott C, Blaisdell FW. Vascular complications of drug abuse. *Arch Surg* 1972; 105:875.

55. Rich NM, Hobson RW, Fedde CW. Vascular trauma secondary to diagnostic and therapeutic procedures. *Am J Surg* 1973; 126:639.

56. Geelhoed GW, Joseph WL. Surgical sequelae of drug abuse. *Surg Gynecol Obstet* 1974; 139:749.

57. Neviaser RJ, Butterfield WC, Wieche DR. The puffy hand of drug addiction. *J Bone Joint Surg Am* 1972; 54A:629.

58. Anderson CB. Mycotic aneurysms. In: Rutherford RB, ed. *Vascular Surgery.* 2nd ed. Philadelphia: Saunders; 1984.

59. Farooki MA. Aneurysms in the United States and the United Kingdom. *Int Surg* 1973; 58:475.

60. Anderson CB, Butcher HR, Ballinger WF. Mycotic aneurysms. *Arch Surg* 1974; 109:712.

61. Patel S, Johnston KW. Classification and management of mycotic aneurysms. *Surg Gynecol Obstet* 1977; 144:691.

62. Stengel A, Wolferth CC. Mycotic (bacterial) aneurysms of intravascular origin. *Arch Intern Med* 1923; 31:527.

63. Yellin AE. Ruptured mycotic aneurysm: a complication of parenteral drug abuse. *Arch Surg* 1977; 112:981.

64. Huebl HC, Read RC. Aneurysmal abscess. *Minn Med* 1966; 49:11.

65. Anderson CB. Mycotic aneurysms. In: Rutherford RB, ed. *Vascular Surgery,* 2nd ed. Philadelphia: Saunders; 1984.

66. Feliciano DV, Mattox KL. Traumatic aneurysms. In: Rutherford RB, ed. *Vascular Surgery.* 2nd ed. Philadelphia: Saunders; 1984.

67. Rich NM, Hobson RW II, Collins GJ Jr. Traumatic arteriovenous fistulas and false aneurysms: a review of 558 lesions. *Surgery* 1975; 78:817.

68. Rich NM, Hobson RW II, Fedde CW. Vascular trauma secondary to diagnostic and therapeutic procedures. *Am J Surg* 1973; 126:639.

69. Mumenthaler M, Narakas A, Gilliatt RW. Brachial plexus disorders. In: Dyck PJ, Thomas PK, Lambert EH, Bunge R, eds. *Peripheral Neuropathy.* 2nd ed. Philadelphia: Saunders; 1984:1383.

70. Ilfeld F, Holder H. Winged scapula. Case occurring in soldier from knapsack. *JAMA* 1942; 120:448.

71. Daube JR. Rucksack paralysis. *JAMA* 1969; 208:2447.

72. Kraft GH. Rucksack paralysis and brachial neuritis. *JAMA* 1970; 211:300.

73. Molnar W, Paul DJ. Complications of axillary arteriotomies. An analysis of 1762 consecutive studies. *Radiology* 1972; 104:269.

74. Salam AA. Brachial plexus paralysis: an unusual complication of anticoagulant therapy. *Am Surg* 1972; 38:454.

75. Dhumer KG. Nerve injuries following operations: a survey of cases occurring during a six year period. *Anesthesiology* 1950; 11:289.

76. Dornette WHL. Compression neuropathies: medical aspects and legal implications. In: Hindman BJ, ed. *International Anesthesiology Clinics.* Vol. 24. Boston: Little, Brown; 1986.

77. Challenor Y, Richter RW, Brunn B, Pearson J. Nontraumatic plexitis and heroin addiction. *JAMA* 1973; 225:958.

78. Kori SH, Foley KM, Posner JB. Brachial plexus lesions in patients with cancer: 100 cases. *Neurology (NY)* 1981; 31:45.

79. Thomas JE, Colby MY Jr. Radiation-induced or metastatic brachial plexopathy? *JAMA* 1972; 22:1392.

80. DeSouza FM, Smith PE, Molony TJ. Management of brachial plexus tumors. *J Otolaryngol* 1979; 8:537.

81. Osguthorpe JD, Handler SD, Canalis RF. Neurilemoma of the brachial plexus. *Arch Otolaryngol* 1979; 105:296.

82. Geiger LR, Mancall EL, Penn AS, Tucker SH. Familial neuralgic amytrophy. *Brain* 1974; 97:87.

83. Dunn HG, Daube JR, Gomey MA. Heredofamilial brachial plexus neuropathy (hereditary neuralgia amytrophy with brachial predilection) in childhood. *Dev Med Child Neurol* 1978; 20:28.

84. Jacob JC, Andermann F, Robb JP. Heredofamilial neuritis with brachial predilection. *Neurology* 1961; 11:1025.

85. Windebank AJ. Inherited recurrent focal neuropathies. In: Dyck PJ, Thomas PK, Lambert EH, Bunge R, eds. *Peripheral Neuropathy.* 2nd ed. Philadelphia: Saunders; 1984:1656.

86. Taylor RA. Heredofamilial mononeuritis multiplex with brachial predilection. *Brain* 1960; 83:113.

87. Ungley CC. Recurrent polyneuritis in pregnancy and the puerperium affecting three members of a family. *J Neurol Psychopathol* 1933; 14:15.

88. Asbury AK, Arnason BGW, Adams RD. The inflammatory lesion in acute idiopathic polyneuritis. *Medicine* 1969; 48:173.

89. Adams RD, Victor M. Diseases of peripheral nerve and muscle. In: Adams RD, Victor M, eds. *Principles of Neurology.* 3rd ed. New York: McGraw-Hill; 1986:960–1006.

90. Brady RO. Fabry disease. In: Dyck PJ, Thomas PK, Lambert EH, and Bunge R, eds. *Peripheral Neuropathy.* 2nd ed. Philadelphia: Saunders; 1984:1717.

91. Brady RO, Gal AE, Bradley RM, Martensson E, Warshaw AL, Laster L. Enzymatic defect in Fabry's disease: ceramide trihexosidase deficiency. *N Engl J Med* 1967; 276:1163.

92. Imperial R, Helwig EB. Angiokeratoma, a clinical pathological study. *Arch Dermatol* 1967; 95:166.

93. Cable WJL, Kolodny EH, Adams RD. Fabry's disease: clinical demonstration of impaired autonomic function. *Neurology* 1982; 32:498.

94. Dawson DM, Krarup C. Perioperative nerve lesions. *Arch Neurol* December 1989; 46(12):1355–1360.

95. Halter SK, DeLisa JA, Stolov WC, Scardapane D, Sherrard DJ. Carpal tunnel syndrome in chronic renal dialysis patients. *Muscle Nerve* 1980; 3:438.

96. Potts G, Shahani BT, Young RR. A study of the coincidence of carpal tunnel syndrome and generalized peripheral neuropathy. *Muscle Nerve* 1980; 3:440.

97. Cho DS, Cho MJ. The electrodiagnosis of the carpal tunnel syndrome. *S D J Med* July 1989; 42(7):5–8.

98. Stewart JD, Aguayo AJ. Compression and entrapment neuropathies. In: Dyck PJ, Thomas PK, Lambert EH, Bunge R, eds. *Peripheral Neuropathy,* 2nd ed. Philadelphia: Saunders; 1984:1435.

99. Feindel W, Stratford J. The role of the cubital tunnel in tardy ulnar palsy. *Can J Surg* 1958; 1:287.

100. Brown WF, Yates SK, Fergusen GG. Cubital tunnel and ulnar neuropathy. *Ann Neurol* 1980; 7:289.

101. Payan J. Cubital tunnel syndrome. *Br Med J* 1979; 2:868.

102. Dornette WHL. Compression neuropathies: medical aspects and legal implications. In: Hindman BJ, ed. *International Anesthesiology Clinics.* Vol. 24. Boston: Little, Brown; 1986.

103. Uriburu IJF, Morchio FJ, Marin JC. Compression syndrome of the deep motor branch of the ulnar nerve (pisohamate hiatus syndrome). *J Bone Surg Am* 1976; 58A:145.

104. Trojaborg W. Rate of recovery in motor and sensory fibers of the radial nerve: clinical and electrophysiological aspects. *J. Neurol Neurosurg Psychiatry* 1970; 33:625.

105. Spinner RJ, Bachman JW, Amadio PC. The many faces of carpal tunnel syndrome. *Mayo Clin Proc* July 1989; 64(7):829–836.

106. Toranto IR. Aneurysm of the median artery causing recurrent carpal tunnel syndrome and anatomic review. *Plast Reconstr Surg* September 1989; 84(3):510–512.

107. Gelberman RH, Aronson D, Weisman MH. Carpal tunnel syndrome. *J Bone Joint Surg Am* 1980; 62:1181.

108. Stewart JD, Eisen A. Tinel's sign and the carpal tunnel syndrome. *Br Med J* 1978; 2:1125.

109. Kopell HP, Thompson WAL. Pronator syndrome. A confined case and its diagnosis. *N Engl J Med* 1958; 259:713.

110. Morris HH, Peters BH. Pronator syndrome: clinical and electrophysiological features in seven cases. *J Neurol Neurosurg Psychiatry* 1976; 39:461.

111. O'Brien MD, Upton ARM. Anterior interosseous nerve syndrome. A case report with neurophysiological investigation. *J Neurol Neurosurg Psychiatry* 1972; 35:531.

112. Schmidt H, Eiken O. The anterior interosseous nerve syndrome. *Scand J Plast Reconstr Surg* 1971; 5:53.

113. Rengachary SS, Neff JP, Singer PA, Brackett CE. Suprascapular entrapment neuropathy: a clinical, anatomical and comparative study. *Neurosurgery* 1979; 5:441.

114. Clein LJ. Suprascapular entrapment neuropathy. *J Neurosurg* 1975; 43:337.

115. Bastron JA, Thomas JE. Diabetic polyradiculopathy. *Mayo Clin Proc* 1981; 56:725.

116. Hopper CL, Baker JB. Bilateral femoral neuropathy complicating vaginal hysterectomy. *Obstet Gynecol* 1968; 32:543.

117. Mukherjee SK. Iliacus haematoma. *J Bone Joint Surg Br* 1971; 53B:729.

118. Warfield CW. Meralgia paresthetica: causes and cures. *Hosp Pract Off* 1986; 21:40A.

119. Jefferson D, Eames RA. Subclinical entrapment of the lateral femoral cutaneous nerve: an autopsy study. *Muscle Nerve* 1979; 2:145.

120. Rousseau JJ, Reznik M, Le Jeune GN, Franck G. Sciatic nerve entrapment by pentazocine-induced muscle fibrosis. *Arch Neurol* 1979; 36:723.

121. Baker GS, Parsons WR, Welch JS. Endometriosis within the sheath of the sciatic nerve. *J Neurosurg* 1966; 25:652.

122. Pace JB, Nagel D. Piriform syndrome. *West J Med* 1976; 124:435.

123. Adams JA. The piriformis syndrome—report of four cases and review of the literature. *S Afr J Surg* 1980; 18:13.

124. Sandhu HS, Sandhey BS. Occupational compression of the common peroneal nerve at the neck of the fibula. *Aust N A J Surg* 1976; 46:160.

125. Nagler SH, Rangell L. Peroneal palsy caused by crossing the legs. *JAMA* 1947; 133:755.

126. Edwards WG, Lincoln CR, Bassett FH, Goldner JL. The tarsal tunnel syndrome. Diagnosis and treatment. *JAMA* 1969; 207:716.

127. Lloyd K, Agarwal A. Tarsal tunnel syndrome, a presenting feature of rheumatoid arthritis. *Br Med J* 1970; 3:32.

128. Pringle RM, Protheroe K, Mukherjee SK. Entrapment neuropathy of the sural nerve. *J Bone Joint Surg Br* 1974; 56:465.

129. Bastron JA. Neuropathy in diseases of the thyroid and pituitary glands. In: Dyck PJ, Thomas PK, Lambert EH, Bunge R, eds. *Peripheral Neuropathy.* 2nd ed. Philadelphia: Saunders; 1984:1834.

130. Hurwitz LJ, McCormick D, Allen IV. Reduced muscle alpha-glucosidase (acid-maltase) activity in hypothyroid myopathy. *Lancet* 1970; 1:67.

131. Sheaff HM. Hereditary myokymia: syndrome or disease entity associated with hypoglycemia and disturbed thyroid function. *Arch Neurol Psychiatry* 1952; 68:236.

132. Bastron JA. Neuropathy in diseases of the thyroid and pituitary glands. In: Dyck PJ, Thomas PK, Lambert EH, Bunge R, eds. *Peripheral Neuropathy.* 2nd ed. Philadelphia: Saunders; 1984:1841–1842.

133. Oldberg S. The carpal tunnel syndrome and acromegaly. *Acta Soc Med Ups* 1971; 76:179.

134. Melliere D, Ben Yahia NE, Etienne G, Becquemin JP, de Labareyre H. Thoracic outlet syndrome caused by tumor of the first rib. *J Vasc Surg* August 1991; 14(2):235–240.

135. Winsor T, Winsor D, Mikail A, Sibley A. Thoracic outlet syndromes—application of microcirculation techniques and clinical review. *Angiology* September 1989; 40(9):773–782.

136. Etheredge S, Wilbur B, Storey RJ. Thoracic outlet syndrome. *Am J Surg* 1979; 138:175.

137. Karas SE. Thoracic outlet syndrome. *Clin Sports Med* April 1990; 9(2):297–310.

138. Roos DB. New concepts of thoracic outlet syndrome that explain etiology, symptoms, diagnosis and treatment. *Vasc Surg* 1979; 13:313.

139. Roos DB. Congenital anomalies associated with thoracic outlet syndrome—anatomy, symptoms, diagnosis and treatment. *Am J Surg* 1976; 132:771.

140. Sanders RJ, Haug C. Subclavian vein obstruction and thoracic outlet syndrome: a review of etiology and management. *Ann Vasc Surg* July 1990; 4(4):397–410.

141. Cuetter AC, Bartoszek DM. The thoracic outlet syndrome: controversies, overdiagnosis, overtreatment, and recommendations for management. *Muscle Nerve* May 1989; 12(5):410–419.

142. Urschel HC, Razzuk MA. Management of the thoracic outlet syndrome. *N Engl J Med* 1972; 286:1140.

143. Cherington M. Ulnar conduction velocity in thoracic outlet syndrome. *N Engl J Med* 1976; 294:1185.

144. Brackman R. Cervical spondylotic myelopathy. In: Krayenbuhl, ed. *Advances and Technical Standard in Neurosurgery*. Vol. 6. New York: Springer-Verlag; 1979:137.

145. Bullard DE. Cervical disc lesions. In: Sabiston DC Jr, ed. *Textbook of Surgery: The Biological Basis of Modern Surgical Practice*. 13th ed. Philadelphia: Saunders; 1986:1399.

146. Mumenthaler M, Narakas A, Gilliat RW. Brachial plexus disorders. In: Dyck PJ, Thomas PK, Lambert EH, Bunge R, eds. *Peripheral Neuropathy*. 2nd ed. Philadelphia: Saunders; 1984:1392–1394.

147. Tsairis P, Dyck PJ, Mulder DW. Natural history of brachial plexus neuropathy: report on 99 patients. *Arch Neurol* 1973; 27:109.

148. Waxman SG. The flexion–adduction sign in neuralgia amyotrophy. *Neurology* (Minneapolis) 1979; 29:1301.

149. Flaggman PD, Kelly JJ Jr. Brachial plexus neuropathy. An electrophysiologic evaluation. *Arch Neurol* 1980; 37:160.

150. Igbal A, Arnason BGW. Neuropathy of serum sickness. In: Dyck PJ, Thomas PK, Lambert EH, Bunge R, eds. *Peripheral Neuropathy*. 2nd ed. Philadelphia: Saunders; 1984:2044–2049.

151. Miller HG, Stanton JB. Neurological sequelae of prophylactic inoculation. *Q J Med* 1954; 23:1.

152. Tsairis P, Dyck PJ, Mulder DW. Natural history of brachial plexus neuropathy: report on 99 patients. *Arch Neurol* 1972; 27:109.

153. Conn DL, Dyck PJ. Angiopathic neuropathy in connective tissue diseases. In: Dyck PJ, Thomas PK, Lambert EH, Bunge R, eds. *Peripheral Neuropathy*. 2nd ed. Philadelphia: Saunders; 1984:2027.

154. Irby R, Adams RA, Toone EC Jr. Peripheral neuritis associated with rheumatoid arthritis. *Arthritis Rheum* 1958; 1:44.

155. Dyck PJ, Conn DL, Okazak H. Necrotizing angiopathic neuropathy: three-dimensional morphology of fiber degeneration related to sites of occluded vessels. *Mayo Clin Proc* 1972; 47:461.

156. Lewis DC. Systemic lupus and polyneuropathy. *Arch Intern Med* 1965; 116:518.

157. Warrell DA, Godfrey S, Olsen EGJ. Giant-cell arteritis with peripheral neuropathy. *Lancet* 1968; 1:1010.

158. Ridley A. Porphyric neuropathy. In: Dyck PJ, Thomas PK, Lambert EH, Bunge R, eds. *Peripheral Neuropathy*. 2nd ed. Philadelphia: Saunders; 1984:1704.

159. Hierons R. Acute intermittent porphyria. *Postgrad Med J* 1967; 43:605.

160. Ridley A, Hierons R, Cavanagh JB. Tachycardia and the neuropathy of porphyria. *Lancet* 1968; 2:708.

161. Becker DM, Kramer S. The neurological manifestations of porphyria: a review. *Medicine (Baltimore)* 1977; 56:411.

162. Ridley A. The neuropathy of acute intermittent porphyria. *Q J Med* 1969; 38(151):307.

163. Mustajaki P, Seppalairen AM. Neuropathy in latent hereditary hepatic porphyria. *Br Med J* 1975; 2:310.

164. Asbury AK. Hepatic neuropathy. In: Dyck PJ, Thomas PK, Lambert EH, Bunge R, eds. *Peripheral Neuropathy*. 2nd ed. Philadelphia: Saunders; 1984:1826.

165. Dayan AD, Williams R. Demyelinating peripheral neuropathy and liver diseases. *Lancet* 1967; 2:133.

166. Knill-Jones RP, Goodwill CJ, Dayan AS, Williams R. Peripheral neuropathy in chronic liver disease: clinical electrodiagnostic, and nerve biopsy findings. *J Neurol Neurosurg Psychiatry* 1972; 35:22.

167. Phough JC, Ayerle RS. The Guillian-Barré syndrome associated with acute hepatitis. *N Engl J Med* 1953; 247:61.

168. Niermeijer P, Gips CH. Guillian-Barré syndrome in acute HBS Ag-positive hepatitis. *Br Med J* 1975; 4:732.

169. Thomas PK, Walker JG. Xanthomatous neuropathy in primary biliary cirrhosis. *Brain* 1965; 8:1079.

170. Gammon GD, Burge FW, King G. Neural toxicity in tuberculous patients treated with isoniazid (isonicotinic acid hydrazide). *Arch Neurol Psychiatry* 1953; 70:64.

171. Hughes HB, Biehl JP, Jones AP, Schmidt LH. Metabolism of isoniazid in man as related to the occurrence of peripheral neuritis. *Am Rev Tuberc* 1954; 70:266.

172. Biehl JP, Vilter RW. The effect of isoniazid on vitamin B_6 metabolism and its possible significance in producing isoniazid neuritis. *Proc Soc Exp Biol Med* 1954; 85:389.

173. Raskin NH, Fishman RA. Pyridoxine-deficiency neuropathy due to hydralazine. *N Eng J Med* 1965; 273:1182.

173a. Victor M, Laureno R. Neurologic complications of alcohol abuse: epidemiologic aspects. *Adv Neurol* 1978; 19:603–617.

174. Thomas PK. Clinical features and differential diagnosis. In: Dyck PJ, Thomas PK, Lambert EH, Bunge R, eds. *Peripheral Neuropathy*. 2nd ed. Philadelphia: Saunders; 1984:1169.

175. Adams RD, Victor M. Diseases of the peripheral nerves. In Adams RD, Victor M: *Principles of Neurology*. 3rd ed. New York: McGraw-Hill; 1985:960.

176. O'Hare JA, Warfield CA. The diabetic neuropathies. *Hosp Pract* November 1984; 19(11):41–52.

177. Ellenberg M. Diabetic neuropathy. In: Ellenberg M, Rifkin H, eds. *Diabetes Mellitus: Theory and Practice*. 3rd ed. New Hyde Park, New York: Medical Examination Pub; 1983:777–862.

178. Pirart J. Diabetes mellitus and its degenerative complications: a prospective study of 4,400 patients observed between 1947 and 1973. *Diabetes Care* 1978; 1:168, 252.

179. Pirart J. Diabetes mellitus and its degenerative complications: *Diabetes Care* 1978; 1:168.
180. Root HF, Pate WH, Frehner H. Triopathy of diabetes. Sequence of diabetes, retinopathy and nephropathy in one hundred and fifty-five patients. *Arch Intern Med* 1954; 94:931.
181. Ellenberg M. Diabetic neuropathy: a consideration of factors in onset. *Ann Intern Med* 1960; 52:1067.
182. Brown MJ, Martin JR, Asbury AK. Painful diabetic neuropathy: a morphometric study. *Arch Neurol* 1976; 33:164.
183. Archer A, Watkins PJ, Thomas PK, Sharma AK, Payan J. The natural history of acute painful neuropathy in diabetes mellitus. *J Neurol Neurosurg Psychiatry* 1983; 46:491.
184. Sinha S, Municheodappa CS, Koyak GP. Neuroarthropathy (Charcot's joints) in diabetes mellitus. Clinical study of 101 cases. *Medicine (Baltimore)* 1972; 51:191.
185. Clarke BF, Ewing DJ, Campbell IW. Diabetic autonomic neuropathy. *Diabetologia* 1979; 17:195.
186. Garland H, Taverner D. Diabetic myelopathy. *Br Med J* 1953; 1:1045.
187. Garland H. Diabetic amyotrophy. *Br Med J* 1955; 2:1287.
188. Robson JS. Uraemic neuropathy. In: Robertson RF, ed. *Symposium: Some Aspects of Neurology.* Edinburgh: Royal College of Physicians of Edinburgh; 1968:74.
189. Bolton CF. *N Engl Med* 1980; 302:755. Letter to the editor.
190. Asbury AK. Uremic neuropathy. In: Dyck PJ, Thomas PK, Lambert EH, Bunge R, eds. *Peripheral Neuropathy.* 2nd ed. Philadelphia: Saunders; 1984:1811–1825.
191. Scribner BH. Discussion. *Trans Am Soc Artif Intern Organs* 1965; 11:29.
192. Nielsen VK. The peripheral nerve function in chronic renal failure, I: clinical signs and symptom. *Acta Med Scand* 1971; 190:105.
193. Ekbom KA. Restless leg syndrome. *Neurology* (Minneapolis) 1960; 10:868.
194. Hartfall SJ, Garland HG, Goldie W. Gold treatment of arthritis. A review of 900 cases. *Lancet* 1937; 2:838.
195. Katrak SM, Pollack M, O'Brien CP, et al. Clinical and morphological features of gold neuropathy. *Brain* 1980; 103:671.
196. Wijesekera JC, Critchley EMR, Fahim Y, Lynch PG, Wright JS. Peripheral neuropathy due to perhexiline maleate. *J Neurol Sci* 1980; 46:303.
197. Casey EB, Jelliffe AM, Le Quesne PM, Millett YL. Vincristine neuropathy: clinical and electrophysiological observations. *Brain* 1973; 96:69.
198. Shelanski ML, Wisniewski H. Neurofibrillary degeneration induced by vincristine therapy. *Arch Neurol* 1969; 20:199.
199. Ellis FG. Acute polyneuritis after nitrofurantoin therapy. *Lancet* 1962; 2:1136.
200. Collins H. Polyneuritis associated with nitrofurantoin therapy. *Arch Neurol* 1960; 3:656.
201. Moddel G, Bilbao JM, Payne D, Ashby D. Disulfiram neuropathy. *Arch Neurol* 1978; 35:658.
202. Rainey JM. Disulfiram toxicity and carbon disulfide poisoning. *Am J Psychiatry* 1977; 134:371.
203. Denny-Brown D. Primary sensory neuropathy with muscular changes associated with carcinoma. *J Neurol Neurosurg Psychiatry* 1948; 11:73.
204. Lennox B, Prichard S. Association of bronchial carcinoma and peripheral neuritis. *Q J Med* 1950; 19:97.
205. Morton DL, Itabashi HH, Grimes DF. Nonmetastatic neurological complications of bronchogenic carcinoma. The carcinomatous neuromyopathies. *J Thorac Cardiovasc Surg* 1967; 51:14.
206. Croft PB, Urich H, Wilkinson M. Peripheral neuropathy of sensorimotor type associated with malignant disease. *Brain* 1967; 90:31.
207. Hunder GG, Disney TF, Ward LE. Polymyalgia rheumatica. *Mayo Clin Proc* 1969; 44:849.
208. Chuang TY, Hunder GG, Ilstrup DM, Jurland LT. Polymyalgia rheumatica. A ten-year epidemiologic and clinical study. *Ann Intern Med* 1982; 97:672.
209. Hunder GG, Allen GL. Giant cell arteritis: a review. *Bull Rheum Dis* 1978–1979; 29:980.
210. Hunder GG, Disney TF, Ward LE. Polymyalgia rheumatica. *Mayo Clin Proc* 1969; 44:849.
211. Papaioannou CC, Gupta RC, Hunder GG, McDuffie FC. Circulating immune complexes in giant cell arteritis/polymyalgia rheumatica. *Arthritis Rheum* 1980; 23:1021.
212. Hunder GG, Disney TF, Ward LE. Polymyalgia rheumatica. *Mayo Clin Proc* 1969; 44:849.
213. Fernandez-Herlihy L. Polymyalgia rheumatica. *Semin Arthritis Rheum* 1971; 1:236.
214. Fauchald P, Rygvold O, Oystese B. Temporal arteritis and polymyalgia rheumatica: clinical and biopsy findings. *Ann Intern Med* 1972; 77:845.
215. Wright V. Psoriatic arthritis. In: Kelly W, Harris E, Ruddy S, et al, eds. *Textbook of Rheumatology.* Philadelphia: Saunders; 1985:1021–1031.
216. Wright V. Psoriatic arthritis. In: Kelly W, Harris E, Ruddy S, et al, eds. *Textbook of Rheumatology.* Philadelphia: Saunders; 1985:1021–1031.
217. Calin A. Reiter's syndrome. In: Kelly W, Harris E, Ruddy S, et al, eds. *Textbook of Rheumatology.* Philadelphia: Saunders; 1985:1007–1020.
218. Calin A. Reiter's syndrome. In: Kelly W, Harris E, Ruddy S, et al, eds. *Textbook of Rheumatology.* Philadelphia: Saunders; 1985:1007–1020.
219. Kelly WN. Gout and related disorders of purine metabolism. In: Kelly W, Harris E, Ruddy S, et al, eds. *Textbook of Rheumatology.* Philadelphia: Saunders; 1985:1359–1398.
220. Kelly WN. Gout and related disorders of purine metabolism. In: Kelly W, Harris E, Ruddy S, et al, eds. *Textbook of Rheumatology.* Philadelphia: Saunders; 1985:1359–1398.
221. Kelly W, Harris E, Ruddy S, et al. Gout and related disorders of purine metabolism. In: Kelly W, et al, eds. *Textbook of Rheumatology.* Philadelphia: Saunders; 1985:1359–1398.
222. Howell DS. Diseases due to the deposition of calcium pyrophosphate and hydroxyapatite. In: Kelly W, Harris E, Ruddy S, et al, eds. *Textbook of Rheumatology.* Philadelphia: Saunders; 1985:1398–1416.
223. Howell DS. Diseases due to the deposition of calcium pyrophosphate and hydroxyapatite. In: Kelly W, Harris E, Ruddy S, et al, eds. *Textbook of Rheumatology.* Philadelphia: Saunders; 1985:1398–1416.
224. Howell DS. Diseases due to the deposition of calcium pyrophosphate and hydroxyapatite. In: Kelly W, Harris E, Ruddy S, et al, eds. *Textbook of Rheumatology.* Philadelphia: Saunders; 1985:1398–1416.

225. Brandt KD. Pathogenesis of osteoarthritis. In: Kelly W, Harris E, Ruddy S, et al, eds. *Textbook of Rheumatology.* Philadelphia: Saunders; 1985:1417–1431.

226. Brandt KD. Osteoarthritis: clinical patterns and pathology. In: Kelly W, Harris E, Ruddy S, et al, eds. *Textbook of Rheumatology.* Philadelphia: Saunders; 1985:1432–1458.

227. Brandt KD. Osteoarthritis: clinical patterns and pathology. In: Kelly W, Harris E, Ruddy S, et al, eds. *Textbook of Rheumatology.* Philadelphia: Saunders; 1985:1432–1458.

228. Decker JL, et al. Rheumatoid arthritis: Evolving concepts of pathogenesis and treatment. *Ann Intern Med* 1984; 101;810.

229. Harris ED. Rheumatoid arthritis: the clinical spectrum. In: Kelly W, Harris E, Ruddy S, et al, eds. *Textbook of Rheumatology.* Philadelphia: Saunders; 1985:915–950.

230. Gerr F, Letz R, Landrigan PJ. Upper-extremity musculoskeletal disorders of occupational origin. *Annu Rev Public Health* 1991; 12:543–566.

231. Knighton ES, Dumke PR. *Pain.* Boston: Little, Brown; 1966.

232. Mense S, Schmidt RF. Muscle pain: which receptors are responsible for the transmission of noxious stimuli? In: Clifford Rose F, ed. *Physiological Aspects of Clinical Neurology.* Oxford: Blackwell Scientific Publications; 1977:265–278.

233. Kumazawa T, Mizumara K. Thin fibre receptors responding to mechanical chemical and thermal stimulation in the skeletal muscle of the dog. *J Physiol* 1977; 273: 179–194.

234. Mense S. Reduction of the bradykinin induced activation of feline Group III and IV muscle receptors by acetylsalicylic acid. *J Physiol* 1982; 376:269–283.

235. Layzer RB, Rowland LP. Cramps. *New Engl J Med* 1971; 285:31–40.

236. Penn AS. Myoglobin and myoglobinuria. In: Vynken PJ, Bruhn GW, eds. *Handbook of Clinical Neurology.* Holland: Elsevier; 1980.

237. Demos MA, Gitlin EL, Kagen LJ. Exercise myoglobinuria and acute exertional rhabdomyolysis. *Arch Int Med* 1974; 134:669–673.

238. Edwards RHT, Wiles CM, Mills KR. Quantitation of human muscle function. In: Dyck P, Thomas PK, Lambert EH, eds. *Peripheral Neuropathy.* Philadelphia: Saunders; 1985.

239. Mills KR, Newham DJ, Edwards RHT. Force, contraction frequency and energy metabolism as determinants of ischemic muscle pain. *Pain* 1982; 14:149–154.

240. Abraham WM. Factors in delayed muscle soreness. *Med Sci Sports* 1977; 9:11–26.

241. Newham DJ, Mills KR, McPhail G, Edwards RHT. Muscle damage following eccentric contractions. *Eur J Clin Invest* 1982; 12:29.

242. Moersch FP, Woltman HW. Progressive fluctuating muscular rigidity ("stiff-man syndrome"): report of a case and some observations in 13 other cases. *Mayo Clinic Proc* 1956; 31:421.

243. Valli G, Barbrieri S, Stefano C, et al. Syndromes of abnormal muscular activity: overlap between continuous muscle fiber activity and the stiff-man syndrome. *J Neurol Neurosurg Psychiatry* 1983; 46:241.

244. Isaacs H. A syndrome of continuous muscle fiber activity. *J Neurol Neurosurg Psychiatry* 1961; 24:319–325.

245. Lane RJ, Mastaglia FL. Drug-induced myopathies in man. *Lancet* 1978; 2:562–566.

246. Bohan A, Peter JB. Polymyositis and dermatomyositis. *N Engl J Med* 1975; 292:344, 1227.

247. Whitaker JN. Inflammatory myopathy: a review of etiologic and pathogenetic factors. *Muscle Nerve* 1982; 5:573.

248. Bohan A, Peter JB. Polymyositis and dermatomyositis. *N Engl J Med* 1975; 292:344.

249. Riddoch J, Morgan-Hughes JA. Prognosis in adult polymyositis. *J Neurol Sci* 1975; 26:71–80.

250. Keil H. The manifestations in the skin and mucous membranes in dermatomyositis with special reference to the differential diagnosis from systemic lupus erythematosus. *Ann Intern Med* 1975; 16:828.

251. Bohan A, Peter JB, Bowman RL, Pearson CM. A computer assisted analysis of 153 patients with polymyositis and dermatomyositis. *Medicine* 1977; 56:255.

252. Bitnum S, Daeschner CW, Travis LB, Dodge WF, Hopps HC. Dermatomyositis. *J Pediatr* 1964; 64:101.

253. Buchthal F, Pinelli P. Muscle action potentials in polymyositis. *Neurology* 1953; 3:424.

254. Bohan A, Peter JB, Bowman RL, Pearson CM. A computer assisted analysis of 153 patients with polymyositis and dermatomyositis. *Medicine* 1977; 56:255.

255. Gould SE. *Trichinosis in Man and Animals.* Springfield, IL: Charles C. Thomas; 1970.

256. Gross B, Ochoa J. Trichinosis: a clinical report and histochemistry of muscle. *Muscle Nerve* 1979; 2:394.

257. Adams RD, Victor M. Polymyositis and other acute and subacute myopathic paralyses. In: Adams RD, Victor M, eds. *Principles of Neurology.* 3rd ed. New York: McGraw-Hill; 1965.

258. Layzer RB, Shearn MA, Satya-Murti S. Eosinophilic polymyositis. *Ann Neurol* 1977; 1:65.

259. Stark RJ. Eosinophilic polymyositis. *Arch Neurol* 1979; 36:721.

CHAPTER 15

Foot Pain

René Cailliet

The painful foot is amenable to accurate diagnosis because every joint, nerve, ligament, blood vessel, and tendon is palpable or visible.[1] The history often is specific, and the examination, therefore, can focus on the precise anatomic site and confirm the particular tissue injured that is producing the pain.

The ankle also is amenable to proper diagnosis but to a lesser degree. This is unfortunate because ankle injuries of soft tissue (ligaments and joint capsules) may be overlooked and minimized, leading to less than optimal treatment.

ANKLE JOINT INJURIES

The ankle joint refers specifically to the talotibial joint. The talus articulates primarily on the tibia in a mortice formed by the malleoli of the tibia medially and fibula laterally.[2] Movement of the ankle is principally plantar flexion and dorsiflexion because the talus moves on a hinge. There is limited motion in the lateral or rotatory direction of the talus in the mortice, except when the foot is markedly plantar flexed. At this point, the narrow width of the talus is in the ankle mortice, and the ankle can move in a lateral or medial direction.

The tissues that restrict lateral–medial motion are the ankle ligaments. There are two major groups of ligaments. The medial group is composed of the deltoid ligaments; the lateral group includes the anterior and posterior talofibular ligaments and the calcaneofibular ligaments (Fig. 15-1). The medial ligaments rarely are injured because they radiate equally around a central axis of attachment. The lateral ligaments are unequal, eccentric, and subject to injury.

The most common injury is caused by an inversion with the foot plantar flexed; this results in a ligamentous sprain.[3,4] The force of the inversion determines the seriousness of the injury. The least severe is a sprain. In this type of injury, the ligaments are overstretched but not disrupted or torn. (A *sprain*, by orthopedic definition, suggests damage to a muscle or tendon. A moderate sprain results from a small partial tear that causes increased laxity. A severe sprain results from a complete or larger partial tear.)

Symptoms

The history usually reveals an episode of trauma during which the ankle joint was forced beyond its normal range of motion. Pain and swelling are the major complaints.

Examination

Tenderness can be elicited over the affected ligament, and swelling usually is present with or without ecchymosis. Comparing the involved ankle with the opposite normal ankle, the degree of inversion can be measured, and the degree of pain elicited by this maneuver can be observed.

In addition to testing inversion, a so-called drawer sign always is tested. The foot is anterior–posterior sheared or translated against the fixed lower leg with the foot at a 90° angle. Excessive movement indicates a severe or moderate sprain of the talocalcaneal ligament.

Tenderness over the medial or lateral malleolus may signify a fracture or avulsion of the bone from the ligamentous insertion. X-rays are indicated.

In a severe injury, the malleoli may be separated if the interosseous ligament is torn. This can be diagnosed by inversion stress x-rays that reveal a widened mortice and/or a talar tilt. An increased talar tilt also may indicate tearing of the lateral or medial ligaments.

Treatment

This depends on the severity of the injury. A mild sprain may respond well to immediate elevation, compression dressing, ice packs, and avoidance of weight bearing and walking. As soon as tolerated, the ankle can be put through gentle active (not passive) range-of-motion exercises. Weight bearing should be allowed using crutches with the ankle taped or wrapped with an elastic bandage to keep it in a neutral dorsiplantar flexion and slightly everted. In 10 to 14 days, normal walking can be anticipated.

Moderate sprains are treated similarly except that active range-of-motion exercises should be delayed for 1 week and the ankle taped or bandaged for 2 to 4 weeks. If any question arises that the sprain may be more severe, a walking cast may be applied for 10 to 14 days.

Severe sprains associated with an avulsion fracture should be treated with a cast applied with compression as soon as the edema permits. If a cast is applied early and then becomes loose in 1 to 3 days, a snugger cast should be applied. With no avulsion but with ligamentous tearing, casting for 4 weeks may stabilize the ankle. Open reduction is advocated by some and refuted by others in favor of casting. Any of these sprains will benefit from the administration of oral nonsteroidal anti-inflammatory drugs.

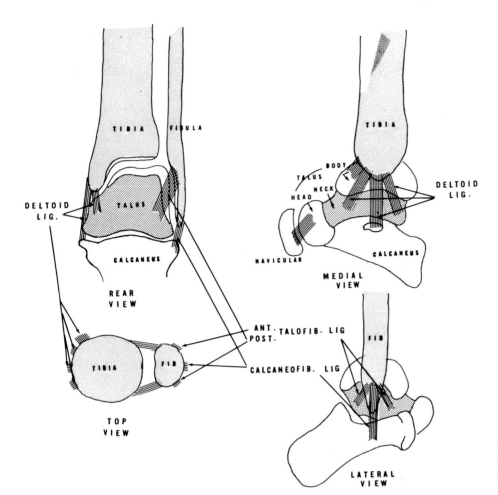

FIGURE 15-1. Ligaments of the ankle. (From Cailliet R. *Foot and Ankle Pain.* Philadelphia: Davis; 1968.)

After the ankle ligaments have healed (as determined by manual testing for stability, loss of edema, and minimal or no pain), rehabilitation can be started. Rehabilitation attempts to strengthen the ankle muscles (that is, the anticus, peronei, posterior tibialis, and gastrocsoleus) and improve proprioception by balancing exercises. The so-called weak ankle is an ankle whose ligaments have sustained a moderate or severe ligamentous sprain, has been treated inadequately, and has excessive laxity and impaired proprioception.[5]

FOOT PAIN

Hind Foot

The hind foot is the weight-bearing portion or the talocalcaneal portion of the foot. The common sites of pain are: (1) the Achilles tendon, (2) the bursal area behind the tendon, (3) the bursa between the tibia and the Achilles tendon, (4) the bottom of the calcaneus, (5) the anterior portion of the calcaneus (the so-called spur area), and (6) the talocalcaneal joint (Fig. 15-2).

Achilles Tendon Injuries

As in any tendon, the injury can be mild, moderate, or severe. It can be a result of chronic stress from running or jumping or acute stress from a direct blow.

Examination. There is tenderness and possibly thickening of the tendon. With the patient kneeling and observed from behind with their feet over the edge of the table, the degree of dorsiflexion is noted. This tests the range of motion of the ankle and the resilience of the Achilles tendon.

A mild sprain will not allow excessive dorsiflexion; there is tenderness of the tendon and pain on stretching. A moderate sprain allows greater dorsiflexion. A severe sprain allows excessive motion compared with the other normal side; often, a tear of the tendon is palpable and retraction of the gastrocsoleus muscle gives a "bunched-up" appearance.

Treatment. A mild sprain usually responds to ice packs, minimizing walking, and avoiding stretching and high-heeled shoes for 7 to 10 days. Administration of oral anti-inflammatory medication is valuable. A slight elevation of the heel also is useful.

A moderate sprain is treated similarly but for a longer period. Avoidance of stretching, such as occurs in exercise, jumping, or running is stressed.

A severe sprain with partial or complete tearing of the tendon is a more controversial treatment problem with regard to early surgical repair versus casting in a full plantar flexed position. Both have their proponents, and both are effective. The important aspect of a complete tear of the Achilles tendon is that it must receive prompt acute care and

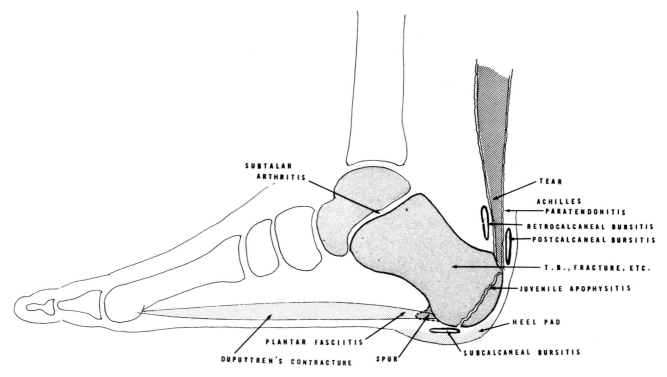

FIGURE 15-2. Common sites of foot pain. (From Cailliet R. *Foot and Ankle Pain.* Philadelphia: Davis; 1968.)

a follow-up rehabilitation program to elongate the gastroc-soleus Achilles complex gradually and strengthen the muscle.

Achilles Tendon Bursitis

Bursitis may occur behind the Achilles tendon under the skin. The most common cause of inflammation is trauma from improper shoe wear (e.g., a high inflexible shoe counter).

Symptoms. Pain, inflammation, and swelling superficially at the level of the shoe counter are the major complaints.

Treatment. The treatment is to remove or modify the offending shoe surface. Apply ice for 1 to 2 days. Then, apply heat. The condition usually is self-limited with no sequelae.

Subtendon Achilles Bursitis

Symptoms and Findings. Pain is most marked on walking or standing up on the toes. Tenderness can be elicited by digital pressure between the tendon and the tibia just above the superior aspect of the calcaneus. Swelling between the tendon and the tibia also occurs.

Treatment. Local heat, rest, and anti-inflammatory oral medication usually suffice. Occasionally, in a persistent inflammation, local injections of an anesthetic agent and a soluble corticosteroid are indicated.

The Heel Spur

This is a condition that causes pain in the anterior–inferior aspect of the calcaneus at the site of attachment of the plantar fascia. The usual initial cause of pain is a traction injury of the plantar fascia with a resultant myofascial periosteal irritation. The fascia pulls the periosteum to which it is attached away from the underlying bone. At first, there is probably tendinitis that then evolves into a tendinitis–periostitis.

There are many causes,[6] such as excessive running or walking, prolonged unaccustomed standing, and gaining excessive weight. Generally, this condition occurs in a person with a pronated foot in which all the stated activities flatten the longitudinal arch, placing a traction strain on the plantar fascia.

Symptoms. Pain while walking or standing is localized by the patient to the sole of the foot three-fourths of the way posteriorly. There is deep tenderness on pressure in the region of the anterior border of the calcaneus. Dorsiflexion of the toes may elicit the pain. X-rays initially do not reveal any disease because the injury is to the soft tissue, but ultimately, the site of traction fills with inflammatory tissue that calcifies to form a spur (an exostosis). The exostosis is not considered the source of the pain, but it is a late sequela of tendoperiosteal traction.

Treatment. Asking a patient to refrain from walking and standing and administering oral anti-inflammatory medication may suffice, but usually an injection of a corticosteroid and local anesthetic directly into the tender area is required. The injection site, carefully localized by deep pressure, is usually at the bony periosteal region. The needle is advanced until contact with the bone is made, then it is withdrawn 1/15 to 1/8 in, and the solution is injected (Fig. 15-3).

A severely or even moderately pronated foot that imposes traction on the plantar facia should be corrected by a proper orthosis and gait correction. The painful heel spur that does not respond to simple conservative measures may benefit from neurotomy of the medial calcaneal nerve,[7] a sensory branch of the posterior tibial nerve. Removal of the exostosis usually is ineffective. In addition, it may produce other problems.

The Bottom of the Calcaneus

A pad usually covers the calcaneus. This cushions the heel during walking and bears weight during standing. In a person whose activities demand frequent heel striking or who has excessive weight impressed on the heel, the bone under the pad becomes inflamed. Some people have a congenitally inadequate heel pad.

Symptoms. Localized pain and tenderness occur around the weight-bearing aspect of the calcaneus. A thin heel pad may be discerned.

Treatment. Rest and administration of anti-inflammatory medication during the acute phase are indicated.

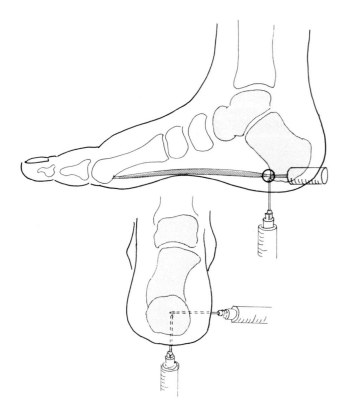

FIGURE 15-3. Injection of heel spur. (From Cailliet R. *Foot and Ankle Pain.* Philadelphia: Davis; 1968.)

Subsequently, insertion of a spongy cushion pad usually is effective, together with weight reduction and proper gait training.

Talocalcaneal Arthralgia

The articulation of the hind foot between the talus and the calcaneus permits limited movement by virtue of the incongruous joint surfaces and the talocalcaneal ligament located in the tarsal tunnel. In a pronated foot with a valgus heel, there may be excessive valgus stress on the tendon and the joint articular surfaces. Prolonged bed rest from a disabling disease or a neuromuscular disease that alters the gait pattern may predispose the joint to excessive stress by causing ligamentous laxity. Systemic collagen disease also may affect this joint.

Symptoms. Pain commonly occurs in the region of the talocalcaneal joint during walking. Passive mobilization of the calcaneus on the talus with the talus locked in the ankle mortice by placing the foot in the dorsiflexed position causes pain. The tarsal tunnel opening is palpable directly under and anterior to the fibular malleolus when the foot is markedly inverted and plantar flexed.

Treatment. An orthosis to prevent heel valgus is indicated. Gait training is valuable. An anti-inflammatory medicine regimen also may be helpful. When these measures fail, an injection of a corticosteroid–local anesthetic solution into the tarsal tunnel to the calcaneotarsal ligament may be useful.

A 1.5 in 20-gauge needle is inserted into the tarsal tunnel of the inverted supinated foot just anterior and inferior to the fibular malleolus. The needle is directed posteriorly and medially to a depth of 1 to 1.5 in. There should be no bony contact if the needle follows the tunnel. Immediate relief after injection of the anesthetic agent is diagnostic and therapeutic.

Midfoot: The Longitudinal Arch

Pronated Foot

The most prevalent painful foot disorder in humans is probably the pronated foot. The so-called flat foot deserves anatomic evaluation. The normal foot is considered to be a slightly supinated (inverted) foot, with a vertical heel and an adequate longitudinal arch. There also is adequate transverse tarsal and transverse metatarsal arches. The supinated foot results from all the articulating bones of the foot being closely packed, giving effortless pain-free support by virtue of the incongruity of the articulations. No capsular, ligamentous, tendinous, or muscular stress is needed to support weight bearing of the supinated inverted foot. Proper gait with this normal foot structure is efficient, nonstressful, and pain-free. However, the pronated foot may cause pain. In pronation, the foot has a valgus heel, everted (pronated) forefoot, and a depressed longitudinal arch. The forefoot (metatarsal bones) are splayed or broadened, and the metatarsal head arch is flattened. The weight-bearing surfaces of the foot during stance and gait are impaired.

Symptoms. Patients complain of aching and fatigue of the feet. The ache is vague, but it is located on the medial aspect of the arch. Walking is awkward, aching, and fatiguing. There is tenderness over the medial aspect of the ankle. The toes feel cramped in the average shoe.

Examination. The heel is in valgus. The foot is pronated, and the forefoot everted with a diminished longitudinal arch. The medial aspect of the midfoot appears closer to the floor. Frequently, there is tenderness over the middle three metatarsal heads. The heel also may be painful. Gait is more wide based with a turnout foot of 8° to 15°. There is no spring in the gait.

Treatment. The acute phase requires rest and anti-inflammatory medications, with the use of local ice packs and contrast baths (that is, alternating between cold baths and warm baths). Ultimately, weight loss and gait training must be instituted, and an orthosis prescribed. The appliance should be custom made with the foot casted in the supinated position. A positive cast is made on which the orthosis is molded.

The pronated foot also may place a strain on the posterior tibial tendon and/or the posterior tibial nerve.

Posterior Tibial Tendinitis

In a pronated foot, the posterior tibial tendon may become inflamed. It can be palpated and pain elicited immediately under and anterior to the medial malleolus. By placing the foot under stressed eversion and then resisting active plantar flexion with inversion, the tendon is stretched. This maneuver will reproduce the pain.

Treatment. The treatment is the same as in the pronated foot with the addition of injecting a corticosteroid–local anesthetic solution into the tendon sheath.

Posterior Tibial Neuritis: Tarsal Tunnel Syndrome

This painful condition is caused by inflammation from entrapment of the posterior tibial nerve under the flexor retinaculum at the medial malleolus.[8]

Symptoms. There are complaints of paresthesias or burning pain over the medial border of the foot in the dermatomal region of the posterior tibial nerve (Fig. 15-4).[9]

Findings. There may be hyperesthesia in the area innervated by the posterior tibial nerve and, ultimately, diminished sensory perception to light touch and pain. The nerve at the retinaculum may be thickened and tender.[10] A Tinel sign often can be seen by gently tapping over the nodular thickening and eliciting the paresthesias.

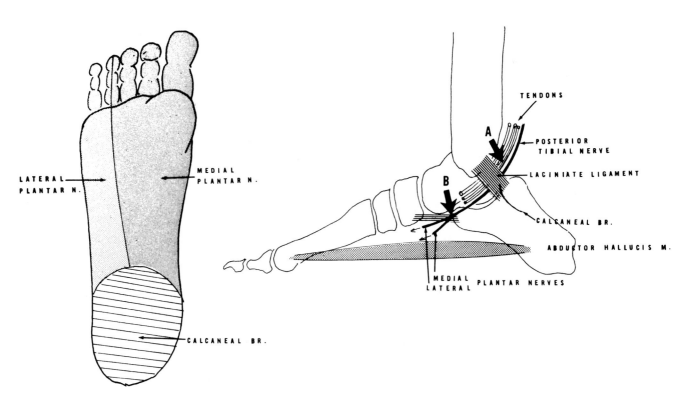

FIGURE 15-4. Sites of pain in tarsal tunnel syndrome. (From Cailliet R. *Foot and Ankle Pain.* Philadelphia: Davis; 1968.)

Painful Forefoot: Toes

The metatarsal bones or their heads can cause pain that can be diagnosed easily by manual palpation and observation.

Metatarsalgia

The patient may complain of pain of the middle metatarsal heads (the second, third, and fourth predominantly). This is termed *metatarsalgia* (that is, pain attributed specifically to the metatarsal heads). The interdigital nerves and interdigital bursas also may cause pain in the same region and must be considered in the differential diagnosis.

Symptoms. The pain is felt by the patient over the balls of the toes predominantly over the middle metatarsal heads. The discomfort has been described as feeling like a stone in the shoe.

Examination. The metatarsal heads are tender on their plantar surfaces. Tenderness may be elicited by the examiner grasping the metatarsal heads separately between the thumb and finger. Pressure is not exerted between the heads because this is where the interdigital nerve and bursa lie. The pronated foot with a splayed broadened forefoot is the most likely to develop metatarsalgia.

Treatment. Pressure on the metatarsal head must be removed or modified. Metatarsal pads should be placed behind (not under) the middle metatarsal heads to elevate the metatarsi and restore the arch (Fig. 15-5).[11] The pronation of the foot also should be corrected with a fitted orthosis, including a metatarsal pad, and gait correction.

Interdigital Bursitis

Between the metatarsal heads are bursas in the compartment that includes the interdigital nerve.

Symptoms. The pain is localized to the metatarsal head region between the heads. It often is produced by weight bearing and/or walking, especially while wearing narrow shoes.

Findings. Digital pressure between the metatarsal heads produces pain and tenderness. Neuritic pain may be elicited in which paresthesias radiate into the phalanges. An injection of a corticosteroid and a local anesthetic agent with the needle inserted from the dorsum of the foot between the metatarsal head is diagnostic and may be therapeutic.

Treatment. General care is indicated, and the treatment is similar to that for metatarsalgia. In addition to pads, an orthosis, oral anti-inflammatory medication, and injection of an anesthetic agent and a corticosteroid into the bursal area may be needed.

Morton Neuroma

This neuroma essentially is an interdigital neuritis or compression neuropathy. The pain is burning, dysesthetic, and

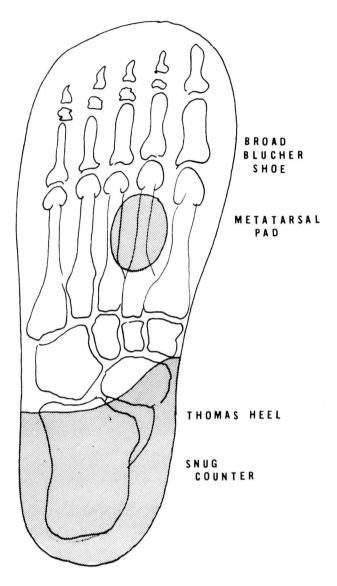

FIGURE 15-5. Correct placement of metatarsal pads. (From Cailliet R. *Foot and Ankle Pain.* Philadelphia: Davis; 1968.)

often accompanied by paresthesias under the metatarsal head region and into the involved toes (usually between the third and fourth or fourth and fifth toes, Fig. 15-6). Paresthesias of the proximal phalanges of the toes also may occur. Patients often claim that removing their shoes relieves the symptoms. This condition frequently occurs in pre- or menopausal women for no known reason.

Diagnosis. The pain may be elicited by pressure of the examiner's thumb and index finger between the metatarsal heads. There may be hypalgesia or hypesthesia of the proximal phalanges of the two toes involved. An interdigital injection of a local anesthetic agent and a soluble corticosteroid relieves symptoms and often is both diagnostic and therapeutic. Proper padding and orthosis is indicated as in treatment of a pronated foot. If there is persistence of pain and/or paresthesias, surgical resection of the neuroma of the

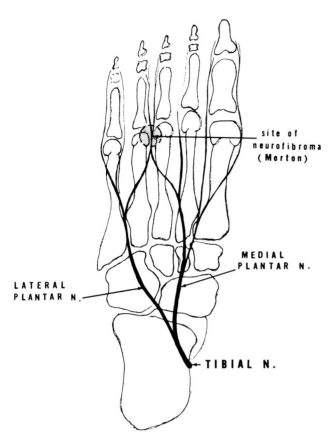

FIGURE 15-6. Common site of Morton neuroma. (From Cailliet R. *Foot and Ankle Pain.* Philadelphia: Davis; 1968.)

interdigital nerve is warranted. Even after surgery, all the conservative techniques should be instituted.

Pain in the Great Toe

The great toe, the hallux, has two bases for pain: (1) hallux valgus with or without a bunion or (2) hallux rigidus.

Hallux Valgus. In this condition, the big toe deviates laterally (into valgus) to compensate for the internal deviation of the first metatarsal bone (metatarsus varus, Fig. 15-7). There are numerous causes postulated for this condition. The patient with a painful hallux valgus has pain, swelling, and tenderness of the joint at the base of the big toe, the articulation of the first metatarsal, and the proximal phalanx. Pain occurs during walking at the toe-off position after the stance phase of gait that dorsiflexes the big toe 60° to 80°. This dorsiflexion occurs 800 to 900 times per mile of walking. Tight shoes, narrow shoes, and high heels promote the pain.

Examination. The forefoot is splayed and the big toe deviates laterally to form an acute angle of the metacarpal–proximal phalangeal joint. There is swelling of the joint with redness and tenderness. Passive and active motion of the joint is painful.

Treatment. Rest, with an anti-inflammatory drug regimen, aborts the acute phase. In the subacute phase, a

chronic recurrent condition, a proper shoe is mandatory to ensure spreading of the forefoot. An orthosis also may be valuable. Intraarticular injection of an anesthetic agent and a soluble corticosteroid into the metacarpal phalangeal joint also is effective. Persistent intractable pain may necessitate surgical intervention. These procedures are numerous, each with its specific indication, benefit, and prognosis.

Hallux Rigidis. Degenerative arthritis of the first metatarsal–proximal phalangeal joint may cause gradual painful ankylosis of the joint. Initially, the painful limited movement of the first metatarsal phalangeal joint is termed hallux limitus. After there is no more movement, there usually is no additional pain, but until ankylosis is complete, pain occurs with any activity that flexes or extends the joint.

Diagnosis. There is marked painful limited motion of the first metatarsal phalangeal joint, frequently with crepitation. X-rays reveal the joint disease.

Treatment. Local means similar to the treatment of hallux valgus are indicated. The shoe must be modified to permit a heel–toe gait without dorsiflexing the big toe. A steel shank in the sole of the shoe prevents flexibility. A rocker bottom is added to the shoe to facilitate gait while still immobilizing the toe. Local intraarticular injections of an anesthetic and corticosteroid may be of temporary value. Surgical intervention, including resection or total replace-

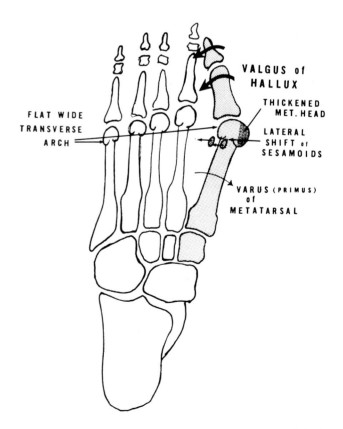

FIGURE 15-7. Hallux valgus. (From Cailliet R. *Foot and Ankle Pain.* Philadelphia: Davis; 1968.)

ment of the joint, may be necessary when the pain is intractable and disabling.

PAINFUL DERMATOLOGIC CONDITIONS OF THE FOOT

Many dermatologic diseases of the foot can be painful and disabling. The most common are corns, calluses, and warts.[12]

Plantar Corn

This usually is a hyperkeratotic area surrounded by callus overlying a bony prominence. Pain is elicited by direct or lateral pressure.

Treatment

The hyperkeratotic tissue can be pared or removed by application of a salicylic acid preparation. Protective padding must be applied, and the foot problem causing the initial pressure must be addressed.

Neurovascular Corn

These resemble warts but last longer and are very painful and tender. They frequently are under the first or fifth metatarsal heads.

Treatment

Paring usually is not effective and may be contraindicated because painful scarring may result. These corns are treated best by applying a 50% to 100% silver nitrate solution and/or a 40% salicyclic acid plaster. Radiation therapy using 10 gray also is therapeutic. Proper pad orthotic correction of the underlying bony prominence is mandatory. In a refractory case, the metatarsal head or its condyles may be resected.

Soft Corns

These usually are found in the interdigital web. Direct pressure on these palpable corns elicits pain. They are usually soft and soggy, hence the term *soft corn*.[13]

Treatment

Relief may be obtained by direct application of a salicylic acid plaster or paring. A pad between the toes to maintain separation is useful; proper shoes are recommended.

Plantar Warts

These may be: (1) single, (2) mother–daughter, or (3) mosaic. The single wart usually occurs under a bony prominence and is the direct result of trauma. Capillary tips often are visible. The mother–daughter types also occur over bony prominences. They are similar to the single wart, and the treatment is the same. The mosaic warts generally are not painful, and they are essentially an academic differentiation.

Treatment

All types of warts are radiation sensitive, but x-ray treatment recently has been condemned. They also can be removed by salicylate paste, cryotherapy, or electrosurgery. Subcuticular injection of an anesthetic agent under the wart that elevates it has been claimed to be remedial.

SUMMARY

In summary, painful conditions of the foot are common,[14] and correct treatment can be ensured easily with proper steps taken toward classification and accurate diagnosis.[15]

References

1. Rosse C, Clawson AK. *The Musculoskeletal System in Health and Disease.* Hagerstown, MD: Harper & Row; 1980.
2. Norkin C, Levangie P. *Joint Structure and Function: A Comprehensive Analysis.* Philadelphia: Davis; 1983.
3. Kulund DN. *The Injured Athlete.* Philadelphia: Lippincott; 1982.
4. Stern Sh. Ankle and foot pain. *Prim Care* December 1988; 15(4):809–826.
5. Cailliet R. *Foot and Ankle Pain.* 2nd ed. Philadelphia: Davis; 1983.
6. Davidson MR, Copoloff JA. Neuromas of the heel. *Clin Podiatr Med Surg* April 1990; 7(2):271–288.
7. Grimes DW, Garner RW. Medial calcaneal neurotomy for painful heel spurs: a preliminary report. *Orthop Rev* 1978; 7:57–58.
8. Lam SJS. A tarsal tunnel syndrome. *Lancet* December 1962:1354–1355.
9. Goodgold J, Kopell HP, Spielholtz HQ. Tarsal-tunnel syndrome: objective diagnostic criteria. *New Engl J Med* 1965; 273:742–745.
10. Keck C. Tarsal-tunnel syndrome. *J Bone Joint Surg* 1962; 44A:180–182.
11. Melgrane JE. Office measures for relief of the painful foot. *J Bone Joint Surg Am* 1964; 46A:1095–1116.
12. Jones FK, Masear VR. Painful syndromes of the foot: diagnosis and management. *Clin Plast Surg* July 1991; 18(3):639–648.
13. Montgomery RM. Dermatologic care of the painful foot. *J Bone Joint Surg* 1964; 46A:1129–1136.
14. Root ML, Oriew WP, Weed JH. Normal and abnormal function of the foot. *Clinical Biomechanics, V. II.* Los Angeles: Clinic Biomech Corp; 1977.
15. Silfverskiold JP. Common foot problems. Relieving the pain of bunions, keratoses, corns, and calluses. *Postgrad Med* April 1991; 89(5):183–188.

PART THREE

Common Painful Syndromes

CHAPTER 16

Sympathetic Dystrophies

Charles H. McLeskey, Francis J. Balestrieri, and Duke B. Weeks

The term *reflex sympathetic dystrophy* includes a range of seemingly unrelated disorders. It is an important clinical entity frequently seen by general practitioners, internists, surgeons, and anesthesiologists. Primarily, it is a neurovascular pain dysfunction complex, most commonly affecting the limbs.[1] If recognized during its early stages of development, it usually can be treated and cured. However, if misdiagnosed or if the treatment is improper or delayed, the condition may progress to a prolonged and sometimes permanent disability. Reflex sympathetic dystrophy represents the most important type of autonomic pain problems.

DEFINITION

In the past, reflex sympathetic dystropy has been described by many different names (Table 16-1). These terms indicate not only the widespread disturbances that may produce sympathetic dystrophy, but also the lack of agreement as to what constitutes the primary physiologic change. Classically, all these syndromes may be grouped under the term *reflex sympathetic dystrophy* because they appear to have the same underlying pathophysiologic mechanism and are similar in clinical manifestation and therapeutic response. Each disorder is a departure from the orderly and predictable response of an extremity to some form of internal or external trauma. This prompted Turf and Bacardi[2] to suggest a more general term, such as *atypical posttraumatic pain syndrome* because it encompasses different forms of disturbances with both distinctive and common clinical characteristics. Similarly, Roberts[3] suggested the use of a more general term, *sympathetically maintained pain*. However, all these related problems will be called *sympathetic dystrophies* in this chapter.

SYMPTOMS

The classic signs and symptoms of the sympathetic dystrophies are pain, hyperesthesia, and swelling in an extremity; trophic skin changes in the affected limb; and a history of a precipitating event that typically involves injury to a peripheral nerve. Perhaps the earliest described type of sympathetic dystrophy was causalgia. The term *causalgia* was introduced first in 1864 by S. Weir Mitchell[4] who described a pain syndrome in wounded soldiers during the Civil War. His classic description follows.

"The seat of burning pain is very various . . . its intensity varies from the most trivial burning to a state of torture, which hardly can be credited, but which reacts on the whole economy until the general health is seriously affected. The part itself is not alone subject to an intense burning sensation, but becomes exquisitely hyperaesthetic, so that a touch or tap of the fingers increases the pain. Exposure to the air is avoided by the patient with a care which seems absurd, and most of the bad cases keep the hand constantly wet, finding relief in the moisture rather than the coldness of the application" (p. 164).

Table 16-1
Terms Describing Conditions Similar to Reflex Sympathetic Dystrophy

Acute atrophy of bone	Posttraumatic sympathetic dysfunction
Causalgia-like states	Posttraumatic sympathetic dystrophy
Chronic segmental arterial spasm	Posttraumatic vasomotor disorders
Chronic traumatic edema	Reflex dystrophy
Homan minor causalgia	Reflex dystrophy of the extremities
Major causalgia	Reflex nervous dystrophy
Minor causalgia	Reflex trophoneurosis
Mitchell causalgia	Shoulder–hand syndrome
Painful osteoporosis	Sudeck syndrome
Peripheral trophoneurosis	Sympathalgia
Posttraumatic dystrophy	Sympathetic neurovascular dystrophy
Posttraumatic pain syndrome	Traumatic angiospasm
Posttraumatic painful osteoporosis	Traumatic edema
Posttraumatic spreading neuralgia	Traumatic neuralgia

As Mitchell noted, the first and most major manifestations of causalgia and the other sympathetic dystrophies are pain (usually of a severe burning nature), hyperalgesia and hyperesthesia, vasomotor and sudomotor disturbances, and skeletal muscle hypotonia. Pain, the most prominent and characteristic feature of the syndrome, is invariable, of a burning quality, and hyperpathic; it is characterized by a prolonged painful sensation after transient contact. The pain also may be described as tearing, throbbing, or aching. It varies in severity from mild discomfort to excruciating unbearable pain. It is usually continuous, but it has recurrent paroxysmal exacerbations provoked by various stimuli including movement, touch (hyperesthesia), pressure (allodynia), a dependent position, noises, breezes, vibrations, changes in temperature, anxiety, and emotional stress. The location of the pain usually is distal; gradually, it moves proximally. It is not limited to a peripheral nerve distribution or dermatome. Rather, the pain seems to be located in areas of the extremities with multiple dermatomes.[5] Hyperesthesia is the second most characteristic manifestation of this disorder. Light stroking or gentle touch of the involved area may elicit severe discomfort. Therefore, the patient postures the extremity to protect it from any contact and avoids moving the limb. An algometer may aid in quantifying the pain and pressure thresholds.[6] Vasomotor disturbances are manifested either by vasodilatation, in which the skin is warm and hyperemic, or more commonly later in the syndrome, by vasoconstriction, in which the skin is cool and there is cyanosis. Temperature differences between the affected and unaffected limbs may vary from 5°C to 10°C in early stages of the disorder. However, in the later stages of the disease process, there may be a similar response in the contralateral originally unaffected extremity, which acts in sympathy with the affected extremity.[7,8] Hyperhidrosis often is present distally in the affected limb, resulting in constant dampness of the skin. Edema also may be observed, and movement disorders have been described.[9] Later stages of the disorder are associated with skeletal changes, including contracture and osteoporosis.

LABORATORY FINDINGS

There is a conspicuous absence of abnormal laboratory findings in patients with sympathetic dystrophies. The best use of laboratory studies is to exclude other diseases. However, in more advanced stages of the disease, soft tissue edema and patchy osteoporosis may be observed radiographically. With fine-detail radiography, juxtaarticular osseous resorption of trabecular, subchondral, subperiosteal, and endosteal bone may be noticed.[10] Karasick and Karasick,[11] using radioisotope scanning, found an increased uptake of technetium-99m by affected juxtaarticular tissues in patients with sympathetic dystrophy. This radionuclide imaging on delayed bone scanning may be observed before pathologic findings are seen using plain-film radiography.[12,13] Specific scintigraphic criteria for diagnosing sympathetic dystrophies are developing. Three-phase radionuclide bone scanning after injection of technetium-99m has been shown to have a 96 percent sensitivity and a 97 percent specificity in diagnosing sympathetic dystrophy and a 99 percent predictability in excluding the diagnosis of sympathetic dystrophy.[14] Magnetic resonance imaging is not useful.[15]

Skin Temperature and Contact Thermography

Skin temperature, measured from the pulp of the digits of upper and lower extremities, provides a crude estimation of the severity of the disorder. Contact thermography is a precise technique that compares the affected and unaffected extremities.[16,17] The extremity is either sprayed with heat-sensitive crystals or is placed against a plate containing similar crystals; these change color in response to different temperatures (Fig. 16-1). Thus, a permanent photographic record of the skin temperature color pattern may be made

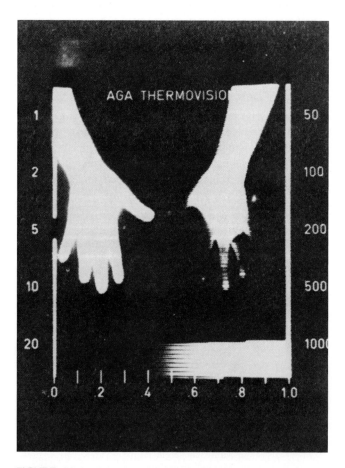

FIGURE 16-1. Thermogram of the hands of a patient with probable sympathetic dystrophy. Dark areas reveal reduced blood flow in the left hand, suggesting increased sympathetic activity. Thermography thus can be used to document cutaneous manifestations of this disorder. (Reproduced with permission from Cousins MJ, Bridenbaugh PO, eds. *Neural Blockade.* Philadelphia: Lippincott; 1980:712.)

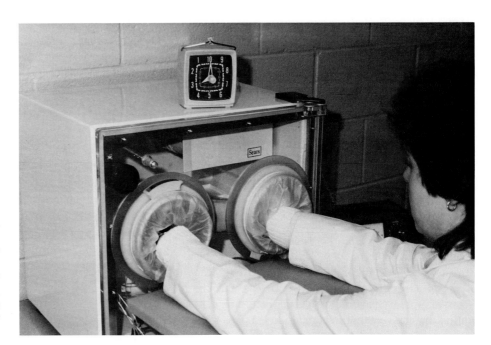

FIGURE 16-2. A modified refrigeration unit for the cold stress test. The ambient temperature inside the refrigeration unit can be varied. With the patient's upper or lower extremities placed inside the unit, digital pulp temperature recordings can be made that are affected by changes in ambient temperature.

and can be used to document the cutaneous manifestation of the disorder and the presence or absence of improvement after therapy.[19]

Cold Stress Test

In this test, the temperature of the skin pulp is measured continuously at all digits on both upper extremities. The hands are placed in a modified refrigerator unit, and control digital temperature measurements are made at room temperature (Fig. 16-2). The temperature of the dry air surrounding the hands in the modified refrigerator unit then is dropped to 10°C for approximately 20 min and subsequently returned to room temperature. A stylized temperature response is shown in Figure 16-3. The stippled area represents the change in ambient temperature in the refrigeration unit, the temperature to which the hands are exposed. The top temperature graph (X–X) shows the temperature change of a normal hand placed in this temporarily cooled environment. The bottom graph (□)–(□) demonstrates a classic pattern that might be observed in a patient with sympathetic dystrophy. Notice that typically the digital temperature of the involved extremity in an affected patient may be slightly lower than that of a normal patient and that the observed temperature fall is more exaggerated in this extremity compared with a normal extremity. In addition, the return of digital temperature toward normal after room temperature is reached in the ambient environment occurs more sluggishly in an affected patient compared with a normal subject. Frequently, the cooling and rewarming phases of ambient temperature cause patients to complain of pain in their affected extremities that is similar to that caused by their disorder.

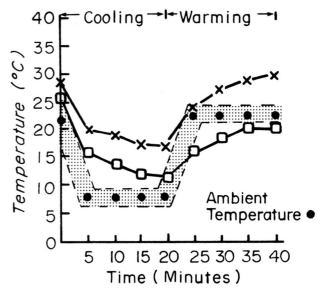

FIGURE 16-3. A stylized temperature response using the cold stress test. The stippled area represents the change in the ambient temperature in the refrigeration unit. The top graph (X–X) represents likely temperature changes in a normal hand when exposed to 20 min of a cooled ambient temperature. The bottom graph (□–□) shows a classic pattern observed in a patient with sympathetic dystrophy. Affected patients have lower digital pulp temperatures at normal ambient temperature, demonstrate a more exaggerated fall in digital pulp temperature during exposure to a cool ambient environment, and rewarm more sluggishly than normal after the return of the ambient environment to room temperature.[20]

Digital Plethysmography

Digital plethysmography and oscillometry permit the clinician to record a magnification of the peripheral pulse waves. We found this technique useful in showing an improvement in peripheral perfusion after a sympathetic block. Frequently, older patients with severe sympathetic hyperactivity who have preexisting peripheral vascular disease may require many minutes before temperature changes in the extremity are observed after a technically adequate sympathetic block is administered. As illustrated in Figure 16-4, plethysmography demonstrates dramatic and progressive changes in peripheral perfusion in a patient after a lumbar sympathetic block. Although no temperature change had occurred 5 min after the block, there was an obvious change observed using digital plethysmography. This is reassuring to the clinician because it demonstrates early the technical adequacy of the block. Also note that the progressive improvement in peripheral perfusion continued during the entire 60-min recording period.

Transcutaneous Oxygen Monitor

Sonneveld and colleagues[21] reported that an extremity with sympathetic dystrophy as a result of sympathetic hyperactivity and reduced peripheral perfusion may have a reduced transcutaneous oxygen content compared with the contralateral unaffected extremity. They also found that effective treatment to correct the sympathetic hyperactivity produces a gradual return of transcutaneous oxygen content in the affected extremity to the levels seen in the contralateral extremity.

STAGES OF DEVELOPMENT

Usually the early signs of reflex sympathetic dystrophy or causalgia occur within 2 or 3 days of the initial injury.

However, this is variable; in some patients, weeks to months may pass before the onset of the syndrome. Sympathetic dystrophy progresses through several identifiable stages of severity as differentiated by Bonica.[22]

Stage 1: The Acute Phase

During the first phase of the development of sympathetic dystrophy, signs of sympathetic denervation or underactivity may be observed. The resultant increase in perfusion of the extremity causes vasodilatation, hyperemia, hyperthermia, and anhidrosis of the extremity. As shown in Figure 16-5 (top), localized edema, dependent rubor, and increased growth of hair and nails also may be observed. The patient complains of burning pain in the extremity that may be constant. It is worsened by changes in environmental conditions and light touch, such as that produced by contact with bed sheets. As a result, the patient protects the extremity from motion and physical contact. The pain is out of all proportion to the severity of the antecedent injury. It is lessened by a quiet environment, sleep, and administration of narcotics.

Stage 2: The Dystrophic Phase

Approximately 2 to 3 months later, the vasoconstrictive stage usually occurs. In this stage, the symptoms are similar to the earlier stage, but the skin becomes pale, cyanotic, cold, sweaty, and frequently is mottled. Edema progresses from a soft to a brawny type with glazed tense overlying skin. As shown in Figure 16-5 (center) and Figure 16-6, cutaneous appendages of the extremity become scant and brittle. The nails become cracked with heavy grooves. Continued limited range of motion secondary to pain causes joint stiffening and contracture; muscular atrophy may develop (Fig. 16-7). Patchy osteoporosis (Sudeck atrophy) may be observed radiographically.[24]

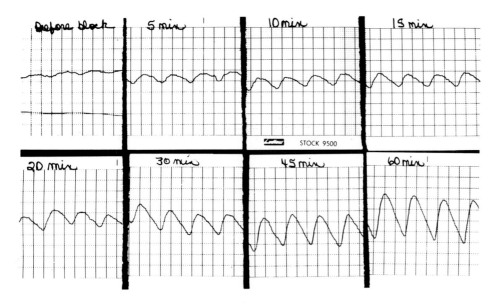

FIGURE 16-4. Digital plethysmography permits us to record the magnification of peripheral pulse waves. It is useful to document the paucity of peripheral perfusion under conditions of sympathetic dystrophy and indicate early improvement in flow after an effective sympathetic block is administered. This recording shows changes in a digital plethysmographic trace at intervals after a technically adequate lumbar sympathetic block in a 46-year-old patient with sympathetic dystrophy.

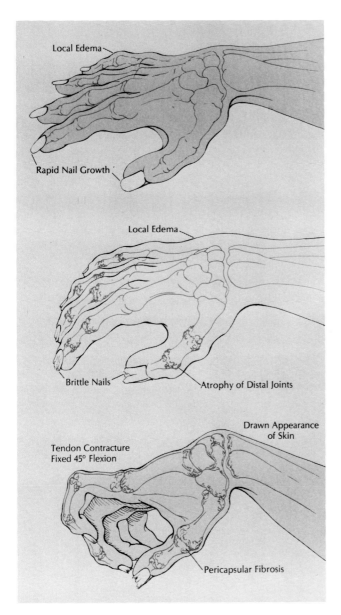

FIGURE 16-5. Classic stages of development of sympathetic dystrophy. The top frame depicts physical findings in the acute phase of sympathetic dystrophy with localized edema, hyperemia, dependent rubor, and increased growth of the hair and nails caused by underactivity of the sympathetic innervation to the affected extremity. The middle frame illustrates the second or dystrophic phase of sympathetic dystrophy; sympathetic hyperactivity is evidenced by pale cyanotic skin with underperfusion of the extremity, resulting in brittle nails and inadequate hair growth. The bottom frame depicts the late stage of sympathetic dystrophy, the atrophic stage. Contracture of the extremity is observed with muscular and bony atrophy. (Reproduced with permission from Warfield CA. The sympathetic dystrophies. *Hosp Pract Off* 1984; 19(5):52g. Illustration by Enid Hatton.)

Stage 3: The Atrophic Phase

During the subsequent months to years, the pain that originally was distal in location spreads proximally. In addition, central nervous system involvement may be shown by bilateral limb involvement[25] and symptoms of diffuse total

body sympathetic dystrophy.[26] Atrophic skin changes and loss of the fat pads of the digit occur; there is resorption of the extremity and the formation of slender narrowed digits (Fig. 16-5, bottom). Muscle wasting and contracture may become severe (Fig. 16-8). During the third stage, generalized systemic responses to this illness include malnutrition, disturbance of diurnal rhythms, and emotional fixation on the pain problem. The intractable pain eventually may cause mental deterioration, chronic invalidism, drug addiction, and possible suicide.[27,28]

INCITING EVENTS

In sympathetic dystrophy, the usual location of the pain is in a traumatized extremity, although symptoms can occur on the trunk,[29] face,[30] or penis.[31] The antecedent event that eventually causes the symptoms of sympathetic dystrophy is usually accidental or surgical trauma, resulting in a crush or laceration injury. The initial event frequently appears trivial in relation to the resulting symptoms. Usually partial nerve interruption is associated with the onset of the syndrome. Other less frequently associated inciting events include bursitis, myocardial ischemia and infarction, cerebrovascular and neurologic lesions,[32] partial spinal cord injuries,[33,34] vertebral crush fractures,[35] venipuncture,[36] and paraplegia or quadriplegia.[37] Other described precipitating factors include cervical osteoarthritis or spondylosis,[38] radiculopathy,[39] carcinoma (the paraneoplastic syndrome),[40,41] excision of impacted teeth,[42] herpes zoster infection,[29] surgery,[43] radiation therapy,[23] renal transplantation,[44] and barbiturate ingestion.[45] Subbarao and Stillwell[46] reported that, in approximately 10 percent of cases, no precipitating event can be identified.

INCIDENCE

In our experience, patients with sympathetic dystrophies may vary in age from their preteen-aged years to an elderly age. Subbarao and Stillwell[46] noticed a peak occurrence in the fifth decade of life. Ruggieri and colleagues[47] observed that it is uncommon to see patients with sympathetic dystrophies younger than 16 years of age.[48] In their large series of 500 cases, no patient was younger than 15 years of age. The disease in children seems to be self-limited and it responds more readily to conservative treatment than that in adults. Drucker and colleagues[49] showed that the disorder occurs more commonly in whites (Fig. 16-9). Women seem to be more predisposed than men; ratios of 2.9:1 frequently are observed.[46] Recent evidence indicates that cigarette smokers may be more likely to have this disorder.[51]

The percentage of patients with sympathetic dystrophy after an injury or accident varies widely from region to region and may have cultural implications. Reports show an incidence rate ranging from 0.05 percent to 15 percent of all trauma cases.[52,53] Why do some patients have sympathetic dystrophy although most who are injured similarly do not?

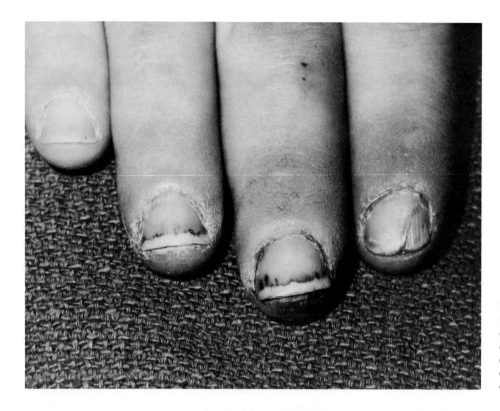

FIGURE 16-6. Close-up view of the hand of a patient in the early dystrophic phase of sympathetic dystrophy. The reduced perfusion of the extremity results in cutaneous changes and grooved and cracked nails.

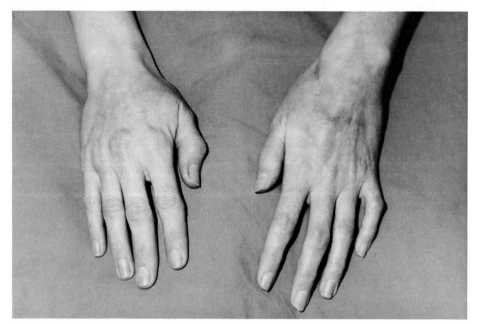

FIGURE 16-7. Observed changes in the affected left upper extremity of a patient during the dystrophic phase of sympathetic dystrophy. The skin of the left hand is shiny with loss of cutaneous appendages. Atrophy of the interosseous musculature has begun. Bony resorption probably would be seen radiographically.

Although psychologically normal patients can be affected, this disorder is seen more often in people with so-called inadequate personality types or those with neurotic tendencies.[54] Subbarao and Stillwell,[46] using the Minnesota Multiple Personality Inventory, found abnormal hysteria, hypochondriasis, and/or depression in 80 percent of 45 patients who had sympathetic dystrophy. Similarly, Bernstein and colleagues[55] found that most children with sympathetic dystrophies had psychological problems, such as overt parental conflict and difficulty expressing anger.

Owens[56] believed patients predisposed to sympathetic dystrophy tend to develop this disorder during times when their sympathetic nervous systems are hyperactive; these patients were called *sympathetic reactors*.

PATHOPHYSIOLOGY

There is no single encompassing pathophysiologic hypothesis that explains sympathetic dystrophies adequately. Most revolve around the notion of an abnormal reverbatory circuit at some level in the nervous system that contributes to a cycle of afferent sensory input and efferent sympathetic hyperactivity. Early explanations of this disorder included the suggestion that the sympathetic nerve fibers themselves transmitted pain impulses to the central nervous system.[57–59] Unfortunately, there is no uniform evidence that afferent fibers occur in sympathetic pathways from extremities.

Mitchell and associates[4] suggested that "irritation of a nerve may impair circulation and nutrition of parts, and these alterations might produce pain" (p. 164). Therefore, it was suggested that the pain and dystrophic changes are caused by alterations in peripheral blood flow resulting from sympathetic hyperactivity. However, plethysmography, oscillometry, and fluorescein injection studies actually show increases in limb blood flow in many affected patients.

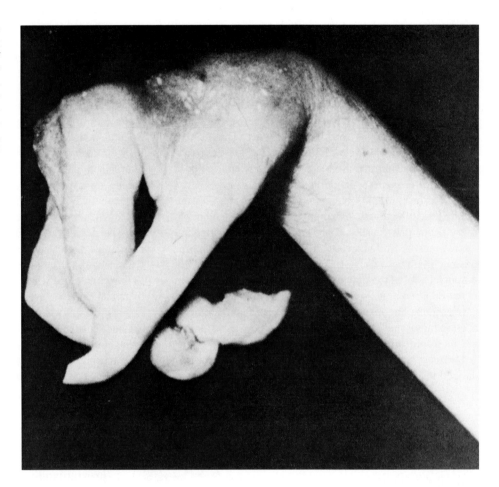

FIGURE 16-8. A classic example of the end result of sympathetic dystrophy. Notice the resorption of the extremity, producing slender shiny digits with marked contracture and total loss of use of the extremity. (Reproduced with permission from Cousins MJ, Bridenbaugh PO, eds. *Neural Blockade.* Philadelphia: Lippincott; 1980:710.)

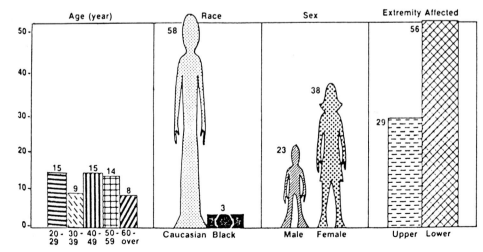

FIGURE 16-9. The epidemiology of sympathetic dystrophy. Patients with sympathetic dystrophy observed by Drucker and colleagues[49] ranged in age from 20 to 60 years or older. Most of those affected were white and female. Although somewhat controversial, in this series, the extremity most likely affected was the lower extremity. (Reproduced with permission from Malaments IB, Glick JB. Sudeck's atrophy—the clinical syndrome. *J Am Podiatry Assn* 1983; 73:363.)

Another hypothesis is that metabolic alterations in the extremity itself activate the autonomic nervous system, producing the characteristic symptoms. It is postulated that excitation of the efferent fibers releases a substance in the peripheral end organs that causes vasodilatation and subsequent sensitization of afferent neuronal pathways.[60] Similarly, as shown in Figure 16-10, after a nerve injury, substances that excite (bradykinin) or sensitize (prostaglandins) skin nociceptors are released in the skin; these enhance the nociceptive loop.[14]

Currently, more popular explanations for this sympathetically mediated syndrome include the idea postulated by Doupe and associates[61] in 1944 and illustrated in Figure 16-10. They proposed that, after a trauma such as a crush injury, there is a loss of myelin insulation around neural structures in the periphery that causes a short circuit in nerve conduction. The loss of neural insulation may create an artificial synapse or so-called ephapse between sensory afferents and efferent sympathetic impulses. Thus, direct cross-stimulation and cycle formation may cause exacerbation of pain during increased sympathetic activity, such as temperature changes or emotional fluctuations.

Livingston[62] in 1944 suggested that three factors were required for sympathetic dystrophy. First, trauma and nerve injury occur that cause chronic irritation of the peripheral sensory nerves and increase afferent traffic to the cord. Second, there is an abnormal state of activity in the internuncial pool of the gray matter of the cord, resulting from increased afferent neuronal traffic. Third, there is increased activity in the internuncial pool and increased stimulation of efferent motor and sympathetic nerves, producing irritation and increased afferent neuronal traffic.

Melzack,[63] cooriginator of the gate-control theory, claimed that changes in the afferent input to the brainstem reticular formation, the so-called central biasing mechanism, resulted in loss of normal inhibitory control over spontaneous sympathetic output at the cord level. This is an example of a centrally oriented hypothesis to explain sympathetic dystrophy in part. Under normal circumstances, the central biasing mechanism exerts a tonic inhibitory influence on neuronal synaptic transmission at all levels of the somatic projection system. A decrease in the inhibitory influence from the biasing mechanism of the reticular formation therefore could produce self-sustaining activity in the closed neuron loops at many spinal levels that is triggered repeatedly by noxious impulses from the site of injury. In part, this may explain how emotional stress can influence sympathetic dystrophy. An impaired inhibitory biasing mechanism produces hyperexcitable neural loops in the cord, which may explain why painful symptoms occur in contralateral extremities or even how a total body complaint of sympathetic dystrophy may follow a remote peripheral injury.

More recently, Roberts[3] suggested that sympathetically maintained pain is a result of tonic activity in mechanoreceptor afferents and that this activity is induced by sympathetic efferent stimulation of these sensory receptors. A possible chronologic development of sympathetic dystrophy is depicted in Figure 16-11. In Figure 16-11a, cutaneous trauma initially generates afferent traffic in the C-nociceptors that travels through the dorsal root ganglion to the spinal cord where it activates and sensitizes the wide dynamic range neurons whose axons subsequently send nociceptive information to higher centers. These neurons remain sensitized and respond to activity in the larger A-mechanoreceptors activated by light touch (Fig. 16-11b). This mechanism produces the condition of allodynia. The same sensitized neurons are hypothesized to transmit, not

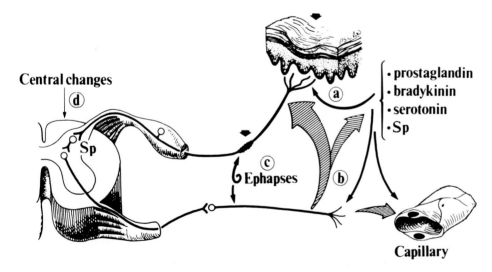

Central changes

(d)

Sp

(a)

· prostaglandin
· bradykinin
· serotonin
· Sp

(c)
Ephapses

(b)

Capillary

FIGURE 16-10. Hypotheses to explain the development of sympathetic dystrophy. A release of substances in the periphery may cause vasodilatation and/or sensitization of afferent neuronal pathways.[14] For example, bradykinin may excite and prostaglandins may sensitize skin nociceptors. Another hypothesis, described by Doupe and associates,[61] suggests that, after a crush injury, a loss of myelin insulation between the nerves creates an artificial neuronal synapse or ephapse. Direct cross-stimulation and cycle formation produces an exacerbation of pain any time increased sympathetic activity is observed. (Reproduced with permission from Holder LE, Mackinnon SE. Reflex sympathetic dystrophy in the hands: clinical and scintigraphic criteria. *Radiology* 1984; 152:522.)

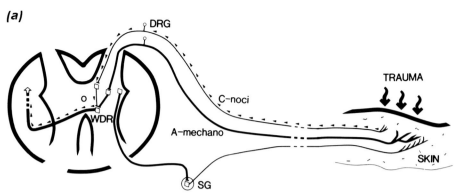

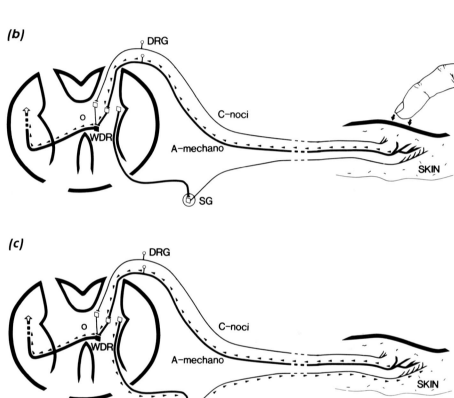

FIGURE 16-11. *Schematic diagram of a model explaining why light touch produces symptoms of severe pain. Chronologic development of this syndrome is depicted. In frame (a), cutaneous trauma generates afferent traffic in the C-nociceptors (C-noci) that travels through the dorsal root ganglion (DRG), enters the spinal cord, and activates and sensitizes the wide dynamic range neurons (WDR), the axons of which subsequently send painful information to higher centers. In frame (b), WDR neurons remain sensitized and respond to activity in larger A-mechanoreceptors (A-mechano) that is activated by light touch. In frame (c), the sensitized WDR neurons are hypothesized to initiate sympathetic efferent activity. This stimulates sensory receptors, inducing a reverberating pain pathway. (Reproduced with permission from Roberts WJ. Review article: A hypothesis on the physiological basis for causalgia and related pains. Pain 1986; 24:300.)*

only painful information to higher centers, but also to initiate the sympathetic efferent activity that may affect the sensory receptors further and induce a circuitous reverberating pain pathway (Fig. 16-11c).

As Schutzer and Gossling[64] have stated, "It appears reasonable to conclude, therefore, that the pathogenesis of reflex sympathetic dystrophy syndrome in any given patient may be related to both peripherally and centrally mediated factors, and this implies that a variety of treatment modalities may be effective."

TREATMENT

Mild cases of reflex sympathetic dystrophy often recover spontaneously or can be treated conservatively only. More

severe cases, however, are resistant to conservative measures and require more aggressive treatment.

Traditional Conservative Treatment Methods

Conservative treatment for sympathetic dystrophy includes administration of oral analgesics and physical therapy[65,66] that concentrates on active range-of-motion exercises. Although physical therapy and occupational therapy seem to be essential, used injudiciously they can exacerbate existing symptoms. Dependent posture must be avoided, and passive range-of-motion exercises may intensify the pain, swelling, and discomfort. It is important that these treatments be restrained but be instituted early after the disorder is recognized. In addition, other relatively conservative methods of treatment, including elevation, acupuncture, and the administration of tricyclic antidepressants, β-adrenergic blockers, and corticosteroids have been used with variable success.[5]

Propranolol in relatively high oral doses has been suggested for patients with reflex sympathetic dystrophy.[67] Although not used generally, this nonselective β-adrenergic blocker occasionally has produced favorable results.

Systemic corticosteroids, however, are used in many centers to treat this disorder. They may be effective if given in short bursts. Christensen and colleagues[68] reported 75 percent relief of pain in patients with reflex sympathetic dystrophy treated with prednisone 10 mg three times a day. These results were superior to those produced by placebo therapy. The corticosteroid was continued until optimal benefit occurred, up to a maximum of 12 weeks. Kozin and coworkers[69] suggest a higher dose range of prednisone 60 to 80 mg or its equivalent that is administered daily in four divided doses for 2 to 4 days. This dose then is tapered over the subsequent 10 to 14 days. Recently, Dirksen and colleagues[70] suggested administering steroids by the cervical epidural route in a fashion analogous to the perispinal route of administration of opioids. They believe that, by giving 60 mg of methylprednisolone acetate in 3 ml of NaCl 0.9%, the steroid is limited to the target organ and does not produce significant systemic effects. The mechanism of action of corticosteroids in the treatment of these disorders is unknown. However, a chronic perivascular inflammatory infiltration has been observed in synovial biopsy specimens from affected extremities.[69] Thus, the potent anti-inflammatory effect of prednisone and other steroids may explain their therapeutic action in affected patients.

Thermal biofeedback[71] and other behavioral approaches also have been valuable.[72]

Traditional Aggressive Treatment Methods

If conservative measures do not improve the symptoms rapidly, there should be no delay before initiating more definitive forms of therapy. More aggressive treatments for affected patients include the application of TENS and regional sympathetic blockade. The former uses an external battery power source to stimulate the painful area electrically. Melzak[73] speculated that TENS could activate transmission in both large and small fibers. He postulated that large fibers might influence and close the pain-control gates and help to abolish cycle activity from afferent noxious stimuli. This may produce definitive improvement in symptoms, but more commonly, it results in transient relief of the syndrome.[74,75] A major advantage of TENS is its apparent lack of morbidity,[76] although Abram[77] cautioned that some patients may have an increase in sympathetic activity when using this device. In more refractory cases, implanted peripheral nerve stimulation and spinal cord stimulation have been used.[78,79]

Currently, the most widely used method is regional sympathetic blockade. As discussed earlier, the sympathetic nervous system is involved intimately in the pathophysiology of sympathetic dystrophy. Thus, regional sympathetic blockade acts both diagnostically and therapeutically. If efferent sympathetic innervation to the involved extremity is interrupted, the cycle of sympathetic overactivity, peripheral ischemia, pain, and further sympathetic efferent response may be broken. Thus, symptomatic improvement may result. Patients who do not obtain pain relief after a technically successful sympathetic block probably should be tested for other medical problems.

Generally, sympathetic dystrophies affecting the upper extremity can be managed using a stellate ganglion block; interruption of sympathetic fibers to the lower extremity and pelvis may be done with a lumbar sympathetic block.

Stellate Ganglion Block

A stellate ganglion block usually is administered on an outpatient basis, using either lidocaine or bupivacaine hydrochloride to bathe the stellate ganglion at the level of C7 to T1 (see Appendix A.I). A technically successful stellate block in a patient with sympathetic dystrophy is manifested by a profound Horner syndrome, rapid onset of pain relief, and a warm dry upper extremity. We find it clinically useful to inject 10 to 20 ml of the local anesthetic with the patient in a semisitting position. Some recent data suggest the inclusion of narcotics in the injection solution, but controlled trials are lacking. With the patient in this position, the solution has a tendency to percolate caudad along the sympathetic chain, anesthetizing sympathetic fibers at the level of the T4 ganglion or below. It is important to anesthetize the nerve of Kuntz.[80] In approximately 10 percent to 20 percent of the population, this nerve is responsible for partial or complete sympathetic innervation to the upper extremity. Fibers in the nerve of Kuntz may originate from the upper thoracic segments and innervate the upper extremity without passing through the stellate ganglion.

In more refractory cases, a continuous block technique may be used to provide continuous sympathetic blockade. The technique of continuous stellate ganglion block, first developed by Betcher and associates[81] recently was revised by Linson and colleagues.[82] An 18-gauge, 15-cm Teflon catheter is inserted by the anterior approach under roentgenographic control to lie on the lateral portion of the anterior surface of the vertebral body of C7. Linson and colleagues[82] administered bupivacaine hydrochloride 0.5% every 8 h for an average of 7 days in hospitalized patients. Approximately one-half of these patients required catheter replacement in 2 to 4 days as a result of catheter migration. Using this aggressive treatment regimen, 27 of 29 patients improved. However, the relapse rate was 25 percent. During long-term follow-up, relief was maintained in only 4 of 29 patients.

Lumbar Sympathetic Block

Lumbar sympathetic block is administered with the patient in the prone position. A pillow or roll is placed under the patient's hips to remove much of the normal lumbar lordotic curve. Because the block is uncomfortable, especially if done repeatedly, sedative or analgesic medication may be administered. Before initiating the block, an intravenous line in inserted to produce adequate hydration in anticipation of subsequent sympathectomy. In addition, we prefer that patients receive nothing by mouth for 6 to 8 h before the block. The site of needle insertion varies from clinic to clinic. The classic three-needle technique using a paravertebral approach with needles inserted at approximately L2, L3, and L4 is described in Moore[83] and other texts of regional anesthesia. With this technique, the needle is advanced until the transverse process of the lumbar vertebra is contacted. At this point, the needle is redirected slightly to pass caudad to the edge of the transverse process and is advanced an additional 1¾ to 2 in until it slides past the vertebral body lying on its anterolateral aspect.

A second technique (and the one we prefer) uses only a single needle advanced at the level of L2 or L3 with the cutaneous insertion site approximately 8 to 10 cm from the midline (see Appendix A.II). With this single-needle technique, the transverse spinous process is not contacted. The needle is directed to contact the vertebral body and then slightly redirected to slide off and remain placed at its anterolateral aspect. This technique seems to be tolerated better by patients, first, because it is only a single needle, and second, because paresthesias are less likely to be produced when the needle approaches the vertebral body from a more lateral position. Initially, 3 to 5 ml of lidocaine 1% is injected as a test to exclude subarachnoid or epidural needle location. Subsequently, an additional 15 to 18 ml of bupivacaine 0.25% with 1:200,000 epinephrine then is injected. Fluoroscopy or cross-table lateral x-rays are useful to document the needle position. Frequently, within 1 to 2 min after injection of the test dose, the temperature of the patient's skin of the lower extremity on the blocked side increases. Sympathetic blocks may be repeated daily or less frequently as required. Generally, the response to a sympathetic block continues from a few hours to many days, and the response lasts progressively longer with subsequent injections. The duration of beneficial effect usually exceeds the duration of the local anesthetic-induced sympathetic nerve blockade. Block therapy may be discontinued when all pain and signs of dystrophy disappear. After the diagnosis has been made, epidural blockade has been used as an alternative to sympathetic block.[84]

Wang and coworkers[85] described a relatively aggressive treatment regimen for patients with lower extremity reflex sympathetic dystrophy. With their technique, lumbar sympathetic blocks are administered every day or every other day for four sessions. If no clinical improvement is observed, the blocks are terminated, but they may be continued until maximal improvement is reached. The same protocol is repeated if pain recurs at a later date. Permanent chemical sympathectomy or surgical sympathectomy alternatively may be recommended. Treated patients were surveyed (with pain levels assessed) 1 month, 6 months, and 3 years after the time of initial treatment. Of the 43 patients treated using this technique, 65 percent were improved at both the 6-month and 3-year evaluations. Seven patients required one additional series of lumbar sympathetic blocks, and four patients needed two additional series during the 3-year follow-up. Three of four patients in whom repeat blocks did not reproduce early signs of improvement and who agreed to undergo surgical sympathectomy also did not obtain long-term benefit. The authors concluded that approximately 65 percent of patients with lower extremity sympathetic dystrophy who receive treatment with lumbar sympathetic block within 12 months of the onset of their syndrome will derive some benefit as a result of this regimen.

Other centers advocate continuous sympathetic or epidural blockade,[86] but the benefit of these techniques over intermittent blockade remains to be proved.

If repeat sympathetic blockade produces complete but only temporary relief, chemical or surgical sympathectomy may be considered. Knowing when to recommend a chemical or surgical sympathectomy is always a clinical dilemma. DeTakats[52] suggested that as few as two successful temporary sympathetic blocks constitute an indication for permanent sympathectomy. However, some authors describe the use of a series of as many as 10 to 15 temporary blocks before trying other techniques.[38] A more commonly accepted practice is that, if a patient has a clinical response but requires more than four to five blocks, consideration should be given to permanent chemical or surgical sympathectomy.[87,88] In our opinion, a more conservative approach usually is preferable. Even if sympathetic blocks are not successful or remain successful only temporarily, other techniques are worth trying before surgical sympathectomy. The decision as to whether chemical or surgical sympathectomy should be recommended to a patient must be individualized on the basis of the patient's age, condition, and consent. Generally, it is accepted that sympathectomy does not guarantee a permanent solution to this disorder. It is less useful when temporary sympathetic blocks are ineffective.

New Treatment Methods

Traditional treatment methods, although frequently efficacious, may be unsuccessful and poorly tolerated by patients. For example, pediatric patients and certain adult populations will not accept repeat stellate ganglion or lumbar sympathetic blocks. As a result, the development of newer techniques to treat reflex sympathetic dystrophy that are better tolerated by the patient and have a higher success rate would be a meaningful contribution. Such new methods include the intravenous regional block (so-called Bier block) technique that uses reserpine or guanethidine and administering the systemic oral calcium-channel blocker, nifedipine.

Intravenous Regional Sympathetic Blocks

The technique of intravenous or intraarterial infusion of ganglionic blocking agents, either reserpine or guanethidine, into affected extremities recently gained prominence.[89–91] There are two reasons why intravenous administration is superior to an intraarterial injection for treatment of sympathetic dystrophy. First, the likelihood of systemic side effects from an injection of these vasodilating agents is significantly greater if administered intraarterially than if administered using an intravenous regional block (Bier block) technique. Second, when these drugs are administered by an intravenous regional anesthetic technique, they may have more protracted contract with the affected extremity; this may allow them to fix to the tissues and produce a more significant and prolonged improvement in symptoms.

Intravenous Regional Reserpine Block

Reserpine is thought to act on the sympathetic nervous system by reducing storage vessel reuptake of cathecholamines, thereby slowly depleting norepinephrine stores in sympathetic nerve endings. Benzon and associates[90] reported the successful treatment of patients with reflex sympathetic dystrophy using intravenous regional reserpine. Experience in the United States with this technique is controversial. Abram[92] and Brown[89] found the results of this technique to be sporadic; we were impressed favorably with the technique.[93] In a series of eight patients (age range, 14 to 57 years) with reflex sympathetic dystrophy of the upper extremity, partial or complete pain relief lasting at least 4 weeks was obtained in seven patients. Reserpine 1 mg was diluted in 40 ml of lidocaine hydrochloride 0.25% and then injected intravenously into an exsanguinated extremity; drug contact to the extremity was permitted for 30 to 45 min using tourniquet inflation (see Appendix A.IV). The side effects include burning pain on injection of the reserpine, postural hypotension lasting 12 to 24 h postblock, and facial flushing persisting 24 h or more postblock. Patient acceptance of repeat blocks is high; we believe that the longer the duration of cuff inflation, the less likely the patient is to have side effects after cuff deflation.

Intravenous Regional Guanethidine Block

In an attempt to improve the results and lessen the side effects during treatment of patients with reflex sympathetic dystrophy using intravenous regional sympathetic blocks, Hannington-Kiff[94] suggested substituting guanethidine for reserpine in the intravenous regional block format. Guanethidine appears to bind to sympathetic nervous tissue, displacing norepinephrine from presynaptic vesicles and preventing its reuptake; this explains its prolonged activity.[95] Complete sympathetic blockade for as long as 3 to 4 days can be achieved. Thomsen and colleagues[96] documented a 300 percent increase in total forearm blood flow after sympathetic blockade using intravenous guanethidine with changes lasting for 48 to 72 h.

The results from Europe and selected North American centers appear to be more consistent and more reliable than those with intravenous regional reserpine.[21,94,97] McKain and coworkers,[98] in a prospective randomized double-blind study, evaluated the sympatholytic effects of intravenous guanethidine and reserpine in asymptomatic volunteers. Guanethidine was better than reserpine in producing selective adrenergic blockade with resultant peripheral vasodilatation.

Our technique is similar to that used for intravenous regional reserpine except that, in place of reserpine, guanethidine 20 mg is diluted in 40 ml of lidocaine 0.25% for upper extremity blocks or 50 ml for lower extremity blocks (see Appendix A.IV). We recently reviewed our results after administering 140 intravenous regional guanethidine blocks in 79 patients (46 women and 33 men; age range, 13 to 60 years). We found partial or complete success in the treatment of painful symptoms in approximately two-thirds of these patients. Repeat block was required in 57 patients. The average duration of symptomatic improvement was 17 days; complete permanent relief of symptoms occurred in 12 patients. Other patients may have had continuous beneficial pain relief, but they were lost to follow-up.

In a prospective study, Driessen and coworkers[99] evaluated 20 patients with reflex sympathetic dystrophy treated similarly. They administered 20 mg of guanethidine diluted in 40 ml of lidocaine 0.25%; tourniquet inflation was maintained for 15 min. The blocks were repeated weekly as long as improvement continued and varied in number from one to eight blocks. They found overall good results in 11 patients, moderate in 2, and poor in 7. Poor results were believed to be the result of an incorrect diagnosis or initiation of therapy too late in the course of the disease process.

Bonelli and colleagues,[97] in a random study of 19 patients with upper extremity reflex sympathetic dystrophy, compared the effectiveness of stellate ganglion blocks with intravenous regional guanethidine block. For intravenous regional guanethidine block, they used the technique described by Bier.[100] Guanethidine 20 mg was diluted in 25 ml of normal saline and injected in the upper extremity with tourniquet inflation for 15 min. For stellate ganglion block, they administered 15 ml of bupivacaine hydrochloride 0.5%. Their patients received a series of stellate ganglion blocks administered every other day for a total of eight blocks or intravenous guanethidine administered every 4 days for a total of four blocks. Both techniques were reasonably successful, both at the end of the treatment period and at the 1- and 3-month follow-ups. Intravenous regional guanethidine block was believed to be superior to stellate ganglion block because it was less risky, was associated with fewer side effects, and provided block of sympathetic activity for a longer duration. In their evaluation, these authors concluded that maximum benefit was most likely to be obtained after a series of three intravenous regional guanethidine blocks administered at 4-day intervals.

A recent study[101] found that the intravenous administration of phentolamine may help predict the efficacy of the intravenous regional guanethidine block.

Although reported complications from guanethidine and reserpine have been few, prolonged orthostatic hypotension, vertigo, nausea, vomiting, and somnolence can occur. Pain during injection seems to be the main complaint. This can be lessened if the drug is injected slowly and diluted in a lidocaine 0.25% solution. The pain after injection of guanethidine probably is caused by the liberation of norepinephrine from sympathetic nerve endings. This pain emulates the pain and hyperesthesia present before the treatment, suggesting that peripheral sensitization to norepinephrine may be the cause of pain in patients with preexisting hyperesthesia.

Although guanethidine block appears to have a minimal complication rate, patients must be observed and counseled appropriately. This drug is used investigationally in the United States and is not available clinically. For this reason, some clinicians use intravenous regional bretylium.[102] A recent study indicates that intravenous regional blockade with saline alone may be beneficial, perhaps related to a tourniquet-induced analgesia.[103] Ketanserin, an S_2 serotonergic antagonist, also is being studied as an alternative intravenous regional agent.[104]

Oral Nifedipine

After the report of the effective use of oral nifedipine in the treatment of Raynaud phenomenon,[105] another condition characterized by vasospasm and cold intolerance, we studied the usefulness of orally administered nifedipine to relieve the symptoms of reflex sympathetic dystrophy.[106] Nifedipine, a calcium-channel blocker, relaxes smooth muscle, increases peripheral blood flow, and antagonizes the effect of norepinephrine on arterial and venous smooth muscle. Thus, it induces peripheral vasodilatation. We initiate nifedipine therapy at 10 mg orally three times a day for approximately 1 week. If the symptoms are not improved adequately, the dose is increased to 20 mg three times a day. It may be increased to 30 mg three times a day during the following week if improvement does not occur. If there is partial or complete improvement, the effective dose is continued for approximately 2 weeks. After this time, the dose is tapered and discontinued over several days. In a series of 13 patients, 7 had complete relief of symptoms, 2 had partial relief, and 1 patient did not respond to this regimen. Nifedipine was withdrawn from three other patients because of the side effect of headache. When the drug is withdrawn, symptoms of lesser intensity may recur. These usually can be relieved by reinstituting the drug.

Although various side effects have been reported with this drug, the only frequent and troubling side effect we observed was headache. Because of its ability to produce cerebral vasodilatation similar to that produced in multiple other organ beds, increased cerebral blood flow may cause the headache that frequently is reported. However, an extreme example of a complication resulting from nifedipine in a patient being treated for reflex sympathetic dystrophy was described by Catchings and colleagues.[107] This unfortunate patient's symptoms of sympathetic dystrophy pain improved after the second oral 10-mg dose of this drug, and he required no further narcotic therapy. Unfortunately, during the next 2 days, weakness, headache, dysarthria, ataxia, and hemiparesis developed. A CT scan showed two previously unsuspected metastatic cerebral lesions. Thus, although rare, significant neurologic complications after nifedipine therapy must be followed by aggressive diagnostic evaluation. Nifedipine treatment may be an alternative to traditional forms of therapy for the management of reflex sympathetic dystrophy, particularly in those who prefer oral therapy to injections.

Intraspinal Narcotics

Several case reports describe the successful use of continuous intraspinal narcotic infusion systems in affected patients.[108] The appropriateness of this therapy in this setting currently is being investigated in a multicenter study.[108]

Other Treatments

Calcitonin has been advocated[109] in the treatment of reflex sympathetic dystrophy, but recent studies have not found it to be beneficial when administered nasally.[110] Topical capsaicin cream also has been reported to be effective in the treatment of this disorder,[111] but controlled trials are lacking.

SUMMARY

Despite the many techniques available to treat patients with sympathetic dystrophies, most clinicians and authors remain frustrated with the results of therapy. For example, in 125 cases, nearly 60 percent of the patients retained some persistent symptoms despite adequate treatment.[46] We and many others believe that difficulty in making the diagnosis may lead to less-than-perfect treatment results. The failure of patients to respond to blocks or other treatment regimens probably means that the presumptive diagnosis of sympathetic dystrophy is incorrect and that a disorder other than this diagnosis is responsible for the patient's pain.

The newer therapeutic techniques to manage patients with reflex sympathetic dystrophy provide options that are less invasive and generally are tolerated better by patients. We find it difficult to predict which technique will be most efficacious in any given patient. Although logically patients who do not respond to one type of therapy similarly might be expected to be unresponsive to other forms of therapy, for unexplained reasons, a patient may not respond to one technique and yet may derive benefits, either transient or permanent, from one of the other alternatives discussed. Although the optimum method of management will be debated for a long time, it is clear that the most promising approach to manage this clinical problem is prevention, early mobilization after an injury, and initiation of aggressive treatment as early as possible after the diagnosis is made.

References

1. Schwartzman RJ, McLellan TL. Reflex sympathetic dystrophy. A review. *Arch Neurol* May 1987; 44(5):555–561.

2. Turf RM, Bacardi BE. Causalgia: clarifications in terminology and a case presentation. *J Foot Surg* 1986; 25:284–295.

3. Roberts WJ. Review article: A hypothesis on the physiological basis for causalgia and related pains. *Pain* 1986; 24:297–311.

4. Mitchell SW, Morehouse GR, Keene WW. *Gunshot Wounds and Other Injuries of Nerves*. Philadelphia: Lippincott; 1864:164.

5. Bonica JJ. Causalgia and other reflex sympathetic dystrophies. *Postgrad Med* 1973; 53:143–148.

6. Bryan AS, Klenerman L, Bowsher D. The diagnosis of reflex sympathetic dystrophy using an algometer. *J Bone Joint Surg Br* July 1991; 73(4):644–646.

7. Karasick S, Karasick D. Case report 193: segmental reflex sympathetic dystrophy syndrome affecting both hands. *Skeletal Radiol* 1982; 8:151–152.

8. Greipp, ME. Reflex sympathetic dystrophy syndrome: a retrospective pain syndrome. *J Adv Nurs* December 1990; 15(12):1452–1456.

9. Schwartzman RJ, Kerrigan J. The movement disorder of reflex sympathetic dystrophy. *Neurology* January 1990; 40(1):57–61.

10. Bickerstaff DR, O'Doherty DP, Kanis JA. Radiographic changes in algodystrophy of the hand. *J Hand Surg Br* February 1991; 16(1):47–52.

11. Karasick S, Karasick D. Case report 193: segmental reflex sympathetic dystrophy syndrome affecting both hands. *Skeletal Radiol* 1982; 8:151–152.

12. Kozin F. Two unique shoulder disorders. Adhesive capsulitis and reflex sympathetic dystrophy syndrome. *Postgrad Med* 1983; 73:207–216.

13. Constantinesco A, Brunot B, Demangeat JL, et al. Three phase bone scanning as an aid to early diagnosis in reflex sympathetic dystrophy of the hand. A study of 89 cases. *Ann Chir Main* 1986; 5(2):93–104.

14. Holder LE, Mackinnon SE. Reflex sympathetic dystrophy in the hands: clinical and scintigraphic criteria. *Radiology* 1984; 152:517–522.

15. Koch E, Hofer HO, Sialer G, Marincej B, von Schulthess GK. Failure of MR imaging to detect reflex sympathetic dystrophy of the extremities. *AJR Am J Roentgenol* January 1991; 156(1):113–115.

16. Ecker A. Thermography in the diagnosis of reflex sympathetic dystrophy. *N Y State J Med* 1984; 84:6.

17. Pochaczevsky R. Thermography in post-traumatic pain. *Am J Sports Med* May–June 1987; 15(3):243–250.

18. Cousins MJ, Glynn CJ. New horizons. In: Cousins MJ, Bridenbaugh PO, eds. *Neural Blockade*. Philadelphia: Lippincott; 1980:710–712.

19. Karstetter KW, Sherman MA. Use of thermography for initial detection of early reflex sympathetic dystrophy. *J Am Podiatr Med Assoc* April 1991; 81(4):198–205.

20. Koman LA, Nunley JA, Goldner JL, Seaber AV, Urbanik JR. Isolated cold stress testing in the assessment of symptoms in the upper extremity. *J Hand Surg* 1984; 9A:305–313.

21. Sonneveld GJ, van der Meulen JC, Smith AR. Quantitative oxygen measurements before and after intravascular guanethidine blocks. *J Hand Surg* 1983; 8:435–442.

22. Bonica JJ. Causalgia and other reflex sympathetic dystrophies. In: Bonica J, Liebeskind J, Albe-Fessard D, et al, eds. *Advances in Pain Research and Therapy*. Vol 3. New York: Raven Press; 1979:141–166.

23. Warfield CA. The sympathetic dystrophies. *Hosp Pract Off* 1984; 19:52c–52.

24. Sudeck P. Ueber die acute ent-zuendliche Knochenatrophic. *Arch fver Chir* 1900; 62:147–156.

25. Kozin F, McCarty D, Sims J, Genant H. The reflex sympathetic dystrophy syndrome, I. *Am J Med* 1976; 60:321–330.

26. Bentley JB, Hameroff SR. Diffuse reflex sympathetic dystrophy. *Anesthesiology* 1980; 53:256–257.

27. Van Houdenhove B. Neuro-algodystrophy: a psychiatrist's view. *Clin Rhuematol* September 1986; 5(3):399–406.

28. Zucchini M, Alberti G, Moretti MP. Algodystrophy and related psychological features. *Funct Neurol* April–June 1989; 4(2):153–156.

29. Grosslight KR, Rowlingson JC, Boaden RW. Herpes zoster and reflex sympathetic dystrophy. *Anesth Analg* 1986; 65:309–311.

30. Jaeger B, Singer E, Kroening R. Reflex sympathetic dystrophy of the face. Report of two cases and a review of the literature. *Arch Neurol* 1986; 43:693–695.

31. Chalkley JE, Lander C, Rowlingson JC. Clinical note—Probable reflex sympathetic dystrophy of the penis. *Pain* 1986; 25:223–225.

32. Tepperman PS, Greyson ND, Hilbert L, Jiminez J, Williams JL. Reflex sympathetic dystrophy in hemiplegia. *Arch Phys Med Rehabil* 1984; 65:442–447.

33. Wainapel SF. Reflex sympathetic dystrophy following traumatic myelopathy. *Pain* 1984; 18:345–349.

34. Gellman H, Eckert RR, Boote MJ, Sakimura I, Waters RL. Reflex sympathetic dystrophy in cervical spinal cord injury patients. *Clin Orthop* August 1988; (233):126–131.

35. Dequeker J, Geusens P, Verstaeten, DeRoo M. Vertebral crush fracture syndrome and reflex sympathetic dystrophy. *Bone* 1986; 7:89–94.

36. Brock TR. Reflex sympathetic dystrophy linked to venipuncture: a case report. *J Oral Maxillofac Surg* December 1989; 47(1):1333–1335.

37. Nepomuceno C, Fine PR, Richards JS, Gowens CA, Stover SL. Pain in patients with spinal cord injury. *Arch Phys Med Rehabil* 1979; 60:605–609.

38. Steinbrocker, O. The shoulder–hand syndrome: present perspective. *Arch Phys Med Rehabil* 1968; 49:338–395.

40. Michaels RM, Sorber JA. Reflex sympathetic dystrophy as a probable paraneoplastic syndrome: case report and literature review. *Arthritis Rheum* 1984; 27:1183–1185.

41. Prowse M, Higgs CM, Forrester-Wood C, McHugh N. Reflex sympathetic dystrophy associated with squamous cell carcinoma of the lung. *Ann Rheum Dis* April 1989; 48(4):399–341.

42. Markoff M, Farole A. Reflex sympathetic dystrophy syndrome. *Oral Surg Oral Med Oral Pathol* 1986; 61:23–28.

43. Weise WJ, Bernard DB. Reflex sympathetic dystrophy syndrome of the hand after placement of an arteriovenous graft for hemodialysis. *Am J Kidney Dis* September 1991; 18(3):406–408.

44. Munoz-Gomez J, Collado A, Gratacos J, et al. Reflex sympathetic dystrophy syndrome of the lower limbs in renal transplant patients treated with cyclosporine. *Arthritis Rheum* May 1991; 34(5):625–630.

45. Horton P, Gerster JC. Reflex sympathetic dystrophy syndrome and barbiturates. A study of 15 cases treated with barbiturates compared with 124 cases treated without barbiturates. *Clin Rheumatol* 1984; 3:493–499.

46. Subbarao J, Stillwell GK. Reflex sympathetic dystrophy syndrome of the upper extremity: analysis of total outcome of management of 125 cases. *Arch Phys Med Rehabil* 1981; 62:549–554.

47. Ruggieri SB, Athreya BH, Doughty R, Gregg JR, Das MM. Reflex sympathetic dystrophy in children. *Clin Orthop* 1982; 163:225–230.

48. Silber TJ, Majd M. Reflex sympathetic dystrophy in children and adolescents. Report of 18 cases and review of the literature. *Am J Dis Child* December 1988; 142(12):1325–1330.

49. Drucker WR, Hubay CA, Holden WD, Buhovhic JA. Pathogenesis of post-traumatic sympathetic dystrophy. *Am J Surg* 1959; 97:454–465.

50. Malaments IB, Glick JB. Sudeck's atrophy—the clinical syndrome. *J Am Podiatr Med Assoc* 1983; 73:362–368.

51. An HS, Hawthorne KB, Jackson WT. Reflex sympathetic dystrophy and cigarette smoking. *J Hand Surg Am* May 1988; 13(3):458–460.

52. DeTakats G. Sympathetic reflex dystrophy. *Med Clin North Am* 1965; 49:117–129.

53. Plawes LW. Sudeck's atrophy in the hand. *J Bone Joint Surg Br* 1956; 38:195–203.

54. Hill GJ. *Outpatient Surgery*. 2nd ed. Philadelphia: Saunders; 1980:624–684.

55. Bernstein BH, Singsen BH, Kent JT, Kornreich H, King R, Hanson V. Reflex neurovascular dystrophy in childhood. *J Pediatr* 1978; 93:211–215.

56. Owens JC. Causalgia. *Am Surg* 1957; 23:636–643.

57. Leriche R; Young A, trans-ed. *The Surgery of Pain*. Baltimore: Williams & Wilkins; 1939.

58. Freeman NE. Treatment of causalgia arising from gunshot wounds of peripheral nerves. *Surgery* 1947; 22:68–82.

59. Bingham JA. Some problems of causalgic pain: a clinical and experimental study. *BMJ* 1948; 62:334–338.

60. Miller DS, DeTakats G. Post-traumatic dystrophy of the extremities: Sudeck's atrophy. *Surg Gynecol Obstet* 1942; 75:558–582.

61. Doupe J, Cullen CH, Chance GQ. Post traumatic pain and the causalgia syndrome. *J Neurol Neurosurg Psychiatr* 1944; 7:33–48.

62. Livingston WK. *Pain Mechanisms: A Physiologic Interpretation of Causalgia and Its Related States*. New York: Macmillan; 1944.

63. Melzack R. Phantom limb pain: implications for treatment of pathological pain. *Anesthesiology* 1971; 35:409–419.

64. Schutzer SF, Gossling HR. Current concepts review—the treatment of reflex sympathetic dystrophy syndrome. *J Bone Joint Surg Am* 1984; 66A:625–629.

65. Portwood MM, Lieberman JS, Taylor RG. Ultrasound treatment of reflex sympathetic dystrophy. *Arch Phys Med Rehabil* February 1987; 68(2):116–118.

66. Watson HK, Carlson L. Treatment of reflex sympathetic dystrophy of the hand with an active "stress loading" program. *Hand Surg Am* September 1987; 12(5 pt 1):779–785.

67. Simson G. Propranolol for causalgia and Sudeck atrophy. *JAMA* 1974; 227:327. Letter.

68. Christensen K, Jensen EM, Noer I. The reflex dystrophy syndrome response to treatment with systemic corticosteroids. *Acta Chir Scand* 1982; 148:653–655.

69. Kozin F, Ryan LM, Carerra GF, Soin JS, Wortmann RL. The reflex sympathetic dystrophy syndrome (RSDS), III: scintigraphic studies, further evidence of the therapeutic efficacy of systemic corticosteroids, and proposed diagnostic criteria. *Am J Med* 1981; 70:23–30.

70. Dirksen R, Rutgers MJ, Coolen JMW. Cervical epidural steroids in reflex sympathetic dystrophy. *Anethesiology* 1987; 66:71–73.

71. Barowsky EI, Zweig JB, Moskowitz J. Thermal biofeedback in the treatment of symptoms associated with reflex sympathetic dystrophy. *J Child Neurol* July 1987; 2(3):229–232.

72. Grunert BK, Devine CA, Sanger JR, Matloub HS, Green D. Thermal self-regulation for pain control in reflex sympathetic dystrophy syndrome. *J Hand Surg Am* July 1990; 15(4):615–618.

73. Melzak R. Prolonged relief of pain by brief, intense transcutaneous somatic stimulation. *Pain* 1975; 1:357–373.

74. Stilz R, Carron H, Sanders D. Reflex sympathetic dystrophy in a 6-year-old: successful treatment by transcutaneous nerve stimulation. *Anesth Analg* 1977; 56:438–441.

75. Richlin DM, Carron H, Rowlingson JC, Sussman MD, Baugher WH, Goldner RD. Reflex sympathetic dystrophy: successful treatment by transcutaneous nerve stimulation. *J Pediatr* 1978; 93:84–86.

76. Kesler RW, Saulsbury FT, Miller LT, Rowlingson JC. Reflex sympathetic dystrophy in children: treatment with transcutaneous electrical nerve stimulation. *Pediatrics* November 1988; 82(5):728–732.

77. Abram SE. Increased sympathetic tone associated with transcutaneous electrical stimulation. *Anesthesiology* 1976; 45:575–577.

78. Robaina FJ, Dominguez M, Diaz M, Rodriguez JL, de Vera JA. Spinal cord stimulation for relief of chronic pain in vasospastic disorders of the upper limbs. *Neurosurgery* January 24, 1989; (1):63–67.

79. Barolat G, Schwartzman R, Woo R. Epidural spinal cord stimulation in the management of reflex sympathetic dystrophy. *Stereotact Funct Neurosurg* 1989; 53(1):29–39.

80. Kuntz A. *The Autonomic Nervous System*. 3rd ed. Philadelphia: Lea & Febiger; 1945.

81. Betcher AM, Bean G, Casten DF. Continuous Procaine

blocks of paravertebral sympathetic ganglions. *JAMA* 1953; 151:288–292.

82. Linson MA, Leffert R, Todd DP. The treatment of upper extremity reflex sympathetic dystrophy with prolonged continuous stellate ganglion blockade. *J Hand Surg Am* 1983; 8:153–159.

83. Moore DC. *Regional Block*. 4th ed. Springfield: CC Thomas; 1971:211–218.

84. Ladd AL, Dehaven KE, Thanik J, Patt RB, Feuerstein M. Reflex sympathetic imbalance. Response to epidural blockade. *Am J Sports Med* September–October 1989; 17(5): 660–667; discussion 667–668.

85. Wang JK, Johnson KA, Ilstrup DM. Sympathetic blocks for reflex sympathetic dystrophy. *Pain* 1985; 23:13–17.

86. Cooper DE, DeLee JC, Ramamurthy S. Reflex sympathetic dystrophy of the knee. Treatment using continuous epidural anesthesia. *J Bone Joint Surg Am* March 1989; 71(3):365–369.

87. Kleinert HE, Cole MN, Wayne L, Harvey R, Kutz JE, Atasoy E. Post-traumatic sympathetic dystrophy. *Orthop Clin North Am* 1973; 4:917–927.

88. Lankford LL, Thompson JE. *Reflex Sympathetic Dystrophy, Upper and Lower Extremity: Diagnosis and Management*. St. Louis: Mosby; 1977: 26:163–178.

89. Brown BR. Intra-arterial reserpine. *Anesth Analg* 1980; 59:889–890.

90. Benzon HT, Chomke CH, Brunner EA. Treatment of reflex sympathetic dystrophy with regional intravenous reserpine. *Anesth Analg* 1980; 59:500–502.

91. Kepes ER, Raj SS, Vemulapalli R, Thomas PS, Kaplan R. Regional intravenous guanethidine for sympathetic blockade. Report of 10 cases. *Reg Anaesth* 1982; 7:52–54.

92. Abram SE. Intravenous reserpine. *Anesth Analg* 1980; 59:889–890.

93. McLesky CH, Weeks MD, Koman KA, Poehling GP. Use of cold stress test and IV regional reserpine block to diagnose and treat reflex sympathetic dystrophy. *Anesthesiology* 1983; 59:A199.

94. Hannington-Kiff JG. Intravenous regional sympathetic block with guanethidine. *Lancet* 1974; 1:1019–1029.

95. Maxwell RA. Guanethidine after twenty years: a pharmacologist's perspective. *Br J Clin Pharmacol* 1982; 13:35–44.

96. Thomsen MB, Bengstsson M, Lassvick C, Lewis DH, Elfstrom J. Changes in human forearm blood flow after intravenous regional sympathetic blockade with guanethidine. *Acta Chir Scand* 1982; 148:656–661.

97. Bonelli S, Conoscente F, Movilia PG, Restelli L, Francucci B, Grossi E. Regional intravenous guanethidine vs. stellate ganglion block in reflex sympathetic dystrophies: a randomized trial. *Pain* 1983; 16:297–307.

98. McKain CW, Urban BJ, Goldner JL. The effects of intravenous regional guanethidine and reserpine. A controlled study. *J Bone Joint Surg Am* 1983; 65A:808–811.

99. Driessen J, van der Werken C, Nicolais PA, Crul JF. Clinical effects of regional intravenous guanethidine (Ismelin®) in reflex sympathetic dystrophy. *Acta Anaesthesiol Scand* 1983; 27:505–509.

100. Bier A. Veber einen neven weg lokalanasthesie an den gludmaassen zu erzeugen. *Vesh Itsch Ges Chir* 1908; 37(2):204.

101. Arner S. Intravenous phentolamine test: diagnostic and prognostic use in reflex sympathetic dystrophy. *Pain* July 1991; 46(1):17–22.

102. Manchikanti L. Role of intravenous regional bretylium in reflex sympathetic dystrophy. *Anesthesiology* September 1990; 73(3):585–586.

103. Blanchard J, Ramamurthy S, Walsh N, Hoffman J, Schoenfeld L. Intravenous regional sympatholysis: a double-blind comparison of guanethidine, reserpine, and normal saline. *J Pain Symptom Manage* December 1990; 5(6):357–361.

104. Hana MH, Peat SJ. Ketanserin in reflex sympathetic dystrophy. A double-blind placebo controlled cross-over trial. *Pain* August 1989; 38(2):145–50.

105. Rodenheffer RJ, Rommer JA, Wigley F, Smith CR. Controlled double-blind trial of nifedipine in the treatment of Raynaud's phenomenon. *N Engl J Med* 1983; 308:880–883.

106. Prough DS, McLeskey CH, Pehling GG, et al. Efficacy of oral nifedipine in the treatment of reflex sympathetic dystrophy. *Anesthesiology* 1985; 62:796–799.

107. Catchings TT, Prough DS, Kelley DL, Higgins AC. Symptoms of clinically silent intracranial mass lesions precipitated by treatment with nifedipine. *Surg Neurol* 1985; 24:151–152.

108. Goodman RR, Brisman R. Treatment of lower extremity reflex sympathetic dystrophy with continuous intrathecal morphine infusion. *Appl Neurophysiol* 1987; 50(1–6):425–426.

109. Rico H, Meono E, Gomez-Castresana F, Torrubiano J, Espinos D, Diaz P. Scintigraphic evaluation of reflex sympathetic dystrophy: comparative study of the course of the disease under two therapeutic regimens. *Clin Rheumatol* June 1987; 6(2):233–237.

110. Bickerstaff DR, Kanis JA. The use of nasal calcitonin in the treatment of post-traumatic algodystrophy. *Br J Rheumatol* August 1991; 30(4):291–294.

111. Cheshire WP, Snyder CR. Treatment of reflex sympathetic dystrophy with topical capsaicin. Case report. *Pain* September 1990; 42(3):307–311.

CHAPTER 17

Medical Management of Cancer Pain

Michael H. Levy

Pain is the most common symptom of patients with advanced cancer.[1–4] Present in 65 percent to 85 percent of such patients,[5–7] pain afflicts thousands of patients[8] and their families.[9] Too often, it is controlled inadequately, especially during the terminal period.[5,6,10–13] Pain is not only the most common symptom of terminally ill patients, but left unrelieved, it is a significant etiologic component of the next most common symptoms: anorexia, weight loss, weakness, nausea, vomiting, and insomnia.[1–4] Nausea and vomiting alternatively may be a toxic effect of the narcotics used to control pain. In addition, narcotics may contribute to a patient's anorexia and may be the most significant cause for one of the most common symptoms, constipation. Finally, narcotics used for pain relief simultaneously may be the most effective means of controlling intractable coughing or intolerable dyspnea, two other common symptoms of patients with advanced cancer.

Cancer pain differs significantly from the so-called chronic pain syndrome (CPS) that occurs in patients with nonmalignant pain.[6,14] The pain of CPS often exists without actual or even likely tissue damage. Cancer pain usually has an organic source. Patients with CPS receive a large secondary gain from their pain, often using it as an excuse to avoid the demands of normal living. Patients with cancer pain derive little or no secondary gain from their discomfort. Their pain impairs their desired life style and only reminds them of their all too often incurable underlying disease. By contrast, the life style of patients with CPS actually depends on the continuation of their pain and the maintenance of their desired sickness role. Patients with cancer have greater psychological and physiological reactions to their pain than do those with CPS. For many patients with cancer, dying in pain often is more feared than death itself. Finally, CPS pain usually resists medical and surgical intervention and often is approached through behavior modification and operant conditioning. Cancer pain, however, usually responds to appropriate pharmacologic therapy, and psychological pain control techniques are of limited benefit.

The reason for the current therapeutic inadequacy in the management of cancer pain appears to be more the improper application of current knowledge than a lack of the adequate knowledge regarding the mechanisms of pain and the methods available for its control.[5,6,15,16] In the highly controlled settings of free-standing hospices or palliative care units, pain can be controlled in 90 percent to 99 percent of patients.[17,18] The purpose of this chapter is to present a practical approach for managing pain in advanced cancer to permit similar success in a wide variety of clinical settings, including the patient's home.[19]

CAUSES OF PAIN

Approximately 70 percent of the pain felt by patients with advanced cancer is caused directly by their cancer (Table 17-1).[20–22] The rest results from their anticancer therapy or from coincidental associated or unassociated medical problems. Cancer-caused pain varies in incidence with the primary site of the tumor,[20,23] but it is related significantly to the location and resulting pathophysiologic changes caused by the primary tumor or its metastases.[20,21,23,24] The main value of delineating the common causes of cancer pain is that specific syndromes often are amenable to specific therapies as alternatives or adjuncts to the administration of systemic narcotics. Prostaglandin metabolism appears to be involved with the pain of bony metastases; therefore, antiprostaglandin nonsteroidal anti-inflammatory drugs may be effective.[25,26] Inflammation also plays a role in tumor compression of nervous structures, such as the brachial plexus, sacral plexus, or spinal cord; this often responds dramatically to corticosteroids.[27,28] Palliative surgery and interventional radiologic techniques often are the most effective means of controlling the pain caused by tumor obstruction of a hollow viscus or the ductal system of a solid viscus. Tumor distension of encapsulated viscera, such as the liver, occasionally is amenable to the anti-inflammatory effects of corticosteroids. It may respond to appropriate palliative anesthesia or neurosurgical procedures. Palliative radiotherapy or appropriately administered chemotherapy or hormonal therapy also may be effective in these cancer-induced pain syndromes if significant tumor debulking can be

Portions of this chapter taken from Levy M. Pain management in advanced cancer. Reprinted with permission form *Semin Oncol* 1985; 12:394–410.

Table 17-1
Pain Syndromes in Patients with Cancer

Pain Caused by Cancer (70 percent)
  Bone metastasis
  Compression or infiltration of nervous structures
  Infiltration or occlusion of blood vessels
  Obstruction of a hollow viscus
  Obstruction of the ductal system of a solid viscus
  Distension of an encapsulated viscus
  Increased intracranial pressure
  Soft tissue infiltration
  Lymphedema
  Myopathy
  Muscle spasm
  Infiltration or ulceration of mucous membranes

Pain Caused by Anticancer therapy (15 percent)
  Surgery
  Chemotherapy
  Radiotherapy

Coincidental Pain (15 percent)
  Related to cancer or its therapy
  Unrelated to cancer or its therapy

SOURCE: Adapted from Foley[20] and Twycross and Lack[21]

achieved. The headache of increased intracranial pressure from primary or secondary malignancies is classically the worst headache ever experienced.[29,30] The combination of palliative radiotherapy and high-dose corticosteroids usually obviates the need for systemic narcotics. Soft tissue infiltration or edema also may show some response to corticosteroid therapy with the possible addition of a diuretic.[27,28] Muscle spasms most often are the result of some underlying pathophysiologic process rather than a direct effect of the cancer. Nevertheless, specific muscle relaxants and physical therapy may be needed as adjuncts for successful palliation.[31] Finally, local necrosis or ulceration of mucous membranes can be treated best by intensive local therapy, including pharmacologic and surgical debridement.

Postsurgical pain is the most common pain associated with anticancer therapy, and other than the expected acute postoperative pains, involves mostly specific pain syndromes.[20,21,32] Postthoracotomy pain is common in patients with lung cancer and often is best treated by paraspinal nerve blockade (see Chap. 8). Postmastectomy pain, a combination of local hyperesthesia and lymphedema, may respond to local anesthetics, corticosteroids, and diuretics. Phantom-limb pain has been studied extensively in patients with or without cancer and seems to be amenable to local nerve blockade or stimulation procedures.[33–36] For patients still receiving chemotherapy, peripheral neuropathies are seen with agents such as vincristine, vinblastine, vindesine, and altretamine.[20,32] Informing the patient that these may occur and providing them with adequate systemic analgesics is an important aspect of therapy. Patients with cancer more often attribute unexplained pains to progressive disease than to a side effect of therapy. Chemotherapy-

induced mucositis from drugs such a 5-fluorouracil or methotrexate can be painful and may not respond to local measures, such as mouthwashes or topical anesthetics. Patients may need oral, rectal, or parenteral narcotics to allow them to ingest enough nutrition to allow healing of this transient chemotherapy-induced side effect. Herpes zoster infections are common in patients immunosuppressed by their malignancy or its treatment. These may be amenable to specific pharmacologic management (see Chap. 21). Finally, postradiotherapy pain has become less common with advancing radiotherapeutic techniques. The most significant adjuncts to systemic narcotics for this type of pain are local anesthesia or neurosurgery.

The coincidental pains[20,21] in patients with advanced cancer are those seen in any chronically debilitated patient with advanced illness. Each requires specific diagnosis, therapy, and prevention when possible. Prevention is especially important in the common coincidental pains of constipation and bed sores. Perhaps the most difficult coincidental pain to relieve is psychogenic pain, the diagnosis of which must always be one of exclusion.

PALLIATIVE CARE CONCEPTS

Successful pain management requires treatment of what has been described as the patient's *total pain,* that is, physical, psychological, social, spiritual, and financial.[14,37] The interdisciplinary hospice team is suited uniquely to diagnose and treat the many pains of terminally ill patients and their families. Patients each have their own thresholds for pain, the point beyond which a physiologic stimulus evokes the sensation of pain.[38,39] Adequate sleep, elevation of mood, diversion, sympathy, and understanding all can raise the patient's pain threshold. Alternatively, fatigue, anxiety, fear, anger, sadness, depression, or isolation can lower the pain threshold. Antidepressants, anxiolytics, and even analgesics exert much of their pharmacologic effect through raising the pain threshold. By contrast, uncontrolled pain is one of the most potent depressors of the pain threshold.

The pain of advanced cancer is more chronic than acute.[5,14,40] As seen in Table 17-2, acute pain (such as that of a fracture or appendicitis) has a specific meaning that informs the patient to seek specific therapy that is usually curative; the pain is linear and ultimately reversible. The chronic pain of advanced cancer, however, usually is irreversible, trapping the patient in a cycle of pain that goes from bad to worse. If chronic cancer pain has any meaning beyond directing the specific palliation mentioned previously, it means that the patient's underlying disease ultimately is incurable and progressive. The therapeutic goal therefore is not simply pain relief but also pain prevention.[41] This can be achieved by giving an individually titrated dose of an analgesic that relieves the pain and then repeating this dose before the pain recurs. In such a model, a rapid onset of effect is not necessary, obviating the need for short-acting parenteral medications, such as meperidine.

Table 17-2
Analgesic Therapy of Acute versus Chronic Pain

Features	Type of Pain	
	Acute	*Chronic*
Pain Character	Meaningful, linear, reversible	Meaningless, cyclic, irreversible
Therapeutic Goal	Pain relief	Pain prevention
Sedation	Often desirable	Usually undesirable
Rapid Onset of Effect	Important	Unnecessary
Desired Duration of Effect	2 to 4 h	As long as possible
Timing	As needed (on demand)	Regularly (in anticipation)
Dose	Usually standard	Individually titrated
Route	Parenteral	Oral
Adjuvant Medication	Uncommon	Common

SOURCE: Adapted from Twycross[40]

To minimize the losses experienced by patients with chronic cancer pain, we should minimize sedation by carefully titrating the dose and increasing the patient's independence through the use of oral medications. As mentioned, the use of adjuvant medications (such as corticosteroids and nonsteroidal anti-inflammatory drugs) is common to achieve specific palliation and reduce the effective dose of systemic narcotics.

Successful pain control requires a precise and complete pain evaluation.[40] Most patients with advanced cancer have more than one pain.[5] Each pain must be evaluated by its site, intensity, quality, variation, and response to therapy. Such an approach allows us to diagnose specific pain syndromes and thereby provide specific palliative treatment. Similarly, it permits individualized treatment, such as increasing the nighttime amount of a narcotic administered every 4 h to a patient whose pain is more intense at night. Assessing the response to earlier therapy allows us to make both a specific diagnosis and appropriate therapeutic change. One of the most difficult aspects of pain control is the accurate measurement of pain intensity.[42] The best research instruments available are the visual analog scale[43–45] and the McGill-Melzack pain questionnaire.[17,46] The visual analog scale is more amenable to clinical practice. It consists of a 10-cm line labeled at one end by "no pain at all" and at the other by "the worst pain imaginable." Even the most debilitated patients are able to indicate where on this line their pain is located. For patients who do not require or cannot use a visual representation of their pain level, a 0 to 10-point scale may be used with the 0 representing no pain and 10 representing the worst pain they can imagine. Alternatively, verbal descriptors may be used instead of the numbers, such as no pain, mild, discomforting, distressing, horrible, and excruciating pain.[42,47] With practice, any one of these scales can provide the clinician with sufficient data to adjust both the dose and dosing interval of the patient's analgesic regimen.

After the cause of the patient's pain(s) has been determined and the intensity assessed, an effective treatment regimen can be developed. Based on a careful pain evaluation, we should choose an appropriate analgesic with or without a coanalgesic and begin treatment. Care should be taken to avoid excessive doses initially to prevent unwanted adverse side effects that could lower the patient's pain threshold further. The most common adverse side effects of narcotics (such as constipation and nausea) must be treated aggressively and prevented. The key to effective pain management is constant reassessment and appropriate treatment modification. It is inappropriate to prescribe a dose of a medication every 4 h without assessing whether that medication is effective at the time of its peak absorption, most commonly 30 to 60 min after administration. Patients must be provided with appropriate dose supplementation recommendations or orders to be sure that they will not be locked into a situation of having to wait 3 h more for an equally ineffective second dose of their initial medication. Narcotics should be taken around the clock to avoid the patient's awakening in pain in the morning. When using morphine dose equivalents of 15 mg every 4 h, some patients can achieve pain-free morning awakening by increasing their bedtime dose by 50 percent to 100 percent and skipping their middle-of-the-night dose. With controlled-release morphine, around-the-clock pain prevention is easier. Even when an effective regular dosing regimen is established, as needed supplements should be available for intercurrent exacerbations or crises. There is no set optimal or maximal dose of narcotics.[48] The right dose is the dose that controls the pain without excessive or intolerable adverse side effects. Most patients achieve pain control with less than 200 mg of morphine orally every 4 h or its equivalent.[1,17,47] I personally have administered 165 mg of hydromorphone every hour using a constant intravenous infusion to a patient who became relatively pain free but remained communicative and oriented. Converted to its oral equivalent, this represents a dose of 1320 mg every 4 h. This large amount obviously would be used in patients with far-advanced malignancy and drug tolerance. It was the result of many weeks of dose escalation. This is by no means a guide for treating the usual patient, but it underscores the irrelevance of the actual milligram amount needed to achieve safe and effective analgesia.

Tolerance and addiction are significant concerns for patients, families, and clinicians; often they are obstacles in achieving adequate pain control.[11,15,48,49] Neither of these two aspects of narcotic use present a real clinical problem in patients with advanced cancer.[40,48–51] Twycross[48] showed that, in large groups of hospice patients, the type of tolerance seen in street addicts that leads to rapid increases in narcotic dosage does not occur. Patients do not become immune to their narcotics. As new information is gained regarding narcotic cell-surface receptors, mechanisms for the development of tolerance are being described.[52–54] As such, cross tolerance between different narcotic agents appears to be incomplete; occasionally, a patient may be switched from a high dose of one narcotic to a less-than-calculated equivalent dose of a second narcotic agent.[52] What usually is achieved by this technique is a reduction in the milligrams, pills, or liquid volume needed to provide comfort rather than an actual improvement in the level of comfort. Nevertheless, in certain situations, such reductions improve patient compliance and therefore might be needed to improve overall patient comfort.

Addiction is psychological dependence on an exogenous substance.[55] Properly treated, patients with advanced cancer pain do not become addicted to their narcotics.[48–51] With pain-preventing regular individually titrated dosing, these patients repeatedly have been able to have their narcotic doses reduced if the specific cause of their pain responds to local specific therapy. These patients are physically dependent on their narcotics just as is a diabetic patient who requires insulin or one with congestive heart failure who is taking digoxin. If a diabetic patient stops taking insulin, the glucose level will rise. If a patient with cancer pain stops taking narcotics, the pain level will recur. At higher doses of narcotics, abrupt cessation may induce withdrawal symptoms. These symptoms usually can be alleviated by replacing 25 percent of the previous day's dose. If the patient's level of pain will allow this, a further gradual titration can be used thereafter. Withdrawal symptoms can be severe in patients given narcotic antagonists for inadvertent overdosing or in those taking regular narcotics who inappropriately are given a mixed narcotic agonist and antagonist, such as pentazocine or nalbuphine.[56] These mixed agents should be avoided in this patient population, and care should be taken to avoid narcotic excesses by individual dose titration and intensive patient and family education. Patient and family education is one of the most important aspects of effective pain control. Not only must patients and their families be convinced that addiction and tolerance are not clinical problems, but they must be informed fully as to the reasons for specific medications and the prevention and treatment of their potential adverse side effects. Assurance by the clinician that the pain can be controlled safely and effectively is itself worth many milligrams of morphine. Beyond a

knowledge of cancer pathophysiology and clinical pharmacology, successful pain management takes time.

A final palliative care concept before specific medications are presented is that of terminal pain. Most patients can have their pain controlled by appropriate doses of orally or rectally administered narcotics until their final hours or days of life.[17,47,48] When a patient is no longer able to tolerate oral or rectal medications, parenteral medications with appropriate dosing equivalents should be administered. When patients cannot communicate verbally whether they are in pain or not, the best approach is to assume that their cancer is still painful and to continue to administer their regular medications unless clinical signs of narcotic excess are apparent. As their vital signs diminish, dosing may be decreased by reducing the amount or lengthening the interval between doses, but a therapeutic narcotic level should be maintained.[57] In this clinical situation, patients often communicate their pain through agitation, which sometimes is treated inappropriately with tranquilizers rather than continued or increased narcotics. Families often are concerned that continued narcotics may hasten the patient's death. Appropriately titrated, this does not occur. Continued narcotics simply ensure that the death will be as peaceful and painless as possible. Similarly, in-patient nurses often are reluctant to give a scheduled injection when they find that the patient's blood pressure is low for fear that the injection may kill the patient. Usually, these patients do not have signs of excessive narcotic dosing, such as myosis or respiratory depression, and their hypotension is merely the harbinger of their impending death. Withholding the appropriately prescribed narcotic will only result in the reemergence of pain and the disruption of what otherwise would have been a satisfactory family vigil. Both family members and nurses must be given adequate information about the pharmacology of the medications they are administering if pain control is to be successful, especially during the final hours of life.

NARCOTIC ANALGESICS

The narcotic analgesics most commonly used for the control of chronic pain in patients with advanced cancer are listed in Table 17-3. Before discussing each agent, three important aspects of this dose-equivalent table must be presented. First, no drug in this list is more effective than morphine. Some drugs are more potent, but none are more effective when given in the equianalgesic doses. Second, there is a hierarchy of potency. When converting from one drug to another, we must be aware of the equianalgesic dosing guidelines presented in this table and be prepared to increase or decrease the dose of the new narcotic as clinically indicated. The third aspect of this table is the dose conversion needed to switch from the oral to the parenteral route of administration. Oral doses essentially are equivalent to rectal suppository doses; intramuscular doses essentially are equivalent to subcutaneous doses. Intravenous doses usual-

Table 17-3
Narcotic Dose Equivalents for the Control of Chronic Pain*

Oral Dose (mg)	Analgesic[†]	Subcutaneous Dose (mg)
150	Meperidine (Demerol)[‡]	50
100	Codeine[‡] (Tylenol #3)	60
90	Pentazocine (Talwin)[‡]	30
15	Morphine (Roxanol, MSIR, MS Contin)[§‖]	5
10	Oxycodone (Percodan, Percocet, Tylox)[¶]	7.5
10	Methadone (Dolophine)[#]	5
5	Oxymorphone (Numorphan)[**]	1
4	Hydromorphone (Dilaudid)[‖]	1.5
2	Levorphanol (Levo-dromoran)	1

*Equianalgesic doses listed were obtained from various, sometimes conflicting, studies and experiences and are meant only as guidelines for around-the-clock standing-order analgesic therapy of chronic pain. No analgesic listed is superior orally to its equianalgesic dose of oral morphine.
[†]Dose interval: Every 3 to 4 h for all except: meperidine, every 2 to 3 h; levorphanol, every 4 to 6 h; methadone, every 6 to 8 h; MS Contin, every 12 h.
[‡]Of little value in severe chronic pain.
[§]Equianalgesic intravenous dose = 3 to 4 mg every 3 to 4 h.
[‖]Rectal suppositories available. Per rectum dose is equal to oral dose. Subcutaneous dose essentially equal to intramuscular dose.
[¶]Oxycodone 10mg in two Percodan, two Percocet, or two Tylox tablets.
[#]Caution: Sedative side effects often accumulate despite inadequate analgesic effect.
[**]Available for nonparenteral use in rectal suppository form only.

ly are a bit more potent than intramuscular or subcutaneous doses.[58] In clinical practice, the subcutaneous dose of morphine is threefold as potent as the oral dose.[17,47,58] This conversion factor of 3:1 has been observed repeatedly in thousands of hospice patients; however, it disagrees with the 6:1 conversion ratio described in many articles and textbooks.[59–65] The higher ratio came from earlier highly controlled single-dose analgesic potency studies,[59] conditions which do not simulate directly the advanced cancer pain-prevention situation. Whether this is a real or apparent contradiction,[66] the treatment recommendation for converting parenteral to oral morphine in patients with advanced cancer who are receiving regular narcotic administration is to use the 3:1 ratio. The use of the 6:1 ratio in these patients will result in over- or underdosing, according to the direction of the conversion. There is good pharmacokinetic data that the parenteral-to-oral conversion of hydromorphone may be 2:1.[67] The key to successful dosing is to convert the dose at a 3:1 ratio and then adjust it using as-needed supplements; these should be dosed at one-third the dose of the 4- or 12-h around-the-clock dose.

Meperidine

Meperidine is not a good drug for this patient population.[68,69] Orally, it has low potency. When it is given in high enough doses around-the-clock to relieve pain, its metabolite, normeperidine, can accumulate and lead to neurologic side effects, including seizures.[70] Its theoretic advantage of not inducing contraction of the sphincter of Oddi has no clinical relevance. Its rapid onset and its short (1 to 2 h) duration of action are inappropriate for patients in

whom the goal of therapy is pain prevention. Finally, meperidine causes less pupillary constriction than other narcotics, removing this useful sign of narcotic excess. The only possible use for meperidine in this patient population is to treat patients who have a true allergy to morphine but cannot tolerate methadone, the only other drug on this list that is sufficiently different biochemically from morphine to avoid a cross-reaction in the morphine-allergic patient.

Codeine

Codeine is an effective narcotic analgesic that may be used safely in mild-to-moderate pain, particularly in elderly or debilitated patients.[71–76] Unfortunately, at a dose equivalent to 15 mg of morphine, codeine 100 mg causes more gastrointestinal and neuropsychiatric side effects than does 15 mg of morphine. The overall utility of codeine in this patient population therefore is limited. Its constipating side effects are so significant that it often is used to control diarrhea that does not respond to antidiarrheals. Hydrocodone, a semisynthetic derivative of codeine, appears to be more potent (5 mg of hydrocodone equals 30 mg of codeine) and less toxic than codeine, but it has not been studied in high doses or in a form other than a fixed combination with acetaminophen.[77]

Pentazocine

Pentazocine is another drug that is of little use in this patient population.[61,71,72,78] It is a mixed narcotic agonist and antagonist initially developed to reduce the risk of addiction and respiratory depression. Not only can these two narcotic adverse effects occur with this agent, but also its use in doses equivalent to 15 mg of morphine causes more gastrointestinal and neuropsychiatric side effects than does codeine. As already mentioned, caution should be taken to prevent patients receiving regular doses of more effective narcotics from being given this drug, nalbuphine, or other mixed agonist–antagonists, to avoid inducing narcotic withdrawal.[56]

Morphine

There is no narcotic that is more effective than morphine. Its most common forms are oral solution, oral tablet, rectal suppository, and injectable solution. Three oral preparations of morphine we should mention are Roxanol, MSIR, and MS Contin. Roxanol (morphine sulfate intensified oral solution, Roxane Laboratories, Inc.) and MSIR (morphine sulfate oral solution concentrate, Purdue Frederick Co.) are high-potency liquid preparations with a morphine concentration of 20 mg/ml of morphine. They are supplied in easy-to-carry and easy-to-titrate plastic dropper bottles that obviate some of the inconvenience of lower potency morphine solutions for ambulatory patients or patients unable to swallow larger volumes of fluid. Their bland taste and lack of accompanying alcohol preservative also enhance their palatability over previously available morphine solutions. MSIR also is available in scored coated 15- and 30-mg tablets for patients who do not like liquid medications. MS Contin (controlled-release morphine sulfate tablets, Purdue Frederick) provides an even more significant advantage to treat patients who require regular narcotic administration. This product is given on a 12-h rather than a 4-h basis.[79] MS Contin has a wax-matrix controlled-release system, therefore, the morphine is absorbed more slowly, resulting in a prolonged therapeutic blood level. It is available as 15-, 30-, 60-, and 100-mg tablets. Significant clinical experience in Europe with this agent under the brand name MST Continus has shown it to be a safe, effective, and advantageous addition to our narcotic therapeutic regimen.[80–82] More recently, several American studies found a clinical advantage for this product over immediate-release morphine.[83–85]

Oxycodone

Oxycodone is the active narcotic component of Percodan, Percocet, and Tylox.[72,86] It also is available as a single entity in a tablet and oral solution. There is little data regarding the use of high doses of oxycodone in patients with advanced cancer because the single-entity forms only recently became available. This dosage form therefore was limited to patients who could tolerate the aspirin in Percodan or the acetaminophen in Percocet or Tylox.[60,87–89] Each tablet of Percodan contains 5 mg of oxycodone and 325 mg of aspirin. The usual maximum dose therefore is three tablets every 3 h; it is limited by either gastric irrita-

tion or salicyclism from this high daily aspirin dose. Percocet contains 5 mg of oxycodone and 325 mg of acetaminophen; Tylox contains 5 mg of oxycodone and 500 mg of acetaminophen. It is unclear whether the 500-mg dose of acetaminophen makes Tylox a more effective analgesic compared with Percocet.[90] The extra acetaminophen, however, limits the usual maximum dose of Tylox to two capsules every 3 h rather than the three tablets of Percocet every 3 h, based on the potential hepatotoxicity of the high daily dose of acetaminophen.

Methadone

Methadone is an effective narcotic agent whose use is complicated by its complex pharmacology.[91–93] In patients who have not received methadone treatment, the primary-phase half-life of methadone is 14.3 h, with a slower secondary half-life of 54.8 h. Repeated doses produce a single half-life of 22.4 h. Clinically, however, methadone must be given on a 8- to 12-h basis for effective analgesia. There is a propensity of patients or clinicians to give methadone on a more frequent basis or increase its dose more frequently than its half-life safely would allow, and it is common to see oversedated methadone-receiving patients who are still in pain.[92,94] When used properly, methadone can be a safe and effective narcotic analgesic.[95,96] Its advantages are that it does not cross react with morphine in patients who have a true morphine allergy, it is less expensive than equianalgesic doses of morphine or hydromorphone, and as mentioned, it can be given on an 8- and sometimes 12-h basis. Since MS Contin was introduced, this last advantage is no longer relevant. We caution that the safe use of methadone requires extensive clinical experience. It should not be administered on an occasional basis or used as an additive to a 4-h program of one of the other narcotic agents simply to "smooth things out." Whether through inadvertent increased dosing or an intercurrent crisis, such use of methadone often results in drug accumulation and unwanted adverse effects.

Heroin

Heroin is a safe and effective narcotic agent has been used extensively in England for patients with advanced cancer.[43,97] Using heroin, Twycross[43] first proved that pain in these patients could be controlled without addiction or tolerance by administering regular oral doses.[43] Subsequent studies, however, have shown that, in equianalgesic doses, morphine is just as effective as heroin, whether given orally or parenterally. Similarly, a simple morphine solution is just as effective as the so-called Brompton's cocktail, a solution containing heroin or morphine, cocaine, chloroform water, alcohol, and sucrose.[47,98] Because of the unavailability of cocaine for medicinal use in this country, dextroamphetamine was added to morphine to offset the narcotic-induced sedation or respiratory depression.[99,100]

Clinical experience has shown that the potentially beneficial effects of the addition of cocaine or dextroamphetamine are overwhelmed by the high doses of morphine required by these patients or quickly lost through rapid development of tolerance to the stimulants themselves. The inclusion of these agents increases the cost of the prescription and often causes significant neuropsychiatric or cardiac adverse side effects, neither of which can be justified. There is continued controversy about the legalization of heroin in this country.[101–105] Most British hospices currently use morphine in their oral preparations. Heroin is used in Britain for parenteral injections because of its greater potency and solubility. Hydromorphone is more potent and almost as soluble as heroin and has time–action characteristics comparable to heroin when given intramuscularly.[106] In the absence of well-controlled studies documenting any clinical superiority of heroin over hydromorphone, the cost and potential negative social consequences of legalizing heroin in this country cannot be justified.

Oxymorphone

Oxymorphone is included in this list because of its availability as a rectal suppository that occasionally is stocked in the community pharmacy. It is not available orally and has no specific intrinsic advantages.

Hydromorphone

Hydromorphone is a potent safe effective narcotic agent that essentially is interchangeable with morphine in its value to treat patients with advanced cancer. It is available in tablet, rectal suppository, and parenteral forms; it has a well-documented parenteral to enteral relative potency ratio of 2:1.[67] The most recent addition to this product line is a high-potency 10-mg/ml injectable solution that allows the clinician to reduce the injection volume, thereby increasing the comfort with which subcutaneous hydromorphone may

be administered. The potency and solubility of this drug also make it an excellent agent for continuous subcutaneous or spinal infusion using pumps with limited reservoir volumes.

Levorphanol

Levorphanol is a potent narcotic agent that has the potential advantage of being clinically effective on a 6- to 8-h basis. It is available orally as a 2-mg tablet. Because of its potency, this occasionally causes difficulty in individualized dosage titration. Its use in patients with advanced cancer is complicated further by its plasma half-life of 12 to 16 h and its high lipid solubility; the latter may result in drug accumulation and excessive sedation.[107]

Fentanyl

Previously available only intravenously for operative anesthesia, fentanyl recently has been introduced in a transdermal form. The fentanyl patch provides 72 h of analgesia, but as a result of depot formation in the subcutaneous tissues, it has a slow onset and elimination. Probably it can be used best to treat patients who have very stable pain and cannot take oral preparations.[108]

RECOMMENDED ANALGESIC THERAPY

Based on the palliative care concepts and narcotic analgesic descriptions, recommended analgesic therapy is presented in Table 17-4. Aspirin or acetaminophen are appropriate agents for the treatment of mild pain.[72,73,87,88] Caution is advised when administering acetaminophen to patients with compromised liver function because of its known toxicity. Alternatively, patients with a history of gastritis, ulcer, allergy to aspirin, chronic rhinitis, blood clotting dysfunction, or low platelet count should not be given aspirin. When the mild pain is caused by inflammation or early bone

Table 17-4
Recommended Analgesic Therapy

Pain	Analgesic(s)	Four Hourly Dose
Mild	Aspirin, Acetaminophen, or	650 mg
	Ibuprofen	400 mg
Moderate	Aspirin or Acetaminophen, and	650 mg
	Codeine	60 mg
	(Tylenol #3)	Two tablets
	Aspirin or Acetaminophen, and	650 mg
	Oxycodone	10 mg
	(Percodan or Percocet)	Two tablets
Severe to overwhelming	Morphine (Roxanol, MSIR, MS Contin*) or	15+ mg
	Hydromorphone (Dilaudid)	4+ mg

*MS Contin 12-h dose = threefold 4-h dose

metastasis, aspirin or other nonsteroidal anti-inflammatory drugs will be more effective than acetaminophen.[25] There is little evidence that propoxyphene is any better than placebo for these patients.[73,74,76]

The addition of codeine to either aspirin or acetaminophen may control moderate or discomforting pain effectively.[72-77] To increase statistically the analgesic effect of 650 mg of aspirin or acetaminophen, we must add 60 mg of codeine. Clinically, however, we may wish to start with 30 mg of codeine and permit doses up to 60 mg if the pain is not relieved after one or two doses. At this dose of codeine, the aspirin or the acetaminophen still provide a significant component of the analgesic regimen and should be used in their full 650-mg dose. Therefore, patients should either be given their appropriate dose of aspirin or acetaminophen and codeine as separate entities or, if using a combined product, should be assured of getting the full dose of aspirin or acetaminophen with the appropriate fixed-combination product or the mixture of a fixed-combination agent and a pure aspirin or acetaminophen tablet.[109]

Severe or distressing pain of 6 on a scale of 0 to 10 often requires a stronger narcotic combination, such as that contained in Percodan, Percocet, or Tylox. Increased pain relief usually is achieved when 10 mg of oxycodone is added to 650 mg of acetaminophen or aspirin instead of the same dose of acetaminophen or aspirin combined with 60 mg of codeine. Some patients may require 15 mg of oxycodone. The choice of Percodan versus Percocet should be made with regard to the advantages or disadvantages of aspirin versus acetaminophen. Percocet is recommended over Tylox because of its lower acetaminophen content. If 10 mg of oxycodone be inadequate, a third Percocet tablet can be added for an additional 5 mg of oxycodone with less risk of hepatotoxicity than using three Tylox.

Most patients with pain from advanced cancer have sensations that are described as very severe/horrible or overwhelming/excruciating. This correlates with a level 8 to 10 on a scale of 0 to 10. Such patients require more potent narcotics that are administered best in pure form to avoid limiting the narcotic dose based on the toxicity of a fixed-dose coanalgesic. For such patients, morphine or hydromorphone are the most commonly used narcotic agents. Unlike the previous doses listed in Table 17-4, the 15-mg dose of morphine and the 4-mg dose of hydromorphone essentially are equal to, rather than the next step up from, two Percodan or two Percocet tablets. For patients not receiving narcotics, a good 4-h starting dose of morphine is 10 to 15 mg. For elderly, cachectic, or narcotic-naive patients, it might be safer to start with a 4-h dose of 5 mg of morphine. Patients already receiving narcotic agents should have their morphine or hydromorphone dose calculated from the dose equivalents listed in Table 17-3 and should receive some additional amount based on the patients' current pain level and their response to their previous narcotic agent. As with most pharmacologic agents, a steady-state plateau morphine level is achieved in five to six drug half-lives (20 to 24 h). If

possible, therefore, dose escalation should be limited to two increases per day for a total increment of 50 percent to 100 percent of the starting dose in any 24-h period. After some amount of pain control is achieved, subsequent titration should proceed more slowly, such as 10 percent to 25 percent increments of the current 4-h dosing regimen with no more than two increments per day. This slower escalation should allow safe and effective pain control and minimize the risk of overshooting the dose, leading to unwanted adverse effects. Some patients with rapidly progressive painful lesions, however, may require and tolerate a more rapid and frequent dose escalation. There are no fixed upper limits for morphine or hydromorphone. As already discussed, the correct dose is the one that relieves pain but does not produce excessive adverse side effects. When converting patients to MS Contin, we should begin with appropriately the calculated 12-h dose and provide a 4-h dose of morphine for breakthrough pain; this technique is similar to the way we begin to treat a diabetic patient with long-acting insulin and as-needed regular insulin supplements. The 4-h morphine dose should be approximately one-third of the 12-h MS Contin dose. The MS Contin dose then should be increased daily until the supplements are no longer needed. A return to 4-h narcotics might be necessary during intercurrent crises and resumption of MS Contin after the patient's condition is stable.

When patients are unable to tolerate oral medications, the rectal suppository route should be considered.[110-112] The appropriateness of this route is limited by the presence of rectal disease or the amount of narcotic required for patient comfort. Commercially available morphine suppositories have a maximum unit dose of 30 mg. Hydromorphone suppositories are available only in a 3-mg size and oxymorphone, in a 5-mg size. Reliable analgesia can be achieved with the insertion of no more than two suppositories at one time. The usefulness of commercially available suppositories therefore is limited to patients who need less than 60 mg of morphine or 6 mg of hydromorphone every 3 to 4 h. Hospice pharmacy is a growing subspecialty, and many communities have individually prepared rectal suppositories available in whatever dose of narcotic the patient requires.[113] Recently, MS Contin has been shown to be effective by the rectal route.[114,115] Delayed pharmacokinetic parameters can be compensated by increasing the dose. As an alternative enteral administration route, sublingual morphine has been shown to be an effective alternative to oral or rectal morphine.[111,116]

Alternatives to the rectal or sublingual routes of narcotic administration are transdermal, intermittent subcutaneous injection, or constant subcutaneous or intravenous infusion. Even in hypotensive poorly perfused patients, the intramuscular route of administration rarely is needed. Subcutaneous injection is less painful for the patient and easier for the family to master. Theoretically, the dose of narcotic in hypoperfused patients might need to be slightly higher when the drug is injected subcutaneously rather than intramuscularly, but this is not clinically significant as long as the dose administered achieves the desired palliative effect. Constant subcutaneous infusion of morphine is useful in patients who have limited injection sites caused by cachexia or who do not have a primary-care person available to them to administer their scheduled injections.[117–119] Hydromorphone has a higher potency and solubility than morphine, it may be preferred for such patients. Fentanyl is the only drug available in a transdermal form, and it can be used when enteral forms of therapy are not feasible.[108]

Constant intravenous infusion of morphine most often is used for inpatients,[120–123] although newly available venous access systems and portable internal or external pumps have begun to make this method of narcotic administration available for select patients at home.[124,125] In the inpatient setting, constant intravenous narcotic infusion is well suited for patients with a low tolerance to the adverse effects of narcotics at the time of peak absorption from intermittent injection. Constant intravenous infusion also economizes on nursing administration and the documentation activities required by intermittent injection. The net result usually is improved pain control, less adverse side effects, and more time for these patients' nurses to attend to their psychosocial and other physical needs. A recent development in the use of intravenous morphine infusion is patient-controlled analgesia (PCA).[126,127] This sophisticated pump system allows the patient to self-administer intravenous narcotics at a preset dose and interval that is titrated to their level and incidence of pain. Patients using PCA postoperatively achieve improved pain relief with a lower total daily narcotic dose than with other forms of intermittent parenteral narcotic therapy. The value of PCA in patients with chronic pain is limited by the inability of many PCA pumps to administer a continuous infusion simultaneously with the intermittent patient-initiated bolus doses. Patients using PCA must either experience or anticipate recurrent pain to maintain an adequate narcotic level. This sustains the undesired operant conditioning of earning or working for comfort that is obviated by an appropriately set constant infusion. Pharmacia (Piscataway, NJ) has a PCA pump that is particularly useful for patients with chronic cancer pain. Their Computerized Ambulatory Drug Delivery Patient Controlled Analgesia™ pump was the first PCA pump that allowed for simultaneous continuous infusion of a prescribed maintenance morphine dose and intermittent infusion of a preset patient-initiated supplemental bolus. The use of PCA pumps without this simultaneous dual-delivery capacity should be limited to brief titrations of intravenous narcotics during intercurrent crises or periods of rapid pain progression with return to the continuous-infusion mode after the new effective narcotic dose has been established. When converting a patient from oral to intravenous morphine, a conservative dose equivalency would be a starting hourly dose of one-quarter that of their calculated hourly oral dose. If a patient has not received narcotics for more than 4 h, the calculated hourly dose may be given by

intravenous bolus as a loading dose immediately before starting the constant infusion. Dose escalation usually may be done with increments of 20 percent to 50 percent of the dose given previously as tolerated; again, we try to avoid more than two dose escalations per day after some pain control has been achieved. A typical dose of intravenous morphine is 0.04 to 0.07 mg/kg/h (2.8 to 4.9 mg/h in a 70-kg adult) with a reported safe range of 0.5 to 200 mg/h.[120] Again, intravenous morphine has been administered at 1000 mg/h safely with 150-mg intravenous bolus doses in selected patients.

A final parenteral application of morphine or narcotics for the control of pain in advanced cancer is that of epidural or intrathecal infusion. (See Chap. 27.)

PREVENTION OF COMMON SIDE EFFECTS OF NARCOTIC THERAPY

Narcotic side effects should be anticipated and prevented or minimized. Pain relief should not be offset by the creation of other distressing symptoms. All patients receiving regular doses of narcotics become constipated and should be maintained on some form of bowel preparation from the beginning of their narcotic therapy.[128,129] Dietary modifications and bulk laxatives alone are seldom tolerable or adequate. Table 17-5 is a protocol for constipation management that has been effective in most such patients. The key to this protocol is to give our patients specific medications with particular directions that include a specific temporal definition of constipation. A reasonable overall goal is for the patient to have a bowel movement at least every 2 days. Another critical element of this protocol is the escalation of the daily treatments in patients who require the use of enemas or manual disimpaction. A typical regimen for a patient receiving 60 mg of morphine every 4 h would be 3 Senokot-S tablets orally three times a day, 10 mg of bisacodyl orally twice a day, and lactulose 30 to 45 ml orally at

Table 17-5
Constipation Management

- Start All Patients on:
  Docusate sodium 50 mg plus senna 187 mg
  (Senokot-S two tablets orally at bedtime,
    range, one tablet at bedtime to four tablets three times a day

- If No Bowel Movement in Any 48-h Period:
  Bisacodyl 10 to 15 mg at bedtime
    range, 5 mg at bedtime to 15 mg three times a day
  If causes cramping, increase daily Senokot-S dose

- If No Bowel Movement in Any 72-h Period:
  Nonimpacted   Magnesium citrate 8 oz orally
          Lactulose 45 to 60 ml orally
          Bisacodyl suppository 10 mg rectally
          Fleet phosphosoda enema rectally
  Impacted   Disimpact
          Enemas until clear
  Increase daily Senokot-S and bisacodyl doses

bedtime as needed for no bowel movement in any 48-h period. When initiating a bowel regimen, patients may take one Senokot-S tablet for every dose of 4 mg of hydromorphone or 15 mg of morphine.[129–131] The exact laxative program depends on the patient's narcotic dose, diet, activity, and concomitant use of other bowel active agents.

Approximately 20 percent of patients receiving narcotic agents develop mild-to-moderate nausea as a result of morphine's stimulation of the chemoreceptor trigger zone and its inhibition of gastrointestinal motility. Recommended antiemetics are listed in Table 17-6. Patients already mildly nauseated or somewhat frail or elderly should begin prophylactic antiemetic therapy at the time of initiation of their narcotic regimen. If they experience no nausea during the first 48 h, their antiemetic may be tapered and then used only on an as-needed basis. Because most of these agents cause sedation that can limit the dose of the narcotic that can be used safely for adequate pain control, attempts should be made to eliminate their use if possible. There is no conclusive data to support the continued use of phenothiazines solely as narcotic potentiators.[132]

Most patients experience drowsiness at the beginning of narcotic therapy or after any significant increase in their previous narcotic dose.[128] This sedation usually wears off in 1 to 3 days. Persistent drowsiness requires a specific diagnosis with respect to the adverse side effects of other medications or the advance of a patient's cancer. Confusion also may occur during these same times; it may respond to small doses of haloperidol. Whenever feasible, a reduction in the dose of morphine should be attempted by adding nonsedating coanalgesics. In some patients, it is impossible to achieve total pain control without sedation or mild confusion. The use of stimulants, such as dextroamphetamine or methylphenidate, is controversial.

Appropriately prescribed narcotics rarely cause clinically significant respiratory depression.[133–135] The threshold for such depression is always above the sedative threshold, which itself is above the analgesic threshold. With around-the-clock narcotic administration, careful individual titration of the dose, and frequent reassessment, respiratory depression should not be a dose-limiting problem. Unexpected respiratory depression in a patient receiving stable analgesic doses suggests metabolic derangement and/or central nervous system damage requiring specific evaluation and treatment. An important clue in the differential diagnosis is the presence or absence of narcotic-induced myosis. Should analgesic-induced respiratory depression occur despite caution, it may be treated with naloxone 0.1 to 0.8 mg.[94] This drug's narcotic antagonist effects usually are immediate and may precipitate reemergence of previously controlled pain and narcotic withdrawal symptoms. We should be aware that the half-life of one dose of naloxone is approximately 20 min, which might be shorter than the half-life of the excessive narcotic agent. Therefore, careful monitoring and repeated or even continuous naloxone administration may be required in severe cases of narcotic overdoses.[94,136]

SPECIFIC PAIN SYNDROMES

Bone Pain

The management of a few specific pain syndromes encountered frequently in patients with advanced cancer will be reviewed before concluding this chapter. As already mentioned, the pain of bony metastasis seems to be mediated, at least in part, by prostaglandins.[24,25] The addition of nonsteroidal anti-inflammatory antiprostaglandin drugs as adjuncts to narcotic analgesia may be helpful in these patients (Table 17-7). Choline magnesium trisalicylate is an excellent drug for patients with cancer because of its lack of antiplatelet[137] or renal failure side effects. Ibuprofen[138,139] is a commonly used well-tolerated agent. Naproxen[23,140] diflunisal,[141,142] and flurbiprofen[126] are other useful drugs. Some patients respond better to indomethacin[143] but may experience a greater amount of gastrointestinal toxicity or confusion.[144,145] This drug recently become available as a 50-mg suppository. Pain from bony metastases is one of the most difficult cancer-induced pains to manage. Nonpharmacologic measures, such as radiotherapy or ortho-

Table 17-6
Nausea Control

- Relieve Constipation

- Provide Prescription for As-Needed Use of:
  Prochlorperazine 5 mg orally every 4 h
    (range, 5 mg every 6 h to 20 mg every 4 h)

- If Too Sedating or Ineffective:
  Haldoperidol 0.5 mg orally every 8 h
    (range, 0.5 mg every 12 h to 1.0 mg every 4 h)

- If Sedation Is Desired in an Agitated Patient:
  Chlorpromazine 10 mg orally every 4 h
    (range, 10 mg every 6 h to 25 mg every 4 h)

- If Gastric Outlet Obstruction Is a Problem, Switch to or Add:
  Metoclopramide 10 mg orally every 6 h
    (range, 10 mg every 8 h to 20 mg every 6 h)

Table 17-7
Recommended Nonsteroidal Anti-Inflammatory Drugs for Pain from Bone Metastasis

Choline magnesium trisalicylate (Trilisate)	1500 mg orally every 8 to 12 h
Ibuprofen (Motrin, Advil)	800 mg orally every 6 to 8 h
Naproxen (Naprosyn)	500 mg orally every 8 to 12 h
Diflunisal (Dolobid)	500 mg orally every 8 to 12 h
Flurbiprofen (Ansaid)	100 mg orally every 8 to 12 h
Indomethacin (Indocin)	50 mg orally every 6 to 8 h

pedic surgery, must be considered carefully. Epidural morphine infusion may help patients with painful low vertebral or pelvic bone metastatic pain. This patient group also benefits from ready access to as-needed injectable narcotic supplements just before times of pain-inducing increased activity.

Nerve Root Compression Pain

Frequently, a significant component of the mass causing nerve compression consists of the body's own inflammatory response to the advancing malignancy.[26,27] The addition of moderately high-dose corticosteroids to narcotic analgesics often provides significant palliation of the pain from acute compression of nerve roots or plexuses by such tumor masses (Table 17-8). A recommended therapeutic trial would be dexamethasone 8 mg orally three times a day for several days. If there is no improvement, the corticosteroid therapy can be discontinued abruptly with no untoward effects. If, however, there is a good palliative response, an attempt should be made to taper the steroid dose gradually to the lowest possible effective dose (often 4 mg of dexamethasone twice a day). The usual side effects of corticosteroid therapy, such as fluid retention, hyperglycemia, and proximal myopathy must be anticipated and managed appropriately. A particularly common adverse effect in this patient population is oral candidiasis. This may be treated with appropriate doses of ketoconazole or clotrimazole.

Headache from Intracranial Tumor

High-dose corticosteroid therapy in conjunction with palliative radiotherapy, when appropriate, is the treatment of choice for the severe headache caused by raised intracranial pressure from primary or secondary brain malignancies.[28,29] Affected patients tend to be sensitive to dose adjustments, with the return of headache or focal neurologic dysfunction after even minimal dose reductions. Corticosteroid doses of more than 100 mg/day of dexamethasone intravenously have been used effectively without any clear-cut evidence of approaching a true dosing plateau.[146,147] Clinically, however, few patients with chronically progressive intracranial malignancy receive benefit from

Table 17-8
Steroid Therapy for Cancer Pain

Dose	Dexamethasone*	Pain
Low	2 to 4 mg orally bid-tid	Soft tissue infiltration
Moderate	4 to 8 mg orally bid-tid	Nerve compression Visceral distension
High	4 to 12 mg orally tid-qid	Increase intracranial pressure

*Alternative Steroid Agents: Methylprednisone (Medrol) 8 mg = Prednisone 10 mg = Dexamethasone (Decadron, Hexadrol) 2 mg

doses in excess of 12 mg of dexamethasone orally four times a day. The ulcerogenic potential of these high doses must be considered, and these patients may benefit from prophylactic therapy with cimetidine 300 mg orally every 6 h or ranitidine 150 mg orally twice a day. Corticosteroid therapy often presents an ethical dilemma because continuating such therapy might have a life-prolonging effect even in the face of advancing symptomatic disease elsewhere in the body. Where cessation of corticosteroid therapy is not achieved naturally by the patient who becomes unable to swallow, the clinician must take an active part in the decision to discontinue such therapy if it is believed only to be prolonging the patient's suffering. This active role is necessary to avoid requiring the patient's family to assume such a responsibility alone. They might be left with difficult-to-manage guilt from the potential outcome of discontinuing steroid therapy.

Visceral and Soft Tissue Infiltration Pain

Painful distension of visceral organs, lymph nodes, and subcutaneous tissue also may be improved by low-to-moderate dose corticosteroid therapy to reduce any inflammatory component that might cause the painful stimuli.[26,27] Occasionally, the addition of diuretics also may reduce any edematous component of soft tissue swelling or lymphedema. Support stockings or pneumatic pumping devices may reduce the pain from such soft tissue distension.[148]

Intestinal Colic from Obstruction

The severe spasmodic pain of partial or complete obstruction often can be relieved by combining an antispasmodic with a stool softener. Diphenoxylate hydrochloride (2.5 mg) with atropine sulfate (0.025 mg) one to two tablets every 4 to 6 h or loperamide hydrochloride 2 to 4 mg every 6 h plus docusate sodium 100 mg two to four times a day are possible treatments for this intense pain. Combined with a limited clear-liquid diet, appropriate systematic antiemetics, and if needed, narcotic analgesics, patients with intestinal colic from bowel obstruction often may remain at home without the need for nasogastric intubation or intravenous hydration.[149]

Rectal or Bladder Spasm Pain

Regular use of belladonna and opium suppositories for severe rectal or bladder spasm from neurologic or infiltrative diseases may reduce the dose or obviate the need for systemic narcotic analgesia.[150] Available in 30- and 60-mg opium doses, these suppositories may be administered rectally every 4 to 6 h. Chlorpromazine 10 to 25 mg orally every 4–6 h also may be useful, particularly in painful rectal tenesmus.[151]

Postherpetic Neuralgic (See Chap. 21)

Patients with advanced cancer are susceptible to herpes zoster infection. The use of moderate-dose corticosteroids during the infection may shorten its course and reduce the incidence or intensity of postherpetic neuralgia. Amitriptyline 25 to 150 mg orally at bedtime is a useful adjunct to narcotic analgesic in patients with severe pain from postherpetic neuralgia.[152,153] Levodopa 100 mg and carbidopa 25 mg two tablets orally three times a day[154] and the combination of clomipramine and carbamazepine[155] also have been reported to be effective. The reader is referred to recent reviews of the role of antidepressants in chronic pain for further information regarding the usefulness of this class of drugs in chronic pain other than postherpetic neuralgia.[156,157]

Intermittent Stabbing Pains (Tics)

Along with severe bony metastasis pain, intermittent stabbing pains of presumed neuritic cause are difficult to control.[151] Their sporadic, unpredictable, and often intense character makes tics poorly controlled by constant-dose narcotic therapy. Agents that have been tried with variable success include carbamazepine 200 to 600 mg orally twice a day, phenytoin sodium 100 mg orally three times a day, and valproic acid 200 orally two to three times a day.[151,158] When using carbamazepine, we should begin with a 100-mg dose twice daily and increase by 100 mg per dose per day until the pain is relieved or the maximum dose is achieved. When using carbamazepine or phenytoin, the dose should be titrated to achieve a therapeutic blood level.

Muscle Spasm Pain

The most common cause for muscle spasm in this patient population is an underlying adjacent pain-producing process, such as a soft tissue mass, a compressed nerve, or a bony metastasis.[30] Treatment with a narcotic analgesic usually disrupts the pain-spasm cycle. Massage, physical therapy, and heat also may be beneficial. If painful muscle spasm is not relieved, direct muscle-relaxing agents may be considered. Their efficacy is limited by the sedative side effects; these may be particularly problematic in patients already receiving high-dose narcotics. Diazepam 2 to 10 mg orally every 6 to 12 h is the best oral muscle relaxant. Baclofen 5 to 20 mg orally three times a day (increased by 5 mg per dose every 3 days as needed) or dantrolene sodium 25 to 100 mg orally three to four times a day (increased by 25 mg per dose every 3 days as needed) also may be effective. For severe acute spasm, methocarbamol 1000 to 3000 mg intramuscularly every 6 to 12 h is best. This drug may be given also intravenously as can diazepam. The latter may be given intramuscularly, but its absorption is unreliable.

NONPHARMACOLOGIC MANAGEMENT OF PAIN

The palliative benefits of appropriate surgery,[159] radiotherapy,[160] chemotherapy, and hormonal therapy[161] go beyond the scope of this chapter but should be considered for each pain in each patient. Useful anesthesic[162] and neurosurgical[163] techniques also should be considered and are covered elsewhere in this text. Various psychotherapeutic techniques, such as hypnosis and biofeedback, also have been helpful in patients with advanced cancer and require further study.[164-166]

CONCLUSION

The control of pain in patients with advanced cancer has been the subject of many articles and books. The recommendations included in this chapter are a clinical distillation of many resources from various health care professions and treatment settings. These recommendations are guidelines not inviolable protocols. There is no magic to successful pain control. Beyond a sound knowledge of the causes of cancer pain and the pharmacology of narcotic and nonnarcotic analgesics, successful pain management requires a positive, patient, yet aggressive approach on the part of the practicing clinician. The patient and family must be engaged as, not only the focus of therapy, but also as integral participants in the palliative care team. Recent advances in the research of the body's own opiates, endorphins and enkephalins, may lead to new understandings and new safer more effective analgesic agents.[52-54] Nevertheless, without a rational approach to the control of the patient's total pain, the value of such new ideal agents will go unrealized. Pain management in advanced cancer is both an art and a science. It owes much of its current level of success to the hospice movement. Expanded research and education are needed to further this success to realize the goal of making patients relatively pain free[167] to permit patients with advanced cancer to end their lives with as much dignity and purpose as possible.[61]

References

1. Walsh TD, Saunder CM. Hospice care: the treatment of pain in advanced cancer. *Recent Results Cancer Res* 1984; 89:201–211.
2. Kaiser CB. Hospice inpatient care: characteristics of an institution and its patients. *Conn Med* 1984; 48:146–151.
3. Norton WS, Lack SA. Control of symptoms other than pain. In: Twycross RG, Ventafridda V, eds. *The Continuing Care of Terminal Cancer Patients*. Oxford: Pergamon; 1980:167.
4. Wilkes E. Some problems in cancer management. *Proc R Soc Med* 1974; 67:1001–1005.
5. Twycross RG. Incidence of pain. *Clin Oncol* 1984; 3:5–15.
6. Bonica JJ. Management of cancer pain. *Recent Results Cancer Res* 1984; 89:13–27.

7. Daut RL, Cleeland CS. The prevalence and severity of pain in cancer. *Cancer* 1984; 50:1913–1918.

8. Swerdlow M, Stjernsward J. Cancer pain relief—an urgent problem. *World Health Forum* 1984; 3:325–330.

9. Cleeland CS. The impact of pain on the patient with cancer. *Cancer* 1984; 54:2635–2641.

10. Oster MW, Vizel MV, Turgeon LR. Pain of terminal cancer patients. *Arch Intern Med* 1978; 138:1801–1802.

11. Marks RM, Sachar EJ. Undertreatment of medical inpatients with narcotic analgesics. *Ann Intern Med* 1973; 78:173–181.

12. Parkes CM. Home or hospital? Terminal care as seen by surviving spouses. *J R Coll Gen Pract* 1978; 28:19–30.

13. Cartwright A, Hockey L, Anderson JL. *Life Before Death*. London: Routledge & Kegan Paul; 1973.

14. Lack SA. Total pain. *Clin Oncol* 1984; 3:33–34.

15. Bonica JJ. Importance of the problem. In: Bonica JJ, Ventafridda V, eds. *Advances in Pain Research and Therapy*. Vol 2. New York: Raven Press; 1979:115.

16. Charap AD. The knowledge, attitudes, and experience of medical personnel treating pain in the terminally ill. *Mt Sinai J Med* 1978; 45:561–580.

17. Saunders CM. Current views of pain relief and terminal care. In: Swerdlow M, ed. *The Therapy of Pain*. Lancaster: MTP Press Ltd; 1981:215.

18. Melzack R, Ofiesh JG, Mount BM. The Brompton mixture: effects on pain in cancer patients. *Can Med Assoc J* 1979; 115:122–126.

19. Lamerton R. Annual Report of Macmillan Home Care Service. London: St. Joseph's Hospice; 1978.

20. Foley KM. Pain syndromes in patients with cancer. In: Bonica JJ, Ventafridda V, eds. *Advances in Pain Research and Therapy*. Vol 2. New York: Raven Press; 1979:59.

21. Twycross RG, Lack SA. *Symptom Control in Far Advanced Cancer: Pain Relief*. London: Pitman; 1983:20.

22. Banning A, Sjøgren P, Henriksen H. Pain causes in 200 patients referred to a multidisciplinary cancer pain clinic. *Pain* 1991; 45:45–48.

23. Bonica JJ. Cancer pain. In: Bonica JJ, ed. *Pain*. New York: Raven Press; 1980:325.

24. Hill K. Pathological anatomy of cancer pain. *Recent Results Cancer Res* 1984; 89:33–44.

25. Twycross RG, Lack SA. *Symptom Control in Far Advanced Cancer: Pain Relief*. London: Pitman; 1983:119.

26. Pollen JJ, Schmidt JD. Bone pain in metastatic cancer of prostrate. *Urology* 1979; 13:129–134.

27. Twycross RG, Lack SA. *Symptom Control in Far Advanced Cancer: Pain Relief*. London: Pitman; 1983:270.

28. Hanks GW, Trueman T, Twycross RG. Corticosteroids in terminal cancer—a prospective analysis of current practice. *Postgrad Med J* 1983; 59:28–32.

29. Wilson CB, Yorke CH, Levin VA. Intracranial malignant growth, primary and metastatic. *Curr Probl Cancer* 1977; 1:1–46.

30. Black P. Brain metastasis: current status and recommended guidelines for management. *Neurosurg* 1979; 5:617–631.

31. Twycross RG, Lack SA. *Symptom Control in Far Advanced Cancer: Pain Relief*. London: Pitman; 1983:288.

32. Schreml W. Pain in the cancer patient as a consequence of therapy (surgery, radiotherapy, chemotherapy). *Recent Results Cancer Res* 1984; 89:85–99.

33. Omer GE. Nerve, neuroma, and pain problems related to upper limb amputations. *Orthop Clin North Am* 1981; 12:751–762.

34. Steinback TV, Nadvorna H, Arazi D. A five year follow up study of phantom limb pain in post traumatic amputees. *Scand J Rehabil Med* 1982; 14:203–207.

35. Logan TP. Persistent phantom limb pain: dramatic response to chlorpromazine. *South Med J* 1983; 76:1585.

36. Sherman RA, Tippens JK. Suggested guidelines for treatment of phantom limb pain. *Orthopedics* 1982; 5:1595–1600.

37. Saunders CM. *The Management of Terminal Illness*. London: Hospital Medicine Publ; 1967.

38. Twycross RG, Rack SA. *Symptom Control in Far Advanced Cancer: Pain Relief*. London: Pitman; 1983:43.

39. Glynn CJ. Factors that influence the perception of intractable pain. *Med Times* 1980; 108:11S–26S.

40. Twycross RG. Relief of pain. In: Saunders CM, ed. *The Management of Terminal Disease*. London: Edward Arnold Publ Ltd; 1978:65.

41. Mount BM, Ajemian I, Scott JF. Use of the Brompton mixture in treating the chronic pain of malignant disease. *Can Med Assoc J* 1976; 115:122–124.

42. McGuire DB. The measurement of clinical pain. *Nursing Res* 1976; 33:152–156.

43. Twycross RG. 1976. The measurement of pain in terminal cancer. *J Intl Med Res* 1976; 4(suppl 2):58–67.

44. Scott J, Huskisson E. Graphic representation of pain. *Pain* 1976; 2:175–184.

45. Ahles TA, Ruckdeschel JC, Blanchard EB. Cancer-related pain, II: assessment with visual analogue scales. *J Psychosom Res* 1984; 28:121–124.

46. Melzack R. The McGill pain questionnaire: major properties and scoring methods. *Pain* 1975; 1:277–299.

47. Melzack R, Mount BM, Gordon JM. The Brompton mixture versus morphine solution given orally: effects on pain. *Can Med Assoc J* 1979; 120:435–438.

48. Twycross RG. Clinical experience with diamorphine in advanced malignant disease. *Int J Clin Pharmacol* 1974; 9:184–198.

49. Twycross RG, Lack SA. *Symptom Control in Far Advanced Cancer: Pain Relief*. London: Pitman; 1983:226.

50. Porter J, Jick H. Addiction rare in patients treated with narcotics. *New Engl J Med* 1980; 302:123.

51. Evans PJD. Narcotic addiction in patients with chronic pain. *Anesthesia* 1981; 36:597–602.

52. Payne R, Foley KM. Advances in the management of cancer pain. *Cancer Treat Rep* 1984; 68:173–183.

53. Burney WE, Pert CB, Klee W, et al. Basic and clinical studies of endorphins. *Ann Intern Med* 1979; 91:239–250.

54. Hill RG. Endogenous opioids: a review. *J R Soc Med* 1981; 74:448–450.

55. Expert Committe on Drug Dependence. *WHO Tech Rep Ser* 1979; 16(407).

56. Twycross RG, Lack SA. *Symptom Control in Far Advanced Cancer: Pain Relief*. London: Pitman; 1983:253.

57. Twycross RG, Lack SA. *Symptom Control in Far Advanced Cancer: Pain Relief*. London: Pitman; 1983:305.

58. Twycross RG, Lack SA. *Symptom Control in Far Advanced Cancer: Pain Relief*. London: Pitman; 1983:167.

59. Houde RW, Wallenstein SL, Beaver WT. Clinical

measurement of pain. In: de Stevens G, ed. *Analgetics.* New York: Academic Press; 1965:75.

60. Taddeini L, Rotschafer JC. Pain syndromes associated with cancer. Achieving effective relief. *Postgrad Med* 1984; 75:101–108.

61. McGivney WT, Crocks GM. The care of patients with severe chronic pain in terminal illness. *JAMA* 1984; 251:1182–1188.

62. Murphy DH. Update: Relieving the pain of cancer. *Am Pharm* 1984; 24:66–71.

63. Gilman AG, Goodman LS, Gilman A, eds. *Goodman and Gilman's The Pharmacological Basis of Therapeutics.* 6th ed. New York: Macmillan 1980:509.

64. Lewis BJ. Management of pain: Pharmacologic approaches. In: DeVita VT, Hellman S, Rosenberg SA, eds. *Cancer. Principles and Practice of Oncology.* Philadelphia: Lippincott; 1982:1659.

65. Posner JB. Pain. In: Wyngarden JB, Smith LH, eds. *Cecil Textbook of Medicine.* Philadelphia: Saunders; 1982:1945.

66. Kaiko RF. IM/PO morphine equivalency: ⅓ vs ⅙, an apparent contradiction. The 1984 International Symposium on Pain Control. Toronto: Perdue Frederick Co; 1984:17. Abstract.

67. Vallnar JJ, Stewart JT, Kotzan JA, et al. Pharmacokinetics and bioavailability of hydromorphine following intravenous and oral administration to human subjects. *J Clin Pharmacol* 1981; 21:152–156.

68. Twycross RG, Lack SA. *Symptom Control in Far Advanced Cancer: Pain Relief.* London: Pitman; 1983:240.

69. Stambaugh JE, Lane C. Analgesic efficiency and pharmacokinetic evaluation of meperidine and hydroxyzine alone and in combination. *Cancer Invest* 1983; 1:111–117.

70. Szeto HH, Intrurrisi CE, Houde RW, et al. Accumulation of normeperidine, an active metabolite of meperidine in patients with renal failure of cancer. *Ann Intern Med* 1977; 86:738–741.

71. Twycross RG, Lack SA. *Symptom Control in Far Advanced Cancer: Pain Relief.* London: Pitman; 1983:151.

72. Moertal CG, Ahmann DL, Taylor WF, et al. A comparative evaluation of marketed analgesic drugs. *New Engl J Med* 1972; 286:813–815.

73. Moertal CG, Ahmann DL, Taylor WF, et al. Relief of pain by oral medication. A controlled evaluation of analgesic combinations. *JAMA* 1977; 229:55–59.

74. Shimm DS, Logue GL, Maltbie AA, et al. Medical management of chronic cancer pain. *JAMA* 1979; 241:2408–2412.

75. Moertal CG. Treatment of cancer pain with orally administered medication. *JAMA* 1972; 244:2448–2450.

76. Foley KM. The practical use of narcotic analgesics. *Med Clin North Am* 1982; 66:1091–1104.

77. Hopkinson JH. Vicodin, a new analgesic: clinical evaluation of efficacy and safety of repeated doses. *Curr Ther Res* 1978; 24:633–645.

78. Twycross RG, Lack SA. *Symptom Control in Far Advanced Cancer: Pain Relief.* London: Pitman; 1983:261.

79. Homesley HD. Dosing range study of controlled-release morphine in patients with chronic pain. Presented at the Seventh Annual Meeting of the Society of Memorial Gynecologic Oncologists; October 13, 1984; St. Louis, MO.

80. Henriksen H, Knudsen J. MST Continus tablets in pain of advanced cancer: a controlled study. In: Wilkes E, ed. *Advances in Morphine Therapy.* London: The Royal Society of Medicine; 1984:123.

81. Walsh TD. A controlled study of MST Continus tablets for chronic pain in advanced cancer. In: Wilkes E, ed. *Advances in Morphine Therapy.* London: The Royal Society of Medicine; 1984:99.

82. Hanks GW, Twycross RG, Bliss JM. Controlled release morphine tablets: a double-blind trial in patients with advanced cancer. *Anaesthesia* 1987; 42:840–844.

83. Homesley HD, Welander CE, Muss HB, Richards F. Dosage range study of morphine sulfate controlled-release. *Am J Clin Oncol* 1986; 9:449–453.

84. Brescia FJ, Walsh M, Savarese JJ, Kaiko RF. A study of controlled-release oral morphine (MS Contin) in an advanced cancer hospital. *J Pain Symptom Manage* 1987; 2:193–198.

85. Portenoy RK, Maldonado M, Fitzmartin R, Kaiko RF, Kanner R. Oral controlled-release morphine sulfate. Analgesic efficacy and side effects of a 100-mg tablet in cancer pain patients. *Cancer* 1989; 63:2284–2288.

86. Twycross RG, Lack SA. *Symptom Control in Far Advanced Cancer: Pain Relief.* London: Pitman; 1983:156.

87. Cooper SA. Comparative analgesic efficacies of aspirin and acetaminophen. *Arch Intern Med* 1981; 141:282–285.

88. Hollister L. Perspectives and summation of symposium. *Arch Intern Med* 1981; 141:404–406.

89. Goldfrank L, Weisman R. The minor analgesic overdose: salicylates and acetaminophen. *Heart Lung* 1983; 12:215–222.

90. Stambaugh JE. Analgesic equivalence of Tylox and Percodan: double blind crossover study of patients with pain from malignancy. *Curr Ther Res* 1980; 27:302–308.

91. Twycross RG, Lack SA: *Symptom Control in Far Advanced Cancer: Pain Relief.* London: Pitman; 1983:244.

92. Ettinger DS, Vitale PJ, Trump DL. Important clinical pharmacologic considerations in the use of methadone in cancer patients. *Cancer Treat Rep* 1979; 63:457–459.

93. Paalzow L, Nilsson L, Stenberg P. Pharmacokinetic basis for optimal methadone treatment of pain in cancer patients. *Acta Anesthesiol Scand* 1984; 76(suppl 74):55–58.

94. Citron ML. How would you treat . . . narcotic overdoses in cancer patients. *Drug Therapy* 1984; 9:85–90.

95. Maxwell MB. How to use methadone for the cancer patient's pain. *Am J Nurs* 1980; 80:1606–1609.

96. Hansen J, Ginman C, Hartvig P, et al. Clinical evaluation of oral methadone in treatment of cancer pain. *Acta Anesthiol Scand* 1982; 76 (suppl 74):124–127.

97. Twycross RG, Lack SA. *Symptom Control in Far Advanced Cancer: Pain Relief.* London: Pitman; 1983:190.

98. Twycross RG, Lack SA. *Symptom Control in Far Advanced Cancer: Pain Relief.* London: Pitman; 1983:200.

99. Forest WH, Brown BW, Brown CR, et al. Dextroamphetamine with morphine for the treatment of postoperative pain. *N Engl J Med* 1983; 296:712–715.

100. Bourke DL, Allen PD, Rosenberg M, et al. Dextroamphetamine with morphine: respiratory effects. *J Clin Pharmacol* 1983; 23:65–70.

101. Brandt EN. Heroin for the relief of pain. *N Engl J Med* 1984; 311:1634.

102. Monzac AM. Heroin for the relief of pain. *N Engl J Med* 1984; 311:1634.

103. Agnell M. Should heroin be legalized for the treatment of pain? *N Engl J Med* 1984; 311:529–530.

104. Brandt EN. Compassionate pain relief: is heroin the answer? *N Engl J Med* 1984; 311:530–532.

105. Monzac AM. In defense of the reintroduction of heroin into American medical practice and H.R. 5920—The Compassionate Pain Relief Act. *N Engl J Med* 1984; 311:532–535.

106. Houde RW, Wallenstein SL, Beaver WT, et al. Analgesic studies at the Sloan-Kettering Institute for Cancer Research. In: *Proceeding of the 31st Meeting of the NAS-NRC Committee on Problems of Drug Dependence*. Washington, DC: National Academy of Sciences; 1969:5900.

107. Twycross RG, Lack SA. *Symptom Control in Far Advanced Cancer: Pain Relief*. London: Pitman; 1983:250.

108. Roy SD, Flynn GL. Transdermal delivery of narcotic analgesics: pH, anatomical, and subject influences on cutaneous permeability of fentanyl and sufentanil. *Pharmacol Res* August 1990; 7(8):842–847.

109. McCaffery M. How to relieve your patients pain fast and effectively with oral analgesics. *Nursing* 1980; 80 10:58–63.

110. Salkind GD, Angeluicci AJ. Treatment for pain in terminal illness. *JAMA* 1984; 252:1410.

111. Pannuti F, Rossi AP, Iafelice G, et al. Control of chronic pain in very advanced cancer patients with morphine hydrochloride administered by oral, rectal, and sublingual route. Clinical report and preliminary results on morphine pharmacokinetics. *Pharmacol Res Commun* 1982; 14:369–380.

112. Ellison NM, Lewis GO. A pharmacokinetic comparison of rectal morphine sulfate (RMS) suppositories and oral morphine sulfate (OMS) solution. *Proc Am Soc Clin Oncol* 1984; 3:89.

113. Berry JI. Pharmacy services in hospice organizations. *Hospital Formulary* 1982; 17:1333–1338.

114. Kaiko RF, Cronin C, Healey N, Pav J, Thomas G, Goldenheim PD. Bioavailability of rectal and oral MS Contin. *Proc Am Soc Clin Oncol* 1989; 8:336.

115. Maloney CM, Kesner RK, Klein G, Bockenstette J. The rectal administration of MS Contin: clinical implications of use in end-stage cancer. *Am J Hospice Care* 1989; 6:34–35.

116. Whitman HH. Sublingual morphine: a novel route of narcotic administration. *PRN Forum* 1984; 3:1, 8.

117. Miser A, Davis DM, Hughes CS, et al. Continuous subcutaneous infusion of morphine in children with cancer. *Am J Dis Child* 1983; 137:383–385.

118. Campbell CF, Mason JB, Weiler JM. Continuous subcutaneous infusion of morphine for the pain of terminal malignancy. *Ann Intern Med* 1983; 98:51–52.

119. Nahata MC, Miser AW, Miser JS, et al. Analgesic plasma concentrations of morphine in children with terminal malignancy receiving a continuous subcutaneous infusion of morphine sulfate to control severe pain. *Pain* 1984; 18:109–114.

120. Miser AW, Miser JS, Clark BS. Continuous intravenous infusion of morphine sulfate for control of severe pain in children with terminal malignancy. *J Pediatr* 1982; 96:930–932.

121. Boyer MW. Continuous drip morphine. Titrating IV morphine. *Am J Nurs* 1982; 82:602–604.

122. Burnakis T. Treatment of severe chronic pain by continuous parenteral infusion of morphine. *Hospital Pharm* 1983; 18:618–624.

123. Citron ML, Johnston-Early A, Fossiede BF, et al. Safety and efficacy of continuous intravenous morphine for severe cancer pain. *Am J Med* 1984; 77:199–204.

124. Adams JD, Diehl LF, Wilson JP. Ambulatory use of high-dose intravenous morphine for severe pain. *Drug Intell Clin Pharm* 1984; 18:138–140.

125. Dennis EMP. An ambulatory infusion pump for pain control: a nursing approach for home care. *Cancer Nurs* 1989; 7:309–313.

126. Bennett RL, Batenhorst RL, Bivins BA, et al. Patient-controlled analgesia. A new concept of postoperative pain relief. *Ann Surg* 1982; 195:700–705.

127. Graves DA, Foster TS, Batenhorst RL, et al. Patient-controlled analgesia. *Ann Intern Med* 1983; 99:360–366.

128. Twycross RG, Lack SA. *Symptom Control in Far Advanced Cancer: Pain Relief*. London: Pitman; 1983:176.

129. Ruden RA. Prevention of opiate induced constipation. *Curr Concepts Perspect Nutr* 1983; 2:1–6.

130. Izard MW, Ellison FS. Treatment of drug induced constipation with a purified senna derivative. *Conn Med* 1962; 26:589–592.

131. Maquire LC, Yon JL, Miller E. Prevention of narcotic-induced constipation. *N Engl J Med* 1981; 305:1651.

132. McGee JL, Alexander MR. 1979. Phenothiazine analgesia—fact or fantasy. *Am J Hosp Pharm* 36:633–640.

133. Walsh TD. Opiates and respiratory function in advanced cancer. *Recent Results Cancer Res* 1984; 89:115–117.

134. Twycross RG, Lack SA. *Symptom Control in Far Advanced Cancer: Pain Relief*. London: Pitman; 1983:179.

135. Twycross RG, Lack SA. *Symptom Control in Far Advanced Cancer: Pain Relief*. London: Pitman; 1983:223.

136. Bradberry JC, Raebel MA. Continuous infusion of naloxone in the treatment of narcotic overdose. *Drug Intell Clin Pharm* 1981; 15:945–950.

137. Zucker MB, Rothwell KG. Differential influences of salicylates compounds on platelet aggregation and serotonin release. *Nebr Symp Motiv* 1978; 23:194–199.

138. Kantor TG. Ibuprofen. *Ann Intern Med* 1979; 91:877–882.

139. Miller RR. Evaluation of the analgesic efficacy of ibuprofen. *Pharmacotherapy* 1981; 1:21–27.

140. Brodgen RN, Heel RC, Spught TM, et al. Naproxen update: a review of its pharmacological properties and therapeutic efficacy and use in rheumatic diseases and pain. *Drugs* 1979; 18:241–277.

141. Morgan LR, McMillan JE, Donley PJ. Diflunisal (MK-647): its use as an analgesic in advanced cancer. A feasibility study. *Clin Res* 1980; 28:590A.

142. Carratelli C. New system analgesia in treatment of cancer pain. *Gerontologia* 1981; 29:271–274.

143. Reasbeck PG, Rice ML, Reasbeck JC. Double blind controlled trial of indomethacin as an adjunct to narcotic analgesia after major abdominal surgery. *Lancet* 1982; 2:115–118.

144. Scott DL. Prescribing nonsteroidal anti-inflammatory drugs: a prospective study of patients' preference. *Postgrad Med J* 1982; 58:146–148.

145. Clinch D. Banerjee AK, Ostick G, et al. Non-steroidal anti-inflammatory drugs and gastrointestinal adverse effects. *J R Coll Physicians Lond* 1983; 17:228–230.

146. Guitin PH. Corticosteroid therapy in patients with brain tumor. *Natl Cancer Inst Monogr* 1977; 46:151–156.

147. Quandt CM, de los Reyes RA. Pharmacologic management of acute intracranial hypertension. *Drug Intell Clin Pharm* 1984; 18:105–112.

148. Twycross RG, Lack SA. *Symptom Control in Far Advanced Cancer: Pain Relief*. London: Pitman; 1983:146.

149. Baines MJ. Control of other symptoms. In: Saunders CM, ed. *The Management of Terminal Disease*. London: Edward Arnold; 1978:99.

150. Twycross RG, Lack SA. *Symptom Control in Far Advanced Cancer: Pain Relief*. London: Pitman; 1983:220.

151. Twycross RG, Lack SA. *Symptom Control in Far Advanced Cancer: Pain Relief*. London: Pitman; 1983:271.

152. Weiss O, Sriwantanakul K, Weintraub M. Treatment of post herpetic neuralgia and acute herpetic pain with amitriptyline and perphenazine. *S Afr Med J* 1982; 62:274–275.

153. Raftery H. The management of postherpetic pain using sodium valproate and amitriptyline. *Ir Med J* 1979; 72:399–401.

154. Kernbaum S, Hauchecorne J. Administration of levodopa for relief of herpes zoster pain. *JAMA* 1981; 246:132–134.

155. Gerson GR, Jone RB, Luscombe DK. Studies on the concomitant use of carbamazepine and clomipramine for the relief of post herpetic neuralgia. *Postgrad Med J* 1977; 53 (suppl 4):104–109.

156. Walsh TD. Antidepressants in chronic pain. *Clin Neuropharmacol* 1983; 6:271–295.

157. France RD, Houpt JL, Ellinwood EH. Therapeutic effects of antidepressants in chronic pain. *Gen Hosp Pharm* 1984; 6:55–63.

158. Swerdlow M, Cundill JG. Anticonvulsant drugs used in the treatment of lancinating pain. A comparison. *Anaesthesia* 1981; 36:1129–1132.

159. Boraas MC. Palliative surgery. *Semin Oncol* 1985; 12:368–374.

160. Richter MP, Coia LR. Palliative radiation therapy. *Semin Oncol* 1985; 12:375–383.

161. Romond EH, Metcalfe MS, Macdonald JS. Palliative chemotherapy and hormonal therapy. *Semin Oncol* 1985; 12:384–393.

162. Ferrer-Brechner T. Anesthetic management of cancer pain. *Semin Oncol* 1985; 12:431–437.

163. Black P. Neurosurgical management of cancer pain. *Semin Oncol* 1985; 12:438–444.

164. Barber J, Gitelson J. Cancer pain. Psychological management using hypnosis. *CA* 1980; 30:130–136.

165. Spiegel D, Bloom JR. Group therapy and hypnosis reduce metastatic breast carcinoma pain. *Psychosom Med* 1983; 45:333–339.

166. Adler RH, Hemmeler W. Psychological treatment modalities for pain in cancer patients. *Recent Results Cancer Res* 1984; 89:195–200.

167. Health and Public Policy Committee, American College of Physicians. Drug therapy for severe, chronic pain in terminal illness. *Ann Intern Med* 1983; 99:870–873.

CHAPTER 18

Anesthetic Management of Cancer Pain

Mark Mehta and Ashley M. Duthie

"Nothing begins, nothing ends
That is not paid for with a moan.
For we are born in other's pain
And perish in our own."

In this quotation, Milton expressed a defeatist attitude to the problems of pain and suffering that, until recently, was accepted by both the medical profession and the general public. It engendered fear and apprehension at the prospect of old age and terminal illness. Considerable advance has been made in making childbirth safer and less painful, but comparable progress in the treatment of cancer pain has not been as well publicized, despite the pioneer work of Dame Cicely Saunders[1] and her many associates at St. Christopher's Hospice in London. Her contributions were mainly in recognizing the needs of these patients for pain relief using drugs. This is discussed in another chapter in this book (see Chap. 17). It is well known, however, that there are many other problems (such as physical, emotional, and spiritual) to be overcome when essential body mechanisms begin to fail.[2] A coordinated multidisciplinary approach is required, and in this context, an anesthesiologist has much to offer,[3] particularly in the control of pain, which features predominantly in most cases and disturbs the well-being and quality of the patient's remaining life.[4] It has been said with some justification that this is an area in which there have been sporadic, haphazard, and disconnected islands of treatment with many specialists vying with each other to provide different brands of individual expertise.[5] However, common sense dictates that it is really only a question of which method is the most appropriate and acceptable to the patient at the time. Table 18-1 lists techniques currently available for the relief of cancer pain, but in this chapter we will confine our attention to those areas in which the anesthesiologists' expertise is required. Anesthesiologists should recognize that analgesic and allied drugs provide excellent relief in most cases (see Chaps. 17 and 26). However, some of the techniques mentioned here may be required for the few patients whose pain cannot be controlled or in whom there are special reasons why this conservative approach cannot be used.

Table 18-1
Current Methods of Cancer Pain Relief

General Care	Physical, emotional, socioeconomic
Specific Measures	Radiotherapy, deep x-ray treatment Drugs: cytotoxic, hormonal, antibiotic Palliative surgery
Nonspecific Methods of Elevating Pain Threshold	Analgesic and allied drugs Psychotherapy and mental training Biofeedback and muscle relaxation
Neurolytic Blocks (Chemical Neurectomy)	Peripheral nerve blocks Spinal injections Autonomic blocks
Intraspinal Narcotics	Epidural, intrathecal
Radiofrequency Heat Lesions	Percutaneous cordotomy Dorsal root ganglion heat destruction
Cryoablation	Peripheral and central nervous blocks Pituitary ablation (Surgical, chemical, RF, cryoablation)
Neurosurgery	"Open" cordotomy, rhizotomy, myelotomy, thalamotomy, electric stimulation of brain and spinal cord
Noninvasive methods	Stimulation of inhibiting pain control

GENERAL CARE

Before discussing specific techniques, it is essential to have an overall view of the patient's needs and to respect individual wishes about proposed lines of treatment. Each method must be described in clear and simple terms, with a realistic but tactful appraisal of the advantages and a list of complications that may occur. Patients with advanced cancer are often too ill or distressed to take a rational view of their problems and sometimes persistently refuse advice that is given in their best interest. Elderly people, in particular, want to be left alone and are frightened by any form of invasive therapy. It is wrong to persuade them to accept treatment against their own inclinations.

Specific measures usually do not concern the anesthesiologist, but we should be aware of their benefits.[6]

Nonspecific methods are discussed in Chapter 17 and will provide excellent analgesia for most patients with cancer if used appropriately. A small number of patients, however, require other techniques.

NEUROLYTIC BLOCKS

Anesthesiologists, with their proficiency in regional anesthesia, favor this approach because all that is required is a syringe, a needle, and a suitable local anesthetic solution. When indicated, they should be administered early.[7] However, peripheral nerve blocks, even when repeated with a neurolytic agent (phenol or alcohol) play only a limited part in the relief of cancer pain. Their effects are unpredictable because large and small fibers are damaged; all aspects of nerve function may be disorganized.[8] Analgesia often is incomplete or of limited duration; the resulting numbness or paresthesia may be resented more than the original pain.[9]

Several neurolytic agents currently are available (see Chap. 28). A 6% aqueous phenol or absolute alcohol solution, accurately injected under radiographic control or with a block-aid monitor, commonly is used for this purpose. Ammonium sulfate 10% solution also may be used, but the injections are painful, and there is greater incidence of troublesome nerve damage. All these agents may spread into surrounding tissues, causing irritation or even necrosis, but this risk can be minimized by injecting not more than 1.0 ml at any one site and clearing the needle before withdrawal using air from an empty syringe.

Prolonged analgesia can be achieved better with injections into the spinal canal.[10] Intrathecal spinal injection for cancer pain (so-called chemical neurectomy) was introduced by Maher[11] as a simple method to be done at the bedside. However, even with meticulous technique, there is considerable risk of disabling neurologic complications, particularly incontinence, after paralysis of the rectal and bladder sphincters. Generally, it is agreed that the procedure can be done better in a hospital, with radiographic monitoring to check the accuracy of the needle positioning and the flow of the neurolytic mixture into the spinal canal.[10,12] The needle is inserted at the level of the most painful segment, with the painful side uppermost for alcohol and downward for phenol 5% in glycerin (see Appendix A.XII). It is advanced until spinal fluid emerges from the hub, and the needle then is withdrawn gradually until the flow almost stops, when the tip will be just inside the subarachnoid space. Not more than 0.5 ml of phenol

5% in glycerin or alcohol should be injected at any one site, and the operating table should be tilted head down if the solution drifts caudally toward the sacral nerve roots. In this way, there is less likely to be damage to the nerves supplying the sphincters of the bladder and rectum. Backward rotation for phenol or forward rotation for alcohol then is maintained for 0.5 h. This is the basic technique for the lumbar region. Further details regarding injections for pain in other areas are available elsewhere[12–15] (see Chap. 28). Both alcohol and phenol have their advocates, but in our experience, it is more important to be familiar with one agent and the radiologic appearance of the injection when approximately 0.1 to 0.2 ml of absorbable contrast medium is added to the solution.[16]

Similarly there are those who prefer extradural injections, but the solution diffuses widely in this space (see Chap. 28). There is much to be said for the more accurate intrathecal approach with a small volume of the neurolytic agent; this can be repeated on another occasion if the need arises.

Extraarachnoid subdural block is indicated for cervical and upper dorsal root pain, but the technique is difficult and x-ray screening is mandatory.[17,18] Critics of this approach cite the difficulty of ensuring adequate exposure of a sufficient length of the nerve roots to the neurolytic agent because their course in the spinal canal is so short. This is a reasonable comment, but it must be realized that cancer pain in the cervical and upper dorsal region often is severe and may not be controlled even with large doses of potent narcotics. Intraspinal or intraventricular narcotics may be an answer to this dilemma and will be considered in the next section of this chapter and in Chapter 27..

Opinions on the value of chemical neurectomy vary markedly in different centers, and readers are advised to reach their own conclusions only after perusing some of the excellent reviews on this subject.[8,14,19,20] In general, most anesthesiologists would include intrathecal chemical neurectomy in their armamentarium for relief of cancer pain that is severe and localized to a few segments. With small volumes of phenol or alcohol and careful monitoring, the risk of complications is minimized. Better pain control with a steady reduction in analgesic drug requirement is achieved if only two or three segments are treated, and the procedure is repeated on subsequent occasions.

We have only considered somatic nerve blockade. Chemical sympathectomy by neurolytic injection has been a reliable alternative to surgery in many cases, particularly for the elderly or debilitated patient or those with advanced cancer.[20] These techniques are well described elsewhere[9,10,14,21–24] as are the complications.[25] Our comments therefore will be limited in this section to some points of special relevance to clinical practice.

Celiac plexus block (see Appendix A.III) is a useful procedure for upper abdominal cancer pain, particularly of the pancreas.[26–28] It should be done at an early stage, either perioperatively or soon after the laparotomy if severe pain is the main symptom. After the pain is established, the results are poor. The patient's life expectancy is short, and the tumor extends rapidly into neighboring tissues, such as the peritoneum. It may disseminate widely as metastases that are beyond local treatment. X-ray monitoring and, more recently CT scanning, are necessary for accurate placement of the neurolytic solution. Another useful aid to recognizing the celiac plexus is a metal clip left in situ at the original operation. Alcohol is the most popular neurolytic solution, and it is injected only after relief has been obtained with a preliminary diagnostic block. The volume of solution required varies depending on the spread in the retroperitoneal space. The addition of a small amount of contrast medium facilitates this manever and, on occasion, as little as 10 to 15 ml of alcohol 50% is enough to cover the entire plexus.[10] A new transaortic approach has been described using contrast-enhanced CT scans, and further results are awaited with great interest.[29]

Some of the side effects of celiac plexus ablation result from parasympathetic blockade. These may be avoided by substituting the procedure of splanchnic neurectomy. In this, the greater, lesser, and least splanchnic nerves are destroyed by neurolytic injection at the level of T12.[30]

Just as celiac plexus blockade may be a useful treatment for upper abdominal visceral pain, hypogastric plexus blockade at the L5,S1 interspace may be a useful therapy for pain associated with pelvic visceral cancers.[31]

Lumbar sympathectomy (see Appendix A.II) is a relatively easy procedure commonly used for ischemic pain in the lower limb, but it seldom is required for inoperable cancer. Stellate ganglion block (see Appendix A.I) occasionally is required for pain in the head and neck or upper limbs. Smith's anterior tissue displacement technique is recommended.[32] X-ray screening is essential to ensure spread in the pretracheal fascial plane and avoid lateral extension into the brachial plexus. Not more than 3 ml of neurolytic solution, with added contrast medium, should be used. Because of the risks associated with the spread of neurolytic agents to adjacent structures, many practitioners prefer surgical sympathectomy.

INTRASPINAL NARCOTICS (See Chap. 27)

Continuous or intermittent administration of spinal narcotics increasingly is being applied to pain control in advanced malignancy.[33-38] The advantage of this approach is effective analgesia using a smaller dose than would be required systemically with minimal complications.[39,40] The pain relief lasts longer than injections of conventional local anesthetics, without significant changes in the sympathetic outflow or alterations in sensation and motor power.[41,42] However, Bromage and associates[43] showed that minor alterations do occur in these basic functions, but it requires close scrutiny to discover them. The pharmacodynamics of this technique have been reviewed extensively.[44] Fortunately, serious complications have been infrequent. Neverthe-

less, initial enthusiasm has been tempered by occasional, but disturbing, reports of central depression several hours after the initial injection, particularly when the narcotic used was highly water soluble. It is wise to monitor these patients, certainly in the initial stages, carefully.[45] Respiratory depression caused by the opiates administered can be reversed by prompt administration of intravenous naloxone. Pruritus, nausea, and urinary retention are less serious, but troublesome, side effects when they occur. Neurotoxicity, with clinically unsuspected posterior column degeneration, is another possibility. However, a recent review of autopsy findings in seven patients who received prolonged intraspinal opiate administration suggests these changes are more likely caused by the malignant disease than the pain-relieving technique.[46]

On balance, increasing clinical experience confirms that this is a useful advance in the treatment of cancer pain.[47-49] In this group of patients, there is no entirely safe method, and careful vigilance is recommended in every case.[50] Continuous infusion seems to be preferable to intermittent bolus administration, and the morphine solution is prepared without preservatives that may have a deleterious neurolytic effect. The reservoirs are implanted subcutaneously (see Appendix A.VIII) and refilled by periodic injection of the analgesic solution.[51,52] Unfortunately, the apparatus is expensive and can be used for only the one patient.[53] Suitable alternatives are externally worn devices such as the Act-A-Pump (Pharmacia, Piscataway, NJ).[54,55] It is advisable to assess the patients' drug requirements in the hospital, but treatment may be continued with outpatient supervision.[56] Intrathecal somatostatin, a neurotransmitter concerned with pain mechanisms in the dorsal horn of the spinal cord, may be a more effective alternative to morphine and fentanyl, but experience with this agent is limited currently.[57] Other agents that act at different spinal receptor sites are being considered. They include the enkephalins, clonidine,[58-60] and calcitonin.[61] Further information is awaited with interest. Recently, the long-term infusion intraspinally of morphine and bupivacaine has been advocated.[62,63] In the terminal stages of disease, infusions of local anesthetics alone through the epidural, brachial plexus, or interpleural route[64] may be appropriate.

RADIOFREQUENCY HEAT LESIONS

Destruction of the pain-conducting pathways using high-frequency current is more desirable than neurolytic injection because a small, controllable, and consistent lesion can be produced.[65] The electrode can be positioned accurately under the x-ray screen, and its correct placement can be confirmed by the patient's response to electrostimulation. The extent of thermocoagulation is regulated by fine control of the temperature at the electrode tip; in turn, this depends on the output of the lesion generator. The destruction can be confined to the target area, and there is minimal risk to important structures in the neighboring areas. For cancer pain, two techniques should be considered, percutaneous cordotomy and rhizotomy. Percutaneous cordotomy is a useful procedure, particularly for the patient with cancer and severe unilateral pain.[66] It requires a great deal of patience and technical skill, but it is safe if the guidelines for needle positioning and control of the electrical output are observed carefully. Any deviation from these basic rules can lead to serious complications.[67] Nevertheless, good pain relief without untoward effects can be expected in approximately 60 percent of cases; marked improvement with significant reduction in analgesic drug requirements are noted in another 16.5 percent.[68] The percutaneous method is done by some anesthesiologists and is preferable to the open operation in most cases. However, this does require a reasonably stoic and cooperative patient who will report accurately any sensory changes after the preliminary electrostimulation to allow the operator to regulate the extent of the lesion without causing serious damage. It avoids the need for a prolonged general anesthetic and the stress of a major operation. However, the indications for cordotomy have declined sharply in recent years with better drug administration programs and considerable improvements in chemotherapy and radiotherapy. Intraspinal narcotics, with an implanted catheter and refillable subcutaneous reservoirs, may be a more satisfactory alternative.

Technical details are important in cordotomy.[69] In general, a 2-mm exposed tip is relatively safe because it minimizes the possibility of creating too large a lesion and finer adjustment is possible by regulating the output of the RF generator. The dentate ligament must be outlined beyond any doubt. For this purpose, 2 ml of metrizamide or iophendylate emulsified in normal saline or cerebrospinal fluid is satisfactory. The position of the needle point in front of this ligament then is demonstrable radiologically and can be confirmed by electrostimulation. Parameters for motor and sensory tests vary considerably with each machine. A good position is indicated by tingling, temperature changes, or paresthesia in the appropriate anatomic distribution at currents of less than 0.5 V. A greater current suggests the needle point is close but not exactly in the correct place.[70] Neck twitching indicates placement too far anteriorly. A limb motor response means the needle must be withdrawn because it is in the motor tract. After these preliminary tests have been completed satisfactorily, a permanent lesion is made. This is best done by a series of small burns, each of 30-s duration with gradually increasing amperage starting at 30 mA. After each burn, careful clinical examination of motor and sensory function is undertaken. If there is any suspicion of motor weakness, the procedure must stop. The operation can be repeated later or expert neurosurgical advice sought.[71]

Careful selection of patients to be treated is important. Particular emphasis should be placed on the intensity and duration of the pain, the temperament and personality of the patient, and the success or failure of other less invasive means of symptomatic control. Cordotomy is indicated if the patient has severe pain and is likely to survive for more than 6 months.[67,70] The best results are obtained with unilateral leg pain, commonly caused by sarcoma or cancer of the uterus. Treatment of upper leg pain is not as satisfactory, and any muscle weakness may be resented more than the pain. Rectal and bladder tumors rapidly cause bilateral symptoms. Lung cancer already may have caused severe respiratory problems that are likely to get worse after cordotomy. Damage to respiratory fibers is a well-known hazard and precludes the use of this technique, except in experienced hands, for bilateral pain.[72] However, the most common complication is dysesthesia; this occurs in approximately 40 percent of patients, but only one-tenth of these complain of significant discomfort.[70]

Percutaneous rhizotomy or applying radiofrequency electricity to the dorsal root ganglion, is a technique originally devised by Uematsu and associates[73] that was modified in recent years[74] for the treatment of intractable back and neck pain. Pain-conducting fibers are destroyed selectively without jeopardizing large sensory and motor nerves. Like cordotomy, the procedure is conducted mainly under local anesthesia with radiographic monitoring and electrostimulation tests to confirm the accuracy of needle placement. There is a lower incidence of unpleasant dysesthesia, and the method is suitable particularly for pain of limited distribution in elderly and debilitated patients. Unfortunately, the results are unpredictable, possibly as a result of the considerable overlap by nerves above and below the pain segment and the presence of pain fibers in the anterior nerve root. The indications for cancer pain therefore are limited to individual nerve roots in the thoracic and cervical region and for persistent perineal pain that does not respond to any other method.[75]

CRYOABLATION

Freezing a peripheral nerve interrupts the flow of pain impulses but does not alter the gross normal morphology of this structure.[76] Complete return of nerve function is assured within 12 weeks and, at no time, is there any evidence of sensory loss or muscle weakness from this technique.[77] The duration of pain relief is variable, but in a small proportion of cases, it has lasted more than 1 year. The technique is easy to do and can be repeated when required. The cryoprobe is a 12-, 14-, or 18-gauge stainless-steel needle, but different lengths and gauges are available for special cases. The tip of the probe may be used to carry a 100-Hz current to localize the position of the target. For pain relief, it is usual to administer two freezing cycles each at −60°C for 2 min, followed by a pause of 60-s duration. The analgesia is almost immediate and unaccompanied by neuroma formation. The limitations of this method are the variable duration of analgesia and the possibility of secondary infection from a persistent sinus in the track of the frozen tissue. This complication is minimized by observing strict asepsis during the procedure, introducing the instrument through a sterile polythene cannula, and using the new reversed-flow probes.

Cryoanalgesia is a satisfactory alternative to the neurolytic injections of phenol or alcohol that often produce disappointing results from incomplete nerve destruction.[78] Intraneural scarring may be responsible for secondary neuralgia. However, in cancer pain, peripheral nerve block is of limited use, and interruption of the pain-conducting pathways needs to be done at a more central level in the brain or spinal cord where use of a cryoprobe may be impracticable. Modification of this technique for pituitary destruction is described in the next section.

HYPOPHYSECTOMY

There is considerable evidence to show that destruction of the pituitary gland is followed by significant pain relief in 60 percent to 70 percent of patients with advanced cancer.[79–83] In some, there is also tumor regression, but these two effects are not necessarily related. The most favorable outcome is likely when the tumor is hormone dependent, commonly, those in the breast and prostate gland. However, there also have been good results when the pain is caused by other forms of cancer, but tumor regression is unlikely.[84] Some, but not all, patients have almost immediate relief, and the improvement is maintained (usually for 3 to 4 months), although, on occasion, this has extended for more than 1 year.

Surgical hypophysectomy by the transcranial or transphenoidal route almost certainly achieves more complete ablation of anterior pituitary function, but there is considerable debate as to whether such extensive destruction is necessary.[85] Excellent pain relief was obtained in more than 90 percent of patients in one study, figures that have not been matched by others who have, with minor modifications, used the same method.[86–88] The spread of a potent neurolytic agent in the brainstem has deterred many less intrepid operators. Better control is obtained with radiofrequency thermal lesions[89] and cryoablation of the pituitary gland using an x-ray image intensifier.[90,91] Radium implants, with computer-assisted estimation of the dose, may be another excellent method. Overall, however, in terms of efficacy, there seems to be little to choose between these different techniques.

The mechanism of pain relief in these patients is still uncertain.[92] The degree and duration of pain relief do not correlate with the extent of pituitary and hypothalamic damage or with the suppression of their hormonal influence. Transient elevations in blood and cerebrospinal fluid levels of corticotropin and α-endorphin have been observed, but these are not maintained. The pain relief immediately after the operation is not consistent with an endocrine mechanism. X-ray studies after alcohol injection show spreading from the pituitary stalk into the hypothalamus and then into the third ventricle, but the significance of these observations has not been understood fully.[93] However, it is established that pain relief occurs with all the different techniques described.

Anesthesiologists are concerned mainly with using alcohol injection or cryoablation, and a few points of practical importance are stressed for their guidance. No particular preoperative preparation is required, except to administer a vasoconstrictive agent to the nasal mucosa to minimize bleeding.[94] Some prefer antibiotic coverage after nasal culture, particularly if there is evidence of a sinus infection. Although chemical hypophysectomy often is conducted under local anesthesia to observe the pupillary reaction, the procedure is an ordeal for the patient, and most people prefer full general anesthesia. The actual technique is not difficult if the needle and cannula or cryoprobe are advanced into the fossa just above its base within 5 mm of the midline to avoid puncture of the carotid artery or cavernous sinus. The position of the needle is checked carefully in anteroposterior and lateral planes of the x-ray image intensifier. If profuse bleeding occurs, the nose is packed firmly with ribbon gauze containing bismuth and iodine paste or suitable alternative, but this seldom is a problem. Cerebrospinal fluid rhinorrhea is not uncommon and may distress the patient, but it usually resolves spontaneously within 48 h. Appropriate antibiotic coverage is necessary during this period. Although it has not occurred in our experience, a persistent leak can be cured by inserting a silicone plug or surgical repair with a graft of fascia lata. Hormone replacement therapy usually consists of hydrocortisone 200 mg daily that is reduced gradually over 1 to 2 weeks. Thyroid extract (60 mg) also may be given if required. Diabetes insipidus occurs in some patients 2 or 3 days after the operation; it usually subsides in 1 to 2 weeks. Replacement desmopressin nasal spray may be necessary if this complication persists. It is helpful to consult a competent endocrinologist on this and other matters. A much lower incidence of complications has been reported after pituitary cryoablation than occurs after chemical hypophysectomy.[91]

In conclusion, destruction of the pituitary gland is a useful method of controlling severe pain in the head and neck and bilateral pains that are difficult to manage with other techniques.

NEUROSURGERY

Neurosurgical procedures include open cordotomy and hypophysectomy and the destruction or stimulation of peripheral nerves, spinal cord, brainstem, or hypothalamus (see Chap. 35).

NONINVASIVE METHODS

Melzack and Wall, in their gate theory, cited the value of diminishing pain by selective stimulation of inhibitory pathways in the descending columns of the spinal cord and the large lightly myelinated nerve fibers.[98] They coined the term *hyperstimulation analgesia* to explain the paradox of generating mild discomfort to relieve more severe pain.[95] In its simplest form, this is exemplified by vigorous rubbing, massage, counterirritation, and local applications of extreme heat and cold. At the other end of the scale are acupuncture and electrical stimulation. Nerve fatigue by repetitive stimulation and electromagnetism are still in the experimental stage.[96] Peripheral nerve stimulation (TENS) is the most common mode of inhibitory pain control and has been used by clinicians in many different situations.[97] It is particularly useful for pain of mild or moderate intensity emanating from musculoskeletal disorders and peripheral nerve injuries. The technique is relatively inexpensive, has no serious side effects, and allows patients to control their own symptoms. In early cancer pain, TENS may be a useful alternative to potent drugs in a comprehensive treatment program.[98] However, generally it is agreed that it is not ubiquitous in its action nor a panacea for all ills. Success depends on accurate diagnosis, careful psychosocial evaluation, and prior attention to related problems, notably anxiety and depression. The patients must understand the technique, its limitations, and the need to persevere before the full effects are apparent. Those patients whose pain is predominantly psychosomatic or who are addicted to narcotic analgesics are unlikely to benefit.[99] After preliminary screening, each patient participates in a trial of electric stimulation supervised by experienced personnel. Treatment for several weeks is recommended before reassessing the situation and deciding if it is worth continuing. With cancer pain, there may be a need for reinforcement with psychotropic or nonnarcotic analgesic agents. The same approach is recommended for acupuncture.[100,101] Intracranial stimulation of deep brain structures is not recommended for cancer pain unless no alternative approach is available, a rare situation.[102] In general, stimulation techniques have a more limited role in this field than in the relief of nonmalignant pain.

CONCLUSION

Many skills are required to control severe cancer pain, but these should be exercised in a multidisciplinary approach in which anesthesiologists play a significant role. However, courtesy, kindness, and consideration for each patient as an individual are essential ingredients that must be combined with technical competence to achieve good results. Patients with terminal cancer no longer need to endure prolonged suffering and unrelieved pain. Professor Hinton's[103] wise observations provide a fitting end to this chapter.

> "If doctors and nurses set out to relieve discomfort with sincerity and competence, their intention alone brings ease."

References

1. Saunders C, ed. *The Management of Terminal Disease.* London: Edward Arnold; 1978.

2. Twycross RG, ed. *Pain Relief in Cancer. Clinics in Oncology.* Vol. 3, no. 1. Philadelphia: Saunders; 1984.

3. Ferrer-Brechner T. Anesthetic techniques for the management of cancer pain. *Cancer* June 1, 1989; 63(suppl 11):2343–2347.

4. Evans WO. Antitumor, nerve blocks and neuroablative therapies for cancer pain. *Indiana Med* June 1989; 82(6):446–448.

5. Mehta M. *Intractable Pain. Major Problems in Anaesthesia.* Vol. 2. Philadelphia: Saunders; 1973.

6. Foley KM. Treatment of cancer pain. *N Engl J Med* 1985; 313(2):84–95.

7. Lipton S. Pain relief in active patients with cancer: the early use of nerve block improves the quality of life. *BMJ* January 7, 1989; 298:37–38.

8. Wood KM. Peripheral nerve and root chemical lesions. In: Wall PD, Melzack R, eds. *Textbook of Pain.* New York: Churchill Livingstone; 1984:577–580.

9. Cousins MJ, Bridenbaugh PO, eds. *Neural Blockade in Clinical Anesthesia and Management of Pain.* Philadelphia: Lippincott; 1980.

10. Mehta M. Improvements in spinal injection treatment for cancer pain. In: Lipton S, Miles J, eds. *Persistent Pain: Modern Methods of Treatment, II.* New York: Academic Press; 1981:265–278.

11. Maher RM. Relief of pain in incurable cancer. *Lancet* 1955; 1:18.

12. Maher RM, Mehta M. Spinal (intrathecal) and extradural analgesia. In: Lipton S, Miles J, eds. *Persistent Pain: Modern Methods of Treatment, I.* New York: Academic Press; 1977:61–100.

13. Ferrer-Brechner T. Epidural and intrathecal phenol neurolysis for cancer pain. *Anesthesiol Rev* 1981; 8(8):14–20.

14. Swerdlow M. Subarachnoid and extradural neurolytic blocks. In: Bonica JJ, Ventafridda V, eds. *Advances in Pain Research and Therapy.* Vol. 2. New York: Raven Press; 1979:325–337.

15. Hay RC. Subarachnoid alcohol block. *Anesth Analg* 1962; 41:12–16.

16. Mehta M, Salmon N. Extradural block. Confirmation of the injection site by X-ray monitoring. *Anaesthesia* 1985; 40:1009–1012.

17. Mehta M, Maher RM. Injections into the extraarachnoid subdural space. *Anaesthesia* 1977; 32:760–766.

18. Ischia S, Luzzani A, Ischia A, Faggian S. Subdural–arachnoid neurolytic block in cervical pain. *Pain* 1982; 14:347–354.

19. Papo I, Visca A. Phenol subarachnoid rhizotomy for the treatment of cancer pain: a personal account of 290 cases. In: Bonica JJ, and Ventafridda V, eds. *Advances in Pain Research and Therapy.* Vol. 2. New York: Raven Press; 1979:339–346.

20. Katz J. Current role of neurolytic agents. In: Bonica JJ, ed. *Advances in Neurology.* Vol. 4. New York: Raven Press; 1974:471–476.

21. Reid W, Watt JK, Gray TG. Phenol injection of the sympathetic chain. *Br J Surg* 1970; 57:45–50.

22. Cousins MJ, Reeve TS, Glynn CJ, Walsh JA, Cherry DA. Neurolytic lumbar sympathetic blockade. Duration of de-

nervation and relief of rest pain. *Anesth Intensive Care* 1979; 7:121–134.

23. Erikson E, ed. *Illustrated Handbook in Local Anaesthesia.* Philadelphia: Saunders; 1980.

24. Moore DC. *Regional Block. A Handbook for Use in the Clinical Practice of Medicine and Surgery.* 5th ed. Springfield, IL: Charles C. Thomas; 1985.

25. Sett SS, Taylor DC. Aortic pseudoaneurysm secondary to celiac plexus block. *Ann Vasc Surg* January 1991; 5(1):88–91.

26. Thompson GE, Bridenbaugh LD, Moore DC, Artin RY. Abdominal pain and alcohol celiac plexus nerve block. *Anesth Analg* 1977; 56:1–5.

27. Moore DC, Bush WH, Burnett LL. Celiac plexus block: a roentgenographic, anatomic study of technique and spread of solution in patients and corpses. *Anesth Analg* 1981; 60:369–379.

28. Sharfman WH, Walsh TD. Has the analgesic efficacy of neurolytic celiac plexus block been demonstrated in pancreatic cancer pain? *Pain* June 1990; 41(3):267–271.

29. Ischia S, Luzzani A, Ischia A, Faggion S. A new approach to the neurolytic block of the celiac plexus: the transaortic technique. *Pain* 1983; 16:333–341.

30. Saltzburgh D, Foley KM. Management of pain in pancreatic cancer. *Surg Clin North Am* 1989; 69:629–649.

31. Plancarte R, Amescua C, Patt RB, Aldrete JA. Superior hypogastric plexus block for pelvic cancer pain. *Anesthesiology* August 1990; 73(2):236–239.

32. Smith DW. Stellate ganglion block: the tissue displacement method. *Am J Surg* 1951; 57:45–50.

33. Onofrio BM, Yaksh TL, Arnold PG. Continuous low-dose intrathecal morphine administration in treatment of chronic pain of malignant origin. *Mayo Clin Proc* 1981; 56:516–520.

34. Zenz M, Schuppler-Scheele B, Newhaus R. Long-term peridural morphine analgesia in cancer pain. *Lancet* 1981; 1:91.

35. Waldman SD. The role of spinal opioids in the management of cancer pain. *J Pain Symptom Manage* June 1990; 5(3):163–168.

36. Samuelsson H, Hedner T. Pain characterization in cancer patients and the analgetic response to epidural morphine. *Pain* July 1991; 46(1):3–8.

37. Plummer JL, Cherry DA, Cousins MJ, Gourlay GK, Onley MM, Evans KH. Long-term spinal administration of morphine in cancer and non-cancer pain: a retrospective study. *Pain* March 1991; 44(3):215–220.

38. Dennis GC, DeWitty RL. Long-term intraventricular infusion of morphine for intractable pain in cancer of the head and neck. *Neurosurgery* March 1990; 26(3):404–407. Discussion, 407–408.

39. Wang JK, Nauss LW, Thomas JE. Pain relief by intrathecally applied morphine in man. *Anesthesiology* 1979; 50:149–151.

40. Sjogren P, Banning A. Pain, sedation and reaction time during long-term treatment of cancer patients with oral and epidural opioids. *Pain* October 1989; 39(1):5–11.

41. Meynadier J, Blond S, Combelle M. Treatment of intractable pain in patients with advanced cancer. *Pain Suppl* 1984; 2:344S.

42. Sjogren P, Banning AM, Larsen TK, Sorensen CG, Jansen EC. Postural stability during long-term treatment of cancer patients with epidural opioids. *Acta Anaesth Scand* July 1990; 34(5):410–412.

43. Bromage PR, Campores E, Chestnut D. Epidural narcotics for post-operative analgesia. *Anesth Analg* 1980; 59:473–480.

44. Yaksh TL. Spinal opiate analgesia: characteristics and principles of action. *Pain* 1981; 11:293–346.

45. Bromage PR. The price of intraspinal narcotic analgesia: basic constraints. *Anesth Analg* 1981; 60:461–463.

46. Coombs DW, Fratkin JD, Meier FW, Nierenberg DW, Saunders RL. Neuropathic lesions and CSF morphine concentrations during continuous intraspinal morphine infusion. *Pain* 1985; 22:337–351.

47. Arner S, Arner B. Differential effects of epidural morphine in the treatment of cancer-related pain. *Acta Anaesthesiol Scand* 1985; 29:32.

48. Wang JK. Intrathecal morphine for intractable pain secondary to cancer of pelvic organs. *Pain* 1985; 21:99.

49. Shaves M, Barnhill D, Bosscher J, Remmenga S, Hahn M, Park R. Indwelling epidural catheters for pain control in gynecologic cancer patients. *Obstet Gynecol* April 1991; 77(4):642–644.

50. Coombs DW, Saunders, RL, Mroz WT, Pageau MG. Complications of continuous intraspinal narcotic analgesia. *Can J Anaesth* 1983; 30:315–319.

51. Coombs DW, Saunders RL, Gaylor M, Pageau MG. Epidural narcotic infusion reservoir: implantation technique and efficacy. *Anesthesiology* 1982; 56:469–473.

52. Chubrasik J. Low-dose epidural morphine by infusion pump. *Lancet* 1984; 1:738–739.

53. Penn RD. Use and abuse of drug pumps in cancer pain. *Clin Neurosurg* 1989; 35:409–421.

54. Williams AR, Beaulaurier KE, Seal DL. Chronic cancer pain management with the Du Pen epidural catheter. *Cancer Nurs* June 1990; 13(3):176–182.

55. Ali NM, Hanna N, Hoffman JS. Percutaneous epidural catheterization for intractable pain in terminal cancer patients. *Gynecol Oncol* January 1989; 32(1):22–25.

56. Crawford ME, Anderson HB, Augustenborg G. Pain treatment on an outpatient basis utilizing extra-dural opiates. *Pain* 1983; 16:41–49.

57. Meynadier J, Chubrasik J, Dubar M, Wünsch E. Intrathecal somatostatin in terminally ill patients. A report of two cases. *Pain* 1985; 23:9–12.

58. Coombs DW, Saunders RL, La Chance D, Ragnarsson TS, Jensen LE. Intrathecal morphine tolerance: use of intrathecal clonidine, DADLE and intraventricular morphine. *Anesthesiology* 1985; 62:358–363.

59. Onofrio BM, Yaksh TL. Intrathecal delta-receptor ligand produces analgesia in man. *Lancet* 1983; 1:1386–1387.

60. Eisenbach JC, Rauch RL, Buzzanell C, Lysak SZ. Epidural clonidine analgesia for intractable cancer pain: phase I. *Anesthesiology* November 1989; 71(5):647–652.

61. Blanchard J, Menk E, Ramamurthy S, Hoffman J. Subarachnoid and epidural calcitonin in patients with pain due to metastatic cancer. *J Pain Symptom Manage* February 1990; 5(1):42–45.

62. Sjoberg M, Appelgren L, Einarsson S, et al. Long-term

intrathecal morphine and bupivicaine in "refractory" cancer pain, I: results from the first series of 52 patients. *Acta Anaesthesiol Scand* January 1991; 35(1):30–43.

63. Nitescu P, Appelgren L, Linder LE, Sjoberg M, Hultman E, Curelaru I. Epidural versus intrathecal morphine–bupivicaine: assessment of consecutive treatments in advanced cancer pain. *J Pain Symptom Manage* February 1990; 5(1):18–26.

64. Waldman SD, Allen ML, Cronen MC. Subcutaneous tunneled intrapleural catheters in the long-term relief of right upper quadrant pain of malignant origin. *J Pain Symptom Manage* June 1989; 4(2):86–89.

65. Mehta M. Chronic Pain. In: Atkinson RS, Hewer C, eds. *Recent Advances in Anaesthesia and Analgesia*. Vol. 14. New York: Churchill Livingstone; 1982:157–177.

66. Rosomoff HL, Carroll F, Brown J, Sheptak P. Percutaneous radiofrequency cervical cordotomy technique. *Neurosurg* 1965; 23:639–644.

67. Lipton S, McLennon JE. Percutaneous spinothalamic tractotomy. The prototype of neurosurgical pain control. In: Cousins MJ, Bridenbaugh PO, eds. *Neural Blockade*. Philadelphia: Lippincott; 1980.

68. Lipton S. Percutaneous cordotomy. In: Wall PD, Melzack R, eds. *Textbook of Pain*. New York: Churchill Livingstone; 1984.

69. Mullan SF. Percutaneous cordotomy. *J Neurosurg* 1971; 35:360–366.

70. Mullan SF. Cordotomy and rhizotomy for pain. *Clin Neurosurg* 1983; 31:344–350.

71. Wepsic JG. Complications of percutaneous surgery for pain. *Clin Neurosurg* 1976; 23:454–460.

72. Belmusto L, Brown E, Owens G. Clinical observations on respiratory and vasomotor disturbance as related to cervical cordotomies. *J Neurosurg* 1963; 20:225–232.

73. Uematsu S, Undvarhelyei GB, Benson DW, Siebens AA. Percutaneous radio-frequency rhizotomy. *Surg Neurol* 1974; 2(5):319–325.

74. Sluijter ME, Mehta M. Treatment of chronic back and neck pain by percutaneous thermal lesions. In: Lipton S, Miles J, eds. *Persistent Pain: Modern Methods of Treatment*. Vol III. New York: Academic Press 1981.

75. Sluijter ME. Personal communication, 1985.

76. Lloyd JW, Barnard JDW, Glynn CJ. Cryoanalgesia—A new approach to pain relief. *Lancet* 1976; 2:932–934.

77. Evans PJD. Cryoanalgesia. *Anesthesia* 1981; 36:1003–1013.

78. Nathan PW, Sears TA, Smith MC. Effects of phenol solutions on nerve roots of the cat: an electrophysiological and histological study. *J Neurol Sci* 1965; 2:7.

79. West CR, Avellanosa AM, Bremer AM, Yamado K. Hypophysectomy for relief of pain from disseminated carcinoma of the prostate gland. In: Bonica JJ, Ventafridda V, eds. *Advances in Pain Research and Therapy*. Vol. 2. New York: Raven Press; 1979:393–400.

80. Tindall GT, Nettleton S, Payne MD, Nixon DW. Transsphenoidal hypophysectomy for disseminated carcinoma of the prostate gland. *J Neurosurg* 1979; 50:275–282.

81. Moricca G. Chemical hypophysectomy for cancer pain. In: Bonica JJ, ed. *Advances in Neurology*. Vol. 4. New York: Raven Press; 1974:707–714.

82. Hardy J. Transsphenoidal hypophysectomy. *J Neurosurg* 1971; 34:582–594.

83. Takeda D, Uki J, Fuiji T, Kitani Y, Fujita T. Pituitary neuroadenolysis to relieve cancer pain. *Neurol Med Chir (Tokyo)* 1983; 23(1):50–54.

84. Tindall GT, Nixon DW, Christy JH, Neill JH. Pain relief in metastatic cancer other than breast and prostate gland following transsphenoidal hypophysectomy. *J Neurosurg* 1977; 47:659–662.

85. Miles J. Pituitary destruction. In: Wall PD, Melzack R, eds. *Textbook of Pain*. New York: Churchill Livingstone; 1984:656–665.

86. Katz J, Levin AB. Treatment of diffuse metastatic cancer by instillation of alcohol into the sella turcica. *Anesthesiology* 1977; 46:115–121.

87. Lipton S, Miles JB, Williams N, Bark-Jones N. Pituitary injections of alcohol for widespread cancer pain. *Pain* 1978; 5:73–81.

88. Madrid J. Chemical hypophysectomy. In: Bonica JJ, ed. *Advances in Pain Research and Therapy*. Vol. 2. New York: Raven Press; 1979:381–391.

89. Zervas NT. Stereotoxic thermal hypophysectomy. In: Schmidek H, Sweet W, eds. *Current Techniques in Operative Surgery*. New York: Grune & Stratton; 1977:181–186.

90. Bleasal K. Cryogenic hypophysectomy. *Med J Aust* 1965; 2:148–156.

91. Duthie AM, Ingham V, Dell AE, Dennett JE. Pituitary cryoablation. The results of treatment using a transsphenoidal cryoprobe. *Anaesthesia* 1983; 38:448–451.

92. Lloyd JW, Rawlinson WAL, Evans PJD. Selective hypophysectomy for metastatic pain. A review of ethyl alcohol ablation of the anterior pituitary in a regional pain relief unit. *Br J Anaesth* 1981; 53:1129–1133.

93. Miles JB, Lipton S. Mode of action by which pituitary alcohol relieves pain. In: Bonica JJ, Albe-Fessard D, eds. *Advances in Pain Research and Therapy*. Vol. I. New York: Raven Press; 1976:867–869.

94. Duthie AM. Pituitary cryoablation. *Anaesthesia* 1983; 38:495–497.

95. Melzack R. Prolonged relief of pain by brief, intense transcutaneous somatic stimulation. *Pain* 1975; 1:357–373.

96. Mehta M. Current views on non-invasive methods in pain relief. In: Swerdlow M, ed. *The Modern Therapy of Pain*. 2nd ed. Lancaster: MTP Press; 1986.

97. Long DM. Peripheral nervous system and pain control. *Clin Neurosurg* 1983; 31:323–343.

98. Aronoff GM. The use of non-narcotic drugs and other alternatives for analgesia as part of a comprehensive pain management program. *J Med* 1982; 13(3):191–192.

99. Long DM. Cutaneous afferent stimulation for relief of chronic pain. *Clin Neurosurg* 1982; 21:257–268.

100. Lee MHM. Acupuncture for pain control. In: Mork LC, ed. *Pain Control: Practical Aspects for Patient Care*. New York: Masson Publishers; 1981.

101. Mork LC, ed. *Pain Control: Practical Aspects of Patient Care*. New York: Masson Publishers; 1981.

102. Richardson DE. Intracranial stimulation for chronic pain. *Clin Neurosurg* 1983; 31:316–322.

103. Hinton J. *Dying*. Harmondsworth, England: Penguin Books 1975.

CHAPTER 19

Myofascial Syndrome

Burnell R. Brown, Jr.

The myofascial syndrome is one of the more common pain problems physicians encounter.[1] Unfortunately, it is poorly defined, nebulous, and masked by various guises.[2,3] Lack of discrete pathologic definition has hindered its broader acceptance as a true disease entity.[4] In broad terms, a definition of myofascial syndrome encompasses pain problems characterized by discrete circumscribed painful areas in skeletal muscles termed *trigger points*. Stimulation of these points triggers pain sensations that radiate from the points. The myofascial syndrome has masqueraded under many sobriquets. These include fibrositis, myositis, interstitial myositis, acute and chronic muscular sprain and strain, and so-called osteopathic lesions.[5] A number of the trigger points associated with myofascial syndrome are correlated anatomically with many of the gallbladder and bladder meridian points of acupuncture.[6]

The hallmark of identification of the myofascial syndrome is the trigger points.[7-9] Is there a histologic basis for these entities? Some evidence indicates that, in the trigger point areas, there are structural changes observable by electron microscopy. Such morphologic alterations primarily include myofibrillar degeneration, hyalin formation in muscle fibers, and deposition of nonspecific inflammatory residue in the interstices of skeletal muscle. However, it must be stated that such histologic evidence is controversial. The therapist essentially is confined to the myofascial syndrome as a physiologic rather than an anatomic entity. This is not unusual for pain problems.

The trigger points are characteristic on several counts. First, they are remarkably constant anatomically. An experienced observer realizes that there are only certain areas in skeletal muscle topography where these occur. The constancy of location and nature of these trigger points is one of the arcane phenomena associated with the myofascial syndrome. A second characteristic is that stimulation of the trigger points by pressure or electrical current produces a characteristic radiation of pain that, although radicular in nature, is not radicular in anatomy. That is, the radiation of pain triggered by stimulation (usually tactile pressure) of the trigger point, and it radiates in a fashion not associated with large nerve distribution. For example, stimulation of a trigger point in the midarea of the superior border of the trapezius muscle often causes radiation of pain down into the little finger. Obviously, the ulnar nerve does not course through the upper trapezius muscle, and although this particular pain radiation pattern is observed commonly, it does not follow the classic anatomic patterns recognized as true radicular pain. A third characteristic of the myofascial syndrome is that temporary or permanent ablation of the trigger points terminates the focused pain of the trigger and its radiation.

It is probably convenient for therapeutic purposes to divide myofascial syndrome into primary and secondary. Primary myofascial syndrome can be considered caused probably by a traumatic disease of the muscles.[10] Primary myofascial syndrome is defined as pain and disability with no predisposition except skeletal muscle dysfunction per se. A classic example of primary myofascial syndrome is a patient who has skeletal muscle pain from an acute strain caused by lifting or chronic strain. An example of chronic strain is the shoulder girdle muscle pain of secretaries engaged in typing manuscripts for a prolonged period. Obviously, with this type of cause, no neurologic or orthopedic abnormalities can be found. Thus, primary myofascial syndrome is a painful disability of skeletal muscles with no evidence of disease outside the skeletal muscles coupled with trigger points demonstrable in the muscles. Table 19-1 lists several causes of this pain problem. However, secondary myofascial syndrome displays painful foci in skeletal muscles, but the disorder arises outside the skeletal muscles. An example is the failed laminectomy syndrome in which the pathologic entity is scar tissue present in and around the spinal nerves and cord. The pain, however, is manifested in the skeletal muscle and has the characteristics of the myofascial syndrome because trigger points are found. Therapy in either case obviously is symptomatic. The physician can expect a higher percentage of absolute cures in primary myofascial syndrome than in the secondary myofascial syndrome because of the generally more ephemeral nature of the former, regardless of physi-

Table 19-1
Causes of Primary Myofascial Syndrome

Acute muscle strain
Chronic muscle strain (such as postural)
Fatigue or overexertion
Tension headaches

Table 19-2
Some Etiologic Factors in Secondary Myofascial Syndromes

Lumbar or cervical disc disease
Failed laminectomy syndrome
Vertebral collapse (metastasis or osteoporosis)
Chronic headache
Dental occlusive disease (temporomandibular joint syndrome)

cian intervention. Table 19-2 lists some of the many causes of secondary myofascial syndrome.

CAUSE

The cause of myofascial syndrome is not known. Although some observers see alterations in microscopic examination of muscles, these changes probably are not the cause but rather the result of myofascial syndrome.[11] A speculative model can be developed (Fig. 19-1). Assume that the pain stimulus is conferred by A-delta afferent fibers to the spinal cord. These pain fibers enter the spinal cord, are transferred to the contralateral side of the spinal cord, and ascend to the brain primarily by the spinothalamic tract. There synapses occur in the thalamus, an area perceptive to poorly localized protopathic pain. Efferent from the thalamus are numerous fibers that go to the sensory portion of the cortex and others that go to the hypothalamic area, the center of autonomic activity. Each painful impulse produces an autonomic response. For example, with a pinprick, there is hyperhidrosis, dilatation of the pupils, and alterations in the cardiovascular system as a result of a sympathetic response to the pain. The increased autonomic tone causes a vasoconstrictive response in the area of the pain. If perpetuated, such vasoconstriction can lead to a buildup of anerobic metabolites which in and of themselves become irritating. We can imagine that an oscillating circuit can be set up that is autoperpetuating. The oscillation involves both somatic and sympathetic pain fibers. Chronicity causes an activation of the C fibers with opening of the so-called spinal cord gate

in the substantia gelantinosa of Rolando. Again it must be emphasized that such a pathophysiologic mechanism (in light of current knowledge) is speculative, but effective therapy can be predicated on this type of cause. Some recent data indicate that trigger point injection therapy is reversed with naloxone, suggesting an opiate-mediated mechanism.[12]

DIAGNOSIS

Diagnosis of either primary or secondary myofascial syndrome is established by demonstrating the painful trigger points that, when stimulated by pressure, produce radiation of pain. As mentioned, these are constant.[13] They are remarkable for the consistency of their anatomic location. The examining physician presses with their fingers in the appropriate area and elicits local and radiating pain. A secondary encouraging diagnostic clue is the finding that, when these trigger points are infiltrated with a small amount of local anesthetic, all pain ceases. Basically, the clinician should have a high degree of suspicion when approaching the patient with poorly defined pain that myofascial syndrome might be the cause.

Trigger points also can be demonstrated with the help of an algometer[14] or by electrical stimulation. Most commonly used in this circumstance is a machine that produces sinusoidal current, such as a Medcosonalator. At times, the physical therapist informs the clinician that myofascial syndrome may be present. Electrodiagnostic studies are not generally useful.[15]

The constancy of the trigger point should be remembered. Figure 19-2 illustrates the four classic anatomic

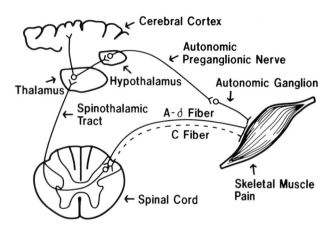

FIGURE 19-1. A speculative model of mechanisms of continuing pain cycles after a skeletal muscle insult.

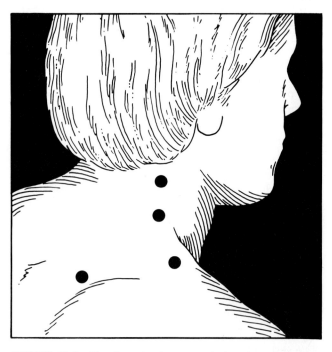

FIGURE 19-2. The four classic anatomic locations for trigger points in the neck and shoulder girdle area.

locations for trigger points in the neck, upper extremity, and shoulder girdle area. Two of these points are located in the neck, the superior one adjacent to the sternocleodomastoid muscle, and the inferior one associated with the scalene muscle group. A third trigger point in the upper extremity is located in the middle portion of the superior border of the trapezius muscle. The last anatomic location for upper extremity myofascial trigger points is at an area just medial to the superior angle of the scapula. It is believed that this trigger point is in the rhomboid muscle mass.

The lower extremity trigger points are three in number (Fig. 19-3). One is located in the area just inferior to the twelfth rib at the lateral part of the paraspinal muscle mass. The other is in the sacroiliac joint area, and the third is located near the center of the gluteus maximus muscle and represents a myofascial trigger zone in the piriformis muscle. An isolated trigger point in the piriformis muscle has been termed *piriformis syndrome*. This entity can mimic sciatic radicular pain and often is confused with herniated disc pain.

Radiation of pain from these points will vary. In addition to increasing the intensity of pain when they are pressed, pain radiation areas may be different from patient to patient. However, their hallmark remains the constancy of their anatomic location, and the finding that they are always present in myofascial syndrome.

THERAPY

Therapy of myofascial syndrome, whether primary or secondary, is similar.[16] In some respects, such therapeutic similarity goes against the grain of traditional treatment. It must be remembered that therapy in such cases, as in many pain syndromes, is aimed at the symptom rather than ablating the basic pathologic condition. In primary myofascial syndrome, where the cause usually is skeletal muscle strain, initial treatment frequently results in total and permanent elimination of pain. Secondary myofascial syndrome, in which there is a recognized cause but one that is not amenable to therapy, must be treated periodically for a prolonged period of time, perhaps for the rest of the patient's life.

Injection Therapy

Injection therapy is the mainstay of therapy of myofascial syndrome.[17] Most commonly, the solution injected is a local anesthetic.[18] The choice of local anesthetic depends on the proclivity and experience of the therapist. Some prefer procaine 1%; others believe that lidocaine 0.5% produces better therapeutic results. Bupivacaine 0.25% ostensibly has advantages because it is the longest acting local anesthetic. Although there are some devotees of this local anesthetic for injection therapy of trigger points, others raise the objection it is the most damaging to the fine myofibrillar structure of skeletal muscle. It is conceivable that additional damage of skeletal muscle can prolong the pain problem. However, this controversy has not been established as scientific dogma, and there is no contraindication to the use of bupivacine. There is no question that the pain relief after bupivacaine administration lasts longer in myofascial syndrome than does that after injection of shorter-acting local anesthetics. Therefore, in many respects, the pain therapist must rely on their own experience in this regard. Because the pathophysiology may involve exacerbation of adrenergic function locally,[19] most physicians treating these trigger points avoid adding epinephrine in the injection solutions. Vasodilatation is one of the goals of therapy and use of a vasoconstrictor in the local anesthetic defeats this purpose.

The following are the details of injection therapy as practiced by the author.[20] A small (3 to 5-ml) syringe is used because this can be handled more deftly than a larger one. I use a 5-ml syringe and fill it with 2 to 3 ml of a local anesthetic solution. For the four upper extremity classic trigger zones, a ¾-in 25-gauge needle is required. This can be used even in obese patients, and I believe that longer needles in this area only increase the incidence of side effects but not the therapeutic efficacy. The trigger zone is identified by pressure over the area with the index finger to a precision of approximately 1-cm diameter. A skin antiseptic then is swabbed over the trigger point. The needle is inserted perpendicular to skin until it contacts the trigger point. This can be determined easily by the fact that the patient will feel an exacerbation of pain and a paresthesia at the time of needle contact with the trigger zone. Holding the needle and syringe in the same site when the trigger is stimulated is an acquired skill. It is important that this be done, because if there is no paresthesia, myofascial syn-

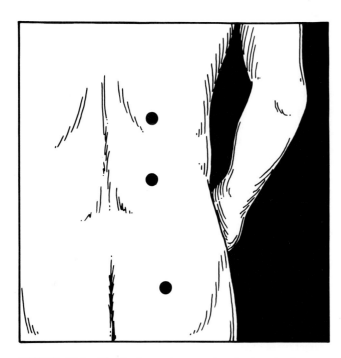

FIGURE 19-3. Classic three trigger points for low back area.

...ablated. When such contact is made, the ...kly is aspirated for blood, and 2 to 3 ml of local ...tic solution is injected. The reader also will notice ..., during the injection, pain and paresthesia are exacerbated. The physician must be careful that the patient does not move abruptly at this time so that needle localization is lost. The needle then is withdrawn quickly. If the diagnosis is correct and the placement of the needle is accurate, there will be an almost immediate relief of pain, not only in the trigger zone, but also in the corresponding referred area. For the lower extremity and back trigger zones, I commonly use a 22-gauge 1½-in needle. The superior trigger of the lumbar area may require a fairly deep needle insertion, almost, if not to, the hub of the needle to detect the trigger located deep in the paraspinal muscle mass. This will occur obviously in the obese patient, but it is rare for a longer needle to be required. The sacroiliac trigger point, however, is relatively superficial and is found at a depth of approximately 15 to 20 mm, regardless of patient size. The trigger in the piriformis muscle is deep. Under certain circumstances, a longer needle may be required, but even in a relatively thin patient, the needle must be inserted fully; at times, indentation of the skin occurs. If the operator is uncomfortable by the total loss of visualization of the needle, a longer needle than a 1½-in can be substituted. I emphasize that paresthesias must be obtained to obtain good relief. Actual sciatic nerve block is a complication of piriformis muscle injection and must be prevented to avoid temporary paralysis of the leg.

The physician must be aware that complications can occur from these blocks. They are rare but have been observed. Some of the more common ones are, first, pneumothorax, particularly from the rhomboid trigger needling. It must be remembered that pneumothorax from a small-gauge needle is not a precipitous event, but rather, it is a tension pneumothorax that takes several hours to develop. Thus the patient must be cautioned that, if any shortness of breath occurs from 6 to 12 h after the block, the physician should be notified immediately. Second, although intravenous injections are possible, the small dose of local anesthetic usually is far below the dose that causes convulsions. However, this must be remembered, and drugs and positive-pressure oxygen equipment for resuscitation must be on hand whenever these blocks are administered. Third, idiosyncratic or allergic reactions to local anesthetics are extremely rare, but they are a possibility. Fourth, sciatic nerve injection with leg paralysis may occur. Fifth, local anesthetic overdose is possible but rare. Injection of all trigger points described bilaterally results in a total volume of local anesthetic of only 30 ml. Use of lidocaine 1% for all these places provides a total dose of 300 mg. Bupivacaine 0.25% gives a dose of 75 mg. Both are below the adult toxic doses of these local anesthetics. Sixth, postinjection muscle pain and spasm may occur. This is probably the most common complication seen with trigger point injection therapy. The patient must be cautioned that there may be an exacerbation of pain after treatment. Usually, this occurs soon after the local anesthetic has worn off, persists for 2 or 3 h, and then for reasons that are unknown, seems to decrease in intensity.

Trigger points may be found occasionally in other sites, and the physician must make a close examination of the patient for these. Many of the satellite triggers, however, are resolved when the primary triggers (those shown in the figures) are treated. The reasons for this, as in so many other phenomena associated with myofascial syndrome, are unknown. Multiple repeat injections in an area usually are not necessary, and injection of the four triggers in the upper area and the three in the lower area (multiplied twice for bilateral pain) usually are all that is required in 80 percent of cases. Trigger points may be found in certain types of facial pain associated with skeletal muscle spasm also. As in any of the other types of this syndrome, careful examination for geographic location of the trigger zone is important. Experience facilitates localization.

The timing of repeat injections is a matter of clinical judgment. Too frequent injection therapy produces residual pain that does not clear between treatments and is counterproductive. In general, injections should be given no more frequently than every 5 to 7 days. In acute injuries, the number of injections will be small. In chronic states, usually secondary myofascial syndrome, injections may have to be repeated at intervals for the duration of the patient's pain, which can be their lifetime.

Refrigerant Therapy

As soon as the trigger point has been injected, refrigerant therapy using fluorimethane can be employed. The exact rationale of this efficacious therapy is unknown. It is speculated that activation of A-delta fibers helps close the spinal cord gate and reduces C-fiber (chronic pain) activity. In addition, stretching and passive manipulation of the sore skeletal muscle groups aids therapy. The spray is applied centripetally. During this period, the neck, shoulder muscles, and back, are moved slowly and actively by the patient in an attempt to reduce the pain and spasm. The spray should be continued for some 2 to 3 min. Spray therapy does not attempt to induce refrigeration anesthesia. Rather, the sharp stinging sensation associated with the spray seems to be conducive to reducing pain and loosening the muscles that have been in spasm.

Medication

There is no single medical regimen for myofascial syndrome. Unanimity of opinion in this regard among clinicians who treat this condition is poor at best. Antispasmotic drugs often are advocated. For the patient with primary myofascial syndrome of an acute nature, use of such drugs probably is justified. One of the difficulties with antispasmotic drugs that work through the polysynaptic reticular formation in the spinal cord is that the primary side effect is central nervous system depression. This should be avoided in most cases of long-standing chronic pain in which there is secondary myofascial syndrome. It is well recognized that these patients frequently are depressed from their chronic pain. Thus, drugs such as diazepam or carisoprodol can play an effective role in relaxing muscle in acute and primary myofascial syndromes caused by overactivity or exertional strain, but they are not indicated in long-term management because they may exacerbate depression.

Mild analgesics, such as diflunisal administered in doses of 500 mg twice a day, often produces excellent results. For more severe cases, codeine 30 mg and aspirin can be administered. Although not proved, it is possible that drugs with anti-inflammatory activity, such as the salicylates, may be more advantageous in these patients than agents, such as acetaminophen, which have no such activity. Aspirin should not be administered if there is a contraindication (such as ulcer).

The long-term medical and psychological effects[21,22] in patients with chronic primary and secondary myofascial syndrome are beyond the scope of this chapter. However, many of these patients may benefit from administration of antidepressants, such as the tricyclics.[23]

Psychological therapy usually is required in chronic cases.[24] However, this issue will not be covered in this chapter. General principles of treatment of this chronic disease are similar to those in other long-standing pain problems.

Physical Therapy

Physical therapy plays an important role in both primary and secondary and acute and chronic myofascial syndrome. Physical therapy methods that can be used in this condition are outlined in Table 19-3. I have had good results with combined sinusoidal electric current and ultrasonic therapy (Medcosonalator). Our aim is to increase the blood supply to the affected muscles to overcome the sympathetic activation produced by pain. The sinusoidal current induces passive skeletal muscle contraction. Both passive and active manipulation of the skeletal muscles during therapy and afterward is advised. A program of exercise should be followed by the patient. It must be understood that these

Table 19-3
Physical Therapy Methods That Are Useful in Treating Myofascial Syndromes

---

Medcosonolater (ultrasound combined with sinusoidal current)
Exercises, passive and active
Deep heat
Manipulation and massage
Traction
Ice packs
Laser therapy[27,28,29]
Electrical stimulation[30]

---

exercises are not a marathon contest. The patient should not exercise to the point of exhaustion because this will make the vulnerable muscles even more painful. Consultation with a physiatrist and/or physical therapist is beneficial to the pain therapist in these conditions. Besides injection therapy, physical therapy is the most useful pain treatment available for these problems.

SUMMARY

The myofascial syndromes are common types of pain conditions that are poorly understood.[25,26] Both primary (from stressed and strained skeletal muscles) and secondary (from an orthopedic or neurologic cause) forms occur. Diagnosis is directed at localizing the trigger points that, when stimulated, produce paresthesias in areas remote from their central focus. Therapy is directed primarily at trigger point injections with local anesthetics to break the cycle of spasm–pain–autonomic reflexes characteristic of this disease. Medication, refrigerant spray therapy, and particularly physical therapy are important adjuvant treatments for alleviation of these common conditions.

References

1. Shootsky SA, Jaeger B, Oye RK. Prevalence of myofascial pain in general internal medicine practice. *West J Med* August 1989; 151(2):157–160.
2. Wolfe F. Fibrositis, fibromyalgia, and musculoskeletal disease, the current status of the fibrositis syndrome. *Arch Phys Med Rehabil* July 1988; 69(7):527–531.
3. Rogers EJ, Rogers R. Pain clinic #14. Fibromyalgia and myofascial pain: either, neither, or both? *Orthop Rev* November 1989; 18(11):1217–1224.
4. Fricton JR. Clinical care for myofascial pain. *Dent Clin North Am* January 1991; 35(1):1–28.
5. Thompson JM. Tension myalgia as a diagnosis at the Mayo Clinic and its relationship to fibrositis, fibromyalgia, and myofascial pain syndrome. *Mayo Clin Proc* September 1990; 65(9):1237–1248. See comments.
6. Melzack R, Stilwell DN, Fox EJ. Trigger points and acupuncture points for pain: correlations and implications. *Pain* 1977; 3:23.
7. Simons EG. Myofascial trigger point: a need for understanding. *Arch Phys Med Rehabil* 1981; 62:97.
8. Travell JG, Rinzler SH. The myofascial genesis of pain. *Postgrad Med* 1952; 11:425.
9. Travell JG, Simons DJ. Myofascial pain and dysfunction: the trigger point manual. Baltimore: Williams & Wilkins; 1983.
10. Yunus MB, Kalyan-Raman UP, Kalyan-Raman K. Primary fibromyalgia syndrome and myofascial pain syndrome: clinical features and muscle pathology. *Arch Phys Med Rehabil* June 1988; 69(6):451–454.
11. Awad EA. Interstitial myofibrositis: hypothesis of the mechanism. *Arch Phys Med Rehabil* 1973; 54:449–453.
12. Fine PG, Milano R, Hare BD. The effects of myofascial trigger point injections are naloxone reversible. *Pain* January 1988; 32(1):15–20.

13. Tunks E, Crook J, Norman G, Kalaher S. Tender points in fibromyalgia. *Pain* July 1988; 34(1):11–19.

14. Fischer AA. Documentation of myofascial trigger points. *Arch Phys Med Rehabil* April 1988; 69(4):286–291.

15. Durette MR, Rodrigues AA, Agre JC, Silverman JL. Needle electromyographic evaluation of patients with myofascial or fibromyalgic pain. *Am J Phys Med Rehabil* June 1991; 70(3):154–156.

16. Friction JR. Myofascial pain syndrome. *Neurol Clin* May 1989; 7(2):413–427.

17. Garvey TA, Marks MR, Wiesel SW. A prospective, randomized, double-blind evaluation of trigger-point injection therapy for low-back pain. *Spine* September 1989; 14(9):962–964.

18. Byrn C, Borenstein P, Linder LE. Treatment of neck and shoulder pain in whip-lash syndrome patients with intracutaneous sterile water injections. *Acta Anaesthesiol Scand* January 1991; 35(1):52–53.

19. Snyder-Mackler L, Barry AJ, Perkins AI, Soucek MD. Effects of helium–neon laser irradiation on skin resistance and pain in patients with trigger points in the neck or back. *Phys Ther* May 1989; 69(5):336–341.

20. Brown BR Jr. Diagnosis and therapy of common myofascial syndromes. *JAMA* 1978; 239:646.

21. Kapel L, Glaros AG, McGlynn FD. Psychophysiological responses to stress in patients with myofascial pain-dysfunction syndrome. *J Behav Med* August 1989; 12(4):397–406.

22. Scudds RA, Trachsel LC, Luckhurst BJ, Percy JS. A comparative study of pain, sleep quality and pain responsiveness in fibrositis and myofascial pain syndrome. *J Rheumatol Suppl* November 1989; 19:120–126.

23. Brown RS, Bottomly WK. Utilization and mechanism of action of tricyclic antidepressants in the treatment of chronic facial pain: a review of the literature. *Anesth Prog* September–October 1990; 37(5):223–229.

24. Fishbain DA, Goldberg M, Steele R, Rosomoff H. DSM-III diagnoses of patients with myofascial pain syndrome (fibrositis). *Arch Phys Med Rehabil* June 1989; 70(6):433–438.

25. Simons DG. Myofascial pain syndromes: Where are we? Where are we going? *Arch Phys Med Rehabil* March 1988; 69(3 pt 1):207–212.

26. Goldenberg DL. Fibromyalgia, chronic fatigue syndrome, and myofascial pain syndrome. *Curr Opin Rheumatol* April 1991; 3(2):247–258.

27. Olavi A, Pekka R, Pertti K, Pekka P. Effects of the infrared laser therapy at treated and non-treated trigger points. *Acupunct Electrother Res* 1989; 14(1):9–14.

28. Waylonis GW, Wilke S, O'Toole D, Waylonis DB. Chronic myofascial pain: management by low-output helium–neon laser therapy. *Arch Phys Med Rehabil* December 1988; 69(12):1017–1020.

29. Perry F, Heller PH, Kayima J, Levine JD. Altered autonomic function in patients with arthritis or with chronic myofascial syndrome. *Pain* October 1989; 39(1):77–84.

30. Graff-Radford SB, Reeves JL, Baker RL, Chiu D. Effects of transcutaneous electrical nerve stimulation on myofascial pain and trigger point sensitivity. *Pain* April 1989; 37(1):1–5.

CHAPTER 20

Acute and Postoperative Pain

Garrett D. Kine and Leonard S. Bushnell

Pain is often the motivation to seek surgery. Although surgical treatment often alleviates the presenting complaint, it paradoxically may produce a pain of greater severity than the original complaint. We, as physicians, have an inherent responsibility to minimize the pain we directly, or indirectly, cause by maximizing the effectiveness with which we use the pharmacologic agents and other techniques available to us.

The field of anesthesiology has made many advances since it began; we now can provide all patients, regardless of their physical condition, a pain-free intraoperative period. Unfortunately, we are not as advanced in our protection of the patient from the discomforts of the postoperative period. The perioperative period places the patient in an infancy-like state of physical and mental dependency and helplessness. It is our responsibility as caretakers of this population to minimize the physical and mental anguish they experience. Postoperative pain may be feared more than surgery and anesthesia. This fear can lead to a delay in surgical intervention, thereby increasing the risks, the extent of surgery, and the postoperative pain. Delay may allow advancement of a pathologic condition, thereby complicating the recovery course.

The tissue damage produced by surgery is similar to that of acute injury. It causes local and systemic noxious stimuli that initiate nociceptive impulses, relays, and reflexes throughout the nervous system. In addition to the disturbances associated with the conscious interpretation of these impulses, there are autonomic effects generated that may disrupt the healing and recovery process. The deleterious physiologic side effects of acute pain are well recognized. In the patient who is breathing spontaneously, muscle splinting (seen in conjunction with discomfort of chest or abdominal origin) may result in decreased vital capacity, decreased functional residual capacity, and ultimately decreased alveolar ventilation. Atelectasis is a frequent postoperative complication. Discomfort experienced during coughing may result in retention of secretions and subsequent pneumonia. The sympathetic response to pain may cause increased cardiovascular demands. This may be apparent clinically by signs of tachycardia, increased peripheral resistance, and hypertension; these are associated with increased cardiac work and myocardial oxygen consumption. The potential for myocardial ischemia and infarction is obvious. Muscle spasm produced by segmental and suprasegmental reflex motor activity may perpetuate pain. In the chest wall and abdomen, pain and muscle spasm may compromise respiratory function. The gastrointestinal tract similarly is affected by increased sympathetic activity. Pain increases intestinal secretions and smooth muscle sphincter tone and decreases intestinal motility. By similar mechanisms, pain may produce urinary retention. Acute injury also has an impact on the endocrine system, causing sodium and water retention and hyperglycemia. Immobility from acute postoperative pain may predispose the patient to deep vein thrombosis and pulmonary embolism as a result of venostasis and platelet aggregation. In a complex intertwined relationship, psychological alterations may occur concomitantly with the physiologic ones.

Since the 1965 report of Melzack and Wall's so-called gate theory of pain,[1] an appropriate increasing emphasis on understanding and determining more effective realistic methods of pain therapy has begun. The predominance of literature on chronic pain should not lead us to believe that medical practitioners have achieved satisfactory acute pain management. This often is a deemphasized or neglected aspect in physician training programs. The importance of acute distress to the patient and society as a whole, and the alleviation thereof, should not be underestimated. Because this text is intended to discuss primarily chronic pain management, only a brief overview of acute pain management will be presented in this chapter. For a more in-depth discussion, the reader is referred to several excellent recent texts that exclusively discuss acute pain management.[2,3]

In this chapter, some of the most common inadequacies and misconceptions in acute pain management will be addressed. Alternative and innovative methods will be presented. Although discussion will be directed toward the management of postoperative pain, the concepts presented are applicable equally to acute nonsurgical pain. The postoperative period more often is used in clinical studies because of the greater consistency in symptoms and the better availability of patients and experimental control subjects.

INADEQUACIES OF TRADITIONAL APPROACHES

Many physicians who have been treated surgically have related experiences that concern the inadequacy of traditional postoperative analgesia and the system in which it is administered. The often quoted 1976 *Lancet*[4] editorial entitled "Tight Fisted Analgesia" was the result of one physician's outcry. The inadequacy of the "as the situation demands" basis for administration of an analgesic was attested personally by another physician.[5] Frequently, it has been proposed that the as-needed nomenclature is misconceived by many care givers who follow the physician's instructions to represent the concept of giving as little, or as infrequent, medication as possible.

Many factors influence our perception of postoperative pain. Determinants of the intensity, quality, and duration of postoperative pain include: (1) the site, nature, and duration of the operation, including the type of incision and the amount of intraoperative trauma; (2) the physiologic and psychological makeup of the patient; (3) the preoperative psychological, physical, and pharmacologic preparation of the patient; (4) the presence of serious related complications; (5) the anesthetic management; and (6) the quality of postoperative care.[6] Cohen[7] attributed some of the ineffectiveness of current medical analgesic therapy to inadequate understanding by nurses of the pharmacology of narcotics.

Inadequate understanding by physicians of the nature of pain also has been demonstrated. A structured interview of 37 medical inpatients showed that 32 percent have severe distress despite a narcotic analgesic regimen; an additional 41 percent declared themselves to be in moderate distress.[8] As part of the study, a questionnaire survey of 102 staff physicians showed an underestimation of effective dose ranges, overestimation of the duration of action, and an exaggerated concern with the addictive potential of meperidine in a therapeutic dosing range. It is thought that the development of addiction in patients with no previous addictive history is rare.[9] Children, perhaps the most dependent group in the hospital population, also bear the burden of postoperative suffering.[10] As a reaction to discomfort, many children withdraw and vegetate. This may be misinterpreted as coping with the pain. Many immature patients fear injections, deny pain, and are unable to realize that a short-term discomfort may grant a longer period of analgesia.

In summary, at least three major factors contribute to the inadequacy of traditional analgesic therapy. Foremost is the incomplete comprehension by medical personnel of analgesic pharmacodynamics. This lack of knowledge coupled with overconcern about respiratory depression and addiction liability leads to the administration of inadequate doses. Secondly, the logistics of administering narcotics often leads to a long lag period between the onset of pain and the administration of pain-relieving drugs. Coupled with the delay in absorption of intramuscularly administered analgesics, this interval may distress the patient greatly. A third barrier to adequate analgesia is a common hospital community attitude that stoicism is a virtue. The suffering patient may sense such an attitude and, rather than attacking this formidable barrier, refrain from requesting appropriate medication.

SYSTEMIC MEDICATIONS (See Chap. 26)

The plethora of drugs available to physicians constantly changes, but concepts supporting their effective use remain relatively static. Some classes of drugs are associated with diminished psychological and hormonal stresses from acute injury. Drugs available to the physician caring for the postoperative patient include: analgesic drugs (narcotic agonists and agonist–antagonists), psychotropic drugs (phenothiazines and butyrophenones), nonsteroidal anti-inflammatory drugs, and the sedative–hypnotics. We hope the use of paralyzing muscle relaxants as a "sedative" is an archaic notion of the past.[11,12] The well-meaning physician must understand, not only the choice of a drug, but also its route and the timing of drug delivery. There is often a large discrepancy between the outward appearance of a traumatic injury and the degree of perceived discomfort. An observed time delay was reported between injury and the perception of pain.[13] Also, in studies of acute injuries in soldiers, local areas of injury were found to be analgesic, and remote areas of the body might convey the sensation of noxious stimuli to the injured soldier.[14]

Narcotic Agonists

Morphine and other opiate agonists are the mainstay of postoperative analgesic care. They are effective, familiar, easy to use, and low cost. Their failure to produce consistently good postoperative pain relief is, as previously mentioned, often related to limitations on the part of the medical staff. One of the most common misconceptions involves the efficacy of routine intramuscular injections. Pharmacologic investigations show large patient-to-patient variability in peak blood levels for meperidine and analgesic efficacy.[15] A given patient's clinical response to a single dose may be anywhere along a bell-shaped curve. Pharmacodynamic variability may be expressed as a different tissue response when exposed to the same concentration of a drug. Pharmacokinetic variability reflects alterations in absorption, distribution, biotransformation, or excretion of the agent. There is a relationship between blood levels of meperidine and its effectiveness in relieving postoperative pain.[15] Variation in local tissue absorption may cause blood concentrations that are insufficient for adequate analgesia.

Methadone traditionally has been administered orally for maintenance therapy of narcotic addicts and analgesia in chronic or terminal pain management. Investigators realize that methadone has potentially desirable pharmacokinetics, including a long half-life and low clearance rate. In an attempt to exploit these characteristics, Gourlay and colleagues[16] administered a 20-mg intravenous bolus dose of methadone during induction of anesthesia in 23 patients undergoing general surgery or orthopedic procedures. The median duration of analgesia resulting from this dose was 27 h. After emergence from anesthesia, the patients were sedated, but their respiratory rates were not depressed significantly. In a subsequent study by Gourlay and colleagues,[17] the authors again administered 20 mg of methadone intravenously as part of the general anesthetic and supplemented the analgesia with additional methadone doses (usually 5 mg intravenously) in the recovery ward until effective postoperative pain was established. Blood methadone concentrations sampled immediately before a supplementary dose provided supporting evidence that there was a relationship between the blood concentration and analgesic response in the patient. Several patients required no additional analgesia during their hospital stay. It should be realized that the use of an analgesic with a slower elimination might allow a patient to maintain an adequate blood level after a single bolus, but this also would decrease our ability to control the medication concentration. If it becomes clinically necessary to antagonize adverse effects of methadone, the exceptionally long half-life of methadone in comparison with naloxone must be remembered. Multiple repeat doses of naloxone may be required because the half-life of naloxone is short compared with that of methadone.

The intravenous route of administration of opioids has been used in an attempt to achieve a more consistent minimal analgesic blood concentration. By this route, we may administer intermittent boluses, a continuous infusion, or a combination of both. The advantages of intravenous injection include a rapid onset of drug action, an earlier and more predictable maximum concentration and resultant clinical effects, and the possibility of rapid tapering should adverse effects occur. When redistribution of a drug is complete, the plateau of the steady-state blood concentrations will be realized. At this point, if the rate of drug elimination is counterbalanced by the rate of drug administration, a consistent drug level will be achieved. Unless a loading dose is used, there may be a long delay before the steady state is reached by a continuous infusion method of administration. Rutter and coworkers[18] studied the continuous intravenous infusion of morphine in 45 patients who had undergone major operations. They concluded that continuous intravenous infusion was superior to intramuscular regimens. Patients who received continuous infusions experienced better pain relief at lower total doses.

Alternative routes of administration of the opioids are possible. The rectal route may be used in patients who cannot take medications by mouth. A study by Goudie and associates[19] concluded that continuous subcutaneous infusion of morphine was equally effective in providing relief of the pain of upper abdominal surgery compared with regular intramuscular injections of morphine. They thought that side effects in the continuous-subcutaneous group appeared to be less frequent.

The newest mode of narcotic administration is the transdermal route. Several studies show that transdermal fentanyl safely and effectively can be used to treat postoperative pain.[20–22] Unfortunately, dose titration is difficult because of its delayed onset and long decay time. Gourlay and colleagues[21] reported a delay in onset time of 12.7 h and a decay time of 16.1 h after the patch was removed; these pharmacokinetic parameters are related to the depot storage of the drug in the skin under the patch.

Patient-Controlled Analgesia (PCA)

More than 20 years ago, it was shown that the use of small intravenous boluses of opioids produced more complete pain relief with lower doses than injection by the intramuscular route.[23] The intravenous route inherently carries the disadvantages of a shorter duration of action as a result of the pharmacokinetic distribution and elimination characteristics of this route, and there is a possibility of an increased incidence of undesirable side effects if larger bolus doses be used in an attempt to achieve longer analgesic effects. During the late 1960s, postoperative analgesia administered by incremental intravenous bolus doses, controlled on a patient-demand basis was evaluated.[24] Sechzer[24] used nursing personnel to administer the narcotics and observe the patient's response. He found that this system provided good postoperative analgesia, and smaller total quantity of narcotic was administered. In addition, he reported a pattern of consistency in each study subject in the quantity of the narcotic and the delivery time between doses. There was, however, great variation in dosage requirements among patients.

In a pioneering study by Bennet and colleagues[25] on a morbidly obese patient population undergoing gastric bypass operations, a PCA group maintained an adequate state of analgesia with greater frequency than the control group that receiving time-sequenced fixed-dose intramuscular analgesia. This study supported the efficacy and safety of PCA in this clinically challenging patient population. Another investigation by Bennet and colleagues[26] found improved postoperative pulmonary function in obese patients receiving PCA.

Studies by other investigators compared PCA with other methods of postoperative pain management. In 1979, White and associates[27] compared a patient-demand infusion system of fentanyl with repeated injections of epidural bupivacaine in patients undergoing major peripheral vascular surgery. Both techniques produced satisfactory analgesia without respiratory depression. They acknowledged that the patient-demand system might have a broader base of application for several reasons. First, the epidural route is not appropriate for all surgical sites. Second, there may be difficulties encountered in the placement of an epidural line as a result of anatomic variations, or its use relatively may be contraindicated (such as in local sepsis or coagulation abnormalities). In addition, epidural analgesia is effective only in a segmental region. Other annoying pain sites must be treated individually. An epidural analgesic would have little effect on some of the distress typically encountered during a hospital stay (such as an irritating nasogastric tube or the discomfort associated with phlebotomy).

The advantages of a patient-demand system through intravenous access became obvious. The technology that offers this therapy coupled with a high degree of patient safety and a minimal burden on the hospital staff took several years of research and development.[28]

The PCA systems in use currently consist of an infusion pump interfaced with a timing device (Fig. 20-1). Administration of an incremental bolus of an analgesic is triggered by the patient through the use of a hand-held switch, similar to a nurse call button. The infusion pump is "piggybacked" into a functioning intravenous access site. In even the simplest devices, two variables require programming into a PCA system. The first is the quantity of analgesic that will be delivered as an intravenous bolus. The second is an inactivation period, often referred to as the so-called lock-out time or refractory period, during which additional activation of the hand switch will not deliver any additional analgesic. This lock-out period (often set at 5 to 15 min) is one of the primary measures to prevent an overdose. It often is set so that the inactivation period is just greater than that which is necessary for the analgesic agent administered to achieve its peak effect. A second indirect safety measure is produced by the inherent sedative effects of the opioids commonly given. A sedated patient will not press the hand switch as readily.

Optimal patient care with opiate agents requires an understanding of the hierarchy of the response to analgesics. The patient's qualitative pain relief correlates with their personal response to a particular serum drug concentration.[15] The feasibility of narcotic therapy stems from the fact that analgesia occurs at serum drug concentrations below those that produce severe sedation and respiratory depression. Optimal analgesic therapy requires maintenance of a serum drug concentration that corresponds to a patient's minute-by-minute changing needs. It has been recognized that postoperative pain is not continuous; it waxes and wanes over various intensities.[29] The PCA devices allow the patient to titrate their own analgesic dose against the experienced discomfort. The individual circadian variation in response to pain,[30] which may complicate the administration of analgesics, could be addressed by a PCA system.

The patient should be educated as to the end point of analgesic therapy. A model proposed by Oxford investigators, Bullingham and coworkers,[31] used the generation of comfort rather than pain relief as the goal of therapy. They stated that analgesic drugs have both positive effects (such as analgesia and feelings of well-being) and negative effects (such as nausea and vomiting). Some properties, such as sedation, may be felt as positive by some patients and negative by others. The analgesic blood level sought should be that which maximizes comfort (positive effects) while maintaining tolerable levels of discomfort (negative

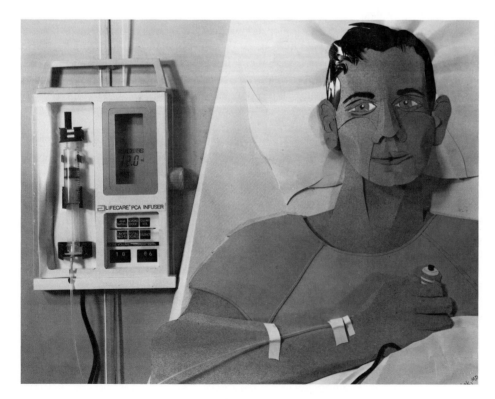

FIGURE 20-1. Typical PCA device (illustration by Stephen Ponchak, M.D.)

effects). Maximal comfort might not correspond with complete pain relief.

An important consideration is a particular patient's psychological profile. Coping styles were found to relate to medication requirements.[32] The ability to cope with pain depends on the patient's psychological propensity. The PCA device offers the patient a partial control that was lost during hospitalization; the importance of this should not be overlooked.

The detrimental effects of pain are well recognized. It would seem reasonable to predict that adequate analgesia might decrease sympathetic tone and thereby enhance bowel recovery after major surgery and trauma, foster early ambulation and return of pulmonary function, and aid cooperation with physical therapy. In one study,[33] investigators reported a 22 percent decrease in the duration of postoperative hospital stay when demand analgesia was used compared with conventional intramuscular therapy.

Morphine and meperidine are the most extensively studied intravenous analgesics for PCA therapy.[34] These agents offer the dual advantage of an intermediate duration of action with a minimal plateau in their analgesic potential. Agonists–antagonists are thought to have a so-called ceiling effect to both analgesia and respiratory depression. A typical recommendation for PCA therapy involves a titrated loading dose (e.g., morphine 2 to 10 mg or meperidine 25 to 100 mg) administered over 15 to 30 min in the recovery room before maintenance PCA therapy.[34] When patients show appropriate levels of awareness, they can assume control of the PCA triggering device. A typical initial bolus dose is 1 mg of morphine or 10 mg of meperidine. This dose then should be tailored to the patient's response and needs; the physical state and idiosyncrasies of the patient must be considered carefully. Often the bolus dose is increased at night to offer an increased interval for a more comfortable sleep.

The benefit of a continuous basal infusion of opioid concurrent with PCA is controversial. Parker and colleagues[35,36] found neither improved pain scores nor improved nighttime sleep patterns in patients receiving PCA plus a continuous infusion versus those receiving PCA alone.

The PCA device is well suited for many acutely painful situations. Experts cite its application to patients with cancer (especially terminal cancer), those in medical wards (e.g., sickle cell crisis), obstetrical patients (labor pain), those in intensive care units (acute traumatic injuries), and patients in coronary care units (myocardial ischemia); it also should be considered in clinical research.[34] In 1986, Tamsen and associates[37] reported the use of PCA for epidural administration of narcotics with partial success. Several studies show that this mode of PCA administration may result in a decreased narcotic requirement while providing the same analgesia as the continuous-infusion technique.[38,39]

Agonists–Antagonists

There may be as many as eight types of opiate receptors in brain and other organ tissues.[40] Although conclusive research evidence is lacking, in the central nervous system, five main categories of receptors, designated as μ, κ, δ, σ, and ϵ, are hypothesized. Attempts have been made to classify generally the opiate compounds based on the drugs interaction with particular receptors. Hence, the morphine-like opiate agonists act primarily at the μ receptor with, perhaps, contributions at the κ and δ receptors. The opiate antagonist naloxone is thought to demonstrate its antagonistic activity at both the μ and κ receptors. The agonist–antagonist compounds appear to be agonists at some receptors and antagonists at others.

The more common agonist–antagonists include pentazocine, nalbuphine, butorphanol, and buprenorphine. In addition, the δ agonist, dezosine is available. There appears to be a ceiling effect to both analgesia and respiratory depression with the agonist–antagonist group of medications.[41] Therefore, their use may be limited in patients with severe pain. Sublingual buprenorphine has been shown to be comparable to intramuscular morphine as a premedicant in those patients who wish to avoid injections.[42] It has been recommended that postoperative pain relief be initiated, however, with an intravenous dose before subsequent subinguinal doses are administered to maintain a comparable efficacy.

Nonnarcotic Analgesics

In the past, nonnarcotic analgesics (such as aspirin, acetaminophen, and the nonsteroidal anti-inflammatory drugs) were of little use in the treatment of pain after major surgery because of the lack of availability of parenteral preparations and the ceiling effect of the analgesia they produce. The recent introduction of ketorolac, however, has abrogated these problems because it is available for intramuscular administration and appears to have a higher analgesic ceiling than the oral nonsteroidal preparations available (see Chap. 26). The combination of such drugs with epidural local anesthesia may provide a new method of so-called balanced analgesia.[43]

Analgesic Adjuvants

Analgesic medications act on the nervous system to minimize or abolish the pain experience. This incorporates more than just the conscious awareness of noxious stimuli. The difference between pain as a specific sensation versus pain as suffering with its concomitant reactions should be realized. There are many secondary psychological associations in the pain experience. Fear, apprehension, anxiety, depression, insomnia, and other negative affective reactions are incorporated. Pharmaceutical therapeutics often are directed toward the psychological manifestations of discomfort.

Skillful therapeutic pharmacologic intervention mandates insight into the pathophysiologic cause of the discomfort. The expected intensity, duration, and secondary characteristics should be anticipated. The primary goal of analgesic medication is pain relief. If pain is severe enough, the narcotic medications generally are given. In the control of pain such as headaches, neuralgias, or rheumatoid disorders, the nonnarcotic or nonsteroidal anti-inflammatory agents may be sufficient. In other circumstances, the discomfort may be of such intensity that attempts are made to prescribe so-called potentiators in addition to narcotics. This strategy stimulated the use of phenothiazines, antihistamines, or minor tranquilizers as potentiating agents. These agents may potentiate the narcotics in ways other than the analgesic action itself. Some phenothiazine derivatives enhance the sedative effects of the narcotics, but an antianalgesic effect has been found for this class of agents.[44] Similarly, barbiturates in small doses are hyperalgesic and increase the reaction to painful stimuli.[45] Unlike the barbiturates, benzodiazepenes do not cause hyperalgesia. If muscle spasms contribute to the pain, anxiolytics could produce analgesia indirectly by causing muscle relaxation of the spasms. A relatively common clinical practice is to prescribe hydroxyzine hydrochloride with a narcotic analgesic. The rationale behind its use is to enhance the analgesia of the narcotic without comparable increase in the respiratory depression that would be experienced by giving a larger dose of the opiate itself. It was concluded by Stambaugh and Wainer[46] that hydroxyzine does not alter the pharmacokinetics or metabolism of meperidine, and it was suggested that, if any analgesic enhancement does occur, it involves a summation of effects in the central nervous system. Also, hydroxyzine appears to potentiate the analgesic effect of narcotics only when given parenterally. Although not currently used clinically, the addition of 10 mg of dextroamphetamine to morphine in postoperative patients was shown to potentiate the analgesic effect twofold over that of morphine alone.[47] In addition, lethargy, sedation, and respiratory depression were minimized. When orally combined with various analgesics, caffeine has been found statistically to be an analgesic adjuvant.[48]

Nausea and vomiting may be produced by morphine through its stimulation of the chemoreceptor trigger zone. The emetic effects may be counteracted by potent dopamine-blocking phenothiazine derivatives. Most neuroleptics have a marked protective action against the nausea produced by apomorhine and certain ergot alkaloids. The nausea caused by vestibular stimulation sometimes may respond to potent piperazines or butyrophenones. With the exception of thioridazine, most neuroleptic agents have antiemetic effects. Phenothiazines can prevent the vomiting caused by opioid analgesics and other etiologic agents. Promethazine also often is useful. Prochlorperazine is thought to produce a high incidence of dystonias, especially if given intramuscularly.[49]

INTRASPINAL OPIATES (See Chap. 27)

The goal of pain management is the reduction or elimination of noxious stimuli reaching the conscious awareness of a patient. Concomitantly, it is desirable to maintain as near a normal physiologic state as possible with minimal untoward effects. To achieve this goal, an encouragingly effective method was developed that involves the application of the opiates, and other related compounds, to the intrathecal and epidural spaces. The rationale for this technique is simple. Receptor activity in the dorsal horn of the spinal cord could block primary afferent transmission and minimize concurrently the systemic effects of the opiates. As the doses of opioid approach those used for intravenous administration (which is often the case with lipid-insoluble agents[50,51]), systemic effects may not be minimized.

Early clinical applications[52,53] of intrathecal and epidural opiates showed the potential for profound and long-lasting analgesia. The preliminary trials prompted trials of many diverse applications with resultant case reports demonstrating that more research was needed. Respectful caution gradually ensued after undesirable side effects, including nausea and vomiting, urinary retention, pruritus, hypotension, and most notably, both early and late respiratory depression, were reported.[54–56] More recent investigations into the pharmacodynamic and pharmacokinetic relationships of opiates in the central nervous system have led to a better comprehension and safer guidelines for optimal therapeutics.

A technical advantage of spinal opiates lies, in part, with their relative analgesic selectivity. Early investigators[57,58] observed no detectable changes in sensory, motor, or sympathetic function. Subsequent studies found sparing of efferent sympathetic vasoconstriction and pseudomotor activity.[59] Touch and proprioception also were not impaired. Both somatic and visceral pain may be obtunded. The practicality of this technique in regard to early ambulation and avoidance of cardiovascular collapse or convulsions easily can be seen, especially in light of the expected effects of local anesthetic blockade.

Rational use of spinal opiates mandates an appreciation of the interaction of the opioid molecules with the components of the central nervous system compartments. The low lipid solubility of morphine coupled with its molecular shape predisposes it to a slower onset of action with delayed peak concentrations in the cerebrospinal fluid.[60] Morphine is thought to have a relatively slower egress from the cerebrospinal fluid with a greater tendency to migrate toward the respiratory centers in the brain. Fentanyl and lofentanil are highly lipid soluble and therefore have a more rapid onset of action with decreased chance of residual late effects. In addition to their liphophilicity and molecular shape, their molecular weights appear to be a factor in the penetration of the dura mater.[61]

Evidence suggests that there is a dose–response relationship between epidural opiates and postoperative analgesia.[62] The dose appears to affect both the quality of the analgesia and its duration.[60] The latter is governed by the initial concentration, rate of systemic absorption, and the rate of dissociation from the receptor.

The choice between epidural opiates versus an intrathecal approach must be based on clinical circumstances. The epidural approach offers the advantage of a decreased likelihood of postdural puncture headache, respiratory depression, and CNS infection.

Recommendations for optimal dosing of epidural opiates have been slow in coming. In part this is associated with discrepancies in suggested doses caused by the concomitant administration of local anesthetics, narcotics, or sedatives by a second route. The operative site appears to influence the quantity of opiate required and the necessary volume of dilution for the opiate solution. In a 1985 prospective study of 1085 patients,[63] where the epidural catheter was placed at a segmental level corresponding to the middle of the operative wound area, morphine 4 mg (diluted in 10 ml of saline or local anesthetic solution) was found to be an optimal initial dose for hip arthroplasty and other major lower extremity operations. After prostatectomies, laparotomies, and thoracotomies, a higher success rate was reported using a 6-mg initial dose of morphine (diluted in 4 ml for high thoracic and 6 ml for low thoracic operations). In addition, a second or third epidural dose often was needed to produce satisfactory analgesia after laparotomies or thoracotomies; a total dose of 10 to 15 mg was not uncommon. Furthermore, a diluting solution of a local anesthetic (bupivacaine) was used if the patient already was experiencing discomfort at the time of the epidural injection.

More recently, in 1991, Ready and colleagues[64] reported their experience with 1106 patients who were treated postoperatively on a surgical ward with epidural morphine. Their patients reported median pain scores of 1 in 10 at rest and 4 in 10 with movement despite considerably lower doses (mean, 3.4 to 4.2 mg of morphine, depending on the site of surgery) than were used earlier.

We emphasize that epidural opiate dosing must be adjusted to the patient's needs, the operation, and the hospital setting; also we must be aware of possible unwanted side effects. Typical guidelines for using the more common opioids in the epidural space have been suggested as follows: morphine 0.1 mg/kg, meperidine 1.0 mg/kg, fentanyl 0.001 mg/kg, hydromorphone 0.01 mg/kg, and methadone 0.1 mg/kg.[65] Intrathecal morphine usually is administered at ⅟₁₅ of the epidural dose.

The merits of combining an opioid with a local anesthetic for epidural administration have been fairly well established. This allows lower doses of both agents to be administered with a consequent lower incidence of side effects, a decrease in the stress response to surgery,[66] im-

proved pulmonary function,[67] and reduced risk of thromboembolic events.[68]

Other agents that produce analgesia when administered by the epidural route include clonidine[69] and ketamine.[70] The value of these agents in the treatment of postoperative pain currently is being investigated.

Epinephrine generally is not used clinically during the administration of epidural opiates. In healthy volunteers, it was found that cutaneous hypalgesia was more intense, faster in onset, and longer in duration after the use of epidural morphine with 1:200,000 epinephrine compared with morphine alone.[71] However, when epinephrine was added, the investigators observed more intense adverse reactions consisting of pruritus, nausea, vomiting, difficulty of micturition, and depressed respiratory sensitivity to carbon dioxide 6 to 16 h after the injection.

The most life-threatening complication of spinal opiates is that of a respiratory depression. The depression may be early (1 to 2 h after the injection) or late (6 to 24 h postinjection). It appears that early respiratory depression is a reflection of vascular absorption.[60] It is influenced by vertebral venous and arterial blood flow and the characteristics of the opiate administered. Late respiratory depression is thought to be caused by rostral migration of the opiate in the cerebrospinal fluid that exerts an influence on the respiratory centers in the brain.[72] There would appear to be a predisposition toward this occurrence related to increased thoracic pressure, advanced age, unusually high subarachnoid dose (as might occur after inadvertent dural puncture), use of the Trendelenburg position, minimal previous exposure to narcotics, or concomitant administration of opiates or other depressant drugs.[56,60,73,74] Recent data[75,76] indicate that the actual clinical incidence of this potentially life-threatening complication is approximately 0.1 percent. With good clinical judgment and a knowledge of potentiating factors, combined with close observation, a disastrous result should be an extremely rare occurrence. Small doses of an opiate antagonist (naloxone, 0.1 to 0.2 mg) should reverse the respiratory depression without severely compromising the analgesia.[76] The dose often should be repeated, however, because of the short duration of action of naloxone compared with intraspinal narcotics. Alternatively, a naloxone drip may be started. Delayed respiratory depression when using fentanyl has not been observed as frequently. In a 1991 series of 1106 patients,[64] a 0.2% incidence rate of respiratory depression, 24% of pruritus, and 29% of nausea were reported.

Other side effects occur with great discrepancy in their incidence. Pruritus has been reported to occur in 0 percent to 90 percent of patients treated with epidural narcotics for the management of postoperative pain.[77] Urinary retention occurs in 3 percent to 100 percent of patients.[77] This retention may respond to naloxone or bethanechol;[48] some percentage of patients requires bladder catheterization. Nausea and vomiting has been reported to occur in 17 percent to 60 percent of patients.[77] The nausea and vomiting may be antagonized by naloxone without significantly affecting the analgesia.[76] Additional side effects might include dysphoria, constipation, headache, interference of thermal regulation, depression of cough reflex, and oliguria. The incidence of complications generally is reported to be higher after intrathecal compared with epidural administration.

Intraspinal narcotics appear to be useful in most postoperative situations, and many centers use epidural fentanyl for the pain after a Caesarean section. There is some controversy about its utility for labor pain.[78]

Several studies compared epidural analgesia with PCA or intramuscular narcotic administration after Caesarean section. Superior analgesia was observed using the epidural technique,[79,80] although patient satisfaction with PCA was high.

Other appropriate acute and chronically painful situations, such as the labor and delivery of a parturient with a single cardiac ventricle,[81] might be handled appropriately using this technique because excellent analgesia is offered with minimal alteration in motor, sensory, or autonomic function.

REGIONAL ANESTHESIA

The availability of the long-acting anesthetics, bupivacaine and etidocaine, have made the use of regional anesthesia more practical for the management of acute and postoperative pain. In general, when the sensory innervation of a traumatized area is accessible readily, it may be prudent to block the afferent input of noxious stimuli by administering these longer acting local anesthetics. A major disadvantage of regional anesthesic techniques is that they are labor intensive. In addition, the regional techniques may be painful, and therefore in postoperative management after a general anesthetic, consideration should be given toward administering the block before emergence. The common types of local anesthetic blockade used postoperatively include central blocks (such as epidurally applied anesthetics) or the more peripheral type (of which the intercostal block is the prototype). Regional techniques should be considered for pain refractory to other methods.

A detailed discussion of epidurally applied anesthetics is not in the scope of this chapter. Patients who are managed with a continuous epidural generally are pleased with the degree of comfort that they experience. However, the difficulties associated with prolonged immobilization, continuous sympathectomy, and urinary retention must be balanced against the benefits. However, many of these effects are dose related; appropriately applied, epidural local anesthetics may facilitate early ambulation. In one study,[82] 81 patients who underwent major abdominal procedures were assigned to one of five treatment groups as follows: (1) epidural morphine, (2) epidural bupivacaine, (3) a combination of morphine and bupivacaine, (4) epidural saline, and (5) no epidural catheter. The results suggest that the patients receiving a combination of morphine and bupivacaine

epidurally did best in measurement of pain intensity and return of respiratory function and ambulation.

Intercostal nerve block is a relatively simple and effective technique that can be used to interrupt the transmission of pain impulses that arise from the superficial structures of the chest wall. It will not relieve discomfort of visceral origin. Intercostal nerve blocks have been done intrathoracically at the time of surgery, or extrapleurally with either an intermittent or continuous technique. An advantage of intercostal blocks, especially in comparison with epidural local anesthetics, is the reduced risk of hypotension. The disadvantages of this technique include the relatively high absorbed blood levels of local anesthetics and the risk of pneumothorax. The effect on measures of pulmonary functions in patients managed by intercostal nerve blocks after thoracotomy is controversial; some clinicians believe that intercostal nerve blocks have less detrimental effects on effort-dependent variables (such as respiratory rate and vital capacity) but no change in the effort-independent variables.[83] Continuous intercostal nerve block has been shown to be successful for the management of multiple fractured ribs.[84]

The appropriate use of wound infiltration with local anesthetics has been thought to delay and lessen the first experience of pain after an operation.[85] The potential benefits of this technique, modified by varying circumstances, have appeared in the literature. The combination of bupivacaine wound infiltration together with efficient esophagogastric decompression and immediate elemental feeding was shown to reduce postoperative analgesia requirements and appeared to decrease the length of hospitalization in patients postcholecystectomy.[86] During laparoscopic tubal occlusion, the use of topical etidocaine 1% (5 ml) dropped on each fallopian tube from the uterus to the fimbria before tubal banding reduced the narcotic requirement, the incidence of vomiting, and the frequency of overnight stay.[87]

Local anesthetic nerve blocks for extremity surgery may be particularly effective. In a report of 167 patients who underwent surgery of the arm, knee, or foot, 80 percent did not require analgesics in the first 4 h postoperatively, and 39 percent did not require them in 8 h.[88]

Interpleural local anesthetics by catheter have been used to manage postoperative pain.[89] The investigators administered 20 ml of bupivacaine 0.5% in patients who had undergone cholecystectomy, renal surgery, and unilateral breast operations. Only three patients in their investigational group of 81 were not satisfied with the total degree of analgesia offered by this technique. Although not occurring in the study, the potential risks for pneumothorax must be addressed. In addition, controlled studies are necessary to determine the most appropriate dose, volume, and concentration of bupivacaine and determine the anesthetic blood levels achieved by this technique.

Cryoanalgesia is a technique useful in both chronic pain situations and postoperative pain management. It is the application of extreme cold (–60°C to –70°C) to a peripheral nerve to produce a reversible interruption of neural transmission. This technique was developed in the wake of an unacceptably high incidence of neuralgia associated with the irreversible techniques of surgical neurectomy, crushing, thermolysis, alcohol neurolysis, and other methods of peripheral nerve destruction. The duration of pain relief is determined by the time taken for normal regeneration of the peripheral nerve that was treated. It may be applied intraoperatively or through a percutaneous route. Cryoanalgesia has received much attention in its use after thoracotomy. In a randomized controlled trial,[90] patients who underwent thoracotomy and received intercostal nerve cryoprobe treatments had less pain at rest than those given intramuscular morphine. More recently, a study[91] of similar patients who underwent intraoperative cryolysis of the intercostal nerves innervating the incision, showed cryoanalgesia can reduce both the analgesic requirement and diminish the impairment of ventilatory capacity. It also was recommended in this study that the sites of drainage be treated. The need for special equipment has hindered the widespread use of cryoanalgesia and prevented the realization of its full potential.

TENS (See Chap. 30)

The search for effective pain relief with minimal undesirable effects continues to challenge our ingenuity. Electricity, which we might consider the most influential energy force since the harnessing of fire, can be used in the production of analgesia. This concept is not new; in fact, there is historic data showing the use of electricity produced by marine and freshwater fish in the therapeutic reduction of suffering during ancient times.[92] Egyptian and Greek healers appreciated that numbing qualities were possible by applying electric eels, rays, or catfish to the skin, and even when they were taken internally. With the development of electrostatic machines in the 18th and 19th centuries, the technology for more consistent electrical analgesia was available. Products were marketed that were useful to alleviate various discomforts and minimize acute procedure-induced pain (such as during dental extractions).

The electrophysiology of stimulation is not understood completely.[93] Major foundations for conceptualization of pain-attenuating interventions were initiated by the gate-control theory of pain transmission by Melzack and Wall[1] in 1965. A practical application of this theory was demonstrated by Wall and Sweet[94] when they used electrical current to stimulate predominantly large-diameter cutaneous afferent fibers and thereby modulate externally the perception of pain.

A TENS stimulator is a device that produces an electrical current through conducive paths on the skin. The current's wave form can be modified in terms of pulse rate, width, and amplitude. Some of the earliest clinical applications of these devices were studied by Long.[95] The concept that a TENS unit can be a useful adjunct for acute postoperative pain management was suggested by Hymes and coworkers[96] in 1973. They reported the reduction of postoperative complications, including ileus and atelectasis. Subsequent studies support the efficacy of a TENS unit in the relief of acute pain, but its role in the reduction of postoperative complications has not been consistent. VanderArk and McGrath,[97] in a prospective randomized placebo-controlled study, reported pain relief in 77 percent of the test patients compared with 17 percent of the control group. In this study population, activating the TENS unit for only 20 min three times per day did not produce a significant decrease in postoperative ileus. Cooperman and colleagues[98] used sham simulators in an attempt to control for a psychological placebo response and found that those patients who were undergoing surgery for malignant disease did not perceive as favorable the pain relief compared with those with a benign disease. In addition, these authors reported no difference between stimulation and control patients regarding ileus, atelectasis, pneumonia, or length of stay in an intensive care unit. Pike[99] reported a decreased subjective index of pain, narcotic requirement, and incidence of nausea and vomiting. In this study of patients undergoing hip surgery, the TENS electrodes were placed in a consistent arrangement away from the immediate incisional area in an attempt to overlie the major innervations of the hip joint. Ali and associates[100] studied the use of TENS in patients undergoing upper abdominal surgery; their data suggested that TENS minimized the changes in postoperative respiratory mechanics and decreased the incidence of pulmonary complications, presumably by alleviating incisional pain. Studies[101,102] confirm the efficacy of TENS in patients undergoing thoracotomy; Warfield and associates[102] observed shorter recovery room stays and better tolerance of chest physical therapy in the TENS group. An observation by Soloman and colleagues[103] was that TENS appeared more effectively to reduce the need for postoperative narcotics in patients who had not been exposed to narcotics during the preoperative period. The dependence of effectiveness of TENS on patient abstinence from narcotics might explain in part some of the earlier conflicting TENS data and offer alternative hypotheses for a TENS mechanism of action.

Many different TENS units, each with their own characteristics, are available. Both the physical hardware and electrical versatility may vary with the particular product. Some units, with increased versatility for contouring the output wave form, may be better suited for a particular pain problem; however, their complexity may increase the possibility of confusing the patient with a large number of control parameters.

A rectangular wave form may be adjusted in rate, width, and amplitude. If a spike wave form is used, then the pulse width is fixed, and the rate and amplitude are adjusted. The rate generally varies from 2 to 150 pulses/s with 80 to 100 pulses/s being most common. The pulse width (duration of each impulse) often ranges between 50 and 200 μs. The lower ranges often are less effective, but the wider pulse widths have an increased probability for stimulating peripheral motor fibers. The amplitude is measured in milliamperes, and together with the pulse width, this determines the total electrical energy of intensity. Generally, a biphasic (alternating) current is used. A full discussion of the advantages of TENS settings for particular pain problems is not in the scope of this chapter.

The side effects of TENS units are generally minimal.[99] Contact dermatitis usually can be avoided with good skin care (applying conductive gel to minimize irregularities in current density beneath the electrode may be helpful) and the use of alternating current rather than direct current. The latter has a greater potential for iontophoresis. Muscle spasms may occur if the intensity is set too high. Safety has not been ascertained in the concomitant use of a TENS unit with a demand cardiac pacemaker. Also, it is not recommended that a TENS unit be placed over the carotid sinus, larynx, trachea, eye, or the uterus of a pregnant woman.[104]

Electrode placement should be tailored to the individual situation. Postoperatively, one set of electrodes often is placed parallel to the incision before sterile dressings are applied. The other set may be placed paravertebrally at the corresponding affected dermatome. If analgesia is not optimal, the unit and setting should be checked, and replacement of the electrodes should be considered.

Preoperative evaluation for proper selection of TENS candidates is recommended highly. A high degree of neuroticism has been shown to have a deleterious effect on TENS efficiency.[105] Also, preoperative explanation may allow determination of initial TENS settings and allay the anxiety of the patient.

In summary, TENS appears to be a relatively low-risk adjunct for acute pain management. When the acute pain is well localized,[106] as in postoperative incisions, it is particularly effective. Selected patients, such as those at increased risk for respiratory compromise, may have additional benefits when TENS is used. Also, the patient will be less sedated and more comfortable; this can be a particularly desirable goal in situations such as that of the post-Caesarean mother who desires a level of alertness for mother–infant bonding.

BEHAVIORAL TECHNIQUES

The patient must be regarded as a whole being. The mind and body interact in many ways that are beyond our current level of comprehension. Relaxation techniques, biofeedback, and hypnosis all have been used in an attempt to exploit the potential of mind control over the body's physiologic state. Although labor intensive, relaxation techniques have been used to deliver a smoother recovery during the postoperative period. Statistical differences have been observed between patients who have been taught relaxation techniques and those not so instructed with re-

gard to reported incisional pain, analgesic consumption, and respiratory rate in patients who have undergone cholecystectomies, herniorrhaphies, and hemorrhoidectomies.[107] Relaxation training has been thought to decrease abdominal muscle tension and influence the psychological variables of anxiety and perceived control.[108] Trial studies have shown its effectiveness in reducing distress.

SUMMARY

Various techniques are available to treat postoperative pain. The selection of an appropriate method must be individualized for each patient. In many cases, a combination of various therapies will provide optimal pain relief. Whatever the situation, application of the available techniques of pain control should ensure a pain-free postoperative period for each patient.

References

1. Melzack R, Wall PD. Pain mechanisms; a new theory. *Science* 1965; 150:971.
2. Sinatra R, ed. *Acute Pain*. St. Louis: Mosby; 1992.
3. Park GR, ed. *Management of Acute Pain*. New York: Oxford University Press; 1991.
4. Tight fisted analgesia. *Lancet* 1976; 1:1338. Editorial.
5. Freed DLJ. Inadequate analgesia at night. *Lancet* 1975; 1:519.
6. Benedetti C, Bonica JJ, Bellucci G. Pathophysiology and therapy of postoperative pain: a review. In: Benedetti C, Chapman CR, Moricca G, et al, eds. *Advances in Pain Research and Therapy*. Vol. 7. New York: Raven Press; 1984:373–407.
7. Cohen FL. Postsurgical pain relief: patient status and nurses' medication choices. *Pain* 1980; 9:265–275.
8. Marks RM, Sachar EJ. Undertreatment of medical inpatients with narcotic analgesics. *Ann Intern Med* 1973; 78:173–181.
9. Porter J, Hershel J. Addiction rare in patients treated with narcotics. *N Engl J Med* 1980; 302:123.
10. Mather L, Mackie J. The incidence of postoperative pain in children. *Pain* 1983; 15:271–282.
11. Miller-Jones CMH, William JH. Sedation for ventilation. A retrospective study of fifty patients. *Anaesthesia* 1980; 35:1104.
12. Paralyzed with fear. *Lancet* 1981; 1:427. Editorial.
13. Ty TZ, Melzack R, Wall PD. Acute trauma. In: Wall P, Melzack R, eds. *Textbook of Pain*. Edinburgh: Churchill-Livingstone; 1984:209–214.
14. Beecher HK. *Measurement of Subjective Responses*. New York: Oxford University Press; 1959.
15. Austin KL, Stapelton JV, Mather LE. Relationship between blood meperidine concentration and analgesic response: a preliminary report. *Anesthesiology* 1980; 53:460–466.
16. Gourlay GK, Wilson PR, Glynn CJ. Pharmacodynamics and pharmacokinetics of methadone during the perioperative period. *Anesthesiology* 1982; 57:458–467.

17. Gourlay GK, Willis RJ, Wilson PR. Postoperative pain control with methadone: influence if supplemental methadone doses on blood concentration–response relationships. *Anesthesiology* 1984; 61:19–26.

18. Rutter PC, Murphey F, Dudley HAF. Morphine: controlled trial of different methods of administration for postoperative pain relief. *Br Med J* 1980; 280:12–13.

19. Goudie TA, Allen MW, Lonsdale M, et al. Continuous subcutaneous infusion of morphine for postoperative pain relief. *Anaesthesia* 1985; 40:1086–1092.

20. Caplan RA, Ready LB, Oden RV, et al. Transdermal fentanyl for postoperative pain management. A double blind placebo study. *JAMA* 1989; 261:1036–1039.

21. Gourlay GK, Kowalski SR, Plummer JL, et al. The transdermal administration of fentanyl in the treatment of postoperative pain: pharmacokinetics and pharmacodynamic effects. *Pain* 1989; 37:193–202.

22. Rowbotham DJ, Wyld R, Peacock JE, et al. Transdermal fentanyl for the relief of pain after upper abdominal surgery. *Br J Anaesth* 1989; 63:56–59.

23. Roe BB. Are postoperative narcotics necessary? *Arch Surg* 1963; 87:912–915.

24. Sechzer PH. Objective measurement of pain. *Anesthesiology* 1968; 29:209–210.

25. Bennet RL, Batenhorst RL, Bivins BA, et al. Patient controlled analgesia. *Ann Surg* 1987; 195:700–704.

26. Bennet RL, Baterhorst RL, Foster TS, et al. Postoperative pulmonary function with patient controlled anesthesia. *Anesth Anal 9* 1982; 6:171.

27. White WD, Pearce DJ, Normal J. Postoperative analgesics: a comparison of intravenous on-demand fentanyl with epidural bupivacaine. *Br Med J* 1979; 2:166–167.

28. Forrest WH Jr, Smethurst PWR, Kienitz ME. Self administration of intravenous analgesics. *Anesthesiology* 1970; 33:363–365.

29. Hull CJ, Sibbald A. Patient controlled analgesia. *Lancet* 1980; 1:1030.

30. Graves DA, Batenhorst RL, Bennett RL, et al. Morphine requirements using patient controlled analgesia—influence of diurnal variation and morbid obesity. *Clin Pharm* 1983; 2:49–53.

31. Bullingham RES, Jacobs OLR, McQuay HJ, et al. The Oxford system of patient controlled analgesia. In: Foley KM, Inturissi CE, eds. *Advances in Pain Research and Therapy*. New York: Raven Press; 1986:319–324.

32. Wilson JF, Bennet RL. Coping styles, medication use, and pain score patients using patient controlled analgesia for postoperative pain. *Anesthesiology* September 1984; 3A:A193.

33. Finley RJ, Keeri-Szanto M, Boyd D. New analgesic agents and techniques shorten postoperative hospital stay. *Pain* 1984; 2:S397.

34. White PF. Patient controlled analgesia: a new approach to the management of postoperative pain. *Semin Anesth* September 1985; 4(3).

35. Parker R, Holtmann B, White P. Patient-controlled analgesia. Does a concurrent opioid infusion improve pain management after surgery? *JAMA* 1991; 266(14)1947–1952.

36. Parker RK, Holtzmann B, White PF. Effects of a nighttime opioid infusion with PCA therapy on patient comfort and analgesic requirements after abdominal hysterectomy. *Anesthesiology* March 1992; 76(3):362–367.

37. Tamsen A, Sjoestroem S, Hartvig P. The Uppsala experience of patient controlled analgesia. In: Foley KM, Inturissi CE, eds. *Advances in Pain Research and Therapy*. Vol. 8. New York: Raven Press; 1986:325–332.

38. Marlowe S, Engstrom R, White P. Epidural patient-controlled analgesia (PCA): an alternative to continuous epidural infusions. *Pain* 1989; 37:97–101.

39. Sjostrom S, Hartvig D, Tamsen A. Patient-controlled analgesia with extradural morphine or pethidine. *Br J Anaesth* 1988; 60:358–366.

40. Jaffe JH, Martin WR. Opioid analgesics and antagonists. In: Goodman LS, Gilman A, eds. *The Pharmacologic Basis of Therapeutics*. 7th ed. New York: Macmillan; 1985:493.

41. Gal TJ, DiFazio CA, Moscick J. Analgesia and respiratory depressant activity of nalbuphine: a comparison with morphine. *Anesthesiology* 1982; 57:376.

42. Risbo AC, Jorgenson B, Kolly P, et al. Subinguinal buprenorphine for premedication and postoperative pain relief in orthopedic surgery. *Acta Anaesthesiol Scand* 1985; 29:180–182.

43. Dahl JB, Rosenberg J, Dirkes WE, et al. Prevention of postoperative pain by balanced analgesia. *Br J Anaesth* 1990; 64:518–520.

44. Moore J, Dundee JW. Alterations in response to somatic pain associated with anesthesia, VII: the effect of nine phenothiazines. *Br J Anaesth* 1981; 33:442.

45. Harvey SC. Hypnotics and sedatives. In: Goodman LS, Gilman A, eds. *The Pharmacologic Basis of Therapeutics*. 7th ed. New York: Macmillan; 1985:353.

46. Stambaugh JE, Wainer IW. Metabolic studies of hydroxyzine and meperidine in human subjects. In: Bonica JJ, ed. *Advances in Pain Research and Therapy*. Vol 1. New York: Raven Press; 1976:559–565.

47. Forrest WH Jr, Brown BWJ, Brown CR, et al. Dextroamphetamine with morphine for the treatment of postoperative pain. *N Engl J Med* 1977; 296:712–715.

48. Laska EM, Sunshine A, Mueller F, et al. Caffeine as an analgesic adjuvant. *JAMA* 1984; 251:1711–1718.

49. Baldessarini RJ. Drugs for the treatment of psychiatric disorders. In: Goodman LS, Gilman A, eds. *The Pharmacologic Basis of Therapeutics*. 7th ed. New York: Macmillan; 1985:411.

50. Camu F, Debucqouy F. Alfentanil infusion for postoperative pain: a comparison of epidural and intravenous routes. *Anesthesiology* 1991; 75:171–178.

51. Loper KA, Ready LB, Downey M, et al. Epidural and intravenous fentanyl infusions are clinically equivalent after knee surgery. *Anesth Analg* 1990; 70:72–75.

52. Wang JK, Nauss LA, Thomas JE. Pain relief by intrathecally applied morphine in man. *Anesthesiology* 1979; 50:149–151.

53. Behar M, Magora F, Olshwang D, et al. Epidural morphine in treatment of pain. *Lancet* 1979; 1:527–529.

54. Reiz S, Westberg M. Side effects of epidural morphine. *Lancet* 1980; 2:203–204.

55. Davies GK, Tolhurst-Cleaver CL, James TL. CNS depression from intrathecal morphine. *Anesthesiology* 1980; 52:280.

56. Glynn CJ, Mather LE, Cousins MJ, et al. Spinal narcotics and respiratory depression. *Lancet* 1979; 2:356–357.

57. Cousins MJ, Mather LE, Glynn CJ. Selective spinal analgesia. *Lancet* 1979; 1:1141–1142.

58. Yaksh TL, Reddy SVR. Studies in the primate on the analgesic effects associated with intrathecal actions of opiates, alpha-adrenergic agonists, and baclofen. *Anesthesiology* 1981; 54:451–467.

59. Glynn CJ, Mather LE, Cousins MJ, et al. Peridural meperidine in humans: analgesic response, pharmacokinetics, and transmission into CSF. *Anesthesiology* 1981; 55:520–526.

60. Cousins MJ, Mather LE. Intrathecal and epidural administration of opioids. *Anesthesiology* 1984; 61:276–310.

61. Moore RA, Bullingham RSJ, McQuay HG, et al. Dural permeability to narcotics: in vitro determination and application to extradural administration. *Br J Anaesth* 1982; 54:1117–1128.

62. Martin R, Salbaing J, Blaise G, et al. Epidural morphine for postoperative pain relief: a dose–response curve. *Anesthesiology* 1982; 56:423–426.

63. Stenseth R, Seltevold O, Breivik H. Epidural morphine for postoperative pain: experience with 1085 patients. *Acta Anaesthesiol Scand* 1985; 29:148–156.

64. Ready B, Loper K, Nessly M, Wild L. Post-operative epidural morphine is safe on surgical wards. *Anesthesiology* 1991; 75:452–456.

65. Raj P. Techniques of postoperative pain relief: intraspinal narcotics. Course syllabus; March 2, 1986; San Antonio, Texas: Dannemiller Memorial Education Foundation.

66. Kehet H. Surgical stress: the role of pain and analgesia. *Br J Anaesth* 1989; 63:189–195.

67. Torda TA. Management of acute and postoperative pain. *Int Anesthesiol Clin* 1983; 21:27–46.

68. Wildsmith JAW. Developments in local anesthetic drugs and techniques for pain relief. *Br J Anaesth* 1989; 63:159–164.

69. Bonnet F, Boico O, Rostaing S, et al. Clonidine-induced analgesia in postoperative patients: epidural versus intramuscular administration. *Anesthesiology* 1990; 72:423–427.

70. Maruset A, Skoglund LA, Hustveit O, et al. Comparison of ketamine and pethidine in experimental and postoperative pain. *Pain* 1989; 36:37–41.

71. Bromage PR, Camporesi EM, Durant PA, et al. Influence of epinephrine as an adjuvant to epidural morphine. *Anesthesiology* 1983; 58:257–262.

72. Bromage PR, Camporesi EM, Durant PA, et al. Rostral spread of epidural morphine. *Anesthesiology* 1982; 156:431–436.

73. Gjessing J, Tomlin PE. Postoperative pain control with intrathecal morphine. *Anaesthesia* 1981; 36:268–276.

74. Welch DB. Epidural narcotics and dural puncture. *Lancet* 1981; 1:55.

75. Rawal N, Arner S, Gustafsson LL, Allvin R. Present state of extradural and intrathecal opioid analgesia in Sweden. A nationwide follow-up survey. *Br J Anaesth* June 1987; 59:791–799.

76. Rawal N, Wattwill M. Respiratory depression following epidural morphine. An experimental and clinical study. *Anesth Analg* 1984; 63:8–14.

77. Staren ED, Cullen ML. Epidural catheter analgesia for the management of postoperative pain. *Surg Gynecol Obstet* 1986; 162:389–404.

78. Husemeyer RF, O'Connor MC, Davenport HT. Aspects of epidural morphine. *Lancet* 1979; 2:583–584.

79. Eisenbach J, Grico S, Dewan D. Patient-controlled analgesia following cesarean section: a comparison with epidural and intramuscular narcotics. *Anesthesiology* 1988; 6:444–448.

80. Harrison D, Sinatra R, Margese L, Chung J. Epidural narcotic and patient-controlled analgesia for post-cesarean section pain relief. *Anesthesiology* 1988; 68:454–457.

81. Ahmad S, Hawes D, Dooley S, et al. Intrathecal morphine in a parturient with a single ventricle. *Anesthesiology* 1981; 54:515–517.

82. Cullen ML, Staren ED, El-Ganzouri A, et al. Continuous epidural infusion for analgesia after major abdominal operations: a randomized, prospective, double-blind study. *Surgery* 1985; 98(4):718–728.

83. Woltering EA, Flye MW, Huntley S, et al. Evaluation of bupivacaine nerve blocks in the modification of pain and pulmonary function changes after thoracotomy. *Ann Thorac Surg* 1980; 30(2):122–127.

84. Murphy DF. Intercostal nerve blockade for fractured ribs and postoperative analgesia: description of a new technique. *Reg Anaesth* 1983; 8(4):151–153.

85. Hashemi K. A review of methods for relief of postoperative pain. *Ann R Coll Surg Engl* 1983; 64(4):274.

86. Moss G, Regal ME, Lichtig L. Reducing postoperative pain, narcotics, and length of hospitalization. *Surgery* 1986; 99(2):206–210.

87. Mckenzie R, Phitayakorn P, Uy NTL, et al. Topical etidocaine during laparoscopic tubal occlusion for postoperative pain relief. *Obstet Gynecol* 1986; 67(3):447–449.

88. Edmonds-Seal J, Paterson GML, Loach AB. Local nerve blocks for postoperative analgesia. *J R Soc Med* 1980; 73:111–114.

89. Reiestad F, Stromskag KE. Interpleural catheter in the management of postoperative pain. A preliminary report. *Reg Anaesth* 1986; 11(2):89–91.

90. Orr IA, Keenan DJ, Dundee JV. Improved pain relief after thoracotomy: use of cryoprobe and morphine infusion. *Br Med J* 1981; 283:945–948.

91. Brynitz S, Schroder M. Intraoperative cryolysis of intercostal nerves in thoracic surgery. *Scand J Thorac Cardiovasc Surg* 1986; 20:85–87.

92. Kane K, Taub A. A history of local electrical analgesia. *Pain* 1975; 1:125–138.

93. Lee KH, Chung JM, Willis WD. Inhibition of primate spinothalamic tract cells by TENS. *J Neurosurg* 1985; 62:276–287.

94. Wall PD, Sweet WH. Temporary abolition of pain in man. *Science* 1967; 155:108–109.

95. Long DM. External electrical stimulation as a treatment of chronic pain. *Minn Med* 1974; 57:195–198.

96. Hymes AC, Rabb DE, Yonehiro EG, et al. Electrical surface stimulation for control of acute postoperative pain and prevention of ileus. *Surg Forum* 1973; 24:447–449.

97. VanderArk GK, McGrath KA. Transcutaneous electrical stimulation in the treatment of postoperative pain. *Am J Surg* 1975; 130:338–340.

98. Cooperman AM, Hall B, Mikalacki K, et al. Use of transcutaneous electrical stimulation in the control of postoperative pain. *Am J Surg* 1977; 133:185–187.

99. Pike PMH. Transcutaneous electrical stimulation. Its use in the management of postoperative pain. *Anaesthesia* 1978; 33:165–171.

100. Ali J, Yaffe CS, Serrette C. The effect of transcutaneous electric nerve stimulation on postoperative pain and pulmonary function. *Surgery* 1981; 89(4):507–512.

101. Rooney SM, Subhash J, Goldiner P. Effect of transcutaneous nerve stimulation on postoperative pain after thoracotomy. *Anesth Analg* 1985; 62:1010–1012.

102. Warfield CA, Stein JM, Frank HA. The effect of transcutaneous electrical nerve stimulation on pain after thoracotomy. *Ann Thorac Surg* 1985; 39(5):462–465.

103. Soloman RA, Viernstein ML, Long DM. Reduction of postoperative pain and narcotic use by transcutaneous electrical nerve stimulation. *Surgery* 1980; 87(2):142–146.

104. Taylor AG, West BA, Simon B, et al. How effective is TENS for acute pain? *Am J Nurs* August 1983:1171–1174.

105. Lim AT, Geraldine E, Kranz H, et al. Postoperative pain control: contribution of psychological factors and transcutaneous electrical stimulation. *Pain* 1983; 17:179–188.

106. Gersh MR, Wolf SL. Applications of transcutaneous electrical nerve stimulation in the management of patients with pain. *Phys Ther* 1985; 65(3):314–336.

107. Flaherty GG, Fitzpatrick JJ. Relaxation techniques to increase comfort level of postoperative patients: a preliminary study. *Nurs Res* November–December 1978; 27(6):352–355.

108. Wells N. The effect of relaxation on postoperative muscle tension and pain. *Nurs Res* 1982; 31(4):236–238.

CHAPTER 21

Herpes Zoster

Prithvi Raj

Herpes zoster, commonly called *shingles,* is an acute infectious viral disease that primarily affects the posterior spinal root ganglia of the spinal nerves. A single posterior spinal root ganglion or a small number of adjacent ones may be affected, usually on the same side. The corresponding ganglia of the cranial nerves also may be involved similarly. The causative virus, varicella-zoster, belongs to a DNA group of viruses that is host specific. The same virus produces chickenpox or varicella in children and young people.[1]

Herpes zoster most frequently occurs in adults who previously have had chickenpox. It is thought that the virus remains dormant in the dorsal root ganglia until, many years later, the virus is reactivated and produces herpes zoster. The fall in immunity that permits the reactivation may be caused by infection or malignancy or it may occur in the iatrogenically immunosuppressed patient. In most cases, there is no known reason.[1] Patients with herpes zoster occasionally relate a history of recent contact with the virus exogenously, but it is rare, if ever, that an infection so develops. The incidence of herpes zoster does not increase during seasonal chickenpox epidemics.[2]

It is thought that after the virus multiplies in the dorsal root ganglion, it is transported along the sensory nerves to the nerve endings where the lesions are formed. In the immunocompetent patient, the disease is confined to a local distribution because there is a rapid mobilization of defense mechanisms.[3]

Although the posterior root ganglia of the spinal and cranial nerves are involved most commonly, any part of the central nervous system can be affected. For example, the anterior motor horn may be involved, or the patient may have myelitis or encephalomyelitis. In rare cases, only the sympathetic ganglia are affected, resulting in a syndrome resembling reflex sympathetic dystrophy.

The location of the herpes zoster infection may be determined by the site of a primary inflammatory disease, malignancy, or trauma. Patients with neoplasms, especially lymphomas, are more susceptible to herpes zoster. It is estimated that as many as 25 percent of patients with Hodgkin disease have herpes zoster. This high incidence may be the result of recent radiation of affected nodes, advanced disease, and possible splenectomy.[2] Other associated diseases include meningitis, spinal cord tumors, anterior poliomyelitis, syringomyelia, tabes dorsalis, intoxication from arsenicals or carbon monoxide, and malignant neoplasms such as breast, lung, or gastrointestinal tumors.[4]

Men are affected more frequently than women. The disease is more common in debilitated patients.

Only recently have important cellular-immune events been investigated in herpes zoster, and our knowledge of this is still scanty.[5] Experimental and clinical studies suggest that symptomatic herpes zoster occurs only when cell-mediated immunity to varicella-zoster is depressed.[6,7] There is an inverse correlation between the capacity of the host to mount a specific cellular immune response and the incidence of zoster. Cell-mediated immune responses to zoster have been difficult to evaluate because the response generally is suppressed during the disease and usually takes time to develop. The function of lymphocytes and monocytes is impaired in herpes zoster.[8] As in other herpetic infections, the normal ratio of helper T-cells to suppressor T-cells is reversed.[9] Immune function has been assessed primarily by measuring the blastogenic response to the peripheral blood mononuclear cells. The transformation index was greater in these patients than in control subjects, but the index did not correlate with the magnitude of the antibody response of the varicella-zoster virus or the interval since the varicella-zoster virus infection had developed, although the index appeared to be fairly specific for the virus.[10,11] The infection is limited by the cell-mediated immune lymphocytic transformation,[12] lymphocyte–monocyte inactivation of the virus,[13] and local host responses of interferon production and polymorphonuclear inflammatory response in the vesicle.[14] Antibody administration also modifies the disease, perhaps by altering membrane antigens and cellular cytotoxicity.[15]

POSTHERPETIC NEURALGIA

Postherpetic neuralgia is a continuation of herpes zoster that generally occurs in older patients. Although spontaneous resolution of herpes zoster may be expected in most patients, a significant number have intractable pain. Postherpetic neuralgia, which persists for months or years after the skin lesions have healed, occurs in approximately 10 percent of patients older than 40 years of age and 20 percent to 50 percent of patients older than 60 years of age.[3,16] Some young patients may have postherpetic neuralgia for 1 or 2 weeks after the lesions have healed, although hypesthesia or hyperesthesia may persist.

This is one of the most difficult problems encountered by physicians. Few other conditions create such agonizing pain and suffering for the patient. Many patients consider suicide as a means of relief from the torturous pain.

DIFFERENTIAL DIAGNOSIS

Acute Herpes Zoster

The diagnosis of herpes zoster usually is difficult to make in the preeruptive stage. After the lesions appear, the clinical features are so typical that the diagnosis is easy. Before eruption, herpes zoster often is mistaken for other pain-causing conditions, such as coronary disease, pleurisy, pleurodynia, cholecystitis, neural disease, appendicitis, peritonitis, and collapsed intervertebral disk. Occasionally, localized herpes simplex may occur. Differentiation between the two herpesvirus conditions can be made by virus isolation procedures in the laboratory.

To confirm the diagnosis of herpes zoster, the virus can be isolated from vesicular, but not usually from pustular or crusting, lesions 7 or 8 days after eruption. Specific antigens also can be found in vesicular fluid and in the crusts of lesions using a simple gel-precipitation technique.

Epithelial cells with eosinophilic intranuclear inclusions and multinucleated giant cells can be identified in material scraped from the base of a vesicular lesion. The leukocyte count is normal in uncomplicated herpes zoster. Mononuclear pleocytosis is present in the cerebrospinal fluid of patients with herpes zoster, particularly those with cranial nerve involvement.

Visceral pain can be differentiated from herpetic pain by a somatic sensory nerve block; this will not relieve visceral pain.

Postherpetic Neuralgia

Postherpetic neuralgia also can be confused with other problems, but the patient usually has a history of a previous unilateral skin eruption, and there may be residual scarring of the skin. Hyperesthesia, dysesthesia, and anesthesia also may be present in the affected areas. Skin eruption may be minimal in some cases, and few or even no scars may be present with postherpetic neuralgia (zoster sine herpete). In these patients, the central nervous system was damaged by the original infection, resulting in neuralgia without producing any scars to the skin. A rising zoster antibody titer in the acute stage confirms the infectious agent.[1]

SIGNS AND SYMPTOMS

Acute Herpes Zoster

The development and course of herpes zoster depends on contributions from both the virus and the host. It can pro-

gress in three stages, with virus and host factors interacting at each stage (Table 21-1).

Acute herpes usually has pain that is localized to the dermatomal distribution of one or more affected posterior root ganglia. The pain may be accompanied by fever and malaise. It usually is mild at first, but it may grow more severe over the succeeding few days. It can be dull, sharp, burning, aching, or shooting. Paresthesia also is present commonly. Skin lesions usually appear 4 to 5 days later, but they may appear immediately.

At first, there is a local redness and swelling followed by red papules that progress through vesicles, blebs, pustules, and then to the crusting stage over the succeeding 2 to 3 weeks. The lesions characteristically are unilateral, running along the dermatome in a band. In mild cases, the skin lesions may not affect the whole dermatome, but sensory involvement of the whole dermatome usually is present. In severe cases, larger blebs usually cover the entire dermatome and tend to coalesce. The area is likely to be extremely painful; the pain is aggravated by contact or movement.

The lesions appear in thoracic dermatomes in more than 50 percent of patients. The next region where they are seen commonly is the trigeminal distribution, with an incidence of 3 percent to 20 percent. The ophthalmic division is involved in 75 percent of these patients. Lumbar and cervical eruptions occur in 10 percent to 20 percent of patients, with a sacral distribution being much less common. With advancing age, the incidence of trigeminal (ophthalmic) zoster increases and that of spinal zoster declines. Bilateral zoster occurs in less than 1 percent of patients. Recurrent zoster has been reported in 1 percent to 8 percent of patients; approximately one-half of the recurrences are at the site of the previous eruption (Table 21-2).

Occasionally, motor paralysis in the intercostal and abdominal muscles, arms, legs, and muscles innervated by cranial nerves may be associated with herpes zoster. These motor deficits may be reversible over a period of years.

If the trigeminal (gasserian) ganglion is affected, the symptoms usually include pain in the nerve distribution, headache, weakness of the eyelid muscles, and occasional-

Table 21-1
Stages of Herpes Zoster

Stage I	Viral replication Loss of immune surveillance

Stage II	Clinical syndrome (acute herpes zoster)
	    Viral effect on ganglion–nerve–dermatome
	    Antiviral immune response by the body
	    Cytolysis from virus and host inflammatory
	        reaction

Stage III	Sequelae of herpes zoster
	    Central nervous system and visceral spread
	    Antiviral immune response

Reproduced with permission from Raj P. Pain due to herpes zoster. In: Raj P, ed. *Practical Management of Pain.* 2nd ed. Chicago: Mosby-Year Book; 1992.

Table 21-2
Site and Incidence of Acute Herpes Zoster

Site of Herpes Zoster	Incidence (percentage)
Thoracic	50
Face (ophthalmic)	3–20
Cervical	10–20
Bilateral	<1
Recurrent	1–8
Recurrent at the site of previous herpes zoster	50

Reproduced with permission from Raj P. Pain due to herpes zoster. In: Raj P, ed. *Practical Management of Pain*. 2nd ed. Chicago: Mosby-Year Book; 1992.

ly, an Argyll Robertson pupil. Lesions may appear on the face, cornea, mouth, and tongue. Scarring and anesthesia of the cornea may occur. The first division of the trigeminal nerve most often is affected. If there is involvement of the geniculate ganglion, there may be Bell's palsy, vertigo, disorders of hearing, and lesions of the external ear and canal and the anterior portion of the tongue.

The crusts generally fall off at approximately 5 weeks, leaving irregular pink scars. These scars eventually become hypopigmented and anesthetic. They form characteristic pocks, which usually are surrounded by mottled pigmentation and may last for years. The hyperesthesia and pain usually subside and disappear at approximately the same time the crusts fall off.

Postherpetic Neuralgia

In 10 percent to 50 percent of patients with herpes zoster, pain and hyperesthesia persist after the lesions are healed. This condition, called *postherpetic neuralgia,* may improve slowly, but after it has been present for 6 months, complete spontaneous cure is unlikely.

The discomfort of postherpetic neuralgia is of two types: pain and dysesthesia. The persistent intractable pain, which is constant and never varies, often is associated with a feeling of heat. It is described variously as burning, shooting, twisting, lancinating, pressing, and gripping. A feeling of tightness also may be present. Relief usually is found during sleep. In chronic postherpetic neuralgia, the patient commonly has hyperpathia. This is associated often with damage to a peripheral nerve, the spinothalamic tract, or the thalamus. It may be caused by a reduction in the number and proportion of conducting nerve fibers.

Dysthesia often is interpreted as pain. Uncomfortable unpleasant sensations make the patient unable to bear the lightest contact with the skin. Some patients even cut holes in their clothing to eliminate the problem. A slight breath of wind can incite a paroxysm of pain. Curiously, most patients can tolerate firm pressure on the affected area but not light pressure. They may wear especially tight clothing or keep their hands pressed over the painful region. Patients

may complain about a feeling of worms under the skin or of ants crawling over the skin (formication).

PATHOPHYSIOLOGY

Acute Herpes Zoster

Early lesions of herpes zoster are minute unilocular vesicles involving the epidermis and corium. There is a ballooning degeneration of the involved epithelial cells, and intranuclear inclusion bodies often are present. Huge giant cells with multiple inclusions are found in mature lesions. There may be necrosis and hemorrhaging into the uppermost portion of the dermis if there is destruction of the germinal layer. The typical varicella vesicles are formed from serum that collects around the damaged cells. The fluid in the vesicle soon becomes cloudy from polymorphonuclear leukocytes, multinucleated giant cells, degenerated cells, and fibrin. A scab is formed when the fluid is absorbed.[3]

The dorsal root ganglion of the affected nerve is hemorrhagic and swollen. There is round cell infiltration and eventually neuronal destruction. Ganglion and satellite cells may have intranuclear inclusions. Maximum degeneration is seen in the posterior nerve root approximately 2 weeks after the dermal lesions first appear. Similar changes may be seen in the posterior column and sensory nerves. Rarely, the anterior horn may be involved and/or a localized meningitis also may occur. Eventually, the ganglion may be replaced by scar tissue.[3]

Postherpetic Neuralgia

Many hypotheses have been postulated to explain the intractable nature of postherpetic neuralgia. Noxious impulses may become established in centrally located closed self-perpetuating loops, and progressive facilitation develops in these synapses. Eventually, pain that is entirely unaffected by surgical section of peripheral pathways occurs spontaneously. There also is a possibility that the infection involves higher pathways in the cord and brain than formerly was believed. If this is true, the infection is outside the reach of extradural and intrathecal medication and possibly beyond cordotomy.

The gate-control theory might explain some of the features involved in the production and persistence of postherpetic neuralgia. It is postulated that pain is carried by small unmyelinated nerve fibers to the central nervous system where the input is modified by pathways in larger myelinated nerve fibers. Nerve impulses are transmitted faster in the large myelinated nerve fibers than in the small unmyelinated nerve fibers. In acute herpes zoster, there is a tendency, proportionately, for more of the larger fibers to be damaged and destroyed than the small fibers. They also regenerate slower than small fibers, and their diameter after regeneration usually is smaller than originally. Hence, there is an increase in the percentage of smaller fibers over large fibers.[17]

According to the gate-control theory, this is the situation in which minimal small fiber stimulation might produce the sensation of pain because the normal modulation of large nerve fiber stimulation is no longer present. It is important to notice that older patients have fewer large fibers initially, and they lose more after herpes zoster infection. Therefore, such patients are more likely to feel a greater degree of pain than younger patients and to be more susceptible to the intractable pain of postherpetic neuralgia.

LABORATORY DIAGNOSIS

Because most viral replication occurs early in the disease process, optimal drug treatment depends on an early and accurate diagnosis. The varicella-zoster virus may be recovered from early vesicles and has been recovered from blood, lung, liver, and cerebrospinal fluid but, only occasionally, from the oropharynx. The virus is cell associated; therefore, scraping the base of the vesicle is more productive than using a fluid overlay. Scrapings also provide cellular material containing multinuclear giant cells. Acidophilic intranuclear inclusions can be seen in the Tzanck smear stained with hematoxylin and eosin, Giemsa, Papanicolaou, or Paragon multiple stain.[18] A punch biopsy for electron microscopic examination provides even more reliable material; the more reliable material may permit a diagnosis before the vesicular stage develops (Table 21-3).

MANAGEMENT

The goals of treatment are early resolution of the acute disease and prevention of postherpetic neuralgia. The earlier the institution of treatment, the less likely the development of postherpetic neuralgia.[19–21]

In attempting to answer the question of whether treating acute herpes zoster prevents postherpetic neuralgia, Pernak and associate[22] reported on a prospective randomized study of 1011 patients. She divided her patients into four groups according to the location of the lesions (333 patients with trigeminal neuralgia and 678 patients with lesions located on the trunk). Methylprednisolone 80 mg was injected around the gasserian ganglion for trigeminal neuralgia; 80 to 160 mg of methylprednisolone with lidocaine 0.5% was injected epidurally at appropriate epidural locations for thoracic neuralgia. Excellent pain relief was obtained in 997 patients. Fourteen patients subsequently had postherpetic neuralgia. All of them had persistent acute herpes zoster pain for 3 weeks. These authors concluded that their data showed that regional application of corticosteroids is effective in producing pain relief and preventing postherpetic neuralgia.

After postherpetic neuralgia is established, there is no reliable treatment for this syndrome. Aggressive management is necessary in patients who are prone to have this disorder (e.g., elderly or immunosuppressed patients). Un-

Table 21-3
Laboratory Diagnosis of Acute Herpes Zoster

Techniques	*Comments*

Virus Recovery from
  Vesicles
  Blood
  Lung
  Liver
  CSF
  Oropharynx (only occasionally)
	Rapid diagnostic tests allows for early diagnosis

Scrapings from the Vesicles contains Cellular Material with Multinucleated Giant Cells	

Tzanck Smear
  Hematoxylin–eosin stain
  Giemsa stain
  Papanicolaou stainn
  Paragon ultiple stain
	Show acidophilic intranuclear inclusions

Punch Biopsy for Electron Microscopy	More reliable and provides diagnosis before vesicular stage develops
Culture Tests (in human epitheloids or fibroblasts) Virus specifically identified in culture by intranuclear inclusions after staining and by gel precipitation techniques	Focal lesion with swollen refractile cells in 3–4 days
Staining of Cellular Material with Direct Fluorescent Antibody of Tzanck smear	Readily identifies infected cells

Reproduced with permission from Raj P. Pain due to herpes zoster. In: Raj P, ed. *Practical Management of Pain*. 2nd ed. Chicago: Mosby-Year Book; 1992.

fortunately, no treatment regimen is fully effective; this has led to many different treatments with varying success rates.

Some physicians do not treat acute herpes zoster because they believe it will resolve spontaneously if left alone. They institute treatment only if postherpetic neuralgia develops. This is a great disservice to the group of patients with intractable pain from postherpetic neuralgia. Treatment during the early stages of acute herpes zoster is the best means of preventing needless pain and suffering.

There is no treatment available which is effective in all cases. Success is limited usually with any method. Many methods of management have been tried for acute herpes zoster and postherpetic neuralgia.

Acute Herpes Zoster

Drug Therapy

The various drugs used in the treatment of the acute stage of herpes zoster are summarized in Table 21-4.

Antiviral Agents. Antiviral agents have been used in the treatment of herpes zoster. The herpes zoster virus, like all viruses, is a parasite that takes over healthy cells and uses their DNA to reproduce itself. It is believed that, if viral DNA synthesis can be slowed or inhibited, then specific host immune systems might have more time to help control the viral infection. Some substances that grossly inhibit DNA synthesis were developed as possible anticancer drugs and have been found to have a more significant antiviral activity than an anticancer activity. Theoretically, these agents could either kill the virus or alter its replication. To be effective, the agents must be given before significant tissue damage occurs.

Such agents include cytarabine, vidarabine, acyclovir,

Table 21-4
Drug Therapy for Acute Herpes Zoster

Antiviral Agents
    Cytarabine
    Vidarabine
    Idoxuridine
    Acyclovir
    Thymidine analogues
    Interferon
    Zoster immune globulin
    Adenosine monophosphate

Analgesics

Anti-Inflammatory Agents
    Prednisone

Antidepressants and Tranquilizers
    Amitriptyline and Fluphenazine
    Doxepin

Other
    Vitamin B_{12}
    B-complex vitamins
    L-tryptophan

and idoxuridine. Experimental trials using systemic administration of cytarabine in various dose schedules gave conflicting results. These results ranged from apparent success in early uncontrolled studies to no benefit or apparent worsening of infection in controlled therapeutic trials.[3] It has been reported that controlled studies of vidarabine in the treatment of herpes zoster in immunosuppressed patients have been promising.[23] Therapy was most successful when administered early and to patients younger than 38 years of age or to those with reticuloendothelial malignancy. Cutaneous healing was accelerated, pain was relieved acutely, and the incidence of postherpetic neuralgia was low.[7] Acyclovir masquerades as one of the building blocks of the DNA needed by the herpes virus to reproduce itself. This stops the chain, and the virus ceases to replicate. Some ophthalmologists have used idoxuridine for treating herpetic lesions of the conjunctiva and cornea. Prompt treatment is necessary, and best results are obtained when used within 4 or 5 days of the onset of infection. This drug's effects are variable, and it will not prevent postherpetic neuralgia.[2] Varying concentration of idoxuridine in dimethyl sulfoxide have been used in New Zealand to treat patients with herpes zoster, and it has been shown that pain decreased faster and that fewer vesicles developed after topical applications. Early initiation of treatment is necessary.[24] Similar positive results have been reported from Denmark.[25] Idoxuridine in dimethyl sulfoxide 35% to 40% has been used in Great Britain on herpes zoster skin lesions. It is reported that there is faster healing of lesions, there is a shorter duration of postherpetic neuralgia, and late sequelas are uncommon. Success depends on early institution of treatment. The solvent decreases inflammation and edema and has a bacteriostatic action. It is an extremely strong solvent that has not been approved by the Food and Drug Administration for this use.[2] Thymidine analogues have been found to have some inhibitory affect on certain strains of varicella-zoster virus.[26]

Interferon, which is produced by the body's immune system, appears to play a role in the control of disease. It seems to work more effectively in tandem with other components of the body's immune system. Large doses, however, can cause adverse effects. It has been reported that interferon production in the vesicle fluid of patients with disseminated herpes zoster is delayed in comparison with that of patients with localized disease.[23] When human leukocyte interferon has been administered, it has been shown to increase circulating interferon.[3] It may, therefore, be used in cases where there might be a risk of herpetic dissemination.

Development of a vaccine against herpes virus currently is underway. Scientists have isolated the gene that makes a major portion of the sheath or coat of the virus. It is hoped that, by introducing a harmless part of the virus into the system, the body will produce antibodies against it. Testing is still in the preliminary stages.

Zoster immune globulin is not effective in altering the

clinical course of herpes zoster in immunocompromised adults. It is used currently, however, for the passive protection of susceptible leukemia patients who have been exposed to chickenpox. It also is recommended for use in immunocompromised children at risk from chickenpox.[16,27]

Adenosine monophosphate given intramuscularly also has been used in the treatment of acute herpes zoster. The exact mechanism by which it provides certain therapeutic benefits is not understood. It may correct underlying biochemical imbalances or defects at the cellular level. Beneficial effects also may occur as a result of the vasodilating effect of the drug and its ability to decrease tissue edema and inflammation.

I believe that the ultimate answer to the problem of herpes zoster and its sequela, postherpetic neuralgia, lies in the field of antiviral therapy. An antiviral agent is needed that will kill the virus safely and reliably before there is neurologic damage. A great deal of investigation still must be done to find suitable antiviral agents against the varicella-zoster virus. Other agents being studied as antiviral agents include isoprinine, ribavirin, and BUDA.

Analgesics. Analgesics are an important adjunctive therapy. They may be categorized as nonaddictive, moderately addictive, or strongly addictive agents.[28] Selecting the optimal agent for a specific patient involves a consideration of various factors, the most important of which are quality, intensity, duration, and distribution of pain.

Nonnarcotic nonaddictive drugs are used for the control of mild pain. Aspirin and acetaminophen are effective drugs with a low incidence of side effects. However, they are not effective in controlling severe pain.

Codeine, propoxyphene, pentazocine, and oxycodone are examples of moderately addicting drugs. The incidence of addiction is relatively low, but dependence may occur with these agents. They are good analgesic agents, but they sometimes produce adverse side effects (such as constipation).

When used properly, the strongly addictive narcotics are effective drugs in the treatment of severe refractory pain. They provide relief to varying degrees. In acute herpes zoster, strong medication may be needed to control severe pain. Because the acute stage is short, strongly addictive drugs may be used for a limited period. In such cases, the narcotic is tapered off as treatment decreases the degree of pain. When pain is at a level that can be controlled by nonnarcotic drugs, the narcotics should be discontinued. Examples of strongly addictive drugs are morphine, hydromorphone, and meperidine.

Anti-Inflammatory Agents. The effects of corticosteroid therapy on herpes zoster are still unclear, but reports are encouraging. Gelfland[29] reported dramatic relief of pain in less than 2 days in patients treated with oral cortisone. Appleman[30] obtained equally good pain relief in the same amount of time with intradermal or intravenous corticotro-

pin. Elliot[31] obtained excellent results treating severely painful zoster with high doses of prednisone. The average duration of pain after early prednisone therapy was 3.5 days; pain averaged 3.5 weeks in untreated control subjects. These studies, however, involved only a small number of patients with few or no controls. Eaglstein and colleagues[32] found that oral corticosteroids did not shorten the course of the infection or affect pain during the first 2 weeks, but they did shorten the duration of postherpetic neuralgia. Best results were obtained when treatment was started early in the course of the disease. Inflammation and scarring are reduced with anti-inflammatory agents. Despite the unclear effects of corticosteroid therapy on herpes zoster, these drugs have been used extensively to treat this infection.[2]

The role of anti-inflammatory drugs in acute herpes zoster is controversial. If host responses contribute significantly to tissue injury, then attenuation of these responses may be beneficial. Unfortunately, the host defenses that cause tissue injury may be inseparable from those that eliminate or prevent the spread of infection. Currently, dissociation of protective from harmful host responses to the virus has not been demonstrated clearly. However, in the immunocompetent individual, a vigorous antiviral response is altered only very mildly by corticosteroids. Similarly, in the presence of potent antiviral therapy, even in the immunosuppressed patient, a reduction in the inflammatory response eventually may be safe and have a salutary effect. These are important issues for future investigation. The area where this issue has been addressed in practical terms is that of postherpetic neuralgia. Two controlled trials suggest that a course of systemic corticosteroids during the acute phase of zoster can prevent postherpetic neuralgia.[27,28] Both studies involved immunologically normal older patients; in neither, were untoward complications of corticosteroid therapy, including dissemination of infection, detected.

In a meta-analysis of the four well-controlled clinical studies conducted, the results indicated a statistically significant decrease in the proportion of patients affected at 6 and 12 weeks compared with usual incidence rates.[33] Standard difference scores were -2.0559 and -4.1442, respectively. At 24 weeks, no differences were detectable between placebo- and corticosteroid-treated groups (standard deviation, 0.6603, $P > 0.05$). The side effects of treatment were rare and mild, affecting only 2.5 percent of patients treated with corticosteroids. No patients had dissemination of disease. Systemic corticosteroid treatment decreased the proportion of patients with postherpetic neuralgia, especially when it was defined as pain occurring 6 or 12 weeks after the acute event.

These drugs usually are administered in the first 10 days and continued for as long as 3 weeks. Prednisone is usually the agent of choice. It may be given orally in doses of 60 mg/day the first week, 30 mg/day the second week, and 15 mg/day the third week.

Corticosteroids also have been administered by subcutaneous injection under affected skin, with and without a local anesthetic. Enthusiastic reports of large numbers of patients claim 80 percent to 100 percent success in treating acute herpes zoster, with a rapid resolution of pain and diminished incidence of postherpetic neuralgia.[34,35] These are anecdotal reports, and the experience of others has been less enthusiastic.

Antidepressants and Tranquilizers. Antidepressants are believed to have two actions: they can relieve pain, and they can relieve depression. Tricyclic drugs are known to block serotonin reuptake. Therefore, they would be expected to enhance the action of this neurotransmitter at synapses, and such enhancement can produce analgesia in laboratory animals. One of the mechanisms active in central pain states is some defect in the transmission system in the neuraxis, specifically, a deficit in serotonin.[36]

There is a strong consensus among clinical investigators that centrally active antidepressants should be tried in any patient who is not obtaining pain relief, whether they appear depressed or not. Tricyclics and anxiolytics frequently are given together because, although depression is not common in acute herpes zoster, many patients experience anxiety along with the severe pain. The most widely used combination is amitriptyline and fluphenazine.

In addition to their antidepressant and analgesic properties, tricyclics are also sedatives (for sleep regulation). Amitriptyline and doxepin may correct the sleep disturbance, frequent awakening, and early morning awakening that is common in severe chronic pain states. Adverse side effects of tricyclic antidepressants include hypo- or hypertension, tachycardia, arrhythmias, drowsiness, confusion, disorientation, dry mouth, blurred vision, increased intraocular pressure, urinary retention, and constipation.

Other Drug Therapies. It is thought that the host immune system is incompetent during the acute outbreak. Vitamins, minerals, and improved general nutrition may help improve the immunologic state or replace a missing element.

Nerve Block

Local Infiltration. In a large group of patients, subcutaneous injections of triamcinolone 0.2% in normal saline were administered under the areas of eruption and the sites of pain and itching.[34,35] Excellent results were obtained that approached 100 percent, and the development of postherpetic neuralgia was reduced to 2 percent. This study suggested that subcutaneous injections of corticosteroids and local anesthetics offer an effective treatment for acute herpes zoster. No significant complications were recorded, the technique is simple and inexpensive, and the response to treatment was fairly predictable. Our own experience with this technique corroborates these results.

Somatic Nerve Blocks. Because nerve root involvement is suspected in acute herpes zoster, somatic nerve

blocks have been used in its treatment. These blocks can include brachial plexus, paravertebral, intercostal, and sciatic blocks. They have been found to be of limited value in the acute phase and of no value in the postherpetic stage.

Sympathetic Nerve Block. As understanding of the pathology of herpes zoster developed, attention was directed toward the sympathetic ganglia. Sympathetic blocks have been done to relieve the vasospasm that was thought to cause the pain and nerve damage. Evidence suggests that sympathetic blockade during the acute phase of herpes zoster can help the immediate pain problem, often dramatically. Of greater value, however, is the possibility that it can prevent the development of postherpetic neuralgia. Although the evidence for this is less compelling, it is probably a worthwhile prophylactic measure that should be used as early as possible.[37]

Trigeminal herpes zoster has been treated with a bupivacaine block of the ipsilateral stellate ganglion in a small study. Dramatic and lasting relief of all dysthesia was obtained in approximately 77 percent of patients; some discomfort and paresthesia of the affected area persisted for several weeks in 22 percent of patients. Pain recurred after initial relief in approximately 22 percent of patients. Vesicular skin lesions dried more quickly than in untreated patients. Transient side effects included hoarseness, paresis of the ipsilateral arm, and paresis of the hemidiaphragm. The investigators were unable to draw any conclusions because of the informality of the study, but they believed that these preliminary results justified further investigation.[38]

In one large study, more than 90 percent of cases of herpes zoster were treated successfully with one sympathetic block. The course of the disease showed definite improvement, and the pain disappeared or diminished within 15 min. The relief lasted 20 to 45 min initially, with spontaneous diminution of pain in 8 h and complete relief in 24 h. The blisters dried within 48 h. Successfully blocked patients did not develop postherpetic neuralgia. Complete failure, in only a few patients, occurred when treatment was begun when the patient had been suffering for 10 days or longer and when the disease extended to a number of segments. A similar study reported complete recovery in 75 percent of cases after one block; the rest responded to a second block 2 days later.[39]

Winnie[40] reported that the incidence of success with sympathetic block depends on how soon after the onset of the disease the block is administered. If a sympathetic block is done within the first 2 or 3 weeks, virtually 100 percent success is achieved. The success rate drops after this point. As postherpetic neuralgia supervenes (after 4 to 6 weeks), the success rate falls to approximately 20 percent. Thereafter, the incidence of success associated with sympathetic blocks decreases even further over the years.

It is clear that, if favorable results are to be obtained, it is necessary for patients to be treated in the first 2 or 3 weeks of their disease. This therapy also apparently prevents the lesions from progressing into the postherpetic syndrome at least in younger patients.

Epidural Blocks. Epidural blocks using local anesthetic have been successful in acute herpes zoster. The duration of the infection is shorter, the lesions dry faster, and the pain is relieved. In patients with herpes zoster of 7 weeks or less duration, in a small series, 70 percent to 100 percent of patients had immediate relief, 90 percent to 100 percent had relief 24 h after treatment, and 100 percent had relief in a 1- to 5-month follow-up. There was no subsequent report of postherpetic neuralgia. Their studies suggested that the local anesthetic alone was effective and that the inclusion of corticosteroids did not increase the benefits.[41]

Spinal Blocks. Spinal blocks usually are not indicated because they are not as specific as epidural blocks. A patient who has had a laminectomy in the affected area would be an exception to this general rule.

Neurolytic Blocks. Neurolytic blocks are not indicated in acute herpes zoster.

Complications. Complications that may result from any nerve block procedure include pain, local hemorrhage, infection, needle soreness, sterile abscess (usually in the immunosuppressed patient), vertigo, and Cushing syndrome.

Psychosocial Therapy

Because the acute phase of herpes zoster is short, psychosocial therapy is not mandatory. Some patients (especially those who have severe anxiety and fright) may benefit from this support program.

Other Therapies

Usually, TENS is not used in the treatment of acute herpes zoster. Ice therapy is a counterirritation technique based on the gate-control therapy. It sometimes is used alone in the acute stage to cool the area. Acupuncture and hypnosis usually are not used in acute herpes zoster because other conventional methods are more appropriate. Surgery and neurosurgery are not indicated. The acute stage is self-limited and does not require such drastic measures.

RECOMMENDED THERAPEUTIC STRATEGY FOR ACUTE HERPES ZOSTER

It is useful to categorize affected patients according to their immune status and age (Table 21-5). This allows the clinician to direct efforts toward all or either antiviral, anti-inflammatory, or antinociceptive effects, based on the probability of success and risk factors involved. These patients can be categorized into four groups: (1) immunocompetent young, (2) immunocompetent old, (3) immunosuppressed young, and (4) immunosuppressed old patients.

Immunocompetent Young Patients

Patients in this group have no defined underlying illness, are younger than 50 years old, and have normal immunologic responsiveness. Although they have acute herpes zoster, their reaction to the infection is brisk, enabling them to confine the rash in the initial unit. Likewise, postherpetic neuralgia does not occur. The acute morbidity is low, and healing is rapid. The rationale for treatment for this group of patients is to relieve their intolerable pain and prevent inflammatory damage of the tissues. Antiviral agents administered during the first 72 h may be helpful in stopping the replication of the virus and spreading the infection to the peripheral nerves. Anti-inflammatory agents (corticosteroids administered locally or systematically) are useful in decreasing tissue damage and keeping the inflammatory reaction of the host to a minimum. The obligatory treatment is to decrease the severe pain of neuralgia. This is done best using sympathetic or epidural blocks in the first 3 to 4 weeks of onset of infection. Antidepressant agents also are helpful as adjuvant agents.

Immunocompetent Old Patients

The major objective of therapy in this group is to prevent postherpetic neuralgia. Although suffering no underlying

Table 21-5
Therapeutic Strategy for Acute Herpes Zoster

Type of Patient	Age (yrs)	Treatment		
		Antiviral	*Anti-inflammatory*	*Pain Relief*
Young immunocompetent	<50	–	–	Sympathetic block
Old immunocompetent	>50	–	+	Epidural, somatic and/or sympathetic block—infiltration block helpful
Young immunosuppressed	<50	++ Within 72 h	–	Systemic narcotics
Old immunosuppressed	>50	+ Within 72 h	±	Nerve blocks + systemic oral analgesics Adjuvant oral analgesics

–, not required; +, useful; ++, necessary
Reproduced with permission from Raj P. Pain due to herpes zoster. In: Raj P, ed. *Practical Management of Pain*. 2nd ed. Chicago: Mosby-Year Book; 1992.

disease, the response to varicella-zoster virus in this group may be less vigorous than in young patients, leading to a slower viral clearance and perhaps a higher incidence of spread beyond the initial unit of infection. Nonetheless, nervous system and visceral complications are still infrequent, and by themselves, they probably do not warrant the use of potentially toxic therapy at this time. However, both antiviral and anti-inflammatory therapies may be valuable in preventing postherpetic neuralgia. Of these, only the latter has been shown prospectively to be effective in this group of patients. In two controlled studies, a course of corticosteroids administered during the acute phase of infection was reported to prevent the development of postherpetic pain in a significant percentage of patients.[42,43] Although this issue deserves further investigation, it is reasonable on the basis of the current evidence to treat older patients with acute herpes zoster who are immunologically normal with a limited course of corticosteroids (e.g., 60 mg of prednisone or its equivalent daily for 5 days, tapering the dose over the following 2 weeks).

The value of antivirals in this group of patients has not been tested carefully, although one trial suggested no effect on the incidence of persistent pain in patients treated with acyclovir despite an effect on acute pain. This issue deserves careful study in the future. A four-treatment arm study of the individual and combined effects of antivirals and corticosteroids is needed. At this point, antiviral therapy is this group probably is indicated only in an investigative setting.

Pain relief should be addressed in these patients. Conventional narcotics should be avoided because the patients in this group are usually older and frail. In addition, there is a high incidence of postherpetic neuralgia. Nonnarcotic analgesics in association with nerve blocks (epidural and sympathetic blocks or local intracutaneous infiltration with bupivacaine and corticosteroids) are recommended.

Immunosuppressed Young Patients

Our principal concern in immunodeficient younger patients is the spread of the virus in and outside the primary ganglion–nerve–dermatome unit. Postherpetic neuralgia is not a major issue. Therapy therefore is directed at confining the viral infection. Currently, acyclovir is available, is of proven efficacy, and can be recommended for patients. It seems reasonable to recommend hospitalization for patients in this group who are at greatest risk of developing complications, particularly those with lymphoproliferative disease or early dissemination. It also must be emphasized that, if therapy is given, every effort should be made to start treatment early. When newer agents become available, they will require similar consideration, with their convenience, cost, and toxicity weighed against the magnitude of their potential benefit. It can be predicted, however, that, when other oral drugs are introduced, their efficacy proved, and their toxicity demonstrated to be low, the indications for treatment will expand. The clinical decision to administer these drugs to this group of patients would be an easy one, with virtually all patients in this group routinely receiving such treatment. Pain relief in such patients should be obtained by the techniques that are common for acute pain management.[44,45]

Immunosuppressed Older Patients

In this group of patients, our therapeutic objectives include prevention of both viral spread and postherpetic pain. As discussed previously, antiviral therapy may be helpful in both respects. Acyclovir has been effective in reducing infection, and it may reduce postherpetic pain. The latter requires additional confirmation. More importantly, because of the risk of viral dissemination, patients in this group require antiviral treatment. However, the use of corticosteroids to prevent postherpetic neuralgia warrants separate comment. In older immunocompetent patients, corticosteroids appear to cause no special risk and to be therapeutically beneficial,[42,46] but in the immunosuppressed individual, greater caution is required. These patients are more susceptible to viral spread and central nervous system and visceral complications. Corticosteroids may impair their remaining defenses below a critical level, increasing the risk of these complications. Data from a collaborative study suggest that corticosteroids did not protect against postherpetic pain in this group. This issue must be investigated separately, particularly to consider the effects of combined antiviral and steroid therapy. If potent antiviral coverage were available, corticosteroids may be safe. Pain relief is best provided by nerve blocks.

MANAGEMENT

Postherpetic Neuralgia

Drug Therapy (Table 21-6)

A threefold purpose governs the role of drug therapy in the patient with postherpetic neuralgia: (1) to provide analgesia for pain, (2) to reduce depression and anxiety, and (3) to decrease insomnia. Because a considerable degree of depression, anxiety, and insomnia accompany all chronic pain syndromes, hypnotics, tranquilizers, antidepressants, and anticonvulsants frequently have been used as analgesic adjuvants in the management of postherpetic neuralgia. These include the barbiturates, rauwolfia alkaloids, phenothiazine

Table 21-6
Drug Therapy for Postherpetic Neuralgia

Analgesics
Antidepressants and Tranquilizers
Anticonvulsants
    Phenytoin
    Carbamazepine
    Sodium valproate and amitriptyline
Topical capsaicin
Oral antiarrhythmics

derivatives, benzodiazepines, amphetamines, tricyclic antidepressants, phenytoin, and carbamazepine.

It is important to warn the patient of the potential side effects of any drug. The patient is less likely to stop taking the prescribed medication if they know that certain unpleasant effects are expected as a normal occurrence and that they usually are not permanent.

However, it is equally important for the physician to adopt a positive approach regarding the medication. On average, 35 percent of patients benefit significantly from the placebo effect.[47] This can be used to advantage by describing enthusiastically the desirable effects of each drug which, with time, may be obtained in some patients. They also are less likely to stop taking their medication before it has had time to provide the desired effect.

Antiviral Agents. As a rule, antiviral agents are inappropriate in the treatment of postherpetic neuralgia. An exception may include their use to prevent the possible recurrence of herpes zoster infection in a susceptible patient. For example, the patient with Hodgkin disease is predisposed to recurrent herpes zoster; antiviral agents may be given before treatment of their primary disease (chemotherapy and radiation therapy) when the reactivation of the virus is most likely.

Analgesics. These may be required to control the severe intractable pain of postherpetic neuralgia. Narcotics should be used with extreme caution, if at all, because (1) they are addictive; (2) the problem is chronic; (3) these patients usually are not terminally ill; (4) the side effects such as nausea, loss of appetite, and constipation usually make these patients miserable; (5) there may be adverse drug interactions with antidepressants and other drugs; and (6) most important, adequate pain relief may be obtained with other drugs. The temporary initial use of narcotics to relieve extreme pain may be necessary, however, until the patient begins to respond to therapy.

Antidepressants and Tranquilizers. Antidepressants and tranquilizers frequently are used in conjunction with analgesics. Some patients become depressed as a reaction to their pain. The signs of depression may be so subtle that they easily are missed. As many as 90 percent of patients seen may be depressed. Approximately 85 percent of these patients will respond to antidepressant drugs.

Tricyclic antidepressants are the most commonly used drugs, and they are the most effective single drug class used in the management of postherpetic neuralgia. Antidepressants may act at a higher level than the neurotransmitters, perhaps on pressure molecules in the hypothalamus or pituitary. This could explain why only some depressed patients fit the catecholamine hypothesis (that is, a deficit of serotonin or norepinephrine is the cause of the problem). Both chronic pain and depression may represent neurotransmitter deficiencies, and the antidepressants may restore these to normal levels. These drugs should be given in appropriate doses, and several different drugs should be tried before concluding that there is no response.

Tricyclics and anxiolytics commonly are given together because many patients have anxiety with their depression. This feeling may be caused by anticipation of painful spasms, social obligations that may exacerbate the pain by increasing stress, fear of having a painful episode in public, or fear that the pain may never leave. Many patients who did not obtain relief with tricyclics alone may benefit when a phenothiazine is added.[48] For lasting pain relief, treatment must be continued throughout life. Amitriptyline 50 to 75 mg/day and fluphenazine 1 mg three or four times a day is the usual recommended dose.

As a last resort, immediate relief was obtained in approximately one-third of hospitalized patients who had not responded to any other therapy.[49] A short course of high-dose chlorprothixene 50 mg every 6 h for 5 days was used. The prominent side effects of this high dose made hospitalization during the course of therapy necessary, and many patients stopped taking the medication because they were unable to tolerate the side effects. This treatment is recommended only if all other methods fail and if the pain is severe because pain often returned in a few weeks or months.

Anticonvulsants. Anticonvulsants sometimes are useful when other medications have failed. Phenytoin 100 mg three to four times a day or carbamazepine 500 to 1000 mg daily in three to four divided doses can be used to relieve sharp pain.[47,50]

Sodium valproate 200 mg twice a day and amitriptyline 10 to 25 mg twice a day have been successful.[51] The pain in this study was characterized in four ways: (1) stabbing or lancinating, (2) burning, (3) dull ache, and (4) hyperesthesia. If the stabbing component of pain continued, the dose of amitriptyline was increased. The dull-ache component of the pain was most resistant to therapy. If it persisted, the scar was infiltrated with a local anesthetic and corticosteroids, or TENS was started.

The side effects of anticonvulsants tend to limit their use. These effects include bone marrow depression, ataxia, diplopia, nystagmus, abnormal liver function tests, nausea, lymphanadenopathy, confusion, and vertigo.[25]

Topical Capsaicin. This drug depletes substance P from sensory nerve endings in the skin, and capsaicin has been used topically for various dermatologic diseases.[52] In a double-blind study, Bernstein and associates[53] reported that 80 percent of elderly patients with postherpetic neuralgia obtained pain relief. Watson and colleagues[54] reported some relief in 78 percent of patients and good-to-excellent relief in 56 percent of them after topical capsaicin application for 4 weeks.

Antiarrhythmics. Intravenous lidocaine has been advocated for the treatment of many types of chronic neurogenic pain,[55,56] including postherpetic neuralgia. As a result of these data, the oral antiarrhythmics (such as mexiletine) have been tried, and early reports are encouraging.[57,58] However, definitive studies on the efficacy or oral antiarrhythmics for the treatment of postherpetic neuralgia are lacking.

Nerve Blocks

The pathogenesis of postherpetic pain is unknown. Autopsy studies have shown that the entire sensory pathway, including the brain and sympathetic ganglia, may be involved.[16] There appear to be multiple areas along this pathway that can initiate pain. This provides a rationale for the various methods of treatment and a explanation of treatment failures.

Analgesic blocks can be used as prognostic, therapeutic, and prophylactic tools in managing pain. As prognostic tools, blocks help predict the effects of prolonged interruption of nerve pathways achieved through injection of neurolytic agents or surgery. By interrupting pain pathways, therapeutic blocks influence the autonomic response to noxious stimulation. They break the cycle of this disease. Patients with severe intractable pain who are not suited to other treatment regimens may be relieved by blocks with neurolytic agents.[59]

Local Infiltration. Subcutaneous infiltration of corticosteroids was used in one study; pain relief was obtained in approximately 64 percent of patients.[34] A 0.2% solution of triamcinolone in normal saline was injected daily under all areas of pain, burning, or itching until the desired effect was obtained. Maximum benefit was achieved in the first 12 treatments. In a comparison study, subcutaneous infiltration of bupivacaine 0.25% and triamcinolone 0.2% was used alone or in conjunction with systemic medication and sympathetic blockade.[59] Overall results showed moderate-to-significant improvement in 70 percent of patients. A difference in response to treatment was noticed in relation to the duration of symptoms; patients with symptoms for less than 1 year responded better (85 percent success) than patients with symptoms for greater than 1 year (55 percent).

These studies suggest that subcutaneous infiltration of corticosteroids can offer an effective treatment for postherpetic neuralgia. No significant complications were recorded; the technique is simple and inexpensive; and the response to treatment is fairly predictable. Most important, it offers relief for some patients with postherpetic neuralgia of many months' duration.

The total number of such treatments ranges from 1 to 10 (average, 4 to 6 injections). In acute herpes zoster, treatments usually are given two or three times weekly and tapered to one per week, if the patient is responding well.

Somatic Nerve Block. Nerve root involvement is an obvious characteristic of postherpetic neuralgia, and sensory nerve blocks were used in early attempts to relieve its pain. The results were limited, depending primarily on the duration of the blocks, although there were some reports of success in managing pain in the early stages of the disease. Coincidental spontaneous resolution may have been responsible. Nerve blocks primarily are used in postherpetic neuralgia for diagnosis and prognosis, especially as a prognostic block before neurolytic block. Corticosteroids injected around the dorsal nerve have had unpredictable and limited success.

Sympathetic Nerve Block. Thirty-four patients with postherpetic neuralgia for an average of 2 years, whose ages ranged from 52 to 82 years, were treated with regional sympathetic blocks. Each patient received an average of three or four blocks. This treatment, however, seemed to be ineffective.[60]

Good, although temporary, results were reported in a series of paravertebral somatic sympathetic blocks using procaine 0.2% at 4-day intervals. The best results were obtained in postherpetic neuralgia of less than 2 months' duration.[4]

Epidural Block. Because epidural corticosteroid administration has been successful in treating various lumbosacral conditions, Forrest[61] experimented with this technique in postherpetic neuralgia. In a well-controlled study, he obtained a progressive decrease in pain. Patients began to have relief after the first injection. One month after the third injection, 57 percent were pain free. At 6 months, 86 percent were pain free. Nine patients were followed for 1 year, and of these, eight were completely pain free. Forrest first identified the affected dorsal roots with segmental epidural injections of bupivacaine 0.5% 2 ml in the lumbar and thoracic regions and 1 ml in the cervical area. This provided complete temporary relief. A series of three epidural steroid injections were then given 1 week apart. Methylprednisolone 80 mg was used for single-root involvement, with 60 mg per root for two roots or three roots, the total dose for any one visit not exceeding 120 mg. The patients were kept in a lateral position for 30 min and discharged 6 h later. Complications included minor weight gain and a slight increase in resting blood pressure. Other studies using a significantly different technique have not had much success with epidural injections.

Neurolytic Block. Neurolytic blocks may be considered when other blocks have not given the patient significant relief. They should only be done after a prognostic block has shown that an effective block of the appropriate area can be achieved. Neurolytic agents are used in cases of prolonged destruction of nerves. These blocks include ethyl alcohol 50% in aqueous solution, absolute alcohol 95% in aqueous solution, and phenol 6%. Ethyl alcohol causes a higher incidence of neuritis than phenol. This is primarily a result of incomplete peripheral nerve block after inaccurate needle placement or spillage of the agent on somatic nerve fibers. The duration of effects may vary from days to years, but usually it ranges from 2 to 6 months.

Ammonium compounds also can be used for peripheral nerve block. Pain relief follows selective destruction of unmyelinated C fibers by the ammonium ion. A solution of ammonium sulfate 10% in lidocaine 1% or ammonium chloride 15% is used. The duration of action ranges from 4 to 24 weeks. Neuritis does not occur with either ammonium sulfate or chloride. The most annoying side effect is numbness, which can be as bad as the pain for some patients.[28]

Cryoanalgesia also has been used as a means of producing long-term neural blockade.

Psychosocial Therapy

It is especially important in patients with postherpetic neuralgia to treat the whole patient and not just an area of the skin. The emotional stability of the patient almost always is affected, and the stresses involved for the patient and all members of the household require thoughtful management.

Severe depression is seen in more than 50 percent of these patients, and as previously noted, suicide commonly is considered by those with long-term intractable pain. Counseling by a psychologist or clinical social worker who is experienced in pain management is a valuable adjunct to drug therapy. Training the patient in stress management and relaxation techniques is important. Anxiety and stress can exacerbate and prolong the pain. By practicing these techniques, the patient may be able to control pain to some degree.

In some patients, the pain–tension–anxiety cycle can convert acute pain symptoms into a chronic condition. Often, no matter what is done to treat these patients, the pain is not relieved unless the stress factors also are removed. Basically, two types of persons are susceptible to chronicity: the tense hard-driving conscientious perfectionist and the dependent individual unable to cope with life but burdened with repressed anger and hostility. Reinforcement of the patient's response to pain (such as moaning, grimacing, asking for medication, and remaining in bed) or favorable consequences of the pain (such as attention and expressions of sympathy, perhaps also the occasion to manipulate others) may lead to chronic behavior which, eventually, is independent of the original underlying pathologic condition.

The most important guideline in preventing chronicity is complete honesty. Make them aware of the relationship between the psyche and pain and relieve them of the fear of organic disease. After the patient fully accepts the emotional causes of pain, they can learn to relieve the pain by controlling anxiety and tension.

Family and friends should be included in counseling sessions. They, too, must cope with the pain a loved one is experiencing. The counselor not only can ease their anxiety but also can teach them how to provide effective emotional support to help the patient endure an extremely difficult period. Concentrating on the special needs of the families may require extra effort on the part of the staff, but it should result in a greater number of patients who recover with the physical and emotional well-being of the family intact.

Many patients are elderly and live alone. They are unable to turn to family and friends to provide the assistance they need to do routine daily tasks. The counselor should contact the appropriate social service agencies to provide transportation and other necessities (such as prepared meals, grocery shopping, housework, and regular contact with the patient to check on their well-being).

Other Therapies

Because many patients continue to have some residual pain of varying degrees that can be aggravating, they may require management with other techniques. The following techniques are used when all others fail (Table 21-7).

TENS. This has been used in an attempt to relieve the intractable pain of postherpetic neuralgia. Winnie[40] reported a success rate of only 20 percent, but relief was sufficient to permit a return to normal activity without analgesic therapy.

Ice and Other Cold Therapies. Ice is applied to the skin for 2 to 3 min several times a day, starting with the least sensitive area and approaching the most sensitive area. A vibrator then is used in the same manner. This is used in conjunction with psychotropic drugs. Ethyl chloride, or other cold sprays, can be used by itself as treatment. The fluid is sprayed over the entire painful area, beginning at the upper area and working down. Evaporation cools the area. The procedure is repeated twice at 1-min intervals until the skin is thoroughly cooled. When beneficial, these treatments will relieve the pain for varying lengths of time. When pain returns to near its former intensity, the treatment can be repeated. If the patient responds satisfactorily, the pain is relieved by two or three sets of sprays per day.[1,50] Good-to-excellent pain relief was maintained in approximately 66 percent of patients with refractory postherpetic pain using cryocautery with a stick of solid carbon dioxide (dry ice) applied directly to the hyperesthesic skin areas of the cutaneous scars.[62]

Acupuncture. A preliminary report shows significant pain relief was obtained in 40 percent of patients with postherpetic neuralgia treated with acupuncture. Further investigation is underway.[63]

Table 21-7
Other Therapies for Postherpetic Neuralgia

TENS
Cold therapies
   Ice
   Ethyl chloride
   Cryocautery with dry ice
Acupuncture
Hypnosis
Surgery and neurosurgery

Hypnosis. Hypnosis acts at the level of the cerebral cortex. Impulses are sent down from higher centers to close the neurophysiologic gate that controls pain. Pain relief through hypnosis is sometimes complete, but more often, it is not. Hypnotism is reported to be helpful in patients with chronic unbearable pain; this changed to bearable discomfort by breaking up patterns of suffering.

Dimethyl Sulfoxide. The treatment value of this agent in postherpetic neuralgia is unknown. It may be tried as a benign last resort. Only a few states have approved this solvent for medical use.

Surgery and Neurosurgery (See Chap. 35)

Surgery is the last resort for the treatment of severe intractable postherpetic pain. It is not always successful. More effective management techniques learned in recent years have limited this option further.

Surgery usually attacks the pain pathway in stages at progressively higher divisions. Because it was suspected that the origin of the pain lay in the scar and peripheral receptors, wide excision and skin grafting was tried. This was not found to be effective and rarely is used today.

Rhizotomy of the somatic afferents and sensory root ganglia also has had poor results. Investigators who have had some success recommended that ablation include several segments above and below the affected area. Sympathectomy has not been successful in treating postherpetic neuralgia.

Cordotomy has been used with good results. In most cases, however, the pain returns. Early recurrence has been blamed on failure to ablate all the nerves in the pathway, which resume function after the swelling has decreased. Stereotactic ablation of the conducting paths in the thalamus and mesencephalon and frontal lobotomy have been used. These should only be tried in patients with short life expectancies who have not had success with any other methods.

Because of the finality of surgery and the unpredictable responses, many surgeons in recent years have taken advantage of the technologic advances in other areas to replace destructive procedures. These include electronic stimulators used to block transmission of nerve impulses. An implantable electrode placed over the dorsal columns of the spinal cord has been tried with some success. More recently, deep brain stimulators, which are patient activated, have been applied to the mesencephalic medial lemniscus.[64] The purpose was to block the pain-conducting systems and stimulate endorphin secretion, the body's natural pain reliever. Good pain relief was found in 42 percent of treated patients.

COMPLICATIONS

Acute Herpes Zoster

The most common complications of acute herpes zoster usually appear after eruption of the rash (Table 21-8). They

Table 21-8
Complications of Acute Herpes Zoster

Neuralgia
Facial or oculomotor palsy
Paralysis of motor nerves
Myelitis
Meningoencephalitis
Postherpetic neuralgia
Systemic toxicity or dissemination
Fevers
Chills
Bacteria sepsis
Varicella pneumonia

include neuralgia, facial or oculomotor palsy, paralysis of motor nerves, and myelitis. Meningoencephalitis, which has its onset either during or 2 to 4 days after the rash appears, also can be a complication. Postherpetic neuralgia seems to occur more frequently and is more protracted in immunosuppressed patients, especially in Hodgkin disease or other lymphomas.

There is a marked increase in the incidence of infection in the immunosuppressed or immunoincompetent patient. The clinical course in these patients is exaggerated. It is acutely disabling in many cases, and it may become life-threatening if visceral involvement occurs with dissemination. In the early stages, the infection often spreads segmentally to involve ipsilateral and, less frequently, contralateral dermatomes. It usually is associated with fever and increasing debilitation. While some of the old lesions are healing, new lesions continue to appear. Many patients have dissemination and visceral involvement that ultimately may be fatal.

Generally, patients in whom the disease remains localized for 4 to 6 days do not experience complications. The greatest morbidity and mortality usually occurs with visceral involvement through dissemination, especially in patients older than 40 years of age.

Systemic toxicity, fever, chills, and sometimes secondary bacterial sepsis occur. Varicella pneumonia, which is associated with a high mortality, occurs less frequently.

Postherpetic Neuralgia

Although physical complications occur with acute herpes zoster, the complications from the postherpetic stage primarily are emotional. Depression is common and may include suicidal tendencies. Destruction of the patient's life style (inability to work, break-up of the family, and restricted mobility that prohibits former social activities) may be the tragic human consequences that affect the patient with long-term pain. Physical function may be impaired beyond that seen during the acute stage because of the longer period of immobility.

PROGNOSIS

There is a close relationship between the duration of neuralgia and therapeutic efficacy; prompt treatment shortens the progressive course of the disease and also decreases its severity. There also appears to be a correlation between the age of the patient and the response to therapy. Patients younger than 60 years of age generally respond better to therapy and, even untreated, have a lower incidence of postherpetic neuralgia than older patients. In addition, older patients do not respond as well as young patients to therapy and specifically to sympathetic nerve blocks. For unknown reasons, postherpetic neuralgia lesions in the ophthalmic division of the trigeminal nerve are often the most difficult lesions to treat successfully. The psychological make-up of the individual patient is also important. Lastly, one-fifth of patients with neoplasms who have had herpes zoster will have this disease at least once again.[2]

References

1. Lipton S. Post-herpetic neuralgia. In: Lipton S, ed. *Relief of Pain in Clinical Practice* Oxford: Scientific Publ; 1979:231–248.

2. Raj PP. Herpes zoster: preventing post-herpetic pain. *Consultant* March 1981:71–76.

3. Hines JD, Nankervis GA. Herpes zoster infection. *Hosp Med* 1977; 8:72–84.

4. Bonica JJ. Thoracic segmental and intercostal neuralgia. In: Bonica JJ, ed. *The Management of Pain*. Philadelphia: Lea & Febiger; 1953:861–867.

5. Steele RW. Immunology of varicella-zoster virus. In: Nahmias AJ, O'Reilly RJ, eds. *Immunology of Human Infection*. Part II: Viruses and parasites: Immunodiagnosis and prevention of infectious diseases. New York: Plenum; 1982.

6. Goodman R, Jaffe N, Filler R, et al. Herpes zoster in children with stage. I–II Hodgkin's disease. *Radiology* 1967; 118:429–431.

7. Rand KH, Rasmussen LE, Pollard RB, et al. Cellular immunity and herpesvirus infections in cardiac-transplant patients. *N Engl J Med* 1977; 296:1372–1377.

8. Twomey JJ, Gyorkey F, Norris SM. The monocyte disorder with herpes zoster. *J Lab Clin Med* 1974; 83:786–797.

9. Bertotto A, Gentili F, Vaccaro R. Immunoregulatory T cells in varicella. *N Engl J Med* 1982; 307:1271–1272. Letter.

10. Jordan GW, Merigan TC. Cell-mediated immunity to varicella-zoster virus: in vitro lymphocyte responses. *J Infect Dis* 1974; 130:495–501.

11. Zaia JA, Leary PL, Levin MJ. Specificity of the blastogenic response of human mononuclear cells to herpesvirus antigens. *Infect Immun* 1978; 20:646–651.

12. Russell AS, Maini RA, Bailey M, et al. Cell-mediated immunity to varicella-zoster antigen in acute herpes zoster (shingles). *Clin Exp Immunol* 1973; 14:181–185.

13. Gershon AS, Steinberg S, Smith M. Cell-mediated immunity to varicella-zoster virus demonstrates by viral inactivation with human leukocytes. *Infect Immun* 1976; 13:1549–1553.

14. Stevens DA, Ferrington RA, Jordan GW, et al. Cellular events in zoster vesicles: relation to clinical course and immune parameters. *J Infect Dis* 1975; 131:509–515.

15. Gershon AA, Steinberg SP. Inactivation of varicella zoster virus in vitro: effect of leukocytes and specific antibody. *Infect Immun* 1981; 33:507–511.

16. Frengly JD. Herpes zoster: a challenge in management. *Primary Care* 1981; 8(4):715–731.

17. Haas LF. Postherpetic neuralgia, treatment and prevention. *Trans Opthal Soc N Z* 1977; 29:133–136.

18. Barr RJ, Herten RJ, Graham JH. Rapid method for Tzanck preparations. *JAMA* 1977; 237:1119–1120.

19. Rutgers MJ, Dirksen R. The prevention of post-herpetic neuralgia: a retrospective view of patients treated in the acute phase of herpes zoster. *Br J Clin Pract* 1988; 42:412–414.

20. Raj PP. Herpes zoster: preventing post-herpetic pain. *Consultant* March 1981:71–76.

21. Li WH, Ming ZL, Chen Q, et al. The prevention of post-herpetic neuralgia—a retrospective view of patients treated in the acute phase of herpes zoster. *Clin Med J Engl* 1989; 102:395–399.

22. Pernak JM, Biemans JCH. The treatment of acute herpes zoster in trigeminal nerve for the prevention of post-herpetic neuralgia. In: Edmann W, Oyama T, Pernak MJ, eds. *The Pain Clinic*. Vol 1. Utrecht: VNU Science Press; 1985.

23. Dolin R, Reichman RC, Mazur MH, Whitley RJ. Herpes zoster-varicella infections in immunosuppressed patients. *Ann Intern Med* 1978; 89:375–388.

24. Burton WJ, Gould PW, Hursthouse MW, et al. A multicenter trial of Zostrom (5 percent idoxuridine in dimethyl sulphoxide) in herpes zoster. *N Z Med J* November 25, 1981:384–386.

25. Esmann V, Wildenhoff KE. Idoxuridine for herpes zoster. *Lancet* August 30, 1980:474. Letter to editor.

26. Machida H, Kuninaka A, Yoshino H. Inhibitory effects of antiherpesviral thymidine analogs against varicella-zoster verus. *Antimicrob Agents Chemother* 1982; 21(2):358–361.

27. Gunby P. Leukemia patients to be given varicella vaccine. *JAMA* 1982; 247(17):2340–2341.

28. Tio R, Moya F, Usubiaga L. Management of intractable pain. In: Lichtiger M, Moya F, eds. *Introduction to the Practice of Anesthesia*. Hagerstown, MD: Harper & Row; 1978:485–501.

29. Gelfland ML. Treatment of herpes zoster with cortisone. *JAMA* 1954; 154:911–912.

30. Appleman DH. Treatment of herpes zoster with ACTH. *N Engl J Med* 1955; 253:693–695.

31. Elliot FA. Treatment of herpes zoster with high doses of prednisone. *Lancet* 1964; 2:610–611.

32. Eaglstein WH, Katz R, Brown JA. The effects of early corticosteroid therapy on the skin eruption and pain of herpes zoster. *JAMA* 1970; 211(10):1681–1683.

33. Lycka BA. Postherpetic neuralgia and systemic corticosteroid therapy—efficacy and safety. *Int J Dermatol* 1990; 29:523–527.

34. Epstein E. Triamcinolone in the treatment of zoster and postzoster neuralgia. *Calif Med* 1971; 115(2):6–10.

35. Epstein E. Treatment of herpes zoster and postzoster neuralgia by subcutaneous injection of triamcinolone. *Int J Dermatol* 1981; 20:65–68.

36. Murphy T. Drugs for chronic pain. In: *Advances and Update in Pain Therapy*. ASA Annual Meeting; 1982.

37. Murphy T. Herpes zoster. In: *Advances and Update in Pain Therapy*. ASA Annual Meeting; 1982:40.

38. Olson ER, Ivy HB. Stellate block for trigeminal herpes zoster. *Arch Ophthalmol* 1980; 98:1656. Letter to editor.

39. Rosenek SS. Paravertebral block for the treatment of herpes zoster. *N Y State J Med* September 1, 1965:2684–2687.

40. Winnie AP. The patient with herpetic neuralgia. In: Moya F, Gion H, eds. *Postgraduate Seminar in Anesthesiology*. Program syllabus. Miami Beach; 1983:165–170.

41. Perkins HM, Hanlon PR. Epidural injection of local anesthetic and steroids for relief of pain secondary to herpes zoster. *Arch Surg* 1978; 113:253–254.

42. Eaglstein WH, Katz R, Brown JA. The effect of early corticosteroid therapy on skin eruption and pain of herpes zoster. *JAMA* 1970; 211:1681–1683.

43. Toyama N. Sympathetic ganglion block therapy for herpes zoster. *J Dermatol* 1982; 9:59–62.

44. Tio R, Moya F, Usubiaga L. Management of intractable pain. In: Lichtiger M, Moya F, eds. *Introduction to the Practice of Anesthesia*. Hagerstown, MD: Harper & Row; 1978.

45. Basbaum AL, Fields HL. Endogenous pain control mechanisms: review and hypothesis. *Ann Neurol* 1978; 4:451–462.

46. Bauman J. Treatment of acute herpes zoster neuralgia by epidural injection or stellate ganglion block. *Anesthesiology* 1979; 50(suppl):223.

47. Moore ME. Use of drugs in the management of chronic pain. *Anesthesiol Rev* August 1975:14–18.

48. Taub A. Relief of postherpetic neuralgia with psychotropic drugs. *J Neurosurg* 1973; 39:235–239.

49. Nathan PW. Chlorprothixene (Taractan) in postherpetic neuralgia and other severe chronic pains. *Pain* 1978; 5:367–371.

50. Crue BL Jr, Todd EM, Maline DB. Postherpetic neuralgia—conservative treatment regimen. In: Crue BL Jr, ed. *Pain Research and Treatment*. New York: Academic Press; 1975:289–292.

51. Raftery H. The management of postherpetic pain using sodium valproate and amitriptyline. *J Ir Med Assoc* 1979; 72(9):399–401.

52. Bernstein JE. Capsaicin in the treatment of dermatologic disease. *Cutis* April 1987; 39(4):352–353.

53. Bernstein JE, Korman NJ, Bickers DR, Dahl MV, Millikan LE. Topical capsaicin treatment of chronic postherpetic neuralgia. *J Am Acad Dermatol* August 1989; 21(2 pt 1):265–270.

54. Watson CP, Evans RJ, Watt VR. Post-herpetic neuralgia and topical capsaicin. *Pain* June 1988; 33(3):333–340.

55. Peterson P, Kastrup J, Zeeberg I, Boyson G. Chronic pain treatment with intravenous lidocaine. *Neurol Res* September 1986; 8(3):189–190.

56. Peterson P, Kastrup J. Dercum's disease (adiposis dolorosa). Treatment of the severe pain with intravenous lidocaine. *Pain* January 1987; 28(1):77–80.

57. Tanelian DL, Brose WG. Neuropathic pain can be relieved by drugs that are use-dependent sodium channel blockers: lidocaine, carbamazepine, and mexiletine. *Anesthesiology* May 1991; 74(5):949–951.

58. Dejgard A, Peterson P, Kastrup J. Mexiletine for treatment of chronic painful diabetic neuropathy. *Lancet* January 2–9 1988; 1(8575–8576):9–11.

59. Tio R, Moya F, Vorasaran S. Treatments of postherpetic neuralgia. *Anesth Sin* 1978; 16(4):151–153.

60. Colding A. The effect of regional sympathetic blocks in the treatment of herpes zoster. *Acta Anaesthesiol Scand* 1969; 13:133–141.

61. Forrest JB. Management of chronic dorsal root pain with epidural steroid. *Can Anaesth J* 1978; 25(3):218–225.

62. Suzuki H, Ogawa S, Nakagawa H, et al. Cryocautery of sensitized skin areas for the relief of pain due to postherpetic neuralgia. *Pain* 1980; 9:355–362.

63. Lewith GT, Field J. Acupuncture and postherpetic neuralgia. *Br Med J* August 30, 1980:622. Letter to editor.

64. Mundinger F, Salamao JF. Deep brain stimulation in mesencephalic lemniscus medialis for chronic pain. *Acta Neurochir Suppl* 1980; 30:245–258.

CHAPTER 22

Peripheral Neuropathies and Neuralgias

Peter J. Armstrong and Terence M. Murphy

The study of peripheral neuropathies and neuralgias has become a major area of neurologic endeavor only during the last 30 years. Pain in these conditions is understood poorly and given cursory attention in standard neurologic texts. These sporadic and sometimes tenacious pains can be refractory to treatment. However, a logical therapeutic regimen initiated in a multidisciplinary pain management unit often can offer the best chance of an optimal outcome.

DEFINITIONS AND CLASSIFICATION

Confusion surrounding the semantics of different pain conditions has been helped considerably by the publication of a taxonomy for pain.[1] In this chapter, the following definitions will apply.

1. Neuralgia. Pain in the distribution a nerve or nerves. The term should be used primarily to refer to nonparoxysmal pains, although this is not always the case.
2. Neuropathy. A disturbance of function or a pathologic change in the nerves. It may be in a single nerve (mononeuropathy), in several nerves (mononeuropathy multiplex), or symmetric or bilateral (polyneuropathy).[2] (Neuritis refers to a special type of neuropathy and is reserved primarily for describing inflammatory processes affecting nerves).
3. Peripheral Nervous System. Anatomically, the peripheral nervous system is those parts of the nervous system in which neurons or their processes are related to the Schwann cell. This, therefore, comprises the cranial nerves (except the optic nerve), the spinal nerve roots, the dorsal root ganglia, the peripheral nerve trunks and their ramifications, and the peripheral autonomic nervous system.[3]

Other parts of this text deal with neuralgia and neuropathy in the head and neck; therefore, this chapter will concentrate only on such pains in the limbs and trunk.

The classification of peripheral neuropathy suggested by Dyck[4] is entrapment, leprosy, diabetic[5,6] and other metabolic disorders, inherited, deficiency,[7] inflammatory, demyelinating, toxic,[8] ischemic, and paraneoplastic. A more useful classification for the purposes of a pain management unit would be by anatomic site (e.g., intercostal neuralgia or brachial neuralgia) or by cause (postherpetic neuralgia, diabetic neuropathy, or posttraumatic neuralgia).[9] Howev-

er, even given the best neurologic facilities, it is still only possible to categorize 75 percent of these disorders.[4]

CLINICAL FEATURES

The clinical features of peripheral neuropathy may include weakness, muscle atrophy, fasciculations, cramps, and loss of tendon reflexes. Sensory changes may involve all sensations, or be selective. Pain may present as paresthesias or hyperesthesia. Hyperpathia (characterized by delay, overreaction, and after sensation to a stimulus) often is associated with peripheral nerve injury. Descriptions of pain may include such terms as aching (in diabetic and ischemic neuralgia), burning (in alcoholic neuropathy, causalgia, or meralgia paresthetica) or lancinating (tabetic neuropathy and involvement of peripheral nerves by carcinoma).[10] Autonomic involvement may be heralded by a Horner's syndrome or changes in temperature, color, or sweating in the limbs, disturbances of genitourinary function, or impotence. Confirmation of the diagnosis of peripheral neuropathy is best achieved using nerve conduction studies. If there is difficulty differentiating a myopathy from a peripheral neuropathy, electromyography usually will provide an answer.

MECHANISMS OF PAIN IN NEURALGIA AND PAINFUL NEUROPATHIES

The traditional understanding of pain-generating mechanisms in nociception is that impulses in primary nociceptive afferents result in pain depending on the numbers and frequency of these impulses arriving at the central nervous system. This does not provide a good working model for the pain of neuralgia and neuropathies. Although imperfectly understood, current explanations suggest the removal of normal inhibitory afferent impulses might be a factor, as initially proposed in the gate-control theory of pain.[11,12]

The destruction of large-diameter afferents and their consequent lack of inhibitory input has been suggested as explaining the pain of postherpetic neuralgia.[13] Electrical and physical stimulation affords some relief for these hyperesthetic states; this tends to support the hypothesis that the problem is one of imbalance of afferent sensation. However, the studies of Dyck and associates[4,14] do not provide evidence that the numbers of large myelinated fibers, or their ratio to unmyelinated fibers, explain the pain associated with neuralgias. Therefore, the evidence for nerve fiber imbalance as the sole explanation for pain is not convincing. There are neuropathies in which large-diameter fibers are affected predominantly, such as Friedreich ataxia, which usually are painless. The gate-control theory of pain would predict that this condition is painful. Conditions involving small fibers only (such as the rare inherited polyneuropathy, Fabry disease) are painful. The obverse of this is seen in leprosy. The closest association with pain in Dyck and colleagues'[14] study was in those patients where there was active nerve fiber degeneration. The chronic condition of persistent pain defies adequate explanation on the basis of an active nerve fiber degenerative process causing the pain. Age did not seem to be a major factor in whether or not a patient had pain. Another explanation for the pain often associated with the early stages of neuropathies (such as diabetes) is stimulation of the nervi nervorum (that is the intrinsic innervation) of a freshly damaged nerve, by ischemia.[14,15] Neural demyelination can give rise to spontaneously generating impulses and foci exceptionally sensitive to mechanical and chemical stimuli.[16] The pain associated with peripheral compression mononeuropathies may be ischemic in origin. This can be shown clinically by an increasing discomfort with the application of a pneumatic cuff around an extremity affected by compression mononeuropathy. This often is seen clinically in carpal tunnel syndrome. Asbury and Fields[17] collated data gained in the study of peripheral neuropathies and suggested a hypothesis that dysesthetic pain results from sprouting of neurites at the site of injury but that aching pain is produced by excitation of the nervi nervorum.

An alternative explanation is to think of all these conditions as a form of deafferentation. The term *deafferentation pain* increasingly is being used to denote pain from any part of the body from which the flow of afferent impulses has been interrupted partially or completely. Interruption may occur at any neurologic level, from the periphery to the cortex. Neurodestructive treatments used in attempts to control deafferentation pain have included neurectomy, percutaneous cordotomy, and even cordectomy (that is complete transection of the spinal cord proximal to the initiating lesion). The disappointing results of these procedures prompted a search for an alternative explanation for these types of pain and more effective therapies. A central mechanism first proposed by Livingstone[18] in 1943 has been resurrected to explain these pains rather than a mechanism that depends on transmission in primary nociceptive afferents. This central pain-generating mechanism must still function despite being disconnected from the original site of injury.[19]

Denervation neuronal hypersensitivity may be the mechanism whereby a central cycle is set up by deafferentation in the periphery, resulting in the clinical features of dysesthesia and hyperpathia. Tasker[19] suggested that perturbations in the reticulothalamic pathway are a possible explanation for deafferentation pain. Other authorities conceptualize all these neuralgias as a form of central pain.[20]

Lindblom[21] suggests that ectopic impulses have their origins in neuromas, and nerve sprouts (sometimes intraneurally) may be a possible explanation for neuralgic-type pain. Ephaptic excitation of pain fibers from tactile or thermal afferents may produce nociceptive afferent stimulation. These connections may develop in areas of nerve damage that produce so-called cross talk between regenerating fibers. These self-sustaining nerve impulses may be responsible for continuing pain.

TREATMENT

Prophylaxis

Postherpetic neuralgia (see Chap. 21) is a distressing, often long-term affliction, the treatment of which has confounded physicians for many years. Accordingly, prophylaxis of this condition has been a point of interest. The use of corticosteroids in the treatment of acute herpes zoster has been the subject of two controlled trials.[22,23] These studies suggest that these compounds decrease the incidence of postherpetic neuralgia and promote skin healing. The argument against their use has been the risk of disseminated herpes,[24] although this has been questioned.[25] The administration of levodopa also has been shown to reduce the incidence of postherpetic neuralgia.[26,27]

The effectiveness of antiviral agents in the treatment of acute herpes zoster is not as clear cut in postherpetic neuralgia. Amantadine[19] and acyclovir[28] both reduce healing time in acute herpes zoster. Acyclovir is the less toxic agent, and its use for this condition is now widespread. Whether it has any effect on postherpetic neuralgia is uncertain.

The early recognition and avoidance, if possible, of drugs that can cause peripheral neuropathies is an important part of prophylaxis. The agents most commonly implicated are nitrofurantoin, vincristine, and isoniazid. The incidence of postthoracotomy pain may be lessened by intercostal blocks done at the time of surgery and postoperatively.[29] Surgery on the peripheral nervous system often can result in neuromas, neuralgias, and deafferentation-type pain. Therefore, a careful selection of patients and a trial of conservative therapy is advised before surgery is contemplated for neuralgias and peripheral neuropathy. The use of TENS in the early postoperative or postinjury period also has been advocated.

Medication

Narcotic and nonnarcotic analgesics have been unsuccessful in controlling the pain of peripheral neuralgias and neuropathies. This failure led to the use of centrally acting drugs, such as phenytoin and carbamazepine. Tricyclic antidepressants and substituted phenothiazines also have been used in these conditions. Unfortunately, the success of carbamazepine in treating the episodic neuralgia of tic douloureux in 80 percent to 90 percent of cases has not been repeated in other forms of peripheral neuralgia. However, in those neuralgias characterized by an episodic lancinating pain, it may be successful. For patients with constant pain, the combination of a tricyclic antidepressant and a substituted phenothiazine may be useful.

Although the use of tricyclic antidepressants in the treatment of neuralgia was proposed first more than 20 years ago, there are few well-controlled double-blind studies to support this form of treatment.[30] The initial study of Woodforde and colleagues[31] suggested that, despite an elevation in mood and improved sleep patterns, the background pain frequently persisted unabated. Taub[32,33] suggested the use of a substituted phenothiazine, fluphenazine, combined with the tricyclic antidepressant amitriptyline for the treatment of postherpetic neuralgia. The addition of fluphenazine provided significant amelioration of symptoms in several patients who previously had been unresponsive to amitriptyline alone. Prolonged administration of fluphenazine alone can lead to suicidal depression. Therefore, it was suggested that it be used in combination with a tricyclic antidepressant. The therapeutic effect of the tricyclics seems to be unrelated to their antidepressant effect. In a recent study involving patients with postherpetic neuralgia, a double-blind cross-over administration of amitriptyline produced good relief. The relief was sustained over a 12-month period in approximately one-half of the patients who had an initial good response. Therefore, it appears that, in those patients with postherpetic neuralgia who benefit from the use of tricyclic antidepressants, this effect can be maintained if the patient continues taking the drug.[34]

Why a combination of tricyclic antidepressants and phenothiazines would affect the pain of neuralgias and peripheral neuropathies is unexplained. The response to tricyclics often precedes any antidepressant effect by weeks. There is sometimes a delay in the onset of pain relief. Therefore, patients should take these medications for approximately 3 weeks before abandoning any prospects of improvement with their use.

Chlorprothixene is a medication that has potential for treating neuralgia unresponsive to other forms of treatment. However, the side effects of this drug limit its use (namely, lightheadedness, postural hypotension, and the possibility of psychosis). It is recommended that its use be confined to inpatients. With intensive therapy, Nathan[35] reported that patients obtained weeks of pain relief. Its use may be considered justifiable for those patients with refractory postherpetic neuralgia.

The prolonged use of fluphenazine has been associated with depressive symptoms and confusion. The most common motor side effect is that of parkinsonism, which is characterized by tremor and rigidity. Uncommonly, an acute dystonia can follow shortly after administration of the drug, and rarely, but more seriously, tardive dyskinesia can occur. The latter is a combination of involuntary facial and tongue movements most often seen in elderly patients. The first sign usually is a fine movement of the tongue, and the drug should be stopped if this is suspected.

The most common side effects of tricyclic antidepressants are anticholinergic (dry mouth, exacerbation of narrow-angle glaucoma, and urinary retention). Confusion may result from the central anticholinergic effects of these drugs. Cardiac arrhythmias have been reported, as has worsening of congestive cardiac failure. The dose of carbamazepine has to be titrated carefully. Ideally, plasma drug levels should be monitored and patients frequently reviewed. The side effects predominantly involve the central nervous system, leading to nystagmus, ataxia, sedation, and confusion. Rarely, rashes and agranulocytosis may occur. The drug therefore should be stopped at the first sign of infection. More recently, the oral antiarrythmics, such as mexiletine, have been used to treat some types of neuropathic pain.[36]

The suggested regimens for the administration of these drugs are as follows. Fluphenazine 1 mg twice a day initially can be increased gradually if necessary up to 2 mg four times a day. Amitriptyline therapy is begun with 25 to 50 mg at night and increased as necessary, slowly up to 150 mg. The sedating effect of this drug often can be usefully employed as a hypnotic. Carbamazepine dosing starts with 100 mg per day, increased by 100-mg increments per day until pain relief or side effects occur. If side effects occur, the dose is reduced to that previously tolerated, and a plateau is maintained for several days. Then attempts to increase the dose may be resumed. Monitor the drug serum levels if possible. If there has been no benefit from a daily dose of 1000 mg, further dose increases are unlikely to produce pain relief. The dose of mexiletine is 150 mg at bedtime to start. Then this is increased up to 900 mg per day in divided doses.

Afferent Stimulation

The most common forms of afferent stimulation are by physical means (massage, vibrators, acupuncture, or TENS)[37] (see Chap. 30). Physical therapy with or without the use of TENS should be the first choice of treatment of neuralgic pains. Favorable response rates with TENS in neuralgia can be as high as 60 percent. Therefore, it is essential to instruct patients properly in correct use of the method and encourage them to persist and experiment with the devices to obtain optimal relief. Frequent reassessment by an experienced physical therapist, especially during the early stages of treatment, is important to maximize any benefit that may be obtained. The devices can be used for hours at a time, often with persisting analgesia after use. They are almost devoid of side effects, apart from the possibility of skin irritation from the pads or tape needed to apply them. Hypoallergenic pads are available, and trying different adhesive tapes generally will provide a compatible brand. Sometimes the initial response to the use of the device is an exacerbation of pain, but if the patient persists, the pain may lessen. Electrical stimulation of the dorsal columns through an implanted system has been used for these conditions. Given appropriate patient selection and accurate placement of the leads, this more aggressive form of electrical stimulation can supply relief when all other treatments have failed. The major problems associated with epidural stimulation are lead movement and a potential for infection. This particularly may become a problem if the wounds must be reexplored frequently to reposition the leads. For the most part, the use of TENS is more cost effective and certainly less invasive.

Nerve Blocks

The success of sympathetic nerve blocks in the treatment of causalgia has not been found in the treatment of neuralgias and neuropathies. Several authors,[29,38,39] however, believe that repetitive sympathetic nerve blocks can decrease the incidence of postherpetic neuralgia. However, experience has been mixed.[40] Injection of the vesicles in the acute stage of herpes zoster with a local anesthetic combined with a corticosteroid has been reported to reduce the incidence of pain associated with the acute phase and postherpetic neuralgia.[41] Posttraumatic neuralgias, such as postoperative intercostal neuralgias and stump neuralgias, often respond to intermittent peripheral nerve blocks using a local anesthetic with concomitant physical therapy during the periods of analgesia. Entrapment neuropathies (such as meralgia paresthetica) occasionally can be resolved with intermittent local anesthetic nerve blocks (see Appendix A.X). The use of serial intravenous guanethidine blocks, as described by Hannington-Kiff,[42] has been found to be effective in the treatment of painful neuromas and some posttraumatic peripheral neuropathies.

Topical Treatment

The use of topical agents to treat postherpetic neuralgia recently has been investigated in several centers and has shown promise. Capsaicin is a neurotoxin found naturally in hot peppers. This substance depletes substance P and selectively blocks, and in high concentration destroys, nociceptive sensory afferents. Topical capsaicin 0.025% was used to treat refractory postherpetic neuralgia with modestly good results.[43] The main problem with its use is that the burning caused by the drug is difficult for some patients to tolerate.

Local anesthetic agents penetrate the skin poorly, but a mixture of lidocaine and prilocaine in an emulsion has been used to reduce the pain of venipuncture in children. Stow and colleagues[44] used a 5% cream of this combination in a small group of patients with postherpetic neuralgia. Effec-tive short-term pain relief occurred, especially in those with facial neuralgia. Plasma concentrations of the local anesthetic were minimal. Both these studies await confirmation with placebo-controlled trials.

Surgery

The use of surgery in certain neuralgias (exemplified by the carpal tunnel syndrome) has been proved over the years. However, we should be careful to exclude reversible conditions associated with this syndrome (such as myxedema, pregnancy, and gout) before we operate. The use of neurolytic agents, neurotomy, and neurectomy should be restricted to those patients with neuralgias associated with terminal cancer. The unacceptably high rate of relapse (which is often severe) after such procedures should preclude their use in nonmalignant conditions. The use of dorsal root entry zone lesions in the treatment of refractory neuralgias and deafferentation pain has been described.[45,46] The results of this procedure have been promising in relieving brachial plexus avulsion pain short-to-medium term.

Psychological and Behavioral Sequelae

Sometimes the pain associated with peripheral neuropathies and neuralgia follows a chronic and unrelenting course. In this case, it would be expected that patients will develop significant psychological and learned behavioral problems. Loss of employment and employability may lead to financial hardship, depression, and severe family discord. These patients often can be helped by supportive therapy from a trained psychologist or psychiatrist. A social worker may be able to optimize their financial position and organize patient-support groups. It should be stressed that the skills and time needed to support these patients usually cannot be filled by one therapist. Sometimes the best therapeutic milieu will be engendered by therapy that does not emphasize conventional medical treatment but adopt a supportive approach and deals with the suffering and behavioral sequelae.

In summary, we acknowledge the fact that treatments for refractory neuralgias and neuropathies are disappointing at this time. This almost certainly is related to our incomplete understanding of the mechanisms involved in producing such pains. There is controversy as to the site of the afferent painful stimulus (if any). Does this exist in the peripheral nervous system (at early synapse levels in the dorsal horn and lower spinal cord), or is it some more central mechanism? At this time we cannot answer these questions, nor is there a satisfactory explanation as to why pain occurs in some patients with such neurologic deficits but not in others.

In attempting to help patients with these problems, current therapeutic effort usually is directed toward attempting to find long-term solutions by using some variation of stimulation-produced analgesia, either externally applied by

TENS units or, rarely, by more central applications of dorsal column and thalamic stimulation. Pharmacologic attempts to control the pain are often disappointing. Judicious use of nerve blocks with local anesthetic (but not neurodestructive) agents can help, especially during exacerbations. Usually, these offer only temporary benefit.

It is relatively easy to advise dogmatically against the use of such powerful therapies as narcotic administration or surgical invasion. It is more difficult to suggest specific therapies that can be helpful in this unfortunate group of patients.

References

1. Merskey H, ed. Classification of chronic pain. Descriptions of chronic pain syndromes and definitions of pain terms. *Pain* 1986; 3(suppl):1.

2. Portenoy RK. Painful polyneuropathy. *Neurol Clin* May 1989; 7(2):265–288.

3. Thomas PK. Clinical features and differential diagnosis. In: Dyck PJ, Thomas PK, Lambert EH, eds. *Peripheral Neuropathy*. Philadelphia: Saunders; 1975.

4. Dyck PJ. The causes, classification, and treatment of peripheral neuropathy. *N Engl J Med* 1982; 307:283.

5. Greene DA, Sima AF, Pfeifer MA, Albers JW. Diabetic neuropathy. *Annu Rev Med* 1990; 41:303–317.

6. Ward JD. Diabetic neuropathy. *Br Med Bull* January 1989; 45(10):111–126.

7. Weber GA, Sloan P, Davies D. Nutritionally induced peripheral neuropathies. *Clin Podiatr Med Surg* January 1990; 7(1):107–128.

8. Olesen LL, Jensen TS. Prevention and management of drug-induced peripheral neuropathy. *Drug Saf* July–August 1991; 6(4):302–314.

9. Murphy TM, Kozody R, Yu-Ling Hui. Peripheral neuropathies and neuralgias. In: Stein J, Warfield CA, eds. *International Anesthesiology Clinics. Pain Management 21*. Boston: Little, Brown; 1983.

10. Forman A. Peripheral neuropathy in cancer patients: incidence, features, and pathophysiology [published erratum appears in *Oncology* April 1990; 4(4):16]. *Oncology* January 1990; 4(1):57–62.

11. Melzack R, Wall PD. Pain mechanisms: a new theory. *Science* 1965; 150:971.

12. Rappaport ZH, Devor M. Experimental pathophysiological correlates of clinical symptomatology in peripheral neuropathic pain syndromes. *Stereotact Funct Neurosurg* 1990:54–55, 90–95.

13. Noordenbos W. *Pain*. London: Elsevier; 1959.

14. Dyck PJ, Lambert EH, O'Brien PC. Pain in peripheral neuropathy related to rate and kind of fiber degeneration. *Neurology* 1976; 26:466.

15. Dyck PJ. Hypoxic neuropathy: does hypoxia play a role in diabetic neuropathy? The 1988 Robert Wartenberg lecture. *Neurology* January 1989; 39(1):111–118.

16. Wall PD, Gutnick M. Ongoing activity in peripheral nerves: the physiology and pharmacology of impulses arising from a neuroma. *Exp Neurol* 1974; 43:580.

17. Asbury AK, Fields HL. Pain due to peripheral nerve damage: a hypothesis. *Neurology* 1984; 34:1587.

18. Livingstone WK. *Pain Mechanisms: A Physiological Interpretation of Causalgia and Its Related States*. New York: Macmillan; 1943.

19. Tasker RR. Deafferentation. In: Wall PD, Melzack R, eds. *Textbook of Pain*. Edinburgh: Churchill Livingstone; 1984:119.

20. Agnew DC. Painful neurologic disorders. In: Aronoff GM, ed. *Evaluation and Treatment of Chronic Pain*. Baltimore: Urban & Schwarzenberg; 1985.

21. Lindblom U. Neuralgia: mechanisms and therapeutic prospects. In: Benedetti C, Chapman CR, Moricca G, eds. *Advances in Pain Research and Therapy*. Vol 7. New York: Raven Press; 1984.

22. Eaglestein WH, Katz R, Brown JA. The effects of early corticosteroid therapy on the skin eruption and pain of herpes zoster. *JAMA* 1970; 211:1681.

23. Keczkes K, Basheer AM. Do corticosteroids prevent postherpetic neuralgia? *Br J Dermatol* 1980; 102:551.

24. *BMJ* 1979; 1:5. Editorial.

25. Sutton G. Steroid therapy in the treatment of herpes zoster. *Br J Clin Pract* January 1984:21–24.

26. Kernbaum S, Hauchecorn J. Administration of levodopa for relief of herpes zoster pain. *JAMA* 1981; 246:132.

27. Galbraith AW. Prevention of postherpetic neuralgia by amantadine hydrochloride. *Br J Clin Pract* September 1983:304–306.

28. Loeser JD. Herpes zoster and postherpetic neuralgia. *Pain* 1986; 25:149.

29. Miller RD, Munger WL, Powell PE. Chronic pain and local anesthetic neural blockade. In: Cousins MJ, Bridenbaugh PO, eds. *Neural Blockade in Clinical Anesthesia and Management of Pain*. Philadelphia: Lippincott; 1980.

30. Egbunike IG, Chaffee BJ. Antidepressants in the management of chronic pain syndromes. *Pharmacotherapy* 1990; 10(4):262–270.

31. Woodforde JM, Dwyer B, McEwen BW, et al. Treatment of postherpetic neuralgia. *Med J Aust* 1965; 2:869.

32. Taub A. Relief of postherpetic neuralgia with psychotropic drugs. *J Neurosurg* 1973; 39:235.

33. Taub A, Collins WF. Observations on the treatment of denervation dysesthesia with psychotropic drugs: postherpetic neuralgia, anesthesia dolorosa, peripheral neuropathy. In: Bonica JJ, ed. *International Symposium on Pain (Advances in Neurology, Vol 4)*. New York: Raven Press; 1974.

34. Watson PC, Evens RJ, Reed K, Merskey H, Goldsmith L, Marsh J. Amitriptyline vs. placebo in postherpetic neuralgia. *Neurology* 1982; 32:671.

35. Nathan PW. Chlorprothixene (Taractan) in postherpetic neuralgia and other severe chronic pains. *Pain* 1978; 5:367.

36. Tanelian DL, Brose WG. Neuropathic pain can be relieved by drugs that are use-dependent sodium channel blockers: lidocaine, carbamazepine, and mexiletine. *Anesthesiology* 1991; 74:949–951.

37. Long D, Hagfors N. Electrical stimulation in the nervous system. *Pain* 1975; 1:109.

38. Colding A. The effect of regional sympathetic blocks in the treatment of herpes zoster. *Acta Anesthiol Scand* 1969; 13:113.

39. Kenjiro Dan, Kazuo Higa, Banri Noda. Ten years results of nerve block therapy for herpetic pain. *Pain Suppl* 1984; 2:270S.

40. Riopelle JM, Naraghi M, Grush KP. Chronic neuralgia incidence following local anesthetic therapy for herpes zoster. *Arch Dermatol* 1984; 120:747.

41. Epstein E. Herpes zoster and postzoster neuralgia: intralesional triamcinolone therapy. *Cutis* 1973; 12:898.

42. Hannington-Kiff JG. Antisympathetic drugs in limbs. In: Wall PD, Melzack R, eds. *A Textbook of Pain*. Edinburgh: Churchill Livingstone; 1984.

43. Watson CPN, Evans RJ, Watt VR. Postherpetic neuralgia and topical capsaicin. *Pain* 1988; 33:333.

44. Stow PJ, Glynn CJ, Minor B. EMLA cream in the treatment of postherpetic neuralgia. Efficacy and pharmacokinetic profile. *Pain* 1989; 39:301.

45. Friedman AH, Nashold BS Jr, Ovelmen-Levitt J. Dorsal root entry zone lesions for the treatment of postherpetic neuralgia. *J Neurol* 1984; 60:1258.

46. Nashold BS Jr, Ostdahl RH, Bullitt E, et al. Dorsal root entry zone lesions: a new neurosurgical therapy for deafferentation pain. In: Bonica JJ, Lindblom U, Iggo A, et al, eds. *Advances in Pain Research and Therapy*. Vol 5. New York: Raven Press; 1983.

CHAPTER 23

Peripheral Vascular Disease

Mark Swerdlow and I. G. Schraibman

It is incumbent on the clinician in the pain relief clinic to be familiar with the causes and management of pain from peripheral vascular disease and also to be able to identify conditions that wrongly may be referred or are present incidentally. Pain caused by vascular disease can be divided into two types based on origin: arterial and venous.

PAIN OF ARTERIAL ORIGIN

Arterial insufficiency is most commonly the result of occlusive disease (so-called atheroma), but less commonly it occurs in Buerger disease, Raynaud syndrome, diabetic arteritis, and arteritis associated with collagen disease. Migraine and cluster headache, which have a vascular element as a cause, are discussed in Chapter 5.

Atheroma and Its Consequences

The process of fat deposition in the intima of large arteries and the sequelas of ulceration, embolization, occlusion, and thrombosis have been described exhaustively in pathologic terms, although a definitive hypothesis of the cause still is lacking. A discussion of atherogenesis is beyond the scope of this chapter, but certain adverse risk factors (such as hypertension, excessive blood fat levels, smoking, and lack of exercise) have been identified. In relation to coronary artery disease, it has been estimated, however, that if all known risk factors were eliminated, 70 percent of the incidence would remain unexplained.

Distribution of Atheroma

Atheroma is a systemic condition; pathologically, it affects every artery in the body. Clinically, however, the upper limbs rarely are involved.

Atheromas occur at bifurcations because of the turbulence and increased resistence to flow there. The outstanding exception is disease of the straight femoropopliteal segment; this is involved in 60 percent of lower limb atheromas.

In response to restriction of the lumen of a major artery, volume flow is maintained through two mechanisms as follows: (1) the velocity of blood flow increases automatically so that volume flow does not decrease until 80 percent of the lumen has been lost (Fig. 23-1) and (2) collaterals develop. Enlargement of vessels of arteriolar size can be considerable (e.g., around the knee and hip). It is only when these collaterals themselves become narrow that the patient has symptoms. At first, this occurs only when the circulation is stressed (as in walking); resting levels of blood flow may be normal even in a patient with severe claudication.[1]

Mechanism of Pain from Arterial Disease

Oxygen is the most flow-limited nutrient for the muscle and skin. Muscles normally can metabolize and do work anaerobically, but the oxygen debt must be repaid. Attempts to quantify oxygen debt by measuring lactate and pyruvate levels in ischemic tissue fail because changes are detected only when gross tissue necrosis is present.[1] Modern research techniques allow us to identify reduced oxygen radicals (superoxide oxygen and its derivatives) that are highly reactive and cytotoxic.[2] These radicals are found in ischemic skin.[3] This applies particularly after relief of ischemia—the reperfusion syndrome.

Clinical Picture of Occlusive Arterial Disease

The patient may complain of (1) claudication and (2) rest pain (pedal ischemia). *Claudication* is defined as pain in a muscle group (commonly the calf, and less often, the thigh, instep, or buttock) that occurs while walking and forces the

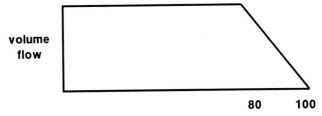

Note: volume flow does not decrease until luminal restriction is 80% or more.

FIGURE 23-1. *Relationship between loss of lumen and volume blood flow.*

patient to stop. The pain is relieved rapidly by rest; after this, walking can be resumed. As the patient's condition deteriorates, the walking distance shortens. If these points are sought in a careful history, it usually is easy to exclude most other causes of the painful leg. Confusion may arise if, through infirmity from another cause (e.g., arthritis), the patient cannot exercise, and evidence of vascular disease may be elicited on examination. In addition, angina may limit walking distance, and the leg symptoms may be masked. The differential diagnosis includes venous and neurogenic claudication. The latter is caused by stenosis of the central spinal canal; this constricts the cauda equina, causing pain in the legs during walking. However, in this condition, walking downhill is more painful than walking uphill, and the peripheral pulses may be good. Myelography CT or MRI will confirm the diagnosis.

If the history is adequate, the site of claudication also indicates the level of occlusion (Table 23-1). Intermittent claudication is more common in men than in women, in whom it is rare before menopause. *Rest pain (pedal ischemia)* consists of pain in the toes or forefoot with or without ulceration or gangrene. The history of ischemic pain is invariably that of pain occurring at night (after a variable recumbent period). This causes the patient to arise and is relieved by dependency of the limb. Patients may volunteer that they prefer to sleep in a chair. As the condition progresses, rest pain becomes more continuous, and the condition of the toes deteriorates. Ulceration or gangrene may occur. When spontaneous in origin, tissue death is as peripheral as possible (on the toes) unless it follows trauma, overzealous chiropody, or orthopedic procedures (such as operations for bunions and ingrown toenails). Rest pain usually is preceded by claudication, but sometimes it appears in patients who have little or no claudication pain.

Other Relevant History

Because atheroma is a generalized disease, the history may provide evidence of myocardial ischemia (infarcts or angina), stroke, hypertension, cardiac irregularities, and transient ischemic attacks (in the form of focal neurologic deficits resolving within 24 h). The patient may be receiving many drugs. Smoking habits must be elicited, and social and psychological aspects should not be ignored.[4]

Table 23-1
Relation of Site of Claudication to Level of Major Arterial Occlusion

Site of Claudication	Level of Occlusion
Instep	Popliteal bifurcation or below
Calf	Femoropopliteal
Thigh	Common femoral
Buttock	Aortoiliac

Table 23-2
An Example of a Pulse Chart

Site	Right	Left
Carotid	+	+
Subclavian	+	+
Radial	+	+
Aorta	[+]	
Femoral	(+)	+
Popliteal	−	+
Dorsalis pedis	−	+
Posterior tibial	−	+
Perforating peroneal	−	−

Note: [ ] indicates aneurysm, ( ) indicates bruit. This patient had an abdominal aortic aneurysm, right iliac stenosis, and right femoropopliteal occlusion.

Physical Examination

The general examination includes blood pressure measurement, cardiac auscultation, and funduscopy. Local examination will reveal ischemic tissue loss and poor capillary circulation. Low input arterial pressure can be enhanced by elevating the legs above the heart for 2 min while the patient repeatedly dorsiplantar flexes the ankles; this will produce elevation pallor.

All accessible pulses should be palpated and large vessels (such as the femoral) should be auscultated for the presence of a bruit as an indication of proximal stenosis. These data should be charted; an example is shown in Table 23-2.

Investigations

The general assessment of the patient is aided by chest radiography, cardiography, complete blood count, and blood chemistries; echocardiography and 24-h monitoring for cardiac irregularity often are invaluable.

The trend in vascular investigations is to avoid, as far as possible, invasive investigations, such as aortography (which can cause morbidity and are expensive), in favor of noninvasive tests (ultrasonography). A relatively cheap portable Doppler instrument can provide more information and be used by anyone with a minimum of training. The standard test is the ankle-to-arm pressure ratio; this relates systolic pressure at the ankle to the systemic arterial pressure. Observed values can be related to the clinical state (Table 23-3). Arteriography is done only as a preliminary before reconstructive surgery.

Table 23-3
Relationship of Severity of Disease to Doppler Ankle-to-Arm Pressure Ratio

Ankle-to-Arm	Severity of Disease
0.85–1.10	Normal
0.60–0.85	Mild claudication
0.30–0.60	Severe claudication
<0.30	Critical ischemia

Management of Major Arterial Occlusion

Management of a patient with an ischemic lower limb is summarized in the flow chart seen below:

Treatment of Claudication

Conservative treatment includes observation and treatment of associated conditions (such as diabetes, anemia, or polycythemia). Efforts must be made to dissuade the patient from smoking because, although there is no evidence to suggest that such secondary intervention influences atherogenesis, nicotine is a vasoconstrictor and smoking causes carboxyhemoglobinemia. This compound cannot bind oxygen, and polycythemia develops and increases the blood viscosity.[5]

The severity of claudication must be weighed in relation to the patient's age, occupation, and life. Younger more active patients will be more disabled than those with a sedentary way of life. When pedal ischemia becomes prominent, this mandates consideration of vascular surgery if it is technically feasible. Arterial reconstruction uses grafting, endarterectomy, or transluminal angioplasty, the technical details of which are beyond the scope of this chapter. Our concern here is to discuss those in whom these procedures have failed or were not applicable.

PAIN RELIEF MEASURES

Sympathectomy

Interruption of the lumbar sympathetic chain has a time-honored place in the treatment of peripheral ischemia. Before the advent of arterial reconstruction, it was the only surgical measure that produced pain relief. The indications for sympathectomy have diminished considerably over the

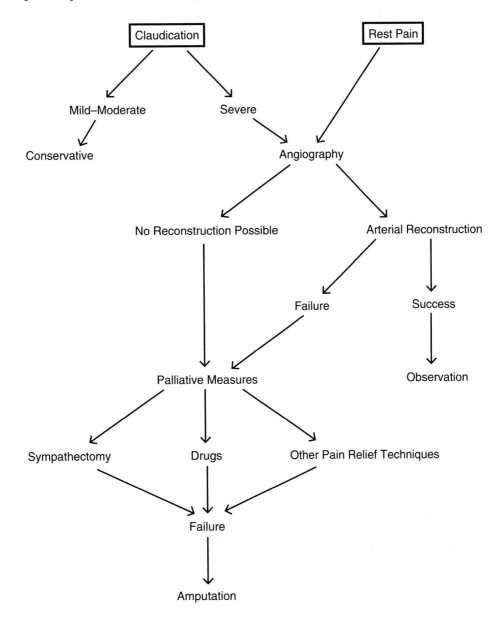

last 30 years, but it still plays a useful role. Currently, it is recognized that sympathectomy is not valuable for claudication,[6] but it is effective in 58 percent of patients with pedal ischemia, a mean figure culled from all large series up to 1970.[1] The effect may result from increased blood flow to the foot, a response that has been shown to persist for 5 years from interruption of afferent nerves that carry the pain sensation. The ideal candidate for sympathectomy has rest pain without gangrene and a cool foot. This procedure also can help to heal ulceration, skin necrosis, and incipient or early gangrene. Kaada[7] claims that healing of ulceration also can be facilitated by TENS. However, Fiume[8] found that, in arteriosclerotic patients with trophic lesions and ulceration of the foot, the results of spinal cord stimulation were disappointing.

If the affected foot is warmer than its fellow, this suggests that autosympathectomy has occurred (especially in diabetic patients) and that the procedure will not be beneficial. However, there are patients who do not respond despite favorable characteristics. If the popliteal inflow index (Doppler inflow pressure in popliteal artery versus arm pressure) is 0.7 or greater, a good response can be predicted.[9] It is unlikely that a favorable response will be obtained if the ankle-to-arm ratio is less than 0.35.[10]

Lumbar sympathectomy can be acheived by injection or operation. The technique of lumbar sympathetic block is well described in the references.[11,12] An accurate block of the sympathetic chain at L3 is adequate; it is not necessary to use multiple needles (see Appendix A.II). However, the use of radiographic control will make the procedure easier and safer. If repeated blocks with dilute local anesthetic solution produce appreciable circulatory improvement, neurolytic block with 5 ml aqueous phenol 5% solution should be considered as an alternative to surgical sympathectomy.[13]

Operative sympathectomy is done by a relatively atraumatic extraperitoneal approach under general anesthesia in which lumbar ganglia 2, 3, and 4 are excised together with the chain connecting them. The only significant postoperative complication is postsympathectomy neuralgia, an aching pain in the femoral nerve distribution that resolves in 6 to 8 weeks.[14]

Other Methods of Improving the Peripheral Circulation

Regional Sympathetic Block (See Appendix A.IV)

An effective alternative means of producing sympathetic block in a limb is to administer intravenous guanethidine.[15] Guanethidine acts on postganglionic neurons, first releasing norepinephrine and then causing noradrenergic block by preventing the reuptake of norepinephrine by the neurons. A tourniquet is placed around the proximal part of the limb and inflated. We inject 20 mg of guanethidine in 50 ml of normal saline into an indwelling intravenous catheter in the leg (10 mg in 30 ml for an arm), and the tourniquet is kept

inflated for 15 min. This method is particularly valuable in patients who are receiving anticoagulant therapy in whom paravertebral lumbar sympathetic block can cause massive hemorrhage. Guanethidine block also can be used in cases where the effects of operative lumbar sympathectomy are receding. If guanethidine is not available, reserpine (2 to 5 mg) may be administered. Bretylium (100 to 200 mg) also has been used for this purpose, but it has the disadvantage of being short acting and, therefore, requires more frequent repetition.

Paravertebral Spinal Block

Feldman and Yeung[16] claim that block of the spinal nerve roots will provide pain relief and improved walking distance in patients with intermittent claudication. They inject 5 to 10 ml of phenol 7.5% in myodil paravertebrally at L1 under x-ray control and claim that almost two-thirds of their patients still had an increased walking distance 6 months after the block. They consider the improvement results from blocking fibers that carry the ischemic pain sensation, which pass into the spinal cord in the gray rami. However, they use this technique only in patients who are not suitable for surgery.

Dorsal Column Electrical Stimulation

During the past few years, several reports of the value of large fiber nerve stimulation have been published.[17–19] Cook and associates[20] studied patients with pain from peripheral arteriosclerotic disease who had not responded to sympathectomy and arterial by-pass surgery. Stimulation of the spinal posterior roots using implanted electrodes produced pain relief together with improved plethysmographic blood flow and increased skin temperature. Dooley and Kasprak[21] reported that, in 16 patients, electrical stimulation of the cord and roots caused arterial vasodilatation in the extremities. Nine patients had varying degrees of vascular insufficiency in a limb. Many had not responded to sympathectomy or by-pass. Dorsal column stimulation at lower thoracic levels produced increased skin temperature, improved plethysmographic blood flow, decreased edema, and pain relief. The effects persisted for 11 months in their first patient. Meglio and colleagues[22] also found that epidural spinal stimulation produced a substantial increase in blood flow in peripheral vascular disease.

According to Augustinsson and coworkers,[23] these vasodilating effects of spinal stimulation could be explained by the following mechanisms: (1) segmental inhibition of vasoconstrictor fibers, (2) antidromic activation of posterior root fibers, and (3) activation of ascending pathways to supraspinal autonomic centers. Stimulation over lumbar spines or peripheral nerves was ineffective in these patients.

Drug Therapy

The search for a noninvasive treatment for peripheral ischemia has highlighted many drugs that, after a brief popularity, have vanished from our treatment armamentarium. Various approaches have been tried, including: (1) vasodilatation, (2) antithrombotic measures, (3) fibrinolysis, (4) antiplatelet drugs, (5) attempts to modify tissue response to anoxia, and (6) prostacyclin.

Vasodilators. Because the regulation of blood flow in the normal foot is affected simply by decreasing or increasing sympathetic tone, α-adrenergic blocking agents have been used, including thymoxamine, phentolamine, and phenoxybenzamine. Other drugs have a local effect on vascular smooth muscle. These include papaverine and derivatives of nicotinic acid. Priscoline is an α-receptor blocker that also has a direct effect.

Vasodilator drugs are not always clinically (as opposed to pharmacologically) active.[24] They have never been shown to influence the outcome of ischemia of the foot. This is hardly surprising to anyone who has handled the stiff, unyielding, and often rigidly calcified arteries in these patients. Systemic use of vasodilators actually may reduce blood flow in the worst affected limb by shunting the blood to healthier areas (the vasodilator paradox).[25] To obtain a local effect, intraarterial injection is feasible, but a long course of treatment logistically is difficult to maintain. Retrograde intravenous infusion (Bier technique) of priscoline has produced remarkable vasodilatation in severely ischemic feet, but the effect is evanescent.[1]

Ketanserin is a serotonin-2 receptor antagonist that antagonizes both the vasoconstricting and platelet aggregating effects of serotonin.[26] DeCree and his colleagues[27] reported a double-blind controlled trial of ketanserin that found both improved claudication distance and peripheral blood flow in patients with intermittent claudication. However, Fonesca and associates,[28] who conducted an open trial of ketanserin in nine diabetic patients with intermittent claudication, report no subjective improvement. Bounameaux and colleagues[29] also could not confirm the beneficial effects of ketanserin therapy.

Antithrombotic Measures. There has been no great enthusiasm for anticoagulant therapy in peripheral vascular disease because thrombosis, when it occurs, is only the final episode in the generation of the ischemic limb. The best available results (in a controlled double-blind trial) did not show any beneficial effect.[30]

Fibrinolysis. Fibrinogen is the substrate for thrombin that converts it to fibrin. Dissolution of fibrin can be achieved using streptokinase, urokinase or tissue plasminogen activator. The only possible application in this disorder would be in acute thrombosis superimposed on atheromatous stenosis. Although it may delay progression, fibrinolysis does not affect atheroma, and rethrombosis will follow cessation of therapy. This is now accepted as useful therapy in acute occlusion but it should be followed by arteriography to assess the need for reconstruction.

Antiplatelet Therapy. Drugs, such as aspirin, dipyridamole, ticlopidine, and prostacyclin, inhibit release of thromboxame A and prevent platelet aggregation. Because the latter only occurs in turbulent flow proximal or distal to atheromatous stenosis or occlusion, such treatment can be only of secondary importance in peripheral arterial disease.

Metabolic Agents. Naftidrofuryl was marketed first as a vasodilator, but it is purported currently to influence muscle metabolism beneficially through the Krebs cycle. Larger studies tend to find this substance ineffective. Boobis and associates[31] found no significant improvement in ischemic rest pain after a controlled trial comparing placebo with high dose intravenous naftidrofuryl followed by oral dosing for 3 months. All objective measurements were unchanged, and the amputation rate was almost identical in control and treated groups.

Prostacyclin. The term prostaglandin was coined by Von Euler[32] who discovered some of the pharmacologic effects of semen. Endoperoxides derived from cell membrane arachidonic acid are converted to thromboxame A_2 in platelets (vasoconstrictor and platelet aggregator) or to prostacyclins in blood vessel endothelium (vasodilator and inhibitor of platelet aggregation). The balance between these two compounds maintains intravascular hemostasis.

The earliest report of the use of prostacyclins in ischemic feet used prostaglandin E by intraarterial infusion; the same workers later administered the drug by the intravenous route. In both instances, they reported dramatic relief of rest pain in small patient groups and healing of some ulcers.[33,34]

There have been three controlled trials of prostacyclin in ischemic limbs. The first[35] reported good subjective improvement but no objective change; the other two found either no effect[36] or a deleterious effect.[37]

Similar to vasodilators, the mode of administration may be important. Hirai and Nakayama[38] demonstrated a steal effect of the drug by the intravenous rather than the intraarterial route. By the latter technique, they were able to use smaller doses with less risk of side effects. Healing of skin ulcers occurred in 3 of 10 patients. This, however, required intraarterial infusion for a mean 30 days (range, 17 to 75 days).

PAIN DUE TO PERIPHERAL ARTERIAL DISEASE

Raynaud Syndrome

This condition differs from all other peripheral arteriopathies because it affects mainly the hands. It was described first by Maurice Raynaud[39] in 1862. Allen and Brown[40] advanced our understanding by separating affected patients into those with and without an underlying cause.

Raynaud syndrome includes the classic clinical picture of pallor in the distal two-thirds of the fingers (a result of arterial shutdown), cyanosis (from partial relaxation of arterial spasm and deoxygenation of blood), and rubor (reactive hyperemia); all occur in response to cold or emotion. As the condition progresses, the pain becomes more severe and continuous. The condition is more common in women than in men; usually, it becomes apparent by the age of 40 years. It occurs much less often in the lower limbs. *Raynaud disease* describes patients in whom no underlying condition can be found. *Raynaud phenomenon* comprises those patients with Raynaud syndrome secondary to underlying pathologic disorders (Table 23-4).

Raynaud phenomenon is particularly important because the associated condition may be treatable. In addition, the prognosis is worse, and these patients may develop pathologic changes of ulceration, subungual infection, and pulp loss after digital arterial occlusion (Fig. 23-2). Porter and Rivers[41] reported 383 patients observed in a 10-year period. Of these, 162 had no associated disease, and 137 had proven or suspected connective tissue disorder (57 of the latter had systemic sclerosis).

Table 23-4
Conditions Associated with Raynaud's Phenomenon

Immunologic and connective tissue disorders (such as systemic sclerosis, systemic lupus erythematosus, rheumatoid dermatomyositis, hepatitis-B associated vasculitis).

Arterial obstruction (such as thoracic outlet syndrome and Buerger disease).

Vibrating tool disease.

Drug induced (such as ergot, β-adrenergic blockers, cytotoxic drugs [vinblastine or bleomycin], or oral contraceptives).

Miscellaneous (such as vinyl chloride disease, cold agglutins, or cryoglobulinemia).

Management

General Measures. Simple avoidance of cold, either of the body or of the hands, may be all that is required in mild cases. A change of occupation may be necessary if vibrating tools are used. Cessation of smoking has been advocated without conclusive evidence to substantiate potential benefit.

Sympathectomy. Because nervous control of digital blood flow occurs simply as a result of increasing or decreasing sympathetic tone, pharmacologic or surgical sympathectomy has been used extensively. Drugs, such as methyldopa, thymoxamine, reserpine, debrisoquine, and phentolamine, have been administered orally and intraarterially. Most of the studies are anecdotal, uncontrolled, or rely on subjective assessment. In one study, reserpine was effective,[42] but another trial in patients with bilateral disease, using one arm as a control against the other, concluded that intrarterial injection of this substance was ineffective.[43] If no effect can be proved when a drug is given intraarterially, it is unlikely that it will work systemically. The pain of Raynaud disease can be controlled adequately by intravenous regional sympathetic block with guanethidine. However, patients with Raynaud disease are sensitive to norepinephrine, and the initial guanethidine block should be preceded by a dose of an α-adrenoreceptor blocker, such as thymoxamine or phentolamine.[15] The injection may need to be repeated once or twice a week. This is probably the method of choice for the management of the pain of Raynaud syndrome.

Surgical sympathectomy can be done using an open

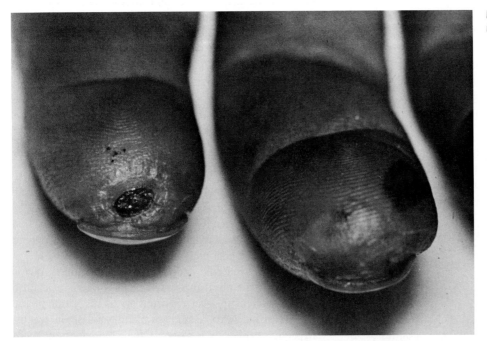

FIGURE 23-2. Digital ulceration in Raynaud disease.

operation, but temporary and permanent Horner syndrome may occur. The approach most favored currently is transaxillary endoscopic coagulation to destroy thoracic ganglia 2 to 5.[44] Although the immediate effect usually is good, the condition invariably recurs in 6 to 24 months; therefore, surgical treatment has been abandoned largely.[14]

A novel but time-consuming approach is to do digital sympathectomy using microvascular techniques. A total of 37 patients have been so treated with excellent results maintained over a follow-up period of up to 4 years.[45]

Sympathetic Blockade. Where the condition is not severe and particularly if it is seasonal, stellate ganglion block can be helpful. The anterior paratracheal approach is recommended[46] (see Appendix A.I). The use of radiographic control and a radiopaque dye such as Conray 280 will facilitate accurate needle placement and help to avoid accidental injection into an elongated dural cuff. Boas[12] found that, although repeated sympathetic block can produce a good result in Raynaud syndrome, it usually is not sustained beyond a few weeks or months. Sheehan and Coray[47] found good results after lumbar sympathetic block in patients with Raynaud syndrome in the legs (see Appendix A.II).

Ketanserin. Stranden and colleagues[48] reported a trial of ketanserin in a dose of 10 mg intravenously in nine patients with Raynaud syndrome. Six of the patients had primary disease, and three had Raynaud phenomenon. The duration of the condition ranged from 3 to 30 years. Blood flow was assessed by photoplethysmography, and skin temperature was measured. Blood flow and temperature increased significantly after ketanserin, but placebo (saline) had no such effect. The dominant effect of ketanserin was on precapillary resistance vessels.

Nerve Stimulation. Groth[49] found that epidural dorsal column stimulation produced increased blood flow and considerable relief of pain in patients with Raynaud syndrome. Kaada[50] also reported that nerve stimulation provided pain relief in these patients.

Biofeedback. Boas[12] believes that patients with Raynaud syndrome may improve to a lesser extent by using temperature biofeedback therapy.

Calcium Blockade. Calcium ions are involved in the transmission of nerve impulses to muscle and in muscle contraction; blockade can be achieved using verapamil or nifedipine. In a study of 20 patients, 11 had favorable responses, particularly those with spastic rather than obstructive disease.[41] These authors advocate the use of nifedipine supplemented by guanethidine.

Antiplatelet Therapy. Because platelet aggregation forms part of the pathologic picture of advanced disease, it was thought logical to prevent this so-called sludging. Our personal experience with aspirin, dipyridamole, and ticlopidine has been disappointing, possibly because the treatment

can influence only a secondary event at a late stage of the disease.

Prostacyclins. There are many, although rather unscientific, reports advocating the use of these substances in Raynaud,[51] but there is no conclusive proof of benefit.

Buerger Disease

Thromboangiitis obliterans was the name Leo Buerger[52] gave to a specific arterial disease he believed was confined largely to Eastern Europeans. This disease subsequently was shown to be prevalent in Sri Lanka, Korea, and Japan, where it is the most common form of arterial pathology. The Japanese have published the world's largest series in one report of 1641 cases of femoropopliteal occlusion; 75 percent of patients were thought to have Buerger disease.[53] They correlated its high incidence to a specific gene found in 10 percent of Japanese people but rare in whites.[54]

Clinical Picture

More than 90 percent of sufferers are men younger than 40 years of age who are smokers. They have instep claudication or painful ischemic changes in the feet. Just less than one-half have manifestations in their upper limbs, usually thrombophlebitis or minor ischemic changes. Foot pulses and, later, popliteal pulses are absent.

Buerger disease is an inflammatory process; the affected artery is surrounded by fibrosis. The pathology is specific with thrombosis in crural arteries and veins. Giant cells are a histologic feature, even in early cases.

Management

Universally, it is accepted that all treatment will be useless if the patient continues to smoke. If patients stop smoking, this alone may be sufficient to provide relief.

Local treatment is directed toward debridement and draining infections. Prostacyclin is reputed to be effective in relieving pain, although it is less effective in healing the lesions.[55] Sympathectomy gives excellent results in 50 percent of patients, and 30 percent[14] are improved. Therefore, it is the main mode of treatment. Groth[49] claims that dorsal column stimulation can reduce pain and improve walking capacity in patients with Buerger disease.

Fortunately, Buerger disease is not a life-threatening illness. More than one-third of patients must undergo amputations, and in approximately one-half of these, it is to a minor extent.[56]

VENOUS DISEASE

This may be acute (deep venous thrombosis [DVT] or thrombophlebitis) or chronic (DVT with recanalization or gravitational disease). DVT occurs when normal venous flow is disturbed in accordance with the Virchow triad: (1) diminished flow velocity after illness, operation, or childbirth; (2) alteration in the characteristics of the contained blood producing increased viscosity, such as polycythemia, abnormal plasma protein fractions, leukemia, or thrombocythemia; and (3) local intimal damage. It has been shown that postoperative DVT begins on the operating table, and this may be associated with the widespread use of paralyzing anesthetic agents since the middle 1950s.

In most cases, more than one factor is responsible. Many cases apparently arise spontaneously in healthy people; however, a search for an underlying malignant condition or collagenosis is mandatory. Some cases are proved over time to arise de novo and resolve without further harm.

Acute Venous Disease

The clinical diagnosis of DVT is made by the triad of local tenderness, swelling, and color change. Clinical diagnosis alone does not detect the subtler changes and may overdiagnose the condition in the presence of atheroma; false-positive and false-negative results comprise 50 percent of all cases.

When edema is present, it implies that the deep veins are occluded; embolization is less likely, but local sequelae are more likely. The clinical picture is either the white leg (milk leg), which is pale and shows infragenicular pitting edema, or the blue leg, which involves the entire leg as far proximally as the root of the limb. The former is a result of femoropopliteal obstruction; the latter indicates iliac–caval obstruction. The blue leg causes much discomfort, and if tissue pressure continues to rise, peripheral gangrene may supervene.

Acute thrombophlebitis is recognizable easily because there is visible swelling and tenderness along the course of a superficial vein. Apart from the underlying conditions already mentioned, the condition may be the harbinger of carcinoma of the pancreas or lung.

Chronic Venous Disease

Occlusion of the major veins is followed by recanalization with valve destruction. This allows transmission of the full force of the column of blood from the right atrium to the heel (± 80 to 90 mmHg). The patient may complain of a bursting pain in the calf, which, when associated with walking, is called *venous claudication*.

Gravitational changes are more serious because of their reputation for intractability. These changes include pigmentation, distended intracutaneous veins (in the inframalleolar position, so-called venous flare), edema, liposclerosis, and ulceration (Fig. 23-3). The pain of a venous ulcer may be excruciating; it usually is worse at night and is unrelated to ulcer size.

Investigation of venous disease is directed toward the following.

1. Proving the diagnosis. Isotope (iodine-131 fibrinogen) studies may be helpful in acute DVT. Doppler responses may be

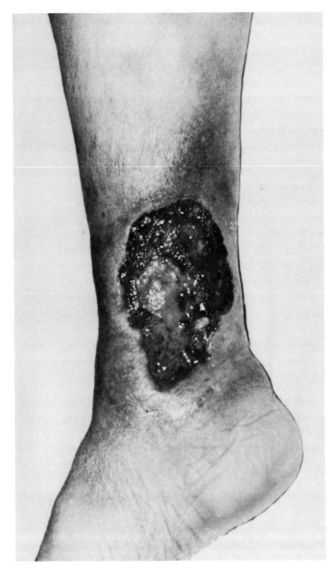

FIGURE 23-3. Typical venous ulcer.

useful, although more to disprove the diagnosis of DVT than to prove it. The "gold standard" investigation is venography, which should be universally available.

2. Demonstrating an underlying cause. A complete blood count, erythrocyte sedimentation rate, chest x-ray, liver diagnostic tests, urinalysis, renal function tests, serum proteins and immunoglobulin levels, tests for lupus erythematosus, and rheumatoid and other collagenoses, may be required.

Management of Venous Disease

Acute Deep Venous Thrombosis

The main-stay of treatment is heparin given by continuous intravenous infusion in a dose of 40,000 units in 24 h, after a loading dose of 5000 units. This will prevent the spread of the thrombus and embolization until the clot becomes adherent and stabilizes. In the absence of bleeding complications, therapy is maintained for 5 days, the last 3 of which overlap with the commencement of oral anticoagulation therapy (coumarin type), which is maintained for 3 months.

Acute Thrombophlebitis

This usually is a self-limited condition that can be treated by local warm compresses and an anti-inflammatory drug (such as ibuprofen). If the process involves the saphenous vein in the thigh, it may be necessary to ligate it at the groin to prevent the thrombosis from spreading into the femoral vein.

Chronic Vein Insufficiency

The venous hypertension that follows extensive valvular obstruction after DVT includes various stigmata in the gaiter area of the leg, the most disabling of which is ulceration. There are many cases of leg ulceration, and it is important to exclude concomitant arterial disease, diabetes, and rheumatoid because these will render standard treatment ineffective. The linchpin of treatment of venous ulcers is effective graded dynamic elastic compression to oppose the harmful effects of venous hypertension. Many topical therapies have been used, including antibiotics, corticosteroids, and enzymes. These testify to the ineffectiveness of them all; they may be expensive and can produce sensitization reactions that are worse than the original condition.

Pain control with analgesic drugs during the healing phase is important; a decreasing need for analgesia is a good indication of progress toward healing.

Acknowledgment

We are grateful to Mr. S. S. Rose, F.R.C.S., for helpful comments.

References

1. Schraibman IG. *The Ischaemic Foot.* Johannesburg, South Africa: University of Witwatersrand; 1971. Thesis.
2. McCord JM, Fridovich I. The biology and pathology of oxygen radicals. *Ann Intern Med* 1978; 89:122–127.
3. Manson PN, Anthinelli RM, Michael J, Bulkley GB, Hoopes JE. The role of oxygen-free radicals in ischemic tissue injury in island skin flaps. *Ann Surg* 1982; 198:87–90.
4. DeBenetittis G, Panerai AA, Villamari MA. Effects of hypnotic analgesia and hypnotizability on experimental ischemic pain. *Int J Clin Exp Hypn* January 1989; 37(1):55–69.
5. Dormandy HA, Hoare E, Colley J, et al. Clinical, haemodynamic, rheological and biochemical findings in 126 patients with intermittent claudication. *Br Med J* 1973; 4:576–581.
6. Baker MH. In: Bergan JJ, Yao J, eds. *Gangrene and Severe Ischemia of the Lower Extremities.* New York: Grune & Stratton; 1978:306.
7. Kaada B. Promoted healing of chronic ulceration by transcutaneous nerve stimulation. *Vasa* 1983; 12:262–269.
8. Fiume D. Spinal cord stimulation in peripheral vascular pain. *Appl Neurophysiol* 1983; 46:290–292.
9. Plecha R, Bounberger RA, Hoffman M, MacPherson K. A new criterion for predicting response to lumbar sympathectomy in patients with severe arteriosclerotic occlusive disease. *Surgery* 1980; 88:357–359.
10. Yao J, Bergan JJ. Predictability of vascular reactivity relative to sympathetic ablation. *Arch Surg* 1973; 107:676–679.
11. Cousins MJ, Bridenbaugh PO. *Neural Blockade.* Philadelphia: Lippincott; 1980.
12. Boas RA. The sympathetic nervous system and pain relief. In: Swerdlow M, ed. *Relief of Intractable Pain.* 3rd ed. Amsterdam: Elsevier; 1983:215–239.
13. McCollum PT, Spence VA, Macrae B, Walker WF. Quantitative assessment of the effectiveness of chemical lumbar sympathectomy. *Brit J Anaesth* 1985; 57:1146–1149.
14. Rose SS, Swerdlow M. Pain due to peripheral vascular disease. In: Lipton S, ed. *Persistent Pain.* Vol. 2. London: Academic Press; 1980.
15. Hannington-Kiff JG. Antisympathetic drugs in limbs. In: Wall PD, Melzack R, eds. *Textbook of Pain.* Edinburgh: Churchill Livingstone; 1984:566–577.
16. Feldman SA, Yeung ML. Treatment of intermittent claudication by lumbar paravertebral block with phenol. *Anaesthesia* 1975; 30:174.
17. Meglio M, Cioni B, Rossi GF. Spinal cord stimulation in management of chronic pain. A 9-year experience. *J Neurosurg* April 1989; 70(4):519–524.
18. Flume D, Palombi M, Sciassa V, Tamorri M. Spinal cord stimulation (SCS) in peripheral ischemic pain. *PACE* April 1989; 12(4 pt 2):698–704.
19. Sampere CT, Guasch JA, Paladino CM, Sanchez Casalongue M, Elencwajg B. Spinal cord stimulation for severely ischemic limbs. *PACE* February 1989; 12(2):273–279.
20. Cook AW, Oygar A, Baggenstos P, Pachecho S, Kleriga E. Vascular disease of extremities. Electrical stimulation of spinal cord and posterior roots. *N Y State J Med* 1976; 76:366–368.
21. Dooley D, Kasprak M. Modification of blood flow to the extremities by electrical stimulation of the nervous system. *South Med J* 1976; 69:1309–1311.
22. Meglio M, Cioni B, Ballago A, A DeSantis M, Polap P, Serricchic Z. Pain control and improvement of peripheral blood flow following epidural spinal cord stimulation. *J Neurosurg* 1981; 54:821–823.
23. Augustinsson LE, Carlson CA, Fall M. Autonomic effects of electrostimulation. *Applied Neurophys* 1982; 45:185–189.
24. Mashiah A, Patel P, Schraibman IG, Charlesworth D. Drug therapy in intermittent claudication and objective assessment of the effect of three drugs on patients with intermittent claudication. *Br J Surg* 1978; 65:342–345.
25. Gillespie JA. The case against vasodilator drugs in occlusive vascular disease of the legs. *Lancet* 1959; 2:955.
26. Janssen PAJ. The pharmacology of specific, pure and potent serotonin 5-HT$_2$ or S$_2$-antagonist. In: Yoshida H, Hagihara Y, Ebashi S, eds. *Advances of Pharmacology and Therapeutics II.* Vol. 4. New York: Pergamon Press; 1982:21–33.
27. DeCree J, Leempoels J, Geukens H, Verhaegen H. Placebo controlled double blind trial of ketanserin in treatment of intermittent claudication. *Lancet* 1984; 2:775–778.
28. Fonesca V, Ramage AG, Mikhailidis DP, Barradas MA,

Jeremy JY, Dandona P. Ketanserin in intermittent claudication. *Lancet* 1984; 2:1212–1213.

29. Bounameaux H, Holditch T, Helleman H, Berent A, Verhaeghe R. Placebo controlled double blind 2-centre trial of ketanserin in intermittent claudication. *Lancet* 1985; 2:1268–1271.

30. DeSmit P, Vroonhaven TH, VanNock H. Long term treatment with oral anticoagulants in patients with peripheral atherosclerosis. *International Vascular Symposium*. London: Macmillan; 1981. Abstract 267.

31. Boobis H, Bell P, Barrie J. In: Bell P, Tilney R, eds. *Vascular Surgery*. London: Butterworths; 1984:39.

32. Von Euler US. Uber der spezifishe blutdrucks enkende substanz des menshilichen Prostata-und samen blasensckretes *Klin Wochenschr* 1935; 14:1182.

33. Carlson LA, Erickson I. Femoral artery infusion of prostaglandin E, in severe peripheral vascular disease. *Lancet* 1973; 1:155–156.

34. Carlson LA, Erickson I. Intravenous prostaglandin E, in severe peripheral vascular disease. *Lancet* 1976; 2:810.

35. Belch JJF, McKay A, McArdle B, et al. Epoprostenol (prostacycline) in severe arterial disease. *Lancet* 1983; 1:315–317.

36. Telles GS, Campbell WB, Wood RF, et al. Prostaglandin E in severe lower limb ischemia; a double blind controlled trial. *Br J Surg* 1984; 71:506–508.

37. Rhodes RS, Heard N. Detrimental effect of high dose prostaglandin E in the treatment of ischemic ulcers. *Surgery* 1983; 93:839–845.

38. Hirai M, Nakayama R. Haemodynamic effects of arterial and intravenous administration of prostacycline in patients with peripheral arterial disease. *Br J Surg* 1986; 73: 20–23.

39. Raynaud M. *De l'asphyxie locale et de la gangrene symmetrique des extremes*. Paris: Righoux; 1862.

40. Allen EV, Brown GE. Raynaud's disease—a critical review of the minimal requirements for diagnosis. *Ann J Med Sci* 1932; 183–187.

41. Porter JM, Rivers SP. Management of Raynaud's syndrome. In: Bergan JJ, Yao J, eds. *Evaluation and Treatment of Upper and Lower Extremity Circulatory Disorders*. Orlando: Grune & Stratton; 1984:182.

42. Peacock JH. The treatment of primary Raynaud's disease of the upper limbs. *Lancet* 1960; 2:65.

43. McFadyen IJ, Housley E, McPherson AIS. Intraarterial reserpine administration in Raynaud's syndrome. *Arch Intern Med* 1973; 132:526–528.

44. Malone RS, Cameron AEP, Rennie JA. Endoscopic thoracic sympathectomy in the treatment of upper limb hyperhidrosis. *Ann R Coll Surg Engl* 1986; 68:93–94.

45. Milgis EFS. Sympathectomy in the hand. In: Bergan JJ, Yao J, eds. *Evaluation and Treatment of Upper and Lower Extremity Circulatory Disorders*. Orlando: Grune & Stratton; 1984.

46. Swerdlow M. Peripheral nerve blocking in the relief of pain. In: Lipton S, ed. *Persistent Pain*. London: Academic Press; 1977.

47. Sheehan TM, Coray PC. Neurolytic lumbar sympathetic block in the treatment of Raynaud's phenomenon. *Anaesthesiology* 1986; 64:119–120.

48. Stranden R, Roald OK, Krohg K. Treatment of Raynaud's phenomenon with the 5-HT$_2$-receptor antagonist ketanserin. *BMJ* 1982; 285:1069–1071.

49. Groth KE. Spinal cord stimulation for the treatment of peripheral vascular disease. In: *Advances in Pain Research and Therapy* Vol. 9. New York: Raven Press; 1985.

50. Kaada B. Mekanismen for akupunkturanalgesia. En oversikt. *Tidsskr Nor Laegeforen* 1982; 102:349.

51. Owen RT. Raynaud's phenomenon current approaches to treatment. *Drugs Today* 1983; 19:403–411.

52. Buerger L. Thrombo-angiitis obliterans. A study of the vascular lesions leading to presenile gangrene. *Ann J Med Sci* 1909; 136:562.

53. Mishima Y. Current status of femoropopliteal occlusion in Japan. *J Cardiovasc Surg Suppl* 1970; 11(3):97.

54. Mishima J, Ishikawa K. Buerger's disease. Current status in Japan. *J Mal Vasc* 1977; 2:121.

55. Saguelle S, Kushaba A, Mishima Y. A multi-clinical double-blind study with PGE, in patients with ischaemic ulcer of the extremities. *VASA* 1978; 7:263.

56. Bastcott HHG. Buerger's disease. In: Bergan JJ, Yao J, eds. *Evaluation and Treatment of Upper and Lower Extremity Circulatory Disorders*. Orlando: Grune & Stratton; 1984: 495.

CHAPTER 24

Central Pain Syndromes

R. R. Tasker

The term *central pain* is used variously to describe pain of psychogenic origin, that caused by stroke or other insults to the brain, that induced by traumatic or other lesions of the spinal cord, and that resulting from damage to the peripheral nervous system, because the latter is thought to be caused by central neuronal changes resulting from deafferentation. Some simple definitions may dispel confusion.

TYPES OF PAIN SYNDROMES

Pain of nonpsychogenic origin often is divided into so-called nociceptive pain (that is, resulting from continual stimulation of nociceptors and continual transmission in nociceptive pathways) and the pain from injury to the nervous system (which we originally termed *dysesthetic pain*).[1] The latter usually is called deafferentation pain if it results from damage to the peripheral nervous system and central pain if it follows damage to the central nervous system.

Current knowledge of the pathophysiology of pain is weighted heavily toward an understanding of nociceptive pain and of pain as a somatosensory input rather than as the suffering the patient experiences. Little is known about the other processes. However, despite our limited knowledge, it may be instructive to speculate that the normal state, absence of pain, is a homeostasis with pain inputs countered by modulatory activities induced either by the pain input itself or by concomitant events, such as distraction, emotion, or other neural inputs. Pain occurs when homeostasis fails, either through excessive input or modulatory failure. Whether the experience of pain ever results from modulatory failure alone is uncertain. It has been postulated that central pain may result from loss of modulation induced by nociceptive input after interruption of the spinothalamic tract.[2] Its potential role in psychogenic pain, as discussed by Sicuteri,[3] is provocative.

Nociceptive Pain

Excessive input is the usual cause of pain. This may be peripheral or central. The excessive firing of nociceptors signaling actual or threatened damage to tissue caused by, for example, a fracture, abscess, long bone metastasis, or herniated intervertebral disk, constitutes a peripheral pain input. This induces the continual transmission in nociceptive pathways, particularly the spinothalamic tract (which projects medially to central lateral-parafascicular nuclei of the thalamus and laterally to ventrobasal complex of the thalamus), that we call nociceptive pain. This signal can be reduced either by interrupting the nociceptive input or transmission or by suppressing it through spontaneous or iatrogenic modulation of the opiate pathways. However, central features (such as fear or the distraction of the battlefield, for example) also play a role in the suffering the patient actually experiences. Nociceptive interruption can be produced by topical anesthesia; interruption of transmission by temporary blockade or section of the peripheral nerves, roots, or spinothalamic tract; stereotactic spinothalamic, especially mesencephalic, tractotomy; medial thalamotomy; or selective thalamotomy of the ventrobasal complex. Available modulatory techniques include acupuncture, low frequency TENS, treatment with opiates (including instillation into the third ventricle, spinal, epidural, and intrathecal spaces), or chronic stimulation of periventricular–periaqueductal gray areas to activate one of the brain's own antinociceptive pathways. Most of the chapters in this book concern themselves with nociceptive pain.

Psychogenic Pain

Pain input also can be central, as in psychogenic pain. It can be affected by many unknown internal modulatory mechanisms and by those applied externally in the form of psychotherapy and medication. However, it is important to realize that whatever or wherever the pain input is and how it is modulated, the net suffering the patient feels uses the same final common pathway as for nociceptive pain. We can hypothesize only about the site of origin of the psychogenic pain. In rare instances of pure hallucinatory or hysteric pain, it is presumably at the cortical level (that is, the result of abnormal activities in higher nervous centers that gain access to the final common pathway for the conscious appreciation of pain). It also may be the result of inhibition of normal pain modulatory activity by such central events. Similar considerations presumably apply in muscle tension pain and psychogenic magnification of pain. This chapter will not address these issues further.

Deafferentation and Central Pain

It is known that injury to the peripheral nervous system induces a so-called cascade of anatomic, physiologic, and neurochemical changes central to the lesion.[4] Some of the more peripheral of such changes could result in spontaneous transmission over nociceptive pathways. For example, they could generate ectopic impulses arising at an injury site. Thus, certain components of a deafferentation pain syndrome could have a peripheral input that might be controlled by interruption of nociceptive transmission. However, the changes caused by deafferentation that induce pain also could be central; although the pathophysiology is uncertain, such changes might not involve nociceptive pathways. Related modulatory activity is even less well understood. Similar, but probably not identical, processes are thought to be operational in central pain caused by lesions of the brain or spinal cord. In other words, both central and peripheral damage to the nervous system can cause pain, either by virtue of ectopic impulses generated at the injury site or by some deafferentation-induced central abnormality of neuronal activities.

Deafferentation and central pain both could result from an excessive central or peripheral pain input. Therefore, its management must include, not only suppression of abnormal input, but also elimination of the abnormal deafferentation-induced central neuronal activity. Possible strategies include drugs, eliminating the abnormal input or abnormal cells themselves (using destructive lesions), or suppression of abnormal cell activity (using modulatory techniques, such as chronic electrical stimulation). Attempts to manage the pain by interrupting nociceptive transmission alone may be disastrous.

Pain caused by an injury to the nervous system is one of the most common problems confronting the pain therapist. Familiar examples include painful neuropathy; minor and major causalgia; postherpetic neuralgia; postcordotomy dysesthesia; the pain that follows brachial plexus avulsion or spinal cord injury; anesthesia dolorosa; phantom pain; some of the pain syndromes associated with chronic lumbar disk disease; the pain of syringomyelia and syringobulbia; that associated with certain neoplasms of nerve, cord, or brain; and the pain associated with stroke, especially supratentorial, but also lateral medullary syndrome. The pathology is protean (e.g., trauma, musculoskeletal abnormalities, inflammation, neoplasia, vascular abnormalities, iatrogenic processes, degenerative lesions) producing either complete or incomplete neural transsection.

Although the pain syndromes caused by this wide diversity of processes have a remarkable clinical homogeneity, suggesting a common pathophysiology in general, there must be underlying individual features in the mechanisms of the different syndromes. However, it is useful to consider all these pain syndromes together in our attempt to discern the main picture, because our knowledge of the underlying process is so poor.

CLINICAL FEATURES OF DEAFFERENTATION AND CENTRAL PAIN IN GENERAL

Let us examine the clinical features that distinguish the pain resulting from nervous system injury. Neurosurgeons have recognized for many years that operations, such as cordotomy, that are designed to control pain, were more successful in patients with cancer than in others. Therefore, the terms benign and malignant pain syndromes were coined, as if chronic pain could ever be benign. Failure was attributed to plasticity in the nervous system that eventually bypassed the surgical interruption or some peculiar feature of the so-called benign pain itself. Currently, it is believed that it is not the benign or cancerous origin of the pain that matters but rather the fact that benign pain usually is the result of nervous damage with a pathophysiology not amenable to treatments used for the usually nociceptive cancer pain.[1,5–7] It is still not realized that damage to the nervous system is not the only cause of what was formerly called "benign pain" and that not all pain syndromes caused by cancer are nociceptive. Cordotomy can be effective in nociceptive pain caused by benign skeletal lesions. Although cancer usually initially causes nociceptive pain by compressing (through an unknown mechanism) the brachial or lumbosacral plexuses, later it adds neural destruction and often deafferentation pain, with all the characteristics of such pain, regardless of whether it is caused by noncancerous or cancerous lesions.

Three features in addition to refractoriness to conventional pain surgery attracted our attention to these types of pain.[1,6,7] We had been taught to use the intravenous sodium thiopental test to identify psychogenic features in patients with chronic pain by the late J. Allan Walters.[8] We were surprised to find patients with undoubted nonpsychogenic pain who were relieved temporarily by this drug. Similarly, we had been taught to believe that infusions of opiates temporarily should relieve pain if it were of organic origin; however, we found many patients who did not seem to have psychogenic pain in whom it did not. Finally, we also believed that local anesthetic blockade could be used as a prognostic test for surgical interruption in the treatment of chronic pain. We found it unreliable. Surgical section of a nerve at a site of effective local blockade often did not relieve pain long term. We noticed that, in all these instances, we were treating patients whose pain appeared to be related to damage to the nervous system.

We therefore reviewed 168 consecutive patients who appeared to have pain resulting from lesions in either the peripheral or central nervous system (Table 24-1).[6,7] It will be noticed that cancerous destruction constituted 10 percent of the series. This list suggested another peculiarity of nerve injury pain. Not all patients with a given lesion had deafferentation or central pain. Herpes zoster did not cause postherpetic neuralgia in all cases. Only 5 percent of patients undergoing cordotomy had postcordotomy dysesthesia.[9] Ten percent of patients with spinal cord injury

Table 24-1
Neural Lesions Causing Pain in 168 Patients

Lesion	Percent of Patients
Postthoracotomy syndrome	5.4
Other peripheral nerve injuries	4.8
Other incisional pain	4.8
Phantom and stump pain	5.4
Trigeminal nerve lesions, including anesthesia dolorosa	1.8
Postdental surgery	0.6
Radiation necrosis peripheral nerves or plexuses	3.0
Cancerous destruction plexuses	10.2
Postherpetic neuralgia	10.8
Brachial plexus avulsion	2.4
Neurologic problems related to disk disease	9.0
Lesions of spinal cord	16.6
Lesions of brain	16.8
Posttraumatic syndrome	8.4

had pain,[10] and 1 in 15,000 patients with strokes did.[11] Laboratory studies suggest that there may be a genetic predisposition to develop pain after neural injury.[12,13]

Our study of 168 patients revealed other peculiar features.[6,7] Pain onset was delayed, often for years, in 61 percent of those in whom the cause could be dated, suggesting the underlying process took time to develop. The pain was described as causalgic or burning in 51 percent, dysesthetic in 43 percent, also sometimes in bizarre or emotional terms, but rarely with adjectives usually used to describe musculoskeletal pain for example. There was no predilection for any part of the body; the representation of body parts in pain syndromes seemed to be proportional to their size. The location of the pain appeared to be related to somatosensory loss, either partial or complete, multimodal or dissociated, in 79 percent of patients and to amputation in 2 percent. In 9 percent, sensory loss was absent at the time the patient sought treatment and was deemed to be subclinical. It either had been documented earlier with subsequent recovery or else other neurologic signs suggested a potential for sensory damage related to the pain that presumably was not detectable clinically. Sometimes blunt trauma or an incision was present in the area in keeping with Livingston's[5] suggestion that damage to small cutaneous nerves insufficient to produce clinical sensory loss could still cause deafferentation pain. In only 5 percent of patients, hyperesthesia was found in an area of potential sensory damage; in 5 percent, data were incomplete. In one patient only, consistent alteration of somatosensory-evoked potentials was found. In 14 percent, evoked pain (that is, hyperesthesia, hyperpathia, or allodynia) was present; rarely was this the only sign of somatosensory damage. An occasional patient had an accompanying sympathetic dystrophy. Subsequent more detailed studies of 335 patients with central and deafferentation pain syndromes[14] revealed a second recurring feature of the pain overlooked in earlier

studies (that is, a lancinating, intermittent, neuralgic element seen in 35 percent of deafferentation syndromes and 25 percent of central syndromes). The incidence of hyperpathia and allodynia was 51 percent and 49 percent, respectively.

Diagnostic Techniques

We investigated various diagnostic measures in patients with central and deafferentation pain. Sodium thiopental was given in 50-mg boluses intravenously to 38 patients in doses of 75 to 300 mg; it abolished pain in 53 percent of these cases and significantly reduced it in 13 percent. Up to 20 mg of morphine sulfate or 300 μg of fentanyl was given in boluses of 5 mg and 50 μg, respectively, to 30 patients; this regimen abolished pain in 13 percent of patients, reduced it in 33 percent, and had no effect in 54 percent. Naloxone 0.4 to 0.8 mg intravenously never reversed any narcotic-induced effect in these patients. Local anesthetic blockade was done proximal to a known neural lesion in 37 patients (nerve, root, or caudal or spinal block); it abolished pain in 65 percent of patients and reduced it in 24 percent.

Effects of Destructive Procedures

We observed that 14 percent to 51 percent of patients had evoked pain, occasionally in the absence of spontaneous pain. By this we meant discomfort induced by somatosensory stimulation, obviously in an area with at least partial preservation of somatosensory function. Although typically occurring with increased threshold for one or more somatosensory modalities and evoked by one or more types of stimulation, evoked pain also can occur in an area of clinically normal but presumed subclinically affected somatosensory function. The confusing term *hyperesthesia* is used to describe the latter phenomenon; this must be distinguished from the hyperesthesia surrounding, for example, an area of inflammation or the hyperesthesia of psychogenic origin. In areas of raised somatosensory threshold, the term *allodynia* is applied to the situation where a nonnoxious stimulus induces a painful effect and the term *hyperpathia* when a painful stimulus is perceived as unnaturally unpleasant, often associated with such features as temporal or spatial spread and autonomic or emotional effects. These evoked pain effects depend on somatosensory receptors and transmission and are the result of abnormal central nervous processing.[15] In contradistinction to spontaneous pain, such effects can be eliminated readily by interrupting the appropriate somatosensory input and/or transmission, using such techniques as by percutaneous neurectomy, rhizotomy,[16] cordotomy, and probably, opiates and chronic stimulation of the periventricular gray areas.[17] However, the more common spontaneous pain seldom is relieved, and often, it is aggravated by such procedures. Such destructive techniques are feasible for the relief of evoked pain only when the accompanying somatosensory function is expendable. Inadvertent damage to motor fibers can be avoided in neurectomy or rhizotomy by careful electrode positioning at sites where stimulation at appropriate thresholds induces only paresthesiae or by using other appropriate physiologic localizing techniques.

In a small number of our patients, changes usually described as sympathetic dystrophy (bluish, cold, shiny, swollen skin; loss of hair; aberrations of sweating; and osteoporosis) may accompany deafferentation pain. In our experience, sympathetic interruption is useful in treating the dystrophy but usually not the pain, even though local anesthetic sympathetic blockade may cause temporary relief.[14] Sympathetic interruption can be done conveniently by percutaneous injection of neurolytic agents[18] or by using the radiofrequency technique.[19] Notable exceptions are the rare cases of so-called major causalgia,[14,20] usually associated with partial transsection of the sciatic nerve, where sympathectomy has eliminated both pain and associated abnormalities. The author is not aware of critical differences between such causalgias and the majority that are not helped by sympathectomy.

The far greater problem in patients with deafferentation and central pain is the spontaneous pain in which the results of permanent deafferenting surgery usually are disappointing. In 35 cases of deafferentation pain involving the chest wall, mostly postthoracotomy syndrome with some cases of postherpetic neuralgia, although local intercostal blockade relieved pain temporarily and completely, percutaneous radiofrequency section of intercostal nerves at the same site provided relief in only 25 percent of patients. In a review of 244 cases of percutaneous cordotomy, significant relief of the pain for which the cordotomy was done was achieved at postdischarge follow-up in 82.3 percent of patients deemed to have nociceptive pain,[9] but only 50.0 percent of patients with deafferentation or central pain reported any relief at all. This figure might be artificially high, depending on the manner in which certain pain syndromes associated with spinal cord injury are classified. In another series of 136 percutaneous cordotomies,[21] we paid particular attention to pain occurring in an area rendered analgesic after the procedure. Such pain was found in 39.8 percent of the 136 patients. In 6.1 percent, it consisted of persistence of the preoperative pain, thought to be of a deafferentation type. In the rest, the preoperative pain was reduced greatly, but some pain persisted in an area of preoperatively recognized sensory loss in 17.3 percent of patients. In 8.2 percent, it persisted in an area with preoperative motor or reflex evidence of neural damage but without clinically detectable sensory loss. In 7.1 percent, it was associated with an area of neural change caused by progression of the cancer developing postoperatively. In 1.1 percent, it appeared to be a result of postcordotomy dysesthesia. Eight of our patients, all with complete or nearly complete thoracic cord transsection, underwent retranssection of the spinal cord at a higher level in an unsuccessful attempt to eliminate diffuse burning pain below their level.[22]

Various reviews of stereotactic mesencephalic, medial, and spinothalamic tractotomy, and medial and ventral caudal thalamotomy, suggest that 25 percent to 50 percent of patients with deafferentation or central pain derive significant relief from these procedures.[1,7,23–26] compared with approximately 70 percent relief in patients with nociceptive pain syndromes. We identified, then, a group of patients with pain caused by neural damage with unusual features (Table 24-2).

However, destructive procedures were not always unsuccessful in the treatment of spontaneous pain. In an effort to gain insight into this observation, we examined the results of different kinds of surgery in our series of patients with central pain caused by lesions of the spinal cord.[27] In particular, we studied the effects on the major components of pain in these patients (that is evoked, spontaneous, steady, usually burning, or spontaneous, intermittent, and lancinating). To our surprise, there appeared to be statistically significantly different roles for modulatory (chronic stimulation of dorsal cord or lemniscal pathway in the brain) and destructive (rhizotomy, cordotomy, dorsal route entry zone, and cordectomy) procedures. Chronic stimulation was effective in 36 percent of patients for spontaneous steady pain, none for spontaneous lancinating pain, and 16 percent for evoked pain. Destructive procedures were effective in 25 percent for spontaneous steady pain, 83 percent for spontaneous lancinating, and 82 percent for evoked pain. Perhaps the smaller but ever-present incidence of reported success in patients with deafferentation and central pain undergoing destructive surgery can be explained by the finding that, in these patients, evoked or spontaneous lancinating pain is the major symptom. A review of the literature suggests that this dichotomy of response has been recognized for decades.[28]

Pathophysiology of Deafferentation and Central Pain

How can such strange properties be explained? Livingston[5] suggested that neural injury caused a central so-called vi-

Table 24-2
Clinical Features of Deafferentation and Central Pain

Caused by central or peripheral neural lesions
Etiology of lesion unimportant
Individual idiosyncrasy for pain
Often, onset delayed
Usually causalgic or dysesthetic
May be accompanied by evoked pain, sympathetic dystrophy, psychic–emotional factors
Usually related to somatosensory loss—partial, complete, multimodal, dissociated spinothalamic, clinical, or subclinical
Usually relieved by thiopental sodium
Not relieved by opiates
Usually not relieved by proximal nociceptive interruption (although evoked pain is)
Usually not relieved by sympathectomy (although sympathetic dystrophy is)

cious cycle that, once established, persisted even after isolation of the cause from the central nervous system. A growing amount of laboratory work documents the neural changes deafferentation causes,[29] although it is difficult to correlate these with the induction of pain in humans. A critical review of this information is beyond the scope of this chapter, but part of it has been reviewed recently by Coderre and colleagues.[30] At the cellular level, loss of synapses, growth of new ones, utilization of previously inactive synapses, sprouting, altered neurohumoral balance, ephaptic connections, reorganized somatotopic maps, disinhibition, and denervation neuronal hypersensitivity all have been postulated or demonstrated.[4,31,32] Such cellular changes could explain the many postulated mechanisms of deafferentation and central pain (e.g., abnormal utilization of hypothalamic, sympathetic, somatosensory, and reticulothalamic pathways, and particularly denervation neuronal hypersensitivity in the somatosensory or reticulothalamic pathways).[1,6,7,22,33–36]

In humans, scattered observations agree with such concepts. Bursting cells, thought to be markers for denervation neuronal hypersensitivity, have been found in the human dorsal horn[37] and human ventrobasal complex[38] in patients with nerve injury-type pain. The observations of Lombard and colleagues[39] in rats that underwent five consecutive brachial dorsal root lesions are interesting. After 195 days, they found thalamic neurons located in central lateral, ventrocaudal, and other thalamic sites that fired repetitively in a manner interpreted as denervation neuronal hypersensitivity and similar to that we recorded[31] in the ventrocaudal and ventral intermediate nucleus in patients with deafferentation and central pain. Such rat neurons seldom had receptive fields, and only one of hundreds of our human thalamic cells did so. We have not had the opportunity to explore human medial thalamic cells, but we have reached the following conclusions concerning lateral thalamic cells.[40] First, bursting cells are common in the lateral thalamus after damage to the peripheral or central nervous system, regardless of whether the patient also feels pain. Second, in deafferented patients who do have pain, the bursting cells tend to lie in the somatosensory relay nucleus and to have receptive fields. Third, the bursting discharges of an individual cell occur in a regular sequence in bursts that are themselves regularly sequenced. Fourth, bursting cells in patients without pain fire more irregularly.

A second observation made possible using microelectrode studies in these patients[41] is that the lemniscal relay nucleus often shows somatotopographic reorganization. However, this phenomenon appears to correlate better with deafferentation than it does with pain. The appearance of unusual receptive fields in neurons of the somatosensory relay nucleus at the margins of areas containing neurons that have been deafferented[42] may correlate better with pain.

Micro- or macrostimulation of the human brain gives curious results in patients with central or deafferentation pain.[1,6,7,34,35,41,43] The pain rarely is elicited by stimulation

of the brain. However, in a substantial number of reports describing operations for the relief of intractable pain, surgeons have induced pain similar to that felt by the patient by electrical stimulation of various structures somatotopically related to the painful body part. It was sometimes noticed that induction of pain was replaced by that of paresthesias as soon as the electrode entered structures somatotopically related to nonpainful body parts. A review of the protocols suggested that this phenomenon of inducing the patient's pain by stimulation occurred in patients with deafferentation and central pain and that it was seen in the ventrobasal complex, thalamic radiations, spinothalamic relay in thalamus, somatosensory cortex, and intralaminar nuclei. In our experience with stereotactic operations on patients with deafferentation or central pain, we observed the same phenomenon in the upper mesencephalon medial to the spinothalamic tract, medial thalamus, spinothalamic tract, and sometimes in the ventrobasal complex. This pain production appeared to be an exclusive feature of deafferentation or central pain; exploration of the same sites in an identical fashion in patients with nociceptive pain caused by cancer never induced this effect. The phenomenon, however, appeared to occur mainly in patients who had allodynia or hyperpathia.

In addition to the phenomenon of pain production, the medial mesencephalon and thalamus (normally insensitive to electrical stimulation at thresholds effective in the somatosensory pathways) were observed to be abnormally excitable in patients with central or deafferentation pain. Their stimulation produced a sensation of burning that was not somatotopically referred to various contralateral body sites, an effect that was not confined to patients with evoked pain.

These physiologic observations combined with clinical ones suggest the following hypothesis to explain the features of central and deafferentation pain. Evoked pain (allodynia and hyperpathia) depends on activities of receptors and their afferent pathways with abnormal central processing of that input.[44,45] The induction of pain by brainstem stimulation highlights the spinoreticulothalamic input in this process. Evoked pain therefore can be controlled by interrupting the input (neurectomy, rhizotomy, cordotomy, stereotactic mesencephalic tractotomy, or thalamotomy) or by administering opiates.

Lancinating spontaneous pain depends on ectopic impulses that originate at neural injury sites and may be transmitted centrally over spinoreticulothalamic pathways. It can be controlled by the same strategies as evoked pain.

Steady spontaneous pain is the result of central aberrations resulting from deafferentation. It may be related to certain types of bursting cells or some kinds of somatotopic reorganization as discussed previously. In addition, it may be associated with stimulation-induced burning in the spinoreticulothalamic pathways and the appearance of bursting cells in the somatosensory relay nucleus. We have not studied neurons in the medial thalamus. Such central aberrations are not likely to be amenable to treatment with destructive surgery unless the entire body of abnormally functioning cells could be eliminated. They do not seem to respond to treatment with opiates, but they may respond in approximately 50 percent of patients to chronic stimulation of peripheral nerves, dorsal spinal cord, or somatosensory pathways in the brain that induce paresthesias in the part(s) of the patient's body affected by pain. Modesti and Waszak[46] and Tsubokawa and Moriyasu[47] presented evidence suggesting that dorsal cord stimulation and ventrocaudal nucleus stimulation, respectively, suppress medial thalamic firing in humans. Whatever processes involving the reticulothalamic system may be identified with central and deafferentation pain, they also must be endowed with somatotopic organization and a channel to consciousness; otherwise deafferentation or central pain would not be felt and could not be localized. Albe-Fessard and associates[48] suggest that the latter is accomplished by a pathway through the medial thalamus to the premotor cortex, but perhaps, the joint involvement of the spinothalamic tract, ventrocaudal nucleus, and somatosensory cortex in the abnormal process may explain the conscious localization of the pain.

PAIN RESULTING FROM PERIPHERAL NEURAL LESIONS

Clinical Picture

Table 24-3 documents types of deafferentation pain caused by lesions of the peripheral nervous system. Major causalgia is listed alone because of its striking clinical picture and the unusual property of relief after sympathectomy that is not shared by other deafferentation pain syndromes. Typically, at a variable interval after a peripheral nerve lesion, the patient may have the illusion that sensation is returning to the numb area. A mild prickling occurs that slowly progresses to stabilize as a steady burning in the denervated area, sometimes with formications or accompanying evoked pain. The affected part may feel swollen or tight as if it were held in a vise; the whole symptom complex usually is aggravated by activity and relieved by rest. The pain most often is constant with unexplained exacerbations.

Therapy

General and Medical

Before administering therapy aimed at the intractable pain itself, we first must be satisfied that all possible specific therapy has been given (e.g., control of diabetes, elimination where possible of compressive elements, optimal repair of injured neural tissue, and attention to skeletal problems). Unfortunately, as Livingston[5] stated, after the process of deafferentation pain has begun, it tends to persist despite removal of the cause.

Having satisfied these requirements, our attention then must be given to every detail of the patient's situation. Although it is the suffering that is being treated, it inevitably is aggravated by coexisting psychic and social prob-

Table 24-3
Pain Caused by Peripheral Neural Lesions

Lesions of peripheral nerves
  Peripheral neuritis, especially diabetic
  Traumatic   Laceration
              Associated with fractures
              Compressive
  Entrapment
  Iatrogenic   Incisional, especially postthoracotomy
              Associated with fractures
              Compressive, especially casts or positioning
              Injections
              Drug-induced neuropathy
              Deliberate section for pain relief, especially trigeminal
  Associated with amputation
              Stump pain
              Phantom pain
  Incisional pain, with or without identifiable nerve injury
  Posttraumatic pain, after blunt trauma, with or without identifiable nerve injury
  Major causalgia

Lesions of plexuses
  Cancerous, especially Pancoast syndrome
  Avulsion of brachial plexus
  Other traumatic
  Thoracic outlet syndrome
  Iatrogenic   Incisional
              Compressive
              Stretch injury
              Radiation necrosis

Lesions of dorsal roots
  Brachial plexus avulsion
  Degenerative disc disease, especially lumbar
  Associated with spinal trauma
  Postherpetic neuralgia
  Iatrogenic   Disc surgery
              Other laminectomy
              After removal of neoplasm
              After deliberate section for pain
              Incisional

lems. Treating accompanying disease, addressing concurrent neural disabilities, assisting with social problems, and helping with the inevitable psychic symptoms are essential.

For established pain, the usual anti-inflammatory and analgesic medications are of little value because the pain generally does not depend on nociceptive processes, although there may be accompanying conditions (such as degenerative disk disease) or evoked or spontaneous lancinating pain that may respond to analgesics. For the treatment of the central or deafferentation pain itself, three other classes of medications may be useful: minor tranquilizers (which generally reduce tension), antidepressants (such as amitriptyline), and antiepileptics (such as carbamazepine in tic douloureux doses, phenytoin sodium in antiepileptic doses, and sodium valproate). Carbamazepine may be more useful in the treatment of spontaneous lancinating than in the other elements of the pain. Recently, other agents such as mexiletene[49] and vasoactive agents, such as clonidine, have been used.

A noninvasive measure frequently used, which probably acts by enhancing modulation of the pain, is TENS. This can also be accomplished by acupuncture, and to TENS,[50] which is more effective when administered at higher frequencies, particularly for the treatment of spontaneous steady pain. Although effective in our experience in only approximately 10 percent of cases, its failure may be largely technical because it is difficult to apply stimulation to a denervated area to produce paresthesias over an extensive area afflicted with pain. When TENS has been effective, dorsal cord stimulation usually is also.

Although Livingston[5] reported relief with repeated anesthetic blockade, this method of treatment has not been successful generally.

Surgical

Surgical treatment, like drug therapy, carries a high incidence of failure and should be used only when the following criteria have been met.

1. The physician is certain that the pain is the result of nerve injury.
2. Primary therapy has been completed.
3. Noninvasive therapy has been exhausted.
4. The disability is caused by the pain and not by the accompanying neurologic deficit.
5. The disability warrants the surgical therapy contemplated with its limitations and complications.
6. A psychogenic magnification syndrome is not the major problem.

The problems of evoked pain and sympathetic dystrophy have been mentioned.

We already explained that, at least in patients with central pain caused by cord lesions, the use of destructive procedures that probably interrupt spinothalamic input (such as neurectomy, rhizotomy, cordotomy, cordectomy, dorsal root entry zone, mesencephalic tractotomy, and thalamotomy), or modulatory procedures (such as opiate instillation or periventricular gray area stimulation) that accomplish the same thing may be effective in controlling hyperpathia, allodynia, and intermittent lancinating pain. The more common spontaneous steady, often burning, pain responds better to chronic stimulation inducing paresthesias in the area of pain. Future studies will have to determine whether the same strategies apply to patients with central pain resulting from brain lesions and to those with deafferentation pain. We believe they do.

Dorsal Root Entry Zone Lesions. Originally introduced by Hyndman[51] to raise the level of analgesia after cordotomy, cuts in the dorsal root entry zone of the cord were employed by Sindou and colleagues[52] to treat nociceptive pain. Nashold and Ostdahl and others[53–55] then advocated the use of tiny carefully controlled radiofrequency lesions in the dorsal root entry zone region to treat deafferentation pain, presumably on the basis that it destroyed abnormally firing neurons. This was particularly successful for the pain that occurred after brachial and lumbosacral plexus avulsion with a 67 percent to 78 percent incidence of reported relief.[53,54,56,57] The main disadvantages of this procedure are that it requires an extensive laminectomy, is time consuming, induces dysesthetic phenomena in the adjacent dermatomes, and carries a significant incidence of leg ataxia or weakness. It remains to be documented whether its success is related to the presence of intermittent lancinating or evoked pain as the chief disability in cases other than cord central pain in which it is effective.

Trigeminal Nucleotomy–Tractotomy. Hitchcock,[58] Crue and coworkers,[59] and Schvarcz[60] reported that percutaneous radiofrequency lesions directed at the caudal nucleus and/or descending tract of the trigeminal nerve were effective in treating trigeminal deafferentation pain of various causes. Schvarcz[60] found that 87.5 percent of patients with postherpetic neuralgia and 57 percent of those with anesthesia dolorosa obtained relief. Presumably, the explanation for success is similar to that of dorsal root entry zone lesions.

Spinal Commissurotomy. It was surprising that Hitchcock[61] reported that spinal commissurotomy done using the percutaneous radiofrequency technique in the cervical region also was effective in controlling deafferentation pain in three patients. His observations[61] and those of Schvarcz[62] agreed with those of Cook and colleagues[63] that pain relief after commissurotomy, by whatever approach, bore no relation to any analgesia produced or to the dermatomal level of the intervention. All authors postulated that some unknown extracommissural structure is being lesioned during this operation.

Cordotomy. Cordotomy is mentioned because we do not recommend it as a means of treating the steady spontaneous element of deafferentation pain. It may be useful in carefully selected cases to treat disabling allodynia or lancinating pain.

Psychosurgery. Although various authors have reported amelioration of deafferentation pain after psychosurgical procedures, such as cingulumotomy,[64] this procedure has not been helpful in the author's limited experience.

Stereotactic Surgery. Of the many stereotactic destructive procedures advocated for the relief of intractable pain, in this author's opinion, only two are major considerations for the treatment of deafferentation pain: medial thalamotomy and medial mesencephalic tractotomy. Both procedures were advocated originally on the grounds that they interrupted nociceptive transmission in the nonsomatotopically organized medial portion of the reticulospinothalamic tract in the upper midbrain or, in the medial thalamus, in the central lateral–parafascicular area. The overall result of 25 percent to 50 percent amelioration of deafferentation pain by such procedures has been discussed. The rate of complications of medial thalamotomy is approximately 25 percent incidence of transient confusion or memory loss. For medial mesencephalotomy, the mortality rate averages 5 percent to 10 percent and the incidence of dysesthesia, 15 percent to 20 percent. Oculomotor palsies affect 15 percent to 20 percent of patients. These procedures may be useful for the management of evoked and spontaneous lancinating pain, but they are disappointing for steady pain.

Modulatory Methods

The two procedures most often used to treat the spontaneous steady element of deafferentation pain are chronic stimulation of the dorsal cord[65,66] and lateral thalamus. They have the advantage of being relatively simple low-risk procedures that should be tried first before more involved or destructive surgery wherever practical. For chronic stimulation to succeed, paresthesias must be delivered to the painful area, and both these induced sensations and the hardware must be acceptable to the patient. For unknown reasons, only one half of the candidates in whom chronic stimulation is considered actually derive relief of their pain. Therefore, it is important to do a trial of stimulation before making a commitment to the hospitalization, surgery, and expense of internalization with a permanent stimulating device. Ideally, an interval of stimulation should be followed by a prolonged suppression of pain; over time, we might expect the patient's pain to lessen. Neither seems to be common. Most patients have a return of pain soon after they turn their stimulator off. Many patients report that, after months to years, the technically adequate stimulation becomes progressively less effective. This is not a matter of tolerance because no strategies, including stimulation holidays lasting for months, recapture pain control in these situations; their function does not involve opiate pathways.

Peripheral Nerve Stimulation. Originally conceived by Wall and Sweet,[67] peripheral nerve stimulation theoretically should be the optimal technique for treating de-afferentation pain of peripheral nerve origin. However, it requires an open procedure and is used little, except for the trigeminal nerve. Chronic trigeminal stimulation by the introduction of an electrode into Meckel's cave, as described by Meyerson and Håkansson,[68] or by an electrode percutaneously introduced through the foramen ovale, as described by Steude,[69] has been a useful means of controlling some cases of trigeminal deafferentation pain as long as it is possible to induce paresthesias in the painful area of the face.

Dorsal Cord Stimulation. Originally introduced by Shealy and colleagues[70] with inter- or intradural insertion of a plate type electrode at laminectomy, dorsal cord stimulation currently should be done by percutaneous insertion of a stimulating electrode, as introduced by Dooley[71] and others, using the same electrode for test stimulation and eventual implantation. Most of the major complications of the procedure were the result of the open operation. Different types of equipment from programable totally implantable to semiimplanted radiofrequency-coupled devices are available. Complications of dorsal cord stimulation using percutaneously inserted leads are low (mainly a 4 percent incidence of infection), but technical problems are significant. Appropriate dorsal column fibers must survive to be stimulated to produce paresthesias in the area of pain. This may be a problem after massive denervation (such as caused by amputation). Furthermore, the appropriate epidural space must not have been obliterated by disease or previous surgery. Electrode migration affects one-quarter to one-third of patients; if the paresthesias abandon the painful area, treatment will fail. Discomfort associated with the implanted hardware is often a nuisance. Lead breakage and failure of receivers is unusual.

It is difficult to find published reports of the use of dorsal cord stimulation in specific deafferentation pain syndromes because the results usually are combined with miscellaneous pain problems. Our experience with chronic epidural stimulation for deafferentation pain is listed in Table 24-4. Although the numbers are small, several facts are noteworthy. First, test stimulation is essential; it is otherwise impossible to predict which patients will have

Table 24-4
Chronic Dorsal Cord Stimulation for Deafferentation Pain

Cause of Pain	No. of Patients	% Passing Test Stimulation	% Obtaining Long-Term Relief
Lesions of peripheral nerve distal to dorsal root	9	67	100
Postthoracotomy syndrome	10	50	40
Cancerous plexus lesion	7	29	0
Other plexus lesions	7	71	100
Amputation or stump pain	12	50	83
Postherpetic neuralgia	4	50	0

successful outcomes. Results in postherpetic, postthoracotomy, and cancer-induced pain syndromes unexplainably are disappointing.

Chronic Brain Stimulation. When the simple expedient of dorsal cord stimulation fails or is technically not feasible, the author next prefers chronic brain stimulation because of its low impact on the patient and low risk. Even when epidural cord stimulation adequately delivered to the painful area fails, brain stimulation still may succeed.[72] Although chronic stimulation of the brain for pain relief has been explored by many investigators for decades, it was Mazars[73] who popularized it as treatment; Adams, Hosobuchi, and their colleagues[74,75] and Turnbull[76] and others added much to our understanding of the technique. The problems and complications are similar to those seen with dorsal cord stimulation, notably a 4 percent infection rate plus up to a 10 percent incidence of neurological effects usually temporary.

The procedure involves the stereotactic introduction of an electrode into the portion of the ventrobasal complex subserving the area of pain. There is no convincing evidence that there are differential advantages from stimulating nucleus as opposed to medial lemniscus or thalamic radiations.[17]

Periventricular–periaqueductal gray stimulation,[77] which modulates nociceptive pathways, is not indicated to treat deafferentation or central pain, except for allodynia or perhaps lancinating pain. In the former, stimulation of the ventrobasal complex is often unpleasant.[17]

CENTRAL PAIN OF CORD ORIGIN

Clinical Features

Table 24-5 lists the lesions responsible for central pain of cord origin; trauma is by far the most common. It accounts for 65 percent of 72 consecutive cases I treated.[22] Iatrogenic causes were second in this series and responsible for 11 percent. The pain onset was delayed more than 1 month in

55 percent of patients and more than 1 year in 15 percent. Although, in general, the pain was similar to that described for deafferentation pain syndromes, there were certain peculiarities (Table 24-6) in our 72 patients. When intermittent pain was present, it tended to be lancinating and was always the most severe. It was seen most often after incomplete lesions, particularly of the conus–cauda. Steady pain alone was more characteristic of high and complete lesions. In regard to hyperpathia and allodynia, in two patients, unpleasant sensations were evoked below the level of injury even though sensation appeared clinically normal, but they were usually found in areas of incomplete sensory loss. A band at the upper level of injury was more common with high complete lesions. Discrete pain below this level, often resembling musculoskeletal or visceral pain and often precipitating extensive investigation, was more common after complete leisons. The pain most often was described as burning, but sensations of pounding, pulling, squeezing, and cutting recurred throughout the clinical records. It accompanied high, low, complete, or incomplete lesions and ones that produced loss of sensation affecting all types. In some instances, there was dissociated sensory loss. The pain tended to change rather significantly over the years, both in its quality and distribution.

Therapy

General and Medical

The introductory remarks under deafferentation pain apply equally well to this disorder. In particular, it is important to investigate concomitant problems of spinal cord injury: infection, nutrition, spasticity, genitourinary function, skin condition, and skeletal instability because these may contribute to the pain. Psychogenic magnification is common, and the central pain of cord injury frequently is accompanied by peripheral deafferentation pain originating from root damage and nociceptive, musculoskeletal, and radicular pain.

Table 24-5
Cause of Central Pain of Cord Origin

Trauma
Herniated disk
Vascular   Infarct
            Hematoma
Neoplasm, especially intramedullary
Syringohydromyelia
Multiple sclerosis
Transverse myelitis
Iatrogenic   Postlaminectomy
              Postthoracic–abdominal vascular surgery
              Postcordotomy dysesthesia
              Radiation necrosis
              Introduction of material into epidural or subarachnoid
                space

Table 24-6
Patterns of Pain Produced by Spinal Cord Lesions

Pain Type	%
Steady pain only	65
Intermittent plus steady	35
Spontaneous only	100
Spontaneous pain plus hyperpathia or allodynia	40
Spontaneous pain plus hyperesthesia	3
Spontaneous pain	
Band at upper margin of lesion	13
Diffuse below level	28
Patchy below level	43
Discrete below level	21
Rectal–perineal	11
Facial	3

Some patients had multiple pain patterns.

Surgical Therapy

Allodynia and Hyperpathia. The general strategies for managing evoked pain have been listed. In the treatment of evoked pain in a radicular distribution where this is a major disability and the subservient sensory function is expendable, the percutaneous radiofrequency technique described by Uematsu[16] is effective. However, it should be preceded by diagnostic local blockade to exclude anomalous innervation. Physiologic monitoring should be done carefully to avoid motor damage. Finally, even a damaged sensory root in a quadriplegic's upper extremity that may be responsible for hyperpathia still may subserve important position-sense function the loss of which might be as disabling as the hyperpathia itself.

There is no effective surgical treatment for generalized evoked pain below the level of a lesion; possibly, treatment with opiates or periventricular gray area stimulation may be successful.

Spontaneous Pain. When lancinating radicular pain is present, rhizotomy again may be useful, provided the subserved sensory function is expendable. Consideration must be given to whether it should best be done using open means to ensure division of the root proximal to the lesion site and avoid important radicular arteries, especially in the low thoracic area. However, rhizotomy has no place in the management of spontaneous deafferentation steady pain after cord injury.

A special plea must be made for considering percutaneous cordotomy in the treatment of pain resulting from cord injury.[9,27] Despite all that has been said about interruptive lesions in the treatment of deafferentation pain syndromes, in keeping with the observations of White and Sweet[10] and others, we found the procedure particularly useful in the management of the intermittent lancinating pain associated with, particularly, cauda–conus lesions, especially if they were incomplete. Seven of our 10 patients with both intermittent lancinating and steady burning pain were relieved of the severe lancinating element by cordotomy. However, we also found that even the steady pain sometimes might be helped (some relief occurred in 8 of 15 patients), mainly in those with cauda–conus or incomplete lesions.

A curious feature of cordotomy in these relatively long-lived patients is that, in time, the induced analgesia may fade, and pain may recur. Then, repetition of the procedure may recapture both the analgesia and the pain relief in approximately one-half of cases.

The remarks applied to cordotomy apply equally well to cordectomy, the retranssection of the cord above the level of injury. Only practical in patients with complete or nearly complete lesions in the thoracic area, its uselessness in the treatment of the common steady, often burning, pain below a complete lesion has been reported by many authors. Both we[27] and Jefferson,[78] however, found the operation effective. Jefferson was successful in 79 percent of 19 paraplegic patients, particularly when the pain was lancinating or lo-

cated anteriorly on the thighs or knees and especially if the lesion was below T10. In this author's opinion, however, percutaneous cordotomy, a simpler procedure, achieves the same results.

Nashold and Bullitt[79] reported that the dorsal root entry zone procedure relieved pain significantly in 10 of 13 paraplegic patients, 10 of whom had cauda–conus lesions. Nashold and colleagues[54,57] reported success in a smaller percentage. It is our impression that this procedure works best in relieving pain other than the steady burning pain below a complete lesion in patients with pain syndromes that are likely to respond to the simpler procedure of percutaneous cordotomy or to cordectomy.

The comments made under peripheral deafferentation pain apply equally well to central pain of cord origin. Various authors report a 25 percent to 50 percent chance of pain relief by either medial mesencephalic tractotomy or medial thalamotomy. This is a treatment for the desperate patient after all else has failed.

Modulatory Treatment

Dorsal Cord Stimulation. Two problems result in a high incidence of failure from this simple technique in the patient with central pain of cord origin. First, the appropriate epidural space often is obliterated by injury or previous surgery, preventing the percutaneous introduction of an electrode. Second, a massive cord injury may result in atrophy of the appropriate dorsal column fibers; therefore, stimulation does not produce paresthesias in the painful area. Nonetheless, the technique should be tried first in patients who do not have a complete lesion above the conus because it is safe and simple and particularly effective in patients with incomplete lesions with burning steady pain rather than the intermittent lancinating pain better handled by other means. Published results of dorsal cord stimulation for pain after cord injury are not promising; most authors suggest a 30 percent effectiveness. We treated 34 patients with pain caused by cord injury. Eleven had significant relief. Many of the failures resulted from our inability to achieve paresthesias in the painful area, and all the successes occurred in patients with clinically incomplete lesions, particularly of the conus–cauda region.

Brain Stimulation. Chronic stimulation of the lemniscal relay is the least risky procedure for the patient who does not respond to or is not a candidate for cordotomy or dorsal cord stimulation (usually these are patients with a complete high lesion and steady burning pain in whom all other techniques have failed).[36,76] Tested in eight of our patients, it was useful in three.

CENTRAL PAIN OF BRAIN ORIGIN

Clinical Features

Table 24-7 lists the brain lesions responsible for central pain. The majority, 90 percent of 50 cases we treated,[22] were strokes, most often occlusive; 76 percent were supratentorial. It is remarkable how rarely craniocerebral injury or craniotomy for tumor cause such pain or, in fact, how rarely cerebral lesions of any kind do so. A small but significant number, chiefly in the parietal zone, have been reported. Brain lesions causing central pain usually produce somatosensory loss, and as is the case with central pain caused by cord lesions, this may be partial or complete and affect all or just spinothalamic types. Rarely, no sensory loss will be detected clinically.

Déjèrine and Roussy[80] originally described this entity in a group of patients with strokes characterized by modest, usually transient, contralateral hemiparesis and more persistent hemihypesthesia, hemiataxia, astereognosis, and sometimes choreoathetosis. After a delay, they had pain in the affected half of their bodies. Although their term *thalamic syndrome* has been associated with this type of pain, modern imaging techniques[81,82] show a poor correlation between the occurrence of pain and involvement of the thalamus.

In our experience, the onset of pain usually is delayed after the causative event (68 percent of 50 cases treated).[22] In 14 percent, this interval exceeded 1 year. The clinical picture consists of spontaneous pain similar to that seen in other deafferentation syndromes, affecting all or part of the bodily region with the somatosensory deficit. This is accompanied by neurologic signs appropriate to the underlying lesion. In the case of lateral medullary syndrome, the pain more often is referred to areas with trigeminal than with spinothalamic sensory loss. The pain was described as burning in 52 percent of our cases, often with additional features, especially paresthesias. Lancinating intermittent pain occurred in 14 percent, and 62 percent had allodynia, hyperpathia, or hyperesthesia. Ten percent had no clinically detectable sensory loss, and one patient had no spontaneous pain but only hyperesthesia.

Of great interest was the relationship of this type of central pain to dyskinesia and epilepsy. As reported by Déjèrine and Roussy,[80] 22 percent of our patients had movement disorders, usually a dystonic process ipsilateral to the pain. Twelve percent had epilepsy, recalling Nashold's[43] experience that epileptic bursts recorded from midbrain tegmentum appeared to coincide with the exacer-

bations of pain, the latter being relieved by a coagulative lesion at the same site that silenced the epileptic activity.

Therapy

General and Medical

The statements made under general and medical treatments in previous sections apply equally well to pain caused by brain lesions.

Surgical

There are few options in the management of central pain of brain origin. It remains one of the most frustrating challenges in contemporary neurology.

Destructive Stereotactic Procedures. As in the case of central pain of cord origin, medial mesencephalotomy and medial thalamotomy offer a limited chance of success and are used in severe cases when all else has failed, particularly if intermittent lancinating pain is present. In keeping with data published by Namba and colleagues[83] and Niizuma and coworkers,[84] partial relief of spontaneous pain occurred in six of nine of our patients; three of them had minor or transient complications.

Modulatory Surgery

Trigeminal Nerve Stimulation. It is logical to consider modulatory therapy in central pain syndromes before resorting to destructive procedures. Obviously, stimulation of peripheral nerves has little application in cases of central pain, except in patients with lateral medullary syndrome and those with supratentorial stroke in whom facial pain is the main problem. Two of three of our patients have gained benefit from this simple procedure.

Dorsal Cord Stimulation. Anecdotal reports in the literature describe useful relief of central pain of brain origin after chronic spinal stimulation; this technique has the great advantage of simplicity. Three of eight of our patients gained short-term relief (and one long-term) using this treatment.

Brain Stimulation. Chronic stimulation of the medial lemniscal pathway remains the chief initial surgical approach to central pain of brain origin, despite the fact that yield is low,[76] because of the low risk and reversibility of this method of treatment. However, some authors have reported encouraging results. Adams,[85] for example, found 8 of 10 patients with so-called thalamic syndrome obtained relief. Siegfried and Demierre[86] cited seven of nine successful cases. The chief technical problem facing the surgeon in such patients is the difficulty of physiologic localization of the electrode because of the diencephalic damage produced by the stroke. Three of six of our patients with central pain of brain origin responded to chronic brain stimulation.

Other Methods. In such a disabling condition, we always are searching for new and more promising methods

Table 24-7
Cause of Central Pain of Brain Origin

Trauma
Vascular
  Supratentorial
    Occlusive
    Hematoma
  Infratentorial, especially lateral medullary syndrome
Neoplasm
Syringobulbia
Multiple sclerosis
Encephalitis and degenerations
Iatrogenic vascular occlusions after deliberate sensory tract lesions

of treating the pain. It is interesting that Levin and colleagues[87] relieved so-called thalamic pain in three patients using intrahypophyseal alcohol injection.

CONCLUSIONS

Central pain is a complex phenomenon requiring careful clinical appraisal to assess the disability from the various component parts of the overall pain syndrome. Only then can therapy be applied intelligently (or withheld). In the course of pain associated with lesions of the peripheral nerves or spinal cord, a reasonable expectation of effective therapy can be predicted; in the case of central pain caused by brain lesions, we are still searching for effective therapy.

References

1. Tasker RR, Organ LW, Hawrylyshyn P. Deafferentation and causalgia. In: Bonica JJ, ed. *Pain Research Publications: A.R.N.M.D. 58.* New York: Raven; 1980:305–329.

2. Bowsher D. The problem of central pain. *Verh Dtsch Ges Inn Med* 1980; 86:1525–1527.

3. Sicuteri F. Persistent non-organic central pain: headache and central paralgesia. In: Lipton S, Miles J, eds. *Persistent Pain.* Vol 3. London: Academic Press; 1981:119–140.

4. Wall PD. Alterations in the central nervous system after deafferentation: connectivity control. In: Bonica JJ, Lindblom U, Iggo A, eds. *Advances in Pain Research and Therapy.* Vol 5. New York: Raven; 1983:677–689.

5. Livingston WK. Pain Mechanisms: *A Physiologic Interpretation of Causalgia and Its Related States.* 2nd ed. New York: Plenum; 1976.

6. Tasker RR, Tsuda T, Hawrylyshyn P. Clinical neurophysiological investigation of deafferentation pain. In: Bonica JJ, Lindblom U, Iggo A, eds. *Advances in Pain Research and Therapy.* Vol. 5. New York: Raven; 1983:713–738.

7. Tasker RR. Deafferentation. In: Wall PD, Melzack R, eds. *Textbook of Pain.* Edinburgh: Churchill Livingstone; 1984:119–132.

8. Walters JA. Psychogenic regional pain alias hysterical pain. *Brain* 1961; 84:1–18.

9. Tasker RR, Organ LW, Hawrylyshyn P. Percutaneous cordotomy: the lateral high cervical technique. In: Schmidek HH, Sweet WH, eds. *Operative Neurosurgical Techniques, Indications, Methods and Results.* New York: Grune & Stratton; 1982:1137–1153.

10. White JC, Sweet WH. *Pain and the Neurosurgeon. A Forty Year Experience.* Springfield: Thomas; 1969:435–447.

11. Gildenberg PL. Stereotactic treatment of head and neck pain. *Res Clin Stud Headache* 1978; 5:102–121.

12. Levitt M, Levitt JH. The deafferentation syndrome in monkeys: dysesthesias of spinal origin. *Pain* 1981; 10:129–147.

13. Inbal R, Devor M, Tuchhenhendler O, Lieblich I. Autonomy following nerve injury: genetic factors in the development of chronic pain. *Pain* 1980; 9:327–337.

14. Tasker RR, Dostrovsky J. Deafferentation and central pain. In: Wall PD, Melzack R, eds. *Textbook of Pain.* 2nd ed. Edinburgh: Churchill Livingstone; 1989:154–180.

15. Lindblom U. Assessment of abnormal evoked pain in neurological patients and its relation to spontaneous pain: a descriptive and conceptual model with some analytical results. In: Fields HL, Dubner R, Cervino F, eds. *Advances in Pain Research and Therapy.* Vol 9. New York: Raven; 1985:409–423.

16. Uematsu S. Percutaneous electrothermocoagulation of spinal nerve trunk, ganglion, and rootlets. In: Schmidek HH, Sweet WH, eds. *Operative Neurosurgical Techniques, Indications, Methods and Results.* New York: Grune & Stratton; 1982:1177–1198.

17. Pitty L, Tasker RR. Experience with chronic stimulation of the brain for the relief of pain. Unpublished observations.

18. Boas RA, Hatangdi VS, Richards EG. Lumbar sympathectomy—a percutaneous chemical technique. In: Bonica JJ, Albe-Fessard DG, eds. *Advances in Pain Research and Therapy.* Vol 1. New York: Raven; 1976:685–689.

19. Wilkinson A. Percutaneous radiofrequency upper thoracic sympathectomy: a new technique. *Neurosurgery* 1984; 15:811–814.

20. Bonica JJ. Causalgia and other reflex sympathetic dystrophies. In: Bonica JJ, Liebeskind JC, Albe-Fessard DG, eds. *Advances in Pain Research and Therapy.* New York: Raven; 1979:141–166.

21. Tasker RR. Percutaneous cordotomy: the lateral high cervical technique. In: Schmidek HH, Sweet WH, eds. *Operative Neurosurgical Techniques, Indications, Methods, and Results.* 2nd ed. New York: Grune & Stratton. In press.

22. Tasker RR. Pain due to central nervous system pathology (central pain). In: Bonica JJ, ed. *Management of Pain in Clinical Practice.* 2nd ed. Philadelphia: Lea & Febiger. In press.

23. Pagni CA. Place of stereotactic technique in surgery for pain. In: Bonica JJ, ed. *Advances in Neurology.* Vol 4. New York: Raven; 1984:699–706.

24. Nashold BS Jr. Brainstem stereotaxic procedures. In: Schalgentbrand G, Walker AE, eds. *Stereotaxy of the Human Brain.* Stuttgart: Thieme Verlag, 1982:475–483.

25. Tasker RR. Thalamic procedures. In: Schaltenbrand G, Walker AE, eds. *Stereotaxy of the Human Brain.* Stuttgart: Thieme Verlag; 1982:484–497.

26. Tasker RR. Stereotaxic surgery. In: Wall PD, Melzack R, eds. *Textbook of Pain.* Edinburgh: Churchill Livingstone; 1984:639–655.

27. Tasker RR, De Carvalho GT. Intractable central pain of cord origin—clinical features and implantations for surgery. Presented at the American Association of Neurological Surgeons Meeting; April 3, 1989; Washington, D.C.

28. Tasker RR. Introduction. In: Nashold BS, Ovelmen-Levitt J, eds. *Deafferentation Pain Syndromes.* New York: Raven; 1990.

29. Rinaldi PC, Young RF, Albe-Fessard D, Chodakiewitz J. Spontaneous neuronal hyperactivity in the medial and intralaminar thalamic nuclei of patients with deafferentation pain. *J Neurosurg* March 1991; 74(3):415–421.

30. Coderre TJ, Grimes RW, Melzack R. Deafferentation and chronic pain in animals: an evaluation of evidence suggestion autonomy is related to pain. *Pain* 1986; 26:61–84.

31. Zimmermann N. Peripheral and central nervous mechanisms of nociception, pain and pain therapy: facts and hypotheses. In: Bonica JJ, Liebeskind JC, Albe-Fessard DG, eds. *Advances in Pain Research and Therapy.* Vol 3. New York: Raven; 1979;3–32.

32. Loeser JD. Definition, etiology, and neurological assessment of pain originating in the nervous system following deafferentation. *Pain Suppl* 1981; 1:81S.

33. Cassinari V, Pagni CA. *Central Pain: A Neurosurgical Survey.* Cambridge: Harvard; 1969.

34. Tasker RR. Identification of pain processing systems by electrical stimulation of the brain. *Hum Neurobiol* 1982; 1:261–272.

35. Tasker RR, Organ LW, Hawrylyshyn P: Wilkins RH, ed. *The Thalamus and Midbrain of Man. A Physiological Atlas Using Electrical Stimulation.* Springfield: Thomas; 1982.

36. Pagni CA. Central pain due to spinal cord and brain damage. In: Wall PD, Melzack R, eds. *Textbook of Pain.* Edinburgh: Churchill Livingstone; 1984;481–495.

37. Loeser JD, Ward AA, White AA, White LE. Chronic deafferentation of human spinal cord neurons. *J Neurosurg* 1968; 29:48–50.

38. Tasker RR. Effets sensitifs et moteurs de la stimulation thalamique chez l'homme. Applications cliniques. *Rev Neurol (Paris)* 1986; 142:316–326.

39. Lombard MC, Nashold BS Jr, Pelissier T. Thalamic recordings in rats with hyperalgesia. In: Bonica JJ, Liebeskind JC, Albe-Fessard DC, eds. *Advances in Pain Research and Therapy.* Vol 3. New York: Raven; 1979:767–772.

40. Hirayama T, Dostrovsky JO, Gorecki J, Tasker RR, Lenz FA. Recordings of abnormal activity in patients with deafferentation and central pain. *Stereotact Funct Neurosurg* 1989; 52:127–135.

41. Gorecki J, Hirayama T, Dostrovsky JO, Tasker RR, Lenz FA. Thalamic stimulation and recording in patients with deafferentation and central pain. *Stereotact Funct Neurosurg* 1989; 52:219–226.

42. Lenz FA, Tasker RR, Dostrovsky JO, Kwan HC, et al. Abnormal single-unit activity recorded in the somatosensory thalamus of a quadriplegic patient with central pain. *Pain* 1987; 31:225–236.

43. Nashold BS Jr, Wilson WP. Central pain: observations in man with chronic implanted electrodes in the midbrain tegmentum. *Confinia Neurol* 1966; 27:30–44.

44. Kayser V, Basbaum AI, Guilbaud G. Deafferentation in the rat increases mechanical nociceptive threshold in the innervated limbs. *Brain Res* February 5 1990; 508(2):329–332.

45. Levitt M. The theory of chronic deafferentation dysesthesias. *J Neurosurg Sci* April–June 1990; 34(2):71–98.

46. Modesti LM, Waszak M. Firing patterns of cells in human thalamus during dorsal column stimulation. *Appl Neurophysiol* 1975; 38:251–258.

47. Tsubokawa T, Moriyasu N. Follow-up results of center median thalamotomy for relief of intractable pain. *Confinia Neurol* 1975; 37:280–284.

48. Albe-Fessard D, Condés-Lara M, Sanderson P, Levante A. Tentative explanation of the special role played by the areas of paleospinothalamic projection in patients with deafferentation pain syndromes. In: Kruger L, Liebeskind JC, eds. *Advances in Pain Research and Therapy.* Vol 6. New York: Raven; 1984:167–182.

49. Awerbuch GI, Sandyk R. Mexiletine for thalamic pain syndrome. *Int J Neurosci* December 1990; 55(2–4):129–33.

50. Tasker RR. Neurostimulation and percutaneous neural destructive techniques. In: Cousins MJ, Bridenbaugh PO, eds. *Neural Blockade in the Management of Pain.* Philadelphia: Lippincott; 1986:748–797.

51. Hyndman OR. Lissauer's tract section. A contribution to chordotomy for the relief of pain. *J Int Coll Surg* 1942; 5:394–400. Preliminary report.

52. Sindou M, Fischer G, Guntelle A, Mansuy L. La radicellotomie postérieure sélective. Premiers résultats dans la chirurgie de la douleur. *Neurochirurgie* 1974; 20:391–408.

53. Nashold BS, Ostdahl RH. Dorsal root entry zone lesions for pain relief. *J Neurosurg* 1979; 51:59–69.

54. Nashold BS Jr, Ostdahl RH, Bullit E, Friedman A, Brophy B. Dorsal root entry zone lesions: a new neurosurgical therapy for deafferentation pain. In: Bonica JJ, Lindblom U, Iggo A, eds. *Advances in Pain Research and Therapy.* Vol 5. New York: Raven; 1983:739–750.

55. Friedman AH, Nashold BS Jr, Ovelmen-Levitt J. Dorsal root entry zone lesions for the treatment of postherpetic neuralgia. *J Neurosurg* 1984; 60:1258–1262.

56. Friedman AH, Bullitt E. Dorsal root entry zone lesions in the treatment of pain following brachial plexus avulsion, spinal cord injury and herpes zoster. *Appl Neurophysiol* 1988; 51:164–169.

57. Moosy JJ, Nashold BS Jr. Dorsal root entry zone lesions for conus medullaris root avulsions. *Appl Neurphysiol* 1988; 51:198–205.

58. Hitchcock ER. Stereotactic trigeminal tractotomy. *Ann Clin Res* 1970; 2:131–135.

59. Crue BL, Todd EM, Carregal EJ. Percutaneous radiofrequency stereotactic trigeminal tractotomy. In: Crue BL, ed. *Pain and Suffering.* Springfield: Thomas; 1970:69–79.

60. Schvarcz JR. Spinal cord stereotactic techniques re trigeminal nucleotomy and extralemniscal myelotomy. *Appl Neurophysiol* 1978; 41:99–112.

61. Hitchcock ER. Stereotactic cervical myelotomy. *J Neurol Neurosurg Psychiatry* 1970; 33:224–230.

62. Schvarcz JR. Stereotactic high cervical extraleminiscal myelotomy for pelvic cancer pain. *Acta Neurochir Suppl (Wien)* 1984; 33:431–435.

63. Cook AW, Nathan PW, Smith MC. Sensory consequences of commissural myelotomy. A challenge to traditional anatomical concepts. *Brain* 1984; 107:547–568.

64. Santo JL, Arias LM, Barolat G, Schwartzman RJ, Grossman K. Bilateral cingulumotomy in the treatment of reflex sympathetic dystrophy. *Pain* April 1990; 41(1):55–59.

65. Simpson BA. Spinal cord stimulation in 60 cases of intractable pain. *J Neurol Neurosurg Psychiatry* March 1991; 54(3):196–199.

66. Spiegelmann R, Friedman WA. Spinal cord stimulation: a contemporary series. *Neurosurgery* January 1991; 28(1):65–70; discussion 70–71.

67. Wall PD, Sweet WH. Temporary abolition of pain in man. *Science* 1967; 155:108–109.

68. Meyerson BA, Håkansson S. Alleviation of atypical trigeminal pain by stimulation of the gasserian ganglion via an implanted electrode. *Acta Neurochir Suppl (Wien)* 1980; 10:303–309.

69. Steude V. Radiofrequency electrical stimulation of the gasserian ganglion in patients with atypical trigeminal pain. *Acta Neurochir Suppl (Wien)* 1984; 33:481.

70. Shealy CN, Mortimer JT, Hagfors NR. Dorsal column electroanalgesia. *J Neurosurg* 1970; 32:560–564.

71. Dooley DM. A technique for the epidural percutaneous stimulation of the spinal cord in man. Presented at the Annual Meeting of the American Association of Neurologic Surgeons; 1975; Miami Beach.

72. Kumar K, Wyant GM, Nath R. Deep brain stimulation for control of intractable pain in humans, present and future: a ten year follow-up. *Neurosurgery* May 1990; 26(5):774–781; discussion 781–782.

73. Mazars GJ. Intermittent stimulation of nucleus ventralis posterolateralis for intractable pain. *Surg Neurol* 1975; 4:93–95.

74. Adams JE, Hosubuchi Y, Fields HL. Stimulation of internal capsule for relief of chronic pain. *J Neurosurg* 1974; 41:740–744.

75. Hosobuchi Y, Adams JE, Rutkin B. Chronic thalamic stimulation for the control of facial anesthesia dolorosa. *Arch Neurol* 1973; 29:158–161.

76. Turnbull IM. Brain stimulation. In: Wall PD, Melzack R, eds. *Textbook of Pain*. Edinburgh: Churchill Livingstone; 1984:706–714.

77. Morgan MM, Gold MS, Liebeskind JC, Stein C. Periaqueductal gray stimulation produces a spinally mediated, opioid antinociception for the inflamed hindpaw of the rat. *Brain Res* April 5 1991; 545(1–2):17–23.

78. Jefferson A. Cordectomy for intractable pain. In: Lipton S, Miles J, eds. *Persistent Pain*. Vol 4. New York: Grune & Stratton; 1983:115–132.

79. Nashold BS Jr, Bullitt E. Dorsal root entry zone lesions to control central pain in paraplegics. *J Neurosurg* 1981; 55:414–419.

80. Déjèrine J, Roussy G. Le syndrome thalamique. *Rev Neurol (Paris)* 1906; 14:521–532.

81. Agnew DC, Shetter AG, Segall HD, Flom RA. Thalamic pain. In: Bonica JJ, Lindblom U, Iggo A, eds. *Advances in Pain Research and Therapy*. Vol 5. New York: Raven; 1983:941–946.

82. Bowsher D, Lahuerta J, Brock L. Twelve cases of central pain, only three with thalamic lesions. *Pain Suppl* 1984; 2:83S.

83. Namba S, Nakao Y, Matsumoto Y, Ohmoto T, Nishimoto A. Electrical stimulation of the posterior limb of the internal capsule for the treatment of thalamic pain. *Appl Neurophysiol* 1984; 47:137–148.

84. Niizuma H, Kwak R, Ikeda S, Ohyama H, Suzuki J, Saso S. Follow-up results of centromedian thalamotomy for central pain. *Appl Neurophysiol* 1982; 45:324–325.

85. Adams JE. Technique and technical problems associated with implantation of neuroaugmentative devices. *Appl Neurophysiol* 1977–1978; 40:111–123.

86. Siegfried J, Demierre B. Thalamic electro-stimulation in the treatment of thalamic pain syndrome. *Pain Suppl* 1984; 2:116S.

87. Levin AB, Ramirez LF, Katz J. The use of stereotaxic chemical hypophysectomy in the treatment of thalamic pain syndrome. *J Neurosurg* 1983; 59:1002–1006.

CHAPTER 25

Pediatric Pain Management

Charles B. Berde, Navil Sethna, and Babu V. Koka

As with adults, our approach to the pediatric patient with acute or chronic pain demands an understanding of the anatomy and physiology of pain pathways; a search for the cause guided by the history, physical examination, and judiciously chosen laboratory studies; and an awareness of the interplay of psychosocial and physiologic factors that determine the patient's response to pain and illness.[1] In this chapter, we consider:

1. The development of pain perception in infancy and childhood and the assessment of pain in infants and children.
2. The diagnostic evaluation, including the history, physical examination, and laboratory studies at different ages and how children of different ages report pain, fear, and anxiety.
3. Behavior-oriented therapies, such as hypnosis, relaxation training, biofeedback, play therapy, and emotional support measures for children of different ages, the psychiatric evaluation, and physical therapies.
4. Physical measures, TENS, and acupuncture.
5. Pharmacologic principles governing the use of analgesics in children.
6. Regional anesthetic techniques, nerve blocks, and neurosurgical approaches.
7. Pain syndromes common in each age group and how differential diagnoses change as a function of age.
8. Our initial experience with a pediatric multidisciplinary pain service.

DEVELOPMENT OF PAIN PERCEPTION AND THE ASSESSMENT OF PAIN IN INFANTS AND CHILDREN

A long-standing controversy surrounds the question of whether or in what manner newborns and infants experience pain. A traditional view has asserted that, because of the immaturity of the newborn's nervous system, they do not experience pain as adults do. Proponents of this view cite the newborn's incomplete myelination of tracts bearing afferent impulses and their responses to painful stimuli, such as pinprick, by a mass withdrawal reflex rather than by isolated withdrawal of a single extremity.[2] Others assert that newborns may experience pain in some fashion but that they do not have emotional suffering or a memory of pain. An alternative view holds that newborns experience pain and suffering in as acute a fashion as adults. Newborns (even premature infants) have a mature capacity to synthe-size the neurotransmitters and neuropeptides commonly associated with pain pathways, including endorphins, enkephalins, and substance P. Because much of nociceptive transmission occurs through small unmyelinated fibers, the argument that incomplete myelination of a newborn's sensory tracts precludes an intense experience of pain appears fallacious. The incomplete myelination of sensory tracts subserving light touch and proprioception may explain in part the newborn's relative inability to localize painful stimulation, but this does not imply a limited capacity of the newborn to experience pain.

Assessment of pain in infants has been difficult, but there have been some preliminary efforts in this direction.[3,4] Using pressure on the tibia as the painful stimulus, Haslam[5] suggested that younger children have a lower threshold for pain than do older children. Levine and Gordon[6] used spectrographic analysis of infant crying patterns to argue that crying as a result of pain can be distinguished from crying caused by hunger or other stresses. Harpin and Rutter[7] noticed that palmar sweating seems to be a specific reaction to painful stimuli in newborns over 37 weeks' gestational age.

Newborns show marked autonomic responses to painful stimulation, and some investigators suggest that these responses may be deleterious. An interesting study by Williamson and Williamson[8] compared babies who received a penile block with a local anesthetic before circumcision with those who did not. Untreated babies showed marked changes in heart rate, blood pressure, and transcutaneous P_{O_2}, suggesting severe stress. They cite follow-up evaluation using a modified Brazelton[9] neonatal assessment scale that showed behavioral changes for a period of weeks, which they and others attribute to the effects of untreated pain.

Newborns may exhibit more dramatic autonomic responses to stress in their pulmonary circulation than in their systemic circulation. A study by Hickey and colleagues[10] examined the effect of analgesia (using fentanyl) on the hemodynamic responses to endotracheal suctioning in newborns after cardiac surgery. Newborns not receiving analgesia often had marked rises in pulmonary artery pressure, with only minor changes in systemic arterial pressure; in those with an open foramen ovale or ductus arteriosus and pulmonary hypertension, this response could lead to marked increases in right-to-left shunting and systemic arterial desaturation.

In summary, although the nature of the newborn pain experience is difficult to assess, there is little evidence to justify concluding that it is less intense than that of older individuals. We prefer to err on the side of treating their pain. It is our custom to administer local anesthetics whenever appropriate for analgesia when procedures are done on newborns and to administer intravenous narcotics to intubated neonates for incisional pain and sedation to permit tolerance of endotracheal tubes.[11] Minor postoperative pain is treated with acetaminophen. When there appears to be significant postoperative pain and where conditions permit sufficiently close observation (including an apnea monitor), we administer small doses of narcotics (morphine, 0.05 to 0.1 mg/kg) to unintubated newborns who do not have specific contraindications (such as severe respiratory disease, apnea, or severe neurologic disease).

In children 6 months of age to at least 7 years, it is apparent that most behavioral measures assess a combination of pain, anxiety, and fear, rather than pain alone.[12] The subjective scales include various versions of a visual analog scale,[13] that may be related to a child's experience such as a graphic representation of a pain thermometer with a scale from 0 to 100 or 0 to 10. Several investigators have found this useful for children ages 8 years and older. A pediatric pain questionnaire was developed by Tesler and colleagues[14] that was based on the model of the McGill pain questionnaire. For younger children, observational scales have been developed, including those of Katz and coworkers[15] and Jay and coworkers.[16] Some of these scales measure distress, regarded as a combination of pain and anxiety, by ranking of behaviors such as crying or flailing. When these scales are used, it appears that, at least regarding the pain of procedures, children younger than 7 years of age have more behavioral manifestations of distress than do older children. This may be related more to age-related differences in anxiety than to age-specific changes in pain threshold or tolerance per se.

Behavioral reactions to chronic pain also differ at different ages. As summarized by Schechter.[17]

"Infants often withdraw, display sad faces, exhibit eating and sleeping disturbances, and have difficulty establishing relationships. Preschoolers often become clingy, immobile, and may lose motor skills, verbal abilities, and sphincter control. They may experience nightmares, chronic anxiety and pain. Because of the limitations of their cognitive abilities, preschoolers often do not understand reasons for their general discomfort or the need for painful medical procedures (e.g. dressing changes). There is often an implicit or explicit assumption that the pain is punishment for some previous wrongdoing. School-aged children often respond to chronic pain with increased aggressiveness, extreme shame (more frequent in burn patients), and nightmares, manifested by withdrawal. Increased anxiety is frequently seen and may relate to concern about loss of control and the potential reaction of peers. In adolescent patients, depression and extreme oppositional behavior are common physiologic responses to chronic pain. . . ."

DIAGNOSTIC EVALUATION

History

Several points may be helpful for taking the history.

1. As much as possible, obtain answers directly from the child in addition to the parent. If questions are asked in a simple nonthreatening manner, most children from age 3 years and older can provide helpful information regarding their pain. In many cases, particularly with adolescents, it is helpful to conduct interviews both in the presence and absence of their parents.
2. It is a common clinical observation that young children may localize their pain inaccurately. For example, hip pain may be ascribed to the knee and vice versa. Despite this clinical experience, a study by Eland and Anderson[18] found that, when children aged 4 to 10 years were asked to make an X on a drawing of a body, 168 of 172 correctly identified the location of their pain. Several investigators confirmed that the use of pictures to describe either the location or the severity of the pain is helpful for smaller children.
3. As with adults, an index of the severity of pain and its effects on functioning can be derived by questions regarding the effects of the pain on eating, sleeping, and activity. If pain keeps the child from doing favorite activities, that is significant, although the clinician should bear in mind that, on occasion, pain complaints permit a child to avoid activities (such as sports) that they are forced to do by their parents.
4. A detailed family and social history is worthwhile in assessing chronic pain. A history of recent stressful events should be sought. Specific inquiry regarding new siblings or marital difficulties must be obtained because many parents will not volunteer such information.
5. Where the pain is considered to have a large psychosomatic component or where the cause of the pain is unclear, it often is illuminating to inquire about the health history of family members. For example, if a youngster has vague chest pain and signs of depression or anxiety, the finding that his grandfather recently had a myocardial infarction with crushing chest pain would be significant.
6. Even where the cause of the child's pain is clear, parents and family members often interpret symptoms in light of their past encounters with illnesses (e.g., headache may mean brain tumor or abdominal pain may mean pancreatic cancer), and a knowledge of the family history may help the clinician anticipate the patient's and parents' worries and provide appropriate reassurance.

Physical Examination

As with adults, when evaluating a part of the body where pain is reported, it is necessary to begin gently to avoid precipitating severe discomfort. In children, this is especially important. If the initial examination causes severe discomfort, then the examiner will find a terrified screaming distrustful child with whom further encounters will be much more difficult. Generally, it is best to begin by examining remote parts of the body first. Pointing to different locations often is helpful in localizing the pain ("Which hurts more, this place or that place?"). Distraction with a game or other activity may permit examination of the painful part without as much guarding or anticipatory reaction.

Laboratory Evaluation

Diagnostic evaluation using laboratory studies should be done parsimoniously to minimize expense, risk to the patient, and generation of false-positive results that are inevitable whenever the test specificity is low or the prevalence of abnormalities in the patient's clinical subgroup is low.

BEHAVIORAL APPROACHES TO PAIN MANAGEMENT IN CHILDREN

For children with many types of pain problems, an approach to pain treatment begins by assessing psychosocial factors and several behavioral interventions. Pain frequently is associated with stress, anxiety, and fear; efforts directed toward relaxation and reduction of anxiety and fear may decrease the distress associated with acute or chronic pain. A detailed discussion of behavioral approaches is given by Masek and associates.[19]

Behavior Modification

Pain behavior may be intensified if it is reinforced or provides a means of obtaining attention or avoiding averse activities. In behavioral approaches to pain management, it frequently is recommended that parents respond positively to well behaviors (engaging in activities, returning to school, or adopting an optimistic and positive demeanor) and that they respond negatively to complaining and avoidance of activities. Although this approach makes sense in the context of behavior modification theory and appears helpful in many cases, it should be apparent that it may be difficult to accomplish in practice by prescription alone. Despite good intentions, if underlying family conflicts are not addressed and this approach is undertaken in an unsupervised fashion, it may backfire. As an example, consider a child whose parents have for a long time shown insufficient love and attention and who begins having recurrent headaches. If pain behavior (complaining or avoidance of school or activities) is ignored or reinforced negatively without other changes in the family dynamics, it seems likely that the child will continue to seek attention either by more extreme pain complaints and behaviors or by other so-called undesirable behaviors. For an unloved child, negative reinforcement of pain behaviors without other changes in parental behavior only may confirm the child's feelings of neglect and lack of worth. Conversely, it seems

sensible to recommend positive reinforcement of well behaviors, resolution of family conflicts, and creation of a context in which the child feels loved and receives attention and approval for normal activities.

Relaxation

Various methods have been used to produce a state of relaxation as a therapy for stress, hypertension, and other psychosomatic disorders. The general approach is outlined by Benson.[20] Techniques, including guided imagery, alternating muscle tension, relaxation, and EMG or temperature biofeedback have been used successfully in children. Depending on how they are approached, these techniques may have aspects in common with hypnosis. They are applicable easily in children age 7 years and older and may be used in younger children in certain cases.

A major application of this method has been in the treatment of recurrent headaches in childhood. Mehagan and colleagues[21] showed that an approach involving relaxation and biofeedback can be used in most children to decrease headache frequency and diminish medication requirements. It is not clear which aspects of the approach are essential; for example, relaxation training alone may be as effective as relaxation with biofeedback.

Hypnosis

Children and adolescents frequently are excellent subjects for hypnosis for the treatment of pain. Readers are urged to consult outstanding works on this subject.[22–24]

Hypnosis has been defined and described in many ways as follows: an altered state of consciousness characterized by dissociation or division of consciousness, focused attention, trance, or profound relaxation. Aspects of these states occur frequently in daily life and in many clinician–therapist interactions without formal induction. After becoming familiar with this condition, many patients practice self-hypnosis (that is, self-induction of a state of trance, relaxation, or focused attention). Hypnotic susceptibility or responsivity appears to be a relatively constant individual characteristic. The nature of the analgesia produced by hypnosis is understood poorly; there is considerable controversy over whether so-called covert pain is perceived but not reported. For the same degree of reduction of subjective pain scores, there appears to be less suppression of autonomic responses (tachycardia and hypertension) to painful stimuli than that produced by narcotics. A fascinating report by Goldstein and Hilgard[25] showed that naloxone does not attenuate the analgesia produced by hypnosis.

Studies by Morgan and Hilgard[26,27] indicate that hypnotizability increases from age 5 years through the school-age years and that a greater fraction of children than adults are highly hypnotizable. Although their formal susceptibility scales extend only from age 5 years and older, clinical reports by others[28,29] suggest that, in certain circumstances, even younger children may be hypnotized. To some degree, hypnotic susceptibility or responsivity measures are influenced by the type of induction used. For example, Morgan and Hilgard[30] showed that induction using guided imagery produces higher response rates in children aged 6 years and younger than induction using relaxation. Also, children and adults vary greatly in the rank order of different tasks under hypnosis (such as posthypnotic suggestion, amnesia, eye closure, and auditory hallucination).[31] Unlike adults, younger children who are susceptible and capable of impressive degrees of hypnoanalgesia rarely keep their eyes closed or remain motionless while in a trance. A conservative interpretation of the literature permits the conclusion that more than 50% of children aged 5 years and older might derive significant reduction of acute or chronic pain using hypnosis.

Gardner and Olness[32] describe induction techniques for various ages. Preschool children frequently do well using story telling or speaking to the child through a doll or stuffed animal. Guided imagery might take the form of imagining a favorite place or activity. School-aged children do well with guided imagery, eye fixation (watching a coin or a point or the image on a hand), and ideomotor (hand levitation) techniques. Adolescents may use imagery techniques or any adult method, including progressive relaxation. With older children and adolescents, who may have negative preconceptions about hypnosis as a loss of control or otherwise fearful activity, use of the term *relaxation* may be less threatening. With familiarity, most children who are susceptible can re-create an induction sequence themselves. The hypnotherapist's style should be permissive not authoritarian.

Anxiety, fear, and anticipation are prominent factors in the distress that children experience from therapeutic procedures, such as bone-marrow aspiration. In older patients, anxiety and pain reduction through hypnosis is correlated positively with hypnotic susceptibility. Two controlled studies[33,34] demonstrate statistically significant reductions in both subjective ratings of pain and observed pain-related behaviors in hypnotized children compared with nonhypnotized children undergoing bone-marrow aspiration. Anecdotal experience suggests that hypnosis also is useful in other situations in children characterized by pain, fear, and anticipation (such as repeated blood drawing, intravenous placement, burn dressing changes, difficult awake intubation, and fiberoptic bronchoscopy).

The advantages of hypnosis as a technique in children include: (1) its efficacy in anxiety, nausea, fear, and pain, (2) its avoidance of the side effects of chemical analgesia, particularly in chronic pain, (3) its promotion of a sense of autonomy and mastery in children who would otherwise feel helpless (4) its provision as a vehicle for effective psychotherapy, and (5) its safety when done by trained therapists. The limitations or disadvantages include: (1) a paucity of therapists with the expertise and commitment to guide hypnotherapy; (2) a lack of susceptibility in some

children and only moderate effectiveness for severe pain in many children; (3) the skepticism, resistance, fear, and lack of information on the part of many health professionals, patients, and families; (4) the difficulty in some children, including the severely retarded, the severely emotionally disturbed, and those who are obtunded or disoriented; and (5) the significant amount of time required in many, but not all, cases.

The Hospital Environment

Hospitalized children have a number of stresses that contribute to fear, anxiety, and focusing on their pain. The environment is threatening, and there is often a seemingly random and unending series of painful procedures, which can create a feeling of helplessness. Support from parents, primary nurses, and activity therapists can be invaluable. Involvement in activities (such as drawing and play with puppets) can permit a young child to confront and express fears that otherwise would be inaccessible to the therapist using classic psychiatric interview techniques.

Efforts also can be made by physicians to diminish the stress of hospital procedures. Even children as young as age 3 years should receive a simple explanation of the need for procedures. The use of a procedure room for inpatient wards is encouraged because it gives order to the child's experience; the hospital room and play room, therefore, remain safe places.

Psychiatric Evaluation and Psychotherapy

As with adults, children with chronic pain occasionally have significant depression and other forms of psychiatric illness. Contrary to a previous belief, depression occurs throughout childhood, and as in adults, it is underdiagnosed. Consultation frequently is helpful to make the diagnosis, including that of a conversion reaction, and for supportive psychotherapy. Conversion symptoms are relatively common in adolescence; they are rare in children younger than age 10 years.

PHYSICAL MEASURES, TENS, AND ACUPUNCTURE

Physical therapy can be helpful to restore mobility and function in chronic limb and back conditions. The use of cooling, heating, whirlpools, and massage also may provide symptomatic relief in many types of chronic pain in children. Case reports suggest the effectiveness of TENS in children as young as age 3 years.[35] Reports on the efficacy of acupuncture in chronic pain in adolescents and children are limited and anecdotal. An advantage of TENS over acupuncture in younger children is the avoidance of needles. Because of its safety, lack of side effects, and sometimes impressive efficacy, we prescribe a trial of TENS for almost all children with localized chronic pain and for many children with acute pain. Exercise programs, such as swimming, are helpful for (1) general aerobic conditioning, (2) restoring limb mobility and strength, (3) relieving tension, and (4) improving the child or adolescent's sense of body image.

PHARMACOLOGY OF AGENTS USED FOR PAIN TREATMENT

General Considerations

The general principles of drug absorption, distribution, action, and elimination are the same for adults and children.[36-38] Some differences in the details are outlined in Table 25-1.

Specific Drugs

Narcotics

Morphine. Dahlstrom and colleagues[35] examined the kinetics of morphine elimination in children and found that, from age 1 year and older, the distribution and elimination are similar to that seen in adults. Lynn and Slattery[39] examined infants between the ages of 1 and 65 days who were receiving morphine during mechanical ventilation in an intensive care unit. They found that the younger infants had

prolonged elimination half-lives. In the first week of life, $t_{1/2\beta}$ averaged 6.8 h, roughly threefold the value for adults reported by Stansky and associates.[40] Because of the delayed clearance, probable higher brain levels, and relatively weak respiratory reflexes, newborns should receive morphine judiciously and only in an environment in which they can be observed closely for respiratory and hemodynamic consequences. As noted by Lynn and Slattery,[41] ". . . the relationship between morphine levels and ventilatory drive in infancy remains to be determined." In our hospital, morphine is used routinely for postoperative pain for patients aged 3 months and older on the infant surgical wards; newborns to 5-month-old children frequently receive apnea monitoring if morphine is used. Morphine is used routinely for newborns, infants, and children of all ages in our intensive care units. Oral morphine elixirs are available in a number of preparations and are used widely and effectively despite the variable bioavailability. Standard initial doses are 0.1 to 0.15 mg/kg intramuscularly or subcutaneously every 3 to 4 h for postoperative pain or 0.06 mg/kg/h by continuous intravenous infusion.

Codeine. Codeine can be administered orally, intramuscularly, or subcutaneously in doses of 0.5 to 1 mg/kg every 4 h. It is an acceptable agent for moderate pain in children of all ages, although contrary to common belief,

Table 25-1
Drug Disposition in Newborns and Children

I. RELATIVE TO ADULTS, NEWBORNS HAVE
  A. Higher fraction of body weight as water.
  B. Different sizes of compartments, that is, larger vessel-rich group (relatively larger central compartment) smaller muscle and fat groups.
  C. Lower albumin concentration and binding affinity or capacity for many drugs.
  D. Variable reductions in glomerular filtration rate that are lower for prematures than term babies and reach adult values per square meter by 3 to 6 months of age
  E. Variable reductions in hepatic metabolism that depend on the particular enzyme pathway, for example, glucuronidation is poor, but sulfonation is good. Metabolism of meperidine to normeperidine is diminished.
  F. Lower values of minimal alveolor concentration for inhalation anesthetics.
  G. Lesser integrity of the blood–brain barrier. This leads to higher brain concentrations of morphine in newborn animals and may explain, in part, the occasional finding of extreme or prolonged responses to morphine in newborn humans.
  H. Pain thresholds as low as or lower than those of adults.
  I. Immaturity of respiratory control, a propensity for respiratory depression, and hypoventilation in response to hypoxemia.
  J. Incomplete myelination of tracts (functionally complete by 2 years of age).
II. RELATIVE TO ADULTS, TODDLERS AND YOUNG CHILDREN HAVE
  A. Efficient hepatic metabolism and glomerular filtration, leading to drug clearance that generally is as rapid as or more rapid than that of adults.
  B. Higher values of MAC than adults.
  C. Intact blood–brain barriers, like adults.
  D. High anxiety regarding procedures.
III. AN APPROXIMATE GUIDELINE FOR ESTIMATION OF DRUG DOSES IN CHILDREN IS (USE AS A CHECK TO AVOID DECIMAL-POINT ERRORS.)

7 Years	½ of adult dose
1 Year	¼ of adult dose
1 Month	⅛ of adult dose
Newborn	⅒ of adult dose

there is no evidence that, at equianalgesic doses, it is less sedating than other opiates.

Methadone. As with adults, two features have made methadone popular as an oral analgesic for children with severe pain: its long duration of action and its reliable absorption. Starting doses of 0.1 mg/kg every 4 h have been used for cancer pain,[42] although this may be excessive for some patients. No detailed kinetic data in children currently are available. Studies of methadone kinetics and intravenous use in children are ongoing in our institution. The prolonged half-life is convenient but demands careful adjustment of doses during the early stages.

Meperidine. Meperidine is used commonly for postoperative pain in children at doses of approximately 1 mg/kg intramuscularly every 3 to 4 h. It also is available as an elixir for oral use. Limited data indicate that the elimination half-life is similar to adult values (2.3 h) in infants and toddlers aged 3 to 18 months,[43] but it can be prolonged dramatically in newborns to 6.5 to 39 h.[44]

Fentanyl. Fentanyl can be used to treat even very sick newborns if there is hemodynamic stability.[45,46] The pharmacokinetics of fentanyl in infants and children has been described in recent reports.[47,48] In newborns, the volume of distribution of the central compartment and the steady-state volume of distribution are greater than those in adults, and the elimination half-life is prolonged to a variable degree. In some newborns, particularly those with increased abdominal pressure, elimination may be prolonged markedly.

Although fentanyl has certain kinetic and hemodynamic properties that make it useful intraoperatively in certain settings, it is used less commonly for pain because of its short duration of action and expense. It is administered commonly in our institution (along with the similar compound sufentanyl) as a continuous infusion for sedation and analgesia in newborns with persistent pulmonary hypertension. We found it useful when given as an infusion to treat some patients with cancer who have severe itching with morphine and hydromorphone. Buccal absorption of fentanyl in lollipops also is being investigated in several centers.

Local Anesthetics

General Considerations. Neonates have lower concentrations of α-1-lipoprotein and albumin than adults. This leads to reduced protein binding of local anesthetics and, in the case of bupivacaine, has been shown to result in increases in the fraction of free drug.[49] This decrease in binding is offset by the increased volume of distribution in neonates. Therefore, free drug concentrations are increased only slightly after equivalent doses.

Myelination of tracts in the spinal cord and peripheral nerves is incomplete in infants and progresses rapidly through the first 2 years of life. Theoretically, this could lead to greater susceptibility to neural blockade by local anesthetic agents,[50] although we are unaware of clinical data addressing this point. The observation of prolonged analgesia from caudal blockade in infants and toddlers compared with older children may be related to this effect.[51]

Esters. Neonates and infants up to 6 months of age have reductions in plasma cholinesterase activity to approximately one-half that of adult levels.[52] Clearance of procaine and chloroprocaine therefore might be diminished. Based on this hypothesis, published recommendations by Singler[53] suggest maximum doses of 7 mg/kg of chloroprocaine and 5 mg/kg of procaine. We are unaware of toxicity data in infants and children reported for these two agents, nor are we aware of any incidence data regarding true allergies to these agents in children. Tetracaine is used mainly for spinal anesthesia. Newborns and infants require larger doses on a per kilogram basis than adults (up to 0.5 mg/kg for prematures), and the duration of action is shorter.

Amides. Lidocaine has been studied in children using several routes of administration. Finholt and coworkers[54] studied children aged 0.5 to 3 years and found that the distribution and elimination of lidocaine after intravenous administration to this age group was the same as that for adults. Neonates have an increased volume of distribution, a slight decrease in hepatic clearance, and a slight increase in urinary excretion of both unmetabolized lidocaine and lidocaine metabolites. The terminal elimination half-life (mean value, 3.2 h) is prolonged for newborns relative to adults (1.8 h).[55] Recommended maximum doses are similar to the adult doses on a per kilogram basis (that is, 5 mg/kg without epinephrine, and 7 mg/kg with epinephrine).[56]

Clinicians using lidocaine ointments, jellies, or sprays for topical use should limit the total dose to these amounts because there are reports of convulsions in children after their use.[57] For small children, more dilute preparations may be required for mucosal use (1%) or infiltration (0.5%). Toxicity as a function of age has been studied systematically in a sheep model by Morishima and associates.[58]

Bupivacaine has achieved great popularity for neural blockade for postoperative pain because of its prolonged duration of action and the availability of concentrations (approximately, 0.25%) that produce greater sensory than motor block. In newborns, particularly sick or premature newborns, diminished levels of albumin and α-1-lipoprotein (α acid glycoprotein) may be present. Because bupivacaine is so highly protein bound, dramatic increases in the effective (unbound) drug concentration may occur. No systemic toxicity data is available, although we are aware of at least two instances of cardiac arrest in neonates attributed to overdosage. Kinetic data in newborns have been obtained by examining plasma levels after epidural administration of bupivacaine to the mothers for elective

Caesarean section.[59] The newborns showed a shorter distribution half-life and the same terminal elimination half-life (mean, 8.1 h) as did their mothers, although these values were longer than those reported by others (3.5 h) for the elimination half-life after intravenous infusion in adults.[60] Eyres and coworkers[61] and Ecoffey and colleagues[62] studied plasma levels after caudal epidural administration of bupivacaine. Toxic levels were not reached after administration of 3 mg/kg.

Nonnarcotic Analgesics

Acetaminophen. Acetaminophen is useful for mild to moderate pain in children of all ages. It can be administered for postoperative pain even to infants. It should not be discontinued automatically when narcotics are added. The standard dose is 10 mg/kg orally or 15 mg/kg rectally every 4 h.

Aspirin. The doses are the same as for acetaminophen. Aspirin should be avoided in children and adolescents during and after acute febrile illnesses because of a statistical association with the development of Reye syndrome.

Nonsteroidal Anti-Inflammatory Drugs. The side effects, efficacy, and indications of these drugs are similar to those for adults. Tolmetin is approved for use in younger children, but naproxen and ibuprofen frequently are used in adolescents and children with equally good efficacy and safety. We usually choose naproxen for those patients who find twice-daily dosing more convenient and ibuprofen for those who prefer a nonprescription medication.

Adjunctive Medications

Amitriptyline. In doses of 0.5 to 1.5 mg/kg at bedtime, amitriptyline frequently is used in several chronic pain conditions in childhood, although with the exception of headache, systematic studies of its efficacy in children are lacking. As with adults, the side effects are diminished by starting at low doses (0.25 mg/kg) and advancing slowly.

Anticonvulsants. Carbamezepine and phenytoin occasionally are useful for painful neuropathies. Carbamezepine is begun at approximately 4 mg/kg/day divided into two equal doses and advanced as tolerated in increments up to 16 mg/kg/day. The smallest effective dose should be used. Phenytoin and phenobarbital frequently are used as prophylactic medications for childhood migraine.[63] They often are effective at levels at the lower end of the anticonvulsant range.

Neuroleptics. Data on the use of butyrophenones and phenothiazines as adjunctive agents in childhood chronic pain are minimal. They frequently are used (and abused) in combination with narcotics to sedate children for procedures.

REGIONAL ANESTHESIA AND OTHER INVASIVE APPROACHES TO PAIN MANAGEMENT IN CHILDREN

General Considerations

In recent years, there has been a resurgence of interest in regional anesthesia for pediatric surgery. Regional anesthesia alone or in conjunction with light general anesthesia has been said to provide several advantages, including postoperative analgesia, with decreased narcotic analgesic use and rapid return of alertness and normal activity. Regional anesthetic techniques (such as diagnostic and therapeutic sympathetic nerve blocks and epidural narcotics) also may be used for chronic pain problems in children.

Regional anesthesia in children should be guided by the same principles and contraindications and done with the same precautions as those that apply to adults. Special attention should be directed to the differences in anatomy and pharmacokinetics of local anesthetics and narcotics in children.

The decision to administer regional anesthesia alone or in combination with general anesthesia depends on the patient's age, psychological makeup, preexisting medical conditions, surgical requirements, and the expectations of patients and their families. Most children younger than age 8 to 10 years will not hold still sufficiently to allow the precise introduction of needles needed for neural blockade. In these children, neural blockade generally is done after heavy sedation or induction of general anesthesia. Placement of an intravenous catheter always precedes major neural blockade. For infants and children aged 6 months to 5 years, their greatest fear is of their separation from their parents and restraint. For these patients, it is convenient to administer methohexital 25 to 30 mg/kg by a rectal catheter using a 10% solution. This typically will render the child unconscious and amnesic, but there still may be movement to stimulation. An alternative used in certain situations, particularly in older children who are hysterical or otherwise uncooperative, is the administration of intramuscular ketamine 3 to 4 mg/kg before induction of anesthesia. The use of ketamine may be associated with dysphoria or bad dreams even in children, and its use must be weighed against this potential adverse effect. Children aged 5 to 10 years generally accept inhalation induction with a face mask, and children older than age 10 years who are cooperative generally tolerate an intravenous catheter for induction of anesthesia or administration of agents for conscious sedation, including fentanyl and diazepam. Teen-aged and cooperative children may benefit from self-administered nitrous oxide during regional blockade and subsequently during the operative procedure.

Many adolescents are fearful of being wide awake and hearing the events during surgery. They may be reassured that it is possible to sedate them as needed during the surgery, or they may be allowed to listen to their favorite music through headphones to provide distraction and prevent them from hearing worrisome noises and conversation. During preoperative evaluation, if the adolescent remains apprehensive and if there is no clear advantage of regional over general anesthesia in regard to the patient's medical condition and proposed surgery, we do not persist in our efforts to convince the patient and parents to permit the use of regional anesthesia.

Combining a regional technique with general anesthesia raises the theoretic concern of exposing the child to the potential risks and complications of both procedures. The anesthesiologist should weigh the risks and benefits in each particular case. For example, we regard some regional techniques (such as thoracic epidural catheters) to have significant potential risk, and therefore we restrict their use to patients with strong indications (e.g., patients with severe lung disease, such as cystic fibrosis, who are undergoing thoracic or upper abdominal procedures).

Caudal Analgesia

Anatomy

In the newborn, the dural sac may extend as low as S3. The dural sac recedes with growth during the first year to its adult extension to the lower border of S2. The sacral hiatus is superficial, and the landmarks can be palpated more readily than in adults.

Technique

Caudal epidural injection can be done easily in infants and children, either with the patient in the prone or lateral decubitus positions.[53,64] After anesthetic induction or sedation and sterile preparation and draping, the sacral hiatus is palpated between the sacral cornu and above the sacrococcygeal joint. For single-shot injection, a short-beveled 21- or 22-gauge needle is advanced 2 to 3 mm through the sacrococcygeal ligament, where a loss of resistance may be felt. Unlike adults, after there is a confirmation of the position, there should be, at most, a minimal cephalad advancement of the needle to avoid dural puncture. The local anesthetic injection is preceded by aspiration tests for blood and cerebrospinal fluid and by observation of the responses to a test dose. Most commonly, bupivacaine 0.5% is used for surgical anesthesia and 0.25% is used for postoperative analgesia. Complications are the same as those described in adults.

Dose

For local anesthetic injection, there are a large number of formulas based on weight, age, number of spinal segments required, and the parameter D, which is the distance from C7 to the sacral hiatus.[65–71] The use of these formulas is more important when caudal anesthesia is used for abdominal surgery than for perineal or lower extremity surgery.

Doses of bupivacaine up to 3.7 mg/kg or lidocaine up to 5.5 mg/kg have resulted in plasma levels in infants and children below the toxic range derived from adult studies.[72–75] The reader is referred to Singler[53] for a summary of the dosing schedules.

Duration of Postoperative Analgesia

Several investigators have shown that caudal analgesia produces excellent and prolonged analgesia in infants and children undergoing a various genitourinary and lower abdominal procedures.[76–78] The duration of effect appears to be prolonged in younger patients and is prolonged substantially in children younger than age 5 years when epinephrine is added to bupivacaine.[78] In this subgroup, the mean duration of analgesia was 22.1 h. In comparing studies or subgroups in a single study, interpretation must be cautious because there is little use of formal criteria for assessing pain and there are marked differences among groups in the nature of the operations done.

Even longer-duration analgesia can be provided either by repeated injections of local anesthetics (using a 21-gauge catheter) or administration of narcotics in the caudal space. The latter technique has the additional advantages of an absence of motor and autonomic blockade and lower morbidity from inadvertent intravenous injection. Jensen[79] administered morphine by the caudal route at doses of 0.1 mg/kg as a 0.5-mg/ml solution (0.2 ml/kg) to children after genital operations. Analgesia was found to range from 10 to 36 h after a single dose. Urinary retention and pruritus can occur similar to lumbar epidural administration. No respiratory depression has been reported, but too few patients have been studied currently to draw firm conclusions in this regard, and careful postoperative observation is indicated if caudal narcotics are administered.

Lumbar and Thoracic Epidural Analgesia

Despite the short distance from the skin to the epidural space in infants and small children,[80] clinicians have reported easy identification of the intervertebral space and ligamentum flavum and easy placement of lumbar and thoracic epidural catheters in infants and small children by standard loss of resistance techniques using 17- to 19-gauge Tuohy needles and 20- to 21-gauge catheters.[81–84] Most commonly, lumbar catheters were placed at L3 to L4 or L4 to L5, and thoracic catheters were placed at several locations ranging from T5 to T6 to T7 to T8.

Meignier and associates[82] administered bupivacaine 0.25% by continuous infusion (4 mg/kg/24 h) through a thoracic epidural catheter to infants and children with severe pulmonary dysfunction undergoing upper abdominal surgery. They were able to extubate all patients postoperatively, and postoperative blood gases were equal to or better than preoperative values.

Ecoffey and colleagues[83] used intermittent injections of bupivacaine 0.25% (1.25 mg/kg) following an intraoperative dose of 4 mg/kg. The mean duration of analgesia for each injection was 8 h. Bupivacaine levels ranged up to 2.2 μg/ml, but no toxic reactions were observed. No postoperative narcotics were required.

Preliminary reports of the use of epidural narcotics for postoperative pain in children after thoracotomy and upper abdominal surgery show favorable results comparable to those reported previously in adults. Glenski and associates[84] found a mean duration of analgesia of 10.8 h after lumbar epidural morphine (average dose, 0.12 mg/kg). Doses of 0.1 mg/kg or less produced a duration of analgesia equal to larger doses with no side effects; patients receiving doses greater than 0.1 mg/kg showed an increasing incidence of minor side effects, such as nausea, vomiting, pruritus, and urinary retention.

All these studies report excellent analgesia for postoperative pain after thoracic and abdominal surgery. The side effects of epidural narcotics include pruritus, nausea, vomiting, and urinary retention. No cases of respiratory depression with epidural narcotics in children were reported in these studies, although sedation did occur. As in adults, either local anesthetics or narcotics can be administered, with similar indications and contraindications. These studies, although promising, include less than 3000 treated children. It is probably too soon to assess the risks and benefits of these techniques compared with standard management (general anesthesia followed by postoperative systemic narcotics). Despite the lack of reported problems, we believe that thoracic epidural analgesia in children should be done only in patients with specific indications, such as severe lung disease, and we believe that it should be administered only by physicians expert in the technique in adults and familiar with lumbar epidural analgesia in children. Because lumbar epidural administration of narcotics is effective even for pain originating from thoracic dermatomes, the primary situation in which thoracic epidural analgesia has a clear advantage is in the use of segmental local anesthetic blockade.

Our practice is to use an apnea device to monitor hourly respiratory rates during sleep for patients receiving neuraxial narcotics. We do not admit these patients automatically to an intensive care unit; however, most of these patients are treated in units that have nurses that are comfortable with the management of children after major surgical problems or who have chronic respiratory conditions.

Peripheral Nerve Blocks

Depending on the child's age and degree of cooperation, peripheral nerve blocks can be administered either while the patient is awake, with light sedation, or after induction of general anesthesia.

Upper Extremity

Although many approaches to the brachial plexus have been used in children,[50] only the axillary approach appears to

have had widespread popularity in younger children.[85,86] It is the safest approach. Recommended volumes for children of different ages (either lidocaine 1% or bupivacaine 0.25%) are approximately: for patients younger than age 1 year, 3 ml; for those 1 to 3 years of age, 6 to 9 ml; for those 4 to 6 years of age, 9 to 11 ml; for those 7 to 9 years of age, 14 to 20 ml; for those 10 to 12 years of age, 21 to 25 ml.

Positioning, technique, complications, and their management are similar to those in adults. The plexus lies more superficially in children, and often the axillary arterial pulsations are visible. The approach can use either paresthesias in awake and cooperative children, location using a nerve stimulator, or location of the axillary sheath by appreciation of a pop on entry and confirmation with the presence of lateral pulsation of the needle.

Lower Extremity

A femoral nerve block can be administered in combination with other blocks for surgery and to provide analgesia for patients with fractures of the femur.[87,88] The needle can be directed either by: (1) paresthesias in older and more cooperative children, (2) use of a nerve stimulator, or (3) recognition of a pop and lateral pulsation of the needle. An appropriate dose is 0.2 ml/kg of bupivacaine 0.25% (0.5 mg/kg). The technique for lateral femoral cutaneous nerve block is similar to that in adults. Singler[53] recommends either 0.1 ml/kg (0.25 mg/kg) of bupivacaine 0.25% or 0.1 ml/kg (1 mg/kg) of lidocaine 1%.

A combination of these two blocks is used along with sedation as our standard technique for muscle biopsy in children with hypotonia, myopathies, or suspected malignant hyperthermia.

Head and Neck Nerve Blocks

Nasal polypectomy and sinus drainage are among the most common operations in patients with cystic fibrosis. Blockade of the maxillary nerve (bupivacaine 0.5% with epinephrine) at the level of the sphenopalatine ganglion and the infraorbital nerve produces prolonged analgesia for these patients and permits a reduction in postoperative narcotic requirements for the first postoperative day (Berde CB and coworkers. Unpublished observations).

Neurosurgical Approaches

Although most children with intractable pain can obtain relief using systemic or neuraxial narcotics, there are situations, mostly in patients with advanced cancer, where consideration should be given to neurosurgical intervention.[89,90] There has been rapid evolution of this subject in adults but only limited experience with several of these methods in children. Technical considerations (for example, in the case of cordotomy, the choice of level, unilateral versus bilateral approach, or percutaneous versus open approach) are beyond the scope of this chapter and are governed by the experience and preference of the consultant neurosurgeon. It is likely that these approaches have been underused in children with intractable cancer pain.

COMMON PAIN SYNDROMES IN CHILDREN AND THEIR TREATMENT

Clinicians commonly state that chronic pain is rare in children or that children are not malingerers or motivated as much as adults by the secondary gain that chronic pain or disability might bring. Although there probably is some truth to the latter view, it is apparent that several types of chronic and recurrent pain are common in children and adolescents and that pain behavior can lead to loss of participation in school and other activities.

Headache

Epidemiology

Several studies confirm that headache is a common complaint in children and adolescents. In a study of 9000 school children in Sweden,[91] 40 percent of children had reported headaches by age 7 years and 75 percent by age 15 years. Migraine is common and may occur as young as 2 years of age. Functional or tension headaches are less common before age 7 years, but they are common in adolescents.

Differential Diagnosis (Table 25-2) and History

The clinician approaching children with these differential diagnoses in mind must have criteria for distinguishing the common and benign causes of headache from the rare and

Table 25-2
Common Causes of Headache in Childhood

Muscle contraction or tension headaches
  Cervical, frontal, or occipital muscle spasm or occipital neuralgia
  Nocturnal bruxism or temporomandibular joint syndrome
  Psychogenic: school phobia or depression
Migraine
  Common, classic, or complicated
Headache associated with mass effect, swelling, or inflammation
  Malignancy: brain tumor or meningeal leukemia
  Trauma: chronic subdural hematoma or postconcussion syndrome
  Cerebrospinal fluid pressure: hydrocephalus or pseudotumor cerebri
  Infection or inflammation: meningitis, brain abscess, sinusitis, or dental abscess
  Hemorrhage: arteriovenous malformation, aneurysm, or subarachnoid
Cluster headaches
Headaches during or after seizures
Eye strain
Metabolic
  Hypoglycemia (controversial)
  Lead intoxication or miscellaneous chronic ingestions
  Hypercarbia: in chronic respiratory failure, including cystic fibrosis

serious ones. In most cases, the history is the best tool for making such distinctions and guiding further evaluation. A history of rapid progression or association with neurologic deficits will direct our attention toward an expanding intracranial process.

Most commonly, headaches are chronic and not associated with progressive neurologic change, although migraine headaches sometimes are associated with frightening transient deficits. The clinician frequently tries to discriminate migraine headaches from functional or tension headaches. Features suggesting migraine include: (1) throbbing quality; (2) bifrontal, occipital, or hemicranial localization, with good reporting of localization; (3) visual aura; (4) positive family history for migraine or car sickness; (5) associated gastrointestinal disturbance, nausea, or vertigo; (6) waxing and waning course; (7) improvement with sleep or medications; and (8) occurrence at younger ages. Functional headaches more commonly are (1) not throbbing but constant aches; (2) localized more poorly; (3) likely to worsen through the day; and (4) poorly responsive to medications such as phenobarbital, propranolol, or ergot derivatives.

Physical Examination

As with adults, a major focus of examination is the search for focal or lateralizing findings or for evidence of an intracranial mass effect. The fundi always should be visualized. Continuous asymmetric bruits may suggest an arteriovenous malformation. Palpation for posterior cervical muscle spasm can be done best with the patient lying supine because these muscles have a high resting tone in the standing position. Testing for neck stiffness is important and may suggest meningitis or subarachnoid hemorrhage. The blood pressure should be measured (often omitted in children). Increasing head circumference may suggest hydrocephalus. Careful examination of the eyes, ears, and teeth may disclose easily treatable causes of headache. Facial tenderness may suggest sinusitis or temporomandibular joint disease.

Laboratory Studies

Most children can have their headaches diagnosed with confidence based on the history and physical examination alone. For those whose evaluation suggests a mass effect, seizures, or infection, additional testing would include CT scan, EEG, or lumbar puncture, as indicated by the particular presentation. Spinal tap should be preceded by examination of the fundi. In ordering these tests, clinicians must be aware of the patient's and parents' hidden fears. Where reassurance fails, there may be situations where nothing short of a CT scan will stop the patient and family from seeking other opinions and diagnoses. In this regard, consultation with a pediatric neurologist often is helpful, both to confirm or reject the diagnostic impressions, particularly in less obvious cases, and to satisfy the parents that expert opinions have found no ominous causes for their child's headaches.

Treatment

Any treatment plan begins with reassurance and education of the patient and parents. Migraine attacks, particularly those associated with transient neurologic deficits, can be frightening; a clear and convincing explanation will relieve patients and their parents, who may fear brain tumors or aneurysms. It is important to inform teachers so that they can cooperate in the child's care.

Attention should be directed toward understanding the contribution made by the child's life-style and home situation to stress and anxiety. Often, instituting regular habits of sleep, exercise, and a healthy diet (including breakfast, which many adolescents omit) may help. Use of sunglasses in direct sunlight may help some children whose headaches worsen during the summer.

Physical measures may be used if the child or adolescent finds them helpful. These may include application of heat or cold or massage of the neck or scalp muscles.

Adolescents and children older than approximately 6 years of age with either functional or muscle spasm or migraine headaches frequently respond well to progressive relaxation training with or without biofeedback training.

Drug therapy for chronic headaches in childhood is of three types. Symptomatic treatment with analgesics (including acetaminophen, aspirin, combinations, and nonsteroidal anti-inflammatory drugs) may be helpful for many children with functional or tension headaches or mild migraine headaches. Abortive treatment with ergotamine derivatives may be indicated when the headaches are too severe to be managed by simple analgesics or relaxation but too infrequent to justify prophylactic therapy. In practical terms, this often is interpreted as less often than twice monthly, although criteria vary.

For prophylactic therapy, amitriptyline, cyproheptadine, propranolol, or anticonvulsants (including phenobarbital and phenytoin) frequently are used. Amitriptyline is effective in childhood migraine, especially but not exclusively, in children with early-morning headaches, depression, or sleep disorders. The anticholinergic side effects can be diminished if treatment is begun with a low dose (12.5 mg at bedtime) and increased slowly over several days. Generally 2 weeks of treatment are required before benefit is seen; frequently there is improvement at doses below those used to treat depression (e.g., as school-aged children may be treated with 25 mg at bedtime or adolescents with 50 mg at bedtime). Propranolol is useful in complicated migraine at doses of 10 mg twice a day in school-aged children and 20 mg twice a day in adolescents, although in both groups larger doses can be administered. A history of asthma or depression are contraindications to the use of propranolol. Cyproheptadine in doses of 2 to 4 mg three or four times a day is effective, although sedation may occur. Frequent dosing makes compliance more difficult.

With any drug regimen, it cannot be overemphasized that patient education is important. There is a tendency for adolescents to become skeptical of any regimen that does not show immediate and complete efficacy, and it requires a strong therapeutic alliance between the clinician and the patient to overcome this assumption. Parents also may be skeptical and need detailed and repeated explanations of the rationale behind a pharmacologic approach. Drug therapy is used best in the setting of an overall approach that emphasizes its administration as an adjunct to the behavioral approaches outlined.

Chest Pain

Epidemiology

In adults, chest pain frequently is a sign of serious disease, particularly angina pectoris and myocardial infarction. In children and adolescents, chest pain is a common complaint, causing more than 650,000 annual physician visits. At least five series have documented that cardiac causes are rare in this age group and that musculoskeletal, functional or psychogenic, or idiopathic causes predominate. The clinician's task usually is first to exclude expeditiously but carefully serious systemic disorders. Often as described by Coleman[92] in his excellent article, the task then is to "acknowledge the pain, provide relief for the symptoms, explain the phenomenology, provide reassurance, and thereby help the patient regain any lost productivity or function".

History

Similar to any sort of pain, questions are directed toward describing the quality of the pain and its location, radiation, temporal association, and factors that relieve or exacerbate it. A careful family and social history may disclose influences on the child's pain. Cardiac pain rarely occurs at rest or on awakening. A history of exertional pain associated with fainting or rhythm disturbance ("It feels like my heart is racing, pounding, or fluttering.") merits further cardiac evaluation.

Physical Examination

A complete cardiac and pulmonary examination is indicated in all patients. Marked irregularity of the pulse, significant murmurs, or stigmata of cyanosis or congestive failure should provoke additional cardiac evaluation. Cough or mild prolongation of exhalation may be the only clues suggesting asthma in patients not experiencing acute episodes. Examination of the chest wall, sternum, xiphoid, and back and finding local tenderness to percussion or palpation may suggest musculoskeletal causes. In evaluating poorly localized pain, knowledge of the dermatomes and patterns of referred pain is essential.[93]

For the differential diagnosis and treatment, see Table 25-3.

Abdominal Pain

Epidemiology

Recurrent abdominal pain is common in school-aged children and adolescents, and may occur in up to 15 percent of the population. As noted by others,[94,95] only a very small fraction of these children have clear-cut organic causes. In most, there is a contribution from functional or psychogenic etiologic factors.

History

In addition to focusing on the quality, location, temporal associations, and exacerbating and ameliorating factors, attention should be directed toward the general review of systems and the child's social milieu, life-style, and habits.[96] Questions regarding diet and toilet habits should be specific.

Table 25-3
Common Causes of Chest Pain in Children and Adolescents

Condition	Diagnostic Clues and Characteristic Features
Musculoskeletal	Reproducible, localized, can be elicited by direct pressure.
Chest wall trauma (bruises, fractures, or muscle strain)	Original injury may have been forgotten; common in athletes; occurs often in patients who cough heavily, including those with cystic fibrosis or asthma; often responds to rest, analgesics, anti-inflammatory agents, or TENS.
Costochondritis	Characteristic localized pain on palpation, commonly at T4 to T6 on the left side; cartilaginous pains also may occur at sternoclavicular joints or xiphoid; often improves with mild analgesics.
Gynecomastia	A source of great anxiety to adolescent boys, usually treated with explanation and reassurance.
Referred vertebral pain	Should be suggested by tenderness over the spine or limited motion.
Pulmonary	Frequently diffuse; should be suggested by the presence of pulmonary signs and symptoms; common with asthma, cystic fibrosis, and pneumonia.
Gastrointestinal Esophageal pain	Esophagitis is relatively common in children and adolescents, classically substernal burning pain increased by supine position, improved by antacids; globus hystericus and aerophagia should be considered where there are indications of anxiety and depression.
Referred abdominal pain	As in adults, diaphragmatic irritation is referred to the shoulders and splenic or biliary tract pain to the costal margins
Cardiac	Rare; suggested by association with exertion, murmurs, syncope, dysrhythmia, palpitations, dyspnea; basic evaluation includes careful cardiac examination with four-extremity blood pressure measurement. Where history or examination are suggestive, chest radiograph, ECG, or oximetry can confirm or exclude most diagnoses. In difficult cases, consultation with a cardiologist, Holter monitoring, exercise ECG, or echocardiography may be helpful.
Congenital	Congenital heart disease usually presents with congestive failure cyanosis, or both but not chest pain. Although mitral prolapse is found in some adolescents with chest pain and/or supraventricular tachyarrythmias, most patients with mitral prolapse are asymptomatic. Valvular aortic stenosis or subaortic stenosis should be considered where there is exertional pain and/or syncope and appropriate murmurs. Coronary artery anomalies and aneurysms can present with exertional chest pain.
Inflammatory	Includes rheumatic carditis (rare in the United States but common in some countries), viral myocarditis or pericarditis (most commonly coxsackievirus B), and Kawasaki disease. In the US, Kawasaki disease is now the most common acquired cause of heart disease in children. Treatment includes aspirin and intravenous gamma globulin.
Idiopathic Precordial catch	Usually sharp stabbing pain of short duration precordially or at the left costal margin. Exacerbated by attempted deep breathing; episodes usually resolve within a few minutes with shallow breathing. Common in adolescents and school-aged children; reassurance is the treatment.
Stitch	Usually dull or crampy pain at costal margin (right more commonly than left) with exertion, such as running. Common home remedies include warming up before exertion and avoidance of food before exercise.
Psychogenic Hyperventilation	Diagnosis can be subtle; paresthesia and tetany may be absent.
Somaticized grief reaction or anxiety	Chest pain is common in children who have unresolved grief, especially in those whose relatives have had angina or myocardial infarction.

Table 25-4
General Classes of Recurrent Abdominal Pains in Children

General Class	Example
Gastrointestinal dysfunctions	Constipation
Intake-related pain	Lactose intolerance
Musculofascial pain	Inguinal hernia
Gynecologic or urologic conditions	Dysmenorrhea
Infections and inflammatory processes	Crohn disease
Neurologic disorders	Migraine
Metabolic disorders	Diabetes mellitus
Hematologic disorders	Sickle cell anemia
Idiopathic	Colic

Physical Examination

Careful abdominal examination should be accompanied by a full examination of the patient, with attention to the chest, back, genital, and rectal examination.

Differential Diagnosis

The reader is encouraged to consult the excellent chapter by Levine and Rappaport[95] for a detailed discussion of their diagnostic approach and a model of the interaction of somatic and psychogenic factors. In broad terms, somatic disorders can be classified as in Table 25-4.

In general, the diagnostic evaluation of abdominal pain will be conducted by a pediatrician or surgeon[97]; it is relatively uncommon for the pain specialist to aid in the diagnosis. On some occasions, local anesthetic infiltration of painful sites or superficial nerves or celiac plexus block may aid in differentiating abdominal wall versus visceral causes for the pain, particularly in cases of chronic pain after an abdominal operation.

Limb Pain

Limb pains also are common during childhood; as with other situations, the clinician frequently is asked to differentiate organic from functional causes. Features useful in making this distinction are listed in Table 25-5.

In most cases, the history and examination will direct the differential diagnosis among orthopedic, collagen vascular, infectious, neoplastic, neurologic, or metabolic causes. For many patients, referral to an orthopedic surgeon, sports-medicine specialist, rheumatologist, or neurologist is indicated for specific treatment.

Two benign diagnoses commonly applied to limb pains in childhood are fibromyalgia (myofibrositis) and growing pains.[98–100] The former term frequently is applied to describe recurrent aching pain and stiffness and points of local tenderness, frequently over tendon insertion sites. These patients often have sleep disturbance, chronic fatigue, and signs of stress. Clinicians have advocated the use of: (1) rest and reassurance, (2) massage, (3) nonsteroidal anti-inflammatory drugs, (4) amitriptyline 25 mg at bedtime, (5) TENS, (6) relaxation and biofeedback training, and (7) local injection of local anesthetics and/or corticosteroids. Because this is a confusing entity often associated with emotional distress, we would advocate treatment with all but the last item listed. There are not enough data on the use of trigger point injections in children to determine their efficacy in these conditions. The term *growing pains* frequently is applied to recurrent deep pains in the limbs, mostly lower limbs, that usually occur bilaterally and may awaken the child from sleep. Naish and Apley[99] and Oster and Nielson[100] stress that these pain syndromes appear to occur more frequently in the setting of emotional upset and in families where other members have pain complaints. Again, reassurance and emotional support seem most important in their treatment.

Reflex sympathetic dystrophy is characterized by limb pain, hyperesthesia, episodic coolness, cyanosis or swelling of the involved extremity, and loss of mobility and functioning. Traditionally, this was regarded as a condition of adults, but in recent years, it has been recognized more commonly in children and adolescents. In our clinic, we have treated 15 children and young adults with this condition during the last 6 months alone. Several patients are competitive athletes or gymnasts, and some seem to have difficult or stressful family situations. Psychosomatic factors often appear to exacerbate the syndrome.

Table 25-5
Differentiation between Organic and Functional Causes of Limb Pain in Children and Adolescents

Organic	Functional
Limp or inability to walk	Normal gait
Occurs day and night, school days and non-school days	Occurs more on school days and at night.
Interferes with play	Does not interfere with play
Associated with signs or symptoms of systemic illness	Appears basically well
Objective signs on examination, such as swelling, redness, localized tenderness, or atrophy	Lack of objective signs on examination

Two small pediatric series suggest that, in children, this syndrome is more benign and self-limited than in adults.[101,102] A study by Bernstein and colleagues[101] indicated that intensive physical therapy resulted in resolution of symptoms in a group of 20 patients over a 2-year period, without resorting to sympathetic blocks or corticosteroids. Our experience has not always been this optimistic. Although some children improved using conservative therapy, several children were referred to us after they did not improve following an extended course of physical therapy or they had pain and immobility sufficiently severe to make participation in therapy difficult.

Our therapeutic approach is outlined in Figure 25-1. Because of the benign character of the condition as seen in other pediatric centers, we begin by introducing the patient to physical therapy, evaluating them using our behavioral medicine and psychology consultants, teaching relaxation training, and administering nonsteroidal anti-inflammatory analgesics, usually either ibuprofen or naproxen. The physical therapists initiate passive range-of-motion exercises, and therapy progresses as tolerated. Because TENS is noninvasive and effective in some cases, we administer a trial course for 1 week in all cases, allowing us time to adjust lead placement, voltages, and pulse characteristics. If the patient shows good improvement in either mobility or pain during this time, then we continue with this program.

If there is no improvement and especially if the pain and immobility are so severe that physical therapy cannot be conducted, then we recommend sympathetic nerve blocks. Sympathetic blockade serves three potential functions.

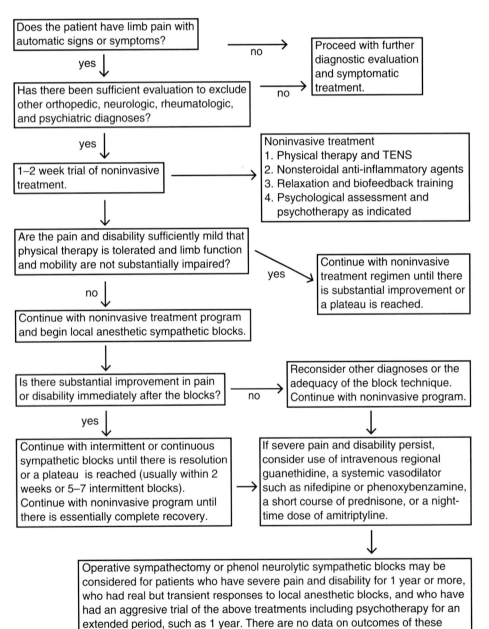

FIGURE 25-1. Reflex sympathetic dystrophy in children and adolescents: a treatment algorithm.

First, showing a loss of pain in the presence of sympathetic block and the absence of somatic block confirms the clinical impression and establishes the diagnosis. In all but one of our patients, our clinical impression was confirmed, but this step is important to show the patient and their family the nature of their condition because many have received several other diagnoses before referral to us. Second, a series of such blocks may break the pain cycle and lead to a prolonged remission or cure. Third, even in patients who have some return of symptoms, the blocks permit enough temporary improvement to allow physical therapy to begin.

The technique of sympathetic blockade is similar to standard techniques used in adults; however, there are a few features pertinent to children. For upper extremity conditions, we use a series of stellate ganglion blocks, typically four or five blocks on alternate days. Light sedation sometimes is administered (typically, fentanyl 1 to 2 μg/kg and diazepam 0.1 mg/kg intravenously or 50% nitrous oxide in oxygen by mask) if the child or adolescent is apprehensive on the first occasion. It is our impression that the block is more scary than painful and that, with adequate rapport and reassurance, sedation may not be needed subsequently or during the first occasion if the child or adolescent is calm. (Adolescents initially may be calm and then lose their composure in the middle of the procedure.) Depending on the size of the patient, we use between 6 to 12 ml of bupivacaine 0.25% after negative aspiration, easy infusion of 1 ml of normal saline, and two test doses of 0.25 ml of lidocaine 1%. For lower extremity conditions, we administer lumbar paravertebral injections of the sympathetic chain at the level of L2 or L3. We prefer to do all injections under fluoroscopic guidance and confirmation of the needle's position by contrast injection. (All adolescent girls should be quizzed without their parents being present regarding their pregnancy or birth control status.) We use the lateral decubitus position; therefore, needle tip location is defined in the medial–lateral direction by walking off the vertebral body and in the anteroposterior direction by visualization of the needle near the anterior edge of the vertebral body on the lateral view using fluoroscopy. The position then is confirmed further by a lack of resistance to injection or demonstration of a linear cephalocaudad spread of contrast material. Older patients and those who are less fearful of needles receive a series of five to seven injections (bupivacaine 0.25%, 10 to 20 ml) typically at alternate-day intervals as outpatients. For younger patients, those who are fearful of needles, and those who have not improved with previous treatments, we have, on seven occasions, placed an indwelling catheter (either a 20-gauge epidural catheter through a 7-in 17-gauge Tuohy needle or a 6-in Bard 18-gauge over-the-needle catheter) adjacent to the sympathetic chain at L2 and L3. These patients are admitted to the hospital and receive injections with bupivacaine through the catheter three to five times daily for 4 to 6 days. Because of needle passage through the psoas muscle and against the vertebral body, this procedure can cause discomfort. We generally use conscious intravenous sedation supplemented by self-administered nitrous oxide 50% in oxygen. Because these catheters tend to migrate, we place two catheters, one each at L2 and L3, under the same sedation and fluoroscopic guidance; if one stops working, then the other can be used.

Our limited experience with 15 children and young adults suggests that, in cases refractory to conservative therapy, sympathetic blockade frequently is helpful in accelerating the patient's improvement. Prospective study will be needed to clarify the indications for sympathetic blockade in children and adolescents with this condition. The reader is referred to Sullivan[103] for a discussion of sports-related limb pain in children and adolescents.

Phantom pain can occur in children of all ages after amputation. It is reasonable to try TENS, relaxation, physical measures, amitriptyline, or anticonvulsants; there are few data regarding the efficacy of these treatments for phantom pain in children.

Back Pain

Epidemiology and Differential Diagnosis

Adults and children differ markedly in the relative frequency and causes of back pain; overall, back pain is much less common in children than in adults.[104]

In children younger than age 10 years, mechanical back pain (such as muscle strain or herniated nucleus pulposus) is uncommon, although they occur rarely in children in highly competitive sports programs or in those with congenital skeletal abnormalities. Infection (osteomyelitis, diskitis, or pyelonephritis) is relatively common, and tumors (primary or metastatic, arising either in the vertebral column or the spinal cord) also can cause back pain. In younger children with back pain, an aggressive search for the cause is indicated.

In adolescents, muscle strain or overuse syndrome can be seen, particularly in athletes involved in vigorous training programs, especially in sports such as football, wrestling, and gymnastics. Scoliosis and other disorders of spinal curvature by themselves generally do not cause severe back pain in children, although they may be associated with mild aching after exertion or fatigue. Patients with Scheuerman disease (juvenile kyphosis secondary to vertebral-body wedging) frequently have aching pain after exertion. Ankylosing spondylitis and other rheumatic disorders can cause low back pain. Spondylolysis and spondylolisthesis are relatively common causes of low back pain in children older than 10 years of age, particularly in gymnasts, football players, and other athletes. Back pain is common in adolescents with sickle cell anemia.

History

As with adults, it is important to inquire regarding precipitating factors (including trauma, recent changes in activity, symptoms of systemic disease, and a detailed description of the location and nature of the pain). Changes in gait or control of bowel and bladder function are significant.

Physical Examination

The general examination should include thorough neurologic, chest, and abdominal examinations. Orthopedic examination should include a brief assessment of upper and lower limb joints for deformity and adequacy of range of motion. Inspection of the back should disclose postural abnormalities (scoliosis, lordosis, or kyphosis) and cutaneous abnormalities suggesting neural tube defects. Detailed palpation of the back discloses sites of local tenderness or muscle spasm. Forward bending from a standing position shows abnormalities of range of motion and spinal curvature. Gait should be assessed carefully.

Laboratory Studies

Where guided by history and physical examination, complete blood count, erythrocyte sedimentation rate, blood culture, urinalysis, and urine culture may aid in the diagnosis of infectious or systemic causes. Specific immunologic or rheumatologic testing (antinuclear antibody, rheumatoid factor, histocompatibility antigen B27 typing) or biopsy of vertebra or disk space may be indicated in certain cases.

Anteroposterior and lateral spine roentgenograms generally are indicated to screen for bony abnormalities, fractures, and dislocations. If there is suspicion of infection or tumor, a radionuclide bone scan is a sensitive indicator. In the presence of neurologic abnormalities, spinal CT scan or myelography can be used to locate sites of compression of spinal cord or nerve roots.

Treatment

The treatment will vary depending on the underlying disorder, and referrals to orthopedic surgeons, rheumatologists, neurologists, and neurosurgeons may be indicated for specific diagnosis and treatment. Symptomatic treatment with rest and nonsteroidal anti-inflammatory agents generally is helpful for pain caused by overuse.

Cancer Pain

Pain is a frequent finding in children with cancer,[105] as in adults. Surveys show significant pain in approximately one-half of children in an inpatient cancer center. Childhood cancers have a different spectrum of sites and different biology from the common adult cancers. In children, leukemias, lymphomas, and primary brain tumors of the posterior fossa are relatively common; carcinomas are relatively rare. As outlined in Table 25-6, the pain may be the result of the tumor directly, or it may be associated with aspects of cancer therapy. Some guidelines for treatment are as follows.

Table 25-6
Pain Syndromes in Children with Cancer

Pain Caused by Tumor Invasion or Infiltration
  Visceral pain
    Liver and spleen may be enlarged and painful in patients with leukemia or lymphoma.
    Intraabdominal tumors (lymphoma, Wilm, neuroblastoma, or rhabdomyosarcoma of the bladder) may cause stretching of any abdominal viscera.

  Bone pain
    Leukemia and lymphoma, particularly in cases resistant to treatment, may pack the marrow and cause pain in the long bones, back, sternum, pelvis, or skull.
    Primary tumors of bone, particularly osteogenic sarcoma, cause pain both at primary and metastatic sites in bone.

  Nerve pain
    Compression of peripheral nerves, plexuses, roots, or spinal cord may cause severe pain in patients with metastatic sarcomas and lymphomas.

  Headache
    May be related to intracranial pressure, hemorrhage, metabolic imbalance, or tension.

Pain Related to Cancer Therapy
  Painful procedures
    Bone marrow aspirate and biopsy.
    Lumbar puncture.
    Venipuncture and intravenous catheter placement.

  Postoperative pain
    Incisional pain from thoracotomy or laparotomy.
    Phantom pain (common after limb amputation for osteogenic sarcoma or Ewing sarcoma).

  Postchemotherapy or postradiotherapy pain
    Neuralgia associated with vincristine.
    Mucositis or esophageal ulceration associated with chemotherapy, radiotherapy or infection.
    Hemorrhagic cystitis.

1. Fear, anxiety, and depression are prominent in children with cancer, and attention should be paid to these factors. Where possible, relaxation, hypnosis, or involvement in activities should be used. Often in younger children, the fear of the disease or dying is either too abstract to be verbalized or is made taboo by equally terrified parents. In this setting, the child's focusing on pain may be intensified by being unable to confront these other fears.

2. Flexibility in routes for narcotic administration is required.[106] For patients with moderate pain who do not have severe nausea, oral narcotics may be effective. In other patients with nausea or severe mucositis, swallowing medications may be impossible, and rectal or parenteral drugs are required. If a patient has an available central line port or other easy intravenous access, then continuous intravenous infusion may be the easiest. If these are unavailable, then continuous subcutaneous infusion may be acceptable. The doses for these two types of infusion are approximately equal.

3. When using oral narcotics, we recommend combining a long-acting agent, methadone, with a short-acting agent, usually either hydromorphone, codeine, or oxycodone while the dose of methadone is being titrated. The methadone is given on a fixed schedule (not as needed) three to five times daily to provide a steady basal level of analgesia. For many patients, this is sufficient. If there is increased pain, then hydromorphone or oxycodone may be taken as needed. If these drugs are required daily for several days, then the fixed methadone dose can be increased. If sedation ensues and this is felt by the patient to be undesirable, the methadone dose can be reduced. This approach helps to combat a common problem with methadone; the prolonged half-life makes titration difficult. The new time-release forms of oral morphine have not been extensively studied in children but hold considerable promise because they require much less frequent dosing.

4. Continuous intravenous or subcutaneous infusions generally are made using morphine or hydromorphone, although methadone or fentanyl also are used. Meperidine should not be administered chronically in high doses because there is a risk of convulsions from the metabolite normeperidine. Good results were reported with continuous narcotic infusions intravenously[107] and subcutaneously[108] in children with cancer. The median effective morphine infusion rate used was 0.06 mg/kg/h for the subcutaneous route and 0.04 to 0.07 mg/kg/h for the intravenous route, although there was substantial individual variation. Patients often may require up to 2 mg/kg/h for pain in terminal cancer. In most children, such infusions will relieve pain adequately. In a small number of cases, even when the infusion is titrated to the point of respiratory depression and sedation, pain relief is not adequate.

5. Adjunctive medications, including antidepressants, antiemetics, and stimulants, are useful, but their administration should be tailored to the individual patient's needs and wishes. For example, some children find phenothiazines, butyrophenones, or cannabinoids so dysphoric that they prefer to experience increased nausea; other children are calmed by these agents and find them helpful for nausea.

   For many children who find narcotics excessively sedating, a small oral dose of dextroamphetamine (0.05 to 0.2 mg/kg) in the morning potentiates narcotic analgesia and combats sedation.

   For many children with anxiety, depression, or disturbed sleep, a small oral dose of amitriptyline (0.5 to 1.5 mg/kg) or another tricyclic or tetracyclic antidepressant at bedtime potentiates narcotic analgesia and appears to improve mood and sleep patterns. Similar to adults, it is best to start at low doses and increase them gradually to diminish the anticholinergic side effects.

   Because children with cancer vary so much in their associated complaints and need for adjunctive medications, we prefer to tailor a regimen individually rather than using a fixed combination, such as the many preparations of so-called Brompton solution.

6. We should anticipate and treat side effects, including nausea, pruritus, constipation, and urinary retention. If tolerance develops, increase doses appropriately.

7. Most children with cancer can be made comfortable if the regimen outlined in Steps 1 to 6 is optimized. Nevertheless, there are a small number of children, usually with widespread bony metastases and nerve root compression, who remain in severe pain despite receiving large doses of narcotics (e.g., hundreds of milligrams of morphine hourly). In these patients, lumbar epidural or subarachnoid catheter placement for administration of narcotics or local anesthetics[109] or neurolytic blocks and neurosurgical procedures may be considered. When the local anesthetic is given initially through an epidural or subarachnoid catheter to patients receiving large doses of narcotic, it should be given in small doses at first. The sudden disappearance of the pain can make the patient rapidly and profoundly narcotized. Epidural and subarachnoid catheters can be placed percutaneously and tunneled subcutaneously in a patient of any age by appropriately experienced personnel; home administration of neuraxial medications by continuous infusion is practical in many areas through home-care companies and visiting nurses familiar with these techniques, which are used widely in adults.

As noted, if these techniques do not provide relief, neurosurgical consultation should be obtained for consideration of ablative procedures.

Painful Crisis in Sickle Cell Anemia

Episodic pain in patients with sickle cell anemia usually is caused by occlusion of small blood vessels by sickled erythrocytes, with infarction or ischemia occurring distally. In young children, this frequently involves the small bones of the extremities (dactylitis or hand–foot syndrome). In older children and adults, common locations of pain are the low back, the abdomen, and the long bones. Vasoocclusion may be precipitated or exacerbated by hypoxemia, acidosis, hypovolemia, hypoperfusion, cold, immobility, or infection.

Although the pain is a result of vasoocclusion, clinicians should understand that bone pain may be secondary to bacterial osteomyelitis, right upper quadrant pain may be caused by cholelithiasis, and left upper quadrant pain may be the result of splenic infarction or sequestration. The severity of the pain and the frequency of episodes are variable. For many patients, rest, oral hydration, and mild analgesics (such as ibuprofen and codeine) are adequate.

For a smaller subgroup of patients, the pain may be severe, and intravenous narcotic analgesics and intravenous hydration are indicated. We agree with Piatt and Nathan[110] and disagree with a standard text[111] that it is appropriate to give adequate doses of narcotics for severe pain in these patients and not to withhold them because of a fear of addiction. Indeed, intermittent and grudging treatment seem to us more likely to predispose the patient to addiction. Initial control of pain by intravenous narcotic infusion should proceed in conjunction with starting oral narcotics (such as methadone) and nonnarcotics (such as ibuprofen and acetaminophen). We encourage TENS use and any other physical measures that the patient finds helpful. In patients with severe crisis pain, adjustment of the narcotic dose may be difficult. Hypoxemia secondary to hypoventilation from narcotic-induced respiratory depression may be especially harmful in these patients because it may precipitate further sickling and vasoocclusion. For a small number of patients in whom it is difficult to find a narcotic regimen that leaves the patient neither in agony nor heavily sedated and in whom the pain is appropriately localized, we recommend either major plexus nerve blocks or epidural analgesia with either narcotics or local anesthetics either by intermittent bolus or continuous infusion techniques. We have administered successfully epidural local anesthetics (bupivacaine) and narcotics (fentanyl or hydromorphone) for leg pain and chest pain (morphine) in this condition. For these severely affected patients, the benefits of hypertransfusion for terminating vasoocclusion must be weighed by the patient and the hematologist against the risks from iron overload, sensitization, and transfusion-acquired infections.

Postoperative and Posttraumatic Pain

Treatment of postoperative pain in infants and children requires an understanding of the differences in reporting pain, pain behaviors, and physiologic responses outlined earlier in this chapter.[112] Children may not be able to report their postoperative pain, either because they are preverbal or frightened, their speech may be restricted by endotracheal tubes or other apparatus, or consciousness is depressed after a general anesthetic. Clinicians caring for infants and children therefore must understand behavioral and physiologic signs of pain and evaluate the entire clinical picture rather than a single sign.[113] For example, a toddler's crying may indicate pain, but it also may indicate missing their mother. Similarly, tachycardia may be secondary to pain, but the clinician also must consider other causes common during the postoperative period, such as hypoxemia and hypovolemia. Children who have been burned are frequently in severe pain and required to undergo recurrent painful dressing changes. Szyfelbein and colleagues[114] studied subjective (visual analog) pain scores, behavioral observations, and plasma endorphin-like immunoreactivity in children undergoing burn dressing changes. There was an inverse relationship between pain

scores and apparent endorphin levels. The visual analog scale (so-called pain thermometer) appeared to these investigators to be an excellent tool for pain assessment in these children.

Treatment Guidelines

1. The experience of postoperative pain in children is exacerbated by fear and can be ameliorated in most cases by a straightforward preoperative description of what the child can expect postoperatively. The presence of parents on the ward, play rooms, and activity therapists can be invaluable to produce a favorable emotional response to the perioperative period.
2. Where feasible, local anesthetic blockade of the incision or appropriate nerves intraoperatively should be used.
3. For mild to moderate pain, oral acetaminophen can be combined with oral narcotics, such as codeine (0.5 to 1 mg/kg every 3 to 4 h) or oxycodone (0.05 to 0.2 mg/kg every 3 to 4 h).
4. For severe pain, standard intramuscular therapy is morphine 0.1 to 0.15 mg/kg every 3 to 4 h. Although fairly effective, this route has disadvantages, such as the pain associated with intramuscular injection that provokes anxiety, the peaks and troughs in levels that can occur with 4-h dosing, and the peak effect that occurs 20 to 30 min after injection, when monitoring may be diminished.

   Alternatives are continuous morphine infusion (median rate, 0.06 mg/kg/h) that provides relatively constant levels, avoids intramuscular injections, and requires infusion pumps and observation for delayed effects as the levels slowly rise. Intermittent intravenous morphine boluses may be given that produce great fluctuation in levels unless given at short intervals (less than every 2 h). Alternatively, intermittent intravenous methadone boluses may be administered. As described by Gourlay and coworkers[115] for adults, the long elimination half-life of methadone permits intermittent intravenous boluses to be used as a so-called poor man's drip. Observations indicate that methadone also produces prolonged postoperative analgesia in children.[116] Patient-controlled analgesia may be used. This is effective and probably ideal for adolescents but not for younger children. An expensive computer-driven pump is required, but the pump can be misprogrammed if the health-care professional is not experienced in its use.

INITIAL EXPERIENCE WITH A PEDIATRIC PAIN TREATMENT SERVICE

In the treatment of adults with chronic pain, clinicians have noticed the advantages of a multidisciplinary approach. Such an approach (1) draws on the expertise of professionals with many different forms of training; (2) encourages concomitant use of medications, physical therapy, and psychologic techniques; (3) discourages the tendency of patients to shop around; and (4) permits practical coverage by a group of physicians who may only be able to devote a portion of their time to pain therapy. This model rarely has been used in children, in part because (1) of a widespread belief that children rarely experience chronic pain, (2) most centers do not have a sufficient volume of pediatric patients, (3) regional anesthetic techniques have been widely used in children only recently; (4) frequently pediatricians and pediatric subspecialists (especially pediatric oncologists), to their credit, are willing to remain generalists and manage their patients' pain problems and psychosocial problems along with treating underlying medical conditions, and (5) although pediatric chronic pain conditions are common, school absenteeism has less of an economic impact than the loss of work time seen in adults with chronic pain.

At Boston's Children's Hospital, one of us recently established a multidisciplinary group for pain management that includes: (1) two psychologists with expertise in relaxation, biofeedback, hypnosis, and psychotherapy; (2) three pediatric anesthesiologists with expertise in pharmacology and nerve blocks; (3) three pediatric hematologist–oncologists who frequently manage pain in children with cancer and sickle cell anemia; (4) two clinical pharmacologist–toxicologists with expertise in therapeutics and techniques of drug assay; (5) eight nurses from the recovery room, orthopedic ward, nursery, and oncology wards who

Table 25-7
Pain Treatment Service Referrals (In a Six-Month Period)

Presenting Diagnoses	No. of Patients
Headache	44
Reflex sympathetic dystrophy	15
Cancer pain	6
Sickle cell crisis pain	7
Perioperative pain with severe respiratory disease	16
Cystic fibrosis (8)	
Bronchopulmonary dysplasia (4)	
Other (4)	
Chest pain (unrelated to cancer or sickle cell anemia)	6
Cystic fibrosis (5)	
Albright disease (1)	
Miscellaneous limb pains	5
Phantom limb (2)	
Rheumatoid arthritis (1)	
Other (2)	
Abdominal pain (unrelated to cancer or sickle cell anemia)	7
Chronic pancreatitis (2)	
Postoperative nerve entrapment (2)	
Crohn disease (1)	
Other (2)	
Back pain unrelated to cancer or sickle cell anemia	1
Psychogenic pain	1
Narcotic dependency or withdrawal	4
Drug interactions	6
Total	118

Procedures		No. Done
Epidural catheters	Thoracic (5 rib fractures in a patient with cystic fibrosis)	1
	Lumbar (perioperative, sickle cell crisis, cancer, and reflex sympathetic dystrophy)	19
	Caudal (perioperative use, bronchopulmonary dysplasia, or apnea of prematurity)	4
Subarachnoid catheter	(terminal malignancy in a patient with widespread epidural and bony metastases)	1
Sympathetic blocks	(reflex sympathetic dystrophy only)	
	Intermittent lumbar	30
	Continuous lumbar	10
	Stellate	24
Peripheral nerve or trigger point diagnostic infiltration		2
Continuous axillary block		2
Pleural catheter		3
Intercostal blocks		4
Total		100

have extensive clinical experience in the care of children with pain; (6) an orthopedic surgeon who directs the sports-medicine program; (7) a pediatric surgeon interested in postoperative pain management; (8) a physical therapist who is expert in the use of TENS and the rehabilitation of patients with reflex sympathetic dystrophies; (9) a pediatric neurologist interested in the treatment of headache; and (10) a general pediatrician interested especially in recurrent abdominal pain. In addition, a pediatric rheumatologist and a neurosurgeon are consulted regularly regarding diagnostic issues. The objectives of the group include: (1) inpatient consultation and treatment for acute and chronic pain; (2) outpatient consultation and treatment; (3) preparation of teaching materials for nurses, residents, and other groups; (4) a biweekly forum for educating members of the group about each other's expertise and about cross referrals of patients; and (5) critical appraisal of clinical research protocols regarding the study of pain in children.

The anesthesiologists of the group typically see approximately three new patients and three to four follow-up patients a week for treatments, including general evaluation and referral, adjustment of drug regimens, TENS, and nerve blocks or perioperative use of epidural catheters for high-risk patients. With rare exceptions, patients receive psychological assessment, relaxation training, physical therapy, TENS, and some type of systemic analgesic agent before consideration of nerve blocks. The psychologists of the group participate in a behavioral medicine service that treats large numbers of children with headache and other chronic pain syndromes using relaxation, biofeedback, and hypnosis techniques. The anesthesiologists, surgeon, orthopedist, and nurses are involved in a prospective study of postoperative pain assessment and treatment in children. Children with chronic abdominal pains are seen in a separate clinic, as described previously by Drs. Levine and Rappaport.[95]

A summary of the referrals during the past 6 months is included in Table 25-7. It is apparent that the distribution of complaints is different from that seen in most adult pain services. It is too early to determine whether such a multidisciplinary approach will be widely applicable in children. Our initial impression is that it will be.[117]

References

1. Weisman SJ, Schecter NL. The management of pain in children. *Pediatr Rev* February; 1991; 12(8):237–243.
2. McGraw MD. Neural maturation as exemplified in the changing reactions of the infant to pinprick. *Child Dev* 1941; 9:31.
3. Schuster A, Lenard HG. Pain in newborns and prematures: current practice and knowledge. *Brain Dev* 1990; 12(5):459–465.
4. Porter F. Pain in the newborn. *Clin Perinatol* June 1989; 16(2):549–564.
5. Haslam DR. Age and the perception of pain. *Psychosom Sci* 1969; 15:86.
6. Levine JD, Gordon NC. Pain in the prelingual children and its evaluation by pain induced vocalization. *Pain* 1982; 14:85–93.
7. Harpin VA, Rutter N. Development of emotional sweating in the newborn infant. *Arch Dis Child* 1982; 57:691–695.
8. Williamson PS, Williamson ML. Physiologic stress reduction by local anesthetic during newborn circumcision. *Pediatrics* 1983; 71:36–40.
9. Brazelton TB. Neonatal behavioral assessment scale re: Brazelton neonatal assessment scale. In: *Clinical and Developmental Medicine*. Vol 50. 2nd ed. Philadelphia: Lippincott; 1984.
10. Hickey PR, Hansen DD, Wessel DL, Lang P, Jonas RA, Elixson EM. Blunting of stress responses in the pulmonary circulation of infants by fentanyl. *Anesth Analg* 1985; 64:1137–1142.
11. Truog R, Anand KJ. Management of pain in the postoperative neonate. *Clin Perinatol* March 1989; 16(1):61–78.
12. Tucker MA, Andrew MF, Ogle SJ, Davison JG. Age-associated change in pain threshold measured by transcutaneous neuronal electrical stimulation. *Age Ageing* July 1989; 18(4):241–246.
13. McGrath PA. Evaluating a child's pain. *J Pain Symptom Manage* December 1989; 4(4):198–214.
14. Tesler M, Ward J, Savedra M. Developing an instrument for eliciting children's description of pain. *Percept Motor Skills* 1983; 56:315–321.
15. Katz ER, Kellerman J, Siegel SE. Behavioral distress in children with cancer undergoing medical procedures: developmental considerations. *J Consult Clin Psychol* 1980; 48:356–365.
16. Jay SM, Ozolins M, Eliot CH. Assessment of children's distress during painful medical procedures. *Health Psychol* 1983; 2:133–147.
17. Schecter NL. Pain and pain control in children. *Curr Probl Pediatr* March 1985; 15(5):1–67.
18. Eland JM, Anderson JE. The experience of pain in children. In: Jacox A, ed. *Pain: A Source Book for Nurses and Other Health Professionals*. Boston: Little, Brown: 1977.
19. Masek BJ, Russo DC, Varni JW. Behavioral approaches to the management of chronic pain in children. Symposium on recurrent pain in children. *Pediatr Clin North Am* October 31 1984; 5:1113–1131.
20. Benson H. *The Relaxation Response*. New York: William Morrow; 1975.
21. Mehagan J, Masek BJ, Harrison W, Russo DC, Leviton A. A multi-component behavioral treatment for pediatric migraine. *Clin J Pain* 1986. In press.
22. Hilgard J, Hilgard E. Hypnosis in the relief of pain. Los Altos, CA: Kaufmann; 1986.
23. Hilgard J, LeBaron S. Hypnotherapy of pain in children with cancer. Los Altos, CA: Kaufmann; 1984.
24. Gardner CG, Olness K. Hypnosis and hypnotherapy with children. Orlando, FL: Grune & Stratton; 1981.
25. Goldstein A, Hilgard E. Lack of influence of the morphine antagonist naloxone on hypnotic analgesia. *Proc Natl Acad Sci U S A,* 1975; 72:2041–2043.
26. Morgan AH, Hilgard ER. Age differences in susceptibility to hypnosis. *Int J Clin Exp Hypn* 1973; 21:78–85.
27. Morgan AH, Hilgard ER. The Stanford hypnotic clinical scale for children. *Am J Clin Hypn* 1978–1979; 21:148–169.

28. Olness K. Imagery (self-hypnosis) as adjunct therapy in childhood cancer. Clinical experience with 25 patients. *J Pediatr Hematol/Oncol* 1981; 3:313–321.

29. Gardner GG. Hypnosis with infants and preschool children. *Am J Clin Hypn* 1977; 19:158–162.

30. Morgan AE, Hilgard E. The Stanford hypnotic clinical scale for children. *Am J Clin Hypn* 1978–1979; 21:148–169.

31. London P, Cooper SA. Norms of hypnotic susceptibility in children. *Dev Psychol* 1969; 1:113–124.

32. Gardner GG, Olness K. Some guidelines for uses of hypnotherapy in pediatrics. *Pediatrics* 1976; 62:228–233.

33. Zelter L, LeBaron S. Hypnotic and nonhypnotic techniques for reduction of pain and anxiety during painful procedures in children and adolescents with cancer. *J Pediatr* 1982; 101:1032–1035.

34. Hilgard JR, LeBaron S. Relief of anxiety and pain in children and adolescents with cancer. Quantitative measures and clinical observations. *Int J Clin Exp Hypn* 1982; 417–442.

35. Dahlstrom B, Bolme P, Feychting H, Noack G, Paalzow L. Morphine kinetics in children. *Clin Pharmacol Ther* September 1979; 354–365.

36. Yaster M, Deshpande JK, Maxwell LG. The pharmacologic management of pain in children. *Compr Ther* October 1989; 15(1):14–26.

37. Gaukroger PB. Pediatric analgesia. Which drug? Which dose? *Drugs* January 1991; 41(1):52–59.

38. Shannon M, Berde CB. Pharmacologic management of pain in children and adolescents. *Pediatr Clin North Am* August 1989; 36(4):855–871.

39. Lynn AM, Slattery JT. Pharmacokinetics of morphine sulfate in early infancy. *Anesthesiology* 1985; 63(3):A349.

40. Stansky DR, Greenblatt DJ, Lowenstein E. The kinetics of intravenous and intramuscular morphine. *Clin Pharmacol Ther* 1978; 24:52–59.

41. Lynn AM, Slattery JT. Pharmacokinetics of morphine sulfate in early infancy. *Anesthesiology* 1985; 63(3A):A349.

42. Ettinger DS, Vitale PJ, Trump DL. Important clinical pharmacological considerations in the use of methadone in cancer patients. *Cancer Treat Rep* 1979; 63:457–459.

43. Atwood GF, Evans MA, Harbison RD. Pharmacokinetics of meperidine in infants. *Pediatr Res* 1976; 10:328.

44. Morselli PL, Rovei V. Placental transfer of pethidine and norpethidine and their pharmacokinetics in the newborn. *Eur J Clin Pharmacol* 1980; 18:25.

45. Robinson SR, Gregory GA. Fentanyl–air oxygen anesthesia for ligation of patent ductus arteriosus in preterm infants. *Anesth Analg* 1981; 60:50.

46. Hickey PR, Hansen DD. Fentanyl and sufentanil–oxygen–pancuronium anesthesia for cardiac surgery in infants. *Anesth Anagl* 1984; 63:117–124.

47. Johnson KL, Erickson JP, Holley FO, Scott JC. Fentanyl pharmacokinetics in the pediatric population. *Anesthesiology* 1984; 61(3A):A441.

48. Koehntop DE, Rodman JH, Brundage DM, Hegland MG, Buckley JJ. Pharmacokinetics of fentanyl in neonates. *Anesth Analg* 1986; 65:227–232.

49. Mather LE, Long GJ, Thomas J. The binding of bupivacaine to maternal and foetal plasma proteins. *J Pharm Pharmacol* 1971; 23:359–365.

50. Cousins MJ, Bridenbaugh PO. *Neural Blockade in Clinical Anesthesia and Management of Pain*. New York: Lippincott; 1983.

51. Warner, et al. *ASA Annual Meeting* September 1985; 63:A464. Abstract.

52. Zsigmond DK, Downs JR. Plasma cholinesterase activity in newborns and infants. *Can Anaesth Soc J* 1971; 18:278.

53. Singler RC. Pediatric regional anesthesia. In: Gregory GA, ed. *Pediatric Anesthesia*. New York: Churchill Livingstone; 1983.

54. Finholt DA, Stirt JA, DiFazio CA, Moscicki JC. Lidocaine pharmacokinetics in children during general anesthesia. *Anesth Analg* 1986; 65:279–282.

55. Mihaly GW, Moore RG, Thomas J, et al. The pharmacokinetics and metabolism of the anilide local anesthetics in neonates. *Eur J Clin Pharmacol* 1978; 13:143–152.

56. Tucker GT, Mather LE. Pharmacokinetics of local anaesthetic agents. *Br J Anaesth* 1975; 47:213.

57. Rothstein P, Dornbusch J, Shaywitz BA. Prolonged seizures associated with the use of viscous lidocaine. *J Pediatr* 1982; 101:461–463.

58. Morishima HO, Pederson H, Finster M, et al. Toxicity of lidocaine in adult, newborn and fetal sheep. *Anesthesiology* 1981; 55:57–61.

59. Magno R, Berlin A, Karlsson K, Kjellmer I. Anesthesia for Caesarean section, IV: placental transfer and neonatal elimination of bupivacaine following epidural analgesia for elective analgesia for elective Caesarean section. *Acta Anaesth Scand* 1976; 20:141–146.

60. Tucker GT, Mather LE. Clinical pharmacokinetics of local anesthetics. *Clin Pharmacokinet* 1979; 4:241–278.

61. Eyres RL, Bishop W, Oppenheim RC, Brown TCK. Plasma bupivacaine concentrations in children during caudal epidural analgesia. *Anaesth Intensive Care* 1983; 11:20–22.

62. Ecoffey C, Desparme J, Maury M, Berdeaux A, Giudicelli J, St-Maurice C. Bupivacaine in children: pharmacokinetics following caudal anesthesia. *Anesthesiology* 1985; 63:447–448.

63. Barlow CF. *Headaches and Migraine in Childhood*. London: Spastics; 1984.

64. Touloukian RJ, Wugmeister M, Pickett LK, Hehre FW. Anesthesia for neonatal anoperineal and rectal operations. *Anesth Analg* 1971; 50:565.

65. Takasaki M, Dohi S, Kawabata Y, Takahashi T. Dosage of lidocaine for caudal anesthesia in infants and children. *Anesthesiology* 1977; 47:527–529.

66. Shulte-Steinberg O, Rahlfs VW. Spread of extradural analgesia following caudal injection in children. *Br J Anaesth* 1977; 49:1027–1034.

67. Schulte-Steinberg O, Rahlfs VW. Caudal anesthesia in children and spread of 1 percent lignocaine. *Br J Anaesth* 1970; 42:1093–1099.

68. Satoyoshi M, Kamiyama Y. Caudal anesthesia for upper abdominal surgery in infants and children: a simple calculation of the volume of local anesthetic. *Acta Anaesth Scand* 1984; 28:57–60.

69. Melman E, Arenas JA, Tandazo WE. Caudal anesthesia for pediatric surgery: an easy and safe method for calculating dose requirements. *Anesthesiology* 1985; 63(3):A463.

70. Spiegel P. Caudal anesthesia in pediatric patients: a preliminary report. *Anesth Analg (Cleve)* 1962; 41:218.

71. Fortuna A. Caudal anesthesia: a simple and safe technique in paediatric surgery. *Br J Anaesth* 1967; 39:165–169.

72. Lourey CS, McDonald IH. Caudal anesthesia in infants and children. *Anaesth Intensive Care* 1973; 1:547–548.

73. Takasaki M, Dohi S, Kawabata Y, et al. Dosage of lidocaine for caudal anesthesia in infants and children. *Anesthesiology* 1977; 47:527.

74. Takasaki M. Blood concentrations of lidocaine, mepivacaine and bupivacaine during caudal analgesia in children. *Acta Anesthesiol Scand* 1984; 28:211–214.

75. Ecoffey C, Desparme J, Maury M, Berdeaux A, Giudicelli J, St-Maurice C. Bupivacaine in children: pharmacokinetics following caudal anesthesia. *Anesthesiology* 1985; 63:447–448.

76. Lourey CJ, McDonald IH. Caudal anesthetic in infants and children. *Anaesth Intensive Care* 1973; 1:547–548.

77. Broadman L. Regional anesthesia and post-operative analgesia in pediatrics. *A S A Ann Refresher Course Lect* 1985; 153:1–6.

78. Warner MA, Kunrel SE, Dawson B, Atchison SR. The effects of age and the addition of epinephrine to bupivacaine for caudal anesthesia in pediatric patients. *Anesthesiology* 1985; 63(3A):A464.

79. Jensen BH. *Acta Anesth Scand* 1981; 25:373–375.

80. Kosaka Y, Sato I, Kawaguchi L. Distance from skin to epidural space in children. *Jpn J Anesthesiol* 1974; 23:874.

81. Ecoffey C, Dubousset AM, Samii K. Lumbar and thoracic epidural anesthesia for urologic and upper abdominal surgery in infants and children. *Anesthesiology* 1986; 65:87–90.

82. Meignier M, Souron R, Leneel J. Postoperative dorsal epidural analgesia in the child with respiratory disabilities. *Anesthesiology* 1983; 59:5:473–475.

83. Ecoffrey C, Dubousset AM, Samii K. Lumbar and thoracic epidural anesthesia for urologic and upper abdominal surgery in infants and children. *Anesthesiology* 1986; 65:87–90.

84. Glenski JA, Warner MA, Dawson B, Kaufman B. Postoperative use of epidurally administered morphine in children and adolescents. *Mayo Clin Proc* 1984; 59:530–533.

85. Eriksson E. Axillary brachial plexus anesthesia in children with Citanest. *Acta Anesthesiol Scand* 1965; 16:291.

86. Niesel HC, Rodrigues P, Wilsmann I. Regional Anesthesie der oberen Extremitat bei Kindern. *Anaesthetist* 1974; 23:176.

87. Berry FR. Analgesia in patients with fractured shaft of femur. *Anaesthesia* 1977; 32:576.

88. Grossbard GD, Love BRT. Femoral nerve block: a simple and safe method of instant analgesia for femoral shaft fractures in children. *Aust N Z Surg* 1979; 49:592.

89. Matson DD. Neurosurgery of infancy and childhood. Springfield: Charles C Thomas; 1969:847–851.

90. Wilkins RH, Rengachary SS. *Neurosurgery III.* Part XIII. New York: McGraw-Hill; 1985:303–334.

91. Bille B. Migraine in schoolchildren. *Acta pediatr Scand* 1962; 51(suppl 136):1–151.

92. Coleman WL. Recurrent chest pain in children. Symposium on recurrent pain in children. *Pediatr Clin North Am* Oct 31, 1984; 5:1007–1026.

93. Selbst SM. Chest pain in children. *Am Fam Physician* January 1990; 41(1):179–186.

94. Barr RG. Recurrent abdominal pain. In: Levine MD, et al, eds. *Developmental Behavioral Pediatric.* Philadelphia: Saunders; 1983.

95. Levine MD, Rappaport LA. Recurrent abdominal pain in children. Symposium on recurrent pain in children. *Pediatr Clin North Am* October 1984; 5:969–991.

96. Buchert GS. Abdominal pain in children: an emergency practitioner's guide. *Emerg Med Clin North Am* August 1989; 7(3):497–517.

97. Silverberg M. Chronic abdominal pain in adolescents. *Pediatr Ann* April 1991; 20(4):179–185.

98. Bowyer SL, Hollister JR. Limb pain in childhood. *Pediatr Clin North Am* 1984; 31:1053–1081.

99. Naish JM, Apley J. Growing pains. A clinical study of non-arthritic limb pains in children. *Arch Dis Child* 1951; 26:134.

100. Oster J, Nielson A. Growing pains: a clinical investigation of a school population. *Acta Pediatr Scand* 1972; 61:329.

101. Bernstein BH, Singsen BH, Kent JT, et al. Reflex neurovascular dystrophy in childhood. *J Pediatr* 1978; 93:211.

102. Ruggieri SB, Arthreya BH, Doughty R, Gregg JR, Das M. Reflex sympathetic dystrophy in children. *Clinical Orthopedics and Related Research* 1980; 225–230.

103. Sullivan JA. Recurring pain in the pediatric athlete. *Pediatr Clin North Am* 1984; 31:1097–1112.

104. Afshani E, Kuhn JP. Common causes of low back pain in children. *Radiographics* March 1991; 11(2):269–291.

105. Miser AW, Miser JS. The treatment of cancer pain in children. *Pediatr Clin North Am* August 1989; 36(4):979–999.

106. Meehan J. Pain control in the terminally ill child at home. *Issues Compr Pediatr Nurs* 1989; 12(2–3):187–197.

107. Miser AW, Miser JS, Clark BS. Continuous intravenous infusion of morphine sulfate for control of severe pain in children with terminal malignancy. *J Pediatr* 1980; 96:930–932.

108. Miser AW, Davis DM, Hughes CS, Mulne AF, Miser JS. Continuous subcutaneous infusion of morphine in children with cancer. *Am J Dis Child* 1983; 137:383–385.

109. McIlvaine WB. Spinal opioids for the pediatric patient. *J Pain Symptom Manage* June 1990; 5(3):183–190.

110. Platt O, Nathan DG. Sickle cell disease. In: Nathan DG, Oski FA, eds. *Hematology of Infancy and Childhood.* 2nd ed. Philadelphia: Saunders; 1981:711.

111. Behrman B, Vaughan V, eds. *Nelson Textbook of Pediatrics.* 12th ed. Philadelphia: Saunders; 1983:1225.

112. McIlvaine WB. Perioperative pain management in children: a review. *J Pain Symptom Manage* December 1989; 4(4):215–229.

113. Beyer JE, Knapp TR. Methodological issues in the measurement of children's pain. *Child Health Care* 1986; 14:233–241.

114. Szyfelbein SK, Osgood PF, Carr DB. The assessment of pain and plasma beta-endorphin immunoreactivity in burned children. *Pain* 1985; 22:173–182.

115. Gourlay GK, Wilson PR, Glynn CJ. Pharmacodynamics and pharmacokinetics of methadone during the perioperative period. *Anesthesiology* 1982; 57:458–467.

116. Berde CB, Beyer JE, Bournaki MC, Levin CR, Sethna NF. Comparison of morphine and methadone for prevention of postoperative pain in 3- to 7-year-old children. *J Pediatr* July 1991; 119(1 pt 1):136–141.

117. Berde C, Sethna NF, Masek B, Fosburg M, Rocklin S. Pediatric pain clinics: recommendations for their development. *Pediatrician* 1989; 16(1–2):94–102.

PART FOUR

Pain Therapy

CHAPTER 26

Systemic Pharmacologic Approaches

W. Thomas Edwards and Christine Peeters-Asdourian

Pain is defined as an unpleasant sensory and emotional experience associated with actual or potential tissue damage or described in terms of such damage.[1] Pain, therefore, does not occur peripherally or even in the spinal cord or thalamus. Nociception may be said to occur at these levels, but pain per se is an experience that can occur only at the cortical level. It is not simply a function of the amount of physical injury sustained by the patient; it is a complex experiential process that is influenced by multiple factors including age, sex, culture, environment, and psychological makeup.

Acute pain is characterized by a well-defined temporal pattern of onset associated with injury. There usually are objective physical signs of hyperactivity of the autonomic nervous system present (such as tachycardia, hypertension, diaphoresis, mydriasis, and pallor). The patient with acute pain usually can give a clear description of its location, character, and timing. By contrast, patients with chronic pain usually lack the objective signs referrable to activity of the autonomic nervous system because adaptation has occurred.[2] The symptoms are less well defined temporally because the pain usually has persisted for more than 6 months, but the existence of a chronic pain state does not imply the absence of nociception. Chronic pain leads to marked changes in personality, life style, and functional ability. Such pain requires an approach that encompasses, not only treatment of the cause of the pain, but also treatment of its psychological and social consequences.

Drug therapy still constitutes the mainstay of medical therapy in the management of patients with acute pain. Patients with acute pain often are treated for the cause of their pain (by surgery, for example) and are likely to respond favorably to analgesic therapy. Importantly, the temporal nature of acute pain makes pharmacologic management comparatively simple.[3]

Sound pharmacologic principles must be used in the management of either acute or chronic pain states by drug therapy. Analgesia must be directed only at those pain states where nociception is significant; adjuvant drugs, such as tricyclic antidepressants, should be used when affective components dominate. The concept of so-called balanced analgesia is the rationale that combines these approaches because all pain states are compounded of multiple parts including nociception and suffering. Basic pharmacokinetic principles must be addressed with the use of any drug. We shall consider both the selection of drugs and the clinical use of drugs for the management of pain in this chapter.

OPIOID ANALGESICS: GENERAL PRINCIPLES

The opioid analgesics, particularly morphine, have been the so-called gold standard against which the effectiveness of all other analgesic agents is measured. Many different classification schemes for opioids have been developed to allow us to apply this standard. Their ability to relieve pain of different intensities has resulted in their classification into categories based on potency. The selectivity of interaction with the various opiate receptors is one of the newer classification schemes. We may characterize morphine-like properties in drugs that interact relatively nonselectively with μ and κ receptors (most strongly with μ) to produce analgesia and euphoria and with σ receptors to produce some of the less desirable effects of opioids, particularly, clouding of the sensorium and dysphoria. Newer opioid-like drugs, such as the synthetic peptide d-alanine-d-leucine enkephalin or ketocyclazine, may interact specifically with one receptor type (δ for the former and κ for the latter), particularly producing selective spinal analgesia. In this chapter, we follow the more classic approach to opioid classification by relative potency because this scheme results in a more usable body of information for clinical application.[3–5]

TECHNIQUES OF OPIOID ADMINISTRATION

In the acute-pain model, there is a minimum analgesic serum concentration for meperidine, below which there is no or little desirable effect in an individual patient.[6,7] The guiding principle in analgesic use should be to achieve a serum concentration that exceeds this level and remains consistently above it. The ideal in this regard is continuous intravenous infusion. Continuous infusion of meperidine is a safe and effective means of controlling postoperative pain. Some assumptions must be made to calculate the proper infusion rate, but these are relatively simple. The time needed to reach steady state (if no loading dose is given) is approximately sixfold the terminal (long) half-life. For meperidine, $t_{1/2}\beta$ equals 4 h. Therefore, the time until steady state is 24 h. If we multiply the volume of distribution of morphine by the desired blood concentration, the loading dose can be calculated. For a 70-kg adult, the initial dose of meperidine is 200 L (V_D) $\times$ 0.5 mg/L or 100 mg as an intravenous bolus where V_D equals the volume of distribution; this can be administered in 25- to 50-mg increments as the infusion is started. The proper infusion rate is calculated by multiplying the liver blood flow (0.6 to 1.0 L/min) by the analgesic concentration (0.5 mg/L) which gives drug clearance (0.3 to 0.5 mg/min or 18 to 30 mg/h). In one study of continuous meperidine infusion (from which these numbers are derived), no patient reported severe pain after the first 3 h, and steady-state concentrations ranged from 0.48 to 0.72 mg/L.[7]

This approach is applicable to any drug administered by continuous infusion and may be applied to morphine or fentanyl. Table 26-1 shows relative potencies, comparative half-lives, suggested loading doses, and infusion rates.[8] The pharmacokinetics of morphine and fentanyl administered by continuous infusion are not defined as clearly currently as those of meperidine. Analgesic levels also are not as well defined, but an understanding of the relative potencies can allow a logical approach to continuous-infusion analgesia with these drugs. A fat-soluble drug, such as fentanyl, accumulates after repeated doses; its kinetics therefore become similar to those of meperidine. The newer fentanyl derivative, alfentanil, has made longer term use of narcotic infusion simpler because of the drug's short terminal half-life and reduced volume of distribution.

Administration of an opioid by continuous infusion is not always feasible because of the equipment required or the monitoring that is necessary. With other routes of administration, fluctuations in plasma levels will occur. When any intermittent dosing scheme is used, drug administration must be on a scheduled, not on an as-needed, basis (Fig. 26-1).

The principle of not allowing levels to drop below a therapeutic range is well accepted with such drugs as antibiotics, cardiac glycosides, and antihypertensives, but analgesics frequently continue to be administered on an as-needed basis. The object of pain therapy is to prevent pain from occurring because this tends to reduce analgesic demand, total dose required, and dependency potential.[9] These goals have been easier to achieve with the introduction of 12-h preparations of morphine.

The exception to the use of as-needed medication is not really an exception. Patient-controlled analgesia (PCA) is a continuous-demand technique whereby the patient is allowed to demand the drug by intravenous self-administration within preset limits. This allows the patient's perception to guide the appropriate therapeutic level of the drug (Fig. 26-2). Because the analgesic threshold for any drug varies from patient to patient, the principle of allowing patients to guide their own analgesic therapy may be ideal.[11-14]

Various approaches and devices have been tested that allow patients to administer their own opioids intravenously. Generally, such techniques are safe and effective. Bennet and colleagues[15] found better pain relief and less total morphine use with PCA compared with intramuscular morphine. Patients select an appropriate dosing rate when drugs of different potency are used or when the concentration is changed. In the studies of Hartvig and associates,[13] PCA rates were constant up to 24 h postoperatively after the first few hours. These were: morphine, 2.6 ± 1.2 mg/h (12 patients); meperidine, 20 mg/h (28 patients); and Ketobemidone, 2.3 ± 0.8 mg/h (16 patients). They reported a high level of patient satisfaction using this technique.

The clinical course for patients receiving PCA has been largely uncomplicated with two exceptions. If the patient has an intercurrent serious disease, the morphine infusion rate calculated as the starting rate must be based on pharmacokinetics derived from acutely ill patients rather than from healthy volunteers to avoid excessive sedation if this is not desirable. Plasma drug clearance is reduced during the

Table 26-1
Guidelines for Continuous Infusion of Opioids

Opioid	Relative Potency	Circulating Half-Life (h)	Loading Dose for 70-kg Patient (mg)*	Suggested Infusion Rate for 70-kg Patient
Morphine	1	2–6	5–10	1–3 mg/h
Fentanyl	50	3–6	100–200	10–50 µg/h
Meperidine	0.1	3–6	100	20–30 mg/h
Methadone	1	15–30	5–10	Not recommended

*The loading dose may be administered during the first 30 min of infusion (rather than as a bolus); this tends to diminish the side effects of nausea and hypotension.
Reproduced with permission from Edwards WT, Burney RG, Kupferber IM: Management of pain, anxiety, and psychosis in the critically ill. In: Rippe JM, Irwin RD, Alpert JS, Dalen JE, eds. *Intensive Care Medicine.* Boston: Little, Brown; 1985.

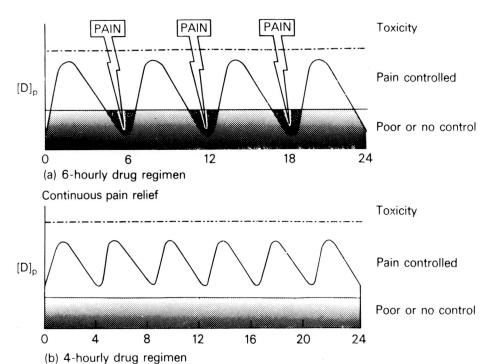

FIGURE 26-1. Diagram to illustrate the results of as-required and overspaced regular medication (a) compared with regular 4-h morphine sulfate (b). $[D]_p$ = plasma concentration of drug. (Reproduced with permission from Twycross RG, Lack SA. *Symptom Control in Far Advanced Cancer.* London: Pitman Publishing Ltd; 1983:110.)

immediate postoperative period (from 12.0 ml/kg/min to 8.9 ml/kg/min for meperidine), and the $t_{1/2}$ will be correspondingly prolonged. Profound respiratory depression may occur in patients who are hypovolemic during any form of intravenous infusion, including PCA, but blood gases will tend to normalize if the circulatory depression is corrected.

Less frequently used routes of administration are sublingual, buccal, transdermal, and rectal routes, which avoid the need for injection and do not subject the drug to the first-pass liver metabolism that can occur after oral administration. This is especially useful for morphine or buprenorphine. Sublingual or buccal administration of buprenorphine is used widely in Europe and is under investigation in this country. Transdermal fentanyl patches are available for the treatment of postoperative and cancer pain.[16] Rectal administration of oxymorphone results in lower and more delayed peak levels but a longer duration of action than intramuscular administration.[17–23] Guidelines for administration of opioid rectal suppositories are presented in Table 26-2.

CHOOSING AN OPIOID ANALGESIC

The choice must be guided, not only by the relative potency of the drug, but also by the effectiveness of a given drug in

FIGURE 26-2. Illustration of the finer control of circulating level of analgesic that is possible with patient-controlled analgesic (PCA) therapy than even with timed intramuscular (IM) administration.

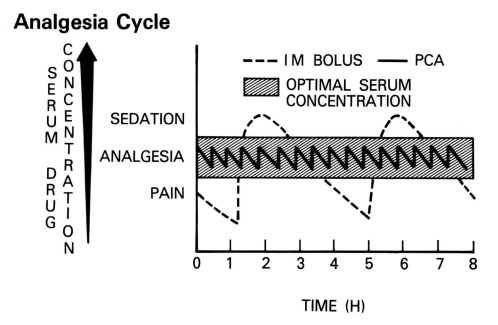

Table 26-2
Available Dosage Forms of Rectal Suppositories

Drug	Dose
Morphine	5, 10, 20 mg
Hydromorphone	3 mg
Oxymorphone	5 mg

managing pain of a given severity. The more potent drugs usually are chosen over less potent agents because of a clinical sense that they are more effective in managing severe pain than the less potent agents. In fact, drugs of low or moderate potency may be effective in managing relatively severe acute pain if the appropriate use is made of their intrinsic pharmacologic properties, and adjustments are made in dose, dosing interval, and route of administration to address these differences.

When we change opioids because of diminished effectiveness, it is important to remember the relative potency and bioavailability related to the route of administration chosen. The relative affinity for opioid receptors also plays a role in effectiveness and may, in part, explain differences in potency. If a patient has inadequate pain relief from 60 mg of codeine orally every 6 h, a change to meperidine 100 mg orally every 6 h may provide some improvement because meperidine is bound more effectively to opioid receptors. In the classic pharmacologic sense, however, meperidine is not much more potent than the so-called weak analgesic codeine.[3–5]

Table 26-3 provides some guidelines for comparing opi-

oids. These doses represent only an average range, and many patients will require less or more depending on the route chosen. An example of the use of this table is as follows. A patient receiving 2 mg/h of morphine by intravenous infusion is to receive oral methadone instead. The total daily dose of morphine is MS 48 mg. The average availability of methadone is 0.80. The equivalent daily dose of methadone orally is 60 mg. Therefore, the appropriate conversion is 20 mg orally every 8 h.

The plasma half-lives of the opioid analgesics vary widely and do not correlate always with their analgesic time courses for a single dose. For example, methadone with a half-life of 15 to 30 h and levorphanol with a half-life of 12 to 16 h reliably produce analgesia for only 4 to 6 h after administration of a single dose at the maintenance level. With repetitive dosing, however, those drugs with long plasma half-lives accumulate, and such accumulation may push plasma levels into the toxic range (this may be manifested by excess sedation and respiratory depression). Several days are required to reach a point of effective analgesia if the dose is begun on a maintenance schedule with longer-acting drugs. Loading (using two- to threefold the maintenance dose as the first dose) therefore is recommended.

The opioid analgesics are eliminated mainly by hepatic biotransformation to their metabolites, some of which are pharmacologically active and may contribute to therapeutic or toxic effects (Table 26-4). High doses of meperidine and propoxyphene may produce central nervous system excitation that can be manifested as convulsions when the metabolites normeperidine and norpropoxyphene accumulate.

Cirrhosis and other liver dysfunction and renal disease

Table 26-3
Practical Guidelines and Characteristics of Most Commonly Used Opioids with Parenteral versus Oral Equivalence

Opioid	Bioavailability (Oral Route)	Slow Half-Life (h)	Usual Period of Effectiveness	Equianalgesic Dose IM	Equianalgesic Dose PO	Comments
Codeine	0.4–0.7	2–4	4–6	32	65	Weak opioid often used in combination with nonopioid
Morphine	0.2–0.4	2–6	4–6	10	30	
Meperidine	0.4–0.6	3–6	4–5	75	300	Metabolized to normeperidine, potentially toxic substance with no analgesic properties
Methadone	0.7–0.9	5–30	4–12	10	20	Highly effective as PO medication, requires careful titration of dose and schedule
Oxycodone	*	*	2–3	30		Formerly available only in 5-mg doses in combination with aspirin or acetaminophen which limited dose. Now available alone.
Hydromorphone	*	*	3–5	1.5	7.5	Available in suppositories, high potency

IM, intramuscular; PO, oral.
Bioavailability = fraction appearing in plasma at peak level after oral administration.
*Data not available.

Table 26-4
Active Metabolites of Opioid Analgesics

Parent Drug	Active Metabolite
Codeine	Morphine
Heroin	Acetylmorphine and morphine
Oxycodone	Oxymorphone
Meperidine	Normeperidine (nonanalgesic, analeptic)
Propoxyphene	Norpropoxyphene (nonanalgesic, hepatotoxic)

may alter the metabolism and disposition of the narcotic drugs and their metabolites. Meperidine, pentazocine, and propoxyphene have increased bioavailability in cirrhotic patients, and there can be accumulation of toxic metabolites in the presence of cirrhosis (Table 26-5).[24–28] With increasing patient age, the clearance of all drugs, including opioids, from the plasma decreases.[29,30] This suggests that elderly patients are more sensitive to opioids and that careful titration of the dose is necessary.

OPIOID AGONIST–ANTAGONIST DRUGS

This group of analgesics was named for its propensity to demonstrate ceiling effects on such opioid properties as production of respiratory depression and its ability to antagonize some μ receptor agonist properties of other opioids. Nalorphine, the archetype of these drugs, was developed in the 1920s and first was thought to be a pure opioid antagonist. Its agonist properties were discovered later.[31] Although the list of drugs in this category has been expanding in recent years, those in common use, except for

pentazocine, still are available only in parenteral formulations in the United States and, therefore, have limited utility in outpatient management programs.

In the literature, it is difficult to distinguish the difference between partial agonist and agonist–antagonist classification schemes. Basically, the partial-agonist drugs (buprenorphine, profadol, propiram, dezocine, and meptazinol) are bound strongly at the μ receptor but have limited activity. Because they are bound so strongly, they may displace more active morphine-like drugs and antagonize their morphine-like effects. The agonist–antagonist drugs (nalorphine, pentazocine, butorphanol, and nalbuphine) show antagonist activity at the μ receptors but are κ receptor agonists (the site responsible for their analgesic properties).[32] Table 26-6 shows the relationship between analgesic and morphine antagonist activity for a group of these drugs.

Among the drugs in this category currently available, buprenorphine is the most potent and longest acting. Although it is not available in an oral formulation (first-pass liver inactivation is high), a sublingual dosage form currently is under investigation in the United States. Butorphanol and nalbuphine, likewise, are available only in parenteral formulations in our country, but 4-mg tablets of butorphanol are available in the United Kingdom. Pentazocine can be used either orally or parenterally, but the oral-to-parenteral dose conversion is 4:1. Dezocine, which has been investigated widely in postoperative pain, seems to offer considerable promise in the management of acute pain.[33]

All mixed-activity drugs can cause acute narcotic withdrawal in addicted patients. Dezocine may be an important exception to this rule,[34] but currently available agonist–antagonists should not be administered to opioid-dependent patients by direct substitution. An appropriate opioid withdrawal schedule must be followed.

Table 26-5
Undesirable Drug or Disease Interactions of Opioid-Type Analgesics

Drug	Interaction	Result
Meperidine	Cirrhosis	↑ Bioavailability and ↓ clearance = accumulation
Pentazocine	Cirrhosis	↑ Bioavailability and ↓ clearance = accumulation
Propoxyphene	Cirrhosis	↑ Bioavailability and ↓ clearance = accumulation
Meperidine	Renal failure	↑ Normeperidine, a toxic metabolite = accumulation
Propoxyphene	Renal failure	↑ Norpropoxyphene, a toxic metabolite = accumulation
Morphine	Older than 50 years	↓ Clearance = accumulation
Meperidine	Phenytoin	↑ Biotransformation = faster elimination
Methadone	Rifampin	↑ Biotransformation = faster elimination
Meperidine	Monoamine oxidase inhibitors	Excitation, hyperpyrexia, and convulsions
Any narcotic	Alcohol or other central nervous system depressants	Enhanced depressant effects

Reproduced with permission from Inturrisi CE. Role of opioid analgesics. *Am J Med* 1984; 77:27–37.

Table 26-6
Guidelines for Use of Opioid Agonist–Antagonist Drugs

Drug	Usual Parenteral Dose (mg)	Relative Antagonist Activity	Comments
Morphine	5–10	0	
Buprenorphine	0.3–0.6	20	Duration of analgesia up to 18 h after single dose
Butorphanol	1–2	0.25	3–4-h duration
Nalbuphine	5–20	0.25	4–5-h duration
Pentazocine	50–150	0.02	No clear ceiling on respiratory depression at higher doses
Dezocine	10–20	—	Data on antagonist activity not available in humans Reversal of respiratory depression > 30 mg/70-kg patient[32]

NONOPIOID ANALGESICS

Aspirin and the nonsteroidal anti-inflammatory agents act peripherally and produce analgesia primarily through their ability to alter enzyme activity of prostaglandin synthetase and prevent the formation of prostaglandin E_2, a compound known to sensitize tissues to the pain-producing effect of substances such as bradykinin.[35] Figure 26-3 shows the relative points of action of steroidal and nonsteroidal anti-inflammatory agents in the cascade of conversion of arachadonic acid to prostaglandins. Indole acetic acid and phenyl propionic acid derivatives act by inhibiting prostaglandin formation relatively high in the cascade, and their effects occur only when the drug is present. Aspirin works in a slightly different fashion to poison the cyclooxygenase system; this action also is responsible for its long-term effect on platelet function.

Full anti-inflammatory aspirin properties are seen only at doses of 3 to 4 g/day. The degree of pain relief that can be produced by aspirin is related to its total dose up to approximately 975 to 1300 mg/day. Beyond this point, increasing the dose in an attempt to produce additional analgesia does not increase the effect, but the duration may increase somewhat. This is known as a *ceiling effect,* and it is seen with all anti-inflammatory agents.

Just as morphine functions as the standard for comparison of opioids, aspirin is the one against which the analgesic action of nonsteroidal anti-inflammatories must be compared. Because of similarities among aspirin and these drugs in mechanism of action, their side effects are similar (Table 26-7), but their pharmacokinetics vary considerably. The Food and Drug Administration has approved several of these drugs for use as analgesics for mild-to-moderate pain (Table 26-8 and Chap. 13). All these appear to have an analgesic potential at least equal to that of aspirin, and in some types of acute pain, they have been shown to be more effective than aspirin in controlled trials.[36,37] Ketarolac is available in a parenteral form with good analgesic prop-

Modulation of Arachidonic Acid Cascade

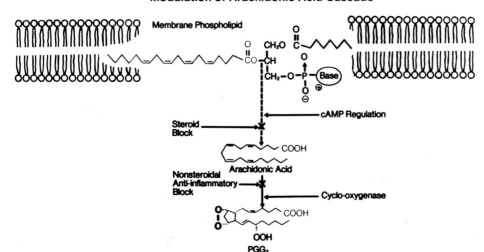

FIGURE 26-3. A simplification of the arachidonic acid to prostaglandin cascade and the points of modulation by corticosteroid and nonsteroidal anti-inflammatory drugs. Aspirin poisons cyclooxygenase, causing irreversible block at this level.

Table 26-7
Comparison of Aspirin and Acetaminophen in Clinical Use

	Aspirin	*Acetaminophen*
Action	Analgesic	Equipotent to aspirin
	Antipyretic	Equipotent to aspirin
	Anti-inflammatory	Less potent than aspirin
	Antiplatelet	None
Usual dose	650 mg	650 mg
Maximum daily dose	Approximately 3 g for analgesic	3 g
	Up to 10 g for anti-inflammatory	Not active
Time action	90-min peak	120 min
	4–6-h duration	4–6 h
Adverse effects	Hypersensitivity	No
	GI upset	No
	Hemostasis	No
	No liver dysfunction	Liver dysfunction
	Associated with Reye syndrome	No

erties.[38–46] With the exception of mefanamic acid, they are somewhat better tolerated than aspirin with regard to gastrointestinal side effects. Ibuprofen is available as an over-the-counter preparation at a reduced dose.

Acetaminophen[47] is similar to aspirin in analgesic and antipyretic potency and duration of analgesia. However, it is less effective than aspirin in the management of pain caused by rheumatoid arthritis and other frankly inflammatory conditions. When it is used as a mild analgesic, it offers some advantages over aspirin. There is no cross sensitivity in aspirin-allergic patients. It does not have serious gastrointestinal side effects or affect platelet function. Also it is available as a stable palatable liquid preparation, which may be important to some patients. Acetaminophen may inhibit prostaglandin synthesis in the central nervous system, but this is not well established. There probably is no central receptor for acetaminophin respons-

ible for the production of analgesia. Hepatotoxicity, the most serious adverse effect, is seen only after ingestion of large doses (10 to 15 g/day); this is above the accepted therapeutic dose. Even patients receiving the extra-strength formulations should not be able to exceed these limits if they follow usual guidelines for use. Table 26-7 shows the principal points of comparison between aspirin and acetaminophen.

ADJUVANTS TO ANALGESICS: THE RATIONALE

Adjuvant medications are drugs that may be combined with analgesics to lessen the experience of pain, either by providing additional antinociceptive effects or lessening the impact of the pain experience on the patient. The use of

Table 26-8
Nonsteroidal Anti-Inflammatory Drugs Approved for Mild to Moderate Pain

Generic Name	Trade Name	Comment
Same duration of action as aspirin (short half-life)		
Mefenamic acid	Ponstel	Use not to exceed 1 week
Fenoprofen	Nalfon	300–1200 mg daily
Ibuprofen	Motrin Advil Nuprin	1600–3200 mg daily
Suprofen	Suprol	800–1200 mg daily (flank pain has been reported)
Longer duration of action than aspirin (long half-life)		
Diflunisal	Dolobid	500 mg twice a day
Naproxen	Naprosyn	Up to 1250 mg daily
Naproxen sodium	Anaprox	275 mg three times a day up to 1375 mg daily

combinations of drugs often enables the physician to increase the patient's analgesic effect without increasing the dose of the specific analgesic drug. This includes, not only the combination of nonopioid analgesics with opioid drugs, but also the addition of tricyclic antidepressants, anticonvulsants, and various psychotropic medications to the opioid or nonopioid analgesic regimen in a balanced-type analgesia.

Adjuvant drugs serve many purposes in the management of chronic pain syndromes. Anxiety and depression may coexist with or result from the chronic pain state. Sleep disturbances or abnormal sleep patterns may contribute to increases in the nocturnal perception of pain and require separate treatment. The simple expedient of combining drugs that treat nociception both centrally and peripherally (or centrally by different mechanisms) may allow more effective analgesia with fewer side effects.

Anticonvulsants

The anticonvulsants (phenytoin, carbamazepine, and sodium valproate) may be useful in the management of patients with trigeminal neuralgia or certain other chronic pain states, such as postherpetic neuralgia, diabetic neuropathy, postamputation pain (stump pain and phantom limb pain), deafferentation pain from brachial plexus avulsion, and lumbar plexopathy all of which are now classified as Neuropathic Pain States. They are thought to be useful because they suppress spontaneous neuronal firing.[48] In addition, sodium valproate increases central levels of γ-aminobutyric acid (GABA); this may depress activity in some nociceptive pathways as may other GABA agonists such as baclofen.[49]

When administering anticonvulsant agents, it is important to ensure that therapeutic levels are attained. Particularly with carbamazepine, this must be achieved gradually, or disturbing side effects will intervene (dizziness, dysphoria, or disorientation). The usual beginning dose of carbamazepine is 200 mg/day in two divided doses with gradual increases over 3 to 4 weeks to 1200 mg/day in divided doses. Phenytoin, however, is a rather benign drug that can be loaded easily by doubling the projected maintenance dose for 2 days, continuing the maintenance dose, and then measuring the serum level in approximately 12 days. Sodium valproate probably should be started at the maintenance level of up to 1 g/day, allowing serum levels to rise slowly to avoid excess gastrointestinal disturbances. It is important to follow liver function in patients receiving valproic acid, and care must be exercised in prescribing carbamazepine with tricyclics because each may inhibit the metabolism of the other, resulting in unexpectedly high concentrations of both.

Antidepressants

The tricyclic antidepressants are the drugs most commonly used as analgesic adjuvants in the management of chronic pain. Patients may be started on low doses of antidepressants and report an improvement in their pain within days. This effect, which is believed to be mediated by enhancing serotonin activity in the central nervous system, occurs at doses below those used in treating depression. This effect seems to be independent of their antidepressant effect because no change in mood is seen when it occurs.[50–52]

The tricyclic antidepressants also seem to restore a more normal sleep pattern in patients with chronic pain. Thus, we favor their use in the treatment of insomnia over the traditional barbiturate sedatives or the benzodiazepines. The disturbances in sleep pattern and depression reinforce each other in a feedback loop. Correcting the sleep pattern also makes treatment of a coexisting depression easier.

Tricyclic antidepressants also may be useful to manage certain painful neuropathic disorders, such as diabetic peripheral neuropathy,[53] particularly if they are combined with certain phenothiazines. Amitriptyline is the drug most commonly prescribed in this way. Guidelines for the use of tricyclics are described in Table 26-9. The newer quad-

Table 26-9
Guidelines for the Use of Antidepressants in Pain Management

Drug	Effect on Serotonin	Anti-cholinergic Properties	Sedative Properties	Daily Dose	Comments
Amitriptyline	+++	+	+++	25–200 mg	10 mg at bedtime sometimes useful if patient unable to tolerate hangover
Nortriptyline	+	++	++	50–200 mg	
Imipramine	++	++	++	50–200 mg	
Desipramine	0	++	+	50–200 mg	
Doxepin	0	+	+	10–150 mg	
Trazodone	+++	0	+++	150–400 mg	Priapism has been reported in men

0 = absent; + = mild; ++ = moderate; +++ = marked.

ricyclic antidepressants do not appear to offer any unique advantages in patients with pain. Anecdotal reports indicate that fluoxetine may play a role in this group of patients[54] and enhance opiate analgesia, but fluoxetine itself has no analgesic properties.[55]

Anxiolytics and Major Tranquilizers

Among the drugs in these categories used as adjuvants to analgesics, chlorpromazine, haloperidol, hydroxyzine, and diazepam are the most popular. The combination of phenothiazines or butyrophenones with opioids gained popularity around the time of the development of neuroleptic analgesia and the introduction of a combination of fentanyl and droperidol into clinical practice in the mid-1960s. The phenothiazines or butyrophenones are believed to spare analgesic use by potentiating opioid-based analgesia. There is little evidence to support this idea, and in one well-controlled trial,[56,57] although chlorpromazine showed some activity on a change-of-pain-intensity scale, there was no difference between morphine alone and morphine plus chlorpromazine. The clinical impression that there is an effect probably is based on the finding that drowsiness is prominent after the combination and patients request medication less frequently. Care must be taken with the use of phenothiazines and butyrophenones in patients receiving tricyclic antidepressants. Perphenazine, chlorpromazine, and haloperidol have been shown to reduce tricyclic elimination by 25 percent to 50 percent while increasing plasma levels (in patients receiving perphenazine) by 10 percent to 30 percent.[58]

When anxiety is a major component of a pain syndrome, however, particularly if agitation is present, one of the major tranquilizers may be useful. Chlorpromazine given at doses of 25 mg three times a day or haloperidol 2 mg two or three times a day may be enough to treat such anxiety. Either drug also may be useful in treating the nausea that may result from opioid therapy.[49]

Hydroxyzine gained popularity as an adjuvant to opioid analgesia after a report of synergy between morphine and hydroxyzine in pain relief.[59] Unfortunately, with oral use, hydroxyzine does not appear to have the effect it has when given parenterally. It is likely that one or more metabolites of hydroxyzine are active pharmacologically as antihistamines, sedatives, and antiemetics, but none have the analgesic activity seen in the parent compound. The opioid-sparing effect often seen in patients receiving oral hydroxyzine, therefore, probably is similar to that seen with phenothiazines (that is, patients request medication less frequently because of drowsiness).

Diazepam also plays a role in pain management similar to that of the phenothiazines. No significant opioid-sparing effect has been reported for this drug. Among those involved in the management of chronic pain syndromes, there is a widespread clinical impression that prolonged use of diazepam is associated with worsening of depression in such patients. It is the practice in our clinic not to administer diazepam to these patients because it does not appear to be particularly useful in patients with chronic pain, either for relief of chronic muscle spasm or sleep regulation. Patients with cancer pain probably are an exception, but again, anxiety is often a major factor.

Other Adjuvant Drugs

Dextroamphetamine has been used to potentiate the analgesic effect of opioids.[60,61] It may be helpful in patients in whom opioid-induced sedation is a problem, but sympathomimetic effects, such as tachycardia, may be difficult. It is not clear whether its apparent opioid potentiation is based on its tendency to produce mood elevation or caused by its α-agonist effect on the descending control of nociception. Cannabinoids (marijuana) have been useful in some patients with cancer to control nausea and stimulate appetite. These substances also may have analgesic effects, but they are not without side effects, including bradycardia, hypotension, and sedation.[62] Several studies investigated the impact of combining caffeine with nonopioid analgesics. Caffeine appears to potentiate the analgesic effects of these drugs, possibly in a manner similar to that seen with dextroamphetamine.[63]

SYSTEMIC LOCAL ANESTHETICS

Systemic local anesthetic infusions have been used in the management of both acute and chronic pain states since 1948. Various reports of their usefulness in different pain states ultimately have resulted in the recommendation that such infusions may be useful in pain syndromes where deafferentation is present. Edwards and associates[64] reported up to 74 percent response rate in patients with monodermatomal radicular pain or peripheral neuropathy. Phero and colleagues[65] reported a gradual decline in pain ratings (measured by visual analog scale) after repeated use of chloroprocaine in a somewhat similar group of patients. Both groups reported relief of pain extending beyond the expected duration of central nervous system effects for either drug.

Edwards's group used 5 mg/kg of lidocaine HCl, Phero's group used up to 1 g of chloroprocaine. However, both groups administered the drugs by continuous infusion pumps to titrate the dose carefully and minimize toxicity. Recently, Edwards's group increased the total dose of lidocaine (Edwards WT. Unpublished data.) up to 8.5 mg/kg with some improvement in responses.

The mechanism of action of systemically administered local anesthetic is not understood currently. Whatever it is, however, the success of this technique in selected patients is undeniable. Another group reported significant improvement in a group of diabetic patients with peripheral neuropathy treated in a double-blind crossover fashion.[66] Patient acceptance of the technique was high, despite the need for repeated infusions because it was the only technique that provided relief without the use of narcotics. Much work remains to be done, including an evaluation of the newer oral antiarrhythmic drugs tocainide and mexiletine in a similar program of pain control. In recent trials, these drugs offered some promise because they have chemical features similar to the local anesthetics.[67–69] Although cocaine has local anesthetic effects, there are no good studies demonstrating its effectiveness as an analgesic or opioid analgesic potentiator.

CHRONIC PAIN: SPECIAL PROBLEMS WITH SYSTEMIC MEDICATIONS

Patients with chronic pain often have not responded to treatment directed at the original cause of their pain (as in patients with terminal malignant disease) or they may have pain resulting from the therapy itself (as in the post laminectomy or so-called failed-back syndrome). They have received many drugs, and therapy often is complicated by tolerance to the opioid analgesics and perhaps dependence on some of the adjuvant drugs, like diazepam. In these patients, too, we must consider the relative importance of such factors as ongoing nociception, fear, stress, depression, the sleep pattern, the home environment, and occupational status before a logical pharmacologic plan can be constructed.[70]

Complications of Long-Term Use of Opioids

Patients with chronic pain who are receiving opioids have a much higher incidence of hospitalization and report substantially more physical impairment than those not using opioids. Patients receiving oxycodone on a chronic basis had a significantly lower treatment success rate than did those who had not used this drug.[71–74]

Narcotic detoxification is often an early goal of comprehensive chronic pain management programs. Any program in which behavior modification is important will require prior opioid detoxification. This usually is accomplished best with an immediate change to timed rigidly controlled administration of the drug, preferably using a long-acting oral opioid (methadone is preferred by our group). Withdrawal begins by changing to methadone (using the same number of morphine equivalents the patient has been receiving regardless of what drug was given (Table 26-3). Detoxification can begin after serum methadone levels are stable, usually after 4 to 6 days. Dose reduction should be done over no more than 6 weeks and can be adjusted depending on the total initial dose of the drug. Supportive psychotherapy is an important concomitant of such a regimen.

In the opioid-dependent patient, opioid withdrawal symptoms can be blocked by administering the α-2-agonist drug, clonidine.[75,76] In its use to rehabilitate drug addicts, it has been shown to be safer, more effective, and less expensive than long-term methadone maintenance. Clonidine is not addicting and alleviates withdrawal symptoms without inducing a withdrawal syndrome.

Clonidine also has some potent analgesic properties.[77] It suppresses central noradrenergic hyperactivity and reduces sympathetic nervous system tone. There seems to be a close overlap of the location of α-2 receptors and opiate binding sites in the brain stem in animals and humans. Clonidine may act at the level of the coerulospinal noradrenergic pathway; this is thought to be involved in the regulation of vigilance and in the processing of nociceptive stimuli, both centrally and at the spinal cord level. This explains, at least in part, the sedative effect and the analgesic effect of clonidine, especially when it is given intrathecally.[78–80] This drug potentiates the effect of the opioid analgesics and is helpful in suppressing the hyperalgesia associated with withdrawal, an important quality when opioid-dependent patients with chronic pain problems are being detoxified. When it is used in small doses, hypotension rarely is a problem, and if clonidine is tapered slowly, rebound hypertension rarely occurs. We often administer as little as 0.1 mg twice a day, but occasionally, daily doses as high as 0.4 mg are necessary.

Narcotic detoxification usually cannot be handled in an outpatient setting without exceedingly strong motivation on the patient's part, and often even then, the conditioned responses learned over years defeat all efforts. Inpatient opioid detoxification is necessary and should be given first priority.

The Choice for Opioid Maintenance

Long-term maintenance with opioid drugs is the rule in the management of chronic cancer pain (see Chap. 17). The term *chronic* is, at least in part, a misnomer for cancer pain because there is frequently a significant ongoing nociceptive component resulting from advancing disease. The chronicity of the problem, however, accentuates the components of fear, anxiety, sleep disturbance, and family and occupational upset alluded to earlier. The problem in opioid maintenance for cancer pain is usually one of appropriate use of the pharmacology of the drug chosen and the appropriate choice of adjuvant medications. Concern about addiction should never be a consideration in the management of malignant pain. Tolerance to analgesic effects can be a problem, however, often requiring dose increases.

All opioids can produce nausea and vomiting, but this appears to vary with the drug and the patient. Sometimes an antiemetic is required concurrently with the opioid. Constipation usually can be prevented if an appropriate bowel regimen (using a stool softener and a mild laxative) is started concurrently with the administration of the opioid. Tolerance to the side effects of sedation, respiratory depression, nausea, and vomiting usually develops more rapidly than to the analgesic effect of the drug. Tolerance to the analgesic effect requires increasing the dose of the opioid.

Switching to an alternative drug also may help because there seems to be a lack of complete cross tolerance among drugs with different pharmacologic profiles (such as morphine, meperidine, methadone, and levorphanol). Increased doses will not always result in an accentuation of side effects, but should this occur, the appropriate selection of adjuvant drugs often will facilitate the opioid maintenance program.

If the patient requires parenteral opioid administration, another convenient route is a continuous subcutaneous infusion by pump. This route avoids repetitive intramuscular or subcutaneous injections and the need for intravenous access. It provides another way of keeping a constant level of pain relief with no peak-level side effects or trough-level pain breakthrough. Both patients and their families find these devices easy to manage. PCA is another alternative and may be used with subcutaneous infusion.

In patients with advanced cancer and chronic pain, it is conventional to administer an oral preparation of liquid morphine at 4-h intervals, and the dose is individualized and titrated against the level of pain. The so-called Brompton mixture (a variable solution often containing morphine, cocaine, ethyl alcohol, syrup, and chloroform water) has long been used to control severe pain in this setting. In a double-blind study comparing this mixture with morphine alone, however, there was no significant difference between Brompton mixture and morphine alone with respect to confusion, nausea, drowsiness, and pain relief.[77] Therefore, liquid morphine has largely replaced the Brompton mixture.

There should be no preconceived upper limit to the dose of morphine required. The availability of newer high concentration (20 mg/ml) liquid preparations makes this approach easier than in the past. An alternative approach for patients who are stable on a steady dose of oral aqueous morphine for at least 48 h can be the use of a controlled-release preparation of morphine sulfate given on a 12-h schedule with no change in the total daily dose. The controlled-release polymer tablet provides effective analgesia, allows for uninterrupted sleep at night, saves appreciably in nursing medication time, and is acceptable to patients. Compliance with an effective analgesic regimen is better when the dosing interval is long.[71] Some pharmacokinetic studies show that controlled-release morphine sulfate produces higher and more prolonged plasma levels than oral morphine sulfate solution, even though the 24-h dose of morphine solution was 50 percent greater.[81,82]

Opioid maintenance of patients with benign chronic pain always has been a controversial area. A recent study indicates that, in certain highly selected patients, this approach may be a humane alternative to no treatment or neurosurgical ablative procedures.[83] Patients selected for this technique must have no prior history of substance abuse, but there seem to be no predictive features common to any one of several psychological measurement scales for the patients who respond. In our clinic, we have managed a small number of patients with chronic nonmalignant pain of such different origins as neurofibromatosis, stable giant cell tumor of the sacrum, multilevel radiculopathy, and de-afferentation with opioid maintenance. With careful monitoring of drug intake and use of long-acting or slow-release opioid preparation by time-contingent dosing schemes, these patients have done well and showed no tendency to increase their opioid intake over time. All had not responded to other approaches, and with this program, they were able to maintain some degree of functioning.

SUMMARY

Although drug therapy remains the foundation of acute pain management, chronic pain states must incorporate multiple approaches. When we choose drug therapy as one of those approaches, a sound pharmacologic basis for the choice of drugs, routes of administration, doses, and dosing intervals must be developed. Then the management of nociception, depression, anxiety, and sleep disturbance by drugs will be a logical building block in a multidisciplinary chronic pain control program.

References

1. Merskey H, Albe-Fessard DG, Bonica JJ, et al. Pain terms: a list with definitions and notes on usage. *Pain* 1979; 6:249–252.
2. Posner JB. Pain. In: Beeson P, McDermott W, eds. *Textbook of Medicine*. Philadelphia: Saunders; 1967:1468–1473.
3. Foley KM. The practical use of narcotic analgesics. *Med Clin North Am* 1982; 66:1091–1104.
4. Inturrisi CE. Narcotic drugs. *Med Clin North Am* 1982; 66:1061–1071.
5. Inturrisi CE. Role of opioid analgesics. *Am J Med* 1984; 77:27–37.
6. Austin KL, Stapleton JV, Mather LE. Multiple intramuscular injections: a major source of variability in analgesic response to meperidine. *Pain* 1980; 8:47–62.
7. Austin KL, Stapleton JV, Mather LE. Relationship between blood meperidine concentrations and analgesic response: a preliminary report. *Anesthesiology* 1980; 53:460–466.
8. Edwards WT, Burney RG, Kupferberg IM. Management of pain, anxiety and psychosis in the critically ill. In: Rippe JM, Irwin RS, Alpert JS, Dalen JE, eds. *Intensive Care Medicine*. Boston: Little, Brown; 1985:1014–1025.
9. Twycross RG, Lack SA. Symptom control in far advanced cancer. London: Pitman Publ; 1983:100–114.
10. Warfield CA. Evaluation of dosing guidelines for the use of oral controlled-release morphine. *Cancer* 1989; 63:2360–2364.
11. Tamsen A, Hartvig P, Fagerlund C, et al. Patient-controlled analgesic therapy, Part II: individual analgesic demand and analgesic plasma concentrations of pethidine in postoperative pain. *Clin Pharmacokinet* 1982; 7:164–175.
12. Tamsen A, Hartvig P, Fagerlund C, et al. Patient-controlled analgesic therapy: clinical experience. *Acta Anaesthesiol Scand Suppl* 1982; 74:157–160.
13. Hartvig P, Tamsen A, Fagerlund C, et al. Pharmacokinetics

of pethidine during anesthesia and patient-controlled analgesic therapy. *Acta Anesthesiol Scand Suppl* 1982; 74:52–54.

14. Ellis R, Haines D, Shah R, et al. Pain relief after abdominal surgery—a comparison of IM morphine, sublingual buprenorphine and self-administered IV pethidine. *Br J Anaesth* 1982; 54:421–428.

15. Bennet R, Batenhorst R, Graves D, et al. Morphine titration in postoperative laparotomy patients using patient-controlled analgesia. *Curr Ther Res* 1982; 32:45–52.

16. Roy SD, Flynn GL. Transdermal delivery of narcotic analgesics: pH, anatomical and subject influences on cutaneous permeability of fentanyl and sufentanil. *Pharm Res* August 1990; 7(8):842–847.

17. Beckett AH, Hossie RD. Buccal absorption of drugs. *Handbook Exp Pharmacol* 1971; 28:24–46.

18. Hirsch JD. Sublingual morphine sulfate in chronic pain management. *Clin Pharm* 1984; 3:585–586.

19. Whitman HH. Sublingual morphine: a novel route of narcotic administration. *PRN Forum* 1984; 3:7–8.

20. Beaver WT, Feise GA. A comparison of the analgesic effect of oxymorphone by rectal suppository and intramuscular injection in patients with postoperative pain. *J Clin Pharmacol* 1977; 17:276–291.

21. Ellison NM, Lewis GO. Plasma concentrations following single doses of morphine sulfate in oral solution and rectal suppository. *Clin Pharm* 1984; 3:614–617.

22. Bell MD, Murray GR, Mishra P, et al. Buccal morphine—a new route for analgesia? *Lancet* 1985; 1:71–73.

23. Pannuti F, Rossi AP, Lafelice G, et al. Control of chronic pain in very advanced cancer patients with morphine hydrochloride administered by oral, rectal, and sublingual route. Clinical report and preliminary results on morphine pharmacokinetics. *Pharmacol Res Commun* 1982; 14:369–380.

24. Neal EA, Meffin PH, Gregory PB, et al. Enhanced bioavailability and decreased clearance of analgesics in patients with cirrhosis. *Gastroenterology* 1979; 77:96–102.

25. Patwardhan RV, Johnson RF, Hoyumpa A Jr, et al. Normal metabolism of morphine in cirrhosis. *Gastroenterology* 1981; 81:1006–1011.

26. Szeto HH, Inturrisi CE, Houde R, et al. Accumulation of normeperidine, an active metabolite of meperidine, in patients with renal failure or cancer. *Ann Intern Med* 1977; 86:738–741.

27. Giacomini KM, Giacomini JC, Gibson TP, et al. Propoxyphene and norproxyphene plasma concentrations after oral propoxyphene in cirrhotic patients with and without surgically constructed portacaval shunt. *Clin Pharmacol Ther* 1980; 28:417–442.

28. Pond SM, Tong T, Benowitz NL, et al. Presystemic metabolism of meperidine to normeperidine in normal and cirrhotic subjects. *Clin Pharmacol Ther* 1981; 30:183–188.

29. Kaiko RF, Wallenstein SL, Rogers AG, et al. Narcotics in the elderly. *Med Clin North Am* 1982; 66:1079–1089.

30. Bellville JW, Forrest WH Jr, Miller E, et al. Influence of age on pain relief from analgesics: a study of postoperative patients. *JAMA* 1971; 217:1835–1841.

31. Lasagna L, Beecher HK. The analgesic effectiveness of nalorphine and nalorphine–morphine combinations in man. *J Pharmacol Exp Ther* 1954; 112:356–363.

32. Rosow CE. Newer synthetic opioid analgesics. In: Smith G, Covino BG, eds. *Acute Pain*. Boston: Butterworths; 1985:68–103.

33. Romongnoli A, Keats AS. Ceiling respiratory depression by dezocine. *Clin Pharmacol Ther* 1984; 35:367–373.

34. Petro DJ. Dezocine. *Clin Anesthesiol* 1983; 1:159–163.

35. Goodwin JS. Mechanism of action of nonsteroidal anti-inflammatory agents. *Am J Med* 1984; 77:57–64.

36. Kantor TG. Nonsteroidal anti-inflammatory agents in the management of cancer pain. In: *Symposium on the Management of Cancer Pain*. New York: Hospital Practice; 1984:30–34.

37. Kantor TG. Anti-inflammatory drug therapy for low back pain. In: Stanton-Hicks M, Boas R, eds. *Chronic Low Back Pain*. New York: Raven Press; 1982:157–169.

38. Estape J, Vinolas N, Gonzales B, et al. Ketorolac, a new non-opioid analgesic: a double-blind trial versus pentazocine in cancer pain. *J Int Med Res* July–August 1990; 18(4):298–304.

39. Goodman E. Use of ketorolac in sickle-cell disease and vaso-occlusive crisis. *Lancet* September 7, 1991; 338(8767):641–642. Letter.

40. Powell H, Smallman JM, Morgan M. Comparison of intramuscular ketorolac and morphine in pain control after laparotomy. *Anaesthesia* July 1990; 45(7):538–542.

41. Kenny GN. Ketorolac trometamol—a new non-opioid analgesic *Br J Anaesth* October 1990; 65(4):445–447. Editorial.

42. Buckley MM, Brodgen RN. Ketorolac. A review of its pharmacodynamic and pharmocokinetic properties, and therapeutic potential. *Drugs* January 1990; 39(1):86–109.

43. Domer F. Characterization of the analgesic activity of ketorolac in mice. *Eur J Pharmacol* February 27, 1990; 177(3):127–135.

44. Brown CR, Mazzulla JP, Mok MS, Nussdorf RT, Rubin PD, Schwesinger WH. Comparison of repeat doses of intramuscular ketorolac tromethamine and morphine sulfate for analgesia after major surgery. *Pharmacotherapy* 1990; 10(suppl 6 pt 2):45S–50S.

45. Ketorolac: a new potent analgesic for parenteral and oral administration. *Pharmacotherapy* 1990; 10(suppl 6 pt 2):29S–131S.

46. Rubin P, Yee JP, Ruoff G. Comparison of long-term safety of ketorolac tromethamine and aspirin in the treatment of chronic pain. *Pharmacotherapy* 1990; 10(suppl 6 pt 2):106S–110S.

47. Bailey BP. Acetaminophen hepatotoxicity and overdose. *Am Fam Physician* 1980; 22:83–87.

48. Maciewicz R, Bouckoms A, Martin JB. Drug therapy of neuropathic pain. *Clin J Pain* 1985; 1:39–49.

49. Atkinson JH Jr, Kremer EF, Garfin SR. Psychopharmacologic agents in the treatment of pain. *J Bone Joint Surg Am* 1985; 67:337–342.

50. Rosenblatt RM, Reich J, Dehring D. Tricyclic antidepressants in treatment of depression and chronic pain: analysis of the supporting evidence. *Anesth Analg* 1984; 63:1025–1032.

51. Clifford DB. Treatment of pain with antidepressants. *Am Fam Physician* 1985; 31:181–185.

52. Pilowsky I, Hallett EC, Bassett DL, et al. A controlled study of amitriptyline in the treatment of chronic pain. *Pain* 1982; 14:169–179.

53. Davis JL, Lewis SB, Gerich JE, et al. Peripheral diabetic neuropathy treated with amitriptyline and fluphenazine. *JAMA* 1977; 238:2291–2292.

54. Theesan KA, Marsh WR. Relief of diabetic neuropathy with fluoxetine. *DICP* July–August 1989; 23(7–8):572–574.

55. Hynes MD, Lochner MA, Bemis KG, Hymos DL. Fluoxetine, a selective inhibitor of serotonin uptake, potentiates morphine analgesia without altering its discriminative stimulus properties or affinity for opioid receptors. *Life Sci* June 17, 1985; 36(24):2317–2323.

56. Houde RW. On assaying analgesics in man. In: Knighton RS, Dumbe R, eds. *Pain.* Boston: Little, Brown; 1966:183–196.

57. Beaver WT. Combination analgesics. *Am J Med* 1984; 77:38–53.

58. Gram LF, Overo KF. Drug interaction: inhibitory effect of neuroleptics on metabolism of tricyclic antidepressants in man. *Br Med J* 1972; 1:463–465.

59. Beaver WT, Feise G. Comparison of the analgesic effects of morphine, hydroxyzine and their combination in patients with post-operative pain. In: Bonica JJ, Albe-Fessard DG, eds. *Advances in Pain Research and Therapy.* Vol. 1. New York: Raven Press; 1976:553–557.

60. Forrest WH Jr, Brown CR, et al. Dextroamphetamine with morphine for the treatment of postoperative pain. *N Engl J Med* 1977; 296:712–715.

61. Izenwasser S, Kornetzky C. Potentiation of morphine analgesia by D-amphetamine is mediated by norepinephrine and not dopamine. *Pain* June 1988; 33(3):363–368.

62. Harris LS. Cannabinoids as analgesics. In: Beers RF, Bassett EG, eds. *Mechanisms of Pain in Analgesics Compounds.* New York: Raven Press; 1979:467–473.

63. Laska EM, Sunshine A, Zighelboim I, et al. Effect of caffeine on acetaminophen analgesia. *Clin Pharmacol Ther* 1983; 33:498–509.

64. Edwards WT, Habib F, Burney RD, et al. Intravenous lidocaine in the management of various chronic pain states: a review of 211 cases. *Reg Anaesth* 1985; 10:1–6.

65. Phero JC, de Jong RH, Devson DD, et al. Intravenous chloroprocaine for intractable pain. *Reg Anaesth* 1983; 8:41.

66. Kastrup J, Petersen P, Dejgard A, et al. Intravenous lidocaine infusion—a new treatment of chronic painful diabetic neuropathy? *Pain* 1987; 23:69–75.

67. Tanelian DL, Brose WG. Neuropathic pain can be relieved by drugs that are use-dependent sodium channel blockers: lidocaine, carbamazepine, and mexiletine. *Anesthesiology* May 1991; 74(5):949–951.

68. Dejgard A, Peterson P, Kastrup J. Mexiletine for treatment of chronic painful diabetic neuropathy. *Lancet* January 2–9, 1988; 1(8575–8576):9–11.

69. Awerbuch GI, Sandyck R. Mexiletine for thalamic pain syndrome. *Int J Neurosci* December 1990; 55(2–4):129–133.

70. Reuler JB, Girard DE, Nardone DA. The chronic pain syndrome: misconceptions and management. *Ann Intern Med* 1980; 93:588–596.

71. Maruta T, Swanson DW. Problems with the use of oxycodone compound in patients with chronic pain. *Pain* 1981; 11:389–396.

72. Houde RW. The use and misuse of narcotics in the treatment of chronic pain. *Adv Neurol* 1974; 4:527–538.

73. Stimmel B. Pain, analgesia, and addiction: an approach to the pharmacologic management of pain. *Clin J Pain* 1985; 1:14–22.

74. Taub A. Opioid analgesics in the treatment of chronic intractable pain of non-neoplastic origin. In: Kitahata LM, Collins JG, eds. *Narcotic Analgesics in Anesthesiology.* Baltimore: Williams & Wilkins; 1982:199–208.

75. Digregorio JG, Budovisky MA. Clonidine for narcotic withdrawal. *Am Fam Physician* 1981; 24:203–204.

76. Washton AM, Resnick RB. Clonidine for opiate detoxification: outpatient clinical trials. *Am J Psychiatry* 1980; 137:1121–1122.

77. Melvack R, Mount BM, Gordon JM. The Brompton mixture vs. morphine solution given orally: effects on pain. *Can Med Assoc J* 1979; 120:435–438.

78. Ghignone M, Quintin L, Duke PC, et al. Effects of clonidine on narcotic requirements and hemodynamic response during induction of fentanyl anesthesia and endotracheal intubation. *Anesthesiology* 1986; 64:36–42.

79. Milne B, Cervenko FW, Jhamandas K, et al. Intrathecal clonidine: analgesia and effect on opiate withdrawal in the rat. *Anesthesiology* 1985; 62:34–38.

80. Coombs DW, Saunders RL, LaChance D, et al. Intrathecal morphine tolerance: use of intrathecal clonidine, DADLE, and intraventricular morphine. *Anesthesiology* 1985; 62:358–363.

81. Walsh TD. A controlled study of MST continus tablets for chronic pain in advanced cancer. In: Wilkes E, Levy J, eds. *Advances in Morphine Therapy, 64.* London: Royal Society of Medicine; 1984:69–72.

82. Welsh J, Stuart JFB, Habeshaw T, et al. A comparative pharmacokinetic study of morphine-sulphate solution and MST continus 30 mg tablets in conditions expected to allow steady-state drug levels. In: Stuart JFB, ed. *Methods of Morphine Estimation in Biological Fluids and the Concept of Free Morphine, 58.* London: Royal Society of Medicine; 1983:9–14.

83. Portenoy RK, Foley KM. Chronic use of opioid analgesics in non-malignant pain: report of 38 cases. *Pain* 1986; 25:171–186.

CHAPTER 27

Intraspinal Opioid Analgesia

Ann-Marie E. Nehme

In our continuing search for methods to relieve disabling pain, one of the most recent advances has been the discovery of the usefulness of intraspinal opioids. It was the recognition of opiate receptors and endogenous opiates that ultimately led to the use of intraspinal opioids in the treatment of pain. In 1973, three reports were published describing binding sites for opioids in the mammalian nervous system.[98,117,125] The spinal cord was one of the areas in which these receptors were found. In 1975, Goldstein and colleagues[49] reported the presence of a substance in the bovine pituitary gland that possessed morphine-like effects. This later was called enkephalin. The discovery of β-endorphin followed shortly afterward.

After these discoveries, it was not surprising that animal studies using intrathecal opiates were reported by 1976.[149] It was found that intrathecal opiates produced analgesia. By 1979, the first controlled study of the analgesic affect of intrathecal morphine in humans was reported.[136] In the same year, epidural morphine was used to treat patients.[8] Many subsequent studies expanded our knowledge and facilitated our clinical use of intraspinal opiates.[2,10,11,46,51,54,68,73,79,106,110,119–121,137]

PHYSIOLOGY

The scientific basis of the opiate receptor system is covered in detail in Chapter 1. To summarize briefly, when nociceptive fibers at the periphery receive noxious stimuli, they generally are transmitted by A-delta and C-fibers to the spinal cord. These primary afferent fibers enter the dorsal horn through the dorsal root ganglia where their cell bodies are located. They then proceed to the Lissauer tract. The second-order neurons have their cell bodies in the substantia gelatinosa (rexed laminae II and III). Input is modulated at the spinal cord level by these afferent inputs and the dorsal horn neurons, which may be excitatory or inhibitory, before ascending.

Studies show that C-fibers, particularly, will evoke a painful response in the wide dynamic range neurons of the dorsal horn.[143,144] This response is inhibited by low dose opiates. This inhibitory response of opiates is not limited to C-fibers but also occurs with input through larger diameter A-fibers. The inhibition of discharge of nociceptive neurons at the spinal level prevents the rostral transmission of these nociceptive impulses. Evidence indicates that intraspinal opiates play their greatest role at the level of the substantia gelatinosa of the dorsal horn of the spinal cord.

Currently, our knowledge of this process is incomplete, but based on animal models, studies, and clinical evidence, much is known. There are several naturally occurring peptides that are known to affect pain. Substance P has been identified at peripheral nerve endings, in dorsal root ganglia, and centrally. Its release is known to be inhibited by morphine.[142] Other peptides (including a peptide similar to cholecystokinin, vasoactive intestinal peptide), prostaglandins, and prostacyclins have each been implicated in the transmission of pain. The inhibitory neurotransmitter γ-aminobutyric acid is found in cells of the substantia gelatinosa presynaptically, and glycine is found postsynaptically.

In recent years, many endogenous opioid peptides have been identified. More than 20 opioid peptides have been found (see Chap. 1 for details). These fall into one of three distinct classes: enkephalins, dynorphins, and β-endorphins, each with affinities for different opiate receptors. The relationship between the opioid peptide and the opiate receptors is neither specific nor simple. Ongoing research will expand our understanding.

Since the discovery of the opiate receptors in the early 1970s,[49,97,126] work has been done to elucidate the issue and provide clinical relevance. The μ, κ, δ, σ, and ε opiate receptors have been demonstrated. The classes of receptors have been named for the drugs or endogenous peptides that bind to them primarily (see Chap. 1). Because morphine binds primarily to the μ receptor and is the most dominant in producing analgesia, it is the one with which we are most interested in this discussion. At least two subclasses of μ receptors are known. The first results in analgesia and the second, respiratory depression. Morphine binds to both. The κ and δ receptors also are believed to play a role in spinal analgesia (as evidenced partly by reversal of their effects by naloxone).[62,130] Some believe that the δ receptors are the strongest at the spinal level and that the primary effect of morphine at the μ receptors is actually at the central medullary level.[111] This area and studies regarding these issues still are controversial.[152]

The discovery of endogenous opioid peptides at the spinal cord level and the identification of opiate receptors with their various affinities for known analgesics led to the clinical use of intraspinal opiates to produce analgesia.[150] The first controlled study[136] showed dramatic pain relief in eight patients with malignancies involving the lumbar plexus, who were treated with intrathecal morphine versus saline. The many subsequent studies and the rapidly widespread clinical use reflected the ongoing need for a method to reduce pain without the many adverse effects of the narcotics administered by other routes. By 1981, many studies had been reported, including an excellent review paper by Yaksh.[142] In 1984, another comprehensive review[34] presented the results of all available controlled human studies to address the efficacy and problems related to spinal opiates. Therefore, the ground work for appropriate clinical application was done early.

PHARMACOLOGY

After the intraspinal opioid is administered, it will enter both the cerebrospinal fluid (CSF) and local blood vessels (Figs. 27-1 and 27-2).[90] If given intrathecally, the route to the CSF is, of course, direct.[35,47] An epidural injection will result in diffusion into the CSF. The rate and amount of opioid that enters the CSF by this indirect route is affected by several factors, including the molecular weight and shape of the opioid and the surface area of the dura exposed to the drug. The latter is related primarily to the volume of the injection and also to anatomic considerations, such as septa, scar tissue, and tumor that may be present in patients who may be considered for this pain therapy.[22] Lipid solubility is a prime factor in the duration of drug action

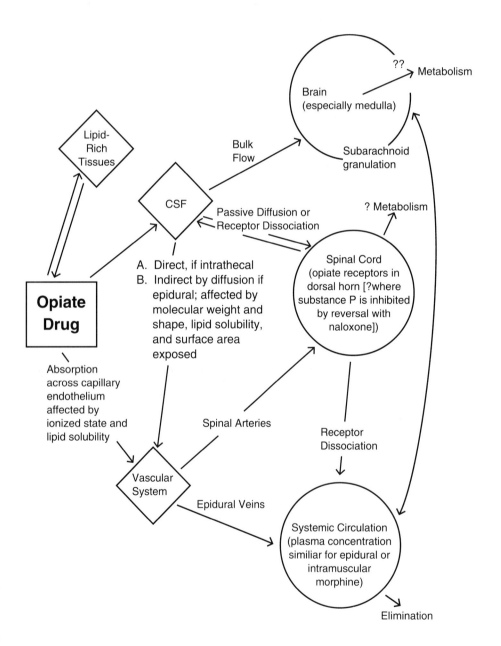

FIGURE 27-1. Distribution of intraspinal opioid after injection.

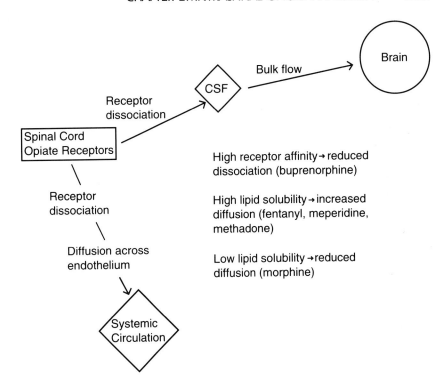

FIGURE 27-2. Methods of distribution of intraspinal opioids.

because of its role in the rate of both dural penetration and escape by the epidural route. The higher the lipid solubility of an agent, that is, the lesser the ionized fraction, the more rapid the diffusion. Therefore, fentanyl, methadone, and meperidine, with their high lipid solubilities, each diffuse quickly and bind to the spinal receptors. They have a rapid onset of action. The disadvantage of this is that they can escape quickly for the same reason and, therefore, have a limited duration of action unless the agent has a particularly high affinity for the receptor, such as occurs with lofentanil. Morphine, however, is much less lipid soluble and therefore is slow to diffuse through the dura, slow to bind to receptor sites, and slow to exit. This results in a slow onset and long duration. It also causes a higher percentage of the dose to be free in the CSF to travel cephalad by bulk flow to the brain and especially to the medullary center with its opiate receptors.[16] Some authors believe this to be the principal mechanism of action of intrathecal morphine.[9]

In addition to the CSF, the second compartment involved with the administration of intraspinal opioids is the hematologic system.[83] Opioids are absorbed across capillary endothelia into both the spinal arteries and epidural veins. After an epidural injection, the absorption into the spinal arteries can lead to an increased amount of drug available at the spinal cord. Systemic absorption into the epidural veins indirectly from drug eliminated by the receptors at the cord level for epidural and intrathecal administration and directly by injection into the epidural space will allow some opioid to be available in the systemic circulation.

Several studies[52,65,89,95,142,147,149,153] examining peak plasma and peak CSF concentrations of morphine after epidural injections have been done in an effort to determine, not only the disposition of morphine after epidural injection, but also to correlate these findings with the clinical effect and, therefore, the mechanism of action. After an epidural injection of morphine, the peak plasma levels are reached in approximately 10 to 30 min (range, 5 to 30 min). After the opiate enters the circulatory system by the azygos vein, its analgesic effects, side effects, and elimination resemble that of an intramuscular dose. The peak CSF levels occur at approximately 60 to 120 min (range, 30 to 120 min), and the CSF concentrations at any given time were up to 100-fold higher than the plasma concentration. The elimination half-life for morphine in CSF was approximately 2 h (range, 60 to 258 min). These studies consistently reported that, although the initial analgesia might be attributed to both systemic and spinal effects, the long duration of analgesia with epidural morphine was secondary to the sustained high concentration of drug in the CSF.

The lipid solubility of the drug used also is important in vascular absorption. High lipid solubility facilitates vascular absorption. Durant and Yaksh[42] found that epidural vascular uptake of morphine in rats was low; fentanyl and lofentanil uptake was high.

The flow rate through the epidural venous plexus is another factor. Increased blood flow increases clearance from the epidural space, although if the volume also is greater, the actual concentration may be lower.

Last, we must mention that the role of actual local metabolism of spinal opioids is still unclear. There is no evidence that it plays a major role.

Tolerance

A limiting factor in the chronic use of intraspinal opioids is drug tolerance. Animal studies show that, with continued use of either intrathecal or epidural opioids, the analgesic effect of a given dose diminishes over time.[123] Tolerance was found during intrathecal morphine therapy in both rats and primates by days 5 to 7.[111,124,131]

Data from human studies give conflicting results.[72,86,94,133,154] There may be interspecies differences although there is no strong evidence to support this. More likely, it may be related to the fact that human clinical studies on chronic pain (usually cancer pain) lack the control group that laboratory studies on normal animals have. Also, there may be factors we do not understand.

Although tolerance is not understood, research studies provide some clinically useful data. First, there is cross tolerance between systemic and intraspinal opiates.[142,146] If a patient was treated previously with parenteral opiate analgesics, then the effective dose needed for intraspinal opiate analgesia would be greater. The human studies in which tolerance occurred early[86,133,154] generally administered a relatively large bolus of epidural drug only once or twice a day. Intermittent smaller injections seem to delay the development of tolerance (up to 280 days in the study of Malone and colleagues,[77]). Reviewing these results, we may conclude that a continuous infusion of low dose opiate is probably the best way to avoid early tolerance. However, it also appears that, after a certain dose of opiate has been reached, the rate of progressive tolerance can be rapid. Therefore, it is advisable to institute intraspinal opioids earlier rather than later in the course of opiate therapy.

When tolerance occurs with intraspinal opioids and pain is not controlled adequately, then several measures can be taken. Increasing the dose of the opioid is generally the first step. It may be useful to switch to another class of narcotics to increase effective analgesia. Ultimately, the system is limited by the volume of drug and, therefore, the dose that physically can be delivered. When a patient's pain is refractory to even massive doses of opioid because of tolerance, then it is useful to "rest" the receptors with the goal of using lower subsequent doses when therapy is resumed. One method is to replace the intraspinal opioid with low dose local anesthetic, for example, bupivacaine 0.0625% to 0.125% at a rate of 10 ml/h to start for 3 to 5 days. This is particularly successful for pain below the T10 level. Another possibility is to administer either clonidine or D-Ala-D-Leu-enkephalin alone or in addition to the local anesthetic. Once the opioid has been substituted, symptoms of withdrawal, hemodynamic stability, and motor blockade should be monitored carefully. The dose of drug must be adjusted accordingly. After 3 to 4 days of this, the spinal opioid is resumed at a lower dose, and the minimum effective dose is calculated based on the patient's level of pain control. The use of intraspinal clonidine alone or with morphine is an established therapy, generally for intractable cancer pain.[28,45,148]

Toxicity

Using preservative-free intraspinal opioids, there is no evidence of neural injury at the spinal cord level. Yaksh[142] studied cats and primates and found no signs of cord disease secondary to either the catheter or the morphine. These catheters had been placed intrathecally and remained in place for 4 to 16 months. Studies by Borner and colleagues[12] revealed that the pH of the opioids used is compatible with CSF, and there was no evidence of precipitation, except for etidocaine and heroin, which became turbid. Autopsies of two terminally ill patients with cancer, whose pain had been treated with epidural morphine for 16 and 21 days, showed no pathologic changes at macro- or microscopic levels.[12] At least two other human studies of such patients treated with intraspinal morphine for 3 weeks to 6 months also found no disease associated with this mode of treatment.[1,81]

DRUG CHOICE

The ideal intraspinal narcotic, like the ideal agent for general anesthesia, has not been discovered. Ideally, we would like the drug to have a rapid onset, long duration, insignificant side effects, and low cost. Fentanyl, meperidine, methadone, sufentanil, alfentanil, diamorphine, hydromorphone, buprenorphine, nalbuphine, butorphanol, and lofentanil all have been used, but preservative-free morphine is administered most commonly and is the best studied drug.

As discussed earlier in this chapter, lipophilicity tends to be the most important factor influencing onset and duration of action, and therefore indirectly, the choice of the drug. In most patients with severe chronic pain, an increased time of onset of analgesia is less important than the longer duration afforded by the less lipophilic drugs. Morphine, therefore, continues to be the most widely used agent in chronic pain because of its long duration of action (usually 12 to 24 h; range, 4 to 36 h). The initial dose of intraspinal morphine generally is calculated by establishing the parenteral morphine or morphine equivalent requirement necessary to maintain reasonable analgesia over a 24 h period. Typically 5 percent to 10 percent of this amount administered epidurally or 0.1 percent of this amount intrathecally will result in an equianalgesic dose in the narcotic-tolerant patient. The dose is more important than the volume administered or the location of the catheter when morphine is used. In acute or postoperative pain, 2 to 5 mg of epidural morphine typically provides good analgesia. Similar to other methods of opioid administration, elderly patients may require smaller doses.

If the goal is short-term rapid onset of analgesia, then the more lipophilic drugs (such as fentanyl, lofentanil, and sufentanil) are better choices. Of these, the most experience has been reported using fentanyl, particularly in obstetric patients.[140] By contrast, lofentanil has a long duration despite its high lipophilicity because of its high receptor affinity.

In addition to the opioids, agonists of other pain neurotransmitter systems have been injected intraspinally. Clonidine and ketamine (as agonists of the norepinephrinergic system), somatostatin, serotonin, baclofen, midazolam, and calcitonin all have been reported to produce analgesia independent of that produced by the opioids.[25,33] This has some exciting implications because cross tolerance among these agents may not occur, and thus patients tolerant to one group may obtain better analgesia from another. Also, in the future, combinations of low doses of these agents may produce good analgesia with limited side effects.

Finally, there are many reports of synergy between opioids and local anesthetics. We administered bupivacaine 0.0625% with epidural morphine chronically and had superior results compared with morphine alone. Trials using lower doses of bupivacaine are in progress in the hope of overcoming the problems associated with this regimen, particularly the patient's inability to ambulate and urinary retention. Whichever drugs are chosen, the preparation must be preservative free.

ADVERSE EFFECTS

Animal studies by Yaksh[142] showed no effect of analgesic doses of spinal opioids on reflexes, light touch, coordinated muscle function, or muscle tone. Autonomic function remained intact. The intraspinal route shares many of the adverse effects seen with other routes of opioid therapy.[85,116,129]

Respiratory Depression

The most ominous adverse effect associated with intraspinal opioid administration is respiratory depression.[36,48,108] This usually has been reported after intrathecal morphine and in the narcotic-naive patient. It is less common in narcotic-tolerant patients, such as those with cancer and chronic pain.[30,34,154]

Respiratory depression may have a fast or a delayed onset with epidural injection and a delayed onset with intrathecal injections.[66] The fast onset seen with epidural injections is believed to result from vascular absorption. Typically, this depression will occur 1 to 2 h postinjection of morphine. A direct route from the epidural plexus to the cerebral venous system is postulated that affects the respiratory centers at the floor of the fourth ventricle.

With delayed respiratory depression, the route to respiratory centers of the brain is probably by rostral spread of CSF by bulk flow to the respiratory centers in the brain. This occurs with intrathecal and epidural injections because the latter diffuse through the dura into the CSF. Some studies indicate that the onset of delayed respiratory depression is sooner with epidural than intrathecal modes. This may mean that vascular absorption also plays a role. Generally, it occurs within 6 to 12 h after treatment with morphine and is not seen after 24 h.

The overall incidence of significant respiratory depression is low (probably 1 percent to 2 percent for epidural and slightly higher for intrathecal administration (Table 27-1). The retrospective nature of most of the studies would tend to underestimate the actual incidence. However, many of these studies were done at a time when large doses of morphine were administered. There is no evidence that there is a greater incidence of respiratory depression with intraspinal opioids than with those given systemically. One study in rats[132] found that epidural opioids, by contrast with subcutaneous ones, produced no significant respiratory depression. This question is still not answered satisfactorily in humans.

Empirically, a few common risk factors appeared in several of the studies of delayed respiratory depression. All patients were postoperative and not normal volunteers or those with chronic pain. Patient age older than 70 years was

Table 27-1
Incidence of Respiratory Depression Related to Delivery Technique

Drug	No. of Patients	Incidence of Respiratory Depression (percent)	Reference
Epidural morphine	>6000	0.3%	Gustafsson et al.[53]
	2000	0.05%	Brownridge[18]
	1085	0.9%*	Stenseth et al.[122]
	> 500	0.2%	Muller et al.[86]
	50	0	Zenz et al.[154]
	90	5.5%	Gustafsson et al.[53]

*The only prospective study of the ones cited.

associated with a higher risk. Concomitant use of parenteral narcotics has been implicated. Intrathecal administration may be associated with a higher risk than the epidural route. When the intrathecal route is used, a supine posture versus a raised head of the bed (up 30 to 40°) seems to increase the risk.

When respiratory depression occurs, administration of 0.1 to 0.4 mg of intravenous naloxone can be used to reverse it, usually without affecting the analgesia. This is presumably because the concentration of opioid at the receptors of the respiratory centers is relatively lower than at those in the spinal cord that are responsible for analgesia. It also may reflect differences in these receptors. It should be remembered that the naloxone has a half-life in the brain of less than 30 min. Therefore, repeated doses or continuous low dose infusion may be necessary. Some clinicians prophylactically infuse 5 μg/kg/h of naloxone into all patients receiving intraspinal opioid. Unless particular risk factors are identified, this probably is unnecessary.

If we look beyond depression of the respiratory rate, we can see changes that may not have obvious clinical significance. Carbon dioxide responsiveness has been studied in six normal volunteers[87] and shown to be decreased an average of 60 percent for 3 to 10 h after 10 mg of epidural morphine. The tidal volume was more diminished than the respiratory rate. A study of seven patients with chronic pain treated with 0.1 mg/kg of lumbar epidural morphine found maximal depression of the slope of the minute ventilatory response to CO_2 at 1 to 2 h posttherapy. At 8 h postinjection, when segmental analgesia and loss of temperature discrimination were greatest, the minute ventilation and average inspiratory flow were reduced statistically significantly.

To summarize, measurable respiratory depression appears to be biphasic with epidural morphine. At 1 to 2 h, it is secondary to vascular absorption and, at 6 to 12 h, to rostral spread of the drug. Intrathecal morphine does not have an early peak. The incidence of clinically significant respiratory depression is low and can be treated successfully with naloxone.

An area of continuing controversy warrants mention here. The question of whether or not epidural opioids after surgery of the upper abdomen or thorax particularly, improve outcome, remains unanswered. There are some strong supporters of each side of this argument. Proponents cite studies indicating early improvement of the forced expiratory volume postoperatively with fewer pulmonary complications and a quicker time to recovery. Opponents claim no significant changes and the added risk of another invasive procedure. The final answer is unknown currently.

Urinary Retention

Another well-known adverse effect of opioid analgesia is urinary retention. Many studies, mostly of epidural mor-

phine use, report an incidence of urinary retention requiring catheterization in 10 percent to 25 percent of men, who may be more susceptible to this effect than women. A prospective study of 1085 postoperative patients managed with epidural morphine found urinary retention in 42 percent.[122] A nationwide study of 6000 to 9150 patients[53] revealed a median 10 percent incidence of urinary retention requiring catheterization (range, 0.3 percent to 25 percent). Another large study of 1200 postoperative patients receiving 10 mg of epidural morphine reported a 15 percent incidence of urinary retention requiring catheterization.[107] There are many studies of smaller numbers of patients with results that also fall into this general range. In studies done on volunteers[15,17,127,128] rather than patients with pain, incidence rates were reported as high as 90 percent of the 10 patients studied[15] and 100 percent of 4 volunteers studied.[128]

The mechanism by which spinal opioids produce urinary retention is unproved, although evidence suggests an effect on opioid receptors at the spinal cord level.[38] Small doses of naloxone are known to reverse this effect, although at least one author contests this finding.[122] In a study of urodynamics in 30 volunteers, increased relaxation of the detrusor muscle and increased bladder capacity were demonstrated.[101] The dose is not a contributing factor; there was no difference in the incidence of urinary retention with doses as low as 0.5 mg compared with 8 or 10 mg of epidural morphine.[78,101] Finally, there seems to be no significant difference in the incidence of urinary retention using epidural morphine versus intramuscular morphine.

Nausea and Vomiting

The most likely incidence of nausea and vomiting after epidural morphine postoperatively is 15 percent to 35 percent.[88,107,122] This is no different from the 30 percent generally quoted for postoperative patients receiving parenteral narcotics. At least one study in volunteers[15] showed a higher value (50 percent) than that seen in patients with pain. The symptoms generally occur at the time when there is evidence of rostral spread and are believed to be caused by stimulation of the chemoreceptors in the floor of the fourth ventricle. Again, naloxone will reverse this effect. Therapy generally consists of an antiemetic (such as transdermal scopolamine, droperidol, a phenothiazine, or metoclopramide).

Pruritus

Intense itching is associated with both epidural and intrathecal opioids.[5] Similar to the other adverse affects, a wide range of incidence is reported. The variability can be explained to some degree by differences in the population under study and possibly by the dose of drug administered and the method of observation (for example, whether patients are asked directly versus whether they volunteer information). In one study of 1200 postoperative patients,[107] an incidence of 15 percent was reported, similar to the finding of 11 percent in 1085 postoperative patients in another trial.[122] Reports vary between an insignificant incidence and 100 percent. Parturients seem to be more susceptible than postoperative patients,[6,18,107,113] and volunteers have high values of 75 percent[128] and 100 percent.[15] There is conflicting evidence as to whether or not a dose–response effect exists.

The mechanism of pruritus production currently is unknown.[67] Parenterally dosed morphine causes histamine release and pruritus in some patients. Because we cannot observe a cutaneous manifestation in patients treated with intraspinal morphine, there is no apparent release of histamine. Administering antihistamines to treat the pruritus has been tried, but conflicting results have been reported. The evidence tends to favor the idea that the mechanism of action is not related to histamine release. This problem has been reported after morphine use with and without preservatives, and there is no indication that the preservative is the culprit. Naloxone relieved this symptom in 90 percent of cases studied by one group.[122]

The pruritus itself generally has an onset near the time of analgesia and a duration that may exceed the analgesia. It is not limited to the segmental distribution of the analgesia but may be generalized. Most often, it affects the head, neck, and palate.

INDICATIONS AND PATIENT SELECTION

Since the first published reports in 1979 of the clinical use of intrathecal[136] and then epidural morphine,[8] there has been widespread use of intraspinal opioids for pain relief.[102,138] The risks associated with the drug and the procedure and the equipment needed limit its use. Appropriate patient selection is crucial for a good outcome. This technique can be used successfully both for acute and chronic pain.

Acute Pain (See Chap. 20)

Use of this technique generally is limited to two groups: surgical or postoperative and obstetric patients. Occasionally, it is used in other acute pain situations, including posttraumatic, postmyocardial infarction, and ischemic leg pain.[13,105]

Surgical or Postoperative Patients

The role of epidural opioid analgesia for pain therapy intraoperatively and postoperatively has been an area of controversy during the last 15 years.[112] Proponents of the technique of combining epidural analgesia with general anesthesia intraoperatively, followed by epidural analgesia postoperatively, claim that, in the patient in whom this technique would be the most valuable (e.g., patients with

ASA status III or IV), undergoing upper abdominal or thoracic surgery, the postoperative morbidity is less. Opponents believe that there is no significant difference in outcome when the patient is given adequate parenteral opioids postoperatively and that, in using this technique, the patient is exposed to the additional risk of another invasive procedure. A well-designed study in 1987[151] attempted to address this question, but the small study group (the study was interrupted for ethical reasons because the investigators believed that combined technique was safer) and the high rate of complications in the general anesthesia group compel us to question this as the definitive study on this subject.

Patients with ASA status III and IV undergoing upper abdominal or thoracic surgery, particularly, generally will receive adequate postoperative analgesia, using the combined epidural and general anesthesia method.[15,17,64,71,78] There is no clear evidence that this method provides better analgesia than properly administered intravenous opioids or patient-controlled analgesia, although it is effective. A prospective but, unfortunately, uncontrolled study of 1085 patients reported a postoperative patient satisfaction of 88 percent (laparotomy group) to 97 percent (hip arthroplasty group) managed with epidural morphine. Postoperative patients undergoing epidural analgesia may have fewer pulmonary complications and improved pulmonary function, early return of peristaltic function, shorter time to ambulation, decreased incidence of deep venous thromboses, and decreased length of hospital stay.[15,103,104,115]

Obstetric Patients

In recent years, the use of epidural fentanyl for labor pain and Caesarean section has become widely used.[37] Used in combination with a local anesthetic, it can provide excellent analgesia and anesthesia. Early studies of low dose (2 to 4 mg) epidural morphine alone generally found unsatisfactory analgesia, whereas bupivacaine alone provided good relief.[6,23,60,141] Subsequent experience and studies have shown that the combination of local anesthetic and opioid provides the best analgesia.[61]

Two recent studies[44,57] randomized patients undergoing Caesarean section into three groups for analgesia: epidural morphine, patient-controlled analgesia with intravenous morphine, and intramuscular morphine. Both studies found that epidural morphine produced statistically significantly better analgesia and patient satisfaction than intramuscular morphine. Epidural morphine was significantly better than patient-controlled analgesia,[57] although this was not found in the other study where they were comparable.[44]

Intrathecal opioids have been used for both labor and delivery, although not as frequently as epidural administration.[6,74,84] One study reported the use of 25 μg of fentanyl plus 0.25 mg of morphine intrathecally in 15 women in labor; 80 percent patient satisfaction was found.[74] We could argue that the risk of spinal headache would outweigh the potential benefit in this group, but this technique at least should be considered.

Chronic Pain

Intraspinal opioids play an important role in the treatment of chronic pain. In patients who have not responded to more traditional pain therapies, this technique offers an alternative that can be successful in alleviating pain and improving the quality of life.[32,91,109,139]

Cancer Pain

Most patients with chronic pain considered for intraspinal analgesics have cancer.[63] This therapy can provide pain relief and afford terminally ill patients and their families relief from suffering in the end stages of painful metastatic disease. In this group, an implanted intraspinal opioid delivery system is indicated for long-term therapy.[19,20,75] As early as 1976, Yaksh and Rudy[149] reported the safety of long-term intrathecal catheters in animal models. The 1979 article by Wang and colleagues[136] described eight patients with cancer whose pain was treated successfully with intrathecal morphine, and Behar and coworker's[8] also reported the use of epidural morphine in the treatment of cancer pain. By 1980, Lazorthes and associates[72] cited three instances of extended relief of cancer pain using the technique of multiple injections daily through an indwelling intrathecal catheter. Onofrio and Yaksh[92] by 1982 had described the use of continuous low dose intrathecal morphine for cancer pain. The use of implanted reservoirs, set to deliver intraspinal morphine at a controlled rate, was reported in 1981.[29,99] In 1990, others used patient-controlled analgesia with intrathecal morphine for a rapid determination of subsequent daily drug scheduling.[56]

When a patient with cancer and uncontrolled pain is evaluated for potential control with an indwelling intraspinal opioid delivery system, several questions must be addressed systematically. First, and in my judgment, foremost, is proper patient selection. This treatment technique, tempting as it is theoretically, is not for everyone. Appropriate patient selection is the key to good outcome. Typically, a patient with cancer presents to the pain clinic with pain refractory to oral or parenteral medications or with a particular intolerance to narcotics, generally manifested as excessive sedation, nausea, or vomiting, that dominates their remaining life. In some cases, a patient's tolerance to opioid analgesics has become so great that there is a practical problem in providing enough drug for successful analgesia.[26] In these instances, a trial of intraspinal opioids may be warranted and may provide an excellent alternative. Both physiologic and psychological considerations must be evaluated before proceeding. The article by Waldman and associates[135] provides a sensible, and I believe, realistic approach to appropriate patient selection. We know from a review of the literature[4,43] and our experience that pain of neuropathic origin generally is difficult to treat with opioids. Physiologic conditions resulting in central nervous system abnormalities may lead to a patient's inability to assess pain or pain relief. The anatomic site of pain obviously will be a factor in outcome. For instance, arm pain secondary to metastatic breast cancer will not respond as well as the pain from a pathologic hip fracture. An important consideration, which may be difficult to assess, is the psychological capability of the patient and family to perceive pain relief. This can be insurmountable in the treatment of chronic pain as those of us in this field know. Another consideration is life expectancy.

After a patient has been deemed to be an appropriate candidate, a trial of the proposed intraspinal opioid must be instituted to demonstrate that this method at least is effective initially. Onofrio and colleagues[92] describe a so-called analgesic index as one method of assessing the sensitivity of the patient to spinal opioids and as a prognostic indicator of outcome. After effectiveness is established, an indwelling system is placed. The basic decision scheme is outlined in Figure 27-3.

The last 12 years has provided us with many articles on this subject, and we have gained experience using this technique. We have much information, if not all the definitive answers. Recent publications describe long-term results of intraspinal morphine primarily for the treatment of cancer pain in a total of 736 patients.[43,76,98,145] Yaksh and Onofrio[145] analyzed data from 163 patients (130 with cancer) from 19 centers using intrathecal morphine. The median number of weeks this therapy was used was 13 (range, 1 to 1215 days; mean, 21 weeks). This compared with a mean of 13.7 weeks in 284 retrospectively reviewed cases[98] and approximately 7 weeks (range, 7 to 420 days) in 255 cases.[43] These reviews substantiate our experience at Beth Israel's Pain Management Center that there is extreme variability in dosing (range, 0.5 mg to > 3 g daily). To a large degree, this reflects how opioid tolerant the patient was when therapy was instituted. Plummer's group[98] reports no dose increase trend over time, although Yaksh and Onofrio[145] note a time-dependent increase, which I suspect exists. The 48 percent of the patients they reviewed who still were using their catheters at 3 months had less than doubled their morphine requirements. Of the 10 patients who reached 52 weeks of use, their average requirements had more than quadrupled (mean, 4.8 ± 0.4 mg/day [n = 130] to 21 ± 9 mg/day [n = 10]). Our group studied one case of a patient with severe hip pain secondary to metastatic cancer who was treated with an implanted reservoir pump and whose requirements eventually exceeded the pump's capabilities. She was admitted to the hospital and changed to low dose bupivacaine plus clonidine to rest her μ receptors; after this time, her morphine was restarted successfully at a lower dose. Tolerance does develop and may be so great as to exceed the system's capabilities to deliver the drug.

It is very difficult to assess the success rate of this technique. In one study,[43] 59.1 percent of 255 patients achieved satisfactory analgesia with intraspinal opioids alone. Because their epidural doses ranged only from 5 to a maximum of 80 mg per day and their average duration of use was less than 2 months, we might suspect this to be an

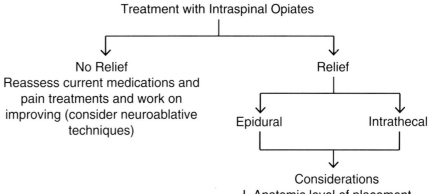

FIGURE 27-3. *Patient selection for permanent intraspinal opioids.*

overestimate. The more severe cases of pain of longer duration might require additional pain therapy.

Failures in this group are secondary to inappropriate patient selection, technical failures, malfunctions, and opioid tolerance.[118] Whether or not this technique is any better than any other well-managed technique, such as subcutaneous morphine infusions,[39] parenteral opioids,[118] or ablative procedures remains to be seen.

Noncancer Pain

There is a limited place for the use of intraspinal opioids in chronic pain unrelated to malignancy. This is caused in part by technical problems involved with a catheter implanted for an indefinite period of time, potential drug tolerance, and evidence suggesting that patients in this group do not respond as well to this approach for analgesia.[31,69] Of the total of 766 patients with chronic pain reported in four recent studies,[43,76,98,145] only 45 or 6 percent had noncancer pain. Intraspinal opiates have been tried in chronic back pain. Cohn and colleagues[27] reported that a single dose of epidural morphine plus corticosteroid effectively provided pain relief in patients with postlaminectomy syndrome. This was not substantiated by subsequent studies, however,[31,98] and rarely is used in the treatment of chronic back pain. Reflex sympathetic dystrophy may be treated with sympathetic blockade using a temporary indwelling catheter, and there are anecdotal reports of epidural and intrathecal morphine used in this group.[50,98] Epidural opioids have been used for vascular surgery and during the postoperative period,[100] but again, this study was not controlled. Therefore, conclusions regarding the advantage of this technique over more conventional methods cannot be reached. Many other diagnoses, including phantom limb pain and periph-

eral ischemia, may warrant consideration of intraspinal opioids, but these drugs are not used regularly because of the risks and practical problems.

CONTRAINDICATIONS

Allergies to the available intraspinal opioids and sepsis would contraindicate this technique. There are relative contraindications for patients with coagulopathies and medical teams who lack experience using this technique, including the pre- and postprocedure evaluations and care. Certain psychological patterns of behavior also would contraindicate this procedure.

PROCEDURE

For acute pain, the standard percutaneous catheter is introduced into the epidural space or intrathecally as desired, the estimated dose of opioid is given, and the patient is monitored in the usual manner. Generally, this is done by the operative anesthesiologist during the perioperative period, the obstetric anesthesiologist, or the acute pain service. Techniques and dosing schedules are well described in any of our standard anesthesia texts. The chronic pain service generally places and manages indwelling systems.

Delivery Systems

In the patient with chronic pain in whom an indwelling catheter is being considered, several delivery systems are available.[82] A percutaneous catheter, such as those commonly used in obstetric patients, first must be placed to ascertain that the patient's pain can be controlled effectively by this method. Untunneled catheters generally are used only for patients with acute or chronic pain and short life expectancies. Zenz and colleagues[154,155] reported the long-term use of percutaneous epidural catheters in 139 patients whose catheters remained implanted for a total of 9716 days. Eighty-seven percent of these patients received adequate relief, and there were two cases of meningitis.

Three general options for indwelling catheters are available: a tunneled catheter with an exterior injection port, an implanted system with a subcutaneous injection port, and an implanted system with a continuous reservoir. Kwan[70] recently reviewed the available infusion systems. The tunneled catheter with an external injection port has the disadvantage of a higher risk of infection, although these probably are rare. In one report of 3891 catheter days of use in 55 patients with cancer, there were no catheter infections using this system.[40] In 1990, Du Pen and colleagues[41] reported their further experience in 350 patients. Thirty had infections of the exit site and superficial catheter track. Eight had catheter track infections beyond the Dacron cuff, and 15 had infections in the epidural space. The superficial infections were treated with daily cleaning and topical or oral antibiotics. In their experience, deep-track infections progressed to infection of the epidural space unless the catheter was removed promptly. Parenteral antibiotics were recommended for deep-track and epidural infections, and catheter reimplantation was considered after completion of antibiotic therapy.

For patients whose life expectancy was weeks to months, a tunneled catheter connected to either a subcutaneous injection port or an external catheter port has been used. Several catheters of Teflon or silastic with prolonged durability are available. They can be implanted percutaneously and tunneled subcutaneously under local anesthesia.

Infusion with any of these systems can be done using a bolus or continuous technique. Bolus injection usually precludes the addition of local anesthetics and probably produces inferior analgesia with higher total doses. In addition, infection may be more likely since the patient or family often are required to manipulate the catheter. Continuous infusion has the disadvantages of requiring that the patient carry an apparatus that may decrease mobility and generally is more expensive. These kits often include an intraspinal catheter with stylet, an external catheter with a Dacron cuff to promote epithelialization, a filter, and a device to connect the two catheters. Some also include a tunneling device.

For patients with life expectancies longer than 6 months, an implanted continuous infusion device may be considered.[21,58,96,114] Implantable devices for the continuous infusion of intraspinal opioids have become increasingly sophisticated during the past decade. The indwelling systems are more difficult to investigate if a problem occurs and can be costly.[59,134]

Some pumps use a chamber filled with freon that expands with body heat as an energy source. Earlier models had a fixed-flow rate, generally about 2 ml/day with a reservoir of 50 ml. Two new models await approval by the Food and Drug Administration. One is a smaller device (63 mm in diameter compared with 87 mm) that will be available with the choice of flow rates of 0.7 or 1.4 ml/day. It will accommodate a volume of 25 ml rather than the older pump's volume of 50 ml. An even newer generation pump awaiting approval will offer the ability to change the flow rate between 1 and 10 ml or vary it throughout the day as needed, using an external programmer.

Other devices employ a small battery as an energy source and currently offer the ability to program the flow rate externally. Unfortunately, the small volume delivered by these devices (maximum, 0.9 ml/h) may pose a problem in patients with large narcotic requirements or when the addition of a local anesthetic is deemed desirable. With increasing sophistication, the costs also are rising (some units cost more than $9000 plus the additional cost for the programmer).

Catheter Implantation Technique

The actual placement procedure typically is done in a chronic pain clinic by the anesthesia team. It can be done in the operating room if no adequate pain clinic facilities are available. The following implantation technique for permanent intraspinal opioid catheters has been used successfully at the Beth Israel Hospital in Boston.

After informed consent is obtained, the patient is given a dose of an antistaphylococcal antibiotic, is positioned in the lateral decubitus position, and the back, flank, and lower lateral abdominal wall are prepared and draped. After infiltration with local anesthetic, a 3-cm paraspinous incision is made at the appropriate lumbar level. A Tuohy needle is introduced through the incision, and the epidural space is identified by a paraspinous approach with a loss of resistance technique. The epidural catheter then is threaded 6 to 8 cm past the tip of the needle. The needle is removed, the catheter is aspirated, and a test dose of local anesthetic is injected to exclude entry into the subarachnoid space or blood vessel. Local anesthetic then is injected through the catheter in a dose and volume to not only confirm positioning in the epidural space, but also to provide anesthesia for the tunneling procedure (15 to 20 ml of chloroprocaine 3%, for example). The catheter is secured with a purse-string suture. Then it is tunneled subcutaneously around the flank to the lower abdominal wall and connected either to an externalized catheter, a subcutaneous injection port, or a subcutaneous continuous-infusion device. The wounds then are closed and dressed aseptically. This technique is well described in the literature.[24,29,30,55,80,88] Companies who make kits for these procedures also detail their own equipment.

Any of the systems discussed may be used with an epidural or intrathecal approach. The choice of intrathecal versus epidural implantation is left up to the practitioner. Intrathecal administration has the potential for cerebrospinal fluid leak; has a higher incidence of respiratory depression, pruritus, urinary retention, and sedation; and is more likely to be associated with meningitis. However, epidural administration more commonly is associated with catheter tip fibrosis, requires larger doses, and produces analgesia that is less predictable, less intense, and of shorter duration than intrathecal administration. The decrease in efficiency as a result of catheter tip fibrosis is of greater consequence with hydrophilic than with lipophilic agents.

Infusion can be done by a bolus or continuous technique.[14,69,93] Bolus injection produces tolerance more rapidly, precludes the addition of local anesthetic, and probably produces inferior analgesia. In addition, infection may be more likely because the patient or family often are required to manipulate the catheter. Continuous infusion has the disadvantage of requiring that the patient carry an apparatus that may decrease mobility. Higher total doses also are required, and greater expense is incurred.

There are complications associated with the catheter and technique. Most frequently reported are infection at the site of the catheter at the skin in the percutaneous systems. Occasional cases of meningitis, which have responded well to antibiotics and catheter removal, have been reported.[154] Catheter tip fibrosis, particularly in the epidural system[42] dislodgement of the catheter, blockage of the catheter or reservoir, and reservoir and pump malfunction all have occurred. Erosion of the catheter through the subcutaneous and cutaneous tissue also have been observed. Results vary considerably in this area and, to some degree, are less frequent when the technique is done by the more experienced teams.

SUMMARY

Anesthesiologists in general, and pain specialists in particular, continually search for better methods to alleviate pain and suffering. There is always a balance between risk and benefit that must be addressed in each individual case. The risk can be significant, and the success limited. With correct patient selection, the benefits can be outstanding. This is particularly true in patients with otherwise refractory cancer-related pain. We hope the future will provide the critical studies needed to address the risks and benefits of this pain technique versus the other less invasive methods of administering opioids. In the meantime, this continues to be an excellent tool for us to use in the treatment of pain.

References

1. Abouleish E, Barmada MA, et al. Acute and chronic effects of intrathecal morphine in monkeys. *Br J Anaesth* 1981; 53:1027.
2. Auld AW, Maki-Jokela A, Murdoch DM, Intraspinal narcotic analgesia in the treatment of chronic pain. *Spine* 1985; 10(8):777.
3. Arner S, Arner B. Differential effects of epidural morphine in the treatment of cancer related pain. *Acta Anaesth Scand* 1985; 29:32.
4. Arner S, Meyerson BA. Lack of analgesic effect of opioids on neuropathic and idiopathic forms of pain. *Pain* 1988; 33:11.
5. Ballantyne JC, Loach AB, Carr DB. Itching after epidural and spinal opiates. *Pain* 1988; 33(2):149.
6. Baraka A, Noueihid R, Hajj S. Intrathecal injection of morphine for obstetric analgesia. *Anesthesiology* 1981; 54:136.
7. Barrow DW, String JE. Postoperative analgesia in major orthopaedic surgery: epidural and intrathecal opiates. *Anaesthesia* 1981; 36:937.
8. Behar M, Magora F, Olshwang D, Davidson JT. Epidural morphine in treatment of pain. *Lancet* 1979; 1:527.
9. Behar M, Orr IA, Dundee JW. Central action of spinal opiates. *Anesthesiology* 1981; 55:334.
10. Benedetti C. Intraspinal analgesia: a historical overview. *Acta Anesthesiol Scand Suppl* 1987; 85:17.
11. Benedetti C, Bonica JJ. Symposium on recent advances in intraspinal pain therapy. *Acta Anaesthesiol Scand Suppl* 1987; 85:31.
12. Borner U, Müller H, et al. Epidural opiate analgesia. Compatibility of opiates with tissue and CSF. *Anesthesiology* 1980; 29:570.
13. Bragg CL. Practical aspects of epidural and intrathecal narcotic analgesia in the intensive care setting. *Heart Lung* 1989; 18(6):599.
14. Brazenor GA. Long-term intrathecal administration of morphine: a comparison of bolus injection via reservoir with continuous infusion by implanted pump. *Neurosurgery* 1987; 21:484.
15. Bromage PR, Camporesi E, Chestnut D. Epidural narcotics for post-operative analgesia. *Anesth Analg Curr Res* 1980; 59:473.
16. Bromage PR, Camporesi EM, Durant PA, et al. Rostral spread of epidural morphine. *Anesthesiology* 1982; 56:431.
17. Bromage PR, Camporesi EM, Durant PAC, Nielson CH. Non-respiratory side effects of epidural morphine. *Anesth Analg* 1982; 61:490.
18. Brownridge PR. Epidural and intrathecal opiates for post-operative pain relief. *Anaesthesia* 1983; 38:74.
19. Bruera E, Brenneis C, MacDonald RN. Continuous SC infusion of narcotics for the treatment of cancer pain: an update. *Cancer Treat Rep* 1987; 71(10):953.
20. Bruera E, Brenneis C, et al. Use of the subcutaneous route for the administration of narcotics in patients with cancer pain. *Cancer* 1988; 62(2):407.
21. Bryant DD III, DeWitty RL Jr, Dennis GC. The Infusaid pump in the management of intractable cancer pain. *J Natl Med Assoc* 1987; 79(3):305.
22. Chauvin M, Samii K, Schermann JM, Sandouk P. Pharmacology of narcotics administered by the epidural or intrathecal route [in French]. *Nouv Presse Med* 1982; 11(13):1003.
23. Chayen MS, Rudick V, Borvine A. Pain control with epidural injected of morphine. *Anesthesiology* 1980, 53:338.
24. Cherry DA. Drug delivery systems for epidural administration of opioids. *Acta Anaesthesiol Scand* 1987; 31:54.
25. Chrubasik J. Spinal infusion of opiates and somatostatin. *Acta Neurochir Suppl (Wien)* 1987; 38:80.
26. Clarke IM, Tempest SM. Opiate doses for terminal cancer. *Lancet* 1980; 1(8164):373.

27. Cohn ML, et al. Computed tomographic and electromyographic evaluation of epidural treatment for chronic low back pain. *Anesthesiology* 1983; 59:A194.

28. Coombs DW, Saunders RL, La Chance D, et al. Intrathecal morphine tolerance: use of intrathecal clonidine, DADLE and intraventricular morphine. *Anesthesiology* 1985; 62:358.

29. Coombs DW, Saunders RL, Gaylor MS, et al. Epidural narcotic infusion reservoir: implantation technique and efficacy. *Anesthesiology* 1981; 55:469.

30. Coombs DW, Saunders RL, Pageau MG. Continuous intraspinal narcotic analgesia: technical aspects of an implantable infusion system. *Reg Anesth* 1982; 7:110.

31. Coombs DW, Saunders RL, Gaylor MS, et al. Relief of continuous chronic pain by intraspinal narcotics infusion via an implanted reservoir. *JAMA* 1983; 250(17):2336.

32. Coombs DW. Management of chronic pain by epidural and intrathecal opioids: newer drugs and delivery systems. *Int Anesthesiol Clin* 1986; 24(2):59.

33. Coombs DW, Allen C, et al. Chronic intraspinal clonidine in sheep. *Reg Anesth* 1984; 19:60.

34. Cousins MJ, Mather LE. Intrathecal and epidural administration of opioids. *Anesthesiology* 1984; 61:276.

35. Crawford JS. Site of action of intrathecal morphine. *Br Med J* 1980; 281:680.

36. Davies GK, Tolhurst-Cleaver CL, James TL. Respiratory depression after intrathecal narcotics. *Anaesthesia.* 1980; 35(11):1080.

37. Donchin Y, Davidson JT, Magora F. Epidural morphine for the control of pain after Cesarean section. *Isr J Med Sci* 1981; 17(5):331.

38. Dray A, Metsch R. Spinal opioid receptors and inhibition of urinary bladder motility in vivo. *Neurosci Lett* 1984; 47(1):81.

39. Drexel H, Dzien A, et al: Treatment of severe cancer pain by low dose continuous subcutaneous morphine. *Pain* 1989; 36:169.

40. DuPen SL, Peterson DG, et al. A new permanent exteriorized epidural catheter for narcotic self-administration to control cancer pain. *Cancer* 1987; 59:986.

41. DuPen SL, Peterson, DG, et al. Infection during chronic epidural catheterization: diagnosis and treatment. *Anesthesiology* 1990; 73:905.

42. Durant PA, Yaksh TL. Epidural injections of bupivacaine, morphine, fentanyl, lofentanil and DADL in chronically implanted rats: a pharmacologic and pathologic study. *Anesthesiology* 1986; 64(1):43.

43. Erdine S, Aldemir T. Long-term results of peridural morphine in 225 patients. *Pain* 1991; 45:155.

44. Eisenach JC, Grice SC, Dewan DM. Patient-controlled analgesia following Cesarean section: a comparison with epidural intramuscular narcotics. *Anesthesiology* 1988; 68(3):444.

45. Eisenach JC, Rauck RL, et al. Epidural clonidine analgesia for intractable cancer pain: Phase I. *Anesthesiology* 1989; 71:647.

46. Finnegan B, Moriarty D. Opiate sensitivity—a case report. *Ir J Med Sci* 1984; 153(3):112.

47. Glass PS. Mechanism of action of extradural compared with intrathecal opiates. *Br J Anesthesia* 1984; 56(6):669. Letter.

48. Glynn CJ, Mather LE, Cousins MJ, Wilson PR, Graham JR. Spinal narcotics and respiratory depression. *Lancet* 1979; 2(8138):356.

49. Goldstein A, Goldstein JS, Cox BM. A synthetic peptide with morphine like pharmacologic action. *Life Sci* 1975; 17(11):1643.

50. Goodman RR, Brisman R. Treatment of lower extremity reflex sympathetic dystrophy with continuous intrathecal morphine infusion. *Appl Neurophys* 1987; 50:425.

51. Gorman ES, Warfield CA. Epidural and spinal opioids. *Hosp Pract* 1986; 21(10A):13.

52. Gustafsson LL, Ackerman S, Adamson H, et al. Disposition of morphine in cerebrospinal fluid after epidural administration. *Lancet* 1982; 1:796.

53. Gustafsson LL, Schildt B, Jacobsen K. Adverse effects of extradural and intrathecal opiates: report of a nationwide survey in Sweden. *Br J Anaesth* 1982; 54(5):479.

54. Gustafsson LL, Wiesenfeld-Hallin Z. Spinal opioid analgesia. A critical update. *Drugs* 1988; 35(6):597.

55. Harbaugh RE, Coombs DW, et al. Implanted continuous epidural morphine infusion system. Preliminary report. *J Neurosurg* 1982; 56:803.

56. Hardy PAJ, Wells JCD. Patient controlled intrathecal morphine for cancer pain. *Clin J Pain* 1990; 6:57.

57. Harrison DM, Sinatra R, Morghese L, Chung JH. Epidural narcotic and patient-controlled analgesia for post-Cesarean section pain relief. *Anesthesiology* 1988; 68(3):454.

58. Hassenbusch S, Pillay PK, et al. Constant infusion of morphine for intractable cancer pain using an implanted pump. *J Neurosurg* 1990; 73:405.

59. Hicks RJ, Kalff V, et al. The radionuclide assessment of a system for slow intrathecal infusion of drugs. *Clin Nucl Med* 1989; 14(4):275.

60. Hughes SC, Abboud TK, et al. Maternal and neonatal effects of epidural morphine for labor. *Anesth Analg* 1982; 61:190.

61. Hughes SC, Rosen MA, et al. Epidural morphine for the relief of post-operative pain after Cesarean section. *Anesth Analg* 1982; 61:190.

62. Hylden JL, Wilcox GL. Intrathecal opioids block a spinal action of substance P in mice: functional importance of both mu- and delta receptors. *Eur J Pharmacol* 1982; 86(1):95.

63. Iacono RP, Linford J, Sandyk, R, Consroe P, Ryan MR, Bamford CR. Intraspinal opiates for treatment of intractable pain in the terminally ill cancer patient. *Int J Neurosci* 1988; 38(1–2):111.

64. Jacobson L. Intrathecal and extradural narcotics. In: Benedetti, C, ed. *Advances in Pain Research and Therapy.* Vol. 7. New York: Raven Press; 1984.

65. Jorgensen BG, Anderson HB, Engkuist A. Influence of epidural morphine on postoperative pain, endocrine, metabolic and renal responses to surgery: a controlled study. *Acta Anesth Scand* 1982; 26:63.

66. Kafer ER, Brown JT, Scott D, et al. Biphasic depression of ventilatory responses to CO_2 following epidural morphine. *Anesthesiology* 1983; 58:418.

67. Kellstein DE, Coghill RC, Frenk H, Bossut DF, Mayer DJ. Opioid inhibition of kainic acid-induced scratching: medication by mu and sigma but not delta and kappa receptors. *Pharmacol Biochem Behav* 1990; 35(1):1.

68. Kitahata LM, Collins JG. Spinal action of narcotic analgesics. *Anesthesiology* 1981; 54:153.

69. Krames ES, Gershow J, et al. Continuous infusion of spinally administered narcotics for the relief of pain due to malignant disorders. *Cancer* 1985; 56:696.

70. Kwan JW. Use of infusion devices for epidural and intrathecal administration of spinal opioids. *Am J Hosp Pharm* 1990; 47(8 suppl):518.

71. Lanz E, Theiss D, Riess W, Sommer V. Epidural morphine for post-operative analgesia: a double-blind study. *Anesth Analg* 1982; 61:236.

72. Lazorthes Y, Gouarderes C, Verdie JC, et al. Analgésie par injection intrathécale de morphine. Etude pharmacocinetique et applicatior aux doulers irreductibles. *Neurochirurgie* 1980; 26:159.

73. Leib RA, Hurtig JB. Epidural and intrathecal narcotics for pain management. *Heart Lung* 1985; 14(2):164.

74. Leighton BL, Desimone CA, et al. Intrathecal narcotics for labor revisited: the combination of fentanyl and morphine intrathecally provides rapid onset of profound, prolonged analgesia. *Anesth Analg* 1989; 69(1):122.

75. Lobato RD, Madrid JL, et al. Intraventricular morphine for intractable cancer pain: rationale, methods, clinical results. *Acta Anaesthiol Scand* 1987; 85(suppl):68.

76. Madrid JL, Fatela LV, Lobato RD, Gozalo A. Intrathecal therapy: rationale, technique, clinical results. *Acta Anesthiol Scand* 1987; 31(suppl 85):60.

77. Malone BT, Beye R, Walker J. Management of cancer pain in the terminally ill by administration of epidural narcotics. *Cancer* 1985; 55:438.

78. Martin R, Salbaing J, et al. Epidural morphine for post-operative pain relief. A dose–response curve. *Anesthesiology* 1982; 56:423.

79. Martin R, Lamarche Y, Tetrault JP. Epidural and intrathecal narcotics. *Can Anaesth Soc J* 1983; 30(6):662.

80. Mather LE, Raj PP. Spinal opiates. In: Raj PP, ed. *Practical Management of Pain*. Chicago: Year Book; 1986.

81. Meier FA, Coombs DW, et al. Pathologic anatomy of constant morphine infusion by intraspinal silastic catheter. *Anesthesiology* 1982; 57:206.

82. Miller BJ, Wyant GM. The epidural opioid internalized system. *Can J Surg* 1987; 30(1):42.

83. Moore RA, Bullingham RE, et al. Dual permeability to narcotics: in vitro determination and application to extradural administration. *Br J Anaesth* 1982; 54:1117.

84. Morgan M. The rational use of intrathecal and extradural opioids. *Br J Anaesth* 1989; 63(2):165.

85. Mott JM, Eisele JH. A survey of monitoring practices following spinal opiate administration. *Anesth Analg* 1986; 65:51.

86. Muller H, Stoyanov M, et al. Epidural opiates for relief of cancer pain. In: Yaksh TL, Muller H, Enguist A, eds. *Anaesthesia Intensive Care Medicine*. Heidelberg: Springer; 1981.

87. Neilson CH, Caomporesi EM, et al. CO_2 sensitivity after epidural and I.V. morphine. *Anesthesiology* 1981; 55: A372.

88. Nitescu P, Appelgren L, et al. Long-term, open catheterization of the spinal subarachnoid space for continuous infusion of narcotic and bupivacaine in patients with "refractory" cancer pain. A technique of catheteriza-

tion and its problems and complications. *Clin J Pain* 1991; 7:143.

89. Nordberg, G. Pharmacokinetic aspects of spinal morphine analgesia. *Acta Anaesth Scand Suppl* 1984; 79(28):1.

90. Nordberg G, Hedner T, Mellstrand T, et al. Pharmacokinetic aspects of epidural morphine analgesia. *Anesthesiology* 1983; 58:545.

91. Onofrio BM, Yaksh, TL. Long term pain relief produced by intrathecal morphine infusion in 53 patients. *J Neurosurg* 1990; 72(2):200.

92. Onofrio BM, Yaksh TL, Arnold PG. Continuous low dose, intrathecal morphine administration in the treatment of chronic pain of malignant origin. *Mayo Clin Proc* 1982; 516.

93. Oyama T, Murakawa T, Baba S, Nagao H. Continuous vs. bolus epidural morphine. *Acta Anaesthesiol Scand* 1987; 31(suppl 85):77.

94. Payne R. Role of epidural and intrathecal narcotics and peptides in the management of cancer pain. *Med Clin North Am* 1987; 71(2):313.

95. Payne R. CSF distribution of opioids in animals and man. *Acta Anaesthesiol Scand Suppl* 1987; 85:38.

96. Penn RD. Use and abuse of drug pumps in cancer pain. *Clin Neurosurg* 1989; 35:409.

97. Pert CB, Snyder SH. Opiate receptor: demonstration in nervous tissue. *Science* 1973; 179:1011.

98. Plummer JL, Cherry DA, et al. Long-term spinal administration of morphine in cancer and non-cancer pain: a retrospective study. *Pain* 1991; 44:215.

99. Poletti CE, Cohen AM, Todd DP, Ojemann RG, Sweet WH, Zervas NT. Cancer pain relieved by long-term epidural morphine with permanent indwelling systems for self-administration. *J Neurosurg* 1981; 55:581.

100. Raggi R, Dardik H, Mauro AL. Continuous epidural anesthesia and post-operative epidural narcotics in vascular surgery. *Am J Surg* 1987; 154(2):192.

101. Rawal N, Mollefors K, et al. An experimental study of urodynamic effects of epidural morphine and of naloxone reversal. *Anesth Analg* 1983; 62:641.

102. Rawal N, Sjostrand UH. Clinical application of epidural and intrathecal opioids for pain management. *Int Anesthesiol Clin* 1986; 24(2):43.

103. Rawal N, Sjostrand UH, et al. Epidural morphine for post-operative pain relief: a comparative study with intramuscular narcotic and intercostal nerve block. *Anesth Analg* 1982; 61:93.

104. Rawal N, Sjostrand U, Dahlstrom B. Postoperative pain relief by epidural morphine. *Anesth Analg* 1981; 60:726.

105. Ready LB. Regional analgesia with intraspinal opioids. In: Bonica JJ, ed. *Management of Pain*. 2nd ed. Philadelphia: Lea Febiger; 1990.

106. Recent advances in intraspinal pain therapy. Papers presented at a symposium; Vincenza, Italy. *Acta Anaesthesiol Scanda Suppl* 1987; 85:1.

107. Reiz S, Westberg M. Side effects of epidural morphine. *Lancet* 1980; 2:203.

108. Respiratory depression after epidural and intrathecal narcotics. *Anaesthesia* 1982; 37(5):600. Letter.

109. Richelson E. Spinal opiate administration for chronic pain: a major advance in therapy. *Mayo Clin Proc* 1981; 56(8):523. Editorial.

110. Rosenberg PH. Spinal analgesia—a modern approach to the treatment of severe pain. *J Intern Med* 1990; 227(5):291.

111. Russell RD, Leslie JB, Su YF, Watkins WD, Chang KJ. Continuous intrathecal opioid analgesia: tolerance and cross-tolerance of mu and delta spinal opioid receptors. *J Pharmacol Exp Ther* 1987; 240(1):150.

112. Samii K. Postoperative spinal analgesia with morphine. *Br J Anaesth* 1981; 53:817.

113. Scott PV, Bowen FE, et al. Intrathecal morphine as sole analgesia during labour. *Br Med J* 1980; 2:351.

114. Sefton MV. Implantable pumps. *Crit Rev Biomed Eng* 1987; 14(3):201.

115. Shulman MS, Brebner J, Sandler A. The effect of epidural morphine in postoperative pain relief and pulmonary function in thoracotomy patients. *Anesthesiology* 1983; 59:192.

116. Sida J, Davidson JT, Behar M, Olshwang D. Spinal narcotics and central nervous system depression. *Anaesthesia* 1981; 36(11):1044.

117. Simon EJ. In search of the opiate receptor. *Am J Med Sci* 1973; 266(3):160.

118. Sjogren P, Banning A. Pain, sedation and reaction time during long-term treatment of cancer patients with oral and epidural opioids. *Pain* 1989; 39(1):5.

119. Sjostrand RH, Rawal N. Regional opioids in anesthesiology and pain management. *Int. Anesthesiol Clin* 1986; 24(2):43.

120. Slattery PJ, Boas RA. Newer methods of delivery of opiates for relief of pain. *Drugs* 1985; 30(6):539.

121. Spinal opiates revisited. *Lancet* 1986; 1(8482):655. Editorial.

122. Stenseth OS, Breivik H. Epidural morphine for postoperative pain: experience with 1085 patients. *Acta Anaesthesiol Scand* 1985; 29:148.

123. Stevens CW, Yaksh TL. Time course characteristics of tolerance development to continuously infused antinociceptive agents in rat spinal cord. *J Pharmacol Exp Ther* 1989; 251(1):216.

124. Stevens CW, Yaksh TL. Magnitude of opioid dependence after continuous intrathecal infusion of mu- and delta-selective opioids in the rat. *Eur J Pharmacol* 1989; 166(3):467.

125. Terenius L. Characteristics of the "receptor" for narcotic analgesics in synaptic plasma membrane fraction from rat brain. *Acta Pharmacol Toxicol (Copenh)* 1973; 33(5):377.

126. Teschemacher H, Opheim KE, Cox BM, Goldstein A. A peptide-like substance from pituitary that acts like morphine, I: isolation. *Life Sci* 1975; 16(12):1771.

127. Thompson WR, Smith PT, et al. Regional analgesic effect of epidural morphine in volunteers. *Can Anesth Soc J* 1981; 28:530.

128. Torda TA, Pybus DA, et al. Experimental comparison of extradural and I.M. morphine. *Br J Anaesth* 1980; 52:939.

129. Tung AS, Tenicela R, Winter PM. Opiate withdrawal syndrome following intrathecal administration of morphine. *Anesthesiology* 1980; 53:340.

130. Tung AS, Yaksh TL. In vivo evidence for multiple opiate receptors mediating analgesia in the rat spinal cord. *Brain Res* 1982; 247:75.

131. Tung AS, Yaksh TL, Wang JY. Tolerance to intrathecal opiates in the rat. *Anesthesiology* 1981; 55:171.

132. Van Den Hoogen RH, Bervoets KJ, Colpaert FC. Respiratory effects of epidural and subcutaneous morphine, meperidine, fentanyl and sufentanil in the rat. *Anesth Analg* 1988; 67(11):1071.

133. Ventafridda V, Figliuzzi M, et al. Clinical observation on analgesia elicited by intrathecal morphine in cancer patients. In Bonica JJ, ed. *Advances in Pain Research and Therapy*. Vol. 3. New York: Raven Press: 1979.

134. Waldman SD, Feldstein GS, Allen ML. A troubleshooting guide to the subcutaneous epidural implantable reservoir. *J Pain Symptom Manage* 1986; 1:217.

135. Waldman SD, Feldstein GS, Allen ML, Turnage G. Selection of patients for implantable intraspinal narcotic delivery systems. *Anesth Analg* 1986; 65(8):883.

136. Wang JK, Nauss LA, Thomas JE. Pain relief by intrathecally applied morphine in man. *Anesthesiology* 1979; 50:149.

137. Warfield CA. Intraspinal narcotics. A new method of pain management. *AORN J* 1985; 41(5):910.

138. Warfield CA, Dohlman LE. Intraspinal narcotics for pain control. *Hosp Pract* 1984; 19(2):148B.

139. Wermeling DP, Foster TS, et al. Drug delivery for intractable cancer pain. Use of a new disposable parenteral infusion device for continuous outpatient epidural narcotic infusion. *Cancer* 1987; 60(4):875.

140. Wolfe MJ, Davies GK. Analgesic action of extradural fentanyl. *Br J Anaesth* 1980; 52:357.

141. Writer WD, James FM, Wheeler AS. Double blind comparison of morphine and bupivacaine for continuous epidural analgesia in labor. *Anesthesiology* 1981; 54:215.

142. Yaksh TL. Spinal opiate analgesia: characteristics and principals of action. *Pain* 1981; 11:293.

143. Yaksh TL. Spinal opiates: a review of their effect on spinal function with emphasis on pain processing. *Acta Anaesthesiol Scand Suppl* 1987; 85:25.

144. Yaksh TL. Opioid receptor systems and the endorphins: a review of their spinal organization. *J Neurosurg* 1987; 67(2):157.

145. Yaksh TL, Onofrio BM. Retrospective consideration of the doses of morphine given intrathecally by chronic infusion in 163 patients by 19 physicians. *Pain* 1987; 31:211.

146. Yaksh TL, Kohl RL, Rudy TA. Induction of tolerance and withdrawal in rats receiving morphine in the spinal subarachnoid space. *Eur J Pharmacol* 1977; 42:275.

147. Yaksh TL, Noueihed R. The physiology and pharmacology of spinal opiates. *Annu Rev Pharmacol Toxicol* 1985; 25:433.

148. Yaksh TL, Reddy SVR. Studies on the analgetic effects of intrathecal opiates, α-adrenergic agonists and baclofen: their pharmacology in the primate. *Anesthesiology* 1981; 54:451.

149. Yaksh TL, Rudy TA. Analgesia mediated by a direct spinal action of narcotics. *Science* 1976; 192:1357.

150. Yaksh TL, Rudy TA. Studies on the direct spinal action of narcotics in the production of analgesia in the rat. *J Pharmacol Exp Ther* 1977; 202(2):411.

151. Yeager MP, Glass DD, et al. Epidural anesthesia and analgesia in high-risk surgical patients. *Anesthesiology* 1987; 66:729.

152. Yeung JC, Rudy TA. Multiplicative interaction between narcotic agonisms expressed at spinal and supraspinal sites

of antinociceptive action as revealed by concurrent intrathecal and intracerebroventricular injections of morphine. *J Pharmacol Exp Ther* 1980; 215:633.

153. Youngstrom PC, Cowan RI, Sutheimer C, et al. Pain relief and plasma concentrations from epidural and intramuscular morphine in post-Cesarean-section patients. *Anesthesiology* 1982; 57:404.

154. Zenz M, Piepenbrock S, Husch M, et al. Experience with long-term peridural catheters: residual morphine analgesia in cancer pain. *Anaesthetist: Reg Anaesth* 1981; 4:26.

155. Zenz M, Piepenbrock S, et al. Epidural opiates: long-term experiences in cancer pain. *Klin Wochenschr* 1985; 63: 225.

CHAPTER 28

Nerve Blocks

Subhash Jain

For a suffering patient, acute or chronic pain becomes one of the most critical aspects of life. Pain is an unpleasant sensory or emotional experience associated with actual or potential tissue damage.[1] Fortunately, pain may be relieved by reducing sensory input from damaged tissues, modulating transmission of sensory impulses through the central nervous system, or altering the patient's emotional responses to actual or perceived stimuli. Unfortunately, despite the many varied methods of abolishing pain, none is always effective. Traditionally, the nonopioid and opioid analgesic drugs are the first line of treatment for all types of pain, but their efficacy may be limited by the fear of addiction, symptoms of chemical dependence, or side effects (including nausea, vomiting, constipation, impairment of consciousness, or the subjective sense of being drugged), any of which may make life unpleasant for the patient. When opioid analgesics are not adequate or not appropriate for pain relief, various alternative therapies are available that offer both short- and long-term benefits for managing pain.[2] These include: nerve blocks,[3] cryoanalgesia,[4] neurectomy,[5] rhizotomy,[6] cordotomy, TENS, and radiofrequency analgesia.[7]

It is also important to remember that no single treatment technique is guaranteed to produce complete pain relief. Advances in diagnostic and treatment methods, coupled with advances in understanding the anatomy, physiology, and pharmacology of pain perception, however, have led to improved control of pain through a multifaceted approach to pain management. An understanding of the nature and origin of the patient's pain is necessary to treat the causes of the pain properly. The purpose of this chapter, however, is to discuss various types of nerve blocks that have been found useful in managing chronic pain states caused by both benign and malignant disease.

For many years, nerve blocks have been useful in managing pain.[8,9] Essentially, a nerve block is the injection of a local anesthetic agent or a neurolytic agent into a peripheral sensory nerve, a sympathetic nerve plexus, or a localized pain-sensitive trigger point. Initially, nerve blocks were plagued by a high incidence of complications, including sepsis and paralysis. Furthermore, the haphazard selection of patients and the performance of blocks by inexperienced and untrained physicians left serious misconceptions about the efficacy of nerve blocks and their apparently poor results.[8–10]

During the last three decades, however, there has been growing evidence of the efficacy of regional nerve blocks in treating carefully selected pain syndromes. Improvements in technology and its application to regional anesthetic techniques have led to better pain relief and fewer disabling complications than occurred previously.

BASIC CONSIDERATIONS FOR USING NERVE BLOCKS

Proper use of nerve blocks in the treatment of pain requires a knowledgeable and experienced physician with a thorough understanding of pain and its syndromes. It is mandatory that a patient be selected for nerve block therapy only after an accurate diagnosis of the origin of pain is made. Thus, a careful workup of the patient should be done, including a complete history, physical examination, appropriate laboratory studies, and a complete psychiatric and psychosomatic assessment, if necessary.

All hospital records, including hospital discharge summaries, workups, and all prior treatments, should be reviewed in an unbiased manner. A patient with multiple disorders, such as a combined motor and sensory weakness, should undergo appropriate laboratory studies and roentgenographic examinations before being considered for nerve block treatment.

Nerve blocks relieve pain by interrupting nociceptive or pain sensory pathways, inducing sympathetic blockade, or causing somatosensory nerve blockade. Interruption of the afferent limb of a reflex mechanism will result in a sensory blockade; the blockade of sympathetic pathways will reduce the vasomotor, visceromotor, and sudomotor overactivity that often is responsible for pain syndromes associated with reflex sympathetic dystrophy.

NEUROPHYSIOLOGIC ASPECT OF IMPULSE CONDUCTION

The nerve membrane is composed of a semipermeable double-thickness wall comprised of lipid molecules with globular protein molecules interspaced throughout.[11,12] Through these lipid molecules are the small channels that permit electrolytic ions to pass between the interior and exterior of the nerve membrane.

As a result of sensory stimulation, there is a sudden

influx of sodium ions.[11,13] The increase in the permeability of the membrane to sodium corresponds to a voltage change and the depolarization of nerve membranes. It is thought that local anesthetics transiently block neuronal transmission by impeding the flow of sodium through the nerve membrane channels.[12]

The neural effects of local anesthetics are temporary and reversible.[11] Neurolytic agents (such as absolute alcohol and phenol), however, produce a permanent block in nerve conduction by the disruption and destruction of neural tissue. Such a block then remains until the nerve tissues regenerate.

The size of nerve fibers plays an important role in their sensitivity to local anesthetics and neurolytic solutions. Although local anesthetics can reduce the excitability of nerve fibers of all sizes, thinner fibers can be blocked more readily than thicker nerve fibers.[14]

Peripheral nerves are comprised of three types of nerve fibers, each of which has a different sensitivity to local anesthetics. The largest myelinated somatic nerve fibers are known as A fibers with a diameter of 4 to 20 μm.[11] The A myelinated fibers are divided further into the α, β, γ, and δ fibers. The α, β, and γ fibers transmit motor and pressure impulses, and the thin A δ fibers subserve pain and temperature functions and signal tissue damage. Their conduction speed varies from 12 to 30 m/s.

B fibers are myelinated preganglionic autonomic nerves with a diameter of between 1 and 3 μm. The preganglionic autonomic sympathetic B fibers, although myelinated, are the most readily blocked nerve fibers.[15,16] The B fibers primarily innervate vascular smooth muscle. Thus, the first sign of a successful nerve block often has the effect of a sympathetectomy, with increased warmth due to increased blood flow and a decrease in sweating. Furthermore, it is the extreme sensitivity of the autonomic B fibers that causes the level of a sympathetectomy to be much higher than the level of analgesia during a subarachnoid or epidural anesthetic.[15,16]

The thinnest nonmyelinated fibers are called C fibers. They have a diameter of 0.5 to 1 μm and are the slowest conducting nerve fibers. They subserve postganglionic temperature and pain transmission. Despite being nonmyelinated, C fibers are more resistant to the effects of local anesthetic agents than are the B fibers.

It is interesting that the body has two types of pain fibers. The A δ myelinated fibers subserve sharp pain, apparently warning the organism of impending danger. The thinnest nonmyelinated C fibers are responsible for dull pain and burning sensations, the sort of pain that becomes a chronic problem in patients with many pain syndromes.[17] A knowledge of the different types of nerve fibers, their role in transmitting pain, and the techniques used to block them, is necessary to achieve pain relief. The anesthesiologist's responsibility is to define the indication and decide whether a nerve block procedure is the appropriate way of treating an individual patient.

INDICATIONS FOR NERVE BLOCKS

It was not until the introduction of the hollow needle in the early 19th century that the pharmacologic interruption of pain pathways became possible. Initially, nerve blocks were reserved for alleviating discomfort. Currently, however, with safe and effective local anesthetic and imaging techniques, every nerve in the body is accessible to pharmacologic blockade. The nerve blocks can be diagnostic, prognostic, or therapeutic.[18]

Types of Nerve Blocks

Diagnostic Nerve Blocks (See Chap. 4)

Diagnostic blocks often are useful in ascertaining what type of pain a patient is having, the possible mechanisms and origins of the pain, and the site of the pain source. Although a thorough analysis of the pain with regard to localization, character, and time pattern is useful in making an appropriate diagnosis, often it is difficult to differentiate pain of somatic origin from visceral pain or pain of sympathetic origin. For example, pain in the upper or lower extremity that is caused by overactivity of sympathetic nerves can be diagnosed easily if pain relief occurs after a sympathetic block. This differentiates the origin of the pain from that of somatic pain; in the latter, a sympathetic block will provide no pain relief. Similarly, a diagnostic celiac blockade with local anesthesia can be used to identify the cause of an unusual abdominal pain syndrome by differentiating an intraperitoneal process from referred pain.[19,20] If the abdominal pain originates from extraabdominal causes (such as pneumonitis, contusions, or radiculitis), there will be no relief from a celiac plexus block.

Prognostic Nerve Blocks

Many patients with pain require comprehensive evaluation and management programs. A substantial number of selected patients obtain long-term relief from semipermanent interruption of nerves either by injecting long-acting agents (such as phenol and absolute alcohol) or surgical interruption using cordotomy or rhizotomy.[6] The prognostic nerve block done before the administration of a neurolytic agent or a neurosurgical procedure will ensure that patients temporarily experience the feeling they will have after the more permanent procedure. For example, a prognostic block temporarily will produce the numbness, strange sensations, effects on sensory and motor function, and the quality of pain relief that ultimately occurs after the irreversible procedure. Occasionally, repeated nerve block may be needed and different levels must be blocked before deciding on surgical or neurolytic interruption of pain pathways. Unfortunately, the prognostic nerve block is only a helpful tool and not a fool-proof device. Loeser[6] suggests that it has limitations in predicting the long-term effect of spinal rhizotomy, but primarily, this is related to the plasticity of the nervous system. If one pathway is interrupted, another often will develop. It is frustrating both for the patient and treating physician when a prognostic block provides a good result, but a permanent procedure leaves the patient with inadequate pain relief. Why does a local anesthetic nerve block produce good relief when surgical or neurolytic procedures do not? This question cannot be answered with certainty, but the development of alternate pain pathways with time seems to be part of the explanation.

Other Local Blocks

Local point blocks are used to infiltrate painful trigger points and in other conditions like bursitis, tendinitis, some local muscle group spasms (such as the scalenus anticus syndrome), and chronic arthritic conditions. In chronic bursitis, infiltration of a local anesthetic usually is combined with an injection of a corticosteroid preparation such as methylprednisolone or dexamethasone.

Occasionally both a diagnostic local anesthetic and a placebo block will be helpful in differentiating pain of an organic nature from that of psychogenic origin.[20] However, if the pain is a result of organic lesions but is affected by psychological factors, then the problems of both diagnosis and treatment become extremely complex.

The diagnostic peripheral nerve block[18] also is useful in pinpointing the location of a pain site. Familiarity with the anatomy of nerve pathways, using a dermatome chart and peripheral nerve map, makes it possible to identify the nerve that carries the painful signals to the central nervous system. A diagnostic block can be done to differentiate central from peripheral pain. If a peripheral nerve block relieves the pain, then a central origin of pain can be excluded.

Therapeutic Nerve Blocks

Therapeutic nerve blocks are done only after diagnostic blocks have established the nature and location of the pain. The efficacy of the block primarily is judged by the patient's subjective responses and the physician's objective observation. Therapeutic nerve blocks can be beneficial in both acute and chronic pain. For instance, a patient with a fracture of the ribs will benefit markedly from an intercostal block, and both intraoperative and postoperative[21] intercostal blocks have been efficacious in relieving postoperative thoracotomy pain.[22,23] Conversely, a patient with chronic pelvic pain from cancer of the rectum or cervix can be treated well with a neurolytic therapeutic block if repeated local anesthetic blocks relieve the pain. Likewise, when sympathetic overactivity causes ischemia and extremity pain, which can be blocked by a lumbar sympathetic or stellate ganglion block, then a more permanent chemical lumbar sympathectomy[24] with alcohol or phenol may be useful.

The therapeutic role of sympathetic blocks also has been well documented for the treatment of sympathetic dystrophies.[24] In this disorder, the pain and swelling from injury or cancer increase efferent sympathetic discharges that lower the peripheral threshold to noxious stimuli. Repeated blocks with local anesthetics have been shown to be helpful in the definitive management of these pain syndromes.

ROLE OF SPECIFIC REGIONAL NERVE BLOCKS

Local Infiltration (Trigger Point) Blocks (See Chap. 19)

The advantages of local infiltration include simplicity and ease of performance; it also can be repeated safely. Of all the regional anesthetic techniques, it probably is the safest and one of the most effective for predictably relieving pain.

One of the most common nerve blocks[3,25] used for pain management is the infiltration of a local anesthetic solution in an isolated somatic focal point that is acting as source of pain and irritation. This simple technique is rewarding in reducing the pain and muscle spasm associated with local trauma, sprain, rib fracture, or other bony fractures. Travell[26] defined a myofascial trigger point in skeletal muscles as a localized area of tenderness in which a palpable firm band of muscle has a positive so-called jump sign.[27] This is a visible shortening of the muscle that occurs when it is stimulated at the point of maximum tenderness.

A myofascial trigger point can produce local tenderness, muscle spasm, stiffness, limitation of movement, and interference with autonomic function.[28–30] Chronic myofascial pain can produce local ischemia with liberation of irritating substances that can aggravate the pain problem further. Histologic examination of trigger points has shown local changes in muscle fibers, such as myofibrillar degeneration, local fatty infiltration, and destruction of muscle fibers,[31,32] although, a typical myofascial pain syndrome is devoid of any demonstrable neurologic or orthopedic deficit. Travell[26] believes that most humans have trigger points irritated by stress and strain.[26]

Trigger point infiltration is done only after proper identification of the specific focal point identified as the most tender spot to palpation. The pain receptors in the skin and other tissues are all free nerve endings. They are widespread in the superficial layers of the skin and also in certain internal tissues and are sensitive to local anesthetics.

The physician must be highly skilled in this procedure and familiar with the safe use of local anesthetics. For example, therapists must be capable of handling complications, such as intravascular injection, pneumothorax, anaphylactic reactions, or systemic toxic reactions to local anesthetics. A common debate is whether a local anesthetic agent should be used plain or in combination with epinephrine. No reliable data is available, but we prefer to use a local anesthetic agent without epinephrine to avoid extreme local vasoconstriction that may aggravate trigger point symptoms.

Local infiltration can include not only an injection of a local anesthetic, but also application of a jet injection,[33] ethyl chloride spray,[34] dry needling[35] of trigger points, local injection of normal isotonic saline, application of TENS, or acupuncture.[36]

A productive local infiltration block can be accomplished with a 22- or 25-gauge 5-cm needle, using a low concentration of a local anesthetic agent such as lidocaine 0.25% to 0.5% or bupivacaine 0.25%. A local subcuticular wheal or so-called peau d'orange is made by injecting 1 to 2 ml of a local anesthetic. After the local area is anesthetized adequately, then 5 to 10 ml of local anesthetic solution is injected into the myofascial plane at the trigger point in a fan-like fashion.

A sudden feeling of loss of resistance often is experienced as the needle enters the myofascial plane. The site of the trigger point is an important consideration in planning the trigger point block. For instance, we must be careful in selecting the size and gauge of the needle when working close to the chest wall, rib cage, cervical, and interscapular region. In these areas, a 25-gauge needle that is 2.5 cm long will be adequate. After local infiltration, it typically takes 3 to 5 min for the pain to subside. Multiple trigger spots require multiple trigger point infiltrations. The absence of pain relief after a trigger point local infiltration indicates that the trigger point was not injected properly and requires reconfirmation of the trigger point and reinjection.

A single infiltration of local anesthetic solution combined with corticosteroids often is effective in treating the severe pain of bursitis, tendinitis, ligamentous sprains, and epicondylitis. Scar tissue pain can be treated effectively with a low concentration of bupivacaine 0.125% injected at intervals of 3 to 5 days.[37]

In acute pain syndromes, the daily infiltration of a local anesthetic two or three times often will produce adequate pain relief.[38] In chronic pain problems, however, injection is recommended initially on a daily basis, followed by alternate-day therapy. When the pain has improved, then twice a week injections followed by an on-demand basis usually are sufficient.

The patient should be cautioned at the initiation of local anesthetic infiltration therapy. After the first treatment when the effect of the local anesthetic has worn off, the pain may be more severe and seem more intense than it was before. The probable causes of this may be local irritation from needle placement, local reaction to the local anesthetic, or perhaps more important, the fear and anxiety of having the pain come back.

SOMATIC NERVE BLOCK

Somatic pain occurs as a result of activation of nociceptors in cutaneous and deep tissues. The pain may be acute or chronic in nature; typically, it is well localized. Usually, it is constant and, frequently, is described as aching or gnawing. Acute pain is characterized by a well-defined pattern of pain onset, often associated with trauma, that generally is accompanied by both subjective and objective physical signs of tissue injury and hyperactivity of the autonomic nervous system. By contrast, chronic pain leads to significant emotional changes and has effects on various systems of the body. It is this latter group of patients that is the most challenging for physicians specializing in the management of pain.

Successful analgesic effects can be achieved by injecting either local anesthetic or neurolytic agents into peripheral nerves or tissues. Knowing the anatomy of peripheral nerves and their distribution, a knowledge of local anesthetics and their mode of action, and experience in regional techniques are necessary for successful regional anesthesia treatment.[39]

Local anesthesia dates back to the application of cocaine as a topical anesthetic agent in 1884 by Koller. Procaine was the most popular local anesthetic until Lofgren's discovery of lidocaine in 1943. It was not until the early 1960s, however, that the concept of regional block was popularized widely by Bonica[8] as a result of the high quality of pain relief obtained and its reliability in comparison with the other available techniques for pain relief. Nerve block techniques depend on the pharmacologic properties of the local anesthetic used and its ability to interrupt specific autonomic, sensory, and motor pathways.[10] Therapeutic neural blockade achieved by local anesthetics offers complete pain relief, with a decrease in stress response and decreased effects of pain on the cardiovascular and respiratory systems. In comparison with systemic analgesics, neural blockade prevents the central effects of sedation, drowsiness, and respiratory depression. Furthermore, a local nerve block can improve local blood flow and restore physiologic function.[12]

Local Anesthetics (See Appendix C)

The basis of local analgesia is the interruption of nociceptive input from peripheral somatic nerves by the local anesthetic. This isolates the focus of stimulation from the central nervous system, thus interrupting the afferent limb of abnormal reflex mechanisms that often contribute to pain syndromes. Local anesthetics inhibit both the excitation and conduction process in a peripheral nerve. Two groups of local anesthetics are available:[12,13] the amino esters and the amino amide compounds. The common ester type local anesthetics are chloroprocaine, procaine, and tetracaine. The amide group includes bupivacaine, etidocaine, lidocaine, and mepivacaine.

The metabolism of injected esters requires hydrolysis by an enzyme, pseudocholinesterase. The amides are metabolized mainly in the liver by microsomal enzymes. Prilocaine is the one amide local anesthetic that is metabolized in extrahepatic tissue.[40] The ester cocaine is metabolized in the liver. The systemic absorption of local anesthetic is influenced by the vascularity of the site of injection, the dose given, the addition of vasoconstricting drugs, and the physiochemical properties of the anesthetic compound.[12,13]

The efficiency of local anesthetics is influenced primarily by their lipid solubility, protein binding, pKa, and intrinsic vasodilator activity. Shames[41] observed that alkaline local anesthetics are more effective in blocking nerve conduction than neutral or acidic solutions. Both the ionization and pH are important with respect to the solubility and activity of local anesthetics. Local anesthetic solutions containing epinephrine have a lower pH; this delays the onset of anesthesia. Similarly, the injection of local anesthetic solution into infected acidic tissue may result in poor nerve penetration. By contrast, carbonated local anesthetic solutions and those made slightly basic result in rapid onset and more extensive spread of blockade. Lipid solubility plays an important role in the duration of blockade. A highly lipid-soluble local anesthetic (like etidocaine) is associated with a long duration of action and higher potency. Etidocaine is 50-fold more lipid soluble and 4-fold more potent than lidocaine. Similarly, an ester drug like tetracaine, which is 10-fold more highly bound to protein than procaine, has a duration that is 3- to 4-fold longer. Bupivacaine and etidocaine are 90 percent protein bound, and thus they are 2- to 3-fold longer acting than lidocaine or mepivacaine.[38,42]

All local anesthetic agents (except cocaine) cause vasodilatation. The addition of a vasoconstrictor to a local anesthetic solution decreases the rate of absorption and results in a lower blood concentration of the drug; a higher concentration of local anesthetic is found if it is injected into highly perfused organs.[42] Systemic effects of local anesthetics can be produced when they are deliberately given intravenously or injected accidentally into a vessel during a regional block. The systemic effects of the local anesthetic may affect the cardiovascular and central nervous systems and smooth and skeletal muscle.[43]

Systemic toxicity, involving the central nervous system, initially results in a general anesthesia-like depression that is followed by excitation and seizures. Additional central nervous system depression may result in coma and respiratory arrest. Signs of cardiovascular depression from high local anesthetic blood levels are seen only after the onset of central nervous system depression. The effect on the cardiovascular system is a result of a high blood concentration of local anesthetic, usually caused by direct vascular injection.[44,45] Bupivacaine is four-fold more toxic than lidocaine and produces ventricular arrhythmia; it may cause death from ventricular fibrillation.[43,45,46] During neural blockade, careful aspiration, use of safe doses of local anesthetic agent, and appropriate premedication of the patient will minimize the likelihood of a patient having local anesthetic toxicity.[47] The latter is influenced by vascular absorption, tissue distribution, metabolism, and excretion. The blood level of the local anesthetic agent is influenced by the total dose of the drug administered rather than the concentration and volume of the anesthetic solution used.[10,12,48,49]

Nerve fiber size plays an important role in the onset of neural blockade. The relationship between sizes of nerve fibers and differential sensitivity to blockade by local anesthetics is well documented. When a local anesthetic is injected near a nerve, the local disposition of anesthetic solution depends on bulk flow of the injected solution along the tissue plane, diffusion across the axonal membrane, and diffusion across the lipid Schwann cell barrier. The initial onset of blockade occurs in the preganglionic sympathetic fibers. The onset of sympathetic block can be rapid, occurring within seconds. Isolated axons are more sensitive to local anesthetic blockade if the frequency of impulse traffic in the nerve is increased.[44]

For common nerve blocks, the amide group of local anesthetic drugs is preferable to the ester group. The duration of block can be prolonged with minimal toxic effect and minimal allergic potential. In therapeutic concentrations, local anesthetics do not produce permanent neuronal injury, but it has been well documented that some preservatives (such as methylparaben) may cause neuronal damage.

Choice of Local Anesthetic

The ideal choice of a local anesthetic agent for neural blockade for pain relief will depend on the type of block; the type of pain; the location of the block; and the patient's general health, weight, height, metabolic status, and organ status. For example, the pain caused by sympathetic dystrophy does not require a large amount of local anesthetic, and a low volume and concentration of local anesthetic agent will be satisfactory. A peripheral nerve block at the fingers or toes should not be done with a vasoconstrictor in the local anesthetic solution because of the risk of inducing distal vascular ischemia. By contrast, the systemic effects of local anesthetics can be avoided during intercostal blocks by adding epinephrine, thus delaying systemic uptake of the local anesthetic agent.[50] The duration of local anesthetic effect may be prolonged by adding epinephrine 1:200,000 to the solution, increasing the volume or concentration of agent, or adding low molecular weight dextran to the anesthetic solution.[36,51,52] The onset of local anesthetic effects can be accelerated by using carbonated solutions of local anesthetics.[52] For diagnostic or prognostic purposes, a short-acting agent may be used. For a prolonged therapeutic effect, a long-acting agent like bupivacaine or etidocaine is desirable.

Cranial Nerve Block

The common cranial nerve blocks include: (1) the trigeminal nerve and its branches, (2) the gasserian ganglion, (3) the glossopharyngeal nerve, and (4) the facial nerve. Cranial nerve blocks are useful in managing severe pain in the head and neck region. Blockade of cranial nerves is valuable diagnostically, therapeutically, and prognostically. The most common indications for cranial nerve blocks are intractable pain syndromes caused by cancer. Pain usually occurs in this group of patients after local spread of the tumor, neural infiltration of the tumor, or tumor-related nerve injury. Tumor-induced pain most commonly is present in the distribution of the involved cranial nerve, depending on the site of tumor infiltration. For example, a tumor infiltrating the mandibular nerve usually presents with pain in the area supplied by the mandibular nerve. Similarly, tumor involvement of the ophthalmic division of the trigeminal nerve will have an effect on the area in the ophthalmic division distribution (that is, mucous membrane of the nasal cavity, skin of the nose, conjunctivae, lacrimal gland, and skin over the lateral canthus).

Trigeminal Nerve Block

The trigeminal nerve is the sensory nerve for the entire face, except the area at the angle of the jaw that is supplied by the second cervical nerve. The trigeminal nerve consists of three divisions: the ophthalmic nerve, maxillary nerve, and mandibular nerve. The trigeminal, or gasserian, ganglion lies in the middle cranial fossa at the upper part of the petrous temporal bone near the apex. The sensory root of the trigeminal nerve arises from the bipolar cells in the gasserian ganglion, and on entering the pons, each fiber is divided into an ascending and descending branch. The gasserian ganglion is covered fully by dura matter anteriorly; the posterior part is in the small recess called the Meckel cave. The cavernous sinus lies medially; the carotid artery lies medially and inferiorly.[53]

Of the three divisions of cranial nerve V, the mandibular nerve, or third division, is the largest. It exits the cranium through the foramen ovale. The first division is the ophthalmic; this is the smallest division of the trigeminal nerve. It enters the orbit through the superior orbital fissure. The second division is the maxillary nerve. It exits by the foramen rotundum and the pterygopalatine fossa. The ophthalmic and maxillary divisions are pure sensory nerves; the mandibular nerve is both sensory and motor.

Mandibular Nerve Block

All three divisions of the trigeminal nerve can be blocked at their anatomic locations. For a successful mandibular nerve block, the aim is to place the needle tip close to the foramen ovale. The block should be done under fluoroscopic control to place the local anesthetic accurately, using a lateral approach. A prior diagnostic block is required if a neurolytic procedure is anticipated. For a diagnostic procedure, 2 to 4 ml of lidocaine 1% is adequate. It is desirable to obtain paresthesias, but this is not always possible. Mandibular nerve block is indicated for malignant conditions of the lower jaw and cancer of the anterior two-thirds of the tongue and mucous membranes of the oral cavity.

Maxillary Nerve Block

This block is indicated for malignancy of the posterior and inferior position of the nasal cavity, the hard palate, the lower part of the nose, the tonsilar fossa, and the middle third of the face. The neurolytic agent commonly used is absolute alcohol or phenol in water. Before an alcohol block, a diagnostic block with 2 ml of a local anesthetic is recommended to ensure proper placement of the neurolytic solution.

Gasserian Ganglion Block

This block is recommended where more than one division of the trigeminal nerve is involved.[54] Intractable pain from cancer or trigeminal neuralgia is the main indication. The block is indicated only when a neurosurgical procedure is contraindicated. An image intensifier should be used for satisfactory placement of the needle in the foramen ovale.

The common complications from trigeminal nerve blocks include accidental subarachnoid injection, hematoma, palsy of other cranial nerves, permanent neurologic sequelae, alcoholic neuritis, paralysis of facial muscles, and deviation of the lower jaw.

Glossopharyngeal Nerve Block

Block of the glossopharyngeal nerve is indicated as a diagnostic or prognostic procedure in patients with severe pain from cancer of the throat, glossopharyngeal neuralgia, or painful conditions of the pharynx.[55] The glossopharyngeal nerve supplies the posterior one-third of the tongue, the palatine tonsils, and the pharyngeal wall. The glossopharyngeal nerve leaves the skull with the vagus nerve through the jugular foramen. Both nerves can be blocked at the base of the skull as they exit from the jugular foramen. This block is done on one side only because a bilateral block will produce complete paralysis of the pharyngeal muscles.

Typical glossopharyngeal neuralgia is characterized by a sudden severe lancinating pain in the throat radiating to the ear and thyroid cartilage.[55] The pain of glossopharyngeal neuralgia is paroxysmal in nature and triggered by swallowing, chewing, talking, yawning, coughing, or sneezing. The diagnosis can be confirmed by palpating the tonsil, which will provoke the pain.

Paravertebral Block (See Appendix A.VII)

Blockade of the paravertebral nerve involves both the somatic and sympathetic divisions. Blockade of paravertebral nerves is done at cervical, thoracic, or lumbar levels according to the type of pain and indication.[56] It is important to know the anatomic landmarks at various levels because the tips of the spinous processes are at a lower level than the corresponding vertebral transverse processes. The most prominent dorsal spine is at the seventh cervical vertebra.

Paravertebral block in the cervical area is indicated in severe pain of the head, neck, and upper arm. The common conditions are whiplash injuries, fibrosis, periarthritis, myositis, and postradical neck pain syndrome.[57] The block also is a diagnostic tool in the patient with neuralgia or a diskogenic problem. Upper cervical blockade and blockade of the greater and lesser occipital nerves are indicated in patients with occipital headache and neuralgia. By contrast, patients with shoulder pain and musculoskeletal disorders are candidates for suprascapular nerve block. After radical neck dissection, patients may present with tight burning sensations in the area of sensory loss.[58] This may indicate injury or interruption of the cervical nerves and can be alleviated by using a local cervical or trigger point block.

Blockade of the thoracic paravertebral region is indicated in managing various pain syndromes involving the upper and lower thoracic region, such as poststernotomy pain, postthoracotomy pain,[51,59] and disorders of the thoracic spine or chest wall. Acute conditions causing thoracic pain and requiring nerve block intervention include surgical procedures on the chest wall,[57] breast surgery, posttraumatic rib and sternal injuries, and acute herpetic neuralgia.[49] Chronic pain[59] conditions include postmastectomy syndrome, postthoracotomy syndrome, postherpetic neuralgia, herniated intervertebral disk, collapsed vertebrae, and metastatic lesions.[58]

The paravertebral block is a simple technique. The needle is inserted a few centimeters lateral to the dorsal spinous process of the vertebral level to be blocked and is directed to touch the corresponding transverse process. The needle is directed further so that it lies medial and caudal to the transverse process. The aim is to have the tip of the needle close to the intervertebral foramen where the corresponding nerve emerges. The duration of relief can be prolonged using drugs like bupivacaine or etidocaine.

Postthoracotomy pain occurs in the distribution of intercostal nerves after surgical interruption or injury.[58] Both retraction and resection of the rib are common causes of nerve injury during surgical procedures on the chest. In patients with cancer, recurrence or metastases of tumor are the most common causes of pain.[58] A small number of postthoracotomy patients also have a traumatic neuroma as a cause of pain. In any case of thoracic pain syndrome, an initial diagnostic paravertebral block is indicated. A neurolytic block is indicated only after repeated successful diagnostic nerve blocks with a local anesthetic. A series of paravertebral blocks also are indicated in patients with segmental neuralgia, radiculitis, nerve root irritation, and postherpetic neuralgia.[60]

Lumbar paravertebral blocks are indicated for painful conditions, such as lumbago, intervertebral disk problems, postherpetic neuralgia, fractures of vertebrae, and postnephrectomy pain syndromes. The relation of the lumbar spines to the transverse processes and intervertebral foramina is different than in the thoracic paravertebral region. At the lumbar area, the upper border of the dorsal spinous process is at the same level as the transverse process of the same vertebra.

Complications of paravertebral blocks include: systemic reaction to local anesthetic; intravascular injection; subdural, epidural, and subarachnoid block; sudden hypotension; cardiorespiratory compromise; and pneumo-

thorax.[61] These complications can best be avoided by taking adequate precautions. An image intensifier may be used because both the level and depth of needle placement can be seen under fluoroscopic control, and this is particularly important if a neurolytic block is planned.

Intercostal Nerve Block (See Appendix)

One of the simplest and most gratifying nerve blocks is the intercostal nerve block.[21] The intercostal nerves are the primary rami at T1 to T12. A typical thoracic nerve divides into ventral and dorsal rami after leaving the intervertebral foramen. The ventral ramus passes to an adjacent rib where it becomes an intercostal nerve and lies with the intercostal artery and vein under the corresponding rib. A typical intercostal nerve has four significant branches. One branch is the gray ramus communicans that passes anteriorly to sympathetic ganglion. The second branch is the posterior cutaneous branch that supplies the skin and muscle in the paravertebral region. The lateral branch, which arises just anterior to the midaxillary line, supplies the skin of the chest and abdominal wall. The terminal branch of the intercostal nerve is the anterior cutaneous branch. The anterior cutaneous branches of the upper six intercostal nerves supply the skin over the anterior chest wall and breast. The lower six anterior cutaneous nerves supply the muscles of the upper abdomen and lower chest wall. The relationships of the nerves vary as they move peripherally. At the posterior angle of the rib, the intercostal nerves lie between the pleura and the intercostal fascia and are accompanied by an intercostal vein and artery that lie superior to the nerve in the inferior groove of the rib. Blockade of a few of these nerves does not affect the muscles of respiration, but the great vascularity in the intercostal space is responsible for a high local anesthetic concentration in the blood when an intercostal block is done.[43,62]

Various techniques have been described for intercostal blocks. Most commonly, the block is done posteriorly at the angle of the rib when the patient is in the prone position.

The analgesic effect of intercostal blocks can be prolonged by using bupivacaine 0.5% or etidocaine 0.5% with epinephrine 1 : 200,000 added.[22] Longer duration of bupivacaine block has been reported after adding dextran 40, a low molecule weight dextran solution.[37,52,60] However, the efficacy of dextran has been questioned by others.[63,64]

Intercostal blockade is indicated both for acute and chronic pain problems. The most common indications for acute pain control include: (1) postoperative pain after thoracotomy, upper abdominal surgery,[49,59] sternotomy, or mediastinal surgery; (2) pleurisy; (3) fractured ribs; (4) traumatic injury of thoracic muscles; and (5) acute herpetic neuralgia, involving thoracic dermatomes.[65] The chronic painful conditions that can be treated by intercostal block include nerve root pain, postthoracotomy pain, pain from tumor infiltration or compression, and postherpetic neuralgia.

The rapid absorption of local anesthetics from the highly vascular intercostal bundle may produce systemic effects. The blood level of the anesthetic is higher after this block than any other block.[47,49] The absorbed drug may have a negative inotropic effect on the myocardium and may produce myocardial depression or heart block. This myocardial depression can be opposed by adding epinephrine to the local anesthetic.[51]

After intercostal block, there is always a possibility of pneumothorax because of the close proximity of the pleura, but the incidence this complication is low. Moore and colleagues[64] reported an incidence of 0.073 percent, and silent pneumothorax has been reported at 0.42 percent.[66] Sudden hypotension often has been reported after intercostal block after inadvertent injection into the intravascular, epidural, or the subarachnoid space.

SYMPATHETIC BLOCKS IN THE MANAGEMENT OF PAIN

The sympathetic system is, by definition, an anatomic part of the autonomic nervous system.[67,68] The sympathetic nerves originate in the spinal cord, where the cell bodies of preganglionic neurons lie in the intermediolateral columns of the spinal cord and pass through the anterior roots of the cord between segments T1 and T2 to form the efferent preganglionic fibers.

As the spinal nerves leave the spinal column, the preganglionic sympathetic fibers separate from the motor nerves and pass through white rami into the ganglia of the sympathetic chain. The sympathetic fiber then can follow one of three courses as follows.

1. It can synapse with postganglionic neurons in the ganglion that it enters.
2. It can pass upward or downward in the chain and synapse in one of the other ganglia of the chain.
3. It can pass for variable distances through the chain and then through one of the nerves radiating outward from the chain to terminate in an outlying sympathetic ganglion.

The post ganglionic neurons then travel to their respective organs. Each spinal nerve contains postganglionic sympathetic fibers that are vasomotor or sudomotor and are adrenergic and cholinergic, respectively. In the upper part of the body (the head), the postganglionic fibers are distributed along the arteries; in the upper abdomen, the celiac plexus receives preganglionic fibers from the splanchic nerve and supplies postganglionic fibers to the upper abdominal viscera.

Most postganglionic fibers pass back from the sympathetic chain into the spinal cord through gray rami. The sympathetic ganglia are divided into three groups: the paravertebral, the prevertebral, and the terminal. The prevertebral ganglia lie in the abdomen and the pelvis near the ventral surface of the vertebral column. They consist of the celiac and the superior mesenteric ganglia. The paravertebral

ganglia consist of 22 pairs that lie on each side of the vertebral column and form the lateral chain of sympathetic ganglia. They lie on the anterolateral aspect of the vertebral column. In the cervical region, the ganglia lie anterior to the transverse processes of the cervical spine; in the thoracic region, they lie anterior to the head of the ribs. In the abdomen, they are located on the sides of the vertebral bodies; in the pelvic region, they are anterior to the sacrum. The sympathetic chain also receives afferent visceral fibers that conduct pain from the head, neck, and upper extremities (cervical thoracic ganglion), the abdominal viscera (celiac plexus), the urogenital system, and the lower extremities (lumbar sympathetic ganglia). The terminal ganglia lie near the organs innervated (such as the urinary bladder and the rectum.[69]

In patients with acute or chronic pain, sympathetic nerve blocks interrupt both visceromotor nerves and specific nociceptive pathways. The conduction block thus will interrupt both efferent and afferent pathways.

Sympathetic blocks commonly are used both for diagnostic and therapeutic purposes. In peripheral pain syndromes, the block helps to differentiate somatic pain from that of sympathetic origin. Repeated sympathetic blocks often will help in predicting the efficacy of surgical or chemical sympathectomy. Loh and Nathan[70] reported the results of sympathetic blockade on selected peripheral nerve lesions that caused chronic pain, showing that such a blockade was most likely to relieve pain associated with hyperpathia. Loh and colleagues[71] further reported that pain induced by central lesions was reduced drastically after sympathetic blockade.

The conditions that are benefited by sympathetic blocks include reflex sympathetic dystrophy,[72,73] phantom limb pain, postamputation stump pain,[74] acute vascular insufficiencies, chronic peripheral arterial disease (rest pain),[75,76] and visceral pain due to malignancy.[77,78] The interruption of the sympathetic pathways can be accomplished at any one of the following sites: prevertebral, paravertebral, epidural, or subarachnoid.

Stellate Ganglion Block (See Appendix A.I)

Blockade of the cervical and upper thoracic sympathetic chain is one of the most common procedures used in managing acute and chronic pain.[79,80] The cervical chain is composed of a superior, middle, and inferior ganglion that are devoid of white rami. The inferior[79] ganglion fuses with the first thoracic ganglion to form the stellate ganglion.

The stellate ganglion is an oval-shaped structure usually 2 to 2.5 cm long, 0.75 to 1 cm wide, and 0.25 to 0.50 cm thick. Usually, it is located behind the subclavian artery and in front of the neck of the first rib near the costovertebral articulation. The caudad part of the ganglion is covered anteriorly by the dome of the pleura, and the cephalad part of ganglia is covered by the vertebral artery. Anterior to the ganglia lies the carotid sheath; medially, the pharynx and larynx are found. The recurrent laryngeal nerves pass between them. Although various techniques have been described for stellate ganglion blocks, the most common and practical technique is the anterior paratracheal approach.[79,81,82] Others include the lateral and posterior approaches. Because this technique is simple and the anatomic landmarks can be identified easily, the upper part of the pleura and the roof of the brachial plexus are avoided.

In the anterior paratracheal approach, the cricoid cartilage and the prominent transverse process of the sixth cervical vertebra or Chassaignac tubercle are identified. The tubercle should be palpated in the sitting position, especially in a patient with a short chubby neck, large neck lesions, or postsurgical changes in neck, such as after radical neck surgery. The patient is placed in the supine position. Before the procedure, the patient must be warned of possible side effects. The patient must not swallow or talk during the procedure and should be told that, if there is any problem, to raise their hand and to wave to the physician if things are not going properly. Ideally, communication must be kept between the patient and physician throughout the procedure. The pulsations of the carotid artery are felt on the side where the block will be done. The carotid artery and sternocleidomastoid muscle then are retracted laterally,[83] and a small skin wheal (a peau d'orange) of 0.5-cm diameter is made at this point. A 22-gauge 5-cm needle is inserted perpendicular to the plane of the skin until it contacts the anterior aspect of the transverse process of the C6 vertebra. The needle then is withdrawn 1 to 2 mm, and after confirming that there is no blood or spinal fluid return after aspirating with a syringe, a test dose of 0.5 to 1 ml of local anesthetic is injected. After reconfirming the correct position of the needle, 5 to 15 ml of lidocaine 1% or bupivicaine 0.25% is injected slowly. During the injection, the patient must be observed closely for any untoward effects.

After the block has been completed, the patient should be instructed to sit up to avoid undue edema of the airway. Correct placement of the local anesthetic in the cervical thoracic ganglion promptly results in injected moistened conjunctiva. The classic triad of Horner syndrome appears, including miosis, ptosis of the upper eye lid, and enophthalmos.[84] In a few minutes, additional signs develop. The face on the blocked side may become flushed, the nostril of the injected side may become blocked, and also anhidrosis of the face is noticeable. The patient, at this point, usually describes a sudden feeling of warmth after an increase in blood flow to the arm.[85,86]

If the block is limited to the stellate ganglion, 5 to 10 ml of local anesthetic are sufficient. However, if a more extensive sympathetic block of the upper extremities is needed, then 10 to 15 ml of local anesthetic should be used because the spread of the local anesthetic cephalad and caudad will bathe surrounding sympathetic fibers and ganglia. A common misconception is that a Horner syndrome is evidence of a successful block. A good sympathetic block must be confirmed by a rise in skin temperature, plethysmographic[87] evidence of increase in blood flow,[85–87] absence of psychogalvanic reflex, or a positive sweat test.[88,89]

Complications

Improperly done blocks can lead to devastating effects.[90,91] During a stellate ganglion block, the most serious complication is an intraarterial injection. If 0.5 to 1 ml of local anesthetic is injected into the vertebral artery, this can result in a grand-mal seizure, with accompanying unconsciousness and respiratory arrest. Accidental injection into the subarachnoid space can lead to high spinal anesthesia with either respiratory arrest or a sudden cardiovascular collapse.[91] Accidental placement of the needle below the C6 level increases the possibility of pneumothorax[90] and air embolism.[92] Inadvertent block of the recurrent laryngeal nerve may lead to hoarseness and occasional stridor after vocal cord paralysis. Occasional cases of local hematoma, osteitis, and mediastinitis also have been reported. Finally, vasovagal attacks probably occur more frequently with this procedure than any other regional block,[93] and they are more common when the right side is blocked. Bilateral stellate blocks should be avoided because this may cause loss of airway response, inhibition of cardioaccelerator activity, and sudden cardiorespiratory embarrassment.

The patient must be advised about proper postblock care. If the upper airway is affected by involvement of the recurrent laryngeal nerve, the patient must be told not to eat or drink until full reflexes return. Orthostatic hypotension must be recognized, and the patient should be advised to remain lying down until the block has worn off.

Indications

A number of acute and chronic disease states can be treated by stellate ganglion block (Table 28-1). Reflex sympathetic dystrophy, however, is one of the prime indications. This syndrome[93–95] is suspected whenever a patient has a history of relatively minor trauma, presents with persistent burning pain, chronic edema, hyperhidrosis, hyperesthesia to light touch, and radiographic evidence of demineralization of bones.[96,97] A typical patient usually requires multiple stellate ganglion blocks.[72,81] Initially, they are done daily, followed by every other day. As the patient improves, the blocks can be repeated twice a week (see Chap. 16). In acute cases, however, the patient may require only a single block. Repeated stellate ganglion blocks have been effective both in reducing the pain of acute herpetic neuralgia and in preventing postherpetic neuralgia.[98–100]

Patients with cancer of the head and neck area often have a burning sensation that usually is not controlled by oral medication or somatic blocks. Occasionally, this pain is relieved by a stellate ganglion block. Patients with postmastectomy brachial plexopathy or postradiation fibrosis also may have burning pain in the arm and may develop disuse atrophy of the muscles, diminished sensory and motor function of the upper arm, hyperpathia, and numbness. These symptoms are characteristic of reflex sympathetic dystrophy, and the pain often can be controlled with repeated stellate blocks.[101]

Circulatory problems of the upper extremity are another group of conditions where stellate ganglian blocks can play an important role, both diagnostically and therapeutically. Conditions such as traumatic injury[95] or embolic occlusion of arteries, chronic arterial occlusive disease, conditions associated with collagen diseases (such as lupus erythematosus or scleroderma), Raynaud disease,[102] thromboangiitis obliterans, and gangrene are all well-documented indications for stellate ganglion block. Additional indications may include management of postamputation pain, acute bursitis, and tendinitis. Chronic nonhealing ulcers from chronic vascular insufficiency often are painful conditions. Stellate ganglion blocks will cause vasodilatation, reduce the pain, increase local blood flow,[76] and promote and speed healing.

We are reluctant to use neurolytic drugs for stellate ganglion blocks. The risks include permanent hoarseness and block of the somatic nerves of the brachial plexus. Surgical sympathectomy probably is a safer technique in this area of the body.

Lumbar Sympathetic Blocks (See Appendix A.II)

Lumbar sympathetic pathway interruption is a useful technique to manage the pain that develops in the lower extremity after trauma, infection, thrombophlebitis, peripheral vascular occlusive disease, or peripheral nerve injury.[95,102–104] Several studies have documented long-term benefit from interruption of nociceptive stimuli.[105–107]

The lumbar sympathetic ganglia[56,108] lie on the anterolateral surface of the lumbar vertebrae along the medial margin of the psoas muscle. The arrangement of these ganglia is variable. Normally, there are five ganglia, but often the T12 and L1 ganglia are fused. The largest ganglia are found at the level of the body of the L2 vertebra. The lumbar sympathetic chain contains both preganglionic and postganglionic efferent neurons that innervate the pelvic viscera and the vessels of the lower extremities. Afferent sensory fibers in the lumbar ganglia transmit sensory information from the uterus, cervix, ipsilateral kidney, ureter, upper part of the urinary bladder, testicle, part of the transverse colon, descending colon, and the rectum. By blocking only the second or third lumbar ganglia, we can produce considerable visceral pain relief in addition to arterial vasodilatation to the lower extremities.

The relationship of the sympathetic chain to the great vessels differs on each side. On the right side, the chain lies posterior to lateral edge of the vena cava. However, on the left side, the chain is 2 to 10 mm lateral to the aorta and usually is covered by lumbar lymph glands and peritoneum. The lumbar sympathetic chain ganglia are inconsistent in their location, shape, size, and position on one side relative to the other. Thus, it is important to do blocks at different levels if it seems that only one or two blocks at the usual site are not producing an adequate result.

There are various approaches to blocking the lumbar sympathetic ganglia. Mandl[109] first described a technique for blocking the lumbar sympathetic chain in 1926. Reid and coworkers[107] reported their experience with more than 5000 procedures, using the paravertebral and lateral approach. Others reported the L2 level as the most important anatomic landmark.[81] For a diagnostic block using a local anesthetic, we use the paravertebral approach described by Moore.[56] If a permanent neurolytic sympathectomy is induced, however, we strongly recommend using x-ray control with the image intensifier. At the lateral edge of the paravertebral muscle opposite the dorsal spine of L2 or L3, a skin wheel is made. A 20-gauge 10- to 12-cm long needle is directed under x-ray control. The anteroposterior and lateral view of the L2 vertebra is important for verifying the depth and location of the needle tip. Similarly, another needle is passed at the L3 level. The position of the needle tips will be satisfactory if they are close to the anterior aspects of the lumbar vertebral bodies. To determine whether the needle is still in the psoas sheath, a small 2- to 3-ml injection of normal saline or local anesthetic is attempted. As long as the needle is in muscle, there will be some resistance to injection. The needle then is advanced slowly until it pierces the fascia; a sudden loss of resistance will be felt. The correct placement of the tip of the needle is verified repeatedly by aspirating with a dry syringe for the presence of blood or spinal fluid. If the

Table 28-1
Therapeutic Indications for Stellate Ganglion Blocks

Acute Conditions
Acute thrombophlebitis
Ischemic contracture
Traumatic vascular occlusion
Acute bursitis
Acute herpes zoster
Frost bite
Acute upper extremity edema
Embolism
Acute retinal artery occlusion
Acute cardiac pain

Chronic Conditions
Reflex sympathetic dystrophy
Causalgia
Central pain
Phantom pain
Posttraumatic pain syndrome
Shoulder–hand syndrome
Sudeck atrophy
Chronic obstructive vascular disease
Rest pain
Chronic herpetic neuralgia
Postamputation pain
Idiopathic neuralgia
Collagen vascular disease
 Scleroderma
 Lupus erythematosus
 Raynaud disease

block is planned for a permanent chemical sympathectomy, then 1 to 2 ml of contrast media is injected, and radiographic evidence of the spread is verified by taking an x-ray to localize the position of the tip of the needle.

For routine diagnostic or therapeutic lumbar sympathetic blocks, radiologic facilities are not required. The block can be done safely using only the anatomic landmarks described. After correct placement of the needle and aspiration with a syringe, a 2-ml test dose of local anesthetic solution (lidocaine 1% or bupivicaine 0.25%) is injected. After waiting a few minutes to observe for untoward effects, 15- to 20-ml of local anesthetic is injected. If the lumbar sympathetic block is done for chemical sympathectomy, the neurolytic solution most commonly used is phenol 6%. A dose of 10 to 15 ml of phenol 6% usually is adequate.[57,110]

After the block has been done, some subjective and objective signs of sympathetic blockade are observed.[111] A good sympathetic block is achieved without any sensory or motor dysfunction.[112] The increase in blood flow can be monitored with plethysmography and temperature sensors. Ideally, the patient should be kept in the same position for 20 to 30 min. During and after the procedure, the patient must be observed carefully for changes in vital signs and any unwarranted side effects (such as postural hypotension).

Premedication before lumbar sympathetic block is controversial. We strongly believe that patients do not require any premedication and that the patient must be fully awake with clear sensory perception to evaluate the effect of the block. Moore,[56] however, recommends relatively heavy premedication for the apprehensive patient.

Indications

The common indications for lumbar sympathetic blocks include reflex sympathetic dystrophy,[112] posttraumatic pain syndrome, compromised peripheral vascular disease,[102] intermittent claudication,[110] circulatory insufficiency, causalgia, renal colic, herpes zoster, intractable urogenital pain,[113] phantom limb, amputation or stump pain, and carcinomatous invasion of nerves and plexi.[114]

In a patient with reflex sympathetic dystrophy of the lower extremities, pain is a predominant symptom, and several authors believe that repeated sympathetic blocks can be used to treat this problem.[112]

We recommend an aggressive regimen of lumbar sympathetic blocks in such patients as follows. Every day for 1 week, blocks are administered followed by every other day, twice a week, and then weekly blocks. Good results depend on early diagnosis and early initiation of the sympathetic blocks combined with early mobilization and aggressive physical and occupational therapy.

In causalgia, if sympathetic blocks are done early, relief often is permanent. However, the analgesic effects of sympathetic blocks are so inconsistent that repeated blocks are recommended before subjecting a patient to chemical or surgical sympathectomy.[105,106]

Phantom limb pain occurs after amputation with an incidence of 35 percent to 70 percent. In 12 percent to 15 percent of these patients, the pain becomes consistently worse over the years and often requires numerous therapies, including sympathetic interruption, physical therapy, psychological support, and group therapy. The burning pain associated with vasomotor and sudomotor changes in the stump derives the greatest benefit from lumbar sympathetic blocks.

In patients with acute herpes zoster, the eruption itself usually is harmless, but the accompanying pain often is so intense that the patients are almost incapacitated for long periods. In some patients, the pain persists after the healing of the eruption and progresses to postherpetic neuralgia. Colding[99] showed the efficacy of lumbar sympathetic blocks in patients with acute herpetic neuralgia involving the back, buttock, and perineal areas of the lower extremity.

Complications

Improperly done lumbar sympathetic block can lead to undesirable side effects. An intravascular injection can result in sudden hypotension[116] and cardiorespiratory compromise. Accidental injection into the subarachnoid space can lead to total spinal anesthesia.[117] Improper placement of the needle introduces the possibility of retroperitoneal hemorrhage[118] and injury to the kidney, ureter, or renal pelvis.

Intravenous Sympathetic Block

Certain conditions preclude the physician from using regional sympathetic blocks. These include anticoagulation, diminished platelets, and postsurgical changes at the site of the block (such as in the neck area after radical surgery). There is an alternate method of sympathetic blockade available consisting of repeated intravenous regional sympathetic blocks with guanethidine. The guanethidine displaces the sympathetic transmitter norepinephrine from its storage sites in the sympathetic nerve endings. Its subsequent accumulation there prevents the usual reuptake of norepinephrine by the sympathetic nerve endings, resulting in a prolonged sympathetic block.

Holland and colleagues[115] reported on the efficacy of intravenous guanethidine and noticed very good to excellent results in 31 of 37 patients with reflex sympathetic dystrophy. Although the technique appears to be simple and permits a new method for sympathetic blockade, further controlled studies to show its efficacy are needed.

NEUROLYTIC BLOCKS

A patient with chronic intractable pain from cancer often will try any treatment to be free of pain. An estimated 440,000 patients die of cancer each year in the United States, and most suffer periods of severe pain during their illness. After several successful diagnostic local anesthetic blocks in these patients, a neurolytic block may be planned, depending on the cause and location of the pain.[119] A careful assessment of the overall situation is the first step in the treatment. It is important to communicate with the patient and family before a neurolytic block is done. Areas where neurolytic agents can be used include peripheral nerves, the epidural and subarachnoid spaces, and the celiac plexus.[120]

Hartel[121] reported the first use of caustic agents on nerve roots for interruption of pain fibers in 1914, and Doppler[122] reported the use of neurolytic agents in destroying nerve tissues in 1926. Initially, neurolytic nerve blocks received adverse publicity because of the lack of knowledge of physicians, inappropriate selection of patients, sepsis, and the lack of technical knowledge and proper facilities. Undesirable side effects and serious complications only made the situation worse. As a result, neurolytic nerve blocks were not considered a viable option for the treatment of intractable pain. It was not until 1931 that Dogliotti[62] used subarachnoid administration of neurolytic agents to achieve prolonged pain relief. After this, various investigations demonstrated neurolysis and pain relief without compromising other structures. The agents used included both hypo- and hypertonic solutions (distilled water, isotonic, and hypertonic saline), local anesthetic solutions in an oil base, ethyl alcohol, and phenol.

During the 1930s, absolute alcohol enjoyed wide popularity. Putnam and Hampton[133] reported the first use of phenol as a neurolytic agent for gasserian ganglion block. Mandle[123] reported successful use of phenol for chemical sympathectomy. Phenol was introduced as an intrathecal hyperbaric solution for intractable pain,[124] and it also was used as an epidural neurolytic agent.[125] Jacob and Howland[126] in 1966 reported a comparison of intrathecal alcohol and phenol.

Patient Selection for Neurolytic Blocks

A perfect nerve block that results in complete pain relief can be gratifying for the physician. Conversely, an adverse complication that results from the wrong selection of a patient, the use of an incorrect technique, or poor choice of neurolytic drug can have adverse consequences for both the patient and treating physician.

Many investigators in this field believe that proper selection of patients for neurolytic procedures is the most important factor. With some exceptions, neurolytic blocks must be restricted to terminally ill patients with cancer who have intractable pain. Several reports describe better results with patients who have cancer compared with those patients without cancer.

The prospective patient for a neurolytic block should undergo a full medical examination, including a thorough history and physical examination, and appropriate laboratory tests and x-ray studies (CT scan or myelogram). Active infection, congenital anomalies, bleeding disorders, or anticoagulant therapy may be relative contraindications.

Before the neurolytic block, an aggressive trial of non-narcotics, narcotics, and repeated temporary nerve blocks should be given in an attempt to obtain pain relief. When available techniques are unsatisfactory (either as a result of inadequate control of pain, failure of therapy, or complications resulting from therapy such as severe nausea, constipation, or heavy sedation, then neurolytic blocks should be considered.

Neurolytic blocks should always be preceded by a temporary diagnostic block using a local anesthetic.[127] Some intractable pain syndromes are more amenable to nerve blocks than others. For example, the pain of upper abdominal tumors (pancreas, stomach, and liver) can be treated readily by celiac plexus blocks.[128] The best results occur in patients who are blocked at an early stage in their illness.

Those who are extremely ill, very weak, or who have other associated medical problems may be at increased risk for surgical pain treatments (such as cordotomy or rhizotomy). In these patients, neurolytic nerve blocks are excellent options. In addition, patients with localized cancer pain involving visceral, somatic, or peripheral nerves are excellent candidates for neurolytic blocks.

Education and Preparation of the Patient and Family

Patients who are candidates for a neurolytic block first must be educated as to the possible advantages, disadvantages, realistic expectations, and complications that may result from the procedure. Such discussions are essential, both for the patient and their relatives, because there is no substitute for patient cooperation and understanding in allaying anxiety and maximizing success.

Most neurolytic blocks can be done on an outpatient basis, and discussions about the results and complications optimally should be undertaken before the date of the scheduled block. On the day of the procedure, the patient then can be as comfortable as possible and arrive with realistic expectations. Because a nerve block close to the central neural axis also may produce a sympathetic block that causes vasodilatation in the vascular bed distal to the block, hypotension should be anticipated. Unless contraindicated for medical reasons, patients should be encouraged to increase their fluid intake for several days before the block. In addition, they are advised not to eat or drink for 6 h before procedures such as celiac plexus, spinal, epidural, and stellate ganglion blocks. Venous access is advised, thus allowing additional prehydration doses of 500 to 1000 ml of balanced salt solutions before the block and affording a route for vasopressors or medications as required. The patient should arrive with a companion who can remain with them and provide safe transport home.

Access to radiologic facilities is advised for all neurolytic blocks.[129] Verification of needle or catheter position is critical as patients often receive blocks only after multiple operations or radiation therapy. These may make surface landmarks no longer accurate for needle placement.

An easily tiltable table and a CT or myelogram suite with biplane fluoroscopy are excellent adjuncts. As in all invasive procedures, adherence to strict aseptic technique is mandatory. The facility must be equipped with adequate cardiovascular monitoring devices and resuscitative equipment.

Neurolytic Agents

There are several neurolytic agents currently used for interrupting axonal conduction (Table 28-2). The commonly used neurolytic agents include absolute ethyl alcohol, phenol, ammonium sulfate, silver nitrate, and chlorocresol.

Absolute Alcohol

Alcohol is available in the United States as a 1-ml single-dose ampule. It is irritating to local tissues and causes considerable temporary pain during injection. The preinjection of a local anesthetic agent prevents this burning. Because absolute alcohol absorbs moisture from the atmosphere, its contents should be used immediately after the ampule is opened. Nathan[130] believes that alcohol exerts a dual action. The initial action is a local anesthetic effect; later, there is a destructive action on nerve tissue.

Absolute alcohol commonly is used as a neurolytic agent for peripheral nerve block, cranial nerve block (trigeminal nerve), sympathetic block in the lumbar region, and celiac plexus block. This drug is a hypobaric solution. Because the solution is lighter than the cerebrospinal fluid, the painful side must be placed uppermost when it is injected into the subarachnoid space. Alcohol used for neurolytic blocks requires a small volume and thus produces none of the systemic side effects of ingested ethanol. It is thought that its neurolytic action is through dehydration of the nerve tissue, producing extraction of cholesterol, phospholipid,

and cerebrosides. Furthermore, it affects the myelin sheath, causing precipitation of mucoprotein and lipoprotein. The uptake of alcohol by neural tissue is rapid. When injected into the subarachnoid space, only 10 percent is present in the spinal fluid after 10 min.[131]

A typical response to alcohol injection in neural tissue includes myelin sheath disruption and inflammatory responses, followed by demyelination and degeneration. Derrick[132] observed that subarachnoid alcohol injection led to degeneration of axis cylinders in the posterior root. The posterior root ganglion near the level of injection showed moderate swelling and chromatolysis, followed by intracellular edema and finally wallerian degeneration. When alcohol is injected, extreme care is required to avoid any local tissue injury or infiltration to prevent cellulitis or necrosis of adjacent tissues. After the injection, the needle should be flushed with a local anesthetic or normal saline solution to avoid depositing residual alcohol along the needle track.

The most common problems after alcohol injection are postinjection neuritis, hyperesthesia, paresthesia, and persistent pain at the site of the injection. If improperly injected, alcohol can cause unwanted effects on motor, sensory, and autonomic nerves. When used for celiac or lumbar sympathetic neurolysis, systemic hypotension may occur after the block.

Phenol

Phenol is the most commonly used neurolytic agent in treating intractable pain. Putnam and Hampton[133] used phenol by injection for neurolysis; Maher[124] deserves credit for the application of phenol as a neurolytic agent. Nathan[134] emphasized a preference for phenol over alcohol, and Maher[135] suggested that phenol has a selective action on C fibers. Nathan and Scott[136] reported that phenol produced a dual action. The initial blockade produced by phenol is

Table 28-2
Neurolytic Agents

Agent	Advantages	Disadvantages
Alcohol (50–100%)	Hypobaricity useful in some cases	Neuritis; solution may spread beyond area desired; can cause sloughing of superficial areas
Phenol (6–12% in saline, glycerine, or contrast dye)	Hyperbaricity of glycerin solutions useful in some cases	Less profound and shorter duration block than alcohol; neuritis, although probably less than alcohol; solution may spread beyond area desired; can cause sloughing of superficial areas
Cryoprobe	Reversible, no neuritis, small area of destruction	Very exact probe placement required, large probe needed (14–18 gauge)
Radiofrequency	Small area of destruction	Neuritis can occur, very accurate probe placement required, large probe needed (12 gauge)

believed to be a conduction blockade similar to a reversible local anesthetic block. Unlike alcohol, phenol injection, therefore, is much less painful. However, the neurolytic action on nerve fibers then leads to an irreversible conduction blockade. Phenol causes indiscriminate destruction depending on its concentration. Iggo and Walsh[137] showed a selective block of smaller nerve fibers using phenol 5%. Nathan and colleagues[138] reported that phenol first blocked the nonmyelinated C fibers and then acted on thinly myelinated A delta fibers; Pedersen and Juul-Jensen[139] reported that the motor effect of intrathecal phenol solution was a result of indiscriminate fiber damage. The primary neurolytic effect appears to be the result of protein degeneration and nonselective destruction. The maximal degeneration occurs at 2 weeks and maximal destruction at 14 weeks. Montoya and coworkers[139a] reported the effect of phenol on conduction and synaptic transmission on the sciatic nerve and the sympathetic system. They noticed that a low concentration of phenol is necessary to block sympathetic transmission. They further observed that an increase in calcium concentration in the phenol solution will decrease the anesthetic effect of the phenol; a decrease in calcium concentration increases the effect of the phenol. Moller and colleagues[140] found that the effect of phenol 5% was equivalent to that of alcohol 40%.

Phenol or carbolic acid is a benzene ring with one hydroxyl group substituted for a hydrogen ion. In its pure state, phenol is colorless and poorly soluble, forming a 6.7% solution in water. On exposure to air, phenol oxidizes to form quinones and other derivatives that give it a reddish tinge. Phenol is highly soluble in glycerin. At higher concentrations, phenol causes tissue injury, protein coagulation, and necrosis. It is excreted by the kidneys as various conjugated derivatives.[141]

Although phenol is not available commercially in an injectable form, it can be prepared by the hospital pharmacy. The solution can be prepared in water in the concentration range from 4% to 6%. The phenol is prepared in glycerin as a hyperbaric solution ranging from 4% to 10%. It is released from glycerin slowly; this is advantageous when used as an intrathecal agent. Because of its hyperbaric nature, spread can be localized, and thus it will have a localized effect. For selected cases of spasticity, a higher concentration of phenol 20% in glycerin can be used.[142] When injected in nonneural tissues, the aqueous phenol solution is a strong sclerotic agent. This drug also may be dissolved in radiocontrast dye, providing a hyperbaric radiopaque solution.

Intrathecal (Subarachnoid) Injection (See Appendix A.XII)

The technique of subarachnoid administration of neurolytic agents was used first by Maher,[62,121,122] who advocated the use of phenol as an intrathecal neurolytic drug. Various authors[124,125] reported good relief of pain in 65 percent to 70 percent of cases after a subarachnoid injection of phenol (see Chap. 18). Maher[135] recommended the use of phenol in glycerin as the drug of choice because it is hyperbaric, minimally diffusable, provides a slow release of phenol, and has a low incidence of complications. Brown[143] reported unsatisfactory results with subarachnoid phenol in patients with chronic pain of benign origin, and Mark and associates[144] confirmed that malignant pain responds better than chronic benign pain. Papo and Visca[145] reported a high failure rate and poor results with cervical and thoracic subarachnoid neurolytic blocks, however.

The duration of relief induced by subarachnoid phenol varies from less than 1 month to 10 months. Mehta[146] reported a higher success rate when the pain was present for less than 4 months before the block was administered. Overall, properly selected patients and techniques are mandatory to provide good quality pain relief in a high proportion of patients.

The choice of neurolytic agent is controversial. Although a solution of absolute alcohol is hypobaric relative to spinal fluid, a combination of phenol with glycerin or contrast dye is hyperbaric. Jacob and Howland[126] compared intrathecal alcohol with phenol for subarachnoid injection. A higher incidence of sphincter impairment was found with alcohol. Both neurolytic agents, however, were efficacious in producing relief of intractable pain.[147-149]

Phenol in glycerin is advantageous when the painful site can be placed in a dependent position to take advantage of the hyperbaric nature of the solution. The diffusion of this solution is slow and the local site of action can be controlled easily. Maher[135] found that 1 ml of phenol in glycerin can treat three nerve roots adequately. The slow release of phenol allows its destructive action to be well controlled in the desired dermatomal distribution.

Alcohol is a hypobaric solution without the localized effect of phenol. Injected into the subarachnoid space, the solution can disperse caudally or cephalad. When alcohol is used, the painful side must be kept upward. This drug has other disadvantages as a neurolytic drug for subarachnoid use. The analgesic effect is not attained for several days, and the chance of tissue sloughing is greater with alcohol than with phenol. Alcohol neuritis is a well-known phenomenon that may occur when alcohol is injected near a somatic nerve. The burning pain caused by alcohol may be worse than the original pain.

Whichever neurolytic agent is used, the position of the patient should be retained for approximately 45 min after injection to allow the neurolytic agent to become fixed to the nerve roots.

Epidural Neurolysis

Injection of a local anesthetic into the epidural space is a widely used procedure in the management of acute pain.[15] Severe intolerable pain (such as lumbar, biliary, renal, thoracic, and postoperative pain), may be managed using segmental epidural analgesia. This method is attractive because the technique is simple and carries minimal risk of spinal cord damage. The currently available literature has little to offer on the role of epidural neurolysis. For example, Maher[135] reported seven cases with excellent results, and others[143,149,150] had small numbers of cases to report. Maher[135] noticed that the epidural approach was safer and achieved better results than the intrathecal route for the relief of pain of cervical segment origin, and Colpitt and colleagues[151] also reported favorable results in treating pain in the cervical and thoracic levels.

Recently Racz and associates[152] reported encouraging results in cervical and thoracic level pain problems. He injected 3 to 4 ml of phenol 6% in saline using a catheter placed at the involved level. Although the number of cases was small, he stressed that single-shot injections often are not adequate, and patients may require three to four injections daily or at longer intervals.

Complications of Neurolysis

Complications after neurolytic procedures have been reported, often related to the spread of the neurolytic agent to adjacent vital organs. During the last two decades, improvements in technical facilities have improved the success rate and lowered the incidence of complications, but neurolytic block should not be attempted by a physician who has not acquired extensive experience or training in this technique. It requires a considerable degree of experience and skill for accurate placement of the solution.

The common complications caused by neurolytic agents can be divided into two categories: transient and permanent. The transient complications include nausea, vomiting, pain at the site of injection, local irritation, headaches, backache, alteration in sensation, localized hematoma, and pneumothorax. These complications most commonly are seen immediately after the block and usually are mild and respond well with minimal interference. Swerdlow[153] reported a 50 percent complication rate after use of chlorocresol. Kuzucu and colleagues[154] reported a 7 percent incidence of complications and a long-term incidence of only 1 percent. There is great variability in the literature concerning the actual incidence of these side effects (range, 6 percent to 50 percent). The major delayed complications include dysfunctions of rectal or bladder sphincters. Retention is common, especially after intrathecal injections. However, paresis of bladder and anal sphincters have been reported more with intrathecal alcohol than with other agents.[126] Nathan[136] reported an overall incidence of sphincter dysfunction of 12 percent. The motor effect of neurolysis varies from simple paresis to paraplegia. Bonica[127] reported an incidence of 25 percent of patients developing rectal, bladder or limb paralysis. Others found cauda equina lesions after intrathecal injections.[155,156] Alcoholic neuritis and arachnoiditis is a known complication when alcohol is used as a neurolytic drug.[157–160]

Neurolytic agents also may compromise spinal cord blood supply.[161–164] Local infiltration or spillage of a neurolytic agent also can result in sloughing and necrosis of local tissue.[165]

Practical Considerations and Results of Neurolysis

A decision to use a neurolytic block requires a clear understanding of the pain pathways involved and an accurate determination of the level at which the block should be done. A lower lumbar or sacral neurolytic block may be indicated in patients with chronic intractable pain from cancer of the bladder, prostate, uterus, cervix, rectum, or perineum.[166–168] The presence of a colostomy, nephrostomy, or ureterostomy will render the risk of sphincter loss less important. However, in the presence of an intact sphincter, extra precautions are recommended. The bladder and rectum are innervated by the sympathetic system through the hypogastric nerve and by the parasympathetic system through the pelvic nerve. Maher and associates[124] reported that making the injection with the tip of the needle, only just penetrating the subarachnoid space, and keeping the patient in the desired position will reduce the incidence of sphincter dysfunction.

Anatomically, cervical and thoracic level blocks are difficult, and the incidence of complications are higher.[169] A small dose and volume of hyperbaric phenol is recommended. Alcohol as a neurolytic agent plays a greater role in celiac plexus block than any other area and, in this case, is the drug of choice.

It is difficult to analyze the results reported in various studies. This lack of consensus is multifactorial. The result of procedures depends on various factors, including the type of disease, extent of lesion, involvement of local tissue, metastases, and the type of therapy the patient received earlier (radiation, chemotherapy, or surgery).

No two studies have identical results because of patient selection and variable criteria. In all major studies, the relief of pain reported varies from 6 to 16 weeks. In our experience, average pain relief lasts for 6 to 8 weeks. The longer intrathecal course of the nerve roots in the lower lumbar region and the larger size of nerve surfaces easily available for the absorption of neurolytic agents makes the technique most suitable for the lower lumbar region where results can be compared better with the upper cervical and thoracic region.

Neurolytic Celiac Plexus Block (See Appendix A.XIII)

Severe upper abdominal and back pain is the most common complaint of patients with upper abdominal malignancy (such as cancer of the pancreas, stomach, duodenum, liver, gall bladder, adrenal glands, and colon).[128,169–172] The overall operative mortality is approximately 20 percent, and

5-year survival is less than 5 percent nationally. Eighty percent of pain is caused by tumor invasion or compression of pain-sensitive areas.[173] The patient with intractable pain from these tumors often requires large amounts of analgesics. The result is poorly controlled pain and unwanted side effects of medications (such as heavy sedation, confusion, changes in consciousness, vomiting, and nausea). The pain[174] usually is well localized and incapacitating. With this background, it is easy to understand why one of the most satisfying and rewarding neurolytic blocks that a physician can administer is the celiac plexus block.[78,175–177] This technique also has been used to treat some benign pain syndromes.[178,179]

The sympathetic system is the primary pathway involved in the abdominal pain of pancreatic cancer. The pain is conveyed through the celiac plexus by the splanchnic sympathetics, vagus, phrenic, and somatic nerves.[170] The size and location of the tumor and its metastases are important etiologic factors.

Anatomic Considerations

In 1919, Kappis[180] first described the role of percutaneous celiac plexus blocks, although during the last 50 years, the technique has been modified with the development of newer medical technology. The easy availability of roentgenographic techniques has led to improvements in results and a simultaneous decrease in the incidence of complications.[169,181,182]

The components of the celiac plexus include the right and left celiac ganglia, the superior mesenteric and aorticorenal ganglia, the terminations of the superior (T5 to T10) and inferior (T10 to T11) splanchnic nerves, and branches of the phrenic, hepatic, gastric, superior mesenteric, suprarenal, and adrenal ganglia. In addition, the plexus also contains parasympathetic fibers from craniosacral nerve roots.[170,183] The cell bodies of the upper abdominal pain fibers lie in the dorsal root ganglion of the spinal nerves, and their course follows the sympathetic system pathways in the upper abdominal organs with dual pathways in the lower abdomen and pelvis through the lumbar ganglion and pelvic splanchnic ganglia.

The celiac plexus is located at the vertebral level of T12 and L1.[183,184] It lies retroperitoneally posterior to the stomach and omental bursa and in front of the crura of the diaphragm. The mean size of the ganglion on the right side is 2.79 × 1.43 cm, and on the left side, it is 2.39 × 1.83 cm. Moore and coworkers[183] showed that the celiac ganglia vary considerably in size, shape, and number. The celiac ganglia are semilunar and irregularly shaped masses located one on each side of the median plane. On the right side, the ganglion lies posterior and medial to the inferior vena cava, and on the left side, it is behind the splenic vessels, anterior to the aorta, and medial to the upper pole of the kidney and adrenal gland.

The celiac ganglia also vary in number and in their relation to the level of the vertebral column. The ganglion on the left side tends to be in a more caudal position, and therefore, it is recommended that the needle be placed on the left side in such a manner that the tip is at the level of the junction of the middle and lower third of the first lumbar vertebra. On the right side, the needle tip should be placed 1 cm cephalad to the L1 vertebral level.

Before the block, a complete physical examination should be done and a history taken and recorded. A patient receiving anticoagulant therapy must discontinue the anticoagulant before the block. In this case, the bleeding and clotting time should be documented before the block. On the day of the procedure, it is preferable to withhold pain medication and sedatives for 4 to 6 h before the block. An intravenous line is established, and 500 to 750 ml of crystalloid balanced salt solution is administered. We prefer to do the procedure in the radiology suite because the anatomic landmarks (such as the body of L1 vertebra and the 12th rib position can be identified easily under fluoroscopic control. After the T12 to L1 interspace is marked, the 12th rib position and diaphragmatic movements are observed closely on the fluoroscopic screen during both the inspiratory and expiratory phases of respirations. A skin wheel is raised 5 to 7 cm lateral to the midline at the L1 vertebral level. The needle most commonly used for celiac plexus block is a 20- to 22-gauge, 10 to 12 cm in length. The tip of the needle is directed toward the lateral side of the body of the first lumbar vertebra. A transaortic approach has been described.[185] Needles are placed on both sides of the vertebra in the same fashion. After the tips of the needles are anterior to the body of the vertebra, then posteroanterior and lateral roentgenograms are taken. Then 1 to 2 ml of metrizamide, a water-soluble radiopaque dye, may be injected to reconfirm the location of the needle. When the position of the needle is satisfactory, a test dose of 2 to 4 ml of lidocaine 1% is injected slowly on each side. The possibility of an intravascular, subarachnoid, or epidural injection must be excluded. When the needle position is verified, 20 to 25 ml of alcohol is injected slowly.[128,169,186] Moore and coworkers[183] observed that the solution spreads primarily cephalad, being 12 cm or more cephalad from the needle tip although only 3 to 5 cm caudally. Singler[181] reported that pain relief occurs from neurolysis of the greater and lesser splanchnic nerves as they approach the celiac plexus and not of the plexus itself. Whatever the mechanism, the success of the procedure varies from 33 percent to 94 percent, although excellent results are reported in only 60 percent of the patient population.[187–189] There are several reasons for unsuccessful blocks, including postoperative changes after surgical procedures, lack of diffusion of the agent through the retroperitoneal space, improper placement of the needle, anatomic variations of the celiac plexus, cancer infiltration,[187] and postradiation changes. Celiac plexus block also has been done by a unilateral approach, using larger volumes of solution.

Similar to any invasive procedure, celiac plexus block is not free of complications, and there may be immediate or late sequelae. The immediate complications include: nausea, vomiting, chest pain, hypotension,[169] pneumothorax, injury to the ureter, injury to the upper pole of the kidney, alcohol intoxication, and pain and burning from local irritation. Aortic or vena caval puncture also may occur but rarely cause clinical problems. In a series of 100 neurolytic celiac plexus blocks, Thompson and colleagues[128] reported only one case with neurologic sequelae. Neurolytic drug spread to undesired areas can lead to motor deficits, paraplegia,[190] myelitis, and neurologic damage. Moore and coworkers[183] showed that the cause of these complications is usually the posterior spread of neurolytic agent toward the sympathetic chain and lumbar plexus. The late complications of celiac block include dysesthesias, alcoholic neuritis, sexual dysfunction, groin neuralgia, local sloughing at the needle site, paresthesias, anesthesia dolorosa, postneurolytic neuralgia, orthostatic hypotension,[169] and pseudoaneurysm.[191]

With improvements in technique[169,181,187] and more use of radiologic facilities during the last decade, the rate of success of celiac block has increased, and the incidence of complications has decreased. Similar to other neurolytic blocks, prior local anesthetic block should be done and may avoid complications and unrealistic patient expectations. Just as a celiac plexus block can provide relief of the pain of upper abdominal visceral cancers, block of the superior hypogastric plexus in a similar fashion at the L5 to S1 interspace can provide relief of the pain produced by pelvic visceral cancers.[192]

CRYOANALGESIA

The application of cold to prevent pain is not a new concept. The oldest anesthetic known to Indian and Greek physicians was refrigeration.[193] Its analgesic effect was recorded by Hippocrates.[194] In the early 11th century, an Anglo-Saxon monk suggested the use of cold to reduce sensation before surgery. Larrey[195] noticed that amputation was much less painful in soldiers with exposure to the snow during the Napoleonic wars. During the 18th and 19th centuries, many famous scientists (including Claude Bernard, John Hunter, Reamur, and Spalianzani) studied the effects of cold. Local application of ether and ethyl chloride[34] as cooling agents were reported in 1866 and 1890.

The modern era of cryotherapy was introduced in 1962 with the introduction of the cryoprobe by Cooper and associates.[196] Various applications of cryo techniques have been used. Cryoanalgesia, however, is a technique in which the extreme low temperature produced by a cryosurgical probe achieves pain relief by blocking peripheral nerves or destroying the nerve endings. The concept of cryoanalgesia was first reported by Lloyd and colleagues.[4]

The cryoprobe currently used works on the principle of the Joule–Thompson effect. It is composed of an inner tube, an outer tube, and a working tip. When a high pressure gas

is allowed to expand in the probe tip, there is a rapid fall in temperature, causing cooling to $-60°C$.

The physiology of cold has been well reviewed by Bierman.[193] Cold application to the skin produces a reduction of local blood flow to tissue, a reduction in tissue metabolism, and an increase in local venous constriction and pressure. The cold also decreases the conduction of peripheral nerves.[197] Brown and colleagues[198] showed that when temperature is reduced to 10°C, an effective nerve blockade is achieved. Sensory fibers are blocked sooner than motor fibers. With the application of a cryoprobe, the local icy lesion produced at the nerve or tissue area is known as a cryolesion.[4] The cryolesion is the formation of intracellular and extracellular ice in the tissue.[199] Various factors play an important role in the extent of tissue damage caused by cryolesions. The most important factors are local temperature, rate of freezing and thawing, and duration of exposed tissue. Carter and colleagues[200] and Beazley and coworkers[201] showed that there is a second-degree burn type of nerve injury after application of a cryoprobe.

After the nerve is frozen, axonal disintegration, wallerian degeneration, and disruption of the myelin sheath occur, although the integrity of the epithelium and perineurium is maintained. Thus the conduction blockade produced by a cryolesion is a temporary effect, and after regeneration of the nerve, the function of the nerve returns to normal.[202] The duration of the block depends on the rate of axonal regrowth and the distance of the cryolesion from the end organ.[201,203] Beazley and coworkers[201] also found that there was no difference clinically in the period of motor or sensory nerve fiber interruption. The duration of conduction interruption can be predicted by controlling the temperature of the freeze injury.[204,205] Considerable damage to vessels was observed when the intact neurovascular bundle was frozen.[197]

Clinical Application of Cryoanalgesia

The application of cryoanalgesia is well reported in the management of acute[4,206–208] postoperative and chronic intractable pain[209,210] syndromes. The simplicity of the technique and the efficacy of the method in reducing postoperative pain without causing permanent damage to peripheral nerve[202] makes it an effective technique for the relief of postthoracotomy pain syndrome, low back pain, and facial pain.[211]

The intractable pain caused by coccydynia, cancer, and peripheral neuralgia also have been studied, with 78 percent of patients improved after cryotherapy.[209] The duration of relief varied, however (mean duration, 30 days). Various facial pain syndromes, nonherpetic neuralgia, tic douloureux, postsurgical neuralgia, atypical facial neuralgia, and postherpetic neuralgia have been treated with cryoanalgesia (mean pain relief duration, 60 days).[210] Although this technique offers advantages,[212] more controlled studies and evaluations are needed.

RADIOFREQUENCY NEUROLYSIS

This technique uses a heat lesion rather than cold to produce neural destruction. It is not reversible and, as in chemical neurolysis, may cause neuritis. (See Chap. 35.)

CONCLUSIONS

Patients with chronic pain often are exhausted physically and emotionally. They are frustrated by the inadequacies of multiple therapeutic options, and they arrive for regional analgesia expecting miracles. Proper patient selection and education therefore is essential. The physician unfamiliar with pain problems must be educated about the various available techniques and alternative approaches to manage pain; these must be used in an unbiased manner. Nerve blocks offer an excellent option in the fight to control chronic pain. Their success depends mostly on proper patient selection, understanding, and cooperation. In addition, the physician must be well trained in doing nerve blocks. It is worthwhile to emphasize the importance of total care of the patient rather than emphasizing just one nerve or a single painful point.

References

1. Merskey H, Albe-Fessard DG, Bonica JJ. International Association for the Study of Pain, Subcommittee on Taxonomy: pain terms: a list with definitions and notes on usage. *Pain* 1979; 6:249–252.
2. Bonica JJ. *The Management of Pain*. Philadelphia: Lea & Febiger; 1953.
3. Bonica JJ. Teaching residents diagnostic and therapeutic nerve blocks. *Anesth Analg* 1955; 34:202–213.
4. Lloyd JW, Barnard JDW, Glynn CJ. Cryoanalgesia. A new approach to pain relief. *Lancet* October 30, 1976; 1:932–934.
5. White JC, Sweet WH. *Pain and the Neurosurgeon: A Forty Year Experience*. Springfield: Thomas; 1969.
6. Loeser JD. Dorsal rhizotomy for the relief of chronic pain. *J Neurosurg* 1972; 36:745–755.
7. Gregg JM, Banerjee T, Ghia JN, Campbell R. Radiofrequency thermoneurolysis of peripheral nerves for control of trigeminal neuralgia. *Pain* 1978; 5:231–243.
8. Bonica JJ. Management of intractable pain with analgesic blocks. *JAMA* 1952; 150:1581–1586.
9. Rovenstive EA, Wertheim HM. Therapeutic nerve blocks. *JAMA* 1941; 117:1599–1603.
10. Vandam LD, Eckenhoff JE. The anesthesiologist and therapeutic nerve block technician or physician (with emphasis on the problems of pain relief). *Anesthesiology* 1954; 15:89–94.
11. Dejong RH. *Local Anesthetics*. Springfield: Thomas; 1971.
12. Covino BG, Vassalo MG. *Local Anesthetics Mechanism of Action and Clinical Use*. New York: Grune & Stratton; 1976.
13. Ritchie JM. Mechanism of action of local anesthetic agents and biotoxins. *Br J Anesth* 1975; 47:191.
14. Franz DN, Perry RS. Mechanism for differential blocks among single myelinate and non-myelinated axons by procaine. *J Physiol* 1974; 235:193.
15. Bromage PR. Physiology and pharmacology of epidural analgesia. *Anesthesiology* 1967; 28:592.
16. Heavner JE, DeJong RM. Lidocaine blocking concentration for B and C nerve fibers. *Anesthesiology* 1974; 40:228–233.
17. Gasser HS, Erlanger J. The role of fiber size in the establishment of a nerve block by pressure of cocaine. *Am J Physiol* 1929; 88:581–591.
18. Jack RD. Regional anesthesia for pain relief. *Br J Anaesth* 1975; 47:278–280.
19. Slelsinger MH, Fordtram JS. *Gastrointestinal Disease*. 2nd. ed. Philadelphia: Saunders; Philadelphia; 1968.
20. Duthie MA, Ingham VAL. Persistent abdominal pain. *Anesthesia* 1981; 36:289–292.
21. Bridenbaugh PO, Dupen SL, Moore DC, Bridenbaugh LD, Thompson GE. Postoperative intercostal nerve block analgesia versus narcotic analgesia. *Anesth Analg* 1973; 52:81.
22. Cronin KD, Davies MJ. Intercostal block for postoperative pain relief. *Anesth Int Care* 1976; 4:259.
23. Delilkan AE, Lee CK, Young WK, Ong SC, Gannendran AI. Postoperative local analgesia for thoracotomy with direct bupivacaine intercostal blocks. *Anesthesia* 1973; 28:561.
24. Boas RA, Hatangdi VS, Richards EG. Lumbar sympathectomy, a percutaneous technique. In: Bonica JJ, Albe-Fessard D, eds. *Advances in Pain Research and Therapy*. Vol. 1. New York: Raven Press; 1976:685–689.
25. Bonica JJ. Management of myofascial pain syndrome in general practice. *JAMA* 1957; 167:732–738.
26. Travell J. Myofascial trigger points. Clinical view. In: Bonica JJ, Albe-Fessard D, eds. *Advances in Pain Research and Therapy*. New York: Raven Press; 1976: 919–926.
27. Simon DG. Electrogenic nature of palpable bands and "jump sign" associated with myofascial trigger points. In: Bonica JJ, Albe-Fessard D, eds. *Advances in Pain Research and Therapy*. New York: Raven Press; 1976:913–918.
28. Long C. Myofascial pain syndrome: general characteristics and treatment. *Henry Ford Hosp Med Bull* 1955; 3:189–192.
29. Brown BR Jr. Diagnosis and therapy of common myofascial syndromes. *JAMA* 1978; 239:646–648.
30. Sola AE, Williams RC. Myofascial pain syndromes. *Neurology* 1956; 6:91.
31. Kraus H. Trigger points. *N Y State J Med* 1973; 73:1310.
32. Awad EA. Interstitial myofibrosis hypothesis of the mechanism. *Arch Phys Med Rehabil* 1973; 54:449–453.
33. Ready LB, Kozody R, Barsa JE, Murphy TM. Trigger point injection us: jet injection in the treatment of myofascial pain. *Pain* 1983; 15:201–206.
34. Travell J. Ethyl chloride spray for painful muscle spasm. *Arch Phys Med Rehabil* 1952; 33:291–298.
35. Lewit K. Needle effect in relief of myofascial pain. *Pain* 1979; 6:83–90.
36. Melzack R, Stillwell DM, Fox EJ. Trigger points and acupuncture points for pain correlations and implications. *Pain* 1977; 3:3.

37. Hannington-Kiff, JG. Treatment of intractable pain by bupivacaine nerve block. *Lancet* 1971; 2:1392–1394.

38. Chinn MA, Wirjoatmadja K. Prolonging local anesthesia. *Lancet* 1967; 2:835.

39. Schneck SA. Peripheral and cranial nerve injuries resulting from general surgical procedure. *Arch Surg* 1960; 81:855–859.

40. Akerman B, Astrom A, Ross S, et al. Studies on the absorption, distribution, and metabolism of labellea prilocaine and lidocaine in some animal species. *Acta Pharmacol Toxicol* 1966; 24:389.

41. Shames AM. Electrochemical aspect of physiological and pharmacological action in excitable cell, II: the action potential and excitation. *Pharmacol Rev* 1958; 10(2):165.

42. Loder RE. A long acting local anesthetic solution for the relief of pain after thoracotomy. *Thorax* 1962; 17:375–376.

43. Mather LE, Bridenbaugh PO, Bridenbaugh LD, Balfour RI, Lyson DF, Horton WG. Arterial and venous plasma levels of bupivacaine following epidural and intercostal nerve blocks. *Anesthesiology* 1976; 45:39–45.

44. Delikan AG, Lee CK, Young WK, Ong SC, Gannendan AI. Post-operative local analgesia for thoracotomy with direct bupivacaine intercostal block. *Anesthesia* 1973; 28:561–567.

45. Bonica JJ. Current role of nerve blocks in diagnosis and therapy of pain. In Bonica JJ, ed. *Advances in Neurology*. Vol. 4. New York: Raven Press; 1974:445–453.

46. Courteny KR, Kending JJ, Cohen EN. Frequency dependent conduction block. The role of nerve impulse pattern in local anesthetic potency. *Anesthesiology* 1978; 48:111.

47. Moore DC, Balfour RI, Fitzgibbons D. Convulsive arterial plasma level of bupivacaine and response to diazepam therapy. *Anesthesiology* 1979; 50:454–456.

48. Kotelko DM, Shnider SM, Daily DA, et al. Bupivacaine induced cardiac arrhythmia in sheep. *Anesthesiology* 1984; 60:10.

49. Liu P, Feldman MS, Covine BM, et al. Acute cardiovascular toxicity in intravenous amide local anesthetic in anesthetized ventilated dogs. *Anesth Analg* 1982; 61:317.

50. Moore DC. Intercostal nerve block for post-operative somatic pain following surgery of thorax and upper abdomen. *Br J Anaesth* 1975; 47:284.

51. Moore DC, Scurlock JG. Possible role of epinephrine in prevention or correction of myocardial depression associated with bupivacaine. *Anesth Analg* 1983; 62:450.

52. Bromage PR, Burfoot MF, Crowell DE, et al. Quality of epidural blockade II carbonated local anesthetic solutions. *Br J Anaesth* 1967; 39:197.

53. Haines SJ, Jannetta PJ, Zorub DS. Microvascular relation of trigeminal nerves. An anatomical study with clinical correlation. *J Neurosurg* 1980; 52:381–386.

54. Onofrio BM. Radiofrequency percutaneous gasserian ganglion lesions result in 140 patients with trigeminal pain. *J Neurosurg* 1975; 42:132–139.

55. Ishii T. Glossopharyngeal neuralgia: surgical treatment and electromicroscopic findings. *Laryngoscope* 1976; 86:577–583.

56. Moore DC. *Regional Block*. 4th ed. Springfield: Thomas; 1965.

57. Kanner RM, Martini N, Foley KM. Nature and incidence of post thoracotomy pain. *Proc Am Soc Clin Oncol* 1982; 1:152.

58. Moore DC, Bush WH, Scurlock JE. Intercostal nerve block; a roentgenographic anatomy study of technique and absorption in humans. *Anesth Analg* 1980; 59:815.

59. Dogliotti AM. Traitment des syndromes douloureux de la peripherie par l'alcoholisation subarachnoidienne. *Presse Med* 1931; 39:1249–1242.

60. Kaplan JA, Miller E Jr, Galagher EG Jr. Post-operative analgesia for thoracotomy patients. *Anesth Analg* 1975; 54:773.

61. Purcell-Jones G, Pither CE, Justins DM. Paravertebral somatic nerve block: a clinical, radiographic, and computed tomographic study in chronic pain patients. *Anesth Analg* January 1989; 68(1):32–39.

62. Yoshikawa K, Mima T, Egawa J. Blood levels of marcaine (LAC-43) in axillary plexus blocks, intercostal nerve blocks, and epidural anaesthesia. *Acta Anesthesiol Scand* 1968; 12:1.

63. Moore DC, Mather LE, Bridenbaugh LD, et al. Arterial and venous plasma level of bupivacaine following peripheral nerve block. *Anesth Analg* 1976; 55:763.

64. Fyf ET, Quin RO. Phenol sympathectomy in the treatment of intermittent claudication. *Br J Surg* 1975; 62:68–71.

65. Findley T, Patzer R. The treatment of herpes zoster by paravertebral procaine block. *JAMA* 1945; 128:1217–1221.

66. Moore DC, Bridenbaugh LD. Pneumothorax: its incidence following intercostal nerve block. *JAMA* 1960; 178:842.

67. Kuntz A. *Autonomic nervous system*. 4th ed. Philadelphia: Lea and Febiger; 1953.

68. Mayers S; Goodman L, Gilman A, eds. Neurohormonal transmission and the autonomic nervous system. In: *The Pharmacological Basis of Therapeutics*. 6th ed. New York: Macmillan; 1980:56–90.

69. Bonica JJ. Autonomic innervation of viscera in relation to nerve blocks. *Anesthesiology* 1968; 29:793–813.

70. Loh L, Nathan PW. Painful peripheral states and sympathetic blocks. *J Neurol Neurosurg Psychiatry* 1978; 41:664–671.

71. Loh L, Nathan PW, Shoot GD. Pain due to lesion of central nervous system removed by sympathetic block. *Br Med J* 1981; 282:1026–1028.

72. Bonica JJ. Causalgia and other reflex sympathetic dystrophies. In: Bonica JJ, Liebeskind JC, Fessard A, eds. *Advances in Pain Research and Therapy*. Vol 3. New York: Raven Press; 1979.

73. Evans JA. Reflex sympathetic dystrophy. *Surg Gynecol Obstet* 1947; 82:36–43.

74. Livingston WK. Post-traumatic pain syndromes. *West J Surg Obstet Gynecol* 1938; 46:341–347.

75. Strandness DE Jr. *Peripheral Arterial Disease: A Physiological Approach*. Boston: Little, Brown; 1969.

76. Cousins MJ, Reeve TS, Glynn CJ, Walsh JA, Cherry DA. Neurolytic sympathetic blockade: Duration of denervation and relief of rest pain. *Anesth Int Care* 1979; 7:2:121–135.

77. Busch EH, Atchison SR. Steroid celiac plexus block for chronic pancreatitis: results in 16 cases. *J Clin Anesth* 1989; 1(6):431–433.

78. Bengstsson M, Lofstrom JB. Nerve block in pancreatic pain. *Acta Chir Scand* April 1990; 156(4):285–291.

79. Moore DC. *Stellate Ganglion Block.* Springfield: Thomas; 1954.

80. Procacci P, Francihi F, Zoppin M, Maresca M. Cutaneous pain threshold changes after sympathetic block in reflex dystrophies. *Pain* 1975; 1:167.

81. Carron H, Litwiller R. Stellate ganglion block. *Anesth Analg* 1975; 54:567–570.

82. Carron H. *Anesth Analg* 1976; 55:451. Letter.

83. Smith DW. Stellate ganglion block: the tissue displacement method. *Am J Surg* 1951; 82:344–345.

84. Horner JF. *Klin Monatsbl Augenheilkd* 1869; 7:193–198.

85. Beene TK, Eggers GWN Jr. Use of the pulse monitor for determining sympathetic block of the arm. *Anesthesiology* 1974; 40:412.

86. Kim JM, Arakawa K, Vonlinter T. Use of the pulse wave monitor as a measurement of diagnostic sympathetic block and surgical sympathectomy. *Anesth Analg* 1975; 54:289.

87. Lynn RB, Barcroft H. Circulating changes in the foot after lumbar sympathectomy. *Lancet* 1950:1105–1108.

88. Lewis LW. Evaluation of sympathetic activity following chemical or surgical sympathectomy. *Anesth Analg* 1955; 34:334.

89. Dhuner KG, Edshage S, Wilhelm A. Ninhydrin test an objective method for testing local anesthetic drugs. *Acta Anaesthesiol Scand* 1960; 4:189.

90. Orkin LR, Papper EM, Rovenstine EA. Complication of stellate and thoracic sympathetic nerve blocks. *J Thorac Surg* 1950; 20:911.

91. Pallin IM, Deutsch EV. Death following stellate ganglion block. *Ann Surg* 1951; 222:226.

92. Adelman MH. Cerebral air embolism complicating stellate ganglion block. *J Mt Sinai Hosp* 1948; 15:28–30.

93. Richards RL. Causalgia: a centennial review. *Arch Neurol* 1967; 16:339–350.

94. Spurling RG. Causalgia of the upper extremity: treatment by dorsal sympathetic ganglionectomy. *Arch Neurol Psychiatry* 1930; 23:784–788.

95. Drucker WR, Hubay CA, Holden WD, Bukovnic JA. Pathogenesis of posttraumatic sympathetic dystrophy. *Am J Surg* 1959; 97:454–465.

96. Gena NT: The reflex sympathetic dystrophy syndrome. *Radiology* 1975; 117:21.

97. Kozin F, Genant JK, Bekerman D, et al. The reflex sympathetic dystrophy syndrome: roentgenographic and scintigraphic evidence of bilaterality and of periarticular accentuation. *Am J Med* 1974; 60:332–338.

98. Giale DA. The management of neuralgias complicating herpes zoster. *Practitioner* 1973; 210:794–798.

99. Colding A. The effect of regional sympathetic blocks in the treatment of herpes zoster. *Acta Anesthesiol Scand* 1969; 13:133–141.

100. Masud KJ, Forster KJ. Sympathetic block in herpes zoster. *Am Fam Physician* 1975; 12:142.

101. Lipton S. *Relief of Pain in Clinical Practice.* London: Blackwell Scientific Publ; 1979.

102. Strandness DE Jr. *Peripheral Arterial Disease: A Physiological Approach.* Boston: Little, Brown; 1969.

103. Myers KA, Irving WT. An objective study of lumbar sympathectomy II skin ischemia. *Br Med J* 1966; 1:943.

104. Sunderland S. *Nerve and Nerve Injuries.* Edinburgh: Churchill Livingstone; 1978:1046.

105. Gillespie JA. Late effects of lumbar sympathectomy. *Lancet* 1960; 891–894.

106. Gillespie JA. Sympathectomy. *Br J Hosp Med* 1975; 14:418–428.

107. Reid W, Watt JK, Gray TG. Phenol injection of the sympathetic chain. *Br J Surg* 1970; 57:45.

108. Threadgill FD. Afferent conduction via the sympathetic ganglia innervate the extremity. *Surgery* 1947; 21:575.

109. Mandl F. *Paravertebral Block in Diagnosis, Prognosis, and Therapy in Minor Sympathetic Surgery.* New York: Grune & Stratton; 1947.

110. Feldman Young. Treatment of intermittent claudication: lumbar paravertebral block with phenol. *Anesthesiology* 1975; 30:174–182.

111. Alexander FAD. Control of pain. In: Hale D, ed. *Anesthesiology.* Philadelphia: Davis; 1963:579–611.

112. Bryce Smith R. Injection of the lumbar sympathetic chain. *Anesthesiology* 1951; 6:150–153.

113. Lloyd JW, Carrie LES. A method for treating renal colic. *Proc R Soc Med* 1965; 58:634.

114. Hupert C. Recognition and treatment of causalgic pain occurring in cancer patients. In: Bonica JJ, Liebeskind J, Albe-Fessard D, eds. *Advances in Pain Research and Therapy.* Vol 3. New York: Raven Press; 1979.

115. Holland AJC, Davies KH, Wallace DH. Sympathetic blockade for isolated limbs by intravenous guanethidine. *Can Anaesth Soc J* 1977; 24:597–602.

116. Moore DC. Complication of regional anesthesia. *Clin Anesth* 1969; 7:217.

117. Gray GR, Evans JA. Total spinal anesthesia following lumbar paravertebral block. A potentially lethal complication. *Anesth Analg* 1971; 50:1344.

118. Learned LO, Calhoun RF. Retroperitoneal hemorrhage as a complication of lumbar paravertebral injection. Report of three cases. *Anesthesiology* 1951; 12:391.

119. Lipton S. Pain relief in active patients with cancer: the early use of nerve blocks improves the quality of life. *BMJ* January 7, 1989; 298(6665):37–38.

120. Ferrer-Brechner T. Anesthetic techniques for the management of cancer pain. *Cancer* June 1, 1989; 63(11 suppl):2343–2347.

121. Hartel F. Die Behandlung der Trigeminus neuralgic mit Intrakraniellen Alkokoleinspritzungen. *Dtsch Z Chir* 1914; 126:429.

122. Doppler K. Die Sympathike Diapttherese. (chemische sympathetic usa uss Chaltung) ander arteria femorales. *Med Klin* 1926; 22:1954–1956.

123. Mandle F. Aqueous solution of phenol as substitute for alcohol in sympathetic block. *J Int Coll Surg* 1950; 13:566–568.

124. Maher RM. Relief of pain in incurable cancer. *Lancet* 1955; 1:18–20.

125. Rodrigues-Bigas M, Petrelli NJ, Herrera L, West C. Intrathecal phenol rhizotomy for management of pain in recurrant unresectable carcinoma of the rectum. *Surg Gynecol Obstet* July 1991; 173(1):41–44.

126. Jacob RG, Howland WS. A comparison of intrathecal alcohol and phenol. *J Ky Med Assoc* 1966; 64:408.

127. Bonica JJ. Diagnostic and therapeutic blocks. A reappraisal based on 15 years experience. *Anesth Analg Curr Res* 1958; 37:58.

128. Thompson G, Moore DC, Bridenbaugh LD, Artin R. Abdominal pain and alcohol celiac plexus nerve block. *Anesth Analg Curr Res* January–February 1977; 56:1–5.

129. Eaton AC, Wriht M, Caullum KG. The use of the image intensifier in phenol lumbar sympathetic block. *Radiography* 1980; XIVI;552:298.

130. Nathan PW. Intrathecal phenol to relieve spasticity in paraplegia. *Lancet* 1959; 2:1099–1102.

131. Matsuki M, Kato Y, Ichiyanagi K. Progressive changes in the concentration of ethyl alcohol in human and canine subarachnoid space. *Anesthesiology* 1972; 36:617–621.

132. Derrick WS. Control of pain in the cancer patient by subarachnoid alcohol block. *Postgrad Med* 1970; 48:232–237.

133. Putnam TJ, Hampton AO. A technique of injection in the gasserian ganglion under roentgenographic control. *Arch Neurol Psychiatry* 1936; 35:92–98.

134. Nathan PW. Pain in cancer: comparison of results of cordotomy and chemical rhizotomy. In: Fusek I, Kunc Z, eds. *Present Limits of Neurosurgery*. Amsterdam: Excerpta Medica; 1972:513–516.

135. Maher RM. Neurone selection in relief of pain. Further experiences with intrathecal injections. *Lancet* 1957; 1:16–19.

136. Nathan PW, Scott G. Intrathecal phenol for intractable pain. Safety and dangers of the method. *Lancet* 1958; 1:76–80.

137. Iggo A, Walsh EG. Selective block of small fibers in the spinal roots by phenol. *Brain* 1960; 83:701–708.

138. Nathan PW, Sears TA, Smith MC. Effects of phenol solution on the nerve roots of the cat. An electrophysiological and histological study. *J Neurol Sci* 1965; 2:7–29.

139. Pederson E, Juul-Jensen P. Intrathecal phenol in the treatment of spasticity. *Acta Neurol Scand* 1962; 3:69–77.

139a. Montoya GA, Soteras RW, Rudolph IM, et al. Effects of phenol on conduction and synoptic transmission block. *Am J Phys Med* August 1980; 59(4):184–195.

140. Moller JE, Helweg Larson J, Jacobson E. Histopathological lesion in the sciatic nerves of rats following perineural application of phenol and alcohol solution. *Dan Med Bull* 1969; 16:116–119.

141. Felsenthal G. Pharmacology of phenol in peripheral nerve blocks: a review. *Arch Phys Med Rehabil* 1974; 55:13–16.

142. Pederson E, Juul-Jensen P. Treatment of spasticity by subarachnoid phenol glycerin. *Neurology (Minneap)* 1965; 15:256.

143. Brown AS. Treatment of intractable pain by nerve block with phenol. *Excerpta Medica* 1961; 36:E59–60.

144. Mark VH, White JC, Zervas NT, Ervin FR, Richardson EP. Intrathecal use of phenol for the relief of chronic severe pain. *N Engl J Med* 1962; 262:589–593.

145. Papo I, Visca A. A phenol rhizotomy in the treatment of cancer pain. *Anesth Analg* 1974; 53:99.

146. Mehta M. *Intractable Pain: Major Problems in Anesthesia II*. London: WB Saunders; 1973.

147. Evans RJ, Mackay IM: Subarachnoid phenol nerve blocks for relief of pain in advanced malignancy. *Can J Surg* 1972; 15:50–53.

148. Wood KA. The use of phenol as a neurolytic agent: a review. *Pain* 1978; 5:205–229.

149. Gentil F, Russo RP, Monti A, Pereira de Almeida, De Fortuna A. Pain relief in cancerous patients by the use of phenol solution. *Acta Univ Int Cancer* 1963; 19:982–985.

150. Finer B. Epidural injection of carbolic acid in incurable cancer. *Lancet* 1958; 2:1179.

151. Colpitt MR, Levy BA, Lawrence M. Treatment of cancer related pain with phenol epidural block. Abstract World Congress on Pain; Montreal; 1978.

152. Racz GB, Sabonghy M, Gintautas J, Klin WM. Intractable pain therapy using a new epidural catheter. *JAMA* 1982; 248:579–581.

153. Swerdlow M. Intrathecal chlorocresol. A comparison with phenol in the treatment of intractable pain. *Anesthesiology* 1973; 281:297–301.

154. Kuzucu EY, Derrick WS, Wilber SA. Control of intractable pain with subarachnoid alcohol block. *JAMA* 1966; 195:541.

155. Tureen LL, Gitt JJ. Cauda equina syndrome following subarachnoid injection of alcohol. *JAMA* 1936; 106:18.

156. Sloane P. Syndrome referable to the cauda equina following the intraspinal injection of alcohol for the relief of the pain. *Arch Neuro Psychiatry* 1935; 34:1120.

157. Gordon RA, Goel SB. Intrathecal phenol block in the treatment of malignant disease. *Can Anaesth Soc J* 1963; 10:357.

158. Superville Sovak B, Rasminsky M, Finlayson MM. Complication of phenol neurolysis. *Arch Neurol* 1975; 32:226.

159. Khalili AA, Bitzler JW. Neurolytic substances in the relief of pain. *Med Clin IV. America* 1968; 52:161–171.

160. Hurst EW. Adhesive arachnoiditis and vascular blockage caused by detergents and chemical irritants. An experimental study. *J Patn Bact Conta* 1955; 70:167–179.

161. Wolfman L. The neuropathological effects resulting from the intrathecal injection of chemical of substances. *Paraplegia* 1966; 4:97–115.

162. Hughes JT. Thrombosis of posterior spinal arteries. A complication of intrathecal injection of phenol. *Neurol* (Minneap) 1970; 20:659–664.

163. Totoki T, Kato T, Nomoto Y, Kura Kazu M, Kanaseki T. Anterior spinal artery syndrome. A complication of cervical intrathecal phenol injection. *Pain* 1979; 6:99–104.

164. Wilkinson MA, Mark VH, White JC. Further experience with intractable phenol for the relief of pain. *J Chron Dis* 1964; 17:1055–1058.

165. Berry K, Olszewski J. Pathology of intrathecal phenol injection in man. *Neurology* 1963; 13:152–154.

166. Stovner J, Endresen R. Intrathecal phenol for cancer pain. *Acta Scand* 1972; 16:17–21.

167. Hay RC. Subarachnoid alcohol block in the control of intractable pain. *Anaesth Analg Curr Res* 1962; 41:12.

168. Wright BD. Treatment of intractable coccygodynia by transsacral ammonium chloride injection. *Anesth Analg* 1971; 50:519.

169. Moore DC. Celiac plexus block with alcohol for cancer pain of the upper intra-abdominal viscera. In: Bonica JJ, Ventafridda V, eds. *Advances in Pain Research and Therapy*. Vol 2. New York: Raven Press; 1979:357–371.

170. Ray BS, Neill CL. Abdominal visceral sensation in man. *Ann Surg* 1974; 126:709–724.

171. Jones RR. A technique for injection of the splanchnic nerve with alcohol. *Anesth Analg* 1975; 36:75–77.

172. Brown DL. A retrospective analysis of neurolytic celiac

plexus block for nonpancreatic intra-abdominal cancer pain. *Reg Anesth* March–April 1989; 14(2):63–65.

173. Drapiewski JR. Carcinoma of the pancreas: a study of neoplastic invasion of nerves and its possible clinical significance. *Am J Clin Pathol* 1944; 14:549–556.

174. Krain LS. The rising incidence of carcinoma of the pancreas: real or apparent. *J Surg Oncol* 1970; 2:115–124.

175. Salzberg D, Foley KM. Management of pain in pancreatic cancer. *Surg Clin North Am* June 1989; 89(3):629–649.

176. Squier R, Morrow JS, Roman R. Pain therapy for pancreatic carcinoma with neurolytic celiac plexus block. *Conn Med* May 1989; 53(5):269–271.

177. Sharfman WH, Walsh TD. Has the analgesic efficacy of neurolytic celiac plexus block been demonstrated in pancreatic cancer pain? *Pain* June 1990; 41(3):267–271.

178. Tanelian D, Cousins MJ. Celiac plexus block following high-dose opiates for chronic noncancer pain in a four-year-old-child. *J Pain Symptom Manage* June 1989; 4(2):82–85.

179. Humbles FF, Mahaffey JE. Teflon epidural catheter placement for intermittent celiac plexus blockade and celiac plexus neurolytic blockade. *Reg Anesth* March–April 1990; 15(2):103–105.

180. Kappis M. Sensibilital und lokale anesthesia im chirurgischen gebiet der bauchhohle mit besondere berucksichtingung der splanchnicus anasthesie. *Bruns Beitraage Zur Klin Cher* 1919; 15:161.

181. Singler RC. An improved technique for alcohol neurolysis of the celiac plexus. *Anesthesiology* 1982; 56:137–141.

182. Ischiastefana Luzzani A, Ischia A, Faggion A. A new approach to the neurolytic block of the coeliac plexus. The transaortic technique. *Pain* 1983; 16:333–341.

183. Moore DC, Bush WH, Burnett LL. Celiac plexus block: a roentgenographic, anatomic study of technique and spread of solution in patients and corpses. *Anesth Analg (Cleve)* 1981; 60:369–379.

184. Ward EM, Rorie DE, Naus LA, et al. The celiac ganglion in man. Normal anatomic variations. *Anesth Analg* 1979; 58:461–465.

185. Lieberman RP, Waldman SD. Celiac plexus neurolysis with the modified transaortic approach. *Radiology* April 1990; 175(1):274–276.

186. Jones J, Gough D. Coeliac plexus block with alcohol for relief of upper abdominal pain due to cancer. *Ann R Coll Surg Engl* 1977; 59:46–49.

187. Buy JN, Moss AA, Singler RC. CT guided celiac plexus and splanchnic nerve neurolysis. *J Comput Assist Tomogr* 1982; 6:315.

188. Filshie JF, Golding S, Robbie DS, Husband J. Unilateral computerized tomography guided coeliac plexus block. A technique for pain relief. *Anaesthesiology* 1983; 38:498–503.

189. Hanowell S, Kennedy S, Macnamara TE, Ericlees D. Celiac plexus block diagnostic and therapeutic applications in abdominal pain. *South Med J* 1980; 73:10:1330–1332.

190. Galizia EJ, Lahira SK: Paraplegia following coeliac plexus block with phenol. *Br J Anaesth* 1974; 46:539–540.

191. Sett SS, Taylor DC. Aortic pseudoaneurysm secondary to celiac plexus block. *Ann Vasc Surg* January 1991; 5(1):88–91.

192. Plancarte R, Amescua C, Patt RB, Aldrete JA. Superior hypogastric plexus block for pelvic cancer pain. *Anesthesiology* August 1990; 73(2):236–239.

193. Bierman W. Therapeutic use of cold. *JAMA* 1955; 157:1189–1192.

194. Jones WHS. Hippocrates, Heraclitus on the universe. *Aphorism* 4:165–167, 201.

195. Larrey DJ. *Surgical Memories of Campaigns of Russia, Germany, and France.* Philadelphia: Carey & Lea; 1832:293.

196. Cooper IS, Grissman F, Johnson R. Principles and rational of cryogenic surgery. *Saint Barnabas Hosp Med Bull* 1962; I:11–16.

197. Marsland AR, Ramamurthy AR, Barnes J. Cryogenic damage to peripheral nerves and blood vessels in the rat. *Br J Anaesth* 1983; 55:555–557.

198. Brown DD, Adams RD, Brenner C, Doherty MM. The pathology of injury to nerve induced by cold. *J Neuropathol Exp Neurol* 1945; 4:305–323.

199. Whittaker DK. Ice crystal formation in tissue during cryosurgery. *Cryobiology* 1974; 11:192.

200. Carter DC, Lee PWR, Gill W, Johnson RJ. The effect of cryosurgery on peripheral nerve functions. *J R Coll Surg Edinb* 1972; 17:25–31.

201. Beazley RM, Bagley DH, Ketcham AS. The effect of cryosurgery on peripheral nerves. *J Surg Res* 1974; 16:231–234.

202. Barnard D. The effect of extreme cold on sensory nerves. *Ann R Coll Surg Engl* 1980; 62:180–187.

203. Savitz MH, Malis LI. Intractable pain treated with intrathecal isotonic iced saline. *J Neurol Neurosurg Psychiatry* 1973; 36:417–420.

204. Whittaker DK. Degeneration and regeneration of nerves following cryosurgery. *Br J Exp Pathol* 1974; 55:595.

205. Hannington-Kiff JG: Cryoanalgesia for postoperative pain. *Lancet* 1980; 1:829.

206. Glynn J, Lloyd JW, Barnard JDW. Cryoanalgesia in the management of pain after thoracotomy. *Thorax* 1980; 35:325–327.

207. Orr IA, Keenan DJM, Dundee JW. Improved pain relief after thoracotomy use of cryoprobe and morphine infusion. *Br Med J* 1981; 281,283:945–947.

208. Maiwand O, Makey AR. Cryonalgesia for relief of pain after thoracotomy. *Br Med J* 1981; 282:1749–1750.

209. Evans PJD, Lloyd JW, Jack TM. Cryoanalgesia for intractable pain. *J R Soc Med* 1981; 74:804–809.

210. Barnard D, Lloyd J, Evans J. Cryonanalgesia in the management of chronic facial pain. *J Maxillofacial Surg* 1981; 9:101–102.

211. Ramamurthy S, Walsh NE, Shoenfeld LS, Hoffman J. Evaluation of neurolytic blocks using phenol and cryogenic block in the management of chronic pain. *J Pain Symptom Manage* June 1989; 4(2):72–75.

212. Rooney S, Jain S, McCormick P, Bains M, Martini N, Goldiner PL. A comparison of pulmonary function test for postthoracotomy pain using cryoanalgesia and transcutaneous nerve stimulation. *Ann Thorac Surg* 1986; 41:204–207.

CHAPTER 29

Epidural Steroids and Facet Injections

Norma J. G. Sandrock and Carol A. Warfield

EPIDURAL STEROIDS

One of the therapeutic options uniquely available to the anesthesiologist in the management of low back pain caused by nerve root compression is the use of epidural injections of corticosteroids. In 1957, Lievre and colleagues[1] reported a 66 percent success rate treating sciatica with epidural hydrocortisone. Brown[2] and Goebert and associates[3] were among the first in the United States to report the use of epidural steroids in the treatment of low back pain and sciatica; this technique has become one of the frequently used conservative options in the management of acute and chronic low back pain.

The natural history of diskogenic low back pain treated with other forms of conservative therapy, such as bed rest[4] and bed rest followed by back support with a brace,[5] generally is encouraging; 68 percent to 82 percent of patients have mild or no pain after 34 to 156 months of follow-up. Only 7 percent to 12 percent of patients eventually undergo laminectomy. Hakelius[6] examined the long-term results of laminectomy for sciatica and compared 166 patients undergoing surgery with 417 patients treated with bed rest and a back brace for up to 2 months; 97 percent of the surgical patients had good results at 1 month compared with 76 percent of the conservatively treated group. However, at 6 months, the results were not significantly different (99 percent versus 93 percent, respectively).

Mechanism of Action

In 1961, Coomes[7] demonstrated that caudal injections of local anesthetic alone—a therapy in use since the turn of the century—could significantly decrease the time to recovery (11 days versus 31 days of bed rest) without any correlation with the duration of symptoms preceding treatment. Several reports suggest that the mechanism of action of epidural anesthetic alone in the treatment of low back pain and sciatica may involve breaking a pain–spasm cycle or reverberating cycle of nociceptive neuronal transmission.[8] Alternatively, the transient analgesia associated with the anesthetic effect may allow a freer range of motion and thereby alter adhesions interfering with the mobility of the dural sleeve of the nerve root. Anesthetics also produce

muscle relaxation, thus allowing proper realignment of facet joints. There also may be some benefit from anesthetic block for the reflex sympathetic dystrophy present in approximately 10 percent of cases.[9,10]

However, many studies show that patients respond better to injections of steroids plus anesthetic than to anesthetic alone.[11–14] Most responders (96 percent) improved within 6 days after epidural steroid injection compared with 11 days for local anesthetic alone and 1 to 4 weeks for bed rest. It is believed that the mechanism of improvement is based on the direct action of the steroid in suppressing both the early (edema, fibrin deposit, capillary dilatation, leukocyte migration, and phagocytic activity) and late (capillary and fibroblast proliferation, deposition of collagen, and cicatrization) inflammatory changes in the nerve root. (Such inflammation is typical and can be seen myelographically, visually at operation, and histologically in biopsy specimens.) Green[15] examined the use of systemic steroids (64 mg of intramuscular dexamethasone tapered over 7 days) in the symptomatic treatment of lumbar disk disease; pain relief occurred in 80 percent of patients. Although symptoms tended to return after the dose was tapered, in most cases, the pain was not as severe as before treatment began. He concluded that inflammation of the nerve root is the origin of the radicular symptoms associated with herniated disks. The theoretic advantage of injection directly into the epidural space compared with systemic administration is our ability to use a much smaller dose with less risk of side effects and longer duration of relief.

The volume of the solution injected has been thought to contribute to the breakdown of adhesions—volumes as large as 120 ml have been injected with this purpose in mind.[16,17] These are potentially dangerous, however, and there is no demonstrated advantage of large volumes over a smaller volume[18] because 6- to 10-ml volumes are more than adequate to ensure spread over several spinal segments.[19]

Indications

Epidural steroid injections are used widely to treat diskogenic disease and spinal stenosis.[20] White and associates[21] conducted a prospective study to determine their efficacy in relation to the diagnosis of low back pain; their results are summarized in Table 29-1. All types of back pain showed a good initial response to epidural steroids. The best long-term results were found in those syndromes in which either nerve root irritation was demonstrable or the natural history was favorable (in which cases the patients studied had not responded to traditional conservative therapies). In addition to the effect of diagnosis in relation to predicting success of therapy, they also noticed higher success rates in patients without psychological overlay and better long-term success in patients with acute (less than 2 weeks' duration) rather than chronic pain.

Warfield and Crews[22] examined 187 patients who underwent lumbar epidural steroid injection, 85 of whom had been told that they would require lumbar surgery. After 1 to 3 years' follow-up, only 34 patients actually required surgery or chymopapain nucleolysis. All patients who improved even transiently after epidural steroid injection improved after chymopapain; 54 of those who did not improve after steroid injection also were unimproved after chemonucleolysis. There was no statistically significant correlation, however, between response to epidural steroids and open surgical outcome. In addition, 161 of these patients were studied retrospectively for any relationship between work status and response to injection.[23] It was found that 68 percent of patients with nonwork-related injuries had favorable outcomes after epidural steroids; only 52 percent of patients whose injuries were work related responded ($P = 0.046$). Epidural steroid injection also has been used suc-

cessfully to treat cervical radiculopathy,[24,25] but the proximity of the spinal cord increases the risk of complications.[26–28]

Efficacy (Table 29-2)

Fifteen studies summarized by Miller and colleagues[29] reported significant or complete relief of pain in 39 percent to 95 percent of patients (mean, 62 percent). A somewhat decreased efficacy in postsurgical patients was observed; this presumably is caused by the prevention of contact between the steroid and the affected root as a result of scar tissue. Five prospective well-controlled studies reviewed by Benzon[30] had success rates ranging from 25 percent to 75 percent; the study with the lowest incidence of successful outcome used a significantly different treatment protocol from the others (the steroid was injected in its undiluted volume of only 2 ml. Benzon also examined reported success rates in relation to the duration of back pain and the cause of the pain, finding success rates of 83 percent to 100 percent of patients when the back pain was present for 3 months or less, 67 percent to 81 percent when the back pain was present for 6 months or less, 69 percent for pain of less than 1 year's duration, and 46 percent for pain of more than 1 year's duration. Longer duration of relief also was associated with earlier treatment.

Dilke and associates,[31] in a prospective randomized double-blind study of 100 consecutive patients with unilateral sciatica from lumbar disk disease who had not undergone previous back surgery, found highly significant differences with respect to both relief of pain and resumption of work. In total, 46 percent of patients who received 80 mg methylprednisolone in 10 ml of normal saline had pain relief, and 92 percent had returned to work after 3 months. Moreover, these patients had a statistically highly significant decrease in analgesic requirements during the rehabilitation period. The control group received injections of 1 ml of normal saline into the interspinous ligament. It was found that 11 percent of these patients had pain relief, and 60 percent returned to work. All patients in the study underwent a program of graded rehabilitation including hydrotherapy, postural exercise classes, and spinal mobilizing exercises, and all patients received diazepam 2 mg three times daily.

Breivik and colleagues[32] studied 35 patients with incapacitating chronic low back pain and sciatica, including 11 patients who had undergone previous back surgery. Each patient was given up to three caudal epidural injections at weekly intervals consisting of either 20 ml of bupivacaine 0.25% with 80 mg of depot methylprednisolone, or 20 ml of bupivacaine 0.25% followed by 100 ml of saline. These authors found 56 percent of the steroid group had considerable pain relief; two-thirds of these patients also had objective neurologic signs of improvement. However, only 26 percent of the saline group had pain relief; all these patients had objective neurologic signs of improvement.

Table 29-1
Effectiveness of a Single Epidural Steroid Injection with Respect to Diagnosis of Back Pain in 304 Patients*

Diagnosis	1 Day	2 Mo	6 Mo
Anulus tear ("back sprain")[†]	+ + + +	+ + +	+ +
Chronic lumbar degenerative disk disease[†]	+ + + +	+ + +	+
Central HNP[†]	+ + + + +	+ +	+
HNP with nerve root irritation[‡]	+ + + + +	+ + + +	+ +
HNP with neurologic deficit	+ + + + +	+ + +	+ +
Spondylolysis	+ + + + +	+ + +	0
Spondylolisthesis	+ + + + +	+ + +	0
Spinal stenosis	+ + + + +	+ + +	+
Postoperative	+ + + + +	+ +	+
Psychological	+ + + + +	0	0
Cancer	+ + + + +	+	0

*Most patients' clinical diagnoses were confirmed by x-ray, EMG, myelogram, epidural venogram, and/or surgery.
[†]No neurologic deficits; straight leg raising, negative results.
[‡]No neurologic deficits; straight leg raising, positive results.
Table derived from results of White and colleagues.[21]

Table 29-2
Percentage of Patients with Relief from Epidural Steroids

Reference	No. of Patients	Control (%)	Steroid				Criteria
			Acute Pain (%)	Chronic Pain (%)	Post-surgical (%)	Overall (%)	
Coomes[7]	40	25*				60	1,2,4
Goebert et al[38]	113				76	72	2
Davidson and Robin[17]		28†			33	14	1,2
Swerdlow and Sayle-Creer[13]	61	57‡	72	67		69	2
Cho[34]	16		83		89		3,5
Warr et al[35]	500					63	2
Winnie et al[9]	20					90	2
Dilke et al[31]	100	60*				92	4
		14*				53	2
		8*				48	6
Breivik[32]	35	25‡				63	1,2
Snoek et al[33]	27	42†				67	5
Arnhoff et al[36]	151					58	5
Brown[37]	56		100	23	15	40	1,2
Heyse-Moore[18]	120		81	45	28	62	1,2

*Bed rest.
†Saline alone.
‡Local anesthetic alone.
Criteria code: (1) improvement in physical examination, (2) improvement in or relief of pain, (3) improvement in straight leg raising, (4) resumption of work, (5) subjective improvement, (6) pain relief obtainable with analgesics.

Of the 14 patients in this group who had no pain relief, 11 subsequently received bupivacaine and steroid caudal injections, with a 73 percent symptomatic response rate. In addition, 63 percent of patients with arachnoiditis after previous disk surgery experienced relief after caudal epidural steroid injection; none of these patients received any benefit from the bupivacaine and saline injection (see Table 29-2).

Klenerman and colleagues[39] reported similar results in patients with unilateral sciatica of less than 6 months' duration who were treated with epidural saline, local anesthetic, steroid, or dry needling.

Cuckler and associates[40] undertook a prospective randomized double-blind study of 73 patients with lumbar radiculopathy and radiographic confirmation of lumbar nerve root compression. Forty-one patients received an epidural injection of 80 mg of methylprednisolone acetate with 5 ml of procaine 1% (total volume, 7 ml) at the L3–4 interspace; the rest received similar injections consisting of 2 ml of saline with 5 ml of procaine. All patients who did not show at least a 50 percent improvement within 24 h of initial injection were given a second injection of steroid and procaine in a nonblinded manner and were designated as having had a failed result. In 61 percent of the patients whose first injec-

tion included the steroid, some degree of improvement occurred. It was found that 20 of 32 (62.5 percent) in the local anesthetic group (including 18 patients who underwent a second injection in 24 h that contained steroid) were improved. Several issues were debated after this report,[41–44] namely, initial assessment at only 24 h (it is well accepted that symptoms may increase during the first 1 to 2 days after injection and that relief of pain may take several days), choice of local anesthetic as a "placebo," and performance of all injections at the same interspace rather than at the level of the involved nerve roots. Nevertheless, this study did show a success rate considerably higher than the expected placebo response, generally considered to be 36 percent.

In 1988, Rosen and colleagues[45] reported an overall efficacy of 50 percent in patients with spinal stenosis or herniated lumbar disk, but the results were temporary. Only 24 percent obtained long-term relief.

Sagar and coworkers,[46] in their study of 107 patients, found that patients younger than 40 years of age with acute symptoms were most responsive to epidural steroid injection.

In summary, five factors seem most important in influencing the outcome of epidural steroid injection as follows: (1) accuracy of diagnosis of root inflammation, (2) duration of symptoms, (3) previous surgery,[47] (4) age, and (5) location of injection (should be made at the level of the affected nerve root).[9]

Technique

Our protocol for the use of epidural steroids begins after complete orthopedic and neurologic evaluation. Nonsteroidal anti-inflammatory drugs that inhibit platelet aggregation are discontinued by some clinicians for an appropriate number of days before the procedure unless there is a medical contraindication for doing so (e.g., aspirin taken by a patient with carotid artery disease). Because many patients with radiculopathy require these agents for pain relief, the risks and benefits of the proposed procedure without discontinuing the drug must be weighed carefully against the risk of discontinuing it; such conversations may include both the patient and the primary care physician. More recently, evidence suggests that these agents need not be discontinued because the risk of epidural hematoma after these injections is similar to the incidence of spontaneous epidural hematoma.[48,49] A similar dilemma is presented by the patient who is chronically systemically anticoagulated; again, management must be coordinated carefully with the patient and primary care physician. If the decision is made to proceed, for example, the patient may be admitted to the hospital several days before the procedure for discontinuation of warfarin while anticoagulation is maintained with intravenous heparin. The latter may be temporarily stopped for several hours during the time the procedure is done. Absolute contraindications are the same as those for any epidural injection (such as preexisting infection at the injection site). These are familiar to the anesthesiologist.

The patient usually is fasted for a minimum of 6 h before the procedure if local anesthetic is included in the injection, and informed consent is obtained, including a discussion of a written information sheet given to every patient (Fig. 29-1). Intravenous access is established if appropriate, and the blood pressure is monitored. The injection is done at the level of the affected nerve roots (Table 29-3) with the patient in the lateral decubitus position with the painful side down to take advantage of the effect of gravity in assisting spread of the steroids to the affected roots. (This position is maintained for 15 min after the injection.) Standard sterile precautions are observed, and local anesthesia of the injection site is obtained by infiltration. A 17- to 20-gauge Tuohy or other needle is used, and the standard technique of loss of resistance (to air or saline, depending on the preference of the operator) is used. Then 50 to 80 mg of a depot formulation of triamcinolone diacetate in 5 to 10 ml of lidocaine 1% without epinephrine or saline is injected slowly, although higher doses have been used. (In general, 5 ml of solution at the L4–5 spreads from L1 to S5, but scarring may inhibit the spread.) It is not unusual for the patient to experience mild discomfort (not a frank paresthe-

sia) during injection as the solution bathes the irritated nerve roots, especially with rapid injection. This is a useful sign for successful placement of the steroid. The needle is cleared of the steroid by flushing with an additional 1 ml of lidocaine or saline before it is removed to avoid leaving a so-called steroid track to the skin, thereby (theoretically), allowing nonhealing of the track with subsequent risk of infection.[50] If a dural tap is obtained, the needle is removed and replaced at the same interspace, and the injection is done only after negative aspiration tests, using saline instead of lidocaine as the diluent for the steroid. (This precaution is taken to avoid the possibility of local anesthetic leakage into the intrathecal space with resultant high spinal effect. Alternatively, some clinicians may choose to minimize this risk by injecting the steroid–local anesthetic mixture at a different interspace from the one at which the tap was obtained, but this may diminish the effect of the steroid.)

The presence or absence of segmental anesthesia resulting from the epidural injection of local anesthetic is determined, and the patient is discharged home (with an escort) after the local anesthetic effect has worn off. Lack of hypesthesia in the affected area after the injection may suggest technical failure because the local anesthetic–steroid mixture might not have been in the epidural space.

The patient returns for follow-up 2 to 3 weeks after the initial injection, which can be repeated up to three times in a 6-month period if there is improvement with a plateau of symptoms or subsequent recurrence of symptoms (Fig. 29-2). If there is no improvement, the procedure is not repeated unless there was some question of technical failure. More than three injections do not provide further improvement.[35] Repeat injections are done using the same technique as described for the initial injection. Some centers advocate a series of three injections at 2-week intervals, regardless of the patient's response.[13,19,32,35] The 2-week interval allows adequate time for the steroid to have an effect and minimizes the potential adverse effects of repeated doses.

Other centers use different local anesthetics and steroid preparations from the ones described. Although the mechanism of pain relief by epidural injection of local anesthetics may suggest a theoretic advantage of a longer-acting agent, this has not been studied. Our choice of lidocaine, therefore, is based on two advantages: decreased time to recovery (and discharge home) in our outpatient population and minimum duration of action in the rare event of an anesthetic-related complication. Hydrocortisone, methylprednisolone acetate, and triamcinolone all have been injected safely into the epidural space, although many preparations contain preservatives. Given intrathecally, methylprednisolone and hydrocortisone have caused meningitis,[51,52] which can be followed by arachnoiditis and even permanent paralysis.[53–55] Bernat and colleagues[54] reported postmortem pathologic evidence that depot methylprednisolone acetate is necrotizing to meningeal tissues. However, Cicala and associates[56] recently reported no inflammatory changes

BETH ISRAEL HOSPITAL PAIN MANAGEMENT CENTER

INFORMATION REGARDING EPIDURAL STEROID INJECTION

Epidural steroid injection has recently been found to be an effective treatment for some patients who are suffering from low back pain or leg pain due to nerve impingement. Commonly, nerves which supply the back or legs are compressed near the spine either by a bulging disk, a bone spur, or scar tissue. This causes the nerve to become irritated, inflamed, and swollen, and the more swollen it becomes, the bigger target it is for whatever is pushing against it. Cortisone is a powerful anti-inflammatory, and its action therefore is to decrease the swelling and inflammation in this nerve—thereby breaking this vicious cycle of swelling and irritation.

Before performing the injection an examination is performed and an intravenous line may be placed in order to provide you with extra fluid and medication, if necessary. You will feel a small pin stick as a local anesthetic is administered to freeze the skin and tissues in your back where the injection takes place. The injection is then performed with little discomfort and the entire procedure takes only 5 or 10 min. After the injection, some patients feel a warmth or numbness in their legs for about 1 h from the effects of the local anesthetic, and for this reason we keep you in our recovery area for a period of observation. You are then free to go home and go about your normal activities, although you should not drive for the remainder of the day since it is possible to have some residual weakness in your legs for a few hours. Relief from the injection generally takes about 3 days although some patients feel relief immediately and others do not feel relief up to 1 week or so. During the first few days after the injection, it is common to feel *increased* back discomfort from the effect of the needle having been placed. Side effects such as headaches occur in less than 1 percent of patients. More serious complications can occur, but they are exceedingly rare. As you may have heard, cortisone itself is sometimes associated with other side effects such as a puffy face, brittle bones, etc. These problems typically occur in patients who are taking cortisone by mouth daily for long periods of time. These problems are very unusual with a single dose of cortisone or with doses widely spaced in time.

In our experience, about 70 percent of patients who have not had previous back surgery obtain relief from epidural steroid injections. For patients who have had previous back surgery, the effectiveness is somewhat less. Many patients obtain permanent relief after one injection, but others find that their pain plateaus or that their pain recurs weeks, months, or years later. It is only in this second group of patients that we repeat the injection. Injections generally are spaced in at least 2-week intervals, and it is rare to receive more than three injections in a 6-month period. Still another group of patients are those who obtain no substantial relief from the injection. Under these circumstances, we do not repeat the injection.

In preparation for your epidural injection we ask that you not eat or drink for 6 h prior and that you arrange for transportation home with a responsible escort since you should not drive until the next day. You can expect to be at the hospital about 1 h.

If you have any further questions, we shall be happy to answer them for you.

BETH ISRAEL HOSPITAL
Pain Management Center
(617) 735-3334

FIGURE 29-1. Patient information on epidural steroids.

Table 29-3
Lumbar Disk Syndromes

Location	Root	Frequency (%)	Reflex	Motor Deficit	Sensory Deficit
L5–S1	S1	50	Ankle jerk	Plantar flexion	Posterolateral leg, lateral foot
L4–L5	L5	40	? Posterior tibial	Dorsiflexion foot, eversion foot, extension toe	Anterolateral leg, dorsum foot, big toe
L3–L4	L4	5	Knee jerk	Quadriceps (slight)	Antero- and posterolateral thigh, anteromedial leg and shin

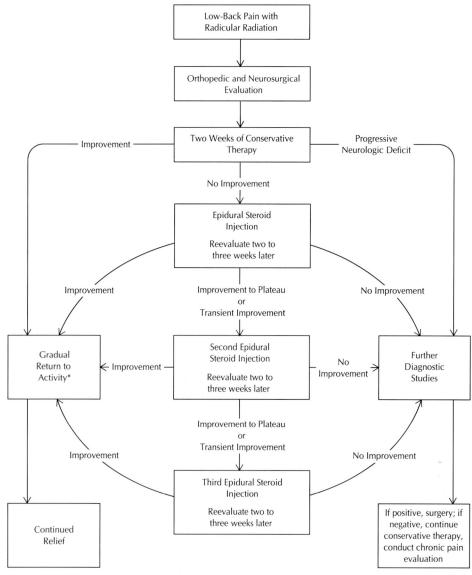

*With recurrence, perform epidural steroid injection, but no more than three in a six-month period.

FIGURE 29-2. Beth Israel Hospital Pain Unit Protocol for Epidural Steroids

after injection of methylprednisolone acetate into the epidural space of rabbits. Animal studies[57] show only minor effects of triamcinolone on the nerves and meninges at the light and electron microscopic levels. Triamcinolone also is more miscible with the local anesthetic or saline solution than methylprednisolone acetate, resulting in less precipitation of the steroid during slow injection and ensuring more reliable distribution of medication. Because of these reports and the reported incidence of delayed hypersensitivity[58] to myristyl-γ-picolinium chloride (a component of some of the available depot preparations), we have adopted triamcinolone as our preparation of choice for administration in the epidural space. None of these preparations is indicated for use in the epidural space; however, after scientific reports of their safe use in hundreds of patients, it has become standard practice to use them in this way. (Lack of explicit Food and Drug Administration approval does not preclude the use

of a drug for other than its original indication; the medicolegal implications of such use are discussed in Chap. 39). Steroids usually are not administered intrathecally for the following reasons: (1) root compression in diskogenic disease is extradural, (2) intrathecal injection is more painful, (3) the undiluted steroid vehicle (specifically, the glycol) may cause neural damage given intrathecally,[54,59] (4) Nelson and colleagues[60] reported adhesive arachnoiditis after intrathecal steroid injection, presumably from the polyethylene glycol in the steroid preparation (no currently marketed steroid preparation is free of both glycols and bacteriostatic agents), (5) in general, complications from intrathecal injection of steroids are not only more numerous but also graver compared with epidural injection,[30,51,61] and (6) the intrathecal route is not more efficacious.[9,51] The caudal route of injection also has been used, but the larger volume required necessitates further dilution of the steroid.[62]

In 1986, Cohn and coworkers,[63] in an uncontrolled study, reported 6 to 24 months of relief in patients receiving epidural injections of methylprednisolone and morphine. Later double-blind studies[64,65] indicated that steroid in combination with morphine was no more effective than steroid alone. In addition, the combination was associated with a higher incidence of respiratory depression than morphine alone, perhaps as a result of an enhanced dural uptake of morphine by the steroid. This practice therefore is not recommended.

Complications

Complications of epidural steroid injection fortunately are rare; the most commonly seen are those associated with any epidural anesthetic. These are familiar to the anesthesiologist, namely, dural puncture, high spinal, intravascular injection, and hypotension from sympathetic blockade. It has been our observation that the incidence of dural tap is slightly higher than the generally accepted 0.5 percent rate.[66] This is not surprising considering the population under treatment and the high anticipated incidence of adhesions of the epidural space, particularly postlaminectomy. However, it is our experience that this population seems to suffer postspinal headache after accidental dural puncture less frequently than generally seen, possibly because adhesions close the potential epidural space leaving no room for leakage of cerebrospinal fluid. Severe headache after epidural steroid injection may be caused by injection of air into the subarachnoid or subdural space.[67]

Complications specific to the epidural injection of steroids for the treatment of low back pain and sciatica include the not uncommon exacerbation of symptoms for the first 24 to 48 h after the injection, presumably caused by mechanical irritation of the inflamed roots. Systemic steroid effects are rare,[68–71] although plasma cortisol suppression by epidural steroids has been observed to last up to 3 weeks after injection.[72] Gorski and colleagues[69,73] examined the adrenal response to stress after epidural steroid injection in dogs and found impairment for 4 weeks after injection with return to normal function at 5 weeks. These data suggest the administration of exogenous steroids during the perioperative period in any patient undergoing surgery within 5 weeks of an epidural steroid injection.

Rare complications that have occurred include fulminant bacterial meningitis,[74,75] Cushing syndrome,[76] epidural abscess,[77–79] and intraocular hemorrhage.[16] We have seen a single case of anaphylactoid reaction after epidural steroid injection, and there has been one other case reported in the literature.[80]

FACET INJECTIONS

The injection of steroid and local anesthetic into the vertebral facet joints is a treatment with a much shorter history than that of epidural steroid injections. As recently as 1963,

Hirsch and coworkers[81] first showed that the facet joint could be a source of low back pain. Rees[82] introduced surgical denervation of these joints to treat back pain in 1971, and the percutaneous denervation of these joints was described first by Shealy[83] in 1975.

The clinical presentation of facet syndrome is variable, and it is often a diagnosis of exclusion. However, there are several findings commonly associated with it as follows: (1) tenderness localized over one or more facet joints, (2) exacerbation of pain with any sustained posture, (3) exacerbation of pain with hyperextension, (4) loss of lumbar lordosis, (5) pain localized to the back with absence of neurologic deficits and with negative straight leg raising, and (6) roentgenologic evidence of degenerative disease of the facet joints (Fig. 29-3).

The pain of the facet syndrome usually is limited to the lower back, but it may refer to the buttocks and posterolateral thighs. It rarely radiates to the lower leg. Facet syndrome may coexist with degenerative disk disease, in which the normal articular mechanics are disrupted. A patient therefore may have symptoms and signs of both nerve root irritation and facet disease. The diagnosis is confirmed by pain relief after injection of a local anesthetic into the joint.

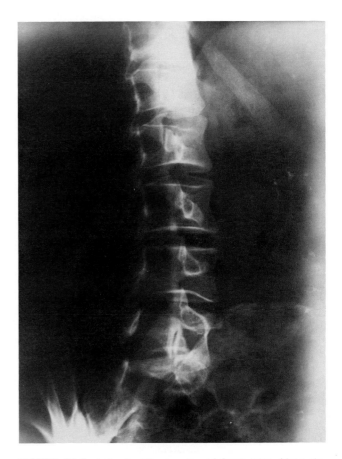

FIGURE 29-3. *Lateral oblique x-ray of facet joint. Note degenerative changes at the L5–S1 facet joint.*

Mechanism of Action

Intraarticular injections of corticosteroids decrease the pain associated with facet syndrome, presumably by reducing inflammation of the joint's small synovial villi (which may become trapped and inflamed, producing pain). Inclusion of local anesthetics in the injection breaks the pain–spasm cycle discussed and also is a diagnostic measure. If 1 to 2 ml of lidocaine 1% injected into the joint produces rapid elimination of pain, the joint itself is likely to be the origin of pain.

Efficacy

Early experience by Destouet and associates[84] and Carrera[85] showed the efficacy of intraarticular steroid and local anesthetic facet injections. In their series of 20 patients, Lewinnek and Warfield[86] found at least a temporary response to injection in 15 patients (75 percent) and lasting relief in 6. (These patients were enrolled in the series after a screening examination for other causes of back pain or sciatica gave negative results, radiologic examination showed degenerative disease in the facet joints, and tenderness was localized over one or more facet joints.) Various factors were examined for a correlation with the response to therapy (Table 29-4). Radiographically demonstrable degenerative disease of the facet joint and pain (which wakes the patient from sleep) were found to correlate most closely with the response to injection. These results were interpreted to suggest that these findings and symptoms might indicate increased severity of facet disease. In his review, Boas[87] cited comparable success rates with both steroid and neurolytic injection in his center and others.

The 1988 Volvo award in clinical sciences was presented

Table 29-4
Correlation of Various Factors with Response to Injection

Characteristic		Percentage of Patients Responding to Injection			
		Initially		*At 3 Mo*	
Facet joint disease on x-ray	+	13/14 (93%)		5/12 (42%)	
	−	0/3 (0%)	P = 0.006	0/3 (0%)	P = 0.26
	Questionable	1/1		0/1	
	N/A	1/2		1/2	
Wakes from sleep	+	7/7 (100%)		4/5 (80%)	
	−	8/13 (62%)	P = 0.08	2/13 (15%)	P = 0.02
Acute onset	+	10/15 (67%)			
	−	5/5 (100%)	P = 0.19	0/5 (0%)	P = 0.23
Pain below knee	+	8/12 (67%)		3/1 (27%)	
	−	7/8 (88%)	P = 0.31	3/7 (43%)	P = 0.43
Sitting increases pain	+	7/8 (88%)		2/7 (29%)	
	−	5/9 (56%)	P = 0.18	1/8 (12%)	P = 0.45
	N/A	3/3		3/3	
Time-dependent positional distress	+	11/13 (85%)		5/12 (42%)	
	−	4/7 (57%)	P = 0.21	1/6 (18%)	P = 0.31
Nonsteroidal anti-inflammatory drug helped	+	3/4 (75%)		2/4 (50%)	
	—	11/14 (79%)	P = 0.67	6/12 (50%)	P = 0.72
	N/A	2		2	
Pain on extension	+	11/12 (92%)		3/1 (27%)	
	−	4/8 (50%)	P = 0.58	3/8 (38%)	P = 0.56
Straight leg raising	+	4/7 (57%)		1/6 (17%)	
	−	10/12 (83%)	P = 0.24	5/11 (45%)	P = 0.26
	N/A	1/1		0/1	

+, characteristic present; −, characteristic absent; N/A, data not available.
Reproduced with permission from Lewinnek GE, Warfield CA. Facet joint degeneration as a cause of low back pain. *Clin Orthop* 1986; 213:216–222.

to Jackson and colleagues[88] for their prospective study on the efficacy of facet injections in 454 patients. They found that factors correlating significantly with more postinjection pain relief were older age; normal gait; history of low back pain; maximum pain on extension; and the absence of leg pain, muscle spasm, and aggravation of pain during a Valsalva maneuver. They added that the facet joints were not the single or primary source of back pain in most patients studied. Lilius and coworkers[89] randomized 109 patients into three groups. One group received cortisone and local anesthetic into two facet joints; the second, the same mixture around two facet joints; and the third, saline into two facet joints. A significant improvement was observed in all groups initially and persisted in 36 percent. Lynch and Taylor,[90] however, studied 50 patients receiving intraarticular and extraarticular facet injections and found that only the intraarticular injections were effective.

A 1990 study suggested that the outcome after facet joint injection could be determined best by evaluating the patient's psychosocial state and motivation for recovery preinjection.[91]

In their 1991 publication in the *New England Journal of Medicine*, Carette and colleagues[92] reported the results of a study in which they injected the L4–5 and L5–S1 facets of all patients who presented to their clinic with low back pain. Those who claimed relief were assigned randomly to receive steroid or saline facet injections. Forty-two percent of the steroid group and 33 percent of the saline group reported marked improvement after 1 month and similarly, after 3 months. At 6 months, the steroid group reported more improvement, less pain, and less physical disability.

Facet injections also have been used successfully in the cervical area,[93] both diagnostically and therapeutically.[94]

Technique (See Appendix A.VI)

The block is done under standard sterile conditions with the patient lying prone and the back slightly flexed over pillows. Intravenous access is established, and the pulse and blood pressure are monitored. Perioperative sedation is minimized so that the patient can communicate continued presence and/or relief of pain. Local anesthesia is obtained by infiltration of the skin over the appropriate levels, approximately 5 to 8 cm lateral to the midline. Under fluoroscopic guidance,[95] a 22-gauge 3.5-in spinal needle is advanced directly into the joint, and 1 to 2 ml of lidocaine 1% is injected. If this produces pain relief, 10 to 20 mg of triamcinolone acetate is injected, and the needle is removed. (A slightly larger volume is used at the L5–S1 joint.) CT guidance also has been advocated.[96]

This procedure is repeated on up to three occasions if pain recurs. If long-term relief is unobtainable after this series of injections, then intraarticular phenol injection or facet denervation (either surgical or percutaneous with radiofrequency or cryoprobe) may be considered. Because each facet joint is innervated by two branches of the posterior primary ramus of the spinal nerves and therefore receives innervation from two levels (Fig. 29-4), denervation must be done both at the affected level and at the level just above. Shealy[97] treated 235 patients with primary low back pain using radiofrequency denervation of the facet joints; 82 percent obtained significant benefit, although the subset of patients who had previous surgery fared less well (40 percent relief). If the previous surgery included fusion, success rates fell to 29 percent. His review of the results of other surgeons reveals success rates ranging from a low of 30 percent to 40 percent to a high of 80 percent. The most

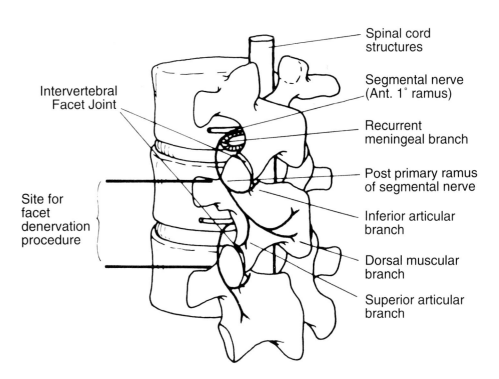

FIGURE 29-4. Segmental innervation of vertebral facet joints. Superior and inferior articular branches from adjacent segmental nerves supply each facet joint. The positions for needle placement to attain denervation at one joint level are shown. (Reproduced with permission from Boas RA. Facet joint injections. In: Stanton-Hicks M, Boas RA, eds. *Chronic Low Back Pain.* New York: Raven Press; 1982:200.

Intervertebral Facet Joint

Site for facet denervation procedure

Spinal cord structures

Segmental nerve (Ant. 1° ramus)

Recurrent meningeal branch

Post primary ramus of segmental nerve

Inferior articular branch

Dorsal muscular branch

Superior articular branch

important factor in prediction of success appeared to be patient selection, especially inclusion or exclusion of patients with previous back surgery. There were no neurologic complications in the more than 800 procedures reviewed.

Complications

Complications associated with injection of the facet joints are rare. Of course, any injection involves the remote risk of infection and/or hematoma formation. Although these events are unusual if standard aseptic precautions are observed, the potential for osteomyelitis of the spine if infection should occur is serious. The anatomic proximity of the facet joint to the nerve roots (and their dural sleeves) and the epidural and radicular vessels may lead to accidental epidural or spinal block or intravascular injection. The small volume of anesthetic used simplifies the management of such events if they occur, but the possibility of motor block should be remembered when allowing the patient to ambulate after the procedure. Rare complications include meningitis after inadvertent dural puncture.[98]

SUMMARY

Both epidural steroid injection and facet injection are useful techniques in the treatment of low back pain.[99] A thorough knowledge of the indications and potential complications involved provides the anesthesiologist with the unique ability to do these procedures safely and effectively.

References

1. Lievre JA, Block-Michel H, Attali P. L'injection transsacree. Etude clinique et radiologique. *Bull Soc Med* 1957; 73:1110–1118.
2. Brown JH. Pressure caudal anesthesia and back manipulation. *Nortwest Med* 1960; 59:905–909.
3. Goebert HW, Jallo SJ, Gardner WJ, Wasmuth CE, Bitte EM. Sciatica: treatment with epidural injections of procaine and hydrocortisone. *Cleve Clin Q* 1960; 27:191–197.
4. Pearce J, Moll JMK. Conservative treatment and natural history of acute lumbar disc lesions. *J Neurol Neurosurg Psychiatry* 1967; 30:13–17.
5. Friedenberg ZB, Shoemaker RC. The results of nonoperative treatment of ruptured lumbar discs. *Am J Surg* 1954; 88:933–935.
6. Hakelius A. Prognosis in sciatica. *Acta Orthop Scand* 1970; 129(suppl):1–76.
7. Coomes EN. A comparison between epidural anaesthesia and bed rest in sciatica. *Br Med J* 1961; 1:20–24.
8. Kirkaldy-Willis WH. Managing Low Back Pain. New York: Churchill Livingstone; 1983:149.
9. Winnie AP, Hartman JT, Meyers HL, Ramamurthy S, Barangan V. Pain Clinic, II: intradural and extradural corticosteroids for sciatica. *Anesth Analg* 1972; 51:990–1003.
10. Kim SI, Sadove MS. Caudal–epidural corticosteroids in

postlaminectomy syndrome: treatment for low back pain. *Compr Ther* 1975; 1:57–60.
11. Beliveau P. A comparison between epidural anesthesia with and without corticosteroid in the treatment of sciatica. *Rheumatol Phys Med* 1971; 11:40–43.
12. Addison RG, Waldstein SA, Benson HT. Relief of back pain following removal of parathyroid adenoma. *Pain* 1979; 7:367–369.
13. Swerdlow M, Sayle-Creer W. A study of extradural medication in the relief of the lumbosciatic syndrome. *Anaesthesia* 1979; 25:341–345.
14. Yates DW. A comparison of the types of epidural injection commonly used in treatment of low back pain and sciatica. *Rheumatol Rehabil* 1978; 17:181–186.
15. Green LN. Dexamethasone in the management of symptoms due to herniated lumbar disc. *J Neurol Neurosurg Psychiatry* 1975; 38:1211–1217.
16. Clark CJ, Whitwell J. Intraocular hemorrhage after epidural injection. *Br Med J* 1961; 2:1612–1613.
17. Davidson JT, Robin GC. Epidural injections in the lumbosciatic syndrome. *Br J Anaesth* 1961; 33:595–598.
18. Heyse-Moore G. A rational approach to use of epidural medication in the treatment of sciatic pain. *Acta Orthop Scand* 1978; 49:366–370.
19. Harley C. Extradural corticosteroid infiltration: a follow-up study of 50 cases. *Ann Phys Med* 1967; 9:22–28.
20. Hoogmartens M, Morelle P. Epidural injection in the treatment of spinal stenosis. *Acta Orthop Belg* 1987; 53(3):409–411.
21. White AH, Derby R, Wynne G. Epidural injections for the diagnosis and treatment of low-back pain. *Spine* 1980; 5:78–86.
22. Warfield CA, Crews DA. Epidural steroid injection as a predictor of surgical outcome. *Surg Gynecol Obstet* May 1987; 164(5):457–458.
23. Warfield CA, Crews DA. Work status and response to epidural steroid injection. *J Occup Med* April 1987; 29(4):315–316.
24. Rowlingson JC, Kirschenbaum LP. Epidural analgesic techniques in the management of cervical pain. *Anesth Analg* September 1984; 65(9):938–942.
25. Cronen MC, Waldman SD. Cervical steroid epidural nerve blocks in the palliation of pain secondary to intractable tension-type headaches. *J Pain Symptom Manage* December 1990; 5(6):379–381.
26. Waldman SD. Cervical epidural abscess after cervical epidural nerve block with steroids. *Anesth Analg* May 1991; 72(5):7172–7178. Letter.
27. William KL, Jackowski A, Evans PJ. Epidural haematoma requiring surgical decompression following repeated cervical epidural steroid injections for chronic pain. *Pain* August 1990; 42(2):197–199.
28. Waldman SD. Complications of cervical epidural nerve blocks with steroids: a prospective study of 790 consecutive blocks. *Reg Anesth* May–June 1989; 14(3):149–151.
29. Miller RD, Munger WL, Powell PE. Chronic pain and local anesthetic neural blockade. In: Cousins MJ, Bridenbaugh PO, eds. *Neural Blockade in Clinical Anesthesia and Management of Pain*. Philadelphia: Lippincott; 1980:628–629.
30. Benzon, HT. Epidural steroid injections for low back pain and lumbosacral radiculopathy. *Pain* 1986; 24:277–295.

31. Dilke TFW, Burry HC, Grahame R. Extradural corticosteroid injection in management of lumbar nerve root compression. *B Med J* 1973; 2:635–637.

32. Breivik H, Hesla PE, Molnar I, Linda B. Treatment of chronic low back pain and sciatica: comparison of caudal epidural injections of bupivacaine and methylprednisolone with bupivacaine followed by saline. *Adv Pain Res Ther* 1976; 1:927–932.

33. Snoek W, Weber H, Jorgensen B. Double blind evaluation of extradural methylprednisolone for herniated lumbar discs. *Acta Orthop Scand* 1977; 48:635–641.

34. Cho KO. Therapeutic epidural block with a combination of a weak local anesthetic and steroids in management of complicated low back pain. *Am Surg* 1970; 36:303–308.

35. Warr AC, Wilkinson JA, Burn JMB, Langdon L. Chronic lumbosciatic syndrome treated by epidural injection and manipulation. *Practitioner* 1972; 209:53–59.

36. Arnhoff FN, Triplett HB, Pokorney B. Follow-up status of patients treated with nerve blocks for low back pain. *Anesthesiology* 1977; 46:170–178.

37. Brown FW. Management of discogenic pain using epidural and intrathecal steroids. *Clin Orthop* 1977; 129:72–78.

38. Goebert HW, Jallo SJ, Gardner WJ, Wasmuth CE. Painful radiculopathy treated with epidural injections of procaine and hydrocortisone acetate. Results in 113 patients. *Anesth Analg* 1961; 40:130–134.

39. Klenerman L, Greenwood R, Davenport HT, White DC, Peskett S. Lumbar epidural injections in the treatment of sciatica. *Br J Rheumatol* February 1984; 23(1):35–38.

40. Cuckler JM, Bernini PA, Wiesel SW, Booth RE, Rothman RH, Pickens GT. The use of epidural steroids in the treatment of lumbar radicular pain: a prospective, randomized, double-blind study. *J Bone Joint Surg* 1985; 67A:63–66.

41. Warfield CA. Correspondence. *J Bone Joint Surg* 1985; 67A:980–981.

42. Sharrock NE. Correspondence. *J Bone Joint Surg* 1985; 67A:981.

43. Simon D, Carron H, Rowlingson J. Correspondence. *J Bone Joint Surg* 1985; 67A:981.

44. Linson MA. Correspondence. *J Bone Joint Surg* 1985; 67A:982.

45. Rosen CD, Kahanovitz N, Bernstein R, Viola K. A retrospective analysis of the efficacy of epidural steroid injections. *Clin Orthop* March 1988; (228):270–272.

46. Sagar JV, Sharma R, Sharma S. Epidural steroid injection in non-specific low backache. *J Indian Med Assoc* September 1989; 87(9)208–209.

47. Anderson KH, Mosdal C. Epidural application of corticosteroids in low back pain and sciatica. *Acta Neurochir (Wien)* 1987; 87(1–2):52–53.

48. Rao LK, El-Etr AA. Anticoagulation following placement of epidural and subarachnoid catheters. *Anesthesiology* 1981; 55:618–620.

49. Waldman SD, Feldstein GS, Waldman HJ, et al. Caudal administration of morphine sulfate in anticoagulated and thrombocytopenia patients. *Anesth Analg* 1987; 66:267–268.

50. Brown FW. Protocol for management of acute low back pain with or without radiculopathy, including the use of epidural and intrathecal steroids. In: Brown FW, ed. *American Academy of Orthopedic Surgeons Symposium on the Lumbar Spine.* St. Louis: Mosby; 1981:126–136.

51. Stratton I. Dangers of intrathecal hydrocortisone sodium succinate. *Med J Aust* 1975; 2:650.

52. Shealy CN. Dangers of spinal injections without proper diagnosis. *JAMA* 1966; 197:1104–1106.

53. Stratton I. Dangers of intrathecal hydrocortisone sodium succinate. *Med J Aust* 1975; 2:650.

54. Bernat JL, Sadowsky CH, Vincent FM. Sclerosing spinal pachymeningitis, a complication of intrathecal administration of DepoMedrol for multiple sclerosis. *J Neurol Neurosurg Psychiatry* 1976; 39:1124–1128.

55. Cohen F. Conus medullaris syndrome following multiple intrathecal corticosteroid injections. *Arch Neurol* 1979; 36:228–230.

56. Cicala RS, Turner R, Moran E, Henley R, Wong R, Evans J. Methylprednisolone acetate does not cause inflammatory changes in the epidural space. *Anesthesiology* March 1990; 72(3):556–558.

57. Delaney TJ, Rowlingson JC, Carron HC, Butler A. Epidural steroid effects on nerves and meninges. *Anesth Analg* 1980; 59:610–614.

58. Mathias CG, Robertson DB. Delayed hypersensitivity to a corticosteroid suspensions containing methylprednisolone. Two cases of conjunctival inflammation after retrobulbar injection. *Arch Dermatol* 1985; 121:258–261.

59. Wood KM, Arguelles J, Norenberg MD. Degenerative lesions in rat sciatic nerves after local injections of methylprednisolone in aqueous solution. *Reg Anaesth* 1980; 5:13–15.

60. Nelson DA, Vates TS, Thomas RB. Complications from intrathecal steroid therapy in patients with multiple sclerosis. *Acta Neurol Scand* 1973; 49:176–188.

61. Nelson DA. Dangers from methylprednisolone acetate therapy by intraspinal injection *Arch Neurol* July 1988; 45(7):804–806. Comments.

62. Bush K, Hillier S. A controlled study of caudal epidural injections of triamcinolone plus procaine for the management of intractable sciatica. *Spine* May 1991; 16(5):572–575.

63. Cohn ML, Huntington CT, Byrd SE, Machado AF, Cohn M. Epidural morphine and methylprednisolone. New therapy for recurrent low-back pain. *Spine* November 1986; 11(9):960–963.

64. Dallas TL, Lin RL, Wu WH, Wolskee P. Epidural morphine and methylprednisolone for low-back pain. *Anesthesiology* September 1987; 67(3):408–411.

65. Rocco AG, Frank E, Kaul AF, Lipson SJ, Gallo JP. Epidural steroids, epidural morphine and epidural steroids combined with morphine in the treatment of postlaminectomy syndrome. *Pain* March 1989; 36(3):297–303.

66. Bromage P. *Epidural Analgesia.* Philadelphia: Saunders; 1978.

67. Katz JA, Lukin R, Bridenbaugh PO, Gunzenhauser L. Subdural intracranial air: an unusual cause of headache after epidural steroid injection. *Anesthesiology* March 1991; 74(3):615–618.

68. Burn JM, Rao TLK, Glisson SN, McDowell D. Epidural triamcinolone and adrenal responses to stress. *Anesthesiology* 1981; 55:A147.

69. Gorski DW, Rao TLK, Glisson SN, McDowell D. Epidural triamcinolone and adrenal responses to stress. *Anesthesiology* 1981; 55:A147.

70. Stambough JL, Booth RE Jr, Rothman RH. Transient hypercorticism after epidural steroid injection. A case report. *J Bone Joint Surg Am* September 1984; 66(7):1115–1116.

71. Tuel SM, Meythaler JM, Cross LL. Cushing's syndrome from epidural methylprednisolone. *Pain* January 1991; 40(1):81–84.

72. Seghal AD, Tweed DC, Gardner WJ, Foote MK. Laboratory studies after intrathecal steroids. *Arch Neurol* 1963; 9:74–78.

73. Gorski DW, Rao TLK, Glisson SN, Chintagada M, El-Etr A. Epidural triamcinolone and adrenal response to hypoglycemic stress in dogs. *Anesthesiology* 1982; 57:364–366.

74. Dougherty JH, Fraser RAR. Complications following intraspinal injections of steroids: reports of two cases. *J Neurosurg* 1978; 48:1023–1025.

75. Gutknecht DR. Chemical meningitis following epidural injections of corticosteroids. *Am J Med* March 1987; 82(3):570. Letter.

76. Knight CL, Burnell JC. Systemic side-effects of extradural steroids. *Anaesthesia* 1980; 35:593–594.

77. Shealy CN. Dangers of spinal injections without proper diagnosis. *JAMA* 1966; 197:1104–1106.

78. Goucke CR, Graziotto P. Extradural abscess following local anesthetic and steroid injection for chronic low back pain. *Br J Anaesth* September 1990; 65(3):427–429.

79. Chan ST, Leung S. Spinal epidural abscess following steroid injection for sciatica. Case report. *Spine* January 1989; 14(1):106–108.

80. Simon DL, Kunz RD, German JD, Zivkovich V. Allergic or pseudoallergic reaction following epidural steroid deposition and skin testing. *Reg Anaesth* September–October 1989; 14(5):253–255.

81. Hirsch C, Inglemark B, Miller M. The anatomical basis for low back pain. *Acta Orthop Scand* 1963; 33:1–17.

82. Rees WES. Multiple bilateral subcutaneous rhizolysis of segmental nerves in the treatment of the inter-vertebral disc syndrome. *Ann Gen Pract* 1971; 26:126–127.

83. Shealy CN. Percutaneous radiofrequency denervation of spinal facets. *J Neurosurg* 1975; 43:448–451.

84. Destouet JM, Gilula LA, Murphy WA, Monsees B. Lumbar facet joint injection: indication, technique, clinical correlation, and preliminary results. *Radiology* November 1982; 145(2):321–325.

85. Carrera GF. Lumbar facet joint injection in low back pain and sciatica: preliminary results. *Radiology* December 1980; 137(3):665–667.

86. Lewinnek GE, Warfield CA. Facet joint degeneration as a cause of low back pain. *Clin Orthop* 1986; 213:216–222.

87. Boas RA. Facet joint injections. In: Stanton Hicks M, Boas RA, eds. *Chronic Low Back Pain*. New York: Raven Press; 1982:199–211.

88. Jackson RP, Jacobs RR, Montesano PX. 1988 Volvo award in clinical sciences. Facet joint injection in low-back pain. A prospective statistical study. *Spine* September 1988; 13(9):966–971.

89. Lilius G, Laasonen EM, Myllynen P, Harilainen A, Gronlund G. Lumbar facet joint syndrome. A randomized clinical trial. *J Bone Joint Surg Br* August 1989; 71(4):681–684.

90. Lynch MC, Taylor JF. Facet joint injection for low back pain. A clinical study. *J Bone Joint Surgery Br* January 1986; 68(1):138–141.

91. Lilius G, Harilainen A, Laasonen EM, Myllynen P. Chronic unilateral low-back pain. Predictors of outcome of facet joint injections. *Spine* August 1990; 15(8):780–782.

92. Carette S, Marcoux S, Truchon R, et al. A controlled trial of corticosteroid injections into facet joints for chronic low back pain. *N Engl J Med* October 3, 1991; 325(14):1002–1007. Comments.

93. Roy DF, Fluery J, Fontaine SB, Dussault RG. Clinical evaluation of cervical facet joint infiltration. *Can Assoc Radiol J* June 1988; 39(2):118–120.

94. Hove B, Gyldensted C. Cervical analgesic facet joint arthrography. *Neuroradiology* 1990; 32(6):456–459.

95. Carrera GF. Lumbar facet joint injection in low back pain and sciatica: description of technique. *Radiology* December 1980; 137(3):661–664.

96. Murtagh FR. Computed tomography and fluoroscopy guided anesthesia and steroid injection in facet syndrome. *Spine* June 1988; 13(6)686–689.

97. Shealy CN. Facet denervation in the management of back and sciatic pain. *Clin Orthop* 1976; 115:157–164.

98. Thomson SJ, Lomax DM, Collett BJ. Chemical meningism after lumbar facet joint block with local anaesthesia and steroids. *Anaesthesia* July 1991; 46(7):563–564.

99. el-Khoury GY, Renfrew DL. Percutaneous procedures for the diagnosis and treatment of lower back pain: diskography, facet-joint injection, and epidural injection. *AJR Am J Roentgenol* October 1991; 157(4):685–691.

CHAPTER 30

Stimulation-Induced Analgesia

Bonnie McLean and H. Elliott Fives

Stimulation-induced analgesia is analgesia produced by stimulation, most commonly in the form of TENS and acupuncture. Electroacupuncture is the use of acupuncture with stimulation of the needles, generally using a battery-generated source of electricity and tiny wires that can be hooked up to the needles.

ACUPUNCTURE (See Chap. 31)

Acupuncture is a traditional form of Oriental medicine that originated approximately 5000 years ago. In Oriental medicine, the focus is on the whole person and the optimal function of the body's self-regulating systems, including the neurophysiological, biochemical, and endocrine systems. Traditionally, the patient was taught meditative and breathing techniques, therapeutic exercises, and proper nutrition. Body work, such as acupressure, massage and herbal therapy, and acupuncture, were administered. The patient's life style, environment, and relationships were considered during the assessment and treatment.

In Oriental medicine, the body basically is seen as an energetic system around which the physical aspects that we perceive with our senses are built. A so-called life force, known as chi, is thought to be found in all living things. This chi circulates throughout the body in a network of orderly pathways called meridians. If this chi or energy is blocked by stresses, such as congenital weakness, physical injury, emotional or mental experiences, illnesses, or abuses of the body (excessive intake of drugs or alcohol, improper nutrition, and lack of exercise), an imbalance of energy will be manifested by pain and disease. Acupuncture is believed to stimulate the body to heal itself. This is accomplished by the manipulation of specific points along these energy meridians with the purpose of releasing the blocks in the meridians and strengthening and balancing the energy body of the patient. The acupuncture points can be stimulated by heat and cold, pressure (acupressure), electricity (electrotherapy), ultrasound (sonopuncture), and even lasers (laserpuncture) to achieve therapeutic results. The most common and well-known method of stimulation is with the insertion of tiny needles to a depth of a few millimeters. The needles usually are left in place 20 to 40 min. The insertion of the needle feels like a small prick, followed by an ache, tingle, throb, numbness, warmth, or

heaviness around the area. The number of treatments varies according to the patient and the type, chronicity, and seriousness of the problem. Because acupuncture tends to be cumulative,[1] an average course of treatment before significant results occur may be two to three times a week for 3 to 6 weeks.

After 2500 years of popular use in China, acupuncture declined in the 19th century as a result of Western influences and the degeneration of Chinese culture. Mao Zedong encouraged the practice of acupuncture, however, and it is enjoying a renaissance in China, Japan, Europe, North America, Russia, and Australia. There are more than 1 million acupuncturists in practice worldwide. The World Health Organization of the United Nations has indicated that Oriental medicine is effective in treating many common diseases and a large number of difficult degenerative diseases. In the United States, the most common syndromes treated by acupuncture include musculoskeletal and vascular headaches, backache,[2] and other pain syndromes; osteoarthritis; asthma; gastrointestinal disorders; and menstrual problems. It also is used as an adjunctive treatment in the management of chronic stress, obesity, depression,[3] insomnia, withdrawal from addictive substances, and immune dysfunction.[4]

The physiologic basis of acupuncture's effectiveness currently is understood poorly by Western science, although it is known to produce such neurophysiologic and biochemical effects as changes in the heart rate, blood pressure, brain activity, blood chemistry, endocrine function, intestinal activity, and immunologic reactions.[5] The analgesic and sedating effects of acupuncture may be related to the release of endorphins and enkephalins from the brainstem and pituitary gland.[6] The most important confirmation by Western science of this healing technique comes through modern research in energetic physics, bioelectricity, and psychoneuroimmunology.[4]

The following mechanism currently is postulated. Low frequency (4 Hz) electrical stimulation activates the sensory receptors in deep muscle that cause the midbrain to release enkephalins. These enkephalins then activate the raphe nucleus and/or the reticular magnocellular nucleus, which sends descending signals along the dorsolateral funiculus to the spinal cord and inhibits the primary afferent fibers concerned with pain transmission (substance P-containing high threshold A delta and C fibers and Groups III and IV tissue nociceptive fibers). The neurotransmitters serotonin and norepinephrine may play important roles in facilitating this mechanism. Low frequency electrical activation is thought to stimulate the release of β-endorphins from the hypothalamus and β-endorphins and corticotropin from the pituitary. These endorphins then could be released into the systemic circulation, cross the blood–brain barrier, and bind to opiate receptors, causing generalized analgesia. Corticotropin could stimulate the release of cortisol and reduce inflammation. Low frequency electrical activation also may stimulate segmental release of endorphins from the spinal cord interneurons that bind to the opiate receptors in the pain-transmission cells, producing localized analgesia. High frequency (200 Hz) electrical activation is thought to stimulate sensory nerves and the serotonin/norepinephrine descending inhibitory systems and thus induce regional analgesia.[7] The insertion of an acupuncture needle also has a physical effect on the local area into which it is placed. As part of an evolutionary survival mechanism, in which the body attempts to expel, neutralize, or destroy anything foreign, a complex mechanism is set into motion by the insertion of an acupuncture needle. The body mounts an immune response; there is increased blood flow into the area and reduction of the muscular or tissue tension to aid the body in working the object out of the body. This reaction has a therapeutic effect on generalized muscle spasm and trigger points (Fig. 30-1).

Many acupuncture points correspond to motor points. The acupuncture points on the arms and legs usually lie on lines that follow major nerves and blood vessels. The points on the trunk are found at segmental innervation levels where nerves and blood vessels penetrate muscle fascia. On the face and head, they lie near the cranial nerves and blood vessels. Lymphatic vessels also often are present at these locations. On the auricle, there appears to be a relationship between the acupuncture points and the cranial nerves and blood vessels.[8] Acupuncture points may have greater concentrations of pain fibers and vascular structures that explain the enhanced sensitivity and reactivity of these sites.[9]

Several studies have attempted to prove the efficacy of acupuncture in the treatment of chronic pain, but meta-

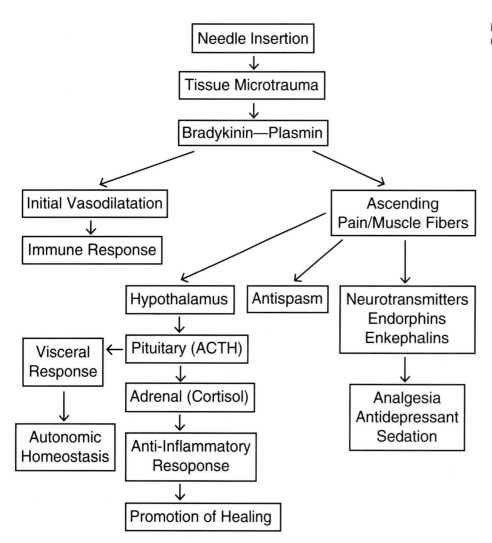

FIGURE 30-1. Body's response to needle insertion.

analyses have produced mixed results.[10,11] One recent study indicated that preoperative acupuncture therapy increased intraoperative pain.[12]

ELECTROMEDICINE

The history of electromedicine begins as early as the 1st century A.D. when Scribonius Largus, a Roman physician, used electric fish to treat gout and headaches. In the 18th century, Luigi Galvani discovered that electrical impulses could cause a muscle contraction through his experiments with frog legs, and Carlo Matteucci showed that injured tissue generates electric current. Since World War II, Dr. Robert Becker[13] of the Veterans' Hospital in Syracuse, New York, has studied the electromagnetic field of living organisms and has determined that bioelectricity plays a major role in the regulation of growth and healing of the body. He particularly investigated the electrical properties of injured tissue and discovered that, immediately after an organism is injured, damaged cells become electrically leaky. Charged atoms (ions) leave the cells, forming a current. Using electricity, Becker stimulated the regrowth of amputated limbs in salamanders and partial regrowth of an amputated limb of a rat. He pioneered the use of electrical stimulation to heal bone fractures. This method is used in many large medical centers across the country. Electricity currently also is used to treat bed sores, burns, and even spinal cord injuries.

Bjorn Nordenstrom,[14] a Swedish radiologist and former Chairman of the Nobel Assembly, postulated a hypothesis of bioelectrical control systems. He proposed that the mechanical blood circulation system is integrated closely anatomically and physiologically with the bioelectric system. He postulated that the vascular interstitial system has two branches. The first branch is the intravenous system. In this system, the blood vessels act as insulators to carry energy, much like battery cables of a car. The intravenous plasma acts as a conductor. Ions, such as sodium, calcium, and chloride, supply immediately available energy to the system by way of electrophoresis. Delayed available energy is carried by blood cells, which bind oxygen and chemicals, such as glucose, fat, and amino acids. These chemicals arrive at specific sites where they undergo oxidation, and energy is released. The second branch is composed of the interstitial system. The interstitial fluid acts as a conductor. The capillary membranes act as junctions between the interstitial and vascular fluids, allowing the exchange of positive and negative ions.[15]

Since the initial pioneering work of Norman Shealy in 1967, low voltage low frequency electrical devices have been used for pain control in the United States. The use of these devices has become increasingly sophisticated and increasingly popular as an adjunctive technique for the management of pain. Currently, there are more than 200 different models of TENS units and bioconductive electrical devices.

Bioconductive Therapy

Many of the bioconductive devices operate on the hypothesis that pathologic areas of the body have a high resistance to electricity. Because electricity follows the path of least resistance, the body's natural energy tends to circumvent these areas. Diseased areas of the body may be located by measuring the electrical conductivity of the skin over suspicious areas with an ohmmeter (point finder). These areas then may be stimulated with an electrical current that helps reestablish the cell membrane potential, the sodium pump. Levels of intracellular metabolic waste, such as lactic acid, are decreased, and a fresh concentration of usable cellular metabolites are allowed to enter the cells. Swelling and inflammation may decrease, pain may be reduced, and cells may become better able to regenerate.[16]

Treatment regimens with these devices will vary according to the severity of pain or injury and the chronicity of the problem. Pain syndromes that reportedly have responded to electrotherapy are sports injuries, whiplash, arthritis, bursitis, tendinitis, headaches, backache, fractures, and premenstrual syndrome.

Auricular Therapy

A highly effective approach using bioconductive therapy is the electrical stimulation of specific points on the ear.[15] Auricular medicine originated in China as part of acupuncture treatments. The Chinese mapped out the auricle in a representation similar to an upside-down fetus. In addition, Egyptians used earrings to treat eye and infertility problems, a technique that later was adopted by the Romans who cauterized a spot on the ear to treat sciatica. In 1957, Paul Nogier, a French neurologist, discovered that some of his patients had scars on the same spot in their ears and learned they had been treated for sciatica by lay practitioners. After much research, he confirmed a system similar to that of the Chinese embryologic model of the ear. It is more complicated and detailed, however, and includes somatic correlations with mesodermal, ectodermal, and endodermal parts of the body. His findings were, in turn, confirmed in China during Mao Zedong's era.

In the late 1970s, Terrence Olesen, Richard Kroening, and David Bresler[17] did extensive research on both the Nogier and Chinese systems. They correlated both systems and obtained impressive results using auricular therapy to treat pain in patients at the University of California, Los Angeles.

Cranial Electrotherapy Stimulation (CES)

Also known as transcranial electrotherapy, alpha sleep, and electrosleep, this form of electrotherapy involves the use of a device similar in size and appearance to a TENS unit. (The amperage is different, however, and these devices cannot be used interchangeably.) Electrodes are placed bi-temporally, front to back, with two bi-temporal electrodes and a third frontal electrode, in the hollow just anterior to the mastoid processes, or simply clipped to the ear lobes. The CES devices vary in the amount of microamperage current from 0.5 to 100 Hz. The intensity gradually is increased until the patient feels a mild tingling sensation at the electrode site. Treatment time is usually 20 to 40 min. This form of therapy is thought to stimulate the production of endorphins and also may involve the hypothalamus and the reticular formation of the brainstem, which plays an important role in attention and alertness. Because of the relaxed and alert state many patients experience, CES is used to relieve anxiety, depression, stress-related disorders (such as hypertension and insomnia), and drug withdrawal. Although relatively new in Europe and the United States, variations of this treatment have been used in Russia for more than 30 years.[15]

The only side effects reported from the use of these forms of electromedicine are dizziness or a slight headache with the CES devices. These devices are contraindicated in patients with epilepsy, brain tumors, and strokes. Patients with infections or blood-clotting disorders are cautioned not to use some of the bioconductive devices. All these devices are contraindicated in patients who are pregnant or have cardiac pacemakers.

TENS UNITS

TENS is the procedure of applying controlled low voltage electrical impulses to the nervous system for the symptomatic relief of pain. This is accomplished by passing electricity through the skin through electrodes placed over strategic loci, often trigger points. The electrical stimulation produces analgesia by modulating the pain impulses that travel from the peripheral nervous system through the spinal cord to the brain. There is evidence that there also may be stimulation of endorphins in the brain that can temporarily modify the pain experience. This device is convenient, portable, and considered to be noninvasive, nonaddictive, and safe (the patient remains completely alert). Because it provides only symptomatic relief, it is best used as an adjunct along with other approaches, such as physical therapy, acupuncture, chiropractic, hypnosis, psychological support systems, and medication.

Hypotheses for Mechanism of Action

Gate-Control Theory

The most popular theory of how TENS works is the gate-control theory, developed by Melzack and Wall.[18,19] In 1965, they published a paper entitled "Pain Mechanisms: A New Theory" in *Science,* which describes the concept of modulation (this is, that incoming pain signals can be controlled and inhibited). The hypothetical gate in this hypoth-

esis was believed to be a complex system found in the dorsal horns of the spinal cord and the thalamus of the brain. This system acted like a switchboard to the brain, allowing some signals to pass through and blocking others. Pain signals thus can be blocked from going to the brain if other messages could be sent through the gate instead.

This hypothesis was expanded to postulate that pain sensations transmitted by smaller diameter sensory C and A delta nerve fibers can be prevented from ascending from the dorsal horn to higher centers. This can occur by stimulating large diameter sensory A beta nerve fibers, which normally convey pressure and touch sensations. The threshold of the large fibers is less than that of the smaller fibers; therefore, it is possible to stimulate the large fibers (e.g., using electricity) to block the sensations of the small fibers and the sensation of pain.

Even though some of the details of the gate-control theory have been proved wrong, much of this hypothesis has been upheld and built on. A major contribution of this work of Melzak and Wall has been that it provided a catalyst for new ways of looking at the mechanism of pain. Pain increasingly is considered a multidimensional phenomenon with emotional and cognitive components that affect the sensory experience. Memories, beliefs, emotions, and attention have an important effect on the perception of pain.[18,19]

Role of Endorphins

Endorphins most commonly are believed to be the members of the family of endogenous transmitter substances that modify pain. It is speculated that morphine-like pentapeptides are manufactured in the brainstem and pituitary gland. This system may be activated by various stimuli, including meditation, exercise, and electrical stimulation of the head and body.[18,20]

Hypothesis of Inhibition

A less known but intriguing theory that has been researched by European and Russian clinicians involves the role of the cortex in dealing with pain perceptions. In general, this hypothesis proposes that counterirritants can suppress cortical responses to pain signals by mechanisms currently unknown. Cortical cells responsive to counterirritation are assumed to be in close proximity with the cells dealing with the pain stimuli. Clinical experience has shown that burn patients tolerate debridement of their wounds much better if a nearby unburned area of their body is rubbed vigorously at the same time.[21]

Stimulation Parameter Settings and Techniques

In using the TENS unit effectively, the therapist must have a working knowledge of the stimulation parameter settings and the mode selections of the unit. There must be a partnership with the patient for the therapist to receive constant feedback about how the patient is feeling when the unit is in operation. The main areas for the therapist to be aware of in determining optimum settings are: (1) is the patient feeling the unit in the painful areas, (2) does the patient experience increased pain relief as the unit is adjusted, and (3) is the pain relief offsetting the pain stimulus and resulting in patient comfort and confidence in the unit?

The total electrical pulse delivered by the TENS unit is determined by the stimulation parameter settings of amplitude, pulse width, and pulse rate. The amplitude translates to the magnitude or intensity of the current being delivered. It is measured in milliamperes and usually ranges from 0 to 60 mA on most TENS units. As the intensity is increased, the patient will experience a wide range of sensations from tingling to pins-and-needles to muscle contraction.

The pulse width is the duration or the length of time each pulse is delivered. It is measured in microseconds and ranges from 40 to 250 μs on most units. The wider the pulse, the larger the increase in the total electrical charge delivered. The patient should report feeling a spreading, deepening, penetrating, radiating sensation that increases in strength as the pulse width widens.

The pulse rate is the frequency or number of pulses delivered per second. It is measured in pulses per second (pps). One cycle per second also is called 1 Hertz (Hz). The range is a low of 1 to 2 pps to 100 pps on most units. For effective stimulation, the electrical currents must be delivered at different rates to match the firing rate of the nerves being treated. The upper level nerve fibers transmit quickly; therefore, high rates (conventional mode) are most effective in these fibers. The lower level nerve fibers transmit more slowly; therefore, low rates are most effective (acupuncture-like TENS). The patient should report an increasing feeling of comfort as the pulse rate approaches its most efficient setting.[21]

Modern TENS units contain varied parameter selections to meet the needs of the patient.[22] Four basic stimulation modes are: (1) conventional, (2) acupuncture-like, (3) burst or pulse train, and (4) brief intense (Table 30-1).

Although it is the therapist who establishes the baseline stimulation parameter settings and the mode connections of the TENS unit, it is important to remember that each patient's needs are unique. To obtain optimal results, the therapist must remember that it is the patient's comfort that ultimately determines the unit settings rather than the unit settings being determined for the patient.[23,24]

Rationale for Selection of Sites

To determine the rationale for selecting sites for optimal TENS stimulation, it is necessary to assess the status of the

Table 30-1
TENS Modes: Optimal Baseline Stimulation Parameter Settings

TENS Modes	Pulse Widths	Pulse Rate	Amplitude	Treatment Time	Onset of Relief	Duration of Relief
Conventional	Narrow, 60 μs	High, 80 pps	Perceptible, paresthesia up to but not causing significant muscle contraction or fasciculation	Average 20 min, but can vary to 60 min; Reassess after each hour	Fast, 20 min	Short, 20–30 min to 2 h. Totally dependent on activities of daily living, posture, and pain level
Low rate, acupuncture-like	Wide, 200–300 μs	Low, 1–4 pps	To patient tolerance, giving rise to strong rhythmic muscle contractions	Average 30 min, but not longer than 1 h	Slow, 20–30 min, or up to 1 h	Usually 2–6 h, totally dependent on activities of daily living, posture, and pain levels
Burst or pulse train	Wide, 200–300 μs	Fixed, 5–7 pulses per burst or 2 bursts/s	To patient tolerance, strong, rhythmic contractions plus background paresthesia	Average 30 min, but not longer than 1 h	Moderate	Somewhere between 20–30 min, up to 6 h, dependent on activities of daily living, posture, and pain level
Brief, intense	Wide, 150 μs	High, highest pps	To patient tolerance, will cause either a tetanic contraction or nonrhythmic fasciculation	Brief, up to 15 min, may repeat after 2–3 min rest	Fast, instantaneous, 10–15 min	Short, usually lasting only as long as stimulation persists

Pulse duration and amplitude ranges are variable and depend on the quality and distribution of pain, interelectrode distance, number of electrodes used, and patient tolerance.

patient completely. This is accomplished by following the specific guidelines for site selection as follows: (1) comprehensive evaluation of the patient; (2) determination of structure involved, that is, the source and location of the pain; (3) innervation, that is, pertinent nerves that innervate the involved structure; (4) palpation to determine optimal stimulation sites; (5) beginning with conventional parameter settings; and (6) eliciting patient feedback regarding sensation.

The rationale for selecting optimal TENS sites begins with an evaluation of the patient with pain. A history of the onset of pain and its current location, quality, and intensity is obtained. Eliciting information about how the patient feels about having pain may be important; emotional issues surrounding the pain experience may be treated by the therapist or another professional. It is important to ask patients about their expectations of TENS treatment. If the patient does not have realistic goals, the TENS experience may be predisposed to failure. Factors in the life style of the patient (such as food, medication, use of alcohol or drugs, posture, movement, activity, rest, friction, straining, and pressure), family and home life situations, stresses and activities at work, and basic beliefs can be catalysts for the fluctuation of the patient's pain. It is important to remember that it is not the pain being treated but the person who is in pain.

After the patient has been evaluated in general, the therapist locates the structure or structures involved in the patient's pain experience and determines the nature and source of the pain. The therapist then ascertains where the spinal cord innervates the involved structure. Knowledge of dermatomes, myotomes, and sclerotomes is important because placing electrodes near the spinal cord to stimulate the central nervous system often enhances the effect of the treatment.

The next step is palpation to determine optimal stimulation sites. Such sites are those regions anatomically and physiologically related to the involved area. These regions must contain the following characteristics: (1) stimulation of the area can be directed to the central nervous system, (2) the region is related segmentally to the source of pain, and (3) the anatomic site can be located distinctly and is accessible easily to a TENS electrode. These optimal stimulation sites may include loci over peripheral nerves, motor points, acupuncture points, and trigger points. The path of referred pain also may be followed or the area of pain may be sandwiched between the electrodes, allowing current to flow through the area. Peripheral nerves usually have one or more regions where they are superficial enough to be stimulated by surface electrodes. Motor points are sites in the muscle where it is innervated by fibers from the motor branches of peripheral nerves. They are characterized by high electrical conductance and low skin resistance. Twitching of the muscle can be achieved by stimulating these points. Acupuncture points are tender areas along

energy pathways of the body. These pathways are invisible to the eye but are depicted in charts as part of traditional Chinese medicine. Many meridians follow peripheral nerve distributions, and most of the commonly used acupuncture points lie over or are innervated by superficial cutaneous nerves. Many acupuncture points are identical to motor and trigger points.

The most commonly used sites for electrode placement are trigger points.[25] Trigger points are hypersensitive regions most often found in muscles, but they also occur in connective tissue, skin, joint capsules, tendons, and ligaments. They are firm to the touch and tender on palpation. When they are pressed, there is a twitch in the muscle and a flinch by the patient. The patient experiences a deep dull ache in the local area, hyperalgesia in the surrounding area, and a referral of discomfort to other areas. Trigger points that remain active for long periods of time may cause satellite trigger points to develop in the area of referred pain. Latent trigger points, which have become inactive when the original cause healed, may become reactivated by stressful conditions. Currently, there is no consensus as to their origin or exact physiology. Theories about their causes include trauma, postural abnormalities, joint dysfunction, spinal and peripheral infection, visceral disease, fatigue, emotional tension, and endocrine imbalance. They are described by some practitioners as areas of fibrous connective tissue created by chronic muscle spasm. (These points are considered excellent stimulation sites for TENS electrodes.)

After the optimal stimulation sites are selected by the therapist, patients then become the primary guides by reporting their sensations as to: (1) when they feel the sensation, (2) what do they feel, and (3) where do they feel it? This information is the basis for the therapist's decision about the unit settings. The first question ("When do you feel it?") determines when the unit is on and which intensity setting is necessary for the patient. "What do you feel?" directs information about the patient's degree of comfort and helps avoid unnecessary uncomfortable sensations such as burning or pricking. "Where do you feel it?" allows the therapist to adjust the unit to provide the maximum amount of concentration and penetration of stimulation into the painful body part. Following these steps encourages the interaction and participation of patients in their own care, an ingredient important for ultimate recovery.[23,26]

Patient Management

The most important aspect in the success of treatment with TENS is patient compliance. This is influenced by the health-related beliefs of patients, the interaction between therapists and patients, the attitude of patients about themselves, and aspects of the regimen itself. Trust in oneself and the therapist and confidence in the technique will enhance the healing process. The therapist can provide important psychological support by (1) communicating a caring attitude and valuing the patient's role as a partner in the treatment; (2) explaining how TENS has been and can be successful; (3) reinforcing a positive attitude and discouraging negative thoughts and feelings; (4) encouraging a balance between exercise within the patient's level of tolerance and rest and relaxation; (5) teaching the patient proper nutrition, including avoidance of nicotine, caffeine, salt, fat, and processed sugar; and (6) periodically evaluating the patient's progress and providing follow-up care.

There are several stages involved in the management of the patient: assessment, periodic evaluation of progress, and follow-up care. Part of the comprehensive evaluation of the patient is the assessment. It is important for the therapist to determine if this technique is appropriate for this patient. Is it possible and indicated to provide systemic relief of pain for this particular patient? As the therapist determines the appropriate stimulation parameter setting and the mode for the patient, other aspects of treatment also will be determined, such as the frequency, the length of time for each treatment, and the projected duration of the treatment program. The patient will need treatments often enough to maintain a state of reduced or absence of pain. Treatments must be long enough for analgesia to persist for a significant amount of time. Postoperative pain usually is treated for 3 to 7 days. Acute pain may require a regimen of weeks or months. A patient in chronic pain needs to establish a protocol that permits a balance between adequate periods of stimulation without overdependence.

As therapists evaluate the progress of their patients they will want to know: (1) how much relief the patients are experiencing, (2) how quickly relief is obtained, (3) how long the pain relief lasts, (4) if their patients still require medication, and (5) if their patients have improved their level of functioning (such as increased range of motion or change in activities of daily living). The use of charts or a diary may be useful because the changes may be subtle. Describing pain levels in terms of a scale of 1 to 10, with 10 being the most severe pain the patient has experienced, may be helpful in evaluation. The focus of follow-up care should be on how well the patient is returning to a normal and independent life.[23]

Electrode Choices

For optimal pain relief, contact between the electrodes and the patient must be secure. Electrodes come in various types, shapes, and sizes to allow adequate conformation to the patient's body. Standard electrodes made of silicone–carbon require tape or foam and paper adhesive tape patches for adherence. Gel or karaya is necessary for activation. These electrodes frequently are used for office treatments. Reusable self-adhering electrodes made of karaya and synthetic polymer require water for activation. Some may require placement of a silicone–carbon electrode. Pregelled self-adhering electrodes are excellent for home use because they can be left in place and used for 2 to 3 days at a time. Sponge electrodes containing carbon are activated by water and are fastened with tape. The most commonly used electrodes are square shaped and approximately 1 to 2 in in diameter. They also may be round or rectangular and may be as small as the diameter of a nickel or as long as 6 in or more.

Contraindications, Precautions, and Complications

The use of TENS is considered safe compared with most other forms of pain control. To date, no documentation of adverse effects has been found; however, TENS would be contraindicated in two situations: (1) for patients with pacemakers and (2) application over the carotid sinuses, which could stimulate the vagovagal reflex and thus a hypotensive response or possibly cardiac arrest.

TENS should be used with considerable caution in the following instances: (1) use near the eyes; (2) placement over the anterior chest wall especially in cardiac patients; (3) use of paired electrodes crossing the midline of the body in the upper torso; (4) pregnancy; (5) patients with cerebrovascular accident, transient ischemic attack, and epilepsy; (6) the incompetent patient; and (7) internal use.

No complications of existing conditions have been recorded with the use of TENS; however, there have been reports of some skin reactions at the electrode sites. Skin problems could be related to the following causes: (1) electrical burns from the use of constant voltage rather than constant current, from excessive stimulation with small-area electrodes or electrodes placed too close to one another (there should be a space the size of the cross-sectional diameter of the electrode), or poor electrical contact between the skin and the stimulation electrode; (2) chemical reactions (electrode gel may contain chemical or abrasive irritants such as silicone oxide); and (3) allergic reactions (some patients react to adhesive tape). Acrylic, cloth, and paper tape may be tolerated better. Some instances of allergic reactions to the electrode gels, especially ones containing propylene glycol, have been reported. Occasionally, a patient may be sensitive to nickel, a component of the metal snap projection in the center of the electrode. Regular washing and periodic changing of the electrodes and the electrode placement sites will help in avoiding these problems. In addition, there may be mechanical reactions. The most common reaction of this kind occurs because of the shearing forces between the tape and skin. To avoid this problem, apply tape in the center first (not at one end and then at the other end, that is, pulled over the electrodes). Consideration must be given to the movement patterns of the area in relation to body movement (for example, parallel tape to the spine causes shearing). The lead wires can be looped approximately 6 to 10 in from the electrode to prevent tugging.

Indications for Use

There are many chronic and acute pain syndromes that may respond to TENS analgesia. They include the following.

I. Musculoskeletal pain.[27]
II. Neurologic and vascular pain.[28]
III. Head and face pain.
IV. Systemic pain.
    A. Cancer pain, usually referred from internal organs or after radiation or surgical therapy.
    B. Multiple sclerosis.
V. Postoperative pain.[29]
VI. Abdominal and pelvic pain (such as dysmenorrhea and bladder pain).

TENS also is being used by pioneers in the medical field to stimulate bone growth.[30] Some recent data indicate that TENS and exercise therapy may provide similar benefits for chronic low back pain.[31] Johnson and colleagues[32] analyzed 179 long-term TENS users and found that therapy reduced pain by more than one-half in 47 percent. Figures 30-2 to 30-18 are some examples of suggested electrode placement sites for common pain syndromes.

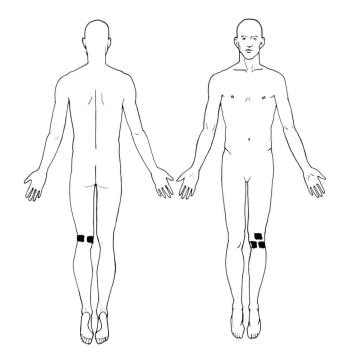

FIGURE 30-3. TENS placement for knee pain.

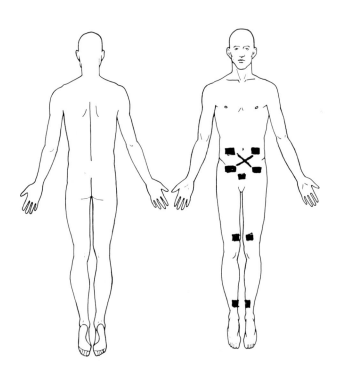

FIGURE 30-2. TENS Placement for dysmenorrhea.

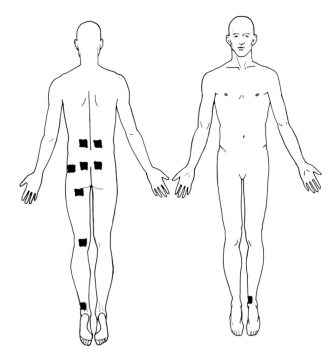

FIGURE 30-4. TENS placement for sciatica.

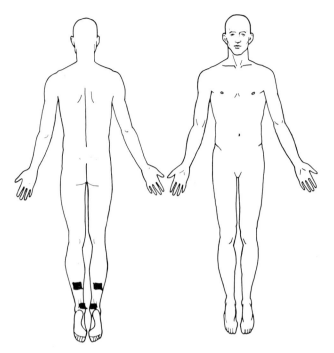

FIGURE 30-5. TENS placement for diabetic neuropathy of both feet.

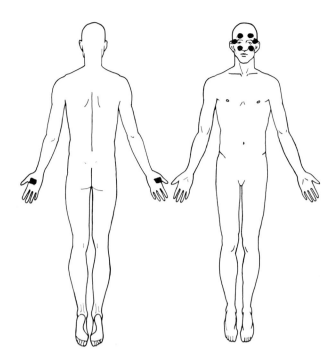

FIGURE 30-7. TENS placement for facial pain.

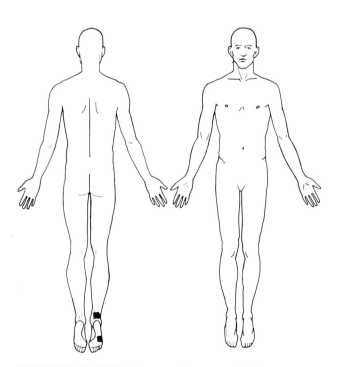

FIGURE 30-6. TENS placement for postpodiatric surgery.

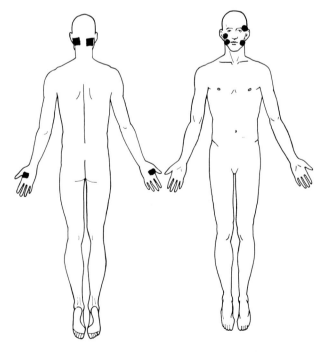

FIGURE 30-8. TENS placement for temporomandibular joint pain.

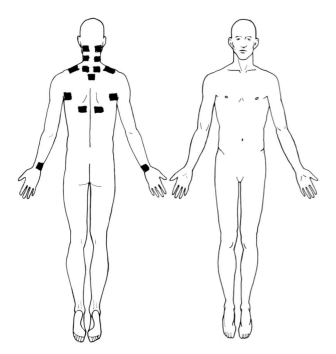

FIGURE 30-9. TENS placement for cervical pain.

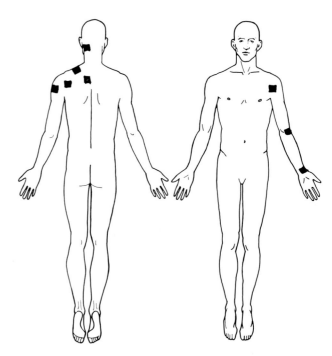

FIGURE 30-11. TENS placement for shoulder pain.

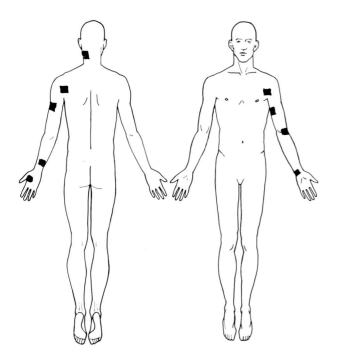

FIGURE 30-10. TENS placement for reflex sympathetic dystrophy.

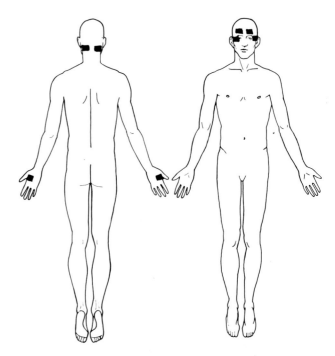

FIGURE 30-12. TENS placement for headaches.

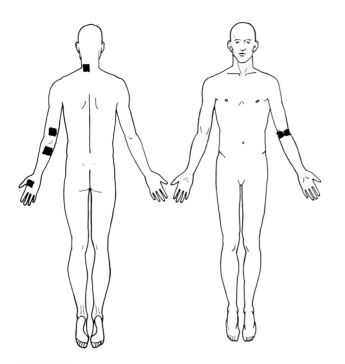

FIGURE 30-13. TENS placement for elbow pain.

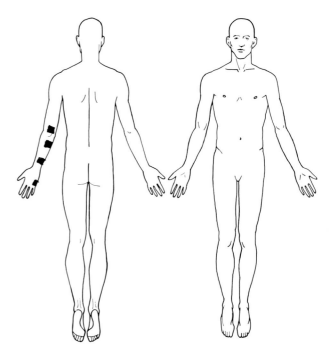

FIGURE 30-15. TENS placement for tendinitis of flexor carpi ulnarus.

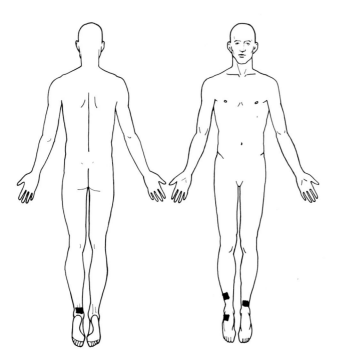

FIGURE 30-14. TENS placement for ankle pain.

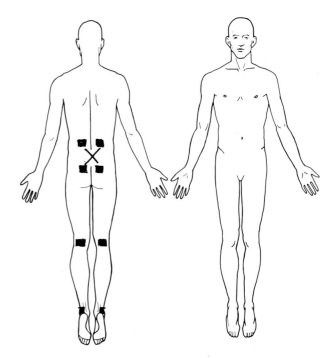

FIGURE 30-16. TENS placement for low back pain.

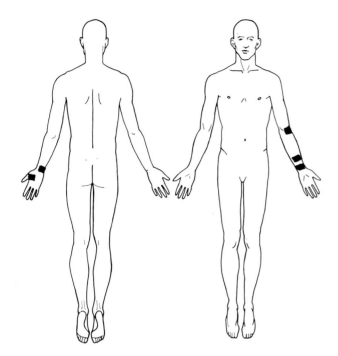

FIGURE 30-17. TENS placement for wrist pain.

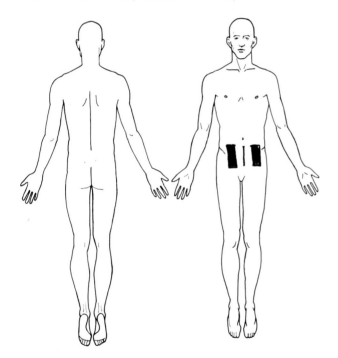

FIGURE 30-18. TENS placement for abdominal surgery.

References

1. Klide AM. An hypothesis for the prolonged effect of acupuncture. *Acupunct Electrother Res* 1989; 14(2):141–147.
2. Arseni A, Valcoreanu-Zbaganu G, Popescu R, Rosca V. Acupuncture treatment of discopathic pain. *Neurol Psychiatr (Bucur)* October–December 1989; 27(4):315–322.
3. Freed S. Acupuncture as therapy of traumatic affective disorders and of phantom limb pain syndrome. *Acupunct Electrother Res* 1989; 14(2):121–129.
4. Pomeranz B. *Scientific Bases of Acupuncture*. New York: Springer-Verlag; 1989:1–2.
5. Williams T, Mueller K, Cornwall MW. Effect of acupuncture—point stimulation on diastolic blood pressure in hypertensive subjects: a preliminary study. *Phys Ther* July 1991; 71(7):523–529.
6. Moret V, Forster A, Laverriere MC, et al. Mechanism of analgesia induced by hypnosis and acupuncture: is there a difference? *Pain* May 1991; 45(2):135–140.
7. Yang ZL, Cai TW, Wu JL. Acupuncture and emotion: the influence of acupuncture anesthesia on the sensory and emotional components of pain. *J Gen Psychol* July 1989; 116(3):132–134, 247–258.
8. Katz J, Melzach R. Auricular transcutaneous electrical nerve stimulation (TENS) reduces phantom limb. *J Pain Symptom Manage* February 1991; 6(2):73–83.
9. Kendall DE. A scientific model for acupuncture. *Am J Acupunct* September–December 1989; 17(3):251–268.
10. Patel M, Gutzwiller F, Paccaud F, Marazzi A. A meta-analysis of acupuncture for chronic pain. *Int J Epidemiol* December 1989; 18(4):900–906.
11. Riet G, Kleijnen J, Knipschild P. Acupuncture and chronic pain: a criteria-based meta-analysis. *J Clin Epidemiol* 1990; 43(11):1191–1199.
12. Ekblom A, Hansson P, Thompson M, Thomas M. Increased postoperative pain and consumption of analgesics following acupuncture. *Pain* March 1991; 44(3):241–247.
13. Becker RO, and Selden G. *The Body Electric: Electromagnetism and the Foundation of Life*. New York: Quill William Morrow; 1985.
14. Nordenstrom BEW. *Biologically Closed Electric Circuits: Clinical, Experimental and Theoretical Evidence for an Additional Circulatory System*. Oslo: Nordic Medical Publications; 1983.
15. Kirsh D, Lerner F. Inovations in pain management: a practical guide for clinicians. In: Weiner RL (ed). *Electromedicine*. Orlando, FL: Paul M. Deutsch Press; 1990:23-1–23-24.
16. Biedebach MC. Accelerated healing of skin ulcers by electrical stimulation and intracellular physiological mechanisms involved. *J Acupunct Electrotherapeutics* 1989; 14:43–60.
17. Olesen T, Kroening R, Bresler DE. Experiental evaluation of auricular diagnosis: the somatrophic mapping of musculoskeletal pain at ear acupuncture points. *Pain* 1980; 8(2):217–229.
18. Melzak R. *The Puzzle of Pain*. New York: Basic Books; 1973.
19. Melzak R, Wall PD. Pain mechanisms: a new theory. *Science* 1965; 150:69–83.
20. Lerner F. The quiet revolution—pain control and electromedicine. *California Health Review*. April–May 1983; 34–37.
21. Mannheimer J, Lampe G. *Clinical Transcutaneous Electric Nerve Stimulation*. Philadelphia: Davis; 1984.
22. Johnson MI, Ashton CH, Thompson JW. The consistency of pulse frequencies and pulse patterns of transcutaneous electrical nerve stimulation (TENS) used by chronic pain patients. *Pain* March 1991; 44(3):231–234.
23. Mannheimer J, Lampe G. *Clinical TENS*. Philadelphia: Davis; 1984.
24. Tapio D, Hymes A. *New Frontiers in Transcutaneous Elec-*

trical Nerve Stimulation. Minnesota: Minnetonka; 1987:53.

25. Travell JG, Simons DG. *Myofascial Pain and Dysfunction: The Trigger Point Manual*. Baltimore: William and Wilkins; 1983.

26. Lampe G. *RPT Presentor Professional Pain Management Seminars, Inc*. Kansas: Shawnee Mission; 1981.

27. Graff-Radford SB, Reeves JL, Baker RL, Chiu D: Effects of transcutaneous electrical nerve stimulation on myofascial pain and trigger point sensitivity. *Pain* April 1989; 37(1): 1–5.

28. Leijon G, Boivie J. Central post-stroke pain—the effect of high and low frequency TENS. *Pain* August 1989; 38(2):187–191.

29. Hargreaves A, Lander J. Use of transcutaneous electrical nerve stimulation for postoperative pain. *Nurs Res* May–June 1989; 38(3):159–161.

30. Sternbach Richard. TENS: *A Pain Management Alternative*. San Diego: La Jolla Technology; 1985:12–16.

31. Deyo RA, Walsh NE, Martin DC, Schoenfeld LS, Ramamurthy S. A controlled trial of transcutaneous electrical nerve stimulation (TENS) and exercise for chronic low back pain. *N Engl J Med* June 7, 1990; 322(23):1627–1634.

32. Johnson MI, Ashton CH, Thompson JW. An in-depth study of long-term users of transcutaneous electrical nerve stimulation (TENS). Implications for clinical use of TENS. *Pain* March 1991; 44(3):221–229.

CHAPTER 31

Physical Measures for Pain Relief

Robert Bengston

Physical measures are useful in the treatment of subacute and chronic pain. The focus of such techniques is to minimize pain to allow therapies and natural healing to proceed uninhibited.[1] In this chapter, physical measures useful in treating pain are divided into three categories. Included are stimulation-produced analgesia (acupuncture, TENS, and iontophoresis), thermotherapy and cryotherapy, and exercise and manual therapies (mobilization, massage, and traction). Physical measures are a powerful tool to provide pain relief if applied in a timely fashion by a skilled therapist. When a multidisciplinary approach to pain management is used, it is critical that the providers work as a coordinated team to optimize outcomes.

STIMULATION-PRODUCED ANALGESIA (See Chap. 30)

Acupuncture has been an integral part of traditional Eastern medicine for more than 5000 years. A Chinese fable tells of a warrior who, shot by an arrow during battle, experienced relief from his wound pain when shot by a second arrow.

Acupuncture stimulation during the Han dynasty (206 BC to 220 AD) was done with a sharp stone that was used to prick the skin to give pain relief. Needles of bone and bamboo eventually were used, until the discovery of metals. How does acupuncture work? In terms of Chinese medicine, on which the therapy of acupuncture originally was based, acupuncture reestablishes the flow of chi or energy coursing through meridian channels. The treatment ultimately would balance the opposing energy forces of yin and yang, resulting in a cure. Western acupuncture treatment for pain reduction currently involves the identification of the appropriate acupuncture points (of which there are more than 600) for the desired result followed by the insertion of a slender needle. (Fig. 31-1). The needle is left in place for minutes to 1 h, rotated between the therapist's fingers, or attached to an electrical current. Hyvarinen and Karlsson[2] found that acupuncture points correlate well with trigger and motor points and areas of increased electrical conductance. In 1825, the French physician Sarlandiers treated back pain using electrical stimulation transmitted through needles inserted into acupuncture points. The recent use of electrical

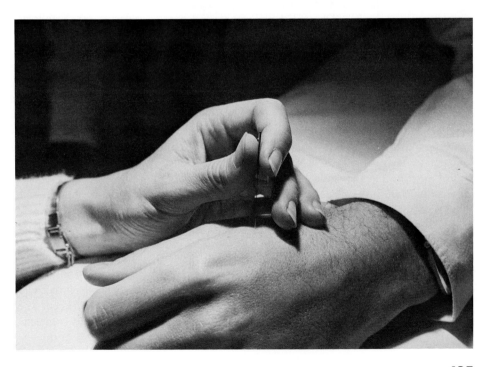

FIGURE 31-1. Classic Chinese acupuncture being applied to the hoku point for treatment of pain in the head.

techniques for pain modulation began with the use of dorsal column stimulator implantation. During the past decade, TENS has played a substantial role in pain therapy.

A change in neuronal activity is the most important physical effect elicited by the use of acupuncture and electrical techniques for pain management. Electrical stimulation acquired widespread clinical application after Melzack and Wall's[3] description of a gating mechanism in the dorsal horn of the spinal cord. They hypothesized that stimulation of large diameter peripheral afferent fibers excites interneurons in the substantia gelatinosa. This presynaptically inhibits the transmission of pain mediated by smaller A delta and C fiber afferents. This was later modified by Wall[4] in 1978. The exact mechanism by which pain is blocked is unclear.

Melzack and Wall[3] reported that, in addition to the segmental gating mechanisms, descending pain-control systems or negative feedback loops further modulate pain. Snyder[5] reported that electrical stimulation of supraspinal brainstem sites, such as the nucleus raphe magnus and the mesencephalic periaqueductal and periventricular gray structures, results in analgesia through the release of endorphins. These substances mediate pain by binding to opiate receptor sites, thereby blocking pain transmission. Endorphins primarily are produced from the breakdown of β-lipotropin in the anterior pituitary to β-endorphin, certain types of enkephalins, and corticotropin. The latter stimulates corticosteroid release from the adrenals that may provide an additional anti-inflammatory effect; the increased endorphin levels stimulate the nucleus raphe magnus and activate a descending pain-control system. Cheng and associates[6] found that stimulation by electroacupuncture caused an increase in blood plasma corticosteroid levels by as much as 50 percent.

One mechanism of analgesia mediated by endorphin stimulation is accomplished through the release of serotonin at the level of the nucleus raphe magnus. This, in turn, may stimulate the release of enkephalins at the spinal cord level to block pain transmission presynaptically. Acupuncture stimulation has been shown to increase levels of serotonin.[7] This substance also may be released by direct stimulation of the nucleus raphe magnus. Analgesic effects after nucleus raphe magnus stimulation are reduced significantly if there is a lesion of the dorsolateral funiculus, implicating this structure as the major vehicle of this descending pain-control system. On the basis of these theories, various nerve-stimulation instruments have been developed to initiate spinal segmental blocking or supraspinal mechanisms of pain modulation.

There are low (0 to 1000 Hz), medium (1000 to 100,000 Hz), and high frequency (>100,000 Hz) modes. Conventional or high frequency TENS (which is a low frequency electrical mode) requires that an AC current be set at a rate of 40 to 400 cycles per second. Pulse widths should be no less than 20 or greater than 250 μs, and the amplitude should be set at a level that will produce paresthesias with-

out muscular contraction. This stimulus is transmitted by large myelinated afferents to the dorsal horn segmentally. The onset of analgesia so produced usually is rapid, within 20 min and has a short period of effectiveness, usually less than 1 h after discontinuing stimulation.

Clinical studies have been done to determine the mechanism of analgesia. Naloxone does not reverse the effectiveness of high frequency TENS, although parachlorophenylalanine (a serotonin synthesis inhibitor) partially blocks high frequency-stimulated analgesia.[6] These studies support the hypothesis that high frequency TENS works, in part, on a segmental gating mechanism at the spinal cord level through the descending serotonin system.

TENS also can be applied at low frequencies. Low and high frequency TENS have both been shown to be effective in relieving pain. Low frequency TENS stimulates at a low frequency of 1 to 5 cycles per second and a longer pulse width of 250 to 500 μs. It should be set at an amplitude of sufficient intensity to cause a strong rhythmic muscular contraction. Low frequency TENS stimulates smaller A delta and C fibers, causing the release of endorphins and serotonin. In clinical trials that attempted to clarify mechanisms by which low frequency TENS was effective in pain relief, β-endorphin and serotonergic-blocking agents diminished the analgesic effect of this technique.[8] This suggests that supraspinal and segmental mechanisms are induced in low frequency TENS. In clinical applications, onset of pain relief usually takes more than 15 min, and the duration of relief is longer than that of high frequency TENS. Low frequency stimulation is effective when used in subacute and chronic pain conditions and conditions with inflammatory causes. One of the greatest clinical advantages of TENS use is that the patient can take this device home and, with proper instruction, maintain full control over its use. This is particularly beneficial in patients with chronic pain.

Brief intense acupuncture-like TENS involves the high intensity pulsed train stimulation of specific acupuncture and trigger points. The current used is a pulsed train at low frequency (1 to 5 cycles per second) with high frequency TENS applied in a burst mode (up to 400·cycles per second). The high frequency bursts stimulate large afferents and elicit the segmental gating mechanism. The bursts of low frequency intervals facilitate the endorphin–corticotropin system at the level of the pituitary, resulting in a systemic anti-inflammatory and analgesic response. It appears that the higher frequency currents act as a carrier current, allowing the low frequency bursts to be carried to greater depths of penetration.

Musculoskeletal pain management with TENS is documented in the literature. Ersek[9] found that TENS reduced both chronic and acute low back pain. Of 35 patients, 23 had 30 percent to 50 percent pain relief; the remainder had close to complete relief. Melzack,[10] applied brief intense TENS at trigger and acupuncture points and showed that the average relief in patients with low back problems was 60 percent. He also observed that the pain relief gained by this type of treatment continued for hours or even days.

In the medium electrical frequency range, interferential units superimpose two currents of 4000 to 5000 cps and 4100 to 5100 cps to bridge skin resistance capacitively to reach the depth of muscle tissue and joint receptors. By superimposing the two currents of medium frequency, the effective stimulation results from the difference between the individual frequencies, thus giving a deeper simulus of 1 to 100 cps. This results in the physiologic effect of low frequency TENS currents (at greater depths of penetration) with decreased superficial noxious stimuli. Whereas the frequency is the difference between the intersecting currents, the amplitude of stimulation is the combination of the currents; each circuit contributing 50 percent of the treatment intensity. This allows greater intensity of endogenous stimulation with minimal unpleasant nociceptor stimulation under the electrodes. This technique is most effective in patients with pain of joint or deep muscle origin. It also can enhance beneficial effects for patients who have thick dry skin, a thick subcutaneous fatty layer, or are adverse to superficial stimulation. Reports indicate that interferential therapy also is effective in reducing edema and increasing vasodilatation.[11]

Interferential therapy requires a treatment time as little as 5 to 10 min for analgesic effects. For edema reduction, 15 to 20 min is necessary. Relative contraindications include: thrombophlebitis, application over a pregnant uterus, artificial pacemakers, or malignant tumors. Brief intense acupuncture-like stimulation is effective in treating conditions similar to those treated by conventional high and low frequency TENS, but it entails lower currents, less discomfort, and substantially longer analgesic effects.

Restoration of pituitary production of endorphins may explain in part the high success rate of acupuncture or TENS. Clinically, it is usual, when treating chronic pain conditions with low frequency TENS, to observe a gradual increase in the duration of pain relief, possibly caused by this restoration of endorphin production. Pain relief may range from only hours, after a 30-min treatment, to eventual total permanent relief, after many weeks of treatment.

Correct electrode placement is essential to the effectiveness of TENS. Electrodes may be placed over the site of tenderness or pain (paravertebrally coinciding with the involved segmental level) or bilaterally on trigger, motor, or acupuncture points. Locating these points is facilitated by the use of a so-called point finder, a unit that measures skin resistance with a probe and also can be used for single-point electrical stimulation. Areas that exhibit a decrease in electrical resistance represent highly innervated tissue, areas close to nerve branches, or areas over neuromuscular points.

The analgesic effects of TENS devices are affected adversely by administration of diazepam, narcotics, and corticosteroids. These devices also are not entirely beneficial in drug-addicted patients. However, tricyclic antidepressants, L-tryptophan, and D-phenylalanine (serotonin precursors) seem to increase the effectiveness of TENS.

A DC application may be used in pain management to drive (iontophoresis) anti-inflammatory or analgesic medication into subcutaneous tissue. Harris[12] reports that, in 1908, LeDuc first showed that ions could be transferred through intact skin by electrical potentials using bipolar electrodes. More recently, Glass and colleagues,[13] using rhesus monkeys, demonstrated quantitatively that dexamethasone was transferred into all tissue layers, including tendinous and cartilaginous structures, under the positive electrode. It was interesting that they found no penetration with a hydrocortisone solution. These findings were supported in human application of dexamethasone administered iontophoretically to patients with various types of tendinitis. Results indicated that iontophoresis was more effective when used in patients younger than 45 years of age and with specific localized cases of tendinitis. Older patients responded poorly as did patients with generalized diagnoses, such as adhesive capsulitis or degenerative joint disease with associated tendinitis.[13] Direct currents used in iontophoresis are from 2 to 5 mA, with a treatment time of 5 to 20 min. Battery-powered units are available for home use and are encouraged in patients with long-term pain.

THERMOTHERAPY AND CRYOTHERAPY

The application of heat or cold are useful therapies in the clinical management of acute and chronic pain. Temperature change (hot or cold) leads to relaxation of underlying muscle tissue. Local application of heat produces reflex vasodilatation and a release of histamine; this increases capillary permeability. Immediately after the application of heat, nerve impulses diminish in number, causing a reduction in skeletal muscle tone.

Local application of cold (Fig. 31-2) produces a pattern of vasoconstriction followed by vasodilatation. The decreased initial vascular flow is accompanied by a reduction in nerve-conduction velocity and skeletal muscle relaxation. When cold is applied and the surrounding tissue becomes sufficiently ischemic, localized reflex vasodilatation occurs to preserve tissue viability, followed again by vasoconstriction to preserve core body temperatures. This alteration of vasoconstriction and vasodilatation induces a so-called milking activity; this may help reduce edema formation.

Control of edema formation is an important part of pain management and one that is amenable to application of heat or cold. In the acute stages of injury or tissue trauma, cold is most effective. Cold-induced vasoconstriction decreases capillary permeability, reduces blood flow and congestion in the area of fragile injured tissue, and retards fluid (plasma) leakage. The vasodilatation sequence of cold application then allows an increase in nutritional supply and en-

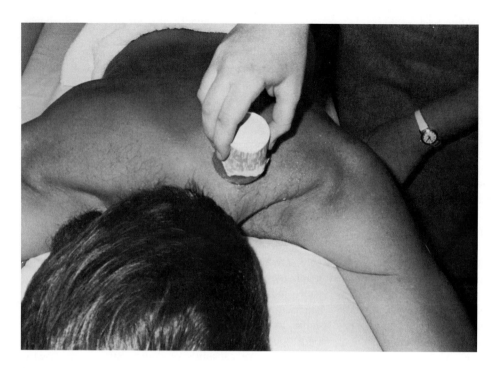

FIGURE 31-2. A convenient method of applying superficial cold massage. Water is frozen in a paper cup, the top of which is then torn off.

hances removal of metabolites. After this short phase of vasodilatation, cold is applied again so that vasoconstriction recurs, with the aforementioned benefits. Cold application may be continued after the acute stages if it is found to be more effective than heat in reducing pain and edema.

Heat application (Fig. 31-3) is most beneficial in the late treatment of edema and painful injury. In the acute stages, heat actually may foster edema formation by increasing blood flow and congestion in an area of capillary fragility. This allows for considerable leakage of plasma into the tissue and an increase in edema formation. After the acute stage, heat application is beneficial because of the increased flow of blood to the area caused by vasodilatation.[14]

Prolonged painful conditions can result in or be aggravated by a decrease in soft tissue extensibility or loss of joint range of motion. The application of heat has a marked influence on connective tissue properties. Through the use of superficial or deep heating, increases in tissue temperature augment the plasticity of connective tissue. Raising connective tissue temperature to approximately 40°C causes a thermal transition of the tissue microstructure to occur, allowing greater plasticity when the tissue is stressed.[15]

During or after heating of deep soft tissue structures, it is necessary to apply prolonged mobilizing forces to induce deformation of the tissues; this will result in increased range of joint motion. Increased tissue temperature, thermal destabilization of intermolecular bonding, and increased viscous flow properties allow collagen deformation to occur more easily and with less external force. It appears that the amount of structural weakening produced by tissue elongation may have an inverse relationship to the temperature of

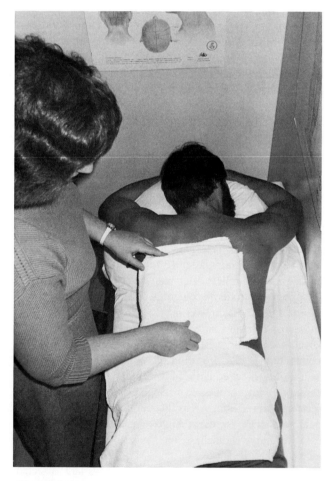

FIGURE 31-3. Hot pack application.

the tissue. Therefore, the use of heating techniques may minimize structural damage.

After the application of heat and prolonged stretching, the stretching force should be maintained while the area is cooled with ice application for approximately 15 min. Force should be maintained until the end of the cooling period, thus promoting the maintenance of the connective tissue in the elongated state. This therapeutic regimen should be done daily, if possible, for a minimum of three times per week. The patient also may be instructed in this method for home use.

Spray and stretch is a technique in which a vapocoolant and reflex inhibitory spray is applied over the area to be stretched, inducing a local anesthetic effect. This is followed by prolonged stretching of the underlying tissue. This is used most frequently for trigger point therapy in myofascial pain syndromes.[16]

Active muscular activity also stimulates an increase in blood flow and an increase in deep tissue temperatures; it should not be overlooked as a method to warm tissue before stretching. For this reason, to avoid aggravating a painful condition, stretching-exercise programs should be preceded by aerobic low resistance exercise for approximately 5 min.

Deep heating with ultrasound (Fig. 31-4) is an effective treatment used to stimulate and accelerate tissue healing. Thermal heating occurs when tissues absorb ultrasonic energy. The flow of sound waves streaming around tissue structures causes a change in membrane permeability, diffusion rate, and metabolic activity in cells. Ultrasound may enhance tissue repair by facilitating anabolic and catabolic processes. Harvey and associates[17] found that exposure to ultrasound at therapeutic levels can increase the rate of fibroblastic protein synthesis. Because of its effect, ultrasound therapy has been used effectively to promote the healing of pressure sores and improve the success rate of skin grafting. Ultrasound also has been proved to be effective as an aid in clearing fibrous adhesions from areas of surgical excision and softening the highly collagenous scar tissue produced after burns or lacerations.

For recent injuries, ultrasound should be applied twice daily for the first 2 days. After this, treatment should be done daily until resolution is achieved. Subacute conditions should be treated daily for the first week and then on alternate days until resolution occurs. Chronic conditions can be treated daily for the first week and then two to three times per week for 2 to 4 weeks.

The temperature after ultrasound application to the human thigh has been recorded at 42.7°C within 1 cm of the femoral shaft.[18] Microwave and short-wave diathermy are effective in elevating muscle temperatures at moderate depths, thus complementing the deep-heating effects of ultrasound and the superficial heating produced by hot packs and whirlpool application. Hydrotherapy, hot packs, and infrared lamps transfer heat to more superficial levels.

MANUAL THERAPIES AND EXERCISE

The exercises most frequently used in clinical practice for pain management are those aimed at improving flexibility, strength, and postural alignment by attempting to reduce those structural asymmetries and muscular imbalances that result in chronic postural stresses. General aerobic conditioning also has been successful in increasing functional levels and has been associated with reduced pain states.[19,20]

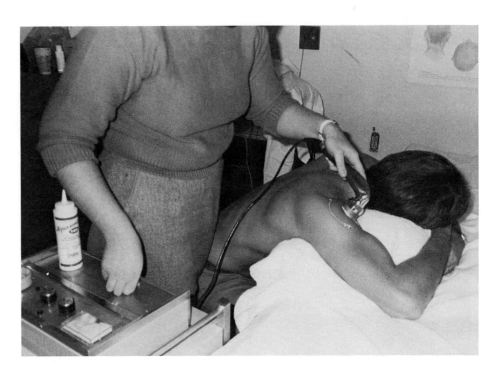

FIGURE 31-4. Therapist applying deep heating ultrasound.

Manual therapies include superficial and deep-tissue massage, traction, and joint mobilization. These therapies reduce pain through the restoration of normal joint and tissue mobility, thereby reducing abnormal forces, and facilitating blood circulation.

Manual Therapies

Traction

Traction is applied while the patient is in a sitting, supine, side lying, or prone position, using electromechanical units, manual techniques, or the application of force by gravitational means. The purpose of spinal traction is to relax spinal musculature and distract and separate the vertebral joint surfaces mechanically. Distraction enlarges the size of the intervertebral foramina and reduces nuclear protrusion, thereby relieving nerve root and facet joint compression.[21] This therapy also may improve vertebral segmental mobility. It has been found that 45 to 225 kg of traction force is most effective in the lumbar spine and 9 to 23 kg in the cervical spine (Fig. 31-5), depending on the patient's body size and pain tolerance.[21] No significant differences have been reported between continuous or intermittent traction. Both methods reduce sacrospinal muscular activity and provide intervertebral distraction.

Gravitational upright axial traction harnesses the gravitational force of the patient's body weight to produce distraction of the spinal column. It is done by securing the upper torso to a rotating bed with straps around the arms and the rib cage and tilting the patient upright with feet unsupported. This allows for the spine to extend without any of the compressive forces caused by standing.

Inverted spinal traction (Fig. 31-6) uses the same principle by fixing the legs to the table and tilting the patient upside down. This technique can be applied in a gradual incremental manner by grading the inclination of the traction unit. Both techniques have been shown to lengthen the lumbar spine, reduce intradiskal pressure, and reduce paraspinal myoelectric activity. Burton[22] reported that, at The Sister Kenney Institute Low Back Pain Clinic in Minneapolis, Minnesota, the upright approach has been beneficial in reducing the duration of bed rest during acute disk prolapse.

Autotraction is a technique whereby the patient lies on an adjustable table, grasps bars at the head of the table, and is secured by a pelvic belt. The patient then does the traction by positioning their body for optimal distraction and pulling with their arms to produce a self-gradation of forces. Larsson and associates[23] found better results at 1 week using this form of traction than by wearing corsets in patients with back pain.

Manual traction is applied by a therapist to the involved body segment (usually to an extremity) to distract joint surfaces. This technique is used to facilitate movement of the affected joint by reducing pain and structural resistance.

Joint Mobilization

Joint mobilization techniques involve therapeutic joint movement (spinal or peripheral) in patterns not possible for the patient to produce independently but critical for normal motion and painless function. Therapeutic movements include very low force rhythmic oscillation (articulation) in the pain-free threshold, sustained forces at maximum range of passive joint motion, and sudden high velocity, short amplitude thrust beyond the passive range (manipulation).

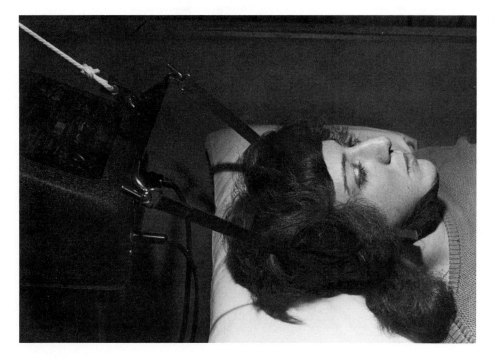

FIGURE 31-5. Cervical traction with the patient supine.

Muscle energy techniques are a form of joint mobilization that can be applied by the patient. The patient uses resisted isometric contractions to act on bony structures to cause changes in articular positioning. This frequently is used in the more stable joints (such as the sacroiliac).

Articulation is employed primarily to elongate soft tissue structures (joint capsules) to restore normal arthrokinematics. Articulation also is intended to stimulate sensory afferents that reduce pain by neurophysiologic mechanisms. Rhythmic mechanical mobilization techniques stimulate large diameter mechanoreceptors that inhibit small fiber nociceptors at the level of the spinal cord (gating) as previously described. This approach is useful when treating disorders such as adhesive capsulitis.

Manipulation

Manipulation involves delivering a thrust at the pathologic limit of the joint's range of motion. This technique is used to alter positional relationships, to sever adhesions, and to produce neurophysiologic effects. Manipulation has been used in treatment regimens for many years. Bone setters, (the original manipulators) have practiced since the beginning of recorded history and still practice in many countries. Bone setting, similar to other trades, appears to have been a

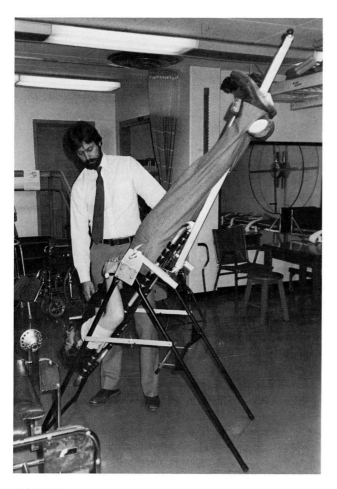

FIGURE 31-6. Inverted spinal traction.

skill passed from father to son. During the past century, two schools of manipulative therapy (the osteopathic school founded by Andrew Still in 1892 and the school of chiropractic founded by D. D. Palmer in 1895 in Davenport, Iowa) have evolved, and their practitioners are numerous and worldwide.

A large number of techniques have been developed in the field of manipulation. The two most commonly used methods are nonspecific, long lever manipulations and specific short lever, high velocity adjustments. The long lever techniques use patient structures (such as the femur, pelvis, shoulder, or arm) to exert a large nonspecific force. Short lever, high velocity adjustments are used more commonly for their specificity of results and improved degree of safety.[24] In the spine, the spinous and transverse processes of the vertebral body are the short levers used to deliver a quick, small amplitude, high velocity thrust.

Clinical trials that have examined the effectiveness of manipulation[25–28] techniques on back dysfunction and pain have found varying results. Potter[29] and Glover and colleagues[30] reported that manipulation appears to be most effective in treating the acute stages of mechanical dysfunction. Rasmussen[31] compared manipulation with short-wave diathermy in a small number of patients and found that, at 7 and 14 days, the manipulation group showed markedly improved spinal mobility and symptoms. Berquist-Ullman and Larsson,[32] in a study comparing manipulation therapy with placebo treatment, reported specific articulation and mobilization therapy to be more effective in reducing pain at 6 weeks. They also found that the treatment group had a higher rate of return to work than control subjects. Other studies have reported that manipulation techniques provide short-term benefit for back dysfunction and pain but no significant differences in long-term improvement of pain compared with placebo therapies.

There are several underlying bone and joint diseases that preclude the application of manipulative therapies. Included are disorders that weaken bone structure, severe or progressive neurologic deficits, acute inflammatory joint disease, severe joint laxity, and bleeding disorders.

Massage

Massage remains one of the oldest forms of therapy for painful conditions. It is described as manipulations of the soft tissues of the body. It is most effective when done with the hands and administered for the purpose of producing effects on the nervous and muscular systems and the local and general circulation of blood and lymph. Superficial massage tends to be relaxing, producing a mild cutaneous hyperemic response that can be a helpful adjunct to other pain therapies. Deep or connective tissue massage is applied to ligaments, tendons, muscle, and fascia. Its purpose is to provide movement in the tissues, restore normal tissue fluid exchange, improve soft tissue pliability and extensibility, and reduce scarring. In acute stages, a deep but gentle massage is used that applies forces which run transverse to the tissue fibers. The tissue movement stimulus encourages fiber realignment and lengthening and also minimizes scar tissue formation. The increased blood flow aids in the removal of metabolic waste products and reduces painful ischemia. In chronic stages, deep tissue massage is used to break up scar tissue and mobilize soft tissue structures. This technique is effective when applied to tissue in which scarring has occurred secondary to trauma (acute or chronic) and inflammatory conditions.

Deep tissue massage also has been effective in the treatment of a condition in which many hypersensitive spots of tenderness in muscle and associated connective tissue (which reproduce pain) are present. Myofascial trigger points may cause weakness, and limited range of motion, and painful dysfunction. When mechanically stimulated, a trigger point will be hypersensitive and often radiate or refer pain. In addition to massage, a spray-and-stretch technique described by Simons and Travell[16] is useful. This technique involves spraying a vapocoolant in parallel sweeps at 10 cm/s to the skin overlying the painful muscle tissue. This is followed by passive stretching and further spraying over the pain reference zone.

Exercise Programs

Exercise programs based on principles of flexibility, strength, and general conditioning should not be overlooked in pain management.[33] The subtle progression of the cumulative deterioration of soft tissue flexibility, muscular strength, and overall cardiovascular condition leads to postural imbalance and relative tissue ischemia, resulting in pain and decreased function.[34] A prospective study ranked the fitness level of 1652 California firefighters, based on flexibility, strength, and cardiovascular endurance, and compared this with the subsequent occurrence of back injuries.[22] These results indicated a protective effect of increased levels of overall fitness (least fit, 7.1 percent injured; intermediate fit, 3.2 percent injured; and most fit, 0.83 percent injured).

In another study, an approach of conditioning, strengthening, and increasing flexibility was used in an intense program with 38 patients who had chronic back pain and were receiving workmen's compensation. Functional capacity measures improved in 80 percent of the patients in 3 weeks. At 1 year, the treatment group had twice the return to work rate and a significantly decreased number of healthcare professional visits, relative to a comparison group.[20]

Aerobic Conditioning

The frequency, intensity, duration (time), and type of exercise program are essential determinants in developing an aerobic conditioning program. It is valuable to use the acronym FITT representing frequency, intensity, time, and type to teach this concept effectively to patients. The program frequency represents the number of workouts per week; the intensity is the effort expressed as a percentage of the patient's maximum capacity; the time is the length of time in each workout session; and the type refers to the exercise mode itself. The following have been shown to be the minimally acceptable guidelines for developing an exercise program that will achieve a conditioning response.

Frequency. Generally, it is accepted that an exercise program must have a frequency of at least three times per week to achieve results.[35]

Intensity. Sixty to 65 percent of maximal aerobic capacity is required. At this point in prescribing a program, it becomes necessary to determine a patient's maximal aerobic capacity. If the patient is older than 35 years of age and/or has been previously sedentary, aerobic capacity should be assessed by a medically supervised exercise tolerance test. If an exercise tolerance test is not obtained, the Karvonen formula[36] can be used to determine the training intensity.

$$\text{Training heart rate} = \text{resting heart} + 0.6 \text{ (maximal heart rate-resting heart rate)}.$$

The maximal heart rate is predicted by subtracting the patient's age from 220. If we apply the formula to a 30-year-old patient with a resting heart rate of 70 beats/min, the age-predicted maximal heart rate = 220 − 30 = 190 beats/min.

$$\begin{aligned}\text{Training heart rate} &= 70 \text{ beats/min} + 0.6 \text{ (190 beats/min} - \\ &\quad 70 \text{ beats/min)} \\ &= 142 \text{ beats/min.}\end{aligned}$$

Time. The time duration of each exercise session should be 15 to 60 min.[37] In a patient with chronic pain, it often is necessary to set 15 to 20 min as a goal to work toward, but this must be attained to achieve the desired outcomes.

Type. Guidelines for the mode of exercise include (1) exercise with large muscle masses, such as the legs; (2) select an exercise that can be done continuously; and (3) above all, select an exercise that is enjoyable to the patient and has the lowest risk of increasing pain. It may take some trial and error to determine which activity best suits the patient. Some activities that satisfy these criteria are swimming, running, fast walking, cross country skiing, bicycling, aerobic dance, and rowing.

In summary, the goal for patients with pain is to choose an aerobic activity and slowly progress to 3 or more days per week for 15 to 60 min per session, at a minimal level of 60 percent of their maximal aerobic capacity. Adequate instruction is essential to achieve the desired results from a fitness program. The participants should be provided with an explanation of the beneficial effects that general conditioning will have. They also must be given specific instruction for exercise, monitoring parameters, and physiologic cues. The group instruction approach has been used in most chronic pain units and in the increasingly popular so-called back school approach.

BACK SCHOOLS

Back pain schools incorporate a holistic educational approach, using the latest information on the prevention, treatment, and management of back disorders. The educational concept of a back pain school addresses a patient's back pain and functional disability, dependence on healthcare providers, and the tremendous financial and psychosocial burden associated with back pain. The underlying premise of back schools is that, if participants understand the physiology, psychology, and anatomy of back pain, they will manage their back problem more independently and effectively. Back school programs have been characterized as intervention programs that provide instruction to participants who have function-limiting back pain and prevention programs that provide instruction for participants who are at risk for experiencing back pain and dysfunction.

Prevention Programs

In general, prevention programs incorporate instruction in the anatomy and pathology of back pain, body mechanics and principles of lifting, positioning techniques, stress management, nutritional guidelines, symptom management, and an exercise program directed toward improving trunk strength and flexibility. Slide tapes, films, model skeletons, and other audiovisual aids are used to reinforce the content.

Prevention programs are one to six sessions in length and involve groups of six or more participants. A maximum group size of 25 participants is recommended to ensure group interaction. Prevention programs frequently are conducted in fitness centers or industrial settings. Educational goals for participants in industrial settings include an increased knowledge of the anatomy and causes of back pain and increased skills in managing back pain symptoms to result in (1) increased employee responsibility for their own health, (2) decreased pain and dysfunction, (3) increased productivity, (4) decreased absenteeism, (5) reduced workmen's compensation costs, and (6) decreased insurance premiums.

Intervention Programs

Intervention programs involve patients with function-limiting back pain and may average from 1 week to several weeks or more in duration. Group size is smaller than in the prevention program, consisting of approximately 4 to 12 patients per instructor. This allows more individualized care. The program consists of a series of classes extending over several weeks to 6 months.

Intervention programs usually are interdisciplinary and involve physicians, physical therapists, occupational health nurses, psychologists, ergonomists, and rehabilitation counselors. These programs may incorporate a physical assessment and an assessment of the participants work site. Recommendations are made to the candidate and the employer regarding the candidate's rehabilitation potential and the necessary intervention programming.

Back pain education programs (known as back schools) prove the benefits of providing knowledge for self-assessment and self-care. Berquist-Ullman and Larsson[32] studied the impact of group education in the back school on pain and return-to-work status in 217 Volvo employees with back pain of acute onset. One of the treatment groups received traditional physical therapy, including mobilization therapies and exercise. Another treatment group consisted of only the back school program, and this program included education on anatomy and causes of back pain, biomechanics, and ergonomics. It also provided the patient with guidelines for trunk strengthening, flexibility, and general conditioning. The control group received low intensity short-wave diathermy in a dose that would not produce any physiologic change. The results showed that the physical therapy and back school groups had significantly decreased duration of symptoms compared with the control group. Furthermore, the back school group returned to work earlier than the physical therapy and placebo groups. This study found that manual therapy and exercise-conditioning programs are effective in decreasing the duration of pain symptoms. It also showed that the education focus and group process incorporated into the back school enabled the patient to return to work at an earlier date. There are several explanations for this, but perhaps the group support engendered by this approach and the emphasis on self-assessment and control of the cause and effect of back pain are the most effective aspects of this approach.

CONCLUSION

Physical measures produce beneficial patient outcomes in both subacute and chronic pain management; however, they are maximally effective when applied in early stages. These measures aid in the reduction of pain and promote healing. Therefore, the chances of subacute pain progressing to a chronic pain syndrome are minimized. In my experience, the best results occur when electrical and temperature techniques are combined with gentle exercise and mobilization, in conjunction with rest.

If pain progresses to the chronic stage, the rate of subsequent improvement is much slower, predisposing the patient to the development of dependent pain behaviors. At this point, physical measures should shift to those in which the patient has direct control and is able to function independently. Superficial hot and cold and home electrical units are techniques that the patient can use effectively to aid in pain management. After a careful evaluation, specific exercise programs that the patient can follow with minimal professional monitoring are tailored to the patient's needs. This approach has been effective, not only in controlling the physiologic sequelae of pain, but also in involving patients in their own care, which is, in itself, useful in treating the psychosocial sequelae of pain.

References

1. Moncur C, Shields MN. Physiotherapy methods of relieving pain. *Baillieres Clin Rheumatol* April 1987; 1(1):183–193.
2. Hyvarinen J, Karlsson M. Low resistance skin points that may coincide with acupuncture loci. *Med Biol* 1977; 55(2)88–94.
3. Melzack R, Wall P. Pain mechanisms: a new theory. *Science* 1965; 150:971.
4. Wall PD. The gate theory of pain mechanisms: a re-examination and restatement. *Brain* 1978; 101, 1–18.
5. Snyder S. Opiate receptors and internal opiates. *Sci Am* 1977; 236:44.
6. Cheng R, McKibben L, Roy B, Pomeranz B. Electroacupuncture elevates blood cortisol levels in native horses. *J Neurosci* 1980; 10:95.
7. Han J, Terenius L. Neurochemical basis of acupuncture analgesia. *Annu Rev Pharmacol Toxicol* 1982; 22:193–220.
8. Cheng R, Pomeranz B. Electroacupuncture analgesia could be mediated by at least two pain relieving mechanisms: endorphin and non-endorphin systems. *Life Sci* 1979; 25, 1957–1962.
9. Ersek RS. Low back pain: prompt relief with transcutaneous electrical nerve stimulation. *Orthop Rev* 1976; 5:12.
10. Melzack R. Prolonged relief of pain by brief, intense transcutaneous electrical stimulation. *Pain* 1975; 1:357.
11. Kinsman A. Clinical effects and uses of inferential current therapy. Presentation at the Australian Physiotherapy Association Congress; August 1975; Sydney, Australia.
12. Harris P. Iontophoresis: clinical research in musculoskeletal inflammatory conditions. *J Orthop Sports Phys Ther* 1982:109–112.
13. Glass J, Stephen R, Jacobson C. The quantity and distribution of radiolabeled dexamethasone delivered to tissue by iontophoresis. *Int J Dermatol* 1980; 19(9):519–525.
14. Goats GC. Microwave diathermy. *Br J Sports Med* December 1990; Dec;24(4):212–218.
15. Sapega A, Quedenfeld J, Moyer R, Butler R. Biophysical factors in range of motion exercises. *Physician Sports Med* 1981; 9:157.
16. Simons D, Travell T. Myofascial origins of low back pain. *Postgrad Med* 1983; 73(2)66–108.
17. Harvey W, Dyson M, Pond J, Graham R. The in vitro stimulation of protein in human fibroblasts by therapeutic levels of ultrasound. In: *Proceedings of the Second European Congress of Ultrasound in Medicine (International Congress Series 363)*. Princeton: Excerpta Medica; 1975:10–21.
18. Lehman J, Stonebridge J, Delateur B, Warren G, Halar J. Temperature in human thighs after hot pack treatment followed by ultrasound. *Arch Phys Med* 1978; 59:470.
19. Cady L, Bischoft D, O'Connell E, Thomas P, Allan J. Strength and fitness and subsequent back injuries in firefighters. *J Occup Med* 1979; 21:269.
20. Mayer TG, Gatchel RJ, Kishino N, et al. Assessment of spine function following industrial injury. *Spine* 1985; 10(6):482–493.
21. Judovich B, Nobel G. Traction therapy, a study of resistive forces: preliminary report on new method of lumbar traction. *Am J Surg* 1957; 93:108.
22. Burton C. The Sister Kenney Institute, gravity lumbar reduction program in low back pain. In: Finneson B, ed. *Low Back Pain*. 2nd ed. Philadelphia: Lippincott; 1980:277–280.
23. Larsson U, Choler U, Lidstrom A, et al. Auto traction for treatment of lumbago-sciatica: a multicentre controlled investigations. *Acta Orthop Scand* 1980; 51:791–798.
24. Kleynhaus AM. Complications of and contraindications to spinal manipulative therapy. In: Haldeman S, ed. *Modern Developments in the Principles and Practice of Chiropractic*. New York: Appleton-Century-Crofts; 1980.
25. Klinoski B, Lebouf C. A review of the research papers published by the International College of Applied Kinesiology from 1981 to 1987. *J Manipulative Physiol Ther* May 1990; 13(4):190–194.
26. Lumbar intervertebral disc herniation: treatment by rotational manipulative. *J Manipulative Physiol Ther* January 1990; 13(1):36–42.
27. Fitz-Ritson D. The chiropractic management and rehabilitation of cervical trauma. *J Manipulative Physiol Ther* January 1990; 13(1):17–25.
28. Lebouf C. A review of data reports published in the *Journal of Manipulative and Physiological Therapeutic* from 1986 to 1988. *J Manipulative Physiol Ther* February 1990; 13(2):89–95.
29. Potter G. A study of 744 cases of neck and back pain treated with spinal manipulation. *J Can Chiropract Assoc* 1977; 21:154.
30. Glover J, Morris J, Khosla T. Back pain: a randomized clinical trial of rotational manipulation of trunk. *Br J Ind Med* 1974; 31:59.
31. Rasmussen G. Manipulations in low back pain: a randomized clinical trial. *Manuelle Med* 1977; 1:8.
32. Berquist-Ullman M, Larsson U. Acute low back pain in industry. *Acta Orthop Scand* 1977; 170:1.
33. Koes BW, Boeter LM, Beckerman H, Van der Heijdan GJ, Knipschild PG. Physiotherapy exercises and back pain: a blinded review. *BMJ* June 29 1991; 302(6792):1572–1576.
34. Hicks JE. Rehabilitation and biomechanics. *Curr Opin Rheumatol* April 1990; 2(2):320–326.
35. Lamb D. *Physiology of Exercise: Responses and Adaptations*. New York: Macmillan; 1978.
36. Karvonen M, Kentala J, Mustula O. The effects of training on heart rate: a longitudinal study. *Ann Med Exp Biol Fenniae* 1957; 35:305.
37. Fox E, Mathews D. *Physiological Basis of Physical Education and Athletics*. Philadelphia: Saunders; 1981.

CHAPTER 32

Behavioral Therapy

Alice D. Domar, Richard Friedman, and Herbert Benson

The prevalence, persistence, and the all too often refractory nature of chronic pain syndromes is well known. Clinicians responsible for the treatment of chronic pain are acutely aware of the need to address the psychosocial and the physical aspects of pain. Pain is not simply an index of organic disease or tissue damage, but it also represents an experience resulting from a complex interaction of biochemical, physiological, behavioral, emotional, and cognitive factors. The almost universal acceptance of this multifactorial conceptualization for the cause and exacerbation of pain has resulted logically in treatment programs that attempt to remediate pain by addressing all these factors[1] and provide assessment strategies that separate the sensory and reactive components of the pain experience.[2]

In this chapter, the behavioral methods used as an adjunct to traditional pharmacotherapy, surgery, and other pain treatments will be reviewed. The rationale for the incorporation of such methods into a comprehensive pain-management program is compelling. Despite considerable efforts, medical and surgical approaches often have been unsuccessful in relieving chronic pain.[3–6] Long-term use of pharmacologic agents usually is contraindicated in patients with chronic pain because of the dangers of habituation, addiction, precipitation of withdrawal, and fibrosis of muscle sites associated with frequent injections.[3] More invasive procedures are costly and only may eliminate nociception in a small selection of patients.[7]

Anxiety and its attendant physiologic arousal increases the pain experience, leading to more anxiety and more arousal. Behavioral methods can reduce anxiety and arousal, thereby reversing this cycle.[8] The behavioral approaches to pain management can produce beneficial alterations in both psychological and physiologic functioning.[9] There are five basic behavioral interventions used for chronic pain. They are: (1) relaxation training, (2) hypnosis, (3) biofeedback, (4) operant conditioning, and (5) cognitive-behavioral therapy. Each intervention will be discussed in the following sections. However, one must remember that these interventions are not mutually exclusive.

RELAXATION TECHNIQUES

There is a basic incompatibility between the emotional response to relaxation and the emotional reactive component of pain, commonly referred to as suffering. Based on the premise that it is impossible simultaneously to be relaxed and anxious, it has been hypothesized that, if a patient can become relaxed and tranquil, then suffering should abate.[10] In addition, it is believed that muscular relaxation can break the pain cycle. When bodily injury occurs, causing pain, the natural tendency is to tense muscles to immobilize the site and protect against further trauma. Although this has value in minimizing acute pain, chronic muscle tension can produce more pain, then more tension, and the initiation of a self-sustaining cycle. Relaxation techniques can terminate this cycle.[4]

Various relaxation techniques have been used in the treatment of chronic pain, including progressive relaxation, autogenic training, and meditation. Progressive relaxation attempts to achieve increased discriminative control over skeletal muscle. It is practiced in a supine position in a quiet room. A passive attitude is essential because mental images induce slight measurable tensions in the muscle, especially those of the eyes and face. The subject is taught to recognize even slight muscle contractions so that they can be avoided to achieve the deepest degree of relaxation possible.[11]

Most investigations of relaxation training for chronic pain have been conducted with tension headaches. These show significant decreases in headache frequency after relaxation training. The treatment effects generally are maintained at follow-up.[6] In a review of behavioral treatments for chronic pain, Turner and Chapman[5] concluded that progressive muscle relaxation leads to significant reductions in tension and migraine headache frequency and, in one study, to some extent, in the suffering of patients with myofascial pain dysfunction. In a representative study of 91 patients with chronic headache (33 tension, 30 migraine, and 28 combined), who attended a 10-session relaxation training program and were instructed to practice progressive muscle relaxation 20 min a day, most had significant reductions in headache activity. Sixty-four percent of the patients with tension headache, 53 percent of those with migraine, and 54 percent of the combined headache group had significant improvement.[12]

Meditative practices, such as yoga, are similar to relaxation and have been an important part of Indian culture for thousands of years. Similar techniques have been described in other cultures, such as Japan and China.[13] Reports in the 1950s and 1960s indicated that yogic meditation could produce various physiologic effects, such as reducing the rate of metabolism and increasing alpha waves on EEGs.[14] The practice of Zen, yoga, or transcendental meditation led to specific physiologic changes, including decreased oxygen consumption, heart rate, and respiratory rate and increased skin resistance and alpha brain waves.[15] Transcendental meditation rapidly became popular in the treatment of stress-related disorders based on its simplicity and apparent effectiveness for achieving deep relaxation.

The regular practice of transcendental meditation had been reported to yield unique physiologic, psychological, medical, and sociologic results, including remediation of chronic pain. In one report of four spinal cord-injured patients with complaints of chronic pain below the level of the spinal lesion, regular practice of a relaxation–meditation procedure resulted in less reported pain and mood improvements.[16] The hospital staff observed improved rehabilitation program attendance and mood. There were no statistical analyses of the reports, however, nor any control group for comparison purposes. In another uncontrolled study, hemophiliac patients with chronic arthritic pain regularly practiced meditation.[17] Again, long-term improvements in sleep,[18] mobility, pain, medication requirements, and reductions in bleeding episodes were reported.[15]

There are two major classes of meditation practice: concentration and mindfulness meditation (which presupposes concentration to maintain steady attention). Thus, although transcendental meditation restricts attention to a single point or object (usually a mental sound), mindfulness meditation emphasizes detached observations from one moment to the next. The expansion of the field of attention is taught gradually during a number of sessions. In a recent study using mindfulness meditation as a treatment for pain,[19] 51 subjects attended a 10-week training course that provided instruction in the technique. All patients had chronic pain, ranging from lower back pain to angina to pelvic pain; pain duration ranged from 6 months to 48 years. After 10 weeks, 65 percent of the patients showed greater than 33 percent reductions on the Melzack–McGill pain questionnaire, and 50 percent of the patients showed greater than 50 percent reductions. There were similar decreases in other pain indexes and in the number of medical symptoms reported. There were large significant decreases in mood disturbances and psychiatric symptoms. These changes were all relatively stable at follow-ups at 2, 4, and 7 months.

HYPNOSIS

Hypnosis is an induced state characterized by increased suggestability. Hypnotized subjects manifest high levels of response to test suggestions, such as muscle rigidity, amnesia, hallucinations, posthypnotic suggestion, and anesthesia.[20] There have been many instances in which hypnosis was the sole anesthetic during procedures ranging

from appendectomies to open heart surgery.[21] That it is possible to do major surgery with the patient under hypnosis as the only anesthesia is a dramatic example of the profound influence that psychological factors can have on the perception of pain. It is important to recognize, however, that patient responsivity to hypnosis for pain relief does not imply that the pain has a psychological cause. Hypnosis is not an appropriate treatment for functional pain; that is, it is not an effective means of modifying the behavior of a patient who is not ready nor willing to modify that behavior.[22]

Hypnosis is used widely for various pain conditions despite the fact that there are few controlled studies examining its efficacy.[23] In one laboratory experiment, hypnosis was compared with acupuncture, placebo point stimulation, morphine, aspirin, diazepam, and a drug placebo in reducing cold-pressor and tourniquet-induced pain.[24] Hypnosis produced significantly more effective levels of anesthesia than any other intervention. In a controlled study that investigated the use of hypnosis in the treatment of chronic pain, 30 patients with chronic pain were assigned randomly to one of three groups.[25] All patients participated in 12 30-min weekly sessions. The first group attended psychotherapy sessions where inter- and intrapersonal problems were discussed. Relaxation was mentioned, but not taught, and no specific instructions for pain relief were provided. The second group was given a placebo drug that was called a "new potent pain drug." The sessions were spent discussing the drug. Patients in the third group were given specific training in relaxation and hypnotherapeutic pain relief. The hypnotherapy was designed individually. After the 12 weeks, placebo patients did not improve on any scale. Sixty-six percent of the psychotherapy group obtained pain relief, but the others became worse. All patients in the hypnosis group improved significantly; 6 of 10 patients had 100 percent improvement. These therapeutic gains were still apparent at a 3-year follow-up.

Various case reports describe how hypnosis has been used to treat acute and chronic pain conditions. It can be used (1) to give direct suggestions for the relief of pain, (2) to facilitate psychotherapeutic treatment intended to help the patient gain understanding as to the meaning of pain and to achieve mastery over it, and (3) to facilitate other behavioral treatments. Sixty to 90 percent of burned patients who used hypnosis during redressing of wounds and debridement achieved substantial relief from the pain. It also was effective in dentistry, especially in patients with severe dental phobias. Terminally ill patients with cancer have used hypnosis to help them gain control over persistent acute pain. This particular application goes beyond mere pain control but also treats the psychological and emotional significance of the disease. Children undergoing bone-marrow aspirations have benefitted from the use of hypnosis, as have a small percentage of obstetric patients.[22]

Unfortunately, not all patients are hypnotizable. There are wide individual differences in the ability to be hypnotized. Some respond to difficult suggestions; others are unable to respond at all. Most individuals fall somewhere in between. In one study on patients undergoing dental treatment under hypnosis, the amount of pain experienced correlated with hypnotizability.[21] This trait is reasonably stable, and motivation does not appear to be particularly important. Therefore, it is difficult to compare hypnoanalgesia with other pain treatments because of the variability of hypnotizability. Most of the cited hypnosis pain research prescreened patients and only included hypnotizable subjects.[22]

The mechanism by which hypnosis alleviates pain is not understood and has been a source of controversy. However, traditional methods of hypnotic induction use the same basic elements employed to achieve deep relaxation or meditational states.[26] Although many different techniques induce hypnosis, most rely on the repetition of a monotonous stimulus, narrowing of the subject's attention, suggestion of relaxation and drowsiness in the subject, closed eyes, a recumbent or semisupine position, and reduction of environmental stimulation. Before hypnotic phenomena are experienced, a physiologic state characterized by reduced heart rate, respiratory rate, and blood pressure, and increased alpha activity on EEG occurs.[26] After these physiologic changes, subjects experience other exclusively hypnotic phenomena (such as perceptual distortions, age regression, posthypnotic suggestion, and amnesia).

In conclusion, hypnosis may be a promising method for treating some patients with pain. Many case studies using hypnosis report good results with various pain syndromes, including cancer pain, neck and shoulder pain, headaches, and phantom limb pain. However, there has been a paucity of clinical research; the research that has been conducted is poor methodologically and uses case history formats, no control groups for comparison purposes, and few subjects. There have been almost no controlled studies that compare hypnosis with a credible control group.[27] Thus, further research is needed before we can recommend definitively the use of hypnosis in the treatment of painful conditions.

THE RELAXATION RESPONSE

Most relaxation interventions have, as an underlying feature, a constellation of predictable and reproducible physiologic alterations. Similarly, before experiencing hypnotic phenomena, the patient first elicits similar physiologic changes. It has been suggested that specific training in the use of relaxation therapy to produce the physiologic alteration might allow even those with minimal hypnotizability to enter a hypnotic state.[21] The persistence of the fairly uniform set of physiologic changes in a wide variety of techniques is striking. It has led to the theory that elicitation of such alterations might be the active and therapeutic aspect of such varied interventions. This set of specific reproducible physiologic changes has been termed the *relaxation response*.[28] Regular elicitation of the relaxation response has been effective in the management of pain.

This response is an innate physiologic response shared by many techniques, and it should not be identified or confused with any one procedure. Several secular techniques have been used to elicit the relaxation response. Two elements appear to be necessary: a passive attitude and a mental device such as a word, sound, phrase, or prayer that is repeated audibly or silently. Many subjective experiences associated with the elicitation of the relaxation response constitute an altered state of consciousness. Subjective experiences have been described as peace of mind, feeling at ease with the world, and a sense of well-being. Despite the diversity of the descriptions of these experiences, there are striking similarities between the techniques used to achieve the same altered states.[29]

The elicitation of the relaxation response results in integrated physiologic changes coincident with decreased activity of the sympathetic nervous system. There is decreased oxygen consumption, carbon dioxide elimination, respiratory rate, heart rate, blood pressure, muscle tonus, minute ventilation, and arterial blood lactate and increased intensity of slow alpha waves, occasional theta wave activity (as seen on EEG), and skin resistance.[13] The relaxation response is believed to be the counterpart of the emergency or so-called fight-or-flight response. The emergency response is mediated by the sympathetic nervous system. When stimulated, it produces dilatation of the pupils and increased blood pressure, respiratory rate, and motor excitability.[30] The relaxation response leads to generalized decreased sympathetic nervous system activity, thereby directly opposing the emergency reaction. Both responses probably are mediated through activation of the hypothalamic areas of the brain.[26] The relaxation response, when elicited in humans, resembles the trophotropic syndrome described by Hess[28] after electrical stimulation of the hypothalamus in cats. This author postulated that this response functioned as a protective mechanism against overstress and that it countered the emergency fight-or-flight response described earlier.[29]

Patients with chronic pain often show abnormal psychophysiologic response patterns. Sympathetic nervous system hyperactivity is considered one of the major psychophysiologic mechanisms of chronic pain.[3] Thus far, however, it has been difficult to determine the exact mechanism(s) by which the relaxation response produces analgesia. Recent studies revealed that stimulation of the anterior hypothalamus produces powerful inhibition of spinal cord dorsal horn responses to nociception.[31] The close proximity of many of the hypothalamic stimulation sites to the arcuate nucleus and the location of β-endorphin cells in the brain raises the possibility that Hess was evoking an endorphinergic mechanism. However, currently, to our knowledge, no one has tested this hypothesis explicitly by examining the effects of endorphin-blocking drugs, such as naloxone, on the trophotropic syndrome. In humans, naloxone interferes with the ability to focus thinking and inhibits the ability to elicit the relaxation response. Thus, attempts to test the possible endorphinergic mediation of relaxation response-induced pain suppression have been inconclusive. The effects of naloxone on clinical hypnotic analgesia have been contradictory as are the studies investigating naloxone's effects on placebo analgesia.[29] A neurochemical basis for the effectiveness of the elicitation of the relaxation response in pain management has not been established.

One physiologic feature of the relaxation response that might be related to pain management is the presence of increased alpha waves in EEGs.[14] Painful experiences can cause decreased alpha activity. This reduction may be related to increased cortical arousal, although the precise nature of this relationship is not clear. Because elicitation of the relaxation response combines increased alpha activity with attentional modification and suggestion, the synergistic effects may explain the successful use of this response in the treatment of pain.

Another hypothesis postulated to explain the efficacy of the relaxation response in the treatment of chronic pain is based on studies of mindfulness meditation.[19] When patients assume the attentional stance of mindfulness meditation, a spontaneous and momentary uncoupling of the sensory component of pain from the affective and cognitive dimensions appears to occur. When the technique is practiced regularly, a deconditioning of the alarm reaction to the primary pain sensation occurs. The nociceptive signals appear to be undiminished, but the emotional and cognitive components of the pain experience (hurt and suffering) are reduced.

One of the most important features of the relaxation response is that the changes in sympathetic reactivity have carry-over effects that last longer than the actual period during which the mental exercise is done. This is important and helpful in the treatment of patients with chronic pain because the benefits are not limited to the exercise periods but instead can last throughout the day.

In conclusion, techniques that elicit the relaxation response for the treatment of chronic pain appear to be efficient and pragmatic. Instruction in the various techniques are relatively simple, and it only requires one therapist, usually for one session. The techniques can be learned easily, and the transfer of practice from the hospital to home environment does not present any problem.

Our laboratory has incorporated elements common to many historic relaxation techniques into a simple nonreligious technique.[32] Instruction in the technique takes approximately 5 min. The instructions are as follows.

1. Sit quietly in a comfortable position with your back straight. Close your eyes.
2. Deeply relax all your muscles, beginning at your feet and progressing up to your face. Keep them deeply relaxed.
3. Breathe through your nose. Become aware of your breathing. As you breathe out, say a particular word or phrase silently to yourself. For example, if your word was one, you would breathe in . . . out, one; in . . . out, one; etc. Continue for 20 min. You may open your eyes to check the time but do not use an alarm clock. When you finish, sit quietly for several minutes with your eyes closed and then with your eyes open.
4. Do not worry about whether or not you are successful in achieving a deep level of relaxation. Maintain a passive attitude and permit relaxation to occur at its own pace. You should expect other thoughts. When distracting thoughts occur, ignore them by thinking "Oh well" and continue to be aware of your breathing and the silent repetition of your word or phrase. With practice, the response should come with little effort.
5. Practice the technique once or twice per day. Do not practice the technique within 2 h after a meal because digestive processes seem to interfere with the subjective changes.

BIOFEEDBACK

Biofeedback is another behavioral treatment often with a more circumscribed approach than that using relaxational, meditational, and hypnotic procedures. During the past 15 years, there has been a proliferation of articles, books, workshops, training programs, and research centers devoted to biofeedback and the regulation of pain. It is one of the most widely publicized behavioral treatments.[33] In 1962, two articles presented evidence that autonomic nervous system responses in animals could be shaped by instrumental methods and that EEG alpha rhythms could be altered by operant procedures in humans. This preliminary research led to the core concept of biofeedback (that is, accurate and salient feedback will enable a patient to gain at least partial voluntary control over normally autonomic physiologic changes.[34] However, the seminal preliminary data still have not been replicated. Furthermore, the efficacy of biofeedback training in general and its viability in the treatment of pain in particular has not been documented.[33,35]

Biofeedback uses physiologic instrumentation to provide information about changes in otherwise nonconscious biologic processes. Generally, a distinctive visual or auditory signal is provided to the patient, indicating that a particular physiologic event has occurred. Through a process of trial and error, the subject presumably learns to recognize a particular subjective state and subtle internal changes associated with alterations of the particular physiologic response. As the subject becomes more proficient at such recognition and alteration, the instrument sensitivity is adjusted to permit gradual shaping of the desired physiologic response. The intent is to provide patients with information that will enable them to control voluntarily an aspect of their physiology that purportedly is linked causally to the pathogenesis of a given disease. Such strategies have been used to reduce the pain experience. The most obvious assumption in this instance is that the patient can learn to control some physiologic factors that are either producing or exacerbating the pain.[7,33] Physiologic indexes vary from study to study and have included electromyograms (EMGs) of various muscles in different parts of the body, skin temperature, pulse volume, and EEG wave forms.[36]

Although biofeedback has been used to treat many pain syndromes,[37] the most common by far has been EMG feedback for muscle contraction headache. There also have been reports of the efficacy of biofeedback in the treatment of vascular headache, Raynaud syndrome, arthritis, and low back pain.[36] The preponderance of actual research studies, however, do not support the unique effectiveness of biofeedback. Critics of the biofeedback techniques claim that the principles on which biofeedback is based grossly oversimplify the nature of chronic pain and that there is little support for these concepts. For example, in studies of EMG biofeedback in patients with headaches, muscle tension levels were not associated strongly with changes in headache activity. Furthermore, decreases in muscle tension did not seem to mediate improvement.[5,6] Several biofeedback studies produced seemingly paradoxic results; for example, hand warming and cooling both were equally effective in treating headaches. Pseudobiofeedback also has been as effective as "real" biofeedback in the treatment of chronic pain, leading researchers to conclude that the beneficial effects of biofeedback stem from nonspecific effects (such as the placebo effect).[36,38]

There has been a lack of consistency in biofeedback research. These include the study of many different pain syndromes, variations in pain history; a lack of collection of baseline rates of pain, and different biofeedback procedures. There also have been many methodologic problems such as lack of control conditions, potential biases in subject selection, lack of evaluation of experimenter attention, and inadequate follow-up. Some processes have been proposed as mediators for improvement during biofeedback: measurement artifacts, personality treatment interactions, anxiety reduction, enhanced sense of self-control, therapist contact, and the relaxation instructions themselves.[7,36]

Thus, there remain many unknowns about the efficacy of biofeedback in the treatment of pain. The evidence in support of using biofeedback for the treatment of pain is marginal at best, resting mainly on case studies and poorly controlled research. Biofeedback in pain management seems less well grounded theoretically, and hence, its lack of empiric substantiation is particularly significant.[34] In addition, the emphasis on unitary physiologic aspects tends to ignore the complex psychological, affective, and behavioral components that frequently are involved in the pain experience.[7] In an extensive review of the literature on biofeedback and pain, Turk and colleagues[33] concluded that biofeedback should be considered a research tool only. In addition, numerous controlled direct comparisons of biofeedback and relaxation training have shown them to be equally efficacious.[12,34–36,39] Relaxation training is simpler to administer and more cost-effective. Because relaxation is transferred more easily from the hospital environment to the home and biofeedback requires extensive practice, relaxation training would be the treatment of choice.[25,38] Furthermore, despite the relatively circumscribed nature of biofeedback training protocols, such training, especially when it is successful, actually may result in the set of physiologic changes described in the relaxation response. In the authors' experience, the use of biofeedback training often produces patient reports of increased ability to focus mentally and to ignore intrusive thoughts passively. Hence, biofeedback may represent an automated indirect method for achieving the relaxation response.

With this caveat in mind, the evidence supports the efficacy of biofeedback in conjunction with other behavioral treatments. For example, when patients with chronic pain were trained in either hypnosis, alpha EEG biofeedback, or a combination of the two methods, only the patients who received both kinds of interventions had significant decreases in pain ratings over baseline.[40] There is also some indication that biofeedback may be an adjunct to relaxation-response training in migraine and tension headache pain.[21] Finally, one study found that biofeedback could be used as the second treatment of choice for headache pain.[12] Patients who did not achieve at least a 60 percent reduction in headache activity after relaxation-response training were offered biofeedback. Of the patients who then did attend the biofeedback sessions, 53 percent of those with tension, 50 percent of those with migraine, and 78 percent of those with combined headaches had markedly lessened headache activity. Thus, biofeedback may have potential use as an adjunctive treatment.

THE OPERANT APPROACH

The operant approach for the treatment of pain consists of the therapist's providing attention and affection when the patient engages in healthy or adaptive behaviors.[41] When the patient engages in pain behaviors, such as moaning or taking medications, the therapist remains neutral and undemonstrative. The essence of the approach is that we can extinguish pain behavior through negative reinforcement while simultaneously shaping well behaviors through positive reinforcement. The core of this therapy is the acquisition of desired skills by the patient using the skillful and systematic application of the principles of reinforcement.[4,42–44]

Operant programs usually are initiated in an inpatient hospital setting, and hence, their utility may be limited. The goals are to decrease pain medications, levels, and behaviors and to increase physical activity and other constructive behaviors. Medications are given on a time-contingent rather than pain-contingent schedule and gradually are decreased. Hospital staff and family members are trained not to reinforce pain behaviors with sympathy but instead to ignore such behavior and reinforce well behavior. Every study of operant treatments has reported increases in activity levels and large decreases in medication needs, but there have only been minor reductions in pain ratings.

The improvements tend to lessen slightly at follow-up, although the increased activity and decreased medications are, for the most part, maintained for 1 to 8 years. However, patients have been selected carefully for such programs and the rejection, refusal, and drop-out rates often are as high as 40 percent. There is little information as to whether these programs reduce pain.[4,27,43]

The operant management research often has several inadequacies: small numbers of patients, no control groups, no follow-ups in many studies, retrospective reports of pain, no isolation of operant treatments from other treatments, no pain ratings, a select population of patients, and no physiologic measurements. Thus, the impact of operant conditioning on the experience of pain has not been determined. It is also the most expensive behavioral approach because the treatment typically involves several weeks of inpatient care.[4,6,43]

THE COGNITIVE-BEHAVIORAL APPROACH

The basic assumption of the cognitive-behavioral approach is that the attitudes, beliefs, and expectations that we maintain in certain situations determine our emotional and behavioral reactions to these situations.[45,46] Because cognitive and emotional variables influence the experience of pain, it seems logical that modifying these cognitions could lead to changes of the experience of pain.[27] The normal well-intentioned and often beneficial bedside interactions between patients and health-care providers is, in a real sense, a cognitive-behavioral approach to pain management. Similarly, the advice, support, and encouragement of friends and relatives falls into this category. What distinguishes the cognitive-behavioral approach from a good bedside manner and the supportive social network is the systematic application of empirically based psychologic principles. These include various treatment strategies and techniques. Patients are taught pain-control strategies (such as relabeling sensations, relaxation, and imagery). They also are taught to become more aware both of events that exacerbate their pain (to avoid or deal more effectively with pain-increasing events), and events that reduce the pain. This approach can give a patient a new sense of control over pain that replaces the feelings of anxiety, helplessness, and hopelessness.[27,47] Cognitive-behavioral treatment programs typically work toward individually prescribed behavioral goals; patients learn to identify cognitive and affective responses to pain and use relaxation techniques, imagery, and coping self-statements to lessen pain and stress.[48]

Cognitive-behavioral approaches enhance tolerance to nociceptive procedures and show promise in the treatment of many pain syndromes, including tension and migraine headaches, abdominal pain, and myofascial pain dysfunction syndrome.[6,27] The exact mechanisms of action are not known, although the data tend to support the importance of modulating pain perception, possibly by "closing" the pain gate. Treatment also might prevent or block abnormal reverberatory neural activity.[1] The treatment can be used in outpatient and group formats. Hence, it is cost-effective.

Because the cognitive behavioral approach is the most recent of the behavioral strategies, there is a paucity of research to confirm the clinical reports. One study compared the cognitive-behavioral approach to relaxation training alone.[40] Thirty-six patients with lower back pain of at least 6 months' duration were recruited into the study and divided into one of three groups. The first group of patients were the control group and received no intervention. The second group of patients attended five weekly 90-min sessions where they were instructed in progressive muscle relaxation. They were provided with audiotapes of the relaxation procedure and instructed to practice at least once daily. The third group of patients received cognitive-behavioral therapy. They also were taught progressive muscle relaxation, but less group time was spent on relaxation instruction. The remaining time was spent on behavioral goals, modification of responses to pain, and learning to use relaxation, imagery, and coping self-statements to handle their pain. At the end of the 5-week training programs, both the relaxation and the cognitive-behavioral patients improved significantly over the control patients on self-reported measures of pain, depression, and disability and on observer's ratings of physical and psychosocial dysfunction. The cognitive-behavioral treatment group rated themselves as having improved more in the ability to tolerate pain and participate in normal activities than the other two groups. The control patients stayed the same or became worse. At the 1-month follow-up, the relaxation patients showed no further improvements, and their pain levels rose slightly. The cognitive-behavioral patients showed further improvement. Both groups of patients reported practicing relaxation approximately once a day. At follow-ups at 1.5 to 2 years, both the relaxation and the cognitive-behavioral patients showed significant pre- to posttreatment improvements. There were no significant differences between the two groups; both were significantly better than the control patients in pain ratings. There were no differences between the two treatment groups in how often they practiced relaxation, how well they learned to relax, and how satisfied they were with their treatment. The relaxation patients had a 74 percent reduction in health-care visits, and the cognitive-behavioral patients had a 79 percent reduction. The only significant difference between the two treatment groups was that the cognitive-behavioral one showed significant increases in the number of hours worked. The number of hours nearly doubled from pre- to posttreatment.

Thus, there is at least preliminary evidence to indicate that the cognitive-behavioral approach may be beneficial for patients with chronic pain. However, there is little evidence to indicate that the technique is superior to the relaxation technique.

CONCLUSIONS

Although the psychological therapies we presented may seem varied and superficially diverse, they share the basic fundamental assumption that reactions to pain can be modified to lessen the pain itself or tolerate the pain experience better.[49] Even modest reductions in pain perception are important because they may provide the opportunity and incentive to increase therapeutic activity levels that lead to improved strength and range of motion and increased general activity levels. In turn, this reduces the additional pain associated with immobilization.[1]

The lack of well-controlled experimental investigations with appropriate follow-ups and outcome measures for virtually all behavioral interventions prevents conclusive statements about their absolute effectiveness. In fairness, however, many of the more traditional pharmacologic and surgical approaches have as small an empiric base, despite a longer history. Some behavioral techniques have potential, based on clinical reports and preliminary research data.[50] Furthermore, the sensory aspects of pain cause psychological reactions (such as anxiety) that produce physiological arousal through the autonomic nervous system, leading to still more pain and anxiety. This cycle of psychophysiologic activation, as any clinician knows, must be disrupted. Traditional medical approaches enter the cycle at the sensory level by alterating nerve conduction and biochemical alterations in the central nervous system. The basic tenet of all behavioral approaches is to enter the cycle at the psychological level, thereby initiating a beneficial downward spiral of less anxiety, less arousal, and in the long run, less actual pain.

The challenge confronting proponents of behavioral approaches to pain management is not to convince the medical and scientific community that behavioral interventions are a necessary component of integrated care. Clinicians do not dispute this. The challenge lies in devising appropriate experiments that will allow some rational distillation of the currently available programs, thereby permitting a more reasonable patient–intervention match. Although questions concerning mechanisms of action, idiosyncratic responsivity, and assessment specificity still must be addressed, clinicians are confronted daily with suffering patients for whom neither medication nor surgery has been completely beneficial. These patients can be treated with behavioral approaches that hold real promise for returning a degree of control and well-being to their lives.

References

1. Turk D, Meichenbaum D, Genest M. *Pain and Behavioral Medicine: A Cognitive-Behavioral Approach.* New York: Guilford Press; 1983.
2. Tursky B, Jamner L, Friedman R. The pain perception profile. A psychophysical approach to the assessment of pain report. *Behav Ther* 1982; 13:376–394.
3. Keefe F. Behavioral assessment and treatment of chronic pain: current status and future directions. *J Consult Clin Psychol* 1982; 50:896–911.
4. Linton S. A critical review of behavioral treatments for chronic benign pain other than headache. *Br J Clin Psychol* 1982; 21:321–337.
5. Turner K, Chapman C. Psychological interventions for chronic pain: a critical review, I: relaxation training and biofeedback. *Pain* 1982; 12:1–21.
6. Turner J, Romano J. Evaluating psychologic interventions for chronic pain: issues and recent developments. In: Benedetti C, Chapman C, Moricca C, eds. *Recent Advances in the Management of Pain.* New York: Raven Press; 1984.
7. Trifletti J. The psychological effectiveness of pain management procedures in the context of behavioral medicine and medical psychology. *Gen Psychol Monogr* 1984:109, 251–278.
8. McKee MG. Behavioral techniques in pain modification. *Cleve Clin J Med* July–August 1989; 56(5):502–508.
9. Turner JA, Clancy S, McQuade KJ, Cardenas DD. Effectiveness of behavioral therapy for chronic low back pain: a component analysis. *J Consult Clin Psychol* October 1990; 58(5):573–579.
10. Aronoff G, Kamen R, Evans W. The relaxation response: a behavioral answer for chronic pain patients. *Behav Med* 1981; 8:20–25.
11. Jacobson E. *You Must Relax.* New York: McGraw-Hill; 1962.
12. Blanchard T, Andrasik F, Neff D, et al. Biofeedback and relaxation training with three kinds of headache: treatment effects and their prediction. *J Consult Clin Psychol* 1982; 50:52–57.
13. Benson H, Beary J, Carol M. The relaxation response. *Psychiatry* 1974; 32:37–46.
14. Wallace R, Benson H. The physiology of meditation. *Sci Am* 1972; 226:84–90.
15. Morse D, Martin S, Furst M, Dublin L. A physiological and subjective evaluation of meditation, hypnosis and relaxation. *Psychosom Med* 1977; 39:304–324.
16. Grzesiak R. Relaxation techniques in treatment of chronic pain. *Arch Phys Med Rehabil* 1977; 58:270–272.
17. Varni J. Self-regulation techniques in the management of chronic arthritic hemiaplasia. *Behav Ther* 1981; 12:185–194.
18. Morin CM, Kowatch RA, Wade JB. Behavioral management of sleep disturbance secondary to chronic pain. *J Behav Ther Exp Psychiatry* December 1989; D; 20(4):295–302.
19. Kabat-Zinn, J. An outpatient program in behavioral medicine for chronic pain patient based on the practice of mindfulness meditation: theoretical considerations and preliminary results. *Gen Hosp Psychiatry* 1982; 4:33–47.
20. Hilgard ER, Hilgard JR. *Hypnosis in the Relief of Pain.* Los Altos, Calif: Kaufman; 1975.
21. Orne Martin T. Nonpharmacological approaches to pain relief: hypnosis, biofeedback, placebo effect. In: Gerald Aronoff, ed. Evaluation and treatment of chronic pain. Baltimore: Urban & Schwarzenberg; 1985.
22. Orne M, Dinges D. Hypnosis. In: Wall P, Melzack R, eds. *Textbook of Pain.* Edinburgh: Churchill Livingstone; 1984:806–816.

23. Edelson J, Fitzpatrick JL. A comparison of cognitive-behavioral and hypnotic treatments of chronic pain. *J Clin Psychol* March 1989; 45(2):316–323.

24. Stern J, Brown M, Ulett C, Sletten I. A comparison of hypnosis, acupuncture, morphine, Valium, aspirin, and placebo in the management of experimentally induced pain. *Ann N Y Acad Sci* 1977; 296:175–193.

25. Elton D, Burrows A, Stanley A. Chronic pain and hypnosis. In: Burrows G, Dennerstein L, eds. *Hand-book of Hypnosis and Psychosomatic Medicine*. Amsterdam: Elsevier; 1980:269–292.

26. Benson H, Arns P, Hoffman J: The relaxation response and hypnosis. *Int J Clin Exp Hypn* 1981; 29:259–270.

27. Turner J, Chapman C. Psychological interventions for chronic pain: a critical review, II: operant conditioning, hypnosis, and cognitive-behavioral therapy. *Pain* 1982; 12:23–46.

28. Hess W, Brugger M. Das subkortikale zentrum der affektiven abwehrreaktion. *Helvetica Physiologica et Pharmacologica Acta* 1943; 1:33–52.

29. Benson H, Pomeranz B, Kutz I. The relaxation response and pain. In: Wall P, Melzack R, eds. *Textbook of Pain*. Edinburgh: Churchill Livingstone; 1984:817–822.

30. Cannon W. The emergency function of the adrenal medulla in pain and the major emotions. *Am J Physiol* 1914; 33:356–372.

31. Fraunhoffer M, Mackimon J, Carstens E. Map of diencephalic sites at which stimulation inhibits spinal nociceptive transmission. *Soc Neurosci Abst* 1982; 8:767.

32. Beary J, Benson H. A simple psychophysiologic technique which elicits the hypometabolic changes of the relaxation response. *Psychosom Med* 1974; 36:115–120.

33. Turk D, Meichenbaum D, Berman W. Application of biofeedback for the regulation of pain: a critical review. *Psychol Bull* 1979; 86:1322–1338.

34. Jessup B, Neufeld R, Merksen H. Biofeedback therapy for headache and other pain: an evaluative review. *Pain* 1979; 7:225–270.

35. Roberts A. Biofeedback. Research, training, and clinical roles. *Am Psychol* 1985; 40:938–941.

36. Jessup B. Biofeedback. In: Wall P, Melzack R, eds. *Textbook of Pain*. Edinburgh: Churchill Livingstone; 1984:776–786.

37. Grunert BK, Devine CA, Sanger JR, Matloub HS, Green D. Thermal self-regulation for pain control in reflex sympathetic dystrophy. *J Hand Surg* July 1990; 15(4):615–618.

38. Zitman R. Biofeedback and chronic pain. In: Bonica JJ, ed. *Advances in Pain Research and Therapy*. Vol 5. New York: Raven Press; 1983.

39. Brooke R, Stenn P. Myofascial pain dysfunction syndrome—how effective is biofeedback-assisted relaxation training. In: Bonica JJ, ed. *Advances in Pain Research and Therapy*. Vol 5. New York: Raven Press; 1983.

40. Melzack R, Perry C. Self-regulation of pain: the use of alpha feedback and hypnotic training for the control of chronic pain. *Exp Neurol* 1975; 46:452–469.

41. Nicholas MK, Wilson PH, Goyen J. Operant-behavioral and cognitive-behavioral treatment for chronic low back pain. *Behav Res Ther* 1991; 29(3):225–238.

42. Fordyce W. Behavioral conditioning concepts in chronic pain. Bonica JJ, ed. *Advances in Pain Research and Therapy*. Vol 5. New York: Raven Press; 1983.

43. Latimer P. External contingency management for chronic pain: critical review of the evidence. *Am J Psychiatry* 1982; 139:1308–1312.

44. Sternbach R. Behavior therapy. In: Wall P, Melzack R, eds. *Textbook of Pain*. Edinburgh: Churchill Livingstone; 1984:800–805.

45. Fernandez E, Turk DC. The utility of cognitive coping strategies for altering pain perception: a meta-analysis. *Pain* August 1989; 38(2):123–135.

46. Skinner JB, Erskine A, Pearce S, Rubenstein I, Taylor M, Foster C. The evaluation of a cognitive behavioral treatment programme in outpatient with chronic pain. *J Psychosom Res* 1990; 34(1):13–19.

47. Turk D, Meichenbaum D: A cognitive-behavioral approach to pain management. In: Wall P, Melzack R, eds. *Textbook of Pain*. Edinburgh: Churchill Livingstone; 1984.

48. Turner J. Comparison of group progressive-relaxation training and cognitive behavioral group therapy for chronic low back pain. *J Consult Clin Psychol* 1982; 50:757–765.

49. Sternbach R. Fundamentals of psychological methods in chronic pain. In: Bonica JJ, ed. *Advances in Pain Research and Therapy*. Vol 5. New York: Raven Press; 1983.

50. Caudill M, Schnable R, Zuttermeister P, Benson H, Friedman R. Decreased clinic utilization by chronic pain patients after behavioral medicine intervention. *Pain* June 1991; 45(3):334–335.

CHAPTER 33

Nutrition

Stuart Berger

Chronic pain is a phenomenon about which much remains unknown. Because of this, the patient's capacity to function productively is challenged continuously by chronic pain. The devastating effects of chronic pain are reflected economically, socially, and psychologically for the patient, their family, and society in general.[1-3]

Recently, controlling chronic pain by nutritional manipulation was investigated. This dietary approach offers a new therapeutic tool for both the physician and patient.[4] Certain foods and dietary deficiencies can provoke some well-known painful syndromes, such as migraine headache, premenstrual syndrome, dysmenorrhea, hypoglycemia, muscle aches, and chronic muscle pain. Pain from other causes also has been linked to diet.[3,5,6] Although some foods can provoke pain syndromes, other nutrients (such as tryptophan, phenylalanine, leucine, vitamin C, and B complex vitamins) can be used to treat pain.[3,7]

The vital role of nutrients in preserving functions of the nervous system is recognized. A high degree of homeostasis is needed continuously for both the central nervous system and peripheral nerves. An abundant supply of oxygen must be combined with a readily available source of energy. Vitamins and minerals act in the nervous system's numerous enzyme systems and metabolic functions.[8] The physiology of the nervous system is influenced in different ways by nutritional factors. Various nutritional deficits produce functional derangements in the highly susceptible nervous system, particularly in the brain.

Controversy continues regarding the effects on the brain and behavior of various food additives (primarily preservatives and artificial colors and flavors, which are phenol derivatives). These substances have produced toxic effects in children, including the so-called hyperkinetic syndrome (hyperactive, inattentive, short attention span, unable to concentrate, aggressive, destructive, and abusive). This condition improves by avoiding all foods that contain additives and are related chemically to aspirin and salicylates. Further research is needed to clarify the chemical basis for the mechanism of action of hyperkinesis.[8]

A recent new approach in orthomolecular psychiatry uses so-called megavitamin therapy for mental disorders. The reported benefits of this approach still are controversial. In 1975, Ch'ien and associates[9] showed that large doses of folic acid can interfere with the anticonvulsant action of phenytoin in patients with epilepsy.

Epidemiologists suggest that the combination of dietary sodium chloride, saturated fats, and cholesterol can contribute to hypertension, vascular headache, and cerebral vascular occlusion. Although diets high in saturated fat and cholesterol favor platelet aggregation, the reverse effect may occur with small amounts of saturated fat and cholesterol. Adding linoleic acid, an essential fatty acid, to the diet appears to have an antiaggregation effect on platelets.[8,9]

Moderate amounts of polyunsaturated fats were advocated by some (10 percent of total calories) to lower plasma levels of cholesterol. However, insufficient data do not justify recommending a specific optimal amount of linoleic acid in the diet. As an essential fatty acid, the recommended intake is 1 to 2 percent of total kilocalories (kcal) or up to 7 g for a person consuming 3000 kcal/day. However, this amount of linoleic acid is much lower than the amount of total polyunsaturates recommended as a preventive measure.[10]

DIET AND COMMON PAINFUL SYNDROMES

Migraine

A relationship between diet and vascular headache often has been suggested. These headaches may be related to changes in certain neurotransmitters (serotonin, catecholamines [chiefly norepinephrine], and certain polypeptides [mainly bradykinin]). During an attack, patients with migraine have lower than normal serotonin levels.[11] Because tryptophan is the precursor for serotonin synthesis, patients were treated with tryptophan supplements; this agent was effective in relieving pain in almost 50 percent of patients with migraine headaches. During the migraine attack, an increase in free fatty acid blood levels occurs. Some patients relate migraine attacks to fasting, starting a weight-loss diet, emotional stress, and alcohol consumption; all these conditions produce elevated free fatty acid blood levels. These free fatty acids may be responsible for the low serotonin levels during a migraine attack.

Friedman[12] noticed that, in most patients with migraine, neither tyramine in food nor lack of food (hypoglycemia) caused the headache. Although a few such patients were food sensitive to tyramine in foods, most of them were not.[12] Tyramine-rich foods include: (1) dairy products (aged cheeses, sour cream, and yogurt), (2) meats and fish (beef, chicken livers, sausages, pickled herring, and salted dried fish), (3) vegetables (sauerkraut and Italian fava beans), (4) alcoholic beverages (red wines, sauterne, champagne, sherry, beer, and ale), and (5) other foods (chocolate, vanilla, yeast and yeast extract, and soy sauce).[13]

The controversy still continues over the effects of certain foods that induce migraine headaches. Some specialists endorse, as a standard treatment for migraine, a diet that does not include foods containing nitrites or nitrates (preservatives), alcohol, monosodium glutamate (MSG), and tyramine. All these substances vasoactive and cause blood vessels to dilate or constrict. Thus, they may initiate the migraine process.[13] One treatment for migraine includes caffeine (which constricts blood vessels). This presents a paradox because some patients have migraine headaches after ingestion of coffee, tea, and chocolate, all of which contain caffeine.[13]

Nitrites and nitrates are preservatives found in cured and lunch meats. Patients with migraine should avoid ham, bacon, salami, sausage, hot dogs, lunch loaves, and other packaged meats and most Chinese food, which contains MSG as a flavor enhancer.[13] In addition to causing headaches, MSG may be responsible for burning chest pain in adults.[14]

The seven foods that have the best established reputation for producing headaches, either alone or in combination with other foods, are: milk, chocolate, wheat, eggs, citrus fruits (including tomatoes), peanuts, and pork.[13] An increased salt intake and nitroglycerin also can trigger a migraine attack. Certain drugs (oral contraceptives, corticosteroids, amphetamines, and nitrates) also may precipitate headaches. However, the mechanisms whereby foods cause headaches still are understood poorly.[15]

Musculoskeletal Disorders

Patients with chronic muscle tension, pain, and stiffness may have dietary-induced subclinical vitamin and mineral deficiencies that are not evident clinically. These patients need to make a critical dietary change by increasing their intake of B vitamins (especially B_1, B_6, and B_{12}), folic acid, vitamin C, and chelated calcium and magnesium. If patients have one vitamin B deficiency, then usually all B vitamins are deficient. Poor personal habits (such as modest alcohol consumption) cause excessively rapid metabolism of vitamin B_1, and smoking depletes vitamin C. Symptoms of vitamin C deficiency include aching muscles.[6]

Caffeine causes increased urination with subsequent vitamin and mineral depletion. Also, it increases muscle tension by direct action on the nervous system. Therefore, caffeine elimination should be advised in patients with chronic muscle tension and pain. Calcium (which is essential for muscle tone) often is deficient in the diet. Calcium starvation occurs more often in women who are less efficient than men in calcium absorption and retention. The slender dieting woman who has muscle tension in the neck and shoulders often is surprised that calcium supplementation solves her problem.[6]

Initiating vitamin and mineral supplements will not produce immediate relief from muscular aches, pain, and tension. Structural or skeletal disorders and poor postural or work habits that contribute to muscle dysfunction first must be corrected.[16] Within a month, if taken regularly, the effect of vitamin and mineral supplements should be apparent. For the average person, a high potency multi-B supplement with folate (100 to 150 mg of each B vitamin), 1000 to 2000 mg of vitamin C, and 800 to 1200 mg of calcium daily is adequate. Vitamin and mineral supplements must become a regular part of the patient's daily intake if relief from chronic muscle tension and pain is to be permanent.[6]

To prevent pain, food additives and artificial flavors should be eliminated from the diet. When ingested over 10 to 20 years, food additives that contain chemical preservatives and stabilizers accumulate in the body. This can affect the nervous system adversely and influence the onset and severity of pain.[14] Studies show that artificial flavors in food can cause everything from headache to asthma. One man developed severe anaphylactic shock when he ate ice cream artifically flavored with chocolatin and strawberrin.[14]

Premenstrual Syndrome

Some studies show a relationship between premenstrual syndrome and dysmenorrhea and increased salt consumption. Fluid retention may be relieved by limiting salt intake and giving a diuretic (e.g., hydrochlorothiazide 50 mg to 100 mg/day, orally, during the last 10 days of the menstrual cycle or, preferably, 24 to 36 h before the expected onset of symptoms). The addition of vitamin B_6 (pyridoxine) is recommended in a dose of 50 to 100 mg/day orally to correct the deficiency that often is present. Vitamin B_6 converts tryptophan to niacin, a vasodilator, and thereby, it may relieve the pain from spasm in uterine blood vessels.[14]

Gout

Gout is one of the most common diseases of the joints. This genetic or acquired disorder of purine metabolism primarily affects men aged 40 years and older. The severe pain of gout occurs when uric acid accumulates in the body and forms crystals in the joints (knuckles, knees, toes—especially the big toe) and ear lobes. Overeating, drinking, eating rich foods, and losing weight all trigger a gout attack. To prevent attacks, the patient should be advised to avoid excess alcohol or food, heavy beers, red wines, port, and foods high in uric acid (fish roes and offal).[17]

The dietary sources of uric acid are not the basic cause of gout. Patients have a uric acid reaction to orange juice, mushrooms, cauliflower, organ meats (such as calf's liver), and beef. Some seafoods (shrimp and lobster) contain uric

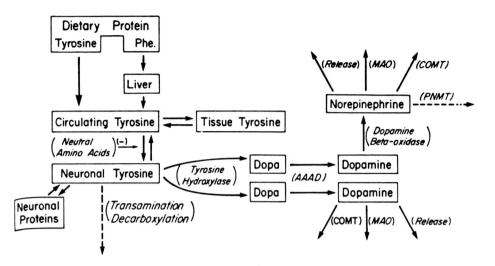

FIGURE 33-1. Control of catecholamine synthesis in brain neurons. Phe = phenylalanine, MAO = monoamine oxidase, COMT = catechol-O-methyl transferase, PNMT = phenylethanolamine-N-methyl transferase, AAAD = aromatic L-amino acid decarboxylase, ---- indicates unproved pathway. (Reproduced with permission from Wurtman RJ, Fernstrom JD. Control of brain monoamine synthesis by diet and plasma amino acids. *Am J Clin Nutr* 1975; 28(6):638–647.)

acid. Therefore, if the patient produces uric acid at a faster than normal rate, eating these foods can trigger the crystallization process and cause an attack of gout.[17,18]

DIETARY MANIPULATION FOR PAIN RELIEF

Tryptophan

Most tissues in the body require that amino acid intake be proportional to the rate of cellular regeneration. However, the brain and possibly the spinal cord use certain amino acids (tryptophan, tyrosine, and phenylalanine) as substrates from which three primary monoamine neurotransmitters (the indoleamine serotonin and the catecholamines dopamine and norepinephrine) are synthesized (Figs. 33-1, 33-2, and 33-3).[8,19]

Tryptophan, an essential amino acid, cannot be made in the body. Therefore, brain tryptophan can originate only from the lysis of brain proteins, and circulating tryptophan must be obtained from the diet or other tissue pools.[8,19] Therapeutic amounts of tryptophan have been used for pain, depression, obesity, and insomnia.[20,21] Another interesting dietary substance (found in plant and animal foods, including milk and lecithin) is choline, a quaternary ammonium base. Thus, the two dietary substances, tryptophan and choline, can be converted by neurons in the brain to the neurotransmitters, serotonin and acetylcholine, respectively. The formation and concentration of these neurotrans-

mitters (serotonin and acetylcholine) are influenced by the nutritional status of the patient. Furthermore, brain tyrosine levels may control the synthesis of other catecholamines (dopamine and norepinephrine); this also may be related to nutritional factors. On a metabolic basis, treatment with choline may reverse tardive dyskinesia, a serious neurologic disorder caused by neuroleptic drugs. Therefore, tardive dyskinesia may be a cholinergic transmission disorder that might be reversed by dietary manipulation.[4,22,23]

To some extent, diet controls the synthesis of monoamine neurotransmitters in the brain. By giving tryptophan and then injecting insulin, the amount of brain tryptophan is increased. Almost the same result occurs after a carbohydrate meal. However, a protein meal decreases the concentration of both tryptophan and serotonin in the brain. The effects of various neurotransmitters on mental illness require more research, but there is agreement that most antipsychotic drugs act by increasing or decreasing specific neurotransmitters.[19]

Recent studies indicate that ingesting the essential amino acid, L-tryptophan, may relieve pain significantly. Tryptophan appears to be effective for treatment of depression, obesity, insomnia, and migraine headaches. Also tryptophan helps the antibody-forming response in B-lymphocytes and is essential for the synthesis of nicotinic acid. Investigation into the dietary control of pain has been directed toward manipulation of central neurotransmitters.[14,24]

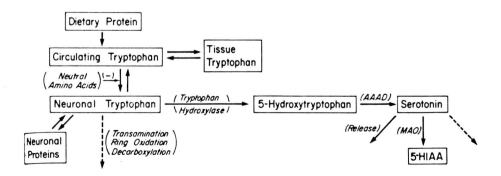

FIGURE 33-2. Control of serotonin synthesis in brain neurons. AAAD = aromatic L-amino acid decarboxylase, MAO = monoamine oxidase, ---- indicates unproved pathway. (Reproduced with permission from Wurtman RJ, Fernstrom JD. Control of brain monoamine synthesis by diet and plasma amino acids. *Am J Clin Nutr* 1975; 28(6):638–647.)

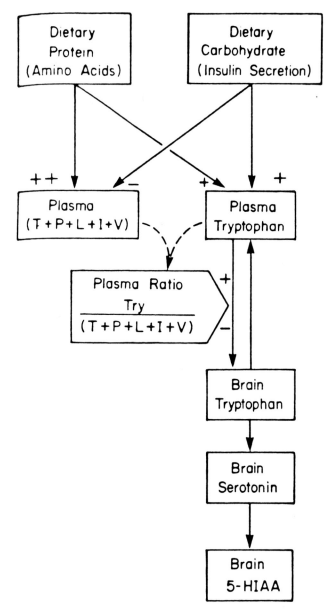

FIGURE 33-3. Proposed sequence describing diet-induced changes in brain serotonin concentration in the rat. The ratio of tryptophan to the combined levels of tyrosine, phenylalanine, leucine, isoleucine, and valine in the plasma is thought to control the tryptophan level in the brain. (Reproduced with permission from Wurtman RJ, Fernstrom JD. Control of brain monoamine synthesis by diet and plasma amino acids. *Am J Clin Nutr* 1975; 28(6):638–647.)

Some dietary substances, such as tryptophan, can be converted into neurotransmitters (serotonin) by brain neurons. Thus, brain serotonin levels can be altered by tryptophan ingestion used to treat chronic pain. Many natural foods (Table 33-1) contain rich sources of tryptophan, including red meat, fish, chicken, liver, lamb, soybeans, cottage cheese, mixed nuts, peanuts, baked beans, lentils, soya protein, bananas, green leafy vegetables, milk, eggs, brown rice (uncooked), pumpkin and sesame seeds, avocados, and pineapples.[4,14,24]

In 1983, the Food and Agriculture Organization of the World Health Organization estimated the daily amino acid requirements for infants to be 17 mg/kg body weight/day; for 2-year-old children, 12.5 mg/kg/day; for school-aged boys (10 to 12 years old), 4 mg/kg/day; and for adults, 3.5 mg/kg/day (262 mg for a 75-kg man). However, most persons do not consume adequate amounts of tryptophan in their daily diets. With deficient tryptophan intake, especially during stress, serotonin blood levels can decrease, resulting in anxiety, depression, poor appetite, migraine headache, agitation, insecurity, hyperactivity, insomnia, and pain. In high quality animal and plant protein, tryptophan constitutes approximately 11 mg/g.[14,24]

Tryptophan is one of 22 amino acids, and most protein foods contain only approximately 1% tryptophan. Tryptophan competes with other large neutral aromatic or branched-chain amino acids for the common transport mechanism, and not all tryptophan is transported by the blood to the brain.[19]

To eliminate the serotonin deficiency, the diet can be supplemented with L-tryptophan in large doses. Combining L-tryptophan with vitamin supplements (niacin and B_6) that enhance its conversion to serotonin may help to relieve pain and its associated problems of depression, obesity, migraine headache, and insomnia.[14]

Although tryptophan was available, in capsule form, without prescription at drug and health food stores for many years, this is no longer the case. (The Food and Drug Administration recalled tryptophan supplements pending an investigation after they were linked to eosinophilia–myalgia syndrome (EMS), a painful muscle and blood disorder; however, it is now thought that almost all EMS cases could be traced to supplements provided by a single Japanese manufacturer. Therefore, the ban may be lifted in the future.)[25,26] It is therefore imperative that enough foods rich in tryptophan (see Table 33-1) be consumed daily to achieve a therapeutic effect.

A summary of tryptophan therapeutic doses includes: general, 300 mg daily; insomnia, 1 g before sleep plus magnesium and vitamin B_6; pain relief, 2 to 4 g; and depression, 3 g plus 1 g nicotinamide. The maximum therapeutic level is 6 g daily. Tryptophan should always be taken separately from protein meals and at least 1 hour before a meal. Adding vitamin B_6 may increase the serotoninergic effect. Absorption is enhanced with a carbohydrate snack. The effect also may be enhanced by adding niacinamide (the ratio of tryptophan to niacinamide should be 2:1).[24]

Since the early 1970s, the effect of serotonin on pain has been studied. High serotonin levels appear to potentiate morphine analgesia; serotonin antagonists decrease the pain threshold. In one study, a single injection of tryptophan quickly restored the higher pain threshold. Administration of *p*-chlorophenylalanine, a tryptophan hydroxylase inhibitor, potentiated the lower threshold. Reports suggest that tryptophan decreases sensitivity to moderate pain rather than to severe pain in humans.[3]

Table 33-1
Essential Amino Acid Content of Common Foods (Derived from Nutrition Almanac, McGraw Hill, 1979)

Food	Weight (g)	Protein (g)	TRP (mg)	LEU (mg)	LYS (mg)	MET (mg)	PHA (mg)	ISL (mg)	VAL (mg)	THR* (mg)
Wholewheat bread	23	2.1	29	166	71	37	117	106	113	72
Wholewheat flour	120	15	192	1072	432	240	784	688	739	464
Soya flour	110	45	605	3428	2784	650	2179	2380	2339	1734
Oatmeal (cooked)	236	4.7	76	501	221	86	275	275	319	205
Brown rice (raw)	190	14.3	159	1233	558	260	717	675	1004	558
Brown rice (cooked)	150	3.8	41	327	148	68	190	179	266	148
White rice (cooked)	150	3	33	258	117	54	150	141	210	117
Wheatgerm	6	1.8	16	110	99	26	58	76	88	86
Cottage cheese	260	44.2	469	4608	3584	1195	2304	2475	2475	2005
Edam cheese	28	7.7	108	775	591	211	429	523	575	300
Parmesan cheese	28	10	140	980	730	260	540	670	720	370
Egg: boiled/raw	50	6.5	102	559	406	197	369	420	470	318
Buttermilk	246	8.9	90	809	678	188	433	515	613	384
Skim milk	64	23	320	2220	1780	570	1095	1461	1575	1073
Yogurt (part skim)	250	4.3	93	842	706	196	450	536	638	400
Fish, cod (canned)	453	87	870	6609	7655	2523	3216	4435	4611	3742
Shrimp (cooked)	453	92	821	6240	7225	2381	3038	4187	4351	3530
Trout (raw)	453	97	974	7302	8571	2827	3606	6654	6930	5621
Orange	180	1.8	5	—	48	5	—	—	—	—
Peach	100	0.68	4	29	30	31	18	13	40	27
Strawberries	149	1.04	13	63	48	1.5	34	27	34	37
Beef (roast)	453	108	1154	7888	8369	2405	3944	5002	5291	4233
Liver (cooked)	453	120	1354	8398	6772	2167	4515	3786	5689	4334
Lamb	453	80	1525	9075	9543	2884	4832	6131	5768	5421
Chicken (breasts)	358	74.5	894	5438	6630	1937	2980	3948	3800	3204
Almonds	133	25	234	1934	774	344	1524	1161	1495	811
Brazils	167	23	312	1885	740	1571	1030	990	1374	705
Peanuts (roasted)	240	60	800	4432	2592	640	3680	2992	3616	1952
Pumpkin seeds	230	67	1201	5269	3068	1267	3735	3735	3602	2001
Sesame seeds	230	42	711	3461	1256	1382	3181	2052	1925	1548
Walnuts	100	15	175	1228	441	306	767	767	974	589
Lima beans (raw)	100	20	202	1628	1488	250	1212	992	1030	836
Beans (green-cooked)	125	2	28	116	104	30	48	90	96	76
Carrots (cooked)	150	1.35	11	77	62	11	50	54	66	51
Chickpeas dry-raw (garbanzos)	100	20.5	164	1517	1415	266	1004	1189	1004	738
Lentils (cooked)	100	15.6	140	954	898	100	654	540	626	496
Mushrooms (tinned)	200	3.8	12	444	—	266	—	840	596	—
Potato (baked)	100	2.6	26	130	138	31	114	114	138	107
Soybeans	200	22	330	1870	1518	330	1188	1298	1276	846
Tomato (raw)	150	1.65	15	68	69	12	46	48	46	54

*TRP = tryptophan, LEU = leucine, LYS = lysine, MET = methionine, PHA = phenylalanine, ISL = isoleucine, VAL = valine, THR = threonine.
From: Chaitow L. *Amino Acids in Therapy: A Guide to the Therapeutic Application of Protein Constituents.* New York: Thorsons Pub; 1985.

Studies in humans also have shown that tryptophan-enriched diets enhance electrically induced endorphin analgesia, decrease depression, and increase pain tolerance in patients with chronic pain. In several reports, therapy with L-tryptophan for migraine was moderately successful, presumably as a result of an increase of plasma free and total tryptophan levels. However, these studies did not use any dietary manipulation to decrease the total protein intake. Although little data is available on the analgesic effects of such diet regimens, the previously mentioned studies suggest that tryptophan with dietary manipulation may be an effective treatment for chronic maxillofacial pain.[4]

Tryptophan was given orally (3 g/day) with a high carbohydrate, low protein, low fat diet to patients with chronic maxillofacial pain associated with various diseases and induced by electrical stimulation of dental (tooth) pulps. After 1 month of this regimen, the patients showed a marked decrease in pain and increase in pain tolerance threshold. These patients, some with dual diagnoses associated with chronic maxillofacial pain, had (1) temporomandibular joint pain–dysfunction syndrome, (2) atypical facial neuralgia, (3) migrainous neuralgia, (4) trigeminal neuralgia, (5) phantom tooth pain, (6) ciliary neuralgia, and (7) cervical osteoarthritis.[2,4]

In another study, oral tryptophan (4 g/day) was given to patients using narcotics chronically for low back and leg pain for 2 to 9 weeks. Results showed that tryptophan therapy allowed these patients to decrease their narcotic dose significantly. This study suggests that chronic narcotic use lowers brain serotonin turnover, and large doses of tryptophan (the serotonin precursor) may reverse this effect (that is, increase brain serotonin levels).[27]

In another study, tryptophan (2 g/day orally) was given for 1 month to patients who had pain after rhizotomy and cordotomy. Significant pain relief occurred after 1 month of treatment.[28]

In addition to increasing consumption of tryptophan, patients with chronic pain should receive nutritional instruction regarding overeating and obesity; excess weight may cause stress on the structural support of the spine and on the joints of the lower extremities.[3]

Although numerous studies have evaluated tryptophan for treatment of chronic pain, only a few case reports are available. Therefore, we include Warfield and Stein's[3] three brief case reports in their entirety.

Patient 1. A 40-year-old woman was referred for treatment of chronic left shoulder pain. She had previously undergone a left first rib resection for thoracic outlet syndrome and subsequently experienced hyperesthetic pain in her left shoulder in the distribution of C4. Her pain was particularly severe in the evening, and she had considerable difficulty in sleeping. She had a series of nerve blocks, transcutaneous electrical nerve stimulation (TENS), and trials of carbamazepine and phenytoin without relief. We prescribed tryptophan (2 gm PO bid): a month later her pain had been substantialy relieved, and she was sleeping well.

Patient 2. A 32-year-old man was referred for treatment of low back pain. He had injured his back eight years earlier while lifting a heavy object. He subsequently had four surgical procedures, including two laminectomies, one exploration, and a fusion. Transcutaneous electrical nerve stimulation, an epidural steroid injection, physical therapy, and biofeedback provided no relief of pain. He began taking methadone in gradually increasing doses to 20 mg PO q6h, but lately he had not been obtaining his usual relief even on 25 mg PO q6h. He was started on tryptophan (2 gm bid), and within a month he was able to decrease the methadone dose to 20 mg q6h, with substantial relief of his pain.

Patient 3. A 26-year-old woman was referred for evaluation of right knee pain. She had undergone a right medial meniscectomy and re-exploration of the knee for continued pain. Other medical problems included gross obesity. She had tried many types of physical therapy and chiropractic manipulation without relief. Her only medication was a nonsteroidal anti-inflammatory agent, which provided minimal relief. She had tried many diets without success. Tryptophan (2 gm bid) was started, and the patient was encouraged to participate in a structured weight reduction program. On this regimen she managed to lose 40 pounds, and her pain was considerably diminished.

Phenylalanine and Leucine

Phenylalanine and leucine belong to the group of neutral amino acids that include tryptophan, tyrosine, isoleucine, and valine. All these amino acids compete with each other for the same low affinity uptake sites in the brain.[29]

Research by Ehrenpreis and coworkers showed that enkephalin and endorphin analgesia has a short duration because of rapid degradation of endorphin peptides by the enzymes carboxypeptidase A and leucine-aminopeptidase.[4] They also showed that, in rats, analgesia was produced by both the L- and D-forms of phenylalanine and D-leucine. Combinations of D-phenylalanine and D-leucine resulted in analgesia at doses of the individual agents that were insufficient to produce analgesia when administered alone. The analgesic effects of D-phenylalanine were related to inhibition of carboxypeptidase A; D-leucine inhibited leucine aminopeptidase. Naloxone reversed the D-phenylalanine analgesia, indicating that the analgesia was induced by endorphin potentiation.

In humans, orally administered D-phenylalanine was given alone or in combination with aspirin. Within 2 to 3 days, patients were relieved of the long-standing pain associated with whiplash injury, arthritic pain of the extremities, and lower back pain. Patients receiving D-phenylalanine showed neither any adverse effects nor any degree of tolerance (pain relief did not decrease with subsequent use). With D-phenylalanine, peak pain relief occurred within 1 to 4 weeks and often lasted for up to 1 month after stopping the drug.[4,24]

Subsequently, D,L-phenylalanine (DLPA) was used to provide patients with pain relief and supply normal body requirements of phenylalanine. DLPA is especially effective for arthritic conditions. Research shows that DLPA inhibits enzymes that are responsible for the breakdown of endorphins: carboxypeptidase A and enkephalinase enzymes. The endorphins' pain relieving characteristics, therefore, might last longer. Thus, DLPA, or only D-phenylalanine, does not act as an analgesic itself, but rather the endogenous pain control mechanism of the body is permitted to act more advantageously.[24]

In patients with chronic pain, endorphin levels are decreased in the cerebrospinal fluid and serum, and DLPA, or only D-phenylalanine, helps to restore these to normal levels. Because DLPA does not interfere with transmission of normal pain messages, the body's defense mechanism is not compromised, and only the ongoing pain relieving mechanism is enhanced.[24]

Recently, in Balagot's[30] report to the American Pain Society, 50 percent to 75 percent of 43 patients receiving 800 to 1200 mg of D-phenylalanine orally daily obtained relief from chronic painful disorders, including reflex sympathetic dystrophy, osteoarthritis, herpes zoster, and various other neuralgias.

DLPA is available at health food stores as 375- or 500-mg tablets. For pain relief, the usual dose is two tablets taken 15 to 30 min before meals (a total of six tablets daily). If, within 3 weeks, no improvement occurs, the dose is doubled. Then, if there is no response, DLPA is discontinued. Only 5 percent to 15 percent of patients do not respond, and relief usually occurs within 7 days of initiating DLPA. When there is pain relief, the DLPA dose is decreased in stages, until (by trial and error) a minimum maintenance dose is reached. Some patients obtain maintenance of pain relief with DLPA for 1 week per month; others need to receive DLPA continuously in small amounts.[24]

Also, L-phenylalanine has been used for appetite suppression in obesity (dose, 100 to 500 mg per day on an empty stomach at bedtime) and to treat depressive states (100 to 500 mg per day). Phenylalanine produces cholecystokinin (intestinal mucosal hormone) release; this may induce satiety and end eating, either by changing gastrointestinal function (gastric emptying), or by interacting with central nervous system feeding centers (amygdala and hypothalamus) and intact vagal fibers. Phenylalanine also causes more alertness, increased sexual interest, memory enhancement, and within 24 to 48 h, an antidepressant effect.[24]

When treating hypertensive patients or anyone with possible high blood pressure, phenylalanine should be started at low doses (approximately 100 mg/day), and blood pressure should be monitored daily. Phenylalanine should not be combined with monoamine oxidase inhibitor drugs. Currently, there are no reports of contraindications, except these antidepressant drugs, or side effects. Tolerance and addiction do not appear to occur.[24]

The National Academy of Science's adult daily requirement for phenylalanine is 16 mg/kg body weight or 1200 mg/day for a 75-kg man; other studies indicate a range of 420 mg to 2.2 g per day.[24] Foods containing phenylalanine include soybeans, fish, meat, poultry, cottage cheese, pecans, almonds, Brazil nuts, pumpkin and sesame seeds, lentils, lima beans, and chickpeas (garbanzos). In high quality protein, the phenylalanine content is 73 mg/g.

Vitamin C and B Complex Vitamins

Significant pain relief has been claimed with large doses (10 to 29 g/day) of water-soluble vitamin C (ascorbic acid) in patients with cancer, low back pain, headache, arthritis, toothache, and earache. Prostaglandins are involved in the processes that produce inflammation, fever, and pain. Vitamin C, which acts in a manner similar to aspirin, inhibits synthesis of some prostaglandins (PGE_2 and $PGE_{2\alpha}$). This may be the mechanism by which large doses of vitamin C control inflammation, fever, and pain. However, vitamin C is different from aspirin because it increases the rate of synthesis of PGE_1. This prostaglandin is associated with lymphocyte function and other aspects of the immune system; it may play a role in rheumatoid arthritis, various autoimmune diseases, multiple sclerosis, and cancer. Increased intake of vitamin C may provide an anti-inflammatory effect similar to aspirin.[31]

Cancer pain may be caused by the tumor pressing on pain-sensitive structures or invading tissues. Malignant tumors produce an enzyme, hyaluronidase, that attacks and weakens the intercellular "cement" of surrounding tissues, allowing invasion of tissues by the neoplasm. Also, most patients with cancer have decreased levels of ascorbate in their blood, and a known property of ascorbic acid is that it increases the rate of collagen synthesis.[31]

Therefore, we might speculate that large doses of vitamin C strengthen the intercellular cement by increasing the synthesis of collagen fibrils; these are an important part of the intercellular bond. In this way, natural body defense mechanisms then could resist attacks by malignant cells and decrease cancer pain. Studies report vitamin C effectively controlled pain; this permitted patients who were receiving large doses of morphine and diamorphine could stop taking the narcotic drugs.[31]

Good Nutrition

The importance of maintaining adequate nutrition (based on recommended dietary allowances and intakes) is essential in patients who have either acute or chronic pain.[32] Pain in patients produces a stress syndrome called the *general adaptation syndrome*. This is the body's mechanism of defense against stress; it produces changes in the structure and chemical composition of the patient's body.[33]

Frequently, during stress, patients lose their appetite because of gastrointestinal malfunction. Therefore, anorexia may be considered an almost universal accompaniment of disease, and it is the primary reason for most malnutrition observed in patients with acute and chronic pain. Anorexia may be a partial metabolic response to injury but prolonged protein–calorie malnutrition associated with vitamin and mineral deficiencies resulting from semistarvation can be detrimental because the patient's response to disease is impaired.[34,35]

Often, both the protein–calorie malnutrition and the vitamin and mineral deficiencies are not recognized and treated in patients with acute and chronic pain associated with various diseases. In several studies, the percentage of hospitalized patients with malnutrition and vitamin deficiencies was 24 percent to 69 percent for folic acid, 20 percent to 24 percent for vitamin C, 20 percent for riboflavin, and 6 percent for pyridoxine. At hospital admission, most patients were malnourished and generally had a deterioration of nutritional status during the next few weeks. This occurs because the protein–calorie requirements are increased by the metabolic response to the stress of pain, injury, and infection.[34]

The patient's vitamin and mineral status can be evaluated routinely with the following tests: (1) a serum chemical screen, including sodium, potassium, calcium, phosphorus, and alkaline phosphatase; (2) complete blood count to identify nutritional anemia; (3) serum folate and vitamin B_{12} level, commonly low in hospitalized patients; (4) serum magnesium level, essential for normal metabolism of potassium and calcium; (5) serum iron, total iron-binding capacity, and transferrin to assess protein and iron status; and (6) serum zinc level (this chiefly reflects current intake rather than body status). Marginal vitamin and mineral deficiencies caused by pain, injury, and infection are treated either orally or parenterally. If needed, total parenteral nutrition solutions can provide all nutrients for which a recommended daily allowance has been established. Most commercial enteral (oral) formulas do likewise.[34]

SUMMARY

Recent research seems to indicate that diet may have an effect on pain. In addition, certain dietary manipulations have been used successfully to treat painful syndromes. Undoubtedly, as our knowledge of the neurotransmitters involved in pain perception grows, we will understand better the role of diet in causing and treating pain.

References

1. Raimond J, Taylor JW. (1986) *Neurological Emergencies: Effective Nursing Care*. Rockville, MD: Aspen Systems Corp; 1986:288–289, 300, 311.
2. Seltzer S, Dewart D, Pollack RL, et al. The effects of dietary tryptophan on chronic maxillofacial pain and experimental pain tolerance. *J Psychiat Res* 1982–1983; 17(2):181–186.
3. Warfield CA, Stein JM. The nutritional treatment of pain. *Hosp Pract* 1983; 18:100n–100p.
4. Selzter S, Marcus R, Stoch. Perspectives in the control of chronic pain by nutritional manipulation. *Pain* 1981; 11:141–148.
5. Clinical nutrition. Certain foods provoke migraine. *Nutr Rev* 1984; 42(2):41–42.
6. Fickel T. Aches, pain and your diet. *Bestways;* 1985:50–51.
7. Bernstein AL. Vitamins B_6 in clinical neurology. *Ann N Y Acad Sci* 1990; 585:250–260.
8. Hodges RE. Nutrition and the nervous system. In: Hodges RE, Adelman RD, eds. *Nutrition in Medical Practice*. Philadelphia: Saunders; 1980:136–163, 323–331.
9. Ch'ien LT, Krumdieck CL, Scott CW Jr, et al. Harmful effect of megadoses of vitamins: electroencephalogram abnormalities and seizures induced by intravenous folate in drug-treated epileptics. *Am J Clin Nutr* 1975; 28:51–58.
10. Vergroesen AJ. Physiological effects of dietary linoleic acid. *Nutr Rev* 1977; 35(1):1–5.
11. Garrison R Jr. *Lysine, Tryptophan and Other Amino Acids: Food for Our Brains . . . Maintenance for Our Bodies*. New Canaan, CT: Keats; 1982:713.
12. Friedman AP. Metabolic abnormalities in migraine. *Ann Intern Med* 1971; 75(5):801–802. Editorial.
13. Gelb H, Siegel PM. *Killing Pain Without Prescription*. New York: Harper & Row; 1980:56–61, 180–181.
14. Bresler DE, Trubo R. *Free Yourself from Pain*. New York: Simon & Schuster; 1979:76–78, 298–301.
15. Van Den Noort S. Drugs and diet as causes of vascular headaches. *West J Med* 1977; 126(6):459. Abstract.
16. White-O'Connor B, Sobal J, Muncie HL Jr. Dietary habits, weight history, and vitamin supplement use in elderly osteoarthritis patients. *J Am Diet Assoc* March 1989; 89(3):378–382.
17. Lipton S. *Conquering Pain*. New York: Arco; 1984:28–29, 79–80.
18. Berkow R, ed. *The Merck Manual of Diagnosis and Therapy*. 14th ed. Rahway, NJ: Merck; 1982.
19. Wurtman RJ, Fernstrom JD. Control of brain monoamine synthesis by diet and plasma amino acids. *Am J Clin Nutr* 1975; 28(6):638–647.
20. Lieberman HR, Corkin S, Spring BJ, et al. Mood, performance, and pain sensitivity: changes induced by food constituents. *J Psychiat Res* 1982–1983; 17(2):135–145.
21. Lipton MA, Kane FJ Jr. Psychiatry. In: Schneider HA, Anderson CE, Coursin DB, eds. *Nutritional Support of Medical Practice*. 2nd ed. Philadelphia: Harper & Row; 1983:562–580.
22. Olson RE, Broquist HP, Chichester CO, et al, eds. *Nutrition Reviews: Present Knowledge in Nutrition*. 5th ed. Washington, DC: The Nutrition Foundation; 1984.
23. Cohen EL, Wurtman RJ. Brain acetylcholine: control by dietary choline. *Science* 1976; 191(4227):561–562.
24. Chaitow L. *Amino Acids in Therapy: A Guide to the Therapeutic Application of Protein Constituents*. New York: Thorsons Pub; 1985:58–71, 102–109.
25. Martin RW, Duffy J, Engel AG, et al. The clinical spectrum of the eosinophilia–myalgia syndrome associated with L-tryptophan ingestion. Clinical features in 20 patients and aspects of pathophysiology. *Ann Intern Med* July 15, 1990; 113(2):124–134.
26. Dicker RM, James N, Cunha BA. The eosinophilia–myalgia syndrome with neuritis associated with L-tryptophan use. *Ann Intern Med* June 15, 1990; 112(12):957–958.
27. Hosobuchi Y, Lamb S, Bascom D. Tryptophan loading may

reverse tolerance to opiate analgesics in humans. *Pain* 1981; 9(2):161–169.

28. King R. Pain and tryptophan. *J Neurosurg* 1980; 53(1):44–52.

29. Growdon JH, Wurtman RJ. Nutrients and neurotransmitters. *N Y State J Med* 1980; 80(10):1638–1639.

30. Balagot RC. Phenylalanine, a potential therapy in pain relief. *Int Med News* 1979; 12:5.

31. Pauling L. *How to Live Longer and Feel Better*. New York: Freeman; 1986:96–99, 166–171, 238–241.

32. Magni G, Caldieron C, Rigatti-Luchini S, Merskey H. Chronic musculoskeletal pain and depressive symptoms in the general population. An analysis of the 1st National Health and Nutrition Examination Survey data. *Pain* December 1990; 43(3):299–307.

33. Selye H. *The Stress of Life*. New York: McGraw-Hill; 1978.

34. Bistrain BR, Blackburn GL. Assessment of protein-calorie malnutrition in the hospitalized patient. In: Schneider HA, Anderson CE, Coursin DB, eds. *Nutritional Support of Medical Practice*. 2nd ed. Philadelphia: Harper & Row; 1983:128–139.

35. McIlwain H, Bachelard HS. *Biochemistry and the Central Nervous System*. 5th ed. Edinburgh: Churchill Livingstone; 1985.

CHAPTER 34

Psychotherapy

Nelson H. Hendler

Although this is a chapter about the psychotherapy of patients with pain, it must include necessarily a definition of the problem to be solved. Unfortunately, defining pain is elusive, and many attempts to categorize these patients give unsatisfactory results. Subsequently, the definition of what constitutes such a patient not definitive. The following chapter is an attempt to shed some light on the categorization of patients with pain.

There are at least three classifications of pain that a clinician may use. Each has advantages and disadvantages:

1. *The Medical Model.* Using this paradigm, pain is defined as a manifestation of a disease. This approach lends clarity to the problems of pain and offers predictive capabilities for outcome. It may offer a cure where none existed before. As an example, "pain in the back and the leg" is a description but "a herniated disk with radiculopathy" is a diagnosis. Surgery on the disk may cure the pain. However, should the surgery not work, or should there be psychological problems or social problems compounding recovery, the response to surgery may not be as predicted.

2. *The Psychiatric Model.* Using this approach, a clinician tries to establish a psychiatric diagnosis to explain the behavior of a patient with pain who is troublesome or not responding as predicted. Personality disorders, affective disorders, or anxiety traits that might be the source of a patient's complaints are identified and treated.[1] Unfortunately, the use of psychiatric intervention often leads to an either–or type of thinking, with a psychiatric diagnosis being established to the exclusion of a medical diagnosis. A woman with a histrionic personality disorder, who has surgical excision of a disk and does not get well, may not be helped by the system. Her lack of recovery is ascribed to secondary gain or dependency needs, but not to retained disk material missed during the first operation.

3. *The Integrated Response Model.* Using this model, the clinician tries to establish both medical and psychiatric diagnoses, not only from the point in time at which a patient is seen, but also based on the historic perspective of the patient (that is, their premorbid or prepain personality). In this fashion, we can determine the appropriateness of the response to pain and treatment. This technique is time consuming and involves a multidisciplinary approach, with multilevel diagnoses and integration of material. In this model, both medical and psychiatric diagnoses can exist.

Adherence to the medical model often is found in pain treatment centers and clinical practices that use only medical evaluation of the patient. The absence of a psychiatric or psychological professional to assist in evaluation and diagnosis limits the evaluation of the patient with chronic pain to only a medical assessment. It disregards the possibility that a patient may have psychiatric problems as the result of chronic pain that can lead to diagnostic oversights. There are some authors who believe that the incidence of depression in association with chronic pain is remarkably high.[2–4] Others have advanced the hypothesis that chronic pain may be a manifestation of underlying depression.[5,6] Therefore, the medical assessment of chronic pain, without a psychiatric assessment to determine the preexisting personality characteristics and motivations, may lead to an exaggerated response to chronic pain or the expression of psychiatric disease as a chronic pain process. This would compromise any medical diagnostic endeavor. By the same token, severe and chronic illness certainly produces depression and other associated psychiatric disorders that may benefit from therapeutic intervention. The use of a purely medical model cannot be endorsed.

Likewise, the purely psychiatric model has many of the same problems. In a thorough review of the problem, Dr. Charles Ford[7] discussed what has been called the *somatizing disorders*. In this article, the concept of the sick role that allows the ill person to be released from regular duties and obligations was described. He further differentiated illness from disease; the latter is measured objectively, but illness is the change in functioning of a patient. He clarified this point, indicating that disease can occur in the absence of illness; conversely, illness can occur in the absence of disease. Dr. Ford described somatization as "the process by which an individual uses the body, or bodily symptoms, for psychological purpose or personal gain." However, Ford conceded that somatization can occur in the presence of demonstrable physical disease, with amplification of the response to a real physical disorder. He listed nine reasons why people somatize: (1) to avoid unpleasant tasks or achieve primary or secondary gains in the form of payment, (2) to solve family problems, (3) to allow an individual to focus on physical symptoms rather than psychological problems, (4) to communicate displeasure, (5) to express oneself when incapable of expression otherwise, (6) as a culturally determined response, (7) to use a physical symptom because is it more culturally acceptable than a psychiatric one, (8) to focus on physical problems that are manifestations of underlying stress, and (9) to use a fashionable diagnosis to explain underlying psychiatric disease (such as hypoglycemia). Ford believed that patients may use somatic symptoms instead of expressing depression and indicated that these depressions were unrecognized.

Anxiety also may manifest as a somatic complaint; Ford also thought this was commonly undiagnosed. According to Ford, "chronic pain syndromes are one of the more common forms of somatization." Disability syndromes were included under the description of somatizing disorders. He reported that hard-working individuals who have an accident may fall apart. This inability to function allows the patient to obtain support and secondary gains; an underlying dependency may become manifest.

In a superb review article, Dr. Dennis Turk and Dr. Herta Flor[8] reviewed the psychological models contributing to chronic back pain. In this article, theoretical constructs were discussed that explain the transition from acute to chronic back pain, with the exception of the psychoanalytic approach. In this approach, unexplained back pain is considered a conversion neurosis or a manifestation of underlying tension, appearing as increased muscle activity and spasm. Using this model, various authors suggest that pain of unexplained origin should be treated as depression and antidepressant drugs administered. Another explanation for unexplained back pain advances the family systems hypothesis. In this approach, the basic idea is that symptoms of the patient fulfill the emotional needs of other family members. They suggest that the sick role is used for conflict avoidance. Another is the observational learning hypothesis based on cognitive behavioral assumptions. In this model, patients express feelings of helplessness and hopelessness and a loss of control of their environment. Another hypothesis, originally advanced by Flor, discusses the diathesis–stress model of chronic back pain. In this model, biopsychosocial interactions lead to the development of chronic back pain. This is an attempt to integrate the physical, psychological, and social factors that lead to the development of illness. In this diathesis–stress model, hyperactivity of the back muscles may be caused by (1) the existence of a response stereotypy (diathesis) involving the back muscles, (2) recurrent or intense adverse situations perceived as stressful, and/or (3) inadequate coping abilities of the patient.

To explain pain of unknown cause the new diagnostic manual (DSM-III) of the American Psychiatric Association is used. Reich and his group[9] attempted to explain the use of this diagnostic system for patients with chronic pain. In this article, the authors indicate that attempts to categorize such patients "merely in terms of the prime physical complaints has obvious shortcomings." They describe the five categories, or axes in the DSM-III manual that correspond to five major areas of concern: Axis I, used to describe thought disorders (such as schizophrenia, and/or manic depressive disease, and drug abuse problems); Axis II, used to describe personality characteristics; Axis III, used to describe medical diagnoses or physical complaints; Axis IV, used to describe the severity of psychosocial stress; and Axis V, used to describe the highest level of functioning during the past year. Reich and his group[9] believe that an entire category of diagnoses, the so-called somati form disorders, could be used to categorize patients with chronic pain, in whom there is a strong psychological component. This could explain pain unexplained by physical diagnoses. The major diagnosis in this group is psychogenic pain disorder. The criteria for using this diagnosis are (1) the absence of appropriate physical findings and (2) the presence of psychological factors that may explain the cause of the complaint.[10] Combined with this diagnosis are various subjective assessments, such as the severity of the pain, the inability of the pain to conform with an anatomic distribution, and perhaps the most subjective assessment of all, the severity of the pain out of proportion to what we might anticipate.[11,12] Further diagnostic categories under the somatiform disorders are hypochondriasis and conversion disorders. In the former, the patient is concerned with the development of a severe debilitating illness despite the lack of objective findings. In this instance, the patient's concerns are considered inordinate because the organic complaint was not substantiated. In conversion disorders, the physical condition suggests an underlying organic disease, but the basis of the illness is purely psychological. The authors then offer several examples of DSM-III diagnoses in which the predominant feature of Axis III (that is, the physical axis) is the use of words, such as "inconsistent with physical findings," "pain, etiology unknown," and prior surgeries "with residual pain." The authors advocate the use of DSM-III taxonomy because it has achieved better reliability than previous psychiatric diagnostic systems. The κ value for somatization disorders is 0.66, indicating a reasonable degree of reproducibility. However, the validity of these diagnoses remain questionable.

The third approach to diagnosing patients with chronic pain, that is, using an integrated response model, avoids the diagnostic dualism of the previous two models. In this model, an attempt is made to study the normal response to chronic pain in a previously well-adjusted patient and use these responses as a benchmark against which other responses can be measured. Only by thoroughly understanding the normal patterns of response can we determine what is abnormal. For this same reason, a medical student studies anatomy before studying pathology and physiology before pathophysiology. This approach also attempts to integrate responses and considers physical, psychological, and environmental factors, including sociologic and legal considerations. One such attempt at integration was advanced by Richard Black.[13] In his chapter, Dr. Black asserted that a patient with a chronic pain syndrome must be assessed simultaneously for physical, mental, and environmental factors. He believed that sociologic and economic factors rarely are considered, except where litigation was involved. He delineated six factors that should be evaluated in these patients: (1) somatogenic, referring to the physical perception of the pain, divided into both an acute and chronic complaint; (2) anxiety, divided into the psychological state versus the personality traits of the patient; (3) depression, divided into biochemical depression, reactive depression, depression secondary to the use of medications (but, unfortunately, not including any history about preexisting depression before the onset of pain); (4) social factors, divided into problems at work and home; (5) gains, divided into financial and personal gains; and (6) cultural factors, which would allow varying degrees of expression of a patient's pain. Although not complete, this paradigm offered some useful suggestions. First and foremost, Dr. Black recognized that certain psychological problems in chronic pain states are transient; other psychological problems are part of the personality characteristics of the patient and probably preceded the pain. He was one of the first authors to raise the question of cause-and-effect relationships. This is an often neglected consideration because most articles about psychological components of chronic pain do not consider the premorbid state of the patient (what the person was like before they had chronic pain).

In an effort to clarify this issue, Hendler[14–17] formulated a diagnostic system that evaluates (1) the premorbid (prepain) adjustment of the patient (pathologic or well-adjusted), (2) the response to the pain (pathologic or appropriate), and (3) the actual physical diagnosis (the presence or absence of objective findings). Central to his formulation were two basic concepts: (1) chronic pain can create psychological problems in a previously well-adjusted patient, and (2) regardless of the premorbid (prepain) personality characteristics, if a person has a normal response to chronic pain, then the chance of a valid organic basis for the complaint of pain is high. This would be true even in the absence of objective laboratory studies or physical findings. Restated for emphasis, if a patient's response to pain is appropriate, but there are no objective physical findings, it is incumbent on the physician to continue to look for the source of the patient's complaint.

Hindler[14] divided patients with chronic pain into four groups, based on these three factors. These four categories are: (1) objective pain patient, defined as an individual with a good premorbid adjustment, a normal response to chronic pain, and a definable organic lesion; (2) exaggerating pain patient, defined as an individual with psychopathology as part of a premorbid adjustment, an unusual response to pain (for example, there might be an absence of anxiety or depression), and minimal organic findings; (3) an undetermined pain patient, defined as an individual with a good premorbid adjustment, a normal response to pain, and an absence of objective physical findings on physical examination (it is this individual who warrants further in-

vestigation); and (4) affective or associative pain patient, defined as an individual with a poor premorbid adjustment, an unusual response to chronic pain, and a total absence of objective physical findings or positive laboratory studies.

By studying the normal response to chronic pain, we can compare any patient against a known standard. In this case, the objective pain patient serves as the normal model against which all other responses to chronic pain should be judged. The objective pain patient has a good premorbid adjustment, which can be defined as (1) a good work record; (2) a stable family background; (3) a negative psychiatric history, with no previous suicide attempts or depression; (4) the absence of alcohol or drug abuse; (5) a good marital history; (6) lack of financial difficulties before pain; (7) a good sexual adjustment; (8) no sleep difficulties; (9) no radical changes in weight, other than conscious attempts to change it; and (10) the absence of any arrests or sociopathic behavior.[15] Hendler expanded further on the objective pain patient, indicating that there are four stages in response to the chronic pain. The acute stage (0 to 2 months) is when the patient expects to get well and has no psychological problems. Psychological testing administered during this time is normal. In the subacute stage (2 to 6 months), the patient begins to experience somatic concerns and might have elevated Scales 1 and 3 on the MMPI. In the chronic stage of chronic pain, anywhere from 6 months to 8 years after the acquisition of the pain, the previously well-adjusted individual then develops depression, and has elevated Scales 1, 2, and 3 on the Minnesota Multiphasic Personality Inventory (MMPI), with Scale 2 (depression) being higher than Scales 1 and 3 (hypochondriasis and hysteria). From 3 to 12 years after the onset of the pain, the patient enters the subchronic stage of chronic pain, during which time the depression resolves, but hypochondriacal and hysterical scales of the MMPI remain elevated because the patient still has somatic concerns. If all this occurs in an individual with a definable organic lesion and positive objective testing, then we can categorize this type as an objective pain patient. If all the psychological features are present, but no objective tests are positive, then we can consider this individual to be an undetermined pain patient, who still needs further medical investigation.[16]

To facilitate diagnosis, using the four categories described, Hendler and his coworkers[17] devised the Mensana Clinic back pain test. Using a simple 15-question screening test, patients with chronic pain can be divided into the four diagnostic categories. The screening test had good predictive values because women scoring in the objective pain patient category (17 points or less) had positive findings on EMG, nerve conduction velocity studies, thermography, CT scan, myelogram, or x-ray 77 percent of the time. Of those scoring in the exaggerating pain patient category (21 points or greater), none of the 53 women studied had objective physical findings. This is in counterdistinction to the MMPI, which had a great deal of scatter, with only the depression scale correlating with the absence or presence of physical findings. The usefulness of the four diagnostic categories for patients with chronic pain was highlighted by the ability to predict the presence or absence of objective physical findings, based on (1) premorbid adjustment, (2) response to chronic pain, and (3) description of the pain itself. That the MMPI, which measures personality traits, was not a useful predictor of physical abnormalities lent support to the belief that personality characteristics and physical abnormalities are independent events. This reduced the accuracy of the current DMS-III diagnostic manual for validating pain complaints.

The preceding lengthy preamble regarding the psychiatric diagnosis of patients with chronic pain may seem out of place in a chapter on psychotherapy. However, it is appropriate to make a diagnosis of the patient's condition before instituting therapy. By offering the clinician various diagnostic systems from which to choose, the selection of appropriate therapy becomes a less formidable task. Whether we adhere strictly to DSM-III diagnoses or to less conventional diagnostic systems is a matter of which system gives the best results for a particular practitioner. This should facilitate selection of appropriate therapy. Although there are many types of psychotherapy available, this chapter will deal with the more conventional techniques: (1) individual psychotherapy, (2) biofeedback, (3) family therapy, (4) group psychotherapy, (5) pharmacotherapy, (6) narcosynthesis, and (7) hypnosis.[18]

PSYCHOTHERAPY

There are few reports in the psychiatric and medical literature that support the contention that individual psychotherapy is a useful treatment for chronic back problems or pain of any sort.[19,20] For the purpose of definition, we should consider psychotherapy as an individual session conducted between a patient and a therapist, without the use of specialized techniques (such as hypnosis, biofeedback, or narcosynthesis). Likewise, group psychotherapy or conditioning therapy are considered to be separate and distinct from individual, insight-oriented, dynamic psychotherapy. When we impose these parameters on the definition of psychotherapy, reports on its efficacy are sparse indeed. However, there are some components of individual psychotherapy that have therapeutic benefit, even though it is difficult to substantiate their efficacy. Rutrick[21] reports that psychotherapy can be effective if the therapist directs their activity toward understanding the so-called psychosomatic personality, ascribed to those who have (1) difficulty with psychological thinking, (2) difficulty with expressing emotion, and (3) are impulsive. In this abstract, it is suggested that character analysis is a critical element of psychotherapy and "is necessary to assure real emotional insight, and effect integration." So-called digestible interpretations might encourage learning of what component of the pain was thought to be psychological. Furthermore, using countertransference and relationships in the patient's life might help free the expression of emotions. Dr. Rutrick concluded that psychotherapy might overcome major emotional obstacles, facilitate the acceptance of chronic pain, and facilitate functioning despite the presence of chronic pain. He indicated that psychotherapy might generate improved self-esteem and relationships between those in the patient's life. This was attributed to the reordering of so-called narcissistic forces, meaning the patient was encouraged to reprioritize goals and self-perceptions. Unfortunately, there were no substantive data associated with this report, and it is largely anecdotal, using case reports for illustration.

Often, psychotherapy is administered in conjunction with other types of therapy.[22] As such, "eclectic studies, employing numbers of interventions provide some evidence for the usefulness of comprehensive treatment programs. However, the lack of control groups, the lack of a comprehensive pain assessment and the uncertainty about the effective components do not allow definite conclusions to be drawn. Here too, a wide variety of patients has been treated with a lack of or widely divergent sample descriptions. It needs to be determined which patients profit from what treatment. Component analysis of eclectic and cognitive–behavioral treatments are needed to determine the effective interventions and thus reduce cost and treatment time and enhance the effectiveness of the treatment."[23]

One element of psychotherapy, which is present whether an individual therapist recognizes it or not, is the component of modeling. This process occurs when patients observe another person with chronic pain who is functioning despite their physical damage. This other individual serves as a model for the patient's behavior and straddles the bridge between individual psychotherapy and behavioral therapy. Some therapists use videotapes of patients in pain coping with their problem; others use a directive approach, actually instructing the patient about which behaviors are acceptable, and which are not.[24]

BIOFEEDBACK

The use of biofeedback to assist patients with chronic pain has created much controversy.[25,26] Some authors believe that biofeedback does not offer any advantage over relaxation techniques and attribute its efficacy to its placebo effect.[24] Others have conducted more comprehensive reviews and concluded that EMG biofeedback may be a promising treatment for chronic back pain.[23] In the most evenhanded review of biofeedback techniques, Turk and Flor[23] report only the results of EMG biofeedback. This method seems to have the most usefulness for patients with muscle tension-type pain. These authors found that there were three types of reports in the literature: (1) anecdotal or systematic case studies, (2) group outcome or comparison studies, and (3) controlled group studies. The efficacy of

EMG biofeedback was complicated further by the fact that, in a review of more than 20 articles, all researchers, except one, used concomitant medication, not biofeedback exclusively. In the two controlled studies, both showed strong effects of EMG biofeedback on reducing pain and tension levels. In one study, a decrease of 60 percent in pain intensity and duration was noticed. As expected, as muscle tension levels dropped, pain intensity also decreased. However, at the 3-month follow-up, even though muscle tension increased, pain reduction was maintained. In the other study reviewed, EMG biofeedback was compared with medical treatment and pseudotherapy. In this study, EMG biofeedback was more efficacious than pseudotherapy and control consisting of medical treatment alone. EMG readings decreased, and the patients sought less medical attention during EMG biofeedback training. Turk and Flor[23] concluded that muscle relaxation alone does not necessarily contribute to the beneficial effects of EMG biofeedback, but rather a cognitive process is important. Hendler and his coworkers[27] attribute EMG biofeedback effectiveness to another factor. In their study, they evaluated two groups of patients: those who responded to biofeedback and those who did not. Thirteen patients were studied using EMG biofeedback. Six of the 13 reported that they had less pain on at least 4 of 5 days of EMG biofeedback training, but 11 of the 13 were unable to alter EMG biofeedback in the affected muscle group. EMG relaxation consisted of reduction of muscle tension in the forehead. Therefore, we might conclude that specific muscle relaxation was not the therapeutic component of the EMG biofeedback. There were no significant differences between either the starting EMG muscle tension levels or the final levels between the two groups. However, the response rate (6 of 13) was double what we might expect from a placebo effect alone on a consistent basis.[28] The difference between the two groups was thought to be the stages at which the patients were in their chronic pain process (whether they were in the acute stage, subacute stage, chronic stage, or subchronic stage). The difference between the patients who responded and those who did not was the presence of depression in the responders. Those who did not respond did not have elevated depression scales (using the 8CL-90).

Another component that may contribute to the efficacy of biofeedback therapy is the issue of the patient's motivation or preparedness for change. Large[29] measured so-called illness attitudes in an effort to determine which patients might respond to therapeutic interventions. He used an illness behavior questionnaire with a repertory-grid technique. Seven of the 18 patients did not obtain overall relief of symptoms; 11 subjects did. In this report, 48 ratings were analyzed to determine the discrepancy between how patients perceived themselves, and how they wished to be. Correlating these findings with response to biofeedback showed that people who were dissatisfied with their condi-

tion (chronic and persistent pain) were more likely to respond well to biofeedback.

FAMILY THERAPY

The role of the family in the maintenance of chronic pain behavior may be one factor to consider when dealing with treatment failures.[30] The poorest outcome among patients with chronic pain was found in families with the greatest degree of agreement when rating the severity of the patient's pain. Webb[24] interprets this as *tertiary gain,* indicating that the pain is maintained because of the psychological importance to another family member. A more likely explanation is that a patient with severe debilitating disease would have difficulty concealing the deficit from family members, and they would be in agreement with the patient's assessment of the pain. Webb[24] described family studies in which it was clear that the spouse and children of patients with chronic pain experience distress, as might be expected. This is particularly true in families where the patient is unemployed; it is less so in families where the patient is retired. It was concluded that families can reinforce the pain and worsen the prognosis.

In another study, two nurses investigated the impact of pain on 40 spouses of patients with chronic pain (21 men and 19 women).[31] They found that 60 percent of the spouses were uncertain as to the cause or persistence of the pain in their partner. Additionally, 83 percent of the spouses reported experiencing emotional, physical, or social disturbances that they directly attributed to the pain their spouses were feeling. Sixty-nine percent of the spouses believed that they were experiencing emotional difficulties as a result of their partner's pain. The most frequent forms of emotional disturbance were sadness or depression, fear, irritability, and nervousness. Forty percent of the spouses reported that there was a sense of helplessness because they were unable to change their partner's pain, and they were uncertain as to how to do so. They expressed feelings of loss of control. Seventy-five percent of the spouses thought that they could delineate which factors influenced their mate's pain (such as increased activity that reduced or increased the pain and medications that reduced the pain). Rowat and Knafl[31] divided the spouses into two groups: (1) high distress spouses and (2) low distress spouses. The high distress spouses reported feeling stress in the physical, emotional, and social dimensions of their lives. They experienced disturbances of sleep, appetite, physical symptoms, attention, anxiety, fear, sadness, isolation, and loss of freedom. They felt trapped in their relationship. Interestingly, 50 percent of the high distress spouses ranked their mate's pain higher on the McGill pain questionnaire than did the patients. In contradistinction, the low distress spouses denied any major disturbance in their personal or family lives as a result of chronic pain. The major distinction between the two groups was that the low distress spouse's mate had only been in pain for an average of 6.85 years; the high distress group had lived with pain as part of their marital relationship for 12.5 years. Also, only 3 of 13 patients were unemployed in the low stress spouse group; 7 of 12 patients were unemployed in the high stress spouse group. From this study, the authors concluded that the uncertainty of the cause of pain, uncertainty of the family life, uncertainty of pain management, and spousal distress were all factors that contributed to the spouses' distress. The high distress spouse group was unable to recognize factors that influenced the pain experience by their partners. Perhaps this element of loss of control over a particular situation contributed to the distress that they were experiencing. These authors make a strong point for including family members in the psychotherapy of patients with chronic pain.

In an excellent review article, the authors examined the factors influencing family relationships and believed that certain family characteristics and behaviors contributed to the problem of chronic pain and influenced the outcome.[32] It was found that some authors believed that there might be a relationship between the maintenance of pain and large family size. The rationale for this is obvious. In a large family, one of the ways to get attention and reduce tension would be the expression of disability or invalidism. Some authors report that most of their patients come from families with four or more children. Birth order also was considered a factor influencing the complaint of pain. One author found that the youngest or the oldest child complained; another author found that the complaint of pain might reduce tension more effectively for younger children in large families. These findings have not been supported by others. Socioeconomic status also may influence the expression of pain. Most patients with pain are blue-collar workers; this has been interpreted as the inability of working-class people to express emotional conflict, thereby using somatizing terms. Of course, we must consider that there are probably more blue-collar workers than there are professionals and blue-collar workers have manually strenuous jobs that put them at higher risk. Other equivocally substantiated hypotheses have been offered, citing such factors as the quality of relationships with parents, early loss of a family member, incidence of pain or illness in the family, and location of the pain corresponding to that of a family member. Depression in a family member also has been explained in psychodynamic terms; these are equally as difficult to substantiate. No doubt, patients with chronic pain have reduced sexual activity and poor sexual adjustment that may contribute to a poor marital relationship. Unfortunately, most studies in this area discuss only the patient. It is unclear whether marital difficulties develop as the result of the chronic pain or predate the chronic pain; the chronic pain may become a convenient excuse to avoid further sexual contact. When patients with chronic pain and depression were compared with patients with depression alone, the former group had more disturbed marital relationships than the latter. In an-

other study, patients with pain and no documented organic lesion were found to have more frequent so-called upsets, blows, conflicting interests, or separations than those patients with definable organic lesions. Payne and Norfleet[32] further reported that 91 percent of couples interviewed at a chronic pain treatment center reported sexual problems and a decline in their social lives since the onset of their pain problem. This was confirmed by other researchers. These authors concluded that studies on marital relationships involving such patients consistently indicate high rates of sexual and marital maladjustment, even in previously stable relationships. However, they also advanced the notion that the family may maintain the pain of an individual patient. Based on this review of the literature, four factors were found that contribute to the persistence of chronic pain in a patient: (1) the patient's pain is an expression of dysfunction in the family system and it is easier to use the complaint of pain than say there are difficulties with relationships; (2) the family acts as a reinforcer for pain behavior by nurturing and caring for the injured member; (3) the patient may use the symptom of pain to control family members, and pain behavior is reinforced when this works; and (4) the stresses of family life may produce physiologic effects that predispose an individual to stress and disease.

This review article considered three approaches to family therapy: (1) behavioral, (2) transactional, and (3) systems approach of structural family therapy. The behavioral approach was discussed in previous chapters in this book. The transactional approach tries to make family members aware of the ways a patient can use pain for psychological gain and how they might foil these attempts. The systems approach model deals with the family as an organization and tries to change the structure so that no one family member has to take a sick role. Most articles report that family therapy is a combination of behavioral, transactional, and systems approaches. Unfortunately, it is difficult to assess the efficacy of family therapy. However, follow-up studies, designed to reassess the recurrence of symptoms, are the best way of determining efficacy. One study from the Northwest Pain Center compared 25 successful patients with 25 patients who did not maintain gains made at the center. There were more divorced or separated people in the success group; the failure group had done little to change the patterns of behavior in their environment. It was concluded that the role of the family in maintaining pain behavior contributed to the failures. Payne and Norfleet[32] concluded that family members contribute to treatment outcome by reinforcing or not reinforcing pain behavior. They suggested that if a patient had a family who was appropriately supportive and learned not to reinforce pain behavior, the chance of success with pain treatment was improved greatly. If family members have not participated in the program or resist changes in their behavior, then the pain probably will persist. Compared with these resistent family groups, a single patient with pain will probably have a better chance of success even without family support.

GROUP PSYCHOTHERAPY

Group psychotherapy has been an adjunctive treatment for patients with terminal disease, rheumatoid arthritis, and chronic intractable benign pain. These three groups of patients share four common features: (1) they have not had success with conventional therapy, (2) they feel isolated and that they are a burden to their family and friends, (3) they are angry at physicians and disappointed about treatment failure, and (4) they have reactive depression, frustration, and reduced physical activity.[33] Group therapy can be used both on an inpatient and outpatient basis, although the structure and format for these two groups is somewhat different.[34] In the inpatient setting, the patient is involved in group therapy for only a relatively short period of time, usually 8 to 12 sessions. In this context, the group psychotherapy format more closely resembles a mixture of educational and free-interaction group psychotherapy, with a focus on more of the depressive components of the chronic pain process. As described by Hendler,[34] the most common themes of inpatient groups deal with depression and frustration, such as: (1) the feeling that treatment in a pain treatment center is a last resort; (2) expression of displeasure and anger toward physicians for not helping; (3) a willingness to do anything to get rid of the pain; (4) a feeling of helplessness and guilt, compounded by feelings of inadequacy and frustration, because of an inability to function with the pain; (5) indications about a relationship between the patient and family that show whether the family is supportive of the patient's behavior or in conflict with it; (6) questioning of religious faith and the selection process (why me?); (7) feelings of dependency; (8) resentment toward the disbelief of family members, physicians, and associates; and (9) a fear about the origin of the pain and its progression. Outpatient group therapy was more protracted and allowed exploration of different themes: (1) feelings of physical inabilities or handicaps, (2) resentment toward vocational rehabilitation, (3) difficulty readjusting life goals, (4) concern about other group members, (5) frustration regarding the slowness of the process of rehabilitation, and (6) fear regarding the loss of a spouse because of the chronic pain.

As in all forms of psychotherapy, it is difficult to assess the efficacy of group treatment. However, Ford[35] used an objective measure of efficacy (the amount of medical care sought by patients before and after group psychotherapy) and reviewed the literature on this topic. In this chapter, a cogent argument was offered for psychotherapy; it is able to reduce the number of medical visits, on a cost-effective basis, if there is no other reason. Various authors reported a 50 percent to 75 percent reduction in medical clinic visits while patients with somatic illness were undergoing group psychotherapy. Ford's[35] own experience was not as dramatic, but he attributed this to his patients' low socioeconomic group and underscored the need for long-term group treatment before any benefit was noticed. The most important benefit to a patient seemed to be in the area of gaining control over their life. Other authors believe that so-called peer modeling and interaction with other group members allows the patient to express emotion more freely, learn new coping methods, and be more verbal when soliciting help.[36] Although these authors concluded that group psychotherapy was a useful adjunct to their chronic pain treatment program, they did not offer any objective evidence. Hendler and coworkers[33] studied patients assigned to group or individual therapy. In their study, 8 of the 11 patients assigned to group therapy remained in therapy, and 7 of the 8 had abstained from narcotic and hypnotic use. This contrasted with a group of 12 individual-therapy patients, 7 of whom continued to use hypnotics, narcotics, or benzodiazepines prescribed by other physicians. At the end of 3 months, 6 of the 12 had discontinued sessions. In a more comprehensive report, Hall and associates[37] compared the efficacy of combined group therapy and tricyclic antidepressants versus supportive individual therapy, analytically oriented therapy, and management by surgical specialists, using narcotics or antidepressants. Using the Zung rating scales as an indication of the severity of depression, it was found that group psychotherapy, combined with tricyclic antidepressants, was the most efficacious method. Individual psychotherapy and surgical management, using narcotics or antidepressants, were least effective.

Although it is difficult to assess the efficacy of group therapy accurately and many reports do not have objective measures of outcome, the technique is cost-effective and provides a degree of modeling and social reinforcement that is not available from other forms of therapy. The effectiveness of other self-help groups, such as Alcoholics Anonymous, would lend credence to the contention that group therapy is an effective way to treat chronic pain patients.

NARCOSYNTHESIS

There have been many articles in the psychiatric and chronic pain literature suggesting that many undiagnosed chronic pain problems really are conversion reactions or hysterical conversion disorders. Most of these articles are unsubstantiated, or deal with single cases or a few cases. The authors attempt to apply their limited experience to a broad range of patients with chronic pain. The number of conversion disorders presenting as chronic pain problems is probably small. In this author's experience, after treating more than 4000 patients with chronic pain, both at the Chronic Pain Treatment Center of Johns Hopkins Hospital under the direction of the Department of Neurosurgery and at the Mensana Clinic during the past 11 years, the incidence of hysterical conversion disorders was three. These cases were memorable and represented great therapeutic challenges.

We should be careful in making the diagnosis of hysterical conversion reaction. In one of the classic studies, Slater[38] did a 9-year follow-up study on 85 patients originally diagnosed as having hysterical conversion reaction that were treated at Queens Square Hospital in London.[38] At the time of follow-up, only 19 of the 85 patients were free of symptoms. Of these 85 patients, 7 had recurrent endogenous depression, 2 were schizophrenic, 3 had undetected neoplasms, and of the 4 that committed suicide, 2 had atypical myopathy and disseminated sclerosis. Eight died of natural causes. Two patients had trigeminal neuralgia, and one woman's condition finally was diagnosed as thoracic outlet syndrome. Three people had early previously undected dementia; one woman, who had pain in the right shoulder and arm, had Takayasu syndrome. The rest had many organic diseases, including epilepsy, vestibular lesions, and total block of the spinal cord. Of the 85 patients with the original diagnosis of "hysteria," meaning a conversion reaction, only 7 were found to have an acute psychogenic reaction resulting in formation of a conversion symptom. Fourteen had Briquet syndrome, a polysomatic hysterical neurosis more compatible with hypochondriasis or somatizing disorders.

In a thorough review of the literature, encompassing nearly a 50-year period of time at Johns Hopkins Hospital, Stephens and Kamp[39] found that the incidence of hysterical conversion reaction in a psychiatric hospital (Phipps Clinic of Johns Hopkins Hospital) was approximately 2 percent of all psychiatric admissions. Therefore, we must be cautious in assigning the diagnosis of conversion neurosis or hysterical conversion disorder. In addition, many clinicians have difficulty differentiating between histrionic personality disorders and a hysterical personality disorder with many somatic complaints (Briquet syndrome). These two disorders are different than a hysterical conversion reaction because the last of these three disorders can occur in a previously well-adjusted individual subjected to extreme stress.[40] A review of histrionic personality disorders versus hysterical polysomatic Briquet syndrome versus hysterical conversion reactions versus malingering can be found in Hendler's[41] book, *Diagnosis and Nonsurgical Management of Chronic Pain*.

If hysterical conversion reaction is the suspected diagnosis, amobarbital narcosynthesis (or the thiopental challenge test) can be useful in assisting in the diagnosis. One of the leading proponents of this technique, A. Walters,[42] of the University of California School of Medicine, recommended doses between 200 and 500 mg and taking a patient through surgical planes of anesthesia, including loss of corneal reflex; this produces full relaxation of so-called psychogenic tissue pain. Using too small a dose of amobarbital may contribute to many of the failures associated with lack of effectiveness of this technique.[43] In fact, Hendler and Walters specifically found that a diagnostic failure, using amobarbital narcosynthesis, was related directly to an inadequate dose (dose range, 200 to 250 mg). When the dose was increased to 450 to 600 mg, effective narcosynthesis was obtained.

HYPNOSIS

When considering hypnosis for the patient in pain, we must make a distinction between acute and chronic pain. There is no question that hypnosis is an effective treatment for acute pain. Scott[44] discussed the usefulness of hypnotic technique for treating badly burned patients and surgical candidates. However, it was admitted that the effectiveness of this technique was variable and unreliable. In theory, hypnosis can be used to treat the patient with acute pain by altering the perception of the amount of time the pain is experienced. In this fashion, Teitelbaum[45] proposed that hypnosis can be used for hypnoanalgesia and called this phenomenon *time distortion*.

For chronic pain states, generalized relaxation therapy, as described by Jacobson,[46] seems to be useful. As with biofeedback, hypnotic relaxation techniques seem to work best for patients with chronic pain who have myofascial pain or chronic muscle tension. Unfortunately, it is difficult to assess the efficacy of hypnosis, especially in chronic pain states, because the technique does not lend itself to controlled studies. "The question of the efficacy of hypnosis with chronic back pain awaits controlled empirical research."[23] The major objection to hypnosis lies in the fact that it might provide temporary relief for the patient with chronic pain, but long-term relief has not been documented adequately. However, hypnosis may be a useful diagnostic tool for uncovering underlying hysterical conversion reactions, although it may be less reliable than narcosynthesis.

DIAGNOSIS AND TREATMENT OF DEPRESSION

No discussion about the psychotherapy of patients with chronic pain would be complete without a thorough understanding of the depression associated with chronic pain.[47] One of the major difficulties we encounter in diagnosing the cause in such patients with depression pertains to the etiology of the depression. France and Krishnan[48] distinguish between despondency or grief reaction in response to serious physical disease and depression, stating that despondency is similar to grief reaction and must be differentiated from depression in chronic pain states. They also believe that we may be able to differentiate various subtypes of depression in chronic low back pain and distinguish (1) major depression, (2) minor depression, (3) intermittent depression, and (4) chronic low back pain without depression. One way of making this distinction is using the dexamethasone suppression test as a biologic marker of depression. The current Chairman of the Department of Psychiatry at Duke University, Bernard Carroll, along with his coworkers,[49] first advanced the notion of elevated plasma cortisol, resistant to suppression by dexamethasone, in severe depressive illness. Subsequent to this original article in 1968, Dr. Carroll and coworkers published extensively about the use of the so-called dexamethasone suppression test. Randall France, also of Duke University, and his colleagues[48] studied a group of 80 patients with chronic back pain with and without depression, by using the dexamethasone suppression test. They selected a uniform group of such patients (those with chronic low back pain associated with organic disease) and divided them into two groups, based on the presence or absence of major depression, using DSM-III criteria. They then examined the cortisol response to dexamethasone in each group. Of this group of 80 patients, 35 patients had major depression, and 45 patients did not satisfy the criteria for major depression. However, of these 45 patients who did not have major depression, 10 satisfied the criteria for dysthymic disorder. In the group of patients with the diagnosis of major depression, 14 of the 35 had a positive dexamethasone suppression test; none of the 45 patients who did not have a major affective disorder had a positive dexamethasone suppression test. Again, in the group of 45 patients, 10 of them had a dysthymic disorder, which might be described more appropriately as reactive depression. It was concluded that the abnormal dexamethasone suppression test is a response to a major depressive disorder and not to chronic pain itself. In addition, the incidence of abnormal cortisol response to dexamethasone was higher in depressed patients without organic findings. In conclusion, the "difference in the rate of non-suppression in chronic back pain patients with and without depression, suggests that the notion of conceptualizing chronic back pain as a variant of depression or as a marked (sic) (masked) depression might be an oversimplification."[48]

In another study of 63 patients, conducted at the University of Washington Pain Clinic, 49 percent of the sample met the DSM-III criteria for major depression.[50] In this study, depressed patients did not differ significantly from nondepressed patients in the ratio of male to female, use of narcotics, use of sedative–hypnotics or antidepressant medications, number of years in chronic pain, age, or number of surgeries. However, for women, depression was related more closely to subjective reports of pain; in men, depression was related more closely to impairment of activity. In a review of 454 patients with chronic pain at Columbia-Presbyterian Medical Center, Department of Anesthesiology Pain Treatment Service, 100 patients were selected at random.[51] Eventually, 82 patients were contacted by telephone for long-term follow-up of a subsample of the original group. In evaluating the original 454 patients, 79 of these patients were depressed; 375 were not considered depressed. Between the two groups, there was no significant difference in sex, age, marital status, education, or compensation. The only significant differences existed between the percentages of patients undergoing litigation or being employed. The depressed patients had a higher percentage of litigation and a lower percentage of employ-

ment compared with the nondepressed patients. Compared with pain-related characteristics, those with depression more often had constant pain and a higher self-reported scale of pain than the nondepressed patients. In nondepressed patients, significant variables contributing to the ability to predict treatment outcome were number of treatment visits, compensation, number of previous therapies, and the location of pain. In depressed patients, the predictors of treatment outcome were employment and duration of pain.

Atkinson and his group[53] in San Diego defined three subgroups of patients with chronic pain based on MMPI scores and the type of depression they experienced. Using research diagnostic criteria, 44 percent of the 52 patients examined had major depression, 19 percent had minor depression, 13 percent had other psychiatric disorders, and 22 percent had no mental disorder. Patients with major depression had a specific MMPI profile. When the patients were divided by clinical characteristics of somatization, depression, or hypochondriasis, patients with major depression fell into three depression MMPI profile groups. Despite these distinctions there was "an even distribution of objective evidence for pain across all MMPI subgroups." This supports the contention that the MMPI cannot predict the validity of the complaint of pain, and patients with psychiatric problems also can have real physical problems.[17]

By using a psychiatric diagnostic system for delineating the various types of depression in patients with chronic pain and adhering rigorously to DSM-III diagnostic criteria, we can identify a group of such patients that would respond to interventions for depression. There is no doubt that the use of antidepressant medication in these patients with major depression is the most efficacious therapy. To prescribe medication appropriately, physicians should understand the pharmacologic contributions to normal sleep, pain perception, anxiety, and depression. In a review of the literature, Hendler[53] described the common pharmacologic substrate of normal sleep, pain perception, and antidepressant activity in the central nervous system as being an elevation of serotonin levels. Therefore, drugs that enhance serotonin activity in the central nervous system are beneficial; these include tricyclic antidepressants and the newer bicyclic and tetracyclic ones. Thus, an antidepressant, given at bedtime, may promote natural sleep, reduce the perception of pain, and reduce anxiety and depression. The dose should be tailored individually to suit the patient's age and tolerance for medication; as a starting dose, we recommend 50 to 100 mg of amitriptyline or doxepin in patients who are both anxious and depressed. Nortriptyline or desipramine may be administered at doses between 25 and 75 mg in patients who are depressed and report lack of energy or a feeling of sluggishness. The dose can be escalated by 25- to 50-mg increments, depending on the patient's response to the medication. The antianxiety effects of these medications usually occur within the first 2 days, as does enhancement of sleep. However, it may take 2 to 4 weeks before the antidepressant effects of these medications are appreciated fully. If the use of antidepressants is not efficacious by the end of 4 weeks, therapeutic monitoring, using serum levels, will allow adjustment of the dose into the proper range.

Specialized treatments for depression, such as monoamine oxidase inhibitors or electroconvulsive therapy, are best left to psychiatrists, and the selection of patients for these types of therapies should be done only after psychiatric consultation.

SUMMARY

Psychotherapy of patients with chronic pain is a difficult task at best.[54] In part, the process is complicated by the lack of precision of the diagnosis in the realm of psychiatry and medicine. For this reason, such patients are controversial. Improved treatment may be achieved by improved precision of diagnosis. Unfortunately, the efficacy of psychotherapy is difficult to establish, but improved level of functioning, less depression, better family relationships, and improvements in sleep and pain levels all can be achieved with appropriate interventions.

References

1. Rudy TE, Turk DC. Psychological aspects of pain. *Int Anesthesiol Clin* Winter 1991; 29(1):9–21.
2. Krishnan KRR, France RD, Pelton S, McCann UD, Davidson J, Urban BJ. Chronic pain and depression, I: classification of depression and chronic lower back pain patients. *Pain* July 1985; 22(3):279–287.
3. Hendler M. Depression caused by chronic pain. *Clin J Psychiatry* July 1984; 43(3 pt 2):30–36.
4. Pilowsky I, Bassett DL. Pain and depression. *Br J Psychiatry* 1982; 141:30–36.
5. Engel G. Psychogenic pain in the pain prone patient. *Am J Med* 1959; 26:899–918.
6. Maruta E, Swanson D, Swanson W. Pain as a psychiatric symptom: comparison between low back pain and depression. *Psychosomatics* 1976; 17:123–127.
7. Ford CV. Somatisizing disorders. *Psychosomatics* May 1986; 27(5):327–337.
8. Turk D, Flor H. Ideological theories and treatments for chronic back pain, II: psychological models and interventions. *Pain* 1984; 19(3):209–233.
9. Reich J, Rosenblatt R, Tupin J. DSM-III: a new nomenclature for classifying patients with chronic pain. *Pain* June 1983; 16(2):201–206.
10. Corbishley MA, Hendrickson R, Beutler LE, Engle D. Behavior, affect, and cognition among psychogenic pain patients in group expressive psychotherapy. *J Pain Symptom Manage* August 1990; 5(4):241–248.
11. Jenkins PL. Psychogenic abdominal pain. *Gen Hosp Psychiatry* January 1991; 13(1):27–30.
12. Feinmann C. Psychogenic regional pain. *Br J Hosp Med* February 1990; 43(2):123–124, 127.
13. Black RB. The clinical management of chronic pain. In: Hendler N, Long D, Wise T, eds. *Diagnosis and Treatment of Chronic Pain*. Littleton, MA: John Wright; 1982:211–224.
14. Hendler N. *Diagnosis and Nonsurgical Management of Chronic Pain*. New York: Raven Press; 1981; 12–15.
15. Hendler N. The four stages of pain. In: Hendler N, Long D, Wise T, eds. *Diagnosis and Treatment of Chronic Pain*. Littleton, MA: John Wright; 1982:1–8.
16. Hendler N. Validating and treating the complaint of chronic back pain: the Mensana Clinic approach. *Clin Neurosurg* 1989; 35:385–397.
17. Hendler N, Mollett A, Viernstein M, et al. A comparison between the MMPI and the "Mensana Clinic Back Pain Test" for validating the complaint of chronic back pain in women. *Pain* November 1985; 23(3):243–252.
18. Doody SB, Smith C, Webb J. Nonpharmacologic interventions for pain management. *Crit Care Nurs Clin North Am* March 1991; 3(1):69–75.
19. Farquhar CM, Rogers V, Franks S, Pearce S, Wadsworth J, Beard RW. A randomized controlled trial of medroxyprogesterone acetate and psychotherapy for the treatment of pelvic congestion. *Br J Obstet Gynaecol* October 1989; 96(10):1153–1162.
20. Hill D, Beutler LE, Daldrup R. The relationship of process to outcome in brief experiential psychotherapy for chronic pain. *J Clin Psychol* November 1989; 45(6):951–957.
21. Rutrick D. Psychotherapy with chronic intractable benign pain patients. *Pain Suppl* 1981; 1(331):271S.
22. Pilowsky I, Barrow CG. A controlled study in psychotherapy and amitriptyline used individually and in combination in the treatment of chronic intractable, "psychogenic" pain. *Pain* January 1990; 40(1):3–19.
23. Turk D, Flor H. Etiological theories and treatment for chronic back pain, II: psychological models and intervention. *Pain* July 1984; 19(3):209–233.
24. Webb W Jr. Chronic pain. *Psychosomatics* December 1983; 24(2):1053–1063.
25. Grunert BK, Devine CA, Sanger JR, Matloub HS, Green D. Thermal self-regulation for pain control in reflex sympathetic dystrophy syndrome. *J Hand Surg Am* July 1990; 15(4):615–618.
26. Murphy MA, Tosi DJ, Pariser RF. Psychological coping and the management of pain with cognitive restructuring and biofeedback: a case study and variation of cognitive experiential therapy. *Psychol Rep* June 1989; 64(3 pt 2):1343–1350.
27. Hendler N, Derogatis L, Avella J, Long D. EMG biofeedback in patients with chronic pain. *Dis Nerv Syst* 1977; 38:505–509.
28. Hendler N, Fernandez P. Alternative treatments for patients with chronic pain. *Psychiatr Ann* December 1980; 10(12):25–33.
29. Large R. Prediction of treatment response in pain patients: the illness self-concept repertory grid and EMG biofeedback. *Pain* March 1985; 21(3):279–271.
30. Flor H, Turk DC, Rudy TE. Relationship of pain impact and significant other reinforcement of pain behaviors: the mediating role of gender, marital status and marital satisfaction. *Pain* July 1989; 38(1):45–50.
31. Rowat KM, Knafl KA. Living with chronic pain: the spouses' perspective. *Pain* November 1985; 23(3):259–271.
32. Payne B, Norfleet M. Chronic pain and the family: a review. *Pain* July 1986; 26(1):1–22.

33. Hendler N, Viernstein M, Shallanberger C, Long D. Group psychotherapy with chronic pain patients. *Psychosomatics* April 1981; 22(4):332–340.

34. Hendler N. Chronic pain. In: Roback H, ed. *Helping Patients and Their Families Cope with Medical Problems.* San Francisco: Jossey-Bass; 1984:79–106.

35. Ford CV. Somatisizing disorders. In: Roback H, ed. *Helping Patients and Their Families Cope with Medical Problems.* San Francisco: Jossey-Bass; 1984:39–59.

36. Gamsa A, Braha R, Catchlove R. The use of structure group therapy sessions in the treatment of chronic pain patients. *Pain* May 1985; 22(1):91–96.

37. Hall RC, Hall AK, Gardnar ER. Comparison of tricyclic antidepressants, and analgesics. In: *The Management of Chronic Postoperative Surgical Pain.* Read before the Annual Meeting of the Academy of Psychosomatic Medicine; October 31, 1979; San Francisco.

38. Slater E. Diagnosis of "hysteria" *Br Med J* 1965; 1:1395–1399.

39. Stephens J, Kamp. On some aspects of hysteria: a clinical study. *J Nerv Ment Dis* 1962; 134:305–315.

40. Hendler N. *Diagnosis and Nonsurgical Management of Chronic Pain.* New York: Raven Press; 1981:80–92.

41. Hendler N. *Diagnosis and Nonsurgical Management of Chronic Pain.* New York: Raven Press; 1981:64–100.

42. Walters A. Psychiatric Considerations of Pain. In: Youmans J, ed. *Neurological Surgery,* 3. 1st ed. Philadelphia: Saunders; 1973:1516–1645.

43. Hendler N, Filtzer D, Talo S, Panzetta M, Long D. Hysterical scoliosis treated with amorbital narcosynthesis. *Clin J Pain* 1987; 2(3):179–182.

44. Scott DL. *Modern Hospital Hypnosis.* Chicago: Year Book; 1974.

45. Teitelbaum M. *Hypnosis Induction Techniques.* Charles C. Springfield: Charles C. Thomas; 1965:24–29.

46. Jacobson E. *Anxiety and Tension Control.* Philadelphia: Lippincott; 1964:108–111.

47. Covington EC. Depression and chronic fatigue in the patient with chronic pain. *Prim Care* June 1991; 18(2):341–358.

48. France R, Krishnan KRR. The dexamethasone suppression and a biological marker of depression and chronic pain. *Pain* January 1985; 21(1):49–55.

49. Carroll EJ, Martin FIR, Davies B. Resistance to suppression by dexamethasone of plasma II-OHCS in severe depressive illness. *Br Med J* 1968; 3:285–287.

50. Haley W, Turner J, Romano J. Depression in chronic pain patients: relation to pain, activity, and sex difference. *Pain* December 1985; 23(4):337–343.

51. Dworkin R, Richlin D, Handlin D, Brand L. Predicting treatments response in depressed and nondepressed chronic pain patients. *Pain* March 1986; 24(3):343–353.

52. Atkinson JH, Ingram R, Kremer E, Saccuzzo D. MMPI subgroup: and affective disorders in chronic pain patients. *J Nerv Ment Dis* 1986; 174(7):408–413.

53. Hendler N. The anatomy and psychopharmacology of chronic pain. *J Clin Psychiatry* 1982; 43:15–20.

54. Benjamin S. Psychological treatment of chronic pain: a selective review. *J Psychosom Res* 1989; 33(2):121–131.

CHAPTER 35

Neurosurgical Treatment of Pain

David Dubuisson

In this chapter, we consider surgical procedures that are used to relieve pain. There are four categories (Table 35-1).

I. Techniques that attempt to correct the disordered physiology of nerves without creating a lesion.
II. Destructive procedures.
  A. Procedures that transsect primary afferent fibers at the level of peripheral nerve, root, or ganglion.
  B. Operations that interrupt ascending sensory tracts in the spinal cord or brain stem.
  C. Stereotactically placed lesions of deep brain structures.
  D. Operations that inactivate a portion of the sympathetic system.
  E. Destruction of the anterior lobe of the pituitary gland.
III. Procedures in which a device is implanted to deliver narcotic drugs.
IV. Procedures in which a device is implanted to stimulate an analgesia-producing mechanism in the central nervous system.

PROCEDURES TO CORRECT DISORDERED NERVE PHYSIOLOGY

The first category of neurosurgical procedures for pain includes operations designed to relieve constriction of peripheral nerves,[1] spinal nerve roots, or cranial nerves. These decompressive operations are sometimes elegant and often curative. Their use is restricted to specific well-defined syndromes in which the site of disordered nerve physiology can be predicted. The prediction usually is based on radiologic studies, electromyography, nerve conduction studies, and clinical examination. Most procedures of this type have high success rates. Whenever possible, they should be used in preference to destructive lesions.

The reason for the success of nerve decompression is not entirely clear. It is not always understood why pressure on a nerve causes pain. Not all sites of nerve distortion are associated with chronic pain. For example, in a large series

Table 35-1
Neurosurgical Techniques for Pain Relief

Nondestructive procedures	Carpal tunnel release
	Thoracic outlet decompression
	Root decompression
	Cranial nerve decompression
Destructive procedures	
Primary afferent	Peripheral neurectomy
	Excision of neuroma
	Glycerol injection
	Glangliolysis
	Ganglionectomy
	Rhizotomy
	Rhizidiotomy
Spinal cord or brain stem	Cordotomy
	Dorsal root entry zone lesions
Deep brain structures	Stereotactic lesions of thalamus, hypothalamus, or spinal thalamic or spinal reticular tracts
	Psychosurgery
Sympathetic nerves	Thoracic sympathectomy
	Lumbar sympathectomy
Pituitary	Pituitary ablation
Stimulation techniques	Spinal cord stimulation
	Deep brain stimulation
Narcotic delivery systems	Intraspinal narcotic catheters

of patients investigated for possible acoustic nerve tumors, myelograms frequently showed incidental disk protrusions. Asymptomatic lesions severe enough to distort spinal nerve roots were identified in one-third of cases.[2] These well-defined disk protrusions with nerve root compression were not painful, nor were they known to the patients who had them.

From experimental studies, it appears likely that sites of chronic nerve compression undergo demyelination and that spontaneous axonal discharges occur. These sites also become sensitive to mild mechanical distortion. Perhaps the difference between an asymptomatic site of compression and a painful one lies in the extent of demyelination and the amount of mechanical stress placed on the nerve during daily activities. Sometimes the relief of pain using decompression is immediate; in other cases, it may be gradual, suggesting that the initial decompression obviates the mechanical effect, and the passage of time permits recovery from the focal loss of myelin in the afferent fibers.

Peripheral Nerve Decompression

The pain of carpal tunnel syndrome usually is amenable to decompression of the median nerve at the wrist. The procedure is done most often with local or regional anesthesia.[3] Some surgeons use a tourniquet on the forearm, although it is not necessary. The nerve is compressed by the thickened overlying flexor retinaculum of the hand, which yields as it is divided. In some cases, an additional focus of pressure is found above the wrist crease. Similar compression of the ulnar nerve may occur beneath the proximal tendinous attachment of the flexor carpi ulnaris muscle just below the elbow, causing the cubital tunnel syndrome, and in other sites. In most cases, simple division of the overlying ligament suffices. Occasionally, the nerve may benefit from a minor transposition to a location where it is completely free of mechanical distortion.

Thoracic Outlet Syndromes

Chronic pain in the arm, most often in an ulnar distribution, may be accompanied by obliteration of the pulse in certain shoulder positions. This combined neural–vascular compression may be caused by fibrotic changes of the scalene muscles, cervical rib, or a fracture of the clavicle with bony callus compressing the brachial plexus. Adequate treatment in most patients consists of decompression of the lower portion of the plexus; the exact procedure is tailored to correct the anatomic irregularity responsible. A cervical rib may be removed, a fibrous band divided, or the enlarged clavicle and surrounding scar tissue resected. These procedures require a general anesthetic.

Lumbar and Cervical Radiculopathies

A common neurosurgical procedure to relieve pain is decompression of a lumbar or cervical nerve root by excision of an intervertebral disk. Few surgeons currently favor explorations of spinal nerve roots for pain alone; instead, treatment of the associated weakness, sensory loss, or sphincter disturbance assumes greater importance. In cases of lumbar disk disease, if a well-defined lesion is shown by myelogram, CT, or magnetic resonance imaging and the appropriate neurologic signs are present, there is at least a 60 percent chance of relieving back pain and radicular pain.[4]

The cause of lumbar root compression differs from patient to patient. Often, the bulging anulus fibrosis of a degenerated disk protrudes enough to contact an adjacent root, or a firm piece of nucleus pulposus emerges through a rent in the anulus and becomes trapped in the spinal canal. However, the disorder may not be so obvious. Spondylotic changes of the facet joint and ligamentum flavum lead to joint enlargement and ligamentous thickening behind the root; bony osteophytes around the worn disk jut into the canal in front (Fig. 35-1). These changes may require additional surgery, such as partial removal of the facet joint (facetectomy) or unroofing of the intervertebral foramen behind the compressed root (foramenotomy). When the overall dimensions of the canal are too small, all roots of the cauda equina may be compressed or their circulation impeded during erect posture. These cases of lumbar spinal stenosis require complete removal of the lamina bilaterally at every level that is narrowed significantly.

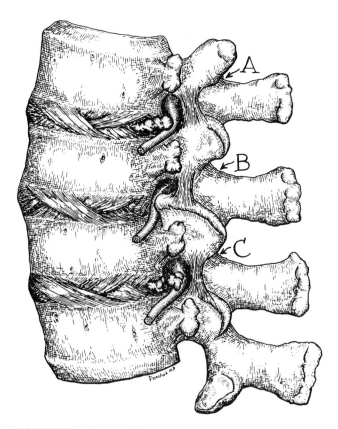

FIGURE 35-1. *Spondylotic changes causing nerve root compression. A: Disk protrusion, B: facet hypertrophy, C: free disk fragment. (Illustration by Stephen Ponchak, M.D.)*

The surgical approach for lumbar disk removal is controversial. Some surgeons advocate a microsurgical approach to diskectomy, with a small skin incision and magnification of the deep structures. There is little doubt that this can be an effective means of treating a fragment of herniated nucleus pulposus; its chief advantages are reduced postoperative pain and shorter hospital stay. Major disadvantages are limitation of the surgeon's view and restricted access of instruments to the disk space itself. Not all cases of root compression consist of simple herniated nucleus pulposus. Lumbar spinal stenosis cannot be treated adequately by the microsurgical approach. It can be argued that diskectomy by a limited exposure may predispose the surgeon to retract harder on the nerve roots and dural tube. Because some of the most intractable cases of sciatica are seen after unsuccessful disk surgery, it is reasonable to ask whether certain surgical approaches may add to the previous degree of nerve root damage. Hard pressure on the root by a surgical instrument could lead to bruising, scar formation, and focal demyelination. In his discussion of the so-called battered root syndrome, Bertrand[5] advocated wider surgical exposure during diskectomy to avoid missing a hidden fragment of material that may have migrated in the epidural space and to visualize all other anatomic features that may be contributing to the patient's symptoms. In some cases, this will require a complete laminectomy. Sometimes it is necessary to explore the adjacent disk if the cause of root compression is not immediately apparent.

As a general rule, if the patient's pain does not resolve after diskectomy, we should suspect that the cause of pain was not identified at the time of operation. If the pain resolves but returns in a slightly different distribution, a second disk protrusion may be present. If the pain is worse and severe numbness or dysesthesia appears, the root may have been damaged by the surgeon. Rarely, a patient may have a fever and severe bilateral cramps and leg spasms during the first few postoperative days; this may be a warning of arachnoiditis.[6] Late recurrences of pain in the original distribution often are associated with prominent scar formation in the epidural space surrounding the nerve root. In some cases, removal of this scar is beneficial, but repeated surgery of this type is risky and often futile.

The decompression of cervical nerve roots usually is done by an anterior approach through the disk space because the roots are located directly behind the disk. Most surgeons who do cervical diskectomies fuse the interspace with a bone plug during the same operation to prevent instability and recurrence of osteophytes at that level. Two disks may be removed in this way. If more than two levels are involved, however, it is preferable to do laminectomies and decompress the nerve roots as necessary by drilling away additional bone posteriorly. In these cases of extensive cervical spondylosis, diskectomy may not be required at all provided an adequate posterior decompression of cord and roots is achieved.

Decompression of Cranial Nerves

In many instances of cranial neuralgia, there is a mechanical factor that can be corrected without sacrificing the involved nerve. Although some older procedures were directed at the peripheral portion of the nerve, as in division of the stylohyoid ligament for glossopharyngeal neuralgia, currently, there is great interest in exploring the posterior cranial fossa. If the patient with typical trigeminal or glossopharyngeal neuralgia is in good enough health to undergo a craniectomy under general anesthesia, local decompression of the fifth or ninth nerve at a focus of constriction may be the definitive means of treating the neuralgia. Jannetta[7] described arteries compressing the trigeminal root near the brain stem in nearly all cases of tic douloureux. It is recognized that veins and tumors may cause similar effects, and separation of the nerve root from the compressing structure will relieve neuralgia long term in 85 percent of patients. This procedure is termed microvascular decompression. The same procedure has been done successfully on the glossopharyngeal root.

Microvascular decompression requires a posterior fossa craniectomy under general anesthesia, with opening of the dura and retraction of the cerebellum. The procedure has a small mortality rate (less than 1 percent) and a morbidity of perhaps 3 percent to 5 percent, consisting primarily of ataxia and facial sensory loss. In cases of trigeminal neuralgia, the typical finding is an ectatic superior cerebellar artery crossing the nerve root close to the pons; this is dissected away and kept separate with a tiny plastic sponge or fragment of muscle. In approximately 10 percent of these patients, a compressive lesion cannot be seen; in this case, the surgeon may have to resort to subtotal rhizotomy.

DESTRUCTIVE PROCEDURES

Surgical Procedures to Interrupt Primary Afferent Fibers

Peripheral Neurectomy and Treatment of Neuromas

Section or avulsion of peripheral nerves as a treatment of neuralgic pain has been done mainly in patients with trigeminal and occipital neuralgia. Although these procedures are simple, they have the obvious disadvantages that complete numbness will occur, and peripheral nerve fibers eventually will regenerate. In the author's opinion, more definitive procedures are available to treat both trigeminal and occipital neuralgia with better long-term success and no greater risk. In elderly or infirm patients, this does not necessarily require craniotomy or spinal surgery; instead, a percutaneous procedure often suffices.

Neuromas, either posttraumatic or after peripheral nerve biopsy, are difficult to treat. Usually, it is easy to detect the presence of a neuroma by palpating directly over the site of nerve injury. Neuromas are often unusually tender, and pressure directly over them is painful. Dozens of procedures have been advocated to prevent the reformation of neuromas after excision. They range from burial of the nerve end in bone or muscle to capping of the cut end with a small metal or plastic sheath. Various toxic and medicinal solutions have been painted onto the cut nerve to little avail. Most surgeons agree that simple excision of the neuroma and avoidance of pressure from surrounding tissues is a worthwhile first attempt at treatment, but if this fails, it is usually worthless to resect the neuroma repeatedly.

Although there is no proven surgical treatment of neuromas, current techniques of interest include (1) the creation of a loop by dividing the cut nerve into fascicles joined end-to-end, (2) sealing individual nerve fascicles by drawing the perineurium over the tip of each and lightly cauterizing it with microsurgical forceps, or (3) ligating each fascicle with fine suture material.[8] To the author's knowledge, the long-term success of microfascicular anastomosis or ligation is not known. Both these procedures have at least anecdotal success, but it is wise to remember that many previous techniques to prevent neuromas have failed after brief initial enthusiasm.

Noordenbos and Wall[9] described seven patients in whom an injured nerve caused local pain and abnormal sensitivity. Resection of the damaged portion and insertion of a sural nerve graft with microsurgical technique was followed inevitably by a recurrence of pain in these patients, suggesting that the peripheral nerve injury had induced changes in the central nervous system that were not reversed by treating the injured nerve itself.

Injection of Glycerol in the Trigeminal Ganglion

Hakanson[10] first reported the procedure of injecting sterile 100 percent glycerol into the Meckel cave to treat trigeminal neuralgia. He reported a 90 percent success rate in 100 patients with no complications and only occasional slight facial numbness. Glycerol injection has been shown to cause some degree of damage to both myelinated and unmyelinated nerve fibers.[11] Since its mechanism of action is still poorly understood and its after effects are usually slight, it might be more appropriate to consider it a means of altering peripheral nerve physiology without a lesion. It is described here as an alternative to percutaneous thermocoagulation of the trigeminal ganglion.[12]

Trigeminal glycerol injection is done by passing a needle through the foramen ovale (Fig. 35-2). A 20-gauge lumbar puncture needle is suitable. The patient is given short-acting or reversible intravenous anesthetics, such as midazolam and/or fentanyl until drowsy. After anesthetizing the cheek with lidocaine, the needle is inserted 1.5-cm lateral to the corner of the mouth and directed posteriorly toward a point 2-cm anterior to the external auditory meatus and medially toward the midpupillary line. The author uses a fluoroscopic C-arm to identify the foramen ovale. The needle tip is positioned 10 to 12 mm below the posterior clinoid processes, and with the stylet withdrawn, cerebrospinal fluid

emerges. Then the patient is placed in a seated position with the head tilted forward slightly, and 0.2 to 0.4 ml of glycerol is injected. The patient is kept upright for 45 min so that the glycerol does not escape rapidly from the trigeminal cistern. The amount of glycerol used determines the extent of the chemical gangliolysis; larger volumes will affect the first division of the nerve and increase the risk of corneal anesthesia. In some cases of first division tic douloureux with a cutaneous trigger zone in the nose or upper cheek, the author has produced excellent relief of pain with 0.25 ml of glycerol, suggesting that the primary effect was on the second division trigger zone. There was no loss of corneal sensation in those cases.

In the author's experience, more than 90 percent of patients with trigeminal neuralgia have either complete relief or marked improvement of their pain after an initial glycerol injection. During the following 18 months, approximately 20 percent return for a second injection; this usually also is successful. In cases of atypical facial pain, there has been only a 40 percent success rate.

One-third of patients who undergo the procedure notice numbness or mild burning sensations in the cheek or mouth, but objective sensory testing rarely shows frank anesthesia in these areas. Careful testing with a wisp of cotton shows the corneal reflex to be blunted initially in most patients, and lubricant eye drops are prescribed. This improves during the first month in nearly all instances. Occasionally, typical cold sores of herpes simplex appear on the lips,

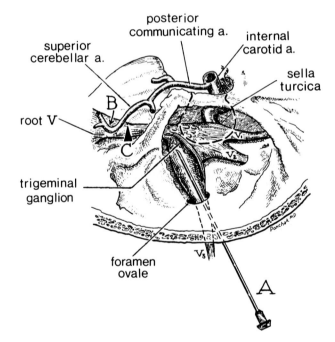

FIGURE 35-2. Surgical treatments of trigeminal neuralgia. The root of the trigeminal nerve is shown at left emerging from the brain stem, and the three major divisions of the nerve are at right. A: Insertion of needle for thermocoagulation or glycerol injection in ganglion, B: separation of vessel from root (microvascular decompression), C: subtotal root section. (Illustration by Stephen Ponchak, M.D.)

nose, or oral mucosa during the first few days after the glycerol injection. This phenomenon may be seen in any surgical procedure on the trigeminal nerve. It is usually transient and of cosmetic importance only, but the sores can be painful, and the patient should be warned beforehand. The author has witnessed one instance of herpetic keratitis in the ipsilateral eye that resolved promptly with treatment. No permanent complications were seen. The author is not aware of any reported deaths from this procedure.

Another percutaneous surgical treatment of tic douloureux still widely used is radiofrequency gangliolysis or thermocoagulation of the trigeminal ganglion. The approach is the same as that described for glycerol injection, except that a larger needle is used. The stylet is modified to serve as a stimulation probe. With the patient moderately sedated, it is feasible to test before the lesion is made by passing electrical pulses through the probe to stimulate different levels of the ganglion and thereby identify the predominant division of the nerve surrounding the probe tip. The patient then is given a short-acting general anesthetic (such as methohexital) while the lesion is made by passing radiofrequency current through the probe tip with temperature control. The patient is awakened to test for sensory deficit and determine whether the lesion is placed suitably. A typical radiofrequency lesion blunts pinprick but not touch in the region of pain. When the trigger zone for trigeminal neuralgia lies in a different division than the area of pain, it is helpful also to destroy the fibers serving the trigger area. Thermocoagulation of the trigeminal ganglion relieves trigeminal neuralgia in 80 percent to 85 percent of cases in various published series. In approximately one-half of cases, a second lesion is required after a variable interval of 1 to 5 years. The second lesion is usually as successful as the first. The mortality rate is less than 0.5 percent, and the rare deaths attributed to the procedure may involve misplacement of the probe with intracranial hemorrhage. The procedure itself can be painful if intravenous sedation is not effective. The author has read anecdotal reports of severe arterial hypertension during the procedure with cerebral hemorrhage in elderly patients. In my experience, the procedure is not tolerated as well as glycerol injection, perhaps because in the latter, the needle is smaller, and electrical stimulation of the ganglion is not used. Moreover, the thermocoagulation lesion itself is painful; the glycerol injection usually can be done with the patient awake. Repeated positioning of the probe for accurate thermocoagulation requires extra sedation.

More cases of thermocoagulation of the ganglion have been reported than of glycerol injection, and neurosurgeons disagree over which procedure is best. The author favors the glycerol technique because it is easier for the patient and it appears to have less risk of permanent facial or corneal anesthesia. In cases of atypical facial pain, neither has the advantage. The percutaneous gangliolysis procedures are preferable for elderly patients or for those who cannot undergo a posterior fossa craniectomy safely. However, the recurrence rate of tic douloureux is significantly greater, especially after the first year.[13]

Cranial Nerve Rhizotomy

When medication trials, percutaneous procedures, and microvascular decompression are unsuccessful, or when decompression is attempted but no constricting lesion can be found, a partial rhizotomy of the trigeminal root can be done with an 80 percent long-term success rate for trigeminal neuralgia. Rhizotomy is believed to have a 1 percent to 2 percent mortality rate and 5 percent to 10 percent morbidity, but these figures may be overly pessimistic, given that most of the reported series were done several decades ago and techniques of microsurgery and intraoperative and postoperative monitoring have improved. Some surgeons are reluctant to do trigeminal rhizotomies because they think that the incidence of anesthesia dolorosa is higher than with other procedures. Rhizotomy produces greater loss of facial sensation than gangliolysis or root decompression. Therefore, it is reasonable to ask whether rhizotomy has a higher incidence of severe postoperative pain than other procedures, and if not, whether the reputedly increased risk of anesthesia dolorosa is a reflection of the greater incidence of numbness in the painful area. Probably, most of the patients with this syndrome would fit the diagnostic category of atypical facial pain preoperatively rather than trigeminal neuralgia. To spare the corneal reflex, the surgeon avoids sectioning the most anterior and superior portion of the trigeminal root. Partly for this reason, some of the most refractory cases of facial pain are those involving the eye and supraorbital region.

Rhizotomy of cranial nerves IX and X remains a standard surgical treatment for glossopharyngeal neuralgia. It has a 75 percent to 80 percent long-term success rate.[14] The operation is done under general anesthesia using a posterior fossa craniectomy. Cardiovascular instability during the operation and immediately afterward is a well-recognized potential complication. The procedure therefore has a higher risk than trigeminal rhizotomy; the reported mortality rate in several series combined was 5 percent for 166 cases.[15] Results of microvascular decompression of the lower cranial nerves[16] were not appreciably different from those of rhizotomy in cases of glossopharyngeal neuralgia, but it would seem desirable to preserve cranial nerves IX and X by decompression when a constricting lesion is present.

Spinal Rhizotomy, Ganglionectomy, and Partial Rhizidiotomy

Pain restricted to the distribution of a few spinal nerve roots sometimes can be treated by dorsal root section or removal of the dorsal root ganglia at levels that encompass the painful area. It is desirable to do this, not only at the corresponding segmental level, but also at one or two segments above and below it as a result of the overlap of dermatomes. Rhizotomy and ganglionectomy have found their greatest use in cases of idiopathic and posttraumatic or postsurgical pain of the neck, trunk, and coccygeal region. The technique of selective partial rhizidiotomy attempts to spare proprioception when roots are sectioned at the level of the extremities. The basic difference between these procedures is illustrated in Figure 35-3.

Dorsal rhizotomy is done intradurally at thoracic and cervical levels; at lumbar and sacral levels, there is the option of sectioning the roots in their sheaths without exposing the spinal cord. An advantage of intradural rhizotomy is that the individual rootlets of each dorsal root (which fan out to enter the cord) can be sectioned separately, avoiding any accompanying blood vessels. With magnification, the vessels can be separated easily and spared. Another advantage is that the ventral roots can be avoided completely; this is not necessarily the case with extradural rhizotomies.

At thoracic levels, it is feasible to excise the dorsal root ganglia without opening the spinal canal. The ganglia lie beneath the most lateral portions of the laminae. Therefore, a small amount of bone removal below the transverse processes will expose them, and there is no need for laminectomies. The theoretic appeal of dorsal root ganglionectomies is that standard dorsal rhizotomy may spare some fine diameter afferent fibers that leave the dorsal root ganglion and reach the cord through the sympathetic chain or the ventral roots. Although there is no anatomic proof of the existence of such afferents in humans, Hosobuchi[17] presented several cases in which dorsal rhizotomy failed but subsequent ganglionectomies succeeded in relieving truncal pain. Multiple spinal rhizotomy or dorsal root ganglionectomy has a 65 percent success rate in reliev-

ing pain of benign origin at thoracic levels. Reported cases include postthoracotomy and posttraumatic intercostal neuralgia and similar idiopathic cases. The author has done multiple thoracic dorsal root ganglionectomies in three cases of intercostal neuralgia with satisfactory long-term pain relief. In all three patients, cutaneous hypersensitivity was noticed at the upper and lower margins of the anesthetic zone, and in one, this was disturbing enough to require repeated spinal nerve blocks at the level of dysesthesia.

Intradural dorsal rhizotomy at the C1 to C3 levels provides satisfactory long-term relief of occipital neuralgia in 70 percent of cases, according to a large number of reported series. My experience shows the procedure to be highly effective for neuralgias associated with severe arthritis or arthrosis of the C1–2 or C2–3 facet joints that impinge on the upper cervical roots as they form the greater occipital nerve. It also has been effective in posttraumatic occipital neuralgia. There is complete anesthesia in the back of the scalp, but these patients usually are gratified by the relief of their neuralgic pain and do not appear to be bothered by the loss of sensation.

Rhizotomy of the third sacral through coccygeal dorsal roots provided long-term relief of coccygodynia in 63 percent of 48 cases reported in the neurosurgical literature.[18] Sacral rhizotomy may be useful for pain caused by malignancies of the pelvis and perineal region by contrast with the relatively poor long-term success rate for pain from malignancy in the trunk, extremities, head, and neck. Dorsal rhizotomy has not been successful for treating sciatica after failed lumbar disk surgery. In 10 cases, there was a 90 percent long-term failure rate with the development of persistent burning or freezing dysesthesias during the subse-

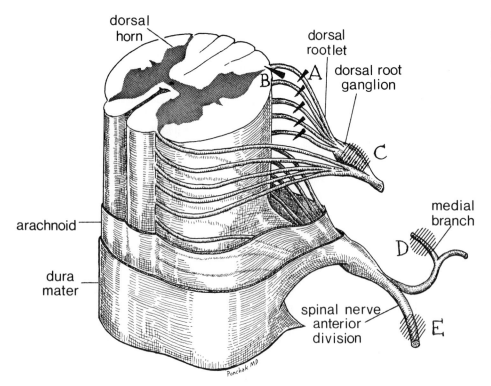

FIGURE 35-3. Surgical procedures at the nerve root and spinal nerve level. A: Intradural dorsal rhizotomy, B: selective posterior rhizidiotomy, C: dorsal root ganglionectomy, D: medial branch coagulation ("facet rhizolysis"), E: coagulation of spinal nerve. (Illustration by Stephen Ponchak, M.D.)

quent 5 years.[5] These dysesthesias also are frequent after dorsal root ganglionectomy at single lumbar or sacral levels.

A microsurgical technique that spares some of the large diameter proprioceptive afferents in individual dorsal rootlets is known as selective posterior rhizidiotomy.[19] Because the small diameter afferent fibers tend to aggregate laterally at the root entry zone and the large fibers tend medially toward the dorsal column, it is feasible to section only the lateral portion of each rootlet. In this way, proprioception in the arm or leg can be saved. This is not the case with complete dorsal rhizotomies at the brachial and lumbosacral plexus levels. This procedure has been used successfully to treat pain of lung apex malignancies.

Percutaneous radiofrequency lesioning of spinal nerves is not as selective as intradural root surgery, but it has the advantage of safety in debilitated patients, particularly those with advanced cancer. Initial rates of pain relief are 40 percent to 65 percent. The long-term success of percutaneous neurotomy seldom is discussed, but this may not be important for patients whose life expectancy is limited. Fairly heavy sedation may be required for percutaneous nerve lesions. In some cases, therefore, an alternative procedure done under general endotracheal anesthesia might have less risk of respiratory complication.

Lesions of the Spinal Cord

Open Cordotomy

This category includes some surgical procedures in which a lesion is made using radiofrequency current and others in which a white matter tract is sectioned directly with a microsurgical blade (Fig. 35-4). All have in common the

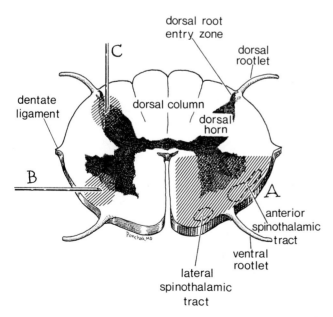

FIGURE 35-4. *Surgical procedures at the spinal cord level. A: Open anterolateral cordotomy, B: percutaneous radiofrequency cordotomy, C: dorsal root entry zone (DREZ) lesion. (Illustration by Stephen Ponchak, M.D.)*

goal of disrupting the neural transmission of nociceptive information from the cord or medulla to the upper brainstem and thalamus. In most instances, the limiting factor will be the proximity of descending pathways of motor control.

The prototype is anterolateral cordotomy, in which the white matter of the cord is sectioned to eliminate a large part of the ascending spinothalamic projection. Open cordotomy usually is done at the T2 or T3 level; this is just below the portion of the cord contributing to the brachial plexus. The spinal cord is exposed by laminectomies and dural incision under general anesthesia. The dentate ligaments are identified on the lateral aspect of the cord. One of them may be sectioned to rotate the cord slightly, exposing the anterior aspect. The pial surface is cauterized lightly with fine microsurgical bipolar cautery forceps, and a small blade is inserted anterior to the dentate ligament to section the anterolateral quadrant of the cord. Bleeding usually is minimal with this procedure, and it can be stopped easily with hemostatic pledgets and microsurgical cautery.

An open T2–3 cordotomy of this sort is expected to produce a level of insensitivity to pinprick and other painful stimuli somewhere on the trunk. The level of analgesia is never as high as T2 because the ascending spinothalamic fibers gradually cross over the midline of the cord for a distance of several segments. Those from the T2–5 segments, perhaps more, have not reached the opposite anterolateral quadrant, and therefore, they are not included in the lesion. The actual level of insensitivity varies from approximately T4 to T10.[20] It is higher when the lesion is extended toward the midline of the cord (see Fig. 35-4). Some spinothalamic and spinoreticular tract fibers lie in the anteromedial white matter near the ventral sulcus of the cord. The anterior spinal artery is found in this sulcus and must be avoided.

Cordotomy can be a highly effective treatment for the pain of cancer in the trunk or legs.[21] The procedure can be done bilaterally, with greater risk of disrupting bowel and bladder control. The best indication for cordotomy is intractable cancer pain in one leg or one side of the pelvis. The major disadvantage of cordotomy is the tendency for pain to recur years later. The initial success rate in patients with cancer, that is, the chance of complete relief or mild residual pain relieved by nonnarcotic medication, varies from 55 percent to 95 percent in different published series; mortality rates in recent series range from 0 to 7.5 percent. In patients with severe pain not caused by cancer, initial success rates were similar. Conditions amenable to cordotomy include tabes dorsalis, cord and cauda equina injuries, and phantom limb pain. In all diagnostic groups, there is a disturbing late recurrence rate that limits long-term success to only 25 percent to 70 percent. Some recurrences are seen during the first 12 months. It has not been possible to predict which patients are susceptible to late failure after cordotomy. Other complications of open cordotomy include weakness or paralysis of the legs, usually transient (in 3 percent to 15 percent of unilateral procedures), and persistent urinary bladder dysfunction in 2 percent to 10 percent. Fecal incontinence and impotence also are possible. The incidence of these complications more than doubles after bilateral cordotomies. Laboratory investigations suggest several reasons why cordotomy might fail. The spinoreticular tracts and, to a lesser extent, the spinothalamic tracts are crossed only partially in primate species. Moreover, there are ascending sensory pathways in the dorsal half of the cord white matter that could assume a more significant role in nociception after disruption of the ventral tracts. Finally, the late effects of central deafferentation are not known completely, and it is tempting to speculate that some late recurrences of pain after cordotomy may be a result of the development of ectopic neuronal discharges in brainstem and thalamic neurons.

Percutaneous Upper Cervical Cordotomy

A lesion similar in location, if not in extent, can be created by radiofrequency thermocoagulation of the anterolateral quadrant of the cord, using a small probe inserted through a spinal needle (see Fig. 35-4). The needle insertion is done using fluoroscopic control and an emulsion of radiographic contrast to outline the dentate ligament. Local anesthetic is injected just behind and below the mastoid process for a straight lateral approach to the cord. Electrical stimulation through the probe is used to elicit paresthesias from the ventral cord white matter to estimate the depth of insertion of the probe tip. Lesions near the cord surface just in front of the dentate ligament tend to produce analgesia in the trunk; deeper lesions affect the sacral region and leg. The patient is sedated heavily with a short-acting intravenous agent (such as methohexital or midazolam) supplemented by a narcotic while the radiofrequency lesion is made. It is feasible to do this procedure in the radiology department if equipment for induction and monitoring of general anesthesia is available. The patient is awakened to determine the extent of sensory deficit, and if necessary, the lesion may be enlarged.

The success rate of percutaneous cordotomy (as reported in several large series) was similar to that of open cordotomy with fewer complications. The percutaneous technique is valuable in debilitated patients. One drawback is the surgeon's inability to be certain of the extent of the lesion. Because there is ample evidence that the ascending sensory pathways relevant to pain are widespread in the cord and the spinothalamic tract itself is diffuse, it may be worthwhile to do an open cordotomy when the patient's general health permits and the life expectancy is long enough to make the surgical procedure and subsequent postoperative hospitalization beneficial. Of course, some patients with cancer are too ill to undergo general anesthesia for an open cordotomy, and the percutaneous procedure then may be appropriate. In many cases of this type, however, alternatives (such as an epidural morphine delivery system or continuous intravenous narcotic infusion) might be simpler.

Percutaneous cordotomy at the C1 to C2 level carries a risk of causing respiratory insufficiency from interference with the spinal axons of the respiratory neurons. The risk definitely increases with bilateral cordotomy at this level, after which there is approximately a 4 percent to 8 percent incidence of sudden respiratory arrest. This typically occurs at night when the patient is asleep. Poor performance on preoperative pulmonary function tests should be considered a relative contraindication to unilateral high cervical cordotomy and an absolute contraindication to bilateral C1 to C2 cordotomy.

Dorsal Root Entry Zone Lesions

The technique of radiofrequency lesioning of the dorsal root entry zone was devised by Nashold. A series of small heat lesions, 2 to 3 mm apart, is created along the line of entry of dorsal rootlets in the segments corresponding to the area of pain and in adjacent segments above and below it. The lesions are made with radiofrequency current passed through a small insulated electrode at a depth of 2 mm; they should be centered in the superficial layers of the dorsal horn (Fig. 35-4).

This procedure has been used to treat pain caused by avulsion of the brachial plexus, pain in paraplegic patients at or below the level of cord injury,[22] postherpetic neuralgia, and various other localized conditions. Nashold and Ostdahl[23] and Thomas and Jones[24] reported that approximately two-thirds of patients with pain from brachial plexus avulsion had significant relief after this procedure. For pain from cord injuries or postherpetic neuralgia, the success rate is slightly less.[25,26] Complications of this operation include mild or moderate lower limb weakness, loss of proprioception in the ipsilateral leg, numbness and paresthesias.[27] These have been reduced substantially by the use of temperature monitoring at the lesioning electrode tip using a thermocouple.

Stereotactic Lesions

With a stereotactic instrument and appropriate radiologic techniques, it is possible to place the tip of a lesioning probe in various nuclei of the thalamus and hypothalamus or in the ascending sensory tracts of the pons and midbrain. Lesions of the ventral and medial thalamus, hypothalamus, and spinothalamic or spinoreticular tracts in the brainstem disrupt ascending connections. Another variety of lesion has the rationale of blunting the patient's affective response to pain. Lesions of the frontal lobe white matter, cingulum,[28] and dorsomedial and anterior thalamus are included in this group. The latter has been termed *psychosurgery* and is practiced infrequently.

Stereotactic lesioning procedures provide an alternative to cordotomy for pain at cervical levels or in the midline of the trunk where bilateral high cervical cordotomy might be ineffective or dangerous because of its risk of respiratory complications. Currently, destructive stereotactic procedures are used less often, partly as a result of newer techniques (such as periventricular gray stimulation and implanted morphine infusion pumps).

One advantage of stereotactic lesions is that they may be effective in cases of deafferentation pain where no good alternative exists. Stereotactic mesencephalic tractotomy is said to relieve deafferentation pain in 40 percent to 50 percent of cases and other types of severe chronic pain in 60 percent to 70 percent of cases.[29,30]

A typical stereotactic destructive procedure for pain relief begins by mounting the stereotactic frame on the skull, using a local anesthetic at pin insertion sites. Then a ventriculogram and perhaps also a CT scan or magnetic resonance imaging scan of the brain is obtained with the frame in place to locate necessary landmarks in the brain (such as the anterior and posterior commissures of the third ventricle). From these landmarks, target coordinates can be given on the frame axes for deep brain structures around the thalamus, upper brainstem, and third ventricle. Coordinates are calculated from maps of the brain in standard atlases, and adjusted according to the dimensions of the patient's brain landmarks. Lesioning of the chosen target is done with a probe inserted to reach the structure through a burr hole in the skull. If a ventriculogram was done for localization, it may be convenient to use the same burr hole. Further localization of the target can be achieved by trials of brief electrical stimulation through the probe tip and recording the patient's subjective responses and any movements produced. To do this requires the patient's attention and cooperation for some time, therefore, heavy sedation would be inappropriate. A lesion is made with radiofrequency electrical current or other means.

Complications of stereotactic lesioning depend on the target, but in general, they include confusion, dysesthesias, eye movement disorders, psychic changes, and infrequent hemorrhages. There is an overall morbidity rate of approximately 10 percent to 40 percent and a mortality rate of 3 percent to 10 percent. In considering these figures, it is wise to remember that these operations usually are done as a last resort when all other treatments fail.

Sympathectomy

Procedures that interrupt the afferent and efferent axons of the sympathetic nervous system are useful for treating pain of peripheral nerve injury when causalgia or painful reflex sympathetic dystrophy is present. Recent physiologic studies of nerve injury and neuroma formation suggest that the sympathetic outflow to the damaged nerve is a factor that produces or aggravates pain, perhaps by augmenting the ectopic discharges that originate peripherally. Sympathectomy occasionally is used for painful conditions of the extremities resembling causalgia but not due to nerve trauma, if temporary sympathetic blocks repeatedly give relief. Sympathectomy has been combined with splanch-

nicectomy to treat pain caused by cancer of the pancreas or other upper abdominal viscera.[31]

Open sympathectomy to treat arm pain is done at the upper thoracic level. The author prefers a posterior approach with removal of the head of the second rib and the corresponding transverse process; two ganglia are excised from the thoracic sympathetic chain and the caudal third of the stellate ganglion. When a true stellate ganglion does not exist, the highest thoracic ganglion is removed instead. The chain also can be approached through the axilla.[32] A percutaneous technique of radiofrequency lesions of the sympathetic chain is described by Wilkinson[33] and may be done bilaterally. Upper thoracic sympathectomy by any approach has a 70 percent to 75 percent chance of relieving arm pain resulting from causalgia or vascular disease initially. Late recurrences are not uncommon, and postoperative hyperesthesia and Horner syndrome are potential complications.

Sympathectomy for leg pain is done by an abdominal approach familiar to most vascular surgeons; the lumbar sympathetic chain is exposed and sectioned anterolateral to the vertebral prominence. Chemical lumbar sympathectomy with phenol injection is a suitable alternative.[34] This is done by lumbar paravertebral block.

The use of lumbar sympathectomy for leg pain caused by vascular claudication or ischemic rest pain, causalgia, and reflex sympathetic dystrophy has an initial success rate of approximately 65 percent to 70 percent; late failures are common, possibly after progressive development of hypersensitivity to circulating catecholamines. The mortality rate for open lumbar sympathectomy is approximately 1 percent to 5 percent. Syndromes of local pain after interruption of the sympathetic nerves are described. These usually occur 7 to 12 days after the operation or injury and may be as unpleasant as the preoperative pain. Postsympathectomy neuralgia typically is felt in the anterior thighs. Sometimes, it can be relieved with carbamazepine or phenytoin.[35] Fortunately, it often remits spontaneously after several weeks or a few months.

Anterior Pituitary Ablation

Operations to ablate or destroy the anterior lobe of the pituitary gland originated from endocrine studies suggesting that some breast and prostate carcinoma metastases may regress after oophorectomy or adrenalectomy. In many instances, there was corresponding relief of pain, which was attributed to a decrease of local pressure and swelling around the metastases, particularly in bone. More recently, as safer simpler techniques of pituitary ablation were developed, it became clear that many patients reported pain relief almost immediately after the operation, sometimes within 30 min. This phenomenon, therefore, could not be explained in terms of tumor regression. There is no satisfactory explanation. One hypothesis states that an unidentified hormonal factor produced by the hypophysis or hypothalamus is disrupted by the procedure. The finding of a large concentration of β-endorphin in the pituitary aroused some interest in this regard, but circulating levels of the peptide did not correlate with pain relief. It appears that neither the extent of the anterior hypophysectomy, the extent of concomitant ventral hypothalamic damage, nor the extent of tumor regression correlates with the degree of immediate pain relief.[36]

Several techniques of pituitary destruction are available. The procedure most certain to ensure selective ablation of the adenohypophysis while sparing the neurohypophysis is transsphenoidal microsurgery.[37] Despite the extremely low morbidity and mortality of this operation in experienced hands and the quick postoperative recovery without disfigurement, patients with advanced malignancy seldom undergo the operation. The emotional barrier to surgery under general anesthesia may be related to the patient's fear of impending death from the underlying disease. Patients with cancer seem more willing to accept the idea of pituitary ablation if it is presented as a simple procedure to relieve pain rather than a major operation. Zervas[38] devised the stereotactic technique of radiofrequency thermocoagulation of the pituitary using a probe inserted through the sphenoid sinus. Moricca[39] and others reported a large clinical experience with the injection of alcohol into the pituitary through a cannula inserted by the sphenoidal approach. Freezing lesions also have been used. Each approach has a high rate of success and a small, but not insignificant, risk of cerebrospinal fluid leak, meningitis, hemorrhage, hypothalamic injury, and death. Pituitary insufficiency after closed ablative procedures (such as alcohol injection) is not inevitable. In many cases, relatively normal corticotropin levels and modest thyroid-stimulating hormone levels can be maintained.

Pituitary ablation is used most commonly for the pain of prostate and breast cancer, but there is good evidence that many kinds of malignancy may respond.[40] The idea that only bone metastases can be treated in this way is probably incorrect; pain due to soft tissue metastases also may subside. Published series indicate that 60 percent to 70 percent of patients have partial or complete relief of pain initially, but the long-term benefits are less. Several months of improvement are seen in most patients with cancer pain. Pituitary ablation has not been shown to increase survival, nor is it useful for pain not caused by cancer.

IMPLANTED DEVICES FOR STIMULATION

This category of neurosurgical procedures includes two devices: spinal cord stimulation units,[41] and deep brain stimulation units.[42] Stimulation of the spinal cord to control pain is based mainly on the concept of a gate-control mechanism in the dorsal horn that could be activated by stimulation of large diameter afferent fibers in the dorsal columns of the cord. Electrical stimulation of the periventricular gray matter of the uppermost brainstem is thought to activate a

descending system of neural connections that reaches the dorsal horn of the spinal cord.[43] In laboratory animals, stimulation of the central gray region causes profound analgesia by various tests.

Spinal Cord Stimulation

Electrical stimulation of the spinal cord through implanted electrodes in the epidural space or on the cord surface may provide relief of pain.[44] The mechanism of action of cord stimulation is not known. Dorsal electrode placements probably produce volleys of afferent impulses in the dorsal columns, with effects in the dorsal horn or possibly in the brainstem.

Stimulating electrodes can be implanted temporarily by percutaneous techniques.[45] Then, if trials of cord stimulation are successful, a permanent system is installed, including a subcutaneous receiver or battery-powered pulse generator. Paresthesias should be felt in the area of pain, indicating activation of large diameter afferents in the appropriate spinal segments. Unfortunately, despite initial indications of a good result, there is considerable risk of late failure of spinal cord stimulation units. In a series of 70 such units followed for 10 years, Erickson and Long[46] reported a 95 percent long-term failure rate. Reasons for failure include migration or breakage of the electrodes, epidural scar formation, infection, and tolerance to the stimulation that may develop for unknown reasons even when the unit appears intact and functional. Intradural electrode placements have additional risks of cord compression and cerebrospinal fluid leakage and, therefore, should be avoided.

Tasker[47] used cord stimulation successfully to treat deafferentation pain syndromes and considered it to be the initial treatment of choice for this type of pain despite the late failure rate. Few effective options are available to patients in this group; therefore, improvement for 1 year or 2 might be a welcome respite.

Periventricular Gray, Internal Capsule, and Thalamic Stimulation

Electrical stimulation of deep brain structures is done by means of stereotactically implanted electrodes connected to a subcutaneous receiver or pulse generator. Stimulation in the somatosensory portion of the thalamus, in the posterior limb of the internal capsule, or medial lemniscus can be effective in suppressing deafferentation pain. Stimulation more medially in the central gray matter lining the posterior third ventricle and rostral portion of the aqueduct may activate a descending analgesia-producing system. It is useful for a wider variety of chronic pains. Opinions are divided over the long-term efficacy of central gray stimulation, and it appears that success rates initially vary from 50 percent to 80 percent. Good results in approximately 55 percent of patients with cancer with relatively long survivals were reported by Meyerson and colleagues.[48] Significant relief of various types of chronic pain of peripheral origin, not caused by cancer, were reported in 70 percent to 80 percent of patients, including those with previously refractory low back pain after failed disk surgery.[49,50] Postherpetic facial pain can be relieved by thalamic stimulation in many cases.[51] Pain of thalamic syndrome is said to be relieved in approximately 50 percent of patients with stimulation near the border of the internal capsule.[52] Amputation stump pain and phantom limb pain respond favorably in more than 90 percent of cases.[53]

Accurate placement of deep brain stimulating electrodes requires, not only radiologic techniques, but also physiologic mapping at the time of surgery. The initial phase of the stereotactic procedure consists of mounting the stereotactic frame on the patient's head. Then, deep brain landmarks are related to frame coordinates by ventriculography and CT scanning. When three-dimensional target coordinates have been calculated, the instrument is used to introduce one or more electrodes. Final targets are chosen after trials of stimulation at different depths. The author has found it useful to do stimulation trials with a probe from the tip of which a stimulating electrode emerges in a curved path. In this way, by retracting the electrode tip and rotating the probe, an area of several cubic centimeters can be explored to find an optimal site that reduces the patient's pain with minimal side effects. Periventricular electrode placements are limited by ocular side effects when the electrode tip is driven ventrally toward the midbrain. Lateral placements near the internal capsule may produce bodily movements and paresthesias.

Potential complications of deep brain stimulation include infection of the electrodes, cerebral hemorrhage, abnormal eye movements induced by stimulation, and unpleasant dysesthesias. Overall, the morbidity rate is 5 percent to 10 percent, and the mortality rate is less than 1 percent.

INTRASPINAL NARCOTIC CANNULAS

Originally, it was demonstrated by Yaksh and Rudy[54] that implantation of a spinal epidural cannula to deliver morphine from a subcutaneous injection port or continuous infusion pump provides a high concentration of narcotic drug at the level of the spinal cord where large numbers of opiate receptor sites can be identified in the dorsal horn and small amounts of morphine instilled around the spinal cord could produce marked analgesia, beyond what would result from a similar dose given systemically. Efforts to take long-term advantage of this phenomenon in humans have been restricted largely to those with pain from advanced malignancies. To minimize the risk of respiratory compromise or cord injury, the spinal catheter usually is placed in the epidural space at the upper lumbar level. Intrathecal placements also have been successful.[55] Low thoracic placements may have a slight advantage because the drug is delivered closer to the conus medullaris of the cord. The use of spinal morphine catheters often has a distinct advantage over intravenous morphine infusion. The daily dose of narcotic is much smaller, and the patient remains more alert with fewer systemic effects. (See Chap. 27.)

Placement begins with the insertion of a suitable indwelling epidural catheter. A small incision in the midline of the lower back facilitates insertion of the Tuohy needle and permits further tunneling of the catheter toward the flank. The catheter then is connected to a rubber injection port that is sutured to the subcutaneous fascia of the abdominal wall. This is done most easily under general anesthesia if the patient's medical condition permits, but it can be accomplished using a combination of spinal and epidural anesthesia through the catheter and local anesthesia. When the abdominal incision heals, percutaneous morphine injections with appropriate needles are given one or two times per day. Single doses of 2 to 8 mg of morphine sulfate in pyrogen-free diluent are satisfactory in most instances.

It is essential to maintain strict sterile technique, not only during the placement of the catheter and port, but also during its subsequent use. In the author's experience, 20 percent to 25 percent of catheters placed in terminally ill patients will be removed because of infection at some time before the patient's death. The presence of a colostomy or urinary diversion system is not an absolute contraindication, but it is wise to choose a position for the injection port at a distance from the colostomy. Some patients and their families can be trusted to adhere to the strict sterile technique of injection for many months, but in most cases, it is necessary to enlist the help of nursing staff, and if possible, a trained nurse–specialist who makes home visits. The staff at nursing homes and even some chronic care hospitals may refuse to employ these catheter systems, even if they have been used successfully in an acute care setting because of lack of familiarity with the system and fear of neurologic complications. The family situation, availability of skilled nurses, plans for home care versus institutional care, and even the patient's life expectancy should all be considered carefully before implanting a morphine injection port.

In some instances, temporary use of an injection port is successful, and the patient's course of illness suggests prolonged need for the device. In these cases, we should consider revising the system to include a continuous infusion pump implanted in the abdominal wall. Pumps of this type deliver morphine at a chosen concentration for intervals of 2 weeks or longer. Similar considerations also apply to infusion pumps. Before deciding to place such a system, it is important to know whether it will be refilled during outpatient hospital visits, at the patient's home, or elsewhere. As in injection port systems, infusion pumps may require periodic increases of the morphine dose.

Continuous infusion of narcotics by epidural catheter was found to be highly effective in controlling cancer pain but not pain of nonmalignant origin.[56,57] Drugs other than morphine can be infused, including meperidine, fentanyl, buprenorphine, and hydromorphone. In one case of progressive tolerance to intrathecal hydromorphone infusion, the addition of clonidine to the infusate was effective.[58]

SUMMARY

The neurosurgical approaches to the management of chronic pain are many and varied. Most commonly, they are used only after more conservative measures fail. In the past, these techniques were used only as a last resort because of a fear of untoward neurologic sequelae, but improvements in our understanding of the pathophysiology of pain and in the neurosurgical techniques themselves have resulted in a high rate of success and a low incidence of complications.

References

1. Williams PH, Trzil KP. Management of meralgia paresthetica. *J Neurosurg* January 1991; 74(1):76–80.
2. Hitselberger WE, Witten RM. Abnormal myelograms in asymptomatic patients. *J Neurosurg* 1968; 28:204–206.
3. Kuschner SH, Brien WW, Johnson D, Gellman H. Complications associated with carpal tunnel release. *Orthop Rev* April 1991; 20(4):346–352.
4. Spangfort EV. The lumbar disc herniation. *Acta Orthop Scand Suppl* 1972; 142:1–95.
5. Bertrand G. The "battered" root problem. *Orthop Clin North Am* 1975; 6:305–309.
6. Auld AW. Chronic spinal arachnoiditis. A postoperative syndrome that may signal its onset. *Spine* 1978; 3:88–91.
7. Jannetta P. Observations on the etiology of trigeminal neuralgia, hemifacial spasm, acoustic nerve dysfunction and glossopharyngeal neuralgia. *Neurochirurgia* 1977; 20:145–154.
8. Battista AD, Cravioto H, Budsilovich GN. Painful neuroma: changes produced in peripheral nerve after fascicle ligation. *Neurosurgery* 1981; 9:589–600.
9. Noordenbos W, Wall PD. Implications of the failure of nerve resection and graft to cure chronic pain produced by nerve lesions. *J Neurol Neurosurg Psychiatr* 1981; 44:1068–1073.
10. Hakanson S. Retrogasserian glycerol injection as a treatment of tic douloureux. In: Bonica JJ, Lindblom U, Iggo A, et al, (eds) *Advances in Pain Research and Therapy*. Vol 5. New York: Raven Press; 1983:927–933.
11. Sweet WH, Poletti CE. Retrogasserian glycerol injection as treatment for trigeminal neuralgia. In: Sweet WH, Schmidek HH, eds. *Operative Neurosurgical Techniques*. New York: Grune & Stratton; 1982:1107–1117.
12. Fujimaki T, Fukushima T, Miyazaki S. Percutaneous retrogasserian glycerol injection in the management of trigeminal neuralgia: long-term follow-up results. *J Neurosurg* August 1990; 73(2):212–216.
13. Burchiel KJ, Steege TD, Howe JF, Loeser JD. Comparison of percutaneous radiofrequency gangliolysis and microvascular decompression for the surgical management of tic douloureux. *Neurosurgery* 1981; 9:111–119.
14. Rushton JG, Stevens JC, Miller RH. Glossopharyngeal (vagoglossopharyngeal) neuralgia. *Arch Neurol* April 1981; 38:201–205.
15. Dubuisson D. Root surgery. In: Wall PD, Melzack R, eds. *Textbook of Pain*. London: Churchill-Livingstone; 1984: 590–600.
16. Laha RK, Jannetta PJ. Glossopharyngeal neuralgia. *J Neurosurg* 1977; 47:316–320.
17. Hosobuchi Y. The majority of unmyelinated axons in human ventral rootlets probably conduct pain. *Pain* 1980; 8:167–180.
18. Albrektsson B. Sacral rhizotomy in cases of anococcygeal pain. *Acta Orthop Scand* 1981; 52:157–190.
19. Sindou M, Fischer G, Mansuy L. Posterior spinal rhizotomy and selective posterior rhizidiotomy. *Prog Neurol Surg* 1976; 7:201–250.
20. White JC, Sweet WH. *Pain and the Neurosurgeon*. Springfield: Charles C. Thomas; 1969.
21. Sundaresan N, DiGiacinto GV, Hughes JE. Neurosurgery in the treatment of cancer pain. *Cancer* June 1, 1989; 63(suppl 11):2365–2377.
22. Sindou M, Jeanmonod D. Microsurgical DREZ-otomy for the treatment of spasticity and pain in the lower limbs. *Neurosurgery* May 1989; 24(5):655–670.
23. Nashold BS, Ostdahl RH. Dorsal root entry zone lesions for pain relief. *J Neurosurg* 1979; 51:59–69.
24. Thomas DGT, Jones SJ. Dorsal root entry zone lesions (Nashold's procedure) in brachial plexus avulsion. *Neurosurgery* 1984; 15:966–967.
25. Nashold BS, Bullitt E. Dorsal root entry zone lesions to control central pain in paraplegics. *J Neurosurg* 1981; 55:414–419.
26. Friedman AH, Nashold BS. Dorsal root entry zone lesions for the treatment of postherpetic neuralgia. *Neurosurgery* 1984; 15:969–970.
27. Jeanmonod D, Sindou M. Somatosensory function following dorsal root entry zone lesions in patients with neurogenic pain or spasticity. *J Neurosurg* June 1991; 74(6):916–932.
28. Hassenbusch SJ, Pillay PK, Barnett GH. Radiofrequency cingulotomy for intractable cancer pain using stereotaxis guided by magnetic resonance imaging. *Neurosurgery* August 1990; 27(2):220–223.
29. Nashold BS. Brainstem stereotaxic procedures. In: Schaltenbrand G, Walker AE, eds. *Stereotaxy of the Human Brain*. Stuttgart: Thieme; 1982:475–483.
30. Tasker RR. Thalamic stereotaxic procedures. In: Schaltenbrand G, Walker AE, eds. *Stereotaxy of the Human Brain*. Stuttgart: Thieme; 1982:484–497.
31. Hardy RW. Surgery of the sympathetic nervous system. In: Sweet WH, Schmidek HH, eds. *Operative Neurosurgical Techniques*. New York: Grune & Stratton; 1982:1045–1061.
32. Berguer R, Smit R. Transaxillary sympathectomy (T2 to T4) for relief of vasospastic/sympathetic pain of upper extremities. *Surgery* 1981; 89:764–769.
33. Wilkinson HA. Percutaneous radiofrequency upper thoracic sympathectomy: a new technique. *Neurosurgery* 1984; 15:811–814.
34. Cross FW, Cotton LT. Chemical lumbar sympathectomy for ischemic rest pain: a randomized, prospective controlled clinical trial. *Am J Surg* 1985; 150:341–345.
35. Raskin NH, Levinson SA, Hoffman PM, et al. Postsympathectomy neuralgia: amelioration with diphenylhydantoin and carbamazepine. *Am J Surg* 1974; 128:75–78.
36. Miles J. Pituitary destruction. In: Wall PD, Melzack R, eds.

Textbook of Pain. London: Churchill Livingstone; 1984:656–665.

37. Hardy J. Transsphenoidal hypophysectomy. *J Neurosurg* 1971; 34:582–594.

38. Zervas N. Stereotactic, radiofrequency surgery of the normal and the abnormal pituitary gland. *N Engl J Med* 1969; 280:429–437.

39. Moricca G. Chemical hypophysectomy for cancer pain. In: Bonica JJ, ed. *Advances in Neurology*. Vol 4. New York: Raven Press; 1974:707–714.

40. Tindall GT, Nixon DW, Christy JH, Neill JD. Pain relief in metastatic cancer other than breast and prostrate gland following transsphenoidal hypophysectomy. *J Neurosurg* 1977; 50:275–282.

41. Spiegelmann R, Friedman WA. Spinal cord stimulation: a contemporary series. *Neurosurgery* January 1991; 28(1):65–70; discussion 70–71.

42. Kumar K, Wyant GM, Nath R. Deep brain stimulation for control of intractable pain in humans, present and future: a ten-year follow-up. *Neurosurgery* May 1990; 26(5):774–781; discussion 781–782.

43. Robaina FJ, Dominiguez M, Diaz M, Rodriguez JL, De Vera JA. Spinal cord stimulation for relief of chronic pain in vasospastic disorders of the upper limbs. *Neurosurgery* January 1989; 24(1):63–67.

44. Shealy CN, Mortimer JT, Resnick J. Electrical inhibition of pain by stimulation of the dorsal column: preliminary clinical reports. *Anesth Analg* 1967; 46:489–491.

45. Erickson DL. Percutaneous trial of stimulation for patient selection for implantable stimulating devices. *J Neurosurg* 1975; 43:440–444.

46. Erickson DL, Long DM. Ten-year follow-up of dorsal column stimulation. In: Bonica JJ, Lindblom U, Iggo A, et al, eds. *Advances in Pain Research and Therapy*. Vol 5. New York: Raven Press; 1983:583–589.

47. Tasker RR. Surgical approaches to the primary afferent and the spinal cord. In: Bonica JJ, Lindblom U, Iggo A, et al, eds. *Advances in Pain Research and Therapy*. Vol 5. New York: Raven Press; 1985:799–824.

48. Meyerson BA, Boethius J, Carlsson AM. Percutaneous central grey stimulation for cancer pain. *Appl Neurophysiol* 1979; 41:57–65.

49. Hosubuchi Y. The current status of analgesic brain stimulation. *Acta Neurochir Suppl* (Wien) 1980; 30:219–227.

50. Plotkin R. Results in 60 cases of deep brain stimulation for chronic intractable pain. *Appl Neurophysiol* 1982; 45:173–178.

51. Siegfried J. Monopolar electrical stimulation of nucleus ventroposterior medialis thalami for postherpetic facial pain. *Appl Neurophysiol* 1982; 45:179–184.

52. Hosubuchi Y. Subcortical electrical stimulation for control of intractable pain in humans. *J Neurosurg* 1986; 64:543–553.

53. Turnbull IM. Brain stimulation. In: Wall PD, Melzack R, eds. *Textbook of Pain*. London: Churchill Livingstone; 1984:706–714.

54. Yaksh TL, Rudy TA. Analgesia mediated by a direct spinal action of narcotics. *Science* 1976; 192:1357–1358.

55. Onofrio BM, Yaksh TL, Arnold PG. Continuous low-dose intrathecal morphine administration in the treatment of chronic pain of malignant origin. *Mayo Clin Proc* 1981; 56:516–520.

56. Coombs DW, Saunders RL, Gaylor MS, et al. Relief of continuous chronic pain by intraspinal narcotics infusion via an implanted reservoir. *JAMA* 1983; 250:2336–2339.

57. Krames ES, Gershow J, Glassberg A, et al. Continuous infusion of spinally administered narcotics for the relief of pain due to malignant disorders. *Cancer* 1985; 56:696–702.

58. Coombs DW, Saunders RL, Fratkin JD, et al. Continuous intrathecal hydromorphone and clonidine for intractable cancer pain. *J Neurosurg* 1986; 64:890–894.

CHAPTER 36

The Role of Pain Clinics

Gerald M. Aronoff

Several factors contributed to the development of the multidisciplinary pain center (MPC). One was the common observation that there was a group of patients who did not respond to conservative treatment measures and surgical intervention. They had chronic pain syndromes with concomitant medication dependency problems, emotional disturbance, work loss, and global life disruption. Another was the increasing recognition of the importance of psychosocial factors in the development and maintenance of the pain syndrome. This clinical observation made by Beecher[1] in 1959 was strengthened further through theoretic formulations.[2]

Pain centers sometimes are regarded as the treatment of last resort. This erroneous impression is beginning to change as more health-care providers recognize that early patient referrals may help eliminate needless or multiple operations, reduce health-care costs, and promote the patient's return to productivity. Insurance carriers ultimately may benefit from chronic pain programs. Ineffective surgical procedures, multiple physician visits, medication dependency, iatrogenic complications, and lost workdays may be reduced.[3,4]

Throughout the development of the MPC, there has been a move away from the model that treats chronic pain as an extension of acute pain. Over time, there has been increasing importance placed on central factors of the cause and maintenance of the pain problem. Current treatment approaches offer strategies for peripheral management of pain and emphasize central factors.[5]

In the 1950s, our methods for treating chronic pain consisted primarily of bed rest, medication, nerve blocks, or surgery. Currently, bed rest generally is thought to be contraindicated for most chronic nonmalignant pain syndromes. Narcotics, often the medications of choice during the 1950s, are used less to treat nonmalignant pain, and the indications for nerve blocks and surgery are being defined better and used more selectively. Whereas pain centers once were considered treatments of last resort; currently, this is often the judgment reserved for invasive treatments. Concepts regarding the treatment of chronic pain have changed dramatically, as has the health-care system generally in the

United States. I hope this represents an improvement in meeting the needs of an unfortunate population, who for years became invalids within the health-care system.

The first multidisciplinary pain centers were founded by Drs. John Bonica and Benjamin Crue 30 years ago. Although different in structure and conceptual framework, both radically changed the treatment of patients with chronic pain syndromes and served as prototypes for the pain centers that followed. As pioneers in the pain movement, both Drs. Bonica and Crue advocated the multidisciplinary team approach to manage intractable chronic pain syndromes. Despite this, there were some fundamental differences in regard to the role of invasive treatments in their pain programs. Dr. Bonica, an anesthesiologist, more frequently used nerve blocks diagnostically or therapeutically. Dr. Crue, a neurosurgeon, viewed chronic nonmalignant pain more as a psychosomatic process, rarely used invasive techniques, and advocated a more behavioral–psychosocial approach. Despite these different viewpoints, both programs were successful. Even now, 30 years after the inception of these programs, it is unclear whether one approach is preferred over the other. We do not have adequate statistical data to condemn or support pain programs that use either invasive techniques or extensive academic evaluations; we need to accumulate such data. In my opinion, this is part of the problem.

Throughout the 1960s, pain centers were rare in the United States and even less common outside this country. These facilities were on the fringes of medical acceptability even during the early 1970s. Patients who had multiple surgeries or numerous nerve blocks were not considered to have been treated radically, and yet, patients treated in pain programs with operant conditioning, biofeedback, and psychotherapy often caused many raised eyebrows.

In 1976, *Medical World News* listed approximately 30 major comprehensive pain centers distributed throughout the United States. By 1979, this number had grown to 278 (according to a questionnaire survey conducted by the American Society of Anesthesiologists). By 1983, the number of alleged pain programs had grown to more than 1000.[6] These numbers represent questionnaire surveys, and there has been no attempt to validate the accuracy of the information provided. Although it is suggested that there are differences in methods, program content, and delivery sys-

Portions of this chapter are reprinted with permission from *Standards Manual for Facilities Serving People with Disabilities*. Tucson, AZ: Commission on Accreditation of Rehabilitation Facilities; 1992:52–56.

tems in these various facilities, details regarding their efficacy are not available. In 1992, it seems that, if people hang up a sign claiming to be able to operate a pain program, they do not need to have any prior experience with the treatment of pain or any specific credentials!

By 1979, the American Pain Society, in an attempt to get a better understanding of the status of formal pain management programs in the United States, established a special committee, which I chaired, to investigate the problem and develop guidelines for classifying pain treatment facilities. The following represents the most complete classification of pain programs currently available. The types of pain programs include:

1. Unidisciplinary, programs having one discipline and including either MDs or non-MDs.
2. Interdisciplinary, programs including at least one physician in an interactional system with nonphysicians as part of the treatment team.
3. Multidisciplinary, programs including two or more physicians and nonphysicians.
4. Pain clinics, pain treatment teams organized in an outpatient setting.
5. Pain units, specialized inpatient programs localized in a separate geographic area specifically for the management of pain.
6. Comprehensive pain center, a program with an inpatient and outpatient pain clinic, facilities for pain research, and teaching programs. Generally treats a heterogeneous population of patients.
7. Syndrome-oriented programs specific to certain types of pain (such as cancer, arthritis, back pain, or headaches).
8. Modality-oriented pain programs, based on the method used, ranging from TENS to acupuncture, physical therapy, psychotherapy, and biofeedback clinics. The types of modality-oriented programs possible are almost endless. Although some of these programs may offer legitimate services, it also was thought that others may use fringe therapies that border on quackery.

In 1982, the American Pain Society established a committee on standards for pain treatment facilities, which I chaired. Our charge was to gather information and develop guidelines to establish national standards for pain facilities in the United States. It was decided, at that time, that the American Pain Society, being a scientific organization, would not be involved in on-site surveys or directly participate in the accreditation process. Concurrently, the Commission on Accreditation of Rehabilitation Facilities (CARF) convened a National Advisory Committee that met in Chicago in July 1982 to develop standards for chronic pain multidisciplinary inpatient and outpatient programs. The committee accomplished its task, and by January 1983, these standards were published. Throughout the development and implementation of these standards, CARF solicited the assistance of the American Pain Society and the American Academy of Pain Medicine (AAPM). I was the liaison member from the board of directors of both these organizations to CARF and remain the liaison member from the AAPM. The standards developed reflect the national advisory view that nonphysicians, especially nurses, psychologists, and physical therapists are often essential team members.

The CARF standards for multidisciplinary and interdisciplinary chronic pain management programs are as follows.[7]

CARF STANDARDS

"CHRONIC PAIN MANAGEMENT PROGRAMS

Program Description

A Chronic Pain Management Program provides coordinated, goal-oriented, interdisciplinary team services to reduce pain, improve functioning, and decrease the dependence on the health care system by persons with chronic pain syndrome. A chronic pain syndrome is any set of verbal and/or nonverbal behaviors which: 1) involves the complaint of enduring pain; 2) differs significantly from the person's premorbid status; 3) has not responded to previous appropriate medical and/or surgical treatment; and 4) interferes with physical, psychological, social, and/or vocational functioning.

The program may operate on an inpatient or outpatient basis or both. If an organization provides both, then both programs must be submitted for accreditation.

Organizations operating Chronic Pain Management Programs for specific syndromes—e.g., headache, low back pain, pain associated with malignancies, temporomandibular joint dysfunction, are expected to meet the chronic pain management standards in this section.

Modality oriented clinics that provide only specific therapies outside of the context of an interdisciplinary team—e.g., psychotherapy, biofeedback, TENS, relaxation therapy, nerve blocks, are not eligible for accreditation under these standards.

The following standards apply to both inpatient and outpatient programs:

1. The program should formulate a written statement of its evaluation and treatment philosophy.
2. The program should specify the functions and responsibilities for clinical program direction and medical direction. The same individual may be responsible for both functions; clinical program direction need not be provided by a physician.
3. The functions of clinical program direction and medical supervision should be provided by identified, designated individual(s) with training and/or experience in dealing with the needs of the persons served.
4. There should be medical supervision of physician-prescribed services.
5. The admission process should identify:
   a. Presenting problem(s).
   b. Goals and expected benefits of the admission.
   c. Initial estimated timeframes for goal accomplishment.
   d. Services needed.
6. A physician who is on the team should obtain a history and conduct a physical examination prior to or immediately following admission of the person to the program.
7. Services should be provided to evaluate and manage the functional, medical, physical, psychological, social, and

vocational needs of each person served from admission through discharge.

8. In order to provide a safe pain program, the scope and intensity of medical services should relate to the person's medical care needs. There should be ready availability of medical services either within the organization or through linkages with other agencies and individuals.

9. Services should be provided by a coordinated interdisciplinary team which includes a core team of individuals who are assigned to the program. The members of the core team, though each may not serve every person, should include:
    a. A clinical psychologist or psychiatrist.
    b. An occupational therapist.
    c. A physical therapist.
    d. A physician.
    e. A rehabilitation nurse.

10. The core team consists of the professional disciplines needed to carry out the pain management program and should:
    a. Provide evaluation and assessment of the needs of each person served.
    b. Guide the development and implementation of the program for the person served.
    c. Provide therapeutic, educational and training services consistent with the needs of the persons served through direct interaction with those persons.
    d. Attend and actively participate in conferences concerning persons served.
    e. Promote interdisciplinary functions and mutual support among all members of the team.
    f. Promote the program's evaluation and treatment philosophy.

11. In addition to the services provided by the core team, the following services should be utilized depending on the needs of the person served:
    a. Alcoholism and other drug dependency treatment.
    b. Audiology.
    c. Biofeedback.
    d. Chaplaincy.
    e. Clinical laboratory.
    f. Dentistry.
    g. Diagnostic radiology.
    h. Dietetics.
    i. Exercise physiology.
    j. Expressive therapies—e.g., movement, dance, art, and/or music therapies, etc.
    k. Medical/surgical subspecialty consultation.
    l. Orthotics/prosthetics.
    m. Pharmacy.
    n. Rehabilitation engineering.
    o. Social services.
    p. Speech-language pathology.
    q. Therapeutic recreation.
    r. Vocational rehabilitation.

12. Services should be provided directly by members of the person's team at least five hours per day, five days per week. At least three of those hours per day should be provided by the core team or under their direct supervision. A significant portion of persons served by the program should be receiving this level of services.

13. A team conference for each person served should be held at least once per week.

14. Appropriate to their needs, the persons served should have the benefit of a consistently assigned staff member from each of the disciplines.

15. A pain program should provide for physician pain management services which meet the following criteria:
    a. Physicians should play an active, meaningful role in the pain management and medical care of persons served with appropriate reliance on and availability of consulting medical specialists to meet the individual needs of the persons served.
    b. The chronic pain physician should provide active management, direction, and supervision of the person's pain program so that it is consistent with the diagnosis(es), presenting problems, and prognosis of the person served. This should include the physician component of decisions for admission, determination of goals, and discharge.
    c. The physician providing medical direction of the pain program should possess training and/or experience in the interdisciplinary management of persons with pain.
    d. The physician providing medical direction should meet the following criteria as specified:

    Category One—All Items

    (1) Three years of experience in the interdisciplinary management of persons with chronic pain.
    (2) Participation in active education on pain management at a local or national level.
    (3) Board certification in a medical specialty or completion of training sufficient to qualify for examination by a member of the American Board of Medical Specialties.
    (4) Two years' experience in medical direction of an interdisciplinary chronic pain program or at least six months of a pain fellowship in an interdisciplinary chronic pain program.

    Category Two—At Least One Item

    (5) Attends one meeting per year of a regional or national pain society.
    (6) Presents an abstract to a regional or national pain society.
    (7) Has published on a pain topic in a peer-reviewed journal.
    (8) Belongs to a pain society at a regional or national level.

    e. A physician should be available to persons served on a 24-hour-per-day, 7-day-per-week basis.
    f. The chronic pain physician should have ongoing and regular participation in efforts to monitor and improve the quality of care and the appropriate utilization of services in a pain program.
    g. The chronic pain physician should prescribe those services which by law must be prescribed and supervised by a physician.

16. The professionals on the core team, other than the physician, should be able to demonstrate training and experience in Chronic Pain Management Programs through at least one of the following:

a. One year of working at least 50% of the time in an interdisciplinary Chronic Pain Management Program.

b. At least three months of a fulltime pain training program in an interdisciplinary Chronic Pain Management Program.

17. The professionals on the core team should participate in educational opportunities in the area of pain management at a local or national level.

18. A multifaceted educational effort should be organized, goal-directed, and appropriate to the needs of the following target groups:

a. The persons served and their families.

b. Personnel.

c. Members of the professional and lay communities, including referral and funding sources.

19. If the person chooses, and when appropriate, there should be provisions for continued contact between the person served and the program after formal exit/discharge.

20. The program evaluation system of the Chronic Pain Management Program should address a variety of measures, at least two of which should be:

a. Appropriate use of medication.

b. Decreased intensity of subjective pain.

c. Increased ability by the person served to manage pain.

d. Increased functional activities.

e. Reduced health care use related to the chronic pain syndrome.

f. Return to gainful employment.

In an inpatient program, the following standards will also apply:

21. The total inpatient program should provide structured therapeutic activities seven days per week.

22. The admission criteria should be written so that persons admitted require the level of intensity provided by an inpatient program.

23. The physician should have direct contact with the person served at least five days per week.

24. The physician and other professionals who are licensed to practice independently in the inpatient setting should have training and experience that is reflected in the privileges granted by the institution.

25. Nursing services should provide for:

a. Nursing coverage 24 hours per day, under supervision of a registered nurse.

b. An intensity of nursing care that corresponds to the needs of persons served.

26. The pain program beds should be in a designated, contiguous area which is organized, staffed, and equipped for the specific purpose of providing a pain program.

a. Designated staff members should be assigned to the pain program.

b. The size of the bed service area should be such as to support a pain treatment environment."

In 1990, the International Association for the Study of Pain published desirable characteristics for pain treatment facilities. In doing so, they defined pain treatment facilities as multidisciplinary pain centers, multidisciplinary pain clinics, pain clinics, and modality-oriented pain clinics. Their guidelines included recommendations for staffing, representation of various specialties and communications among these health professionals, credentials of the director or coordinator, and services that should be offered. They also made recommendations regarding space, record keeping, support staff, licensing, protocols, and educational programs.[8]

NATURE OF THE POPULATION SERVED

Patients with chronic pain, in their desperate search for the elusive cure, often "chase windmills" and convince their doctors to do many invasive tests and procedures. As a result of their pain behavior, many have iatrogenic complications, suffering, and disability. Those involved in the treatment of these patients must find improved ways to detect this highly susceptible population, establish a therapeutic alliance, and short circuit their pain careers. Our health-care system cannot rely solely on the traditional methods of medical and surgical approaches often used with this population.

We should not ask people to live with pain if there is an acceptable treatment to alleviate it and if the potential benefits outweigh the potential risks and side effects. Therefore, I believe that, in all pain treatment facilities, the assessment must begin with a review of the patient's medical status and an updated physical examination to address this issue. This investigation should be done by those experienced in the evaluation of chronic pain. Through the years, I have been distressed by the many clinical recommendations offered by inexperienced consultants. When seeing a patient with chronic pain syndrome, they frequently order extensive diagnostic studies and invasive therapies, whereas more experienced consultants follow a more conservative course. As pain clinicians, our goal should be to develop and provide the most effective therapies for the various pains we treat. Clinical research on the spectrum of pain disorders may help us delineate, not only the treatments of choice, but also the methods involved in their implementation.[9,10]

Regarding the patient's educational level, their average education ranged from a sixth grade level (in a rural environment, University of Virginia Pain Clinic[11]) to more than 12 years of education in the predominantly urban population at the Boston Pain Center.

Back pain was the primary site of pain in most MPCs; this was consistent with chronic pain complaints in the general population.[12] At the Boston Pain Center, 45 percent of recent patient admissions were for back pain; this figure was 50 percent at the University of Virginia.[11] Murphy[13] reported that back and headache together accounted for two-thirds of patients at the University of Washington. Some MPCs focus exclusively on patients with back pain.[14]

Based on a review of more than 1000 patients with pain and back pain treated at pain clinics, I recommended criteria for patients who should have a second opinion before elective surgery (Table 36-1). Because low back operations are being done more selectively and less frequently, pain cen-

Table 36-1
Criteria for Second Opinion before Elective Surgery

Two or more pain-related surgeries without beneficial results.
One or more pain-related surgeries with negative findings.
Attorney-referred patients involved in pain-related litigation.
Known or highly suspected major psychopathology.
History of unjustified overuse of health-care system.

Adapted from Aronoff GM. Chronic pain and the disability epidemic. *Clin J Pain* 1991; 7:333.

ters should be viewed as a positive alternative for treatment, not only by concerned physicians and health-care providers, but also by cost-conscious insurance carriers and employers.[9]

Despite some evidence indicating that narcotic addiction in medical patients is low,[15] many patients with chronic pain are dependent on narcotic medications when admitted to MPCs.[16] Carron and Rowlingson[11] reported that 85 percent of their admissions had received narcotic analgesics. At the Boston Pain Center, 55 percent of patients were admitted to the program while they were taking narcotic medication; this figure was 43 percent at the University of Washington.[13] After narcotic medications, benzodiazepines are administered most frequently. Carron and Rowlingson[11] reported that 85 percent of their patients had received benzodiazepines, resulting in a 60 percent drug dependence that necessitated incorporation of detoxification as a part of treatment. In other programs, the percentage of patients taking sedative–hypnotics was substantially lower, with 9 percent of patients at the Boston Pain Center admitting to having received benzodiazepines. At the University of Washington,[13] 15 percent of patients had taken diazepam.

In terms of surgical treatment, many patients admitted to MPCs have had previous surgery. Murphy[13] reported that 40 percent of admissions have had one or more pain-related operations (average, 2.4 procedures). Gottlieb and coworkers[14] reported an average of two surgical procedures. At the Boston Pain Center, a recent survey indicated an average of 1.29 surgeries, although our previous study of 104 consecutive admissions revealed an average of 1.8 pain-related surgeries per patient.[17] Crue and Pinsky[18] found that 60 percent of their patients had had one or more surgical procedures (average, just under two per patient).

Vocational status is an important consideration when dealing with these patients because the presence of a pain syndrome interferes markedly with vocational functioning. Seres and colleagues[19] reported that 40 percent of their admissions were so-called disabled by pain. At the Boston Pain Center, more than 50 percent of admissions were labeled unemployed due to pain. The average time out of work was 29.4 months.[17]

Most patients at the Boston Pain Center (BPC) are involved in pain-related litigation from work injuries and personal nonindustrial accidents. A pilot study[20,21] at the BPC included a retrospective review of 50 patients who had been discharged between 1985 and 1987 and had returned for follow-up. (All had received Worker's Compensation.) The study suggested that, for those who sustain work-related injuries late in their careers and in whom limited education decreases their retraining potential, secondary gain factors may compromise improvement and return to a functional state. Other factors believed to influence return to work adversely included (1) being out of work more than 1 year; (2) negative treatment course and poor mastery of pain; (3) poor work history with little incentive to return to work; (4) major psychopathology; (5) narcotic dependency; (6) primary, secondary, and tertiary gain; (7) litigation; and (8) delay in return to work after discharge from the pain center.

It is our policy at the BPC that only motivated patients without major conscious secondary gain or suspected malingering are admitted to the pain program. We often recommend to patients who have litigation pending that they resolve these issues and, if their pain problem persists, they contact us. We may be able to structure a treatment program for them at that time. The attrition rate after claims closure and litigation resolution is high.[9]

Malec and associates[22] found that no patients were employed or in training at time of admission. Vasudevan and colleagues[23] reported that only 19 percent of their patients were employed when admitted.

In general, then, the typical MPC admission may be described as a patient in their mid-40s, with slightly less than a high school education, working most probably in a skilled or unskilled occupation but no longer able to work as a result of back pain. The average patient probably is receiving narcotic analgesics on admission and has had more than one surgical procedure.

PSYCHOLOGICAL CHARACTERISTICS

Because chronic pain has such disruptive effects on people's lives and physical functioning, it is not surprising that psychological functioning also is affected. The psychological aspects of pain have been reviewed elsewhere in this volume, and many books have been devoted to this topic.[12,24–26]

We will confine ourselves to delineating the psychological characteristics of patients admitted to MPCs. Keep in mind that patients seen in private practice settings may differ from these patients with regard to their psychological characteristics. Chapman and colleagues[27] compared depression and so-called illness behavior in patients treated in pain clinics or private practices. They found that those treated in private practices were significantly less depressed and showed less conviction of disease, bodily preoccupation, and hypochondriasis. They had less affective disturbance.

Typically, the patient with chronic pain admitted to a MPC is not "psychologically minded" and has little understanding of the role that psychological issues play in the pain problem. The patient often vehemently denies that there is any psychological component to the pain problem and can be rigidly defensive, using most often denial and repression (an unconscious mechanism wherein psychological issues and conflicts are kept out of the patient's awareness). Emotional conflicts often are expressed through somatic symptoms and are discharged in autonomic, vascular, or neuromuscular responses.

Patients may share some or all of the following characteristics: (1) preoccupation with pain, (2) strong needs for dependency and nurturance that may be denied directly and sought through so-called pain behavior, (3) feelings of loneliness and isolation, (4) self-defeating behavior patterns, (5) anger, and (6) hostility.

Seres and coworkers[19] reported that 70 percent of their patients had hysterical features, and more than 50 percent were depressed. Gottlieb and colleagues[14] found that virtually all (71 of 72 patients in their study) had moderate to severe psychopathologic disorders (indicated by significant deviations on standardized psychological tests).

Research using the Minnesota Multiphasic Personality Inventory (MMPI) showed that patients treated in MPCs (any patients with chronic pain in general) achieve significantly elevated scores on the hypochondriasis, depression, and hysteria scales of that test.[28] This profile has been referred to as the *neurotic triad* and suggests a high level of depression, denial of emotional conflicts, and a tendency toward the expression of needs through somatic symptoms. Some investigators suggest that this pattern reflects premorbid neurotic symptoms that contribute to the development of the pain syndrome; others view the pattern as reflecting the emotional problems that result from the chronic pain experience.[29] In support of the latter interpretation, there is evidence to suggest that patients with chronic pain cannot be differentiated from those with chronic disease on the basis of their MMPI profiles.[30]

In looking at the backgrounds of chronic pain admissions, some similarities are found. Some of these were addressed by Engel[31] in his classic treatise on the so-called pain prone patient. They have been updated by Blumer and Heilbronn.[32] These latter authors proposed the term *pain prone disorder* to identify a distinct subgroup of patients with characteristic clinical, psychodynamic, biographic, and genetic features. Some of these features include: continuous pain of obscure origin, hypochondriac preoccupation, desire for surgery, denial of conflicts, prepain workaholism, idealization of self and family relations, and depression. In the family history, there is a high incidence of alcoholism, depression, and relatives with chronic pain. Past abuse by a spouse and sexual abuse by a parent or sibling also may occur.

Whether the psychological dysfunction preceded or followed the onset of the pain problem, by the time the patient is admitted to a MPC, there is tremendous and global life disruption. Addison[33] states that characteristics common on evaluation include:

". . . the perception of one's life being out of one's own control, or a lack of contingencies based on individual behaviors, a sense of helplessness in intervening in one's own behalf is most often the general overlay to all other psychological and emotional changes."

STRUCTURE OF PAIN CENTERS

During the past decade, MPCs have coalesced into similar forms, with common underlying philosophies, assumptions about treatment, and organization.[34,35] A major characteristic is the integration and interdependency of their components.[36] This interdependency means that, despite the diversity of disciplines represented in a MPC, patients are given a message about the nature of their problem and the proposed treatment that is consistent with the philosophy and assumptions of the center as a whole.

The BPC treatment program focuses on several major patient problem areas, including:

1. The pain–depression–insomnia cycle.
2. Medication dependency.
3. Pain-related physical dysfunction.
4. Psychosocial factors affecting the pain syndrome.
5. The distinction between impairment and disability.
6. Early return to work, school, or other productive activity.

It is crucial to the effective functioning of the MPC that staff are aware of these assumptions and can convey the appropriate message to the patient. If a new staff member or consultant arrives whose orientation differs from that of the unit, the nature of the treatment milieu changes. For instance, a common goal of MPCs is analgesic medication reduction. If a consultant unfamiliar with the medication reduction regimen evaluates a patient's particular problem and suggests analgesic medication, the integrity of the MPC message may be compromised, even if the recommendation is not implemented. Inconsistency in communication fosters division of staff (splitting) and may interfere with effective MPC treatment.

Assumptions Underlying MPC Treatment

An assumption of virtually all MPCs is that chronic pain syndromes always involve psychological, social, biologic, and medical factors.[37] This assumption is inherent in the gate-control theory[2] and has been accepted widely throughout the community of pain clinicians. Aronoff[38] emphasized that "any treatment program designed for pain patients must be holistic in its orientation if it is to be effective" (Table 36-2). This assumption does not mean that psychosocial factors are only sequelae to a more fundamentally biologic or medical malady, nor does it mean that patients treated in a MPC have primarily psychogenic pain. The prevalence of somatoform pain disorder in MPCs is remarkably low.[39]

The staff in MPCs generally view the pain syndrome itself as the focal point of treatment, not only as a symptom

Table 36-2
Pain Center Goals

I. Clarify the diagnosis. Review medical records and the need for additional diagnostic studies or invasive procedures.

II. Improve pain control (eliminate pain if possible) through physical therapies:
   A. Help the patient to be more comfortably active, with a return to a functional and productive life.
   B. Promote the use of alternative noninvasive pain-control therapies other than potent medications.
   C. With individually structured exercise programs, reduce the patient's fear of reinjury.
   D. Teach proper body mechanics and postural awareness.
   E. Evaluate limitations and restrictions.

III Improve psychological functioning:
   A. Define and address psychosocial issues influencing chronic pain syndrome.
   B. Relieve drug dependency.
   C. Treat depression and its frequently associated insomnia.
   D. Address primary and secondary gains from pain.
   E. Assess family system.
   F. Strengthen support network (e.g., personal, family and community).

IV. Provide access to occupational and vocational rehabilitation and any other significant health-care personnel and resolve disability when possible.

V. Communicate with the patient's referring physician by discharge summary, telephone, or personal meetings to obtain any information that will assist in the continued management of the patient.

VI. Reduce inappropriate use of the health-care system.

VII. Decrease the cost of medical care associated with chronic pain syndrome.

Adapted from Aronoff GM, McAlary PW. Pain centers: treatment for intractable suffering and disability resulting from chronic pain. In: Aronoff GM, ed. *Evaluation and Treatment of Chronic Pain*. 2nd ed. Baltimore: Williams & Wilkins; 1992:417.

of some underlying pathophysiologic process. Thus, legitimate directions of treatment are to reduce pain behaviors, life disruption, medication dependence, and secondary gain and to increase activity level, physical functioning, and vocational status.

The focus on the syndrome of pain in MPCs can be opposed to the expectation of patients. It is common for patients to expect that pain itself will be the focus of treatment, or perhaps that they will receive another extensive diagnostic evaluation to discover the underlying cause of pain. This discrepancy between patient expectations and MPC orientation needs to be resolved during treatment (as patient and staff come to a common conceptualization of the nature of the pain problem).[26]

Another assumption shared by MPCs is the emphasis on the advantages of a patient taking an active role in rehabilitation. Although research regarding the influence of the so-called locus of control on rehabilitation is equivocal, it is believed that this may reflect difficulties in operationalizing the concept of active responsibility rather than problems with the concept itself.

Active responsibility and independence are orientations shared by many chronic disease specialities, and they differ markedly from those of acute medical care. Patients also may dislike the emphasis placed on independence, seeing this as inadequate caretaking by the staff, who are seen as not understanding the nature of their problem. This discrepancy often is based on patients' (and some clinicians') failure to differentiate acute from chronic pain problems.

A related assumption is that "curing" pain (in the sense of alleviating the cause of nociception) is not always possible. Crue and Pinsky[18] take a centralist, rather than a peripheralist, point of view and argue that, in its chronic form, pain does not require continued nociceptive input. These authors state, "We regard chronic pain syndrome as a result of central nervous system phenomena without the need for an ongoing peripheral nociceptive arm to complete the clinical picture." Not all MPC staff share the centralist viewpoint that cure (in the acute care sense) is not the ultimate focus for treatment of pain syndromes.

Staffing of a Multidisciplinary Pain Center

The core specialities represented at MPCs are usually similar. This similarity occurs because the assumptions are operationalized.[34,35] Also, CARF has delineated staffing guidelines that often are followed by pain centers, not only because of clinical efficacy, but also as a result of the increased importance of certification.

Conformity with CARF guidelines for inpatient multidisciplinary pain centers requires the services of a physician, psychologist or psychiatrist, physical therapist, specialized nursing care, access to a dietician's services, and social services. In addition, many pain centers have relaxation training and biofeedback as an integral part of the program and occupational therapy and/or vocational services.

Medical Director

As noted in the CARF guidelines,[7] the medical director of the pain program does not need to be the clinical director, although frequently the same person serves in both capacities. Current guidelines for qualifications for the medical director include 3 years' experience as a provider, 2 years' experience as a medical director (or a 6-month or greater fellowship in pain management), and board certification or board-eligible status in a specialty approved by the American Board of Medical Specialties.

I believe that the medical director should have adequate clinical skills in the evaluation and treatment of pain to allow for the formulation and implementation of an appropriate treatment plan for the given patient population. With these patients, who are at risk for iatrogenic complications, it may be more important for the physician to know when not to request additional invasive diagnostic studies and procedures than when to request them. Although this clinical decision often is difficult, it must be emphasized that, if we pursue the diagnostic evaluation past a certain point, it often is counterproductive and, therefore, contraindicated. Defining that certain point involves combining the science and art of medicine.

Services Offered at Pain Centers

A similarity of services is also common in MPCs. These usually consist of medical services (including evaluation, supervision, and medication monitoring) and speciality consultation. Psychological services include evaluation and testing and group, individual, and family psychotherapy. The psychologist also can be involved in program development, research, and program management.

Physical therapy is a crucial component to any MPC. Often, a good physical therapy examination can reveal problems that have been overlooked previously. These include biomechanical dysfunctions, myofascial restrictions, diminished endurance, and functional status in relation to the patient's daily vocational and/or leisure activities. Methods offered by physical therapy range from more traditional acute pain treatments (such as heat or cold packs, whirlpool, and ultrasound) to TENS and strength, flexibility, and endurance exercises. Some pain centers, in an attempt to emphasize functional improvement and independence, limit physical therapy involvement to evaluation and active exercise programs; others use all these techniques as needed.

Systematic relaxation training and biofeedback are common features of MPCs because environmental stressors and elevated emotional tension are prevalent in patients with pain and can exacerbate painful conditions. There appears to be little difference in the efficacy between biofeedback and general relaxation training (such as progressive muscle relaxation or autogenic training).[40,41] Both biofeedback and general relaxation training are more effective in pain reduc-

tion than no treatment. Biofeedback methods include EMG, temperature, and electrodermal response (EDR).

The nature of the nursing care often can be the most important way of communicating treatment assumptions to patients, especially if the nursing component in the MPC is strong. Sample and colleagues[42] state

> "The Pain Unit nurse is a unique practitioner. As in all hospitals, the nurse has a major responsibility for the total well-being of the patient. She must exercise accurate clinical judgement and have understanding of pain mechanisms, psychosocial aspects of the chronic pain syndrome, operant conditioning, and behavior modification."

The role of social services in pain programs often is to provide family counseling and educate patients and their families about the relationship between family functioning and the patient who has chronic pain.[43,44] Interventions, in general, assume that chronic pain affects the entire family, not just the patient and that family members can provide both strong support for behavioral change and powerful disincentives to make needed life modifications.

Vocational services are offered by an increasing number of MPCs as return to work or other productive activity becomes a more integral aspect of the patient's rehabilitation. The extent of services varies widely, from referral to state vocational rehabilitation agencies to full-scale vocational evaluation, job analysis or work hardening programs, and job placement. Several professional specialities may take part in MPC vocational services; these include certified vocational counselors, social workers, occupational therapists, and physical therapists.

A formalized educational program also is common in MPCs. Topics are offered that are relevant to patients with chronic pain and include information about medications, depression, body mechanics, and the role of psychological factors in pain. More formalized stress management and assertiveness training programs often are included. The goal of educational programs is to give these patients information that they can use to move out of a position of helplessness[45] to one where they can feel more in control of their lives, with their pain syndrome and its sequelae assuming a less dominant position in their lives.

Although perhaps not accurately considered a service, the milieu and therapeutic community atmosphere is a crucial aspect of treatment in many MPCs. The supportive and sometimes confrontational atmosphere of other community members who also have problems with pain often is one of the most powerful factors in promoting change to a more productive and less pain-focused life. Group interaction is encouraged and activities are managed to maximize socialization among patients and promote group cohesiveness.

REFERRAL PROCESS

Although physicians generally are beginning to recognize the pain center as a community resource, it is equally important to understand which patients may be appropriate for a referral to the MPC. Usually a referred patient has a chronic nonmalignant pain syndrome that has been unresponsive to conventional therapy and is associated with significant life disruption. Often the patient has tried physical therapy, psychological therapy and medication sporadically, all without significant or lasting benefit.

Most comprehensive MPCs treat a heterogeneous population of patients with chronic pain who have problems including intractable headache syndromes, neuropathies, reflex sympathetic dystrophies, and chronic low back, rheumatologic, phantom limb, thalamic, facial, gastrointestinal, and other nonmalignant pains. Many therapeutic techniques used in the management of chronic nonmalignant pain syndromes also may be effective in chronic cancer pain syndromes. Generally, however, these patients are treated in separate programs because of our recognition of the distinct diagnostic and therapeutic challenges in each group.

Pain can disrupt the patient's life, causing prolonged unemployment, medication dependency, or depression. When asked directly, these patients often deny depression, but this can be assessed through questions regarding their vocational, marital, or financial disruptions; possible recent deaths of significant others in their lives; decreased concern about personal appearance; changes in sleeping or eating habits; and the presence of social isolation.

It often may be appropriate to refer a patient to a pain center if there is excessive pain behavior during consultation or examination, pain complaints in excess of that expected from the physical findings, pain that has persisted despite extensive evaluation or treatment, and pain for which surgery or nerve blocks are not believed to be treatments of choice. Despite the ubiquity of psychosocial and economic dysfunction, these patients' chronic pain is real (with the exception of malingering), and they should not be given the impression that you, as their physician, believe it is not. Many patients believe that referral to a pain center means that their pain is "all in their heads." For instance, one patient said he was referred to the BPC because ours was a place for people who "think they have pain."

Treatment at a pain center begins with the referral. Ideally, referring physicians indicate to their patients, positively and supportively, that they would like to try a new approach to the management of the patients' chronic pain. The referring physician then explains that, because the pain clearly is a complex process that does not seem to be resolving adequately, a comprehensive pain center would provide a better setting in which to deal with the many complicated medical, psychological, and social factors that have become intertwined. Many patients may think that, if either medical or surgical intervention has not helped them, then their pain must be imaginary. Reassurance that this is not the case can contribute to a more positive attitude toward pain rehabilitation. The following are criteria for patients appropriate for referral to a pain center:

1. Patient adequately evaluated.
2. Pain refractory to conventional treatments.
3. Significant life disruption.
4. Associated psychosocial difficulties.
5. Medication dependence or substance abuse.
6. Significant pain behavior or poor coping.
7. Patient motivated to change.
8. Resolution of the pain problem more important to the patient than maintaining secondary gains.

It is important that physicians tells their patients that pain centers generally are not primarily involved in looking for a cure for pain through new diagnostic procedures. Although MPCs offer medical evaluation and diagnostic services, many referred patients expect these to be either the only services offered or those that are emphasized most. Patients who expect to have their previous diagnostic evaluations repeated often express considerable anger and hostility; this, in turn, may interfere with rehabilitation.

Finally, it is essential that the patient leave the referral meeting with some sense of hope. Patients are discouraged by the prospect of having to "learn to live with it." They are aware that, for them, treatment has failed, and they often feel discouraged and depressed. Patients may be more hopeful if they realize that, despite previous treatment failures, they can be helped at a pain center equipped to address the complexities of their pain problems.

When determining appropriate candidates for referral, the importance of the patient's motivation cannot be overemphasized. Poorly motivated patients sometimes respond to the pain center milieu, but they often resist demands to participate fully in the active treatment regimen. A patient strongly motivated to return to an active and productive life has a better prognosis for success in a MPC.

Most of this discussion applies to both outpatient and inpatient programs. Having evaluated and treated thousands of patients with chronic pain, Aronoff and McAlary[46] concluded that most of these patients can be treated effectively in a structured outpatient day program. Patients traveling a great distance can be housed in a nearby hotel. This avoids costly hospitalization and more realistically simulates typical activities of daily living. For many patients, there is an easier transition from the treatment program back to their usual lives.

It is my belief that treatment for those with difficult chronic pain problems should be based on a wellness model, recognizing that generally pain does not make them "sick" (in the acute medical sense of the word) but rather that it interferes with their optimal functioning in various areas of their lives. These patients generally do not require around-the-clock medical or nursing care.[4]

Current recommendations for inhospital pain treatment include:

1. Patients requiring diagnostic testing best provided inhospital.
2. Those with unstable medical illness requiring inpatient monitoring and around-the-clock nursing or medical supervision.

3. Those who are not ambulatory or independent in activities of daily living.
4. Patients with major medication dependency, especially with a substance abuse disorder (some of these patients are best treated in chemical dependency centers; others who are highly motivated may be treated as outpatients).
5. Those who are acutely suicidal or have unstable major psychiatric disorders (some are best treated in a psychiatric unit).
6. Those who previously have been unsuccessful with outpatient pain center treatment (assuming the patient was motivated, and the center was credible).

Currently, because hospitals must respond to the economic and administrative pressures of maintaining their patient census, the option of inpatient versus outpatient pain treatment unfortunately may be influenced as much (or more) by these factors as by the best interest of the patient.[4]

If I were to subdivide the chronic pain population we have worked with at the BPC, approximately one-third of the patients truly desire to be involved actively in their health care, with the goal of suffering less with pain, using less medication, and returning to a more active productive life than was the case at the time of their admission. This group generally is reasonably self-motivated and eagerly awaits training in new techniques to help them live better with pain and suffer less. Another one-third of this population consists of those who have learned to be patients with pain—that is, they have developed goal-directed conditioned pain behaviors (learned helplessness), often maintaining these unconsciously. Nonetheless, these patients are "stuck," and investigation has revealed patterns of self-defeating behaviors. Although somewhat more defensive than those in the first group, these patients are at least receptive to participating in a structured program designed to maximize function and minimize dysfunction and to replace maladaptive coping with more adaptive techniques. They can learn not to be disabled by pain. Generally, these two segments of the chronic pain population do well in multidisciplinary pain programs. We have had a major impact on the quality of their lives and also serve society by returning to it more functional members. It is the remaining one-third of this population that is the greatest concern. Although this group tends to be the most "abused" by the health-care system, it is also the group that abuses the health-care system and society.

Increasingly, it appears that there are some patients who cannot be helped, who at some time may not want to be helped, and whose agenda of being enmeshed in the health-care system has nothing to do with receiving health care but, rather, with receiving benefits. We must identify this segment of the population more efficiently and not treat them. Regardless of a patient's complaints, after we have established that the tools at our disposal are unlikely to ameliorate their symptoms, we should establish a series of recommendations, and if the patient is unable or unwilling to consider these, at this point, the system may have ful-filled its responsibility adequately to the patient and should no longer attempt to treat them.[4,47]

We should not underestimate the importance of a physician's authoritative guidance; this can be offered as supportive paternalism. Patients will either live up to our expectations that they need not be disabled or, conversely, become invalids unnecessarily through learned helplessness. It is our ethical responsibility to improve a patient's health whenever possible. Their physical, emotional, social, and spiritual well-being is more likely to be realized with the self-esteem that results from feeling useful (often from gainful employment) rather than from disability (which frequently is preventable).

References

1. Beecher HK. *Measurement of Subjective Responses: Quantitative Effects of Drugs.* New York: Oxford University Press; 1959.
2. Melzack R, Wall PD. Pain mechanisms: a new theory. *Science* 1965; 50:971–979.
3. Aronoff GM, McAlary PW, Witkower A, et al. Pain treatment programs: do they return workers to the workplace? *Spine State Art Rev* 1987; 2(1):123–126.
4. Aronoff GM, McAlary PW. Pain centers: treatment for intractable suffering and disability resulting from chronic pain. In: Aronoff GM, ed. *Evaluation and Treatment of Chronic Pain.* 2nd ed. Baltimore: Williams and Wilkins; 1992:417–420.
5. Hardy PA, Hill P. A multidisciplinary approach to pain management. *Br J Hosp Med* January 1990; 43(1):45–47.
6. Aronoff GM, Crue BL, Seres J. *Pain Centers: Help for the Chronic Pain Patient, Mediguide to Pain.* New York: Della Corte; 1983:1–5.
7. *Standards Manual for Facilities Serving People with Disabilities.* Tucson, AZ: Commission on Accreditation of Rehabilitation Facilities. 1992:52–56.
8. *Desirable Characteristics for Pain Treatment Facilities.* Seattle: International Association for the Study of Pain; 1990.
9. Aronoff GM. *Clin J Pain* 1985; 1:1–3. Editorial.
10. Aronoff GM. Chronic pain and the disability epidemic. *Clin J Pain* 1991; 7:331–333.
11. Carron H, Rowlingson JC. Coordinated outpatient management of chronic pain at the University of Virginia Pain Clinic. In: Ng LKY, ed. *New Approaches to Treatment of Chronic Pain: A Review of Multidisciplinary Pain Clinics and Pain Centers.* Rockville: National Institute on Drug Abuse; 1981.
12. Aronoff GM. Psychological aspects of non-malignant chronic pain: a new nosology. In: Aronoff GM, ed. *Evaluation and Treatment of Chronic Pain.* 2nd ed. Baltimore: Williams and Wilkins; 1992.
13. Murphy TM. Profiles of pain patients, including chronic pelvic pain: University of Washington Clinical Pain Service. In: Ng LKY, ed. *New Approaches to Treatment of Chronic Pain: A Review of Multidisciplinary Pain Clinics and Pain Centers.* Rockville: National Institute on Drug Abuse; 1981.

14. Gottlieb H, Strite L, Koller R, et al. Comprehensive rehabilitation of patients having chronic low back pain. *Arch Phys Med Rehabil* 1977; 58:101–108.

15. Porter J, Jick H. Addiction rate in patients treated with narcotics. *N Engl J Med* 1980; 302:123.

16. Murphy TM, Anderson S. Multidisciplinary approach to managing pain. In: Benedetti C, Chapman CR, Moricca G, eds. *Advances in Pain Research and Therapy*. Vol 7. New York: Raven Press; 1984.

17. Aronoff GM, Evans WO. Evaluation and Treatment of Chronic Pain at the Boston Pain Center. *J Clin Psychiatry* 1982; 43:4–9.

18. Crue BL, Pinsky JJ. Chronic pain syndrome—four aspects of the problem: New Hope Pain Center and Pain Research Foundation. In: Ng LKY, ed. *New Approaches to Treatment of Chronic Pain: A Review of Multidisciplinary Pain Clinics and Pain Centers*. Rockville: National Institute on Drug Abuse; 1981:138.

19. Seres JL, Painter JR, Newman RI. Multidisciplinary treatment of chronic pain at the Northwest Pain Center. In: Ng LKY, ed. *New Approaches to Treatment of Chronic Pain: A Review of Multidisciplinary Pain Clinics and Pain Centers*. Rockville: National Institute on Drug Abuse; 1981.

20. Aronoff GM, McAlary PW, Witkower A, et al. Pain treatment programs: do they return workers to the workplace? *Spine* 1987; 2:123–136.

21. Aronoff GM, McAlary PW, Witkower A, et al. Pain treatment programs: do they return workers to the workplace. *J Occup Med* 1988; 3:123–136.

22. Malec J, Cayner JJ, Harvey RF, Timming RC. Pain management: long term following of an inpatient program. *Arch Phys Med Rehabil* 1981; 62:369–372.

23. Vasudevan SV, Lynch NT, Abram S. Effectiveness of an ambulatory chronic pain management program. *Pain Suppl* 1981; 1:S294. Abstract.

24. Sternback RA. *The Psychology of Pain*. New York: Raven Press; 1978.

25. Barber J, Adrian C. *Psychological Approaches to the Management of Pain*. New York: Brunner/Mazel; 1982.

26. Turk D, Meichenbaum D, Genest M. *Pain and Behavioral Medicine: A Cognitive Behavioral Perspective*. New York: Guilford; 1983.

27. Chapman CR, Sola AR, Bonica JJ. Illness behavior and depression compared in pain center and private practice patients. *Pain* 1979; 6:1–7.

28. Sternbach RA. *Pain Patients: Traits and Treatment*. New York: Academic Press; 1974.

29. McCreary C, Turner J, Dawson E. The MMPI as a predictor of response to conservative treatment for low back pain. *J Clin Psychol* 1979; 35:278–284.

30. Naliboff BD, Cohen MJ, Yellen AN. Does the MMPI differentiate chronic illness from chronic pain? *Pain* 1982; 13(4):333–341.

31. Engel GL. "Psychogenic" pain and the pain-prone patient. *Am J Med* 1959; 26:899–918.

32. Blumer D, Heilbronn M. Chronic pain as a variant of depressive disease. The pain-prone disorder. *J Nerv Ment Dis* 1982; 170(7):381–394.

33. Addison RG. Treatment of chronic pain: The Center for Pain Studies, Rehabilitation Institute of Chicago. In: Ng LKY, ed. *New Approaches to Treatment of Chronic Pain: A Review of Multidisciplinary Pain Clinics and Pain Centers*. Rockville: National Institute on Drug Abuse; 1981:17.

34. Aronoff GM, Wagner JM. The pain center: development, structure and dynamics. In: Burrows GD, Elton D, Stanley GV, eds. *Handbook on Chronic Pain Management*. Amsterdam: Elsevier.

35. Aronoff GM, McAlary PW. Organization and function of the multidisciplinary pain center. In: Aronoff GM, ed. *Pain Centers: A Revolution in Health Care*. New York: Raven Press; 1988:55–74.

36. Rowlingson JC, Hamill RJ. Organization of a multidisciplinary pain center. *Mt Sinai J Med* May 1991; 58(3):267–272.

37. Melzack R. *The Puzzle of Pain*. Harmondsworth, England: Penguin; 1973.

38. Aronoff GM. A holistic approach to pain rehabilitation: the Boston Pain Unit. In: Ng LKY, ed. *New Approaches to Treatment of Chronic Pain: A Review of Multidisciplinary Pain Clinics and Pain Centers*. Rockville: National Institute on Drug Abuse; 1981:34.

39. Fishbain DA, Goldberg M, Meagher BR, Steele R, Rosomoff H. DSM III diagnosis in chronic pain patients. Paper presented at the meeting of the America Pain Society; October 1985; Dallas, Texas.

40. Turner JA, Chapman CR. Psychological interventions for chronic pain: a critical review, I: relaxation training and biofeedback. *Pain* 1982; 12:1–21.

41. Tan SY. Cognitive and cognitive-behavioral methods for pain control: a selective review. *Pain* 1982; 12:201–228.

42. Sample S, Burgess-Page M, Hayes M. Chronic pain management: the nurse's role. In: Aronoff GM, ed. *Evaluation and Treatment of Chronic Pain*. Baltimore: Urban & Schwartzenberg; 1985:565.

43. Hayes MA, McAlary PW, Popovsky J, et al. Alteration in comfort of chronic pain: a nursing challenge. In: Aronoff GM, ed. *Evaluation and Treatment of Chronic Pain*. 2nd ed. Baltimore: Williams and Wilkins; 1992.

44. Goldberg P. The social worker, family systems, and the chronic pain family. In: Aronoff GM, ed. *Evaluation and Treatment of Chronic Pain*. 2nd ed. Baltimore: Williams & Wilkins; 1992.

45. Seligman MEP. *Helplessness: On Depression, Development, and Death*. San Francisco: Freeman; 1975.

46. Aronoff GM, McAlary PW. Multidisciplinary treatment of intractable pain syndromes. In: Liptons, Tunks E, Zuppi M, eds. *Advances in Pain Research and Therapy*. Vol 13. New York: Raven Press; 1990:267–277.

47. Aronoff GM. What is happening to medicine? *Clin J Pain* 1988; 4:65–66. Editorial.

CHAPTER 37

Setting Up a Pain Treatment Facility

Sampson Lipton

Bonica's[1] book *The Management of Pain* was published in 1953. This was the beginning of the systematic treatment of pain in which pain was regarded as a medical entity in itself. Various doctors in different parts of the world had concentrated on treating chronic pain before then, but until this book was published, they worked in isolation and were involved in some other major specialty. In Chapter 6 of this book, Bonica[1] fostered the view that the nerve block clinic was available for other medical practitioners to refer patients to without there being any need to transfer control of the patient. The brief mention of the nerve block clinic was as a forum where like-minded clinicians could discuss difficult pain problems; they came together 1 or 2 half days per week. The book provided a reference work and also a framework within which physicians interested in pain problems could work. Contact and rapport developed between them, and soon the idea of the separate pain clinic developed. The blocking clinic became only one of the possible methods for treating intractable pain.

We can see immediately how advanced this view was at this time and also what great strides have been made in the methods of and organization of centers for pain control during the last 30 years. Throughout this period, Bonica has remained a stalwart and respected figure in the vanguard of the advancing science of chronic pain relief. As time has passed, more and more physicians and other health workers have seen the value and rationale of the separate entity known as the pain clinic. Currently, hospitals large and small regard such a clinic as a necessity.[2-10]

The way a system develops tends to determine the way it progresses. From the foregoing discussion, it can be seen how the proliferation of many types of pain clinics and blocking clinics developed. At one extreme, there is still the basic blocking clinic. This uses nerve blocks of greater or lesser complexity, or it can be confined to one type, for example sympathetic blocks for vascular medicine. Whatever its size, it both treats and diagnoses. At the other extreme, lies the large pain relief center. This contains teaching and training facilities and may provide an information service to other smaller pain clinics, general practitioners, ancillary workers in the pain field and all interested bodies (such as the government or press). It provides diagnostic and treatment services for all types of pain problems arising from either neoplastic or benign sources. A large staff of nurses, physiotherapists, other physical medical experts, clerks, typists, secretaries, and accountants is found in such a center. The medical staff includes those working all or most of their time in the pain clinic and those closely associated with it. This pain clinic can provide outpatient, day ward, and surgical facilities and all the skilled specialists necessary. It will have its own budget and may be independent or a part of another larger department (such as anesthesiology or medical and surgical neurology). It will have close contact with the departments of anesthesia, neurology, psychiatry, orthopedics, and psychology. Most likely, there will be a psychology section in the pain clinic. It will have its own beds where patients can be admitted for observation, diagnosis, and treatment. Many modern methods of pain treatment involve x-ray control; thus radiologic equipment must be readily available or owned. We can continue enumerating the requirements of the large pain clinic. In general terms, what is required is the same as those found in any large hospital department plus the special requirements of a pain clinic.[11]

Only large hospitals or centers can provide the scope of medical personel and equipment for such a facility. Most cannot attain this ideal and therefore will settle for something between the simplest and the most complex. This is what usually happens, complicated, of course, by the individual country's special legislation. It must be remembered that many countries have state-controlled health services and their requirements are different from those where payment per item of service is the norm. Each system requires different working methods, but treatment may be equally difficult to provide and equally frustrating for the administrative, medical, and nursing personnel. For instance, in a state-controlled system such as that in the United Kingdom, a global sum of money is given to each hospital yearly, and this is divided among the different departments. If the pain clinic is part of another department, it will have to fight for its share, along with all the other sections of the department. Because no money is brought in by the services provided (however much they are used), a new piece of necessary equipment (such as an image intensifier) may not be provided because it does not receive a high enough priority or there is not enough money.

In the United States, where payment per item of service is usual, the pain clinic must pay its own way. Any special expensive piece of equipment is bought by the clinic or jointly with another clinic. It must be justified by the expected use and generation of fees. If this x-ray service is provided through the radiologic department, then the charges demanded by that service must be worthwhile to the pain clinic. An added feature is that all nerve-blocking methods potentially may be a source of litigation, and the use of x-ray control is an absolute necessity to minimize this. In addition, the patients' insurance companies and the government agencies may reimburse on two different scales, one for large clinics with rehabilitation facilities and another (a lower scale) for those without. Careful economic decisions must be made in regard to what procedures and expenditure can be undertaken profitably to keep the pain clinic viable.[12]

The availability of the rehabilitation facility is the feature that distinguishes the modern large pain clinic from those that have gone before. Hitherto, it was sufficient to be able to attempt to treat and cure patients with chronic pain problems, but currently, it is necessary, in addition, to be able to treat patients who cannot be cured of their pain problem with the methods available. As mentioned, in the United States, a higher rate of payment may be available to those clinics that have this facility. Rehabilitation units can be accredited by The Commission on Accreditation of Rehabilitation Facilities.[13] In addition, the Committee on Pain Therapy of the American Society of Anesthesiologists keeps a Pain Center and Clinic Directory. This gives abbreviated but comprehensive details of the individual facilities of each clinic. Other countries do not have such a comprehensive record of their pain clinics.

The ability to deal with the patient who does not respond to pain clinic treatment is so important and represents such an advance that it is worthwhile spending a paragraph or two on it. During recent years, based on the pioneering work of Fordyce in Seattle and others,[14,15] it was realized that much chronic pain persisted through factors other than physical damage, although physical damage usually initiated the condition. Fordyce[14] showed that operant conditioning could be applied to train patients with intractable pain to behave in socially accepted ways. To take a simple example, if these patients before becoming ill did not integrate well with others and were somewhat solitary and subsequently had an accident that caused hospitalization and pain, they might find that there was sympathy, acceptance, and communication in such a setting when there had been none before. If the patient appeared to be in pain and kindness was shown (such as the offer to provide an analgesic, bring a cup of tea or coffee, and show concern), this acted as an operant. If a beneficial effect were produced by an operant, then that operant would be used again. When

the patient appeared to be in pain, many things that were unavailable earlier were provided. Such activity might be used again and again. Fordyce[14] found that, by using selected operants in a hospital ward setting, the patient could be taught independence again.

Other patients have conditions that do not respond to treatment. Because of this, they develop an overlay of pain behaviour (grimacing, using strange movements, and holding themselves in awkward postures). These are the operants by which they obtain the sympathy and help they unconsciously need. By these means, they may maintain dominance in their home setting. The Fordyce technique and that of others like it produces a high proportion of patients who can return to normal life and work. There are a number of corollaries. The family of the operant treated patient must be brought into the treatment system because they may be interested in keeping the patient in an ill state. Sometimes these secondary operants are too strong to be overcome. Even the patients' work mates should be brought in to treatment for lasting success. It is not satisfactory using operant conditioning to return someone to a work environment if they are treated there as frail and not fit to work. It is important to obtain the help of the industrial insurance company in finding work for those who have been disabled for a lengthy period. A rehabilitation officer who places patients also is useful.

TYPES OF PAIN TREATMENT FACILITIES

Thus, pain treatment facilities can vary from simple ones treating one type of pain or providing one kind of treatment to complex ones involved with all varieties of chronic pain and treatments available. The former will be run by one or two medical practitioners with a minimum of ancillary help; the latter can call on many specialist physicians and all types of paramedical help. Some of the common types of specialized pain facilities will be mentioned, but this list is not meant to be comprehensive.

Blocking Clinic

As concerns the anesthesiologist, this is the simplest type of pain clinic and is the original prototype from which all pain clinics evolved.[16] There should be a physician who sees the patient and decides whether the blocking injection is diagnostic or therapeutic. An example would be a diagnostic sympathetic block compared with an injection for a tennis elbow. The equipment required is usually simple, involving various local anesthetic solutions (with varying lengths of activity and concentrations), needles, and syringes. There also will be adjuvant substances (such as insoluble corticosteroid solutions). If complicated and deep injections are made (such as a lumbar sypathetic block), an image intensifier is necessary. This requires a suitable radiotransparent table, lead aprons, and a knowledgeable operator. This equipment might be available from the x-ray department in a hospital, but in an independent clinic, care must be taken to conform with the official radiation control authority for such equipment. In the past, many deep injections and injections near the spinal canal were done blindly (without x-ray help), and this was accepted as standard procedure. This is no longer the case. If the injected solution is deposited in the wrong place, the patient has a severe reaction, or there is much pain after the injection and an image intensifier has not been used, the operator may find themselves in litigation, even though all precautions otherwise have been taken. For this reason, no injections should be undertaken without comprehensive resuscitation facilities being immediately available, and no operator should do blocking techniques (even of the simplest kind) without a second person, preferably a nurse, being present.

Blocking techniques can involve the use of neurolytic substances (e.g., phenol solutions 2% to 6%). These[17] are dangerous, especially around the spinal cord, when they are injected through a spinal or epidural needle. The particular danger is that, even though placed perfectly, a sharp needle can move during the injection and become misplaced. Near the spinal cord, an epidural catheter can be placed accurately inside or outside the theca with the aid of the image intensifier. Injection of a water-soluble radiopaque solution then will show the position of its open end accurately.

Much care must be taken in all pain clinics to ensure precautions against wrongly placed injections. Proper protocols should be provided for medical and nursing personnel. There also should be corresponding descriptions of what is being done and what the risks are that are provided to the patient. Because hospitals and clinics are staffed by human beings and they are not perfect, the most stringent precautions sooner or later may fail. This is not recognized sufficiently and allowed for in litigation.

The blocking clinic also provides a service for other hospital departments where this is relevant (such as doing sympathetic blocks or intravenous guanethidine tests for causalgic-type pain for the neurologic department or for atherosclerosis of the lower limb for the vascular surgery department).

TENS and Medical Acupuncture Clinics

TENS and medical acupuncture are two forms of stimulation that are useful in pain relief. They have the added advantage that they are noninvasive. Some pain clinics concentrate on physical methods of pain relief using mobilization (not manipulation), heat, cold, and relaxation techniques. These often include TENS and medical acupuncture. There appears to be a close relationship between trigger points, muscle motor points, and classic acupuncture points that can be used by medical practitioners ethically and easily. These methods, can be separate from the blocking clinic or can extend it.

Relaxation Clinics

Clinics of this type take various forms (from general relaxation to headache or more specifically migraine clinics). Any pain clinic, however limited, must have arrangements for diagnosis before treatment is started. To place this idea in simple terms, is the headache one that can be treated by biofeedback methods[18] and the psychological approach,[19] or does the patient have headaches caused by hypertension or a brain tumor? Ideally, every patient with headache should be examined by a physician skilled in neurologic diagnosis, but in many clinics, the patient first undergoes a psychological assessment. This may save valuable and expensive medical time, but it is not necessarily best. Patients arriving at a pain relief clinic may require one or more diagnostic tests, blocks, or other investigations, followed by straightforward treatment. Only if this and perhaps a subsequent treatment fails should a psychological profile be obtained. In Europe, where there is a shortage of psychologists, the method outlined is the one generally used. In the United States, there are many psychologists available, and in addition, there is a much greater incidence of multiple medication, overdose of medication, and frank drug addiction. This means that many patients must be weaned from their analgesic or narcotic drugs before pain relief can be attempted, and psychological help is of enormous value.

The Pain Rehabilitation Program

This type of pain treatment can be a separate unit or part of a large pain clinic. The methods on which such a program is based already have been mentioned, but briefly, it enables patients with chronic pain that cannot be relieved by any known method to function fairly normally despite their pain. In some patients, where psychological factors are a major consideration, there may be a considerable reduction in pain. One of the features of these programs is that they reduce the pain behavior shown by the patient to near-normal levels.[19] The methods used in these pain management and rehabilitation programs are powerful and have a good record of returning patients to work, even after long layoffs. In the pain management program at the Centre for Pain Relief at Walton Hospital (Liverpool, UK), more than 40 percent of the patients return to work, some after 3 years out of work. These are extremely difficult long-standing chronic patients, and many rehabilitation programs with young or relatively young workers return 50 percent or more of their patients to work. As mentioned, insurance company backing is usually necessary in placing these patients because their previous employers will not take back someone whose back, for instance, is a chronic problem without suitable assurances from their insurers. These programs last 3 to 4 weeks and can be inpatient or outpatient. In either case, accommodation is required in or nearby the clinic. The method is staff and time intensive, but the results justify this effort when done properly. Because the presence of a pain management program may be necessary for full payment by insurers in the United States, we expect to see a proliferation of this type of clinic.

The considerable savings on sick pay, medication, periodic hospitalization, and continuing illness make this type of treatment an economic proposition to the insurers despite the treatment costs (approximately $10,000 to $15,000 or more per patient).

Back Pain Clinic

This type of unit often is organized in tandem with the orthopedic or physical medicine department.[20] However, as these patients only arrive at the pain clinic when standard treatment has failed, it is important for the pain clinic physician to take a proper history and do a complete physical examination. Each physician must determine what the cause of the problem is and decide whether pain clinic treatment is appropriate. The pain clinic must not become a rubber stamp for diagnoses made elsewhere. It is true that, in most cases where the patient has seen reputable and well-trained specialists, the opinion of the pain clinician and the previous specialists will coincide, but this is not invariable. This type of careful examination of both the history and physical examination does not apply only to the back pain unit but to all chronic pain clinics. The apparatus needed at this type of clinic requires physical medicine, whirlpool, relaxation teaching, biofeedback methods, and in the largest units, a swimming pool.[21] The personnel must be borrowed or hired from the other departments or hired by the pain unit and trained there.

SPACE

As in most organizations, the work area expands to take up the available space. In any case, if the clinic is expected to be successful, there should be an expanding input of patients and an increase of treatment and diagnostic procedures; therefore, an increase of personnel of all types is needed. There will be a demand for space, desks, treatment areas, couches, rest rooms, porters, wheel chairs, and so on.[22]

If a pain management course is planned, then there is a minimum space that must be provided, or the course cannot operate. The minimum can be worked out easily. For instance, after the number of patients to be treated together in the course has been decided (e.g., 12 people for 5 days per week for 4 weeks), they will each need a comfortable mattress on the floor with 2 ft of space all round. This is required for relaxation, resting, and exercising. The mattress is 6 ft by nearly 3 ft; therefore, each patient needs a space of approximately 7 ft by 4 ft. A room of approximately 14 ft by 24 ft is absolutely minimal. The therapist must stand in the center of the group, therefore, 18 ft by 24 ft is more reasonable but still tight. When storage space for

apparatus, personal belongings, paper, coffee machine, and the like are added, some sensible ideas about the space required can be calculated.

Each service must be assessed in this way when a large clinic is being started from scratch. The two areas most frequently underassessed are the patients' and relatives' waiting areas and the day treatment area. The experience in Europe suggests that clinics that become well known double in size every 3 to 4 years. This continues until the waiting list (for nonmalignant pain) exceeds 4 months. This suggests that, when setting up this type of large clinic, provision should be made for future expansion.

PERSONNEL

Just as there has to be an assessment of the need for space, so there must be an assessment of personnel requirements. This must involve all workers in the proposed pain relief department. In most hospitals and clinics, there will be no precedent. Therefore, the assessment starts from scratch. Each section of this specialized clinic must be covered for the number, grade, and type of those who will work there. This includes physicians and specialists of different types; nonmedical specialists; head nurses, nurses, and supervisors; secretarial and accounting staff; porters, runners, and cleaners. As far as possible, nothing and no person should be left out, although there should be built into this preliminary scheme a provision for some elasticity because not every eventuality can be foreseen. Just as with space, provision should be made for additional workers as expansion occurs.

The new department should be commissioned in exactly the same way as a new hospital. When a small section confined to one type of pain work is planned, it often is possible to work on an ad hoc basis and incorporate it into the existing setup. If this is done, it will work satisfactorily initially, but acute problems arise as the section grows.

FINANCE

In a similar fashion, plans must be made about the funding that will make all this possible. In those countries where a department is expected to generate all or much of its own finance from fees, a decision[23,24] must be made on the initial capital sum required, where it comes from, and how long it will be before the new unit can be expected to become self-supporting.

In university departments, after a case of need has been made, funds may be provided through the Dean's or Regent's committees. Sometimes there is a committee of departmental chiefs who initiate expenditure. Charitable trusts, charitably minded and philanthropic members of the public, and the League of Friends of the hospital or clinic may raise all or part of the funds.

In those countries where there is a national health service, there will be standing committees that can be approached for the necessary funds. Because all available money is earmarked ahead, there can be long delays with this method. Often, each hospital has some discretionary funds that it is allowed to use as it, or rather its administrative committee, thinks fit. This again tends to be allocated in advance, but determined efforts must be made to secure some or all of this funding. Starting up a new department in such circumstances means obtaining outside funds; getting these depends on the initiative and activity of the clinicians concerned.

The case of need must be prepared carefully. Lists of special medical equipment must be made and up-to-date costs obtained. Previous planning of other new departments will produce useful lists of standard equipment required. Salary scales of the different grades of personnel will be required, and in some cases, a fixed contract may be needed. Probably the simplest method is to plan the whole clinic and then open it in stages using a time table. The danger is that the time table may not be followed.

All these arrangements appear so obvious that they do not need to be printed, but past practice suggests that, if this type of process is not done carefully and completely, difficulties arise, multiply, and much time is required to solve them.[25]

TEACHING

A new unit will start with in-house teaching. The ancillary and medical staff with few exceptions will have little experience in working with patients with intractable pain. Thus there must be general lectures and briefing on the differences between conventional medical and nursing care and the approach required in the pain clinic. All staff (including clerks, accountants, and porters) should attend these briefing sessions. If there is no one in the unit with the necessary experience to do this, then a speaker from another well-established unit should be brought in. When a unit of any size is starting up, there should be at least one doctor and one nurse who have been a part of an established pain clinic and observed and learned the special techniques; they could do the initial briefing. This briefing should be as comprehensive as possible. Not only should it include the differences between general medical and pain clinic practice, but also, the various techniques of treatment (such as detoxification, drugs, and active therapies) should be discussed. It should include the future aim of the program, possible expansion, and the staging of activity as the new clinic gradually starts up and moves into comprehensive clinical work. Some indication of the in-house teaching plan and the system of billing might be discussed. How to handle patients in severe pain physically should be part of this briefing. All of this cannot be discussed in one lecture; therefore, the initial briefing could occupy an entire morning. One of the talks in this session could be geared toward the rest of the hospital or clinic to interest others in it, to state what type of patients are best treated in it, and the methods of treatment used.

There will be a continuing program of mutual learning and teaching in any pain clinic whether newly established or not. This should be aimed at the different levels of experience needed. Medical students require academic information and some demonstration of what can be done. Residents require detailed knowledge, and this can be given by didactic lectures, demonstration on the patient by more senior physicians, and at grand rounds (which should take place at least once a week). The system should be sufficiently flexible for any visiting doctor, senior nurse, psychologist, or others with special knowledge in pain relief to give a talk or demonstration on short notice. There must be special teaching for the special methods of pain relief, such as TENS, relaxation methods, and biofeedback. This is not only for those who use these methods, but for all those in the pain clinic who should have some knowledge of them. Teaching should not only be confined to the junior staff, but it is equally necessary for the senior staff. It is important that each type of specialist connected with the pain clinic should be familiar with what the others do. A talk or demonstration each week after the principal grand rounds is an excellent way of choosing a time when most people are present.

Different clinics require different arrangements, and these may not have been mentioned. It is important that thought should be given to what is needed and that this is then implemented.

PATIENT MANAGEMENT

By this we mean the various arrangements made to get the patient to the clinic; allocate them to the correct specialist; obtain relevant previous medical details; examine and investigate; treat, recall or follow-up by phone or letter when distances are great; arrange visits to other specialists in the clinic or hospital; and arrange for treatments (such as relaxation or counseling). Interim letters to the patient's practitioner must be sent. When all is completed and the patient finally is discharged, the referring clinician or the patient's local practitioner must be informed.

Most of these arrangements are straightforward and are used in any standard clinic. There will usually be a letter from the referring physician to the pain clinic. If this is to a particular pain clinic physician, there is no problem of allocation. Similarly, in small clinics, there is little problem. In large clinics, the initial decision must be made by some authoritative person, usually a physician, as to the initial referral. This decision making can be done on a rotating basis or one physician may do it all the time. It should be possible for either the decision maker or the first pain clinic physician selected to have the important work of following the patient through their subsequent investigation and treatment, even if the patient passes out of their hands temporarily.

The importance of this cannot be overemphasized. It is easy for the patient to be awaiting recall, for instance, and the documents may be mislaid (which can occur in the best units). The patient is left in limbo. There must be some system of automatic review of all patients until they are discharged. If this is done by a physician, it has the added benefit that this physician can be responsible for ensuring that regular letters about the patient are sent to the referring physician and/or the family physician. Also, the patient can be informed at the first appointment that this physician will be in charge. The patient then knows who will answer queries and write to the patient's physician and who they can contact if there appears to be too long a delay in treatment, for example. Most of the follow-up and checking will be done by the clerical staff, but there must be someone the patient can regard as their doctor while attending the clinic.

MEDICOLEGAL CONSIDERATIONS

Finally, a word about litigation.[26] There will always be poor results in a proportion of patients, and this is why it is important to explain thoroughly the risks involved in even the simplest procedures. It is equally important to ensure that the patient has a realistic expectation of what can be achieved. In some countries, the patient must be given written information on what is going to be done to them. These protocols must be comprehensive, and because of this, the patient may not understand them fully and later may sue over a described complication "because the protocol was too difficult to understand." Patients forget easily (particularly unwelcome facts), and therefore, explanation must never be overlooked. Relatives also should be involved. Writing in the case notes (separately from the protocol) that an explanation has been given to the patient and relatives and they appeared to understand it is never wasted time.

Above all, remember that most patients want to get better and rarely start off "gunning" for their physician. They must not be regarded as too foolish to be told the truth early when a procedure has not gone according to plan. Time spent in this way on patient relations rarely is wasted. Information from the medical defense organizations and malpractice insurance companies emphasizes that, in a large proportion of litigation cases, there is a time during the early stages when much litigation can be prevented by straightforward and frank explanations. In view of the huge awards possible in the United States and Europe for successful litigation, it is not surprising that physicians are conscious of it and that some patients take advantage of it.

References

1. Bonica JJ, ed. *The Management of Pain*. Philadelphia: Lea & Febiger; 1953.
2. Bonica JJ. Organization and function of a pain clinic. In: Bonica JJ, ed. *Advances in Neurology*. Vol 4. New York: Raven Press; 1974:433–443.
3. Bonica JJ, Butler SH. The management and functions of pain centers. In: Swerdlow M, ed. *Relief of Intractable Pain*. 2nd ed. Amsterdam: Excerpta Medica; 1978:44–50.
4. Lipton S, ed. *The Control of Chronic Pain*. London: Edward Arnold; 1979:40–43.
5. Swerdlow M. The pain clinic. *Br J Clin Pract* 1972; 25:403.
6. Swerdlow M. The value of clinics for the relief of chronic pain. *J Med Ethics* 1978; 4:117.
7. Mushin WW, Swerdlow M, Lipton S, Mehta MD. The pain centre. *Practitioner* 1977; 218:439.
8. Aronoff GM, Evans WO, Enders PL. A review of follow up studies of multidisciplinary pain units. *Pain* 1983; 16:1–11.
9. Casale FF, Thorogood A. Review of domiciliary consultations for pain relief. *Anaesthesia* 1985; 40:366–368.
10. Guck TP, Skultety FM, Meilman PW, Dowd ET. Multidisciplinary pain center follow-up study; evaluation with a no treatment control group. *Pain* 1985; 21(3):295–306.
11. Aronoff GM. *Clin J Pain* 1985; 1:1–3. Editorial.
12. Crue BJ. Multidisciplinary pain treatment programs: current status. *Clin J Pain* 1985; 1:31–38.
13. *Standards Manual for Facilities Serving People with Disabilities*. Tucson, AZ: Commission on Accreditation of Rehabilitation Facilities.
14. Fordyce W. Learning processes in pain. In: Sternbach R, ed. *The Psychology of Pain*. New York: Raven Press; 1978.
15. Sternbach RA. Behavior therapy. In: Wall PD, Melzack R, eds. *Textbook of Pain*. London: Churchill Livingstone; 1984:800–805.
16. Bisset WI. Pain relief clinics under anaesthetic management in Scotland. *Ann R Coll Surg Engl* November 1988; 70(6):392–394.
17. Hardy PA. The role of the pain clinic in the management of the terminally ill. *Br J Hosp Med* February 1990; 43(2):142–146.
18. Jessup B, Barton A. Biofeedback. In: Wall PD, Melzack R, eds. *Textbook of Pain*. London: Churchill Livingstone; 1984:776–786.
19. Roberts AH, Reinhardt L. The behavioral management of chronic pain: long term follow-up with comparison groups. *Pain* 1980; 8:151–162.
20. Benn RT, Wood PHN. Pain in the back. An attempt to estimate the size of the problem. *Rheumatol Rehabil* 1975; 14:121–130.
21. Simon WH, Gates SJ, Crawford AG, Robinson D. Back school relieves patient's pain. *Pa Med* January 1990; 93(1):40–44.
22. Hannenberg AA, McArthur JD. Establishing a pain clinic. *Int Anesth Clin* 1983; 21(4):1–10.
23. Souhrada L. Pain programs offer opportunities for hospitals. *Hospitals* December 5, 1989; 63(23):52.
24. Simmons JW, Avant WS Jr, Demski J, Parisher D. Determining successful pain clinic treatment through validation of cost effectiveness. *Spine* March 1988; 13(3):342–344.
25. Lipton S. Current views on the management of a pain relief centre. In: Swerdlow M, ed. *The Therapy of Pain*. London: MTP Press; 1981:61–85.
26. Brena SF, Chapman SL. Pain and litigation. In: Wall PD, Melzack R, eds. *Textbook of Pain*. London: Churchill Livingstone: 1984:832–839.

CHAPTER 38

Disability Assessment of Pain-Impaired Patients

Steven F. Brena and Shulim Spektor

The task of determining disability in patients with a wide range of medical diagnoses and physical conditions is difficult. Usually, the disability determination process is based on the assumption that there is a linear relationship between a medical diagnosis, a degree of impairment, and the resulting disability. Unfortunately, the impairment–disability link has not been shown adequately. This is particularly true in patients with chronic pain syndromes where the painful experience is allegedly the main reason for dysfunction. Theoretically, in the traditional medical model, the pain symptoms should correlate clearly with demonstrable pathologic conditions, leading to an impairment judgment. However, the relationship among pain, physical impairment, dysfunctional behaviors, and disability is complex. As Cailliet[1] has written, "[The] evaluation is not of disability; it is [an] evaluation of a patient who claims to be disabled."

This chapter will examine briefly the current definitions of impairment, disability, and residual functional capacity; it will scrutinize the process by which a worker can become disabled and propose a systematic approach to evaluate impairment and residual functional capacity as it has been developed at the Pain Control and Rehabilitation Institute of Georgia.

BASIC DEFINITIONS

As Turk[2] reported, different agencies and systems define impairment and disability somewhat awkwardly. There is a consensus that impairment can be determined objectively, using traditional medical and laboratory tests and physical examination. However, there is no conformity among impairment ratings. Patients with the same degree of physical pathologic findings have different illness behaviors that correlate poorly with the medical findings and create serious problems in assessing disability. The latter is ultimately a

form of behavior, and as such, it depends both on physical and psychological factors. For the sake of clarity, the definitions of impairment, disability, and residual functional capacity accepted will be the ones proposed by the American Medical Association (AMA).[3] Impairment is defined as "an alteration of health, from documented abnormal functioning of an organ of the body and/or of the brain." Disability is defined as "an alteration of the capacity to meet personal, social or occupational demands." Impairment, in most instances, is partial and leads to certain specific limitations of function. This partial impairment always is paired with some unimpaired functional abilities known as the residual functional capacity. This is defined as the patient's performance potential for vocational development and work activities. It is a measure of preserved ability to function.

PATIENTS WITH IMPAIRMENT AND CHRONIC PAIN

According to the AMA definition of impairment, chronic pain can be considered a sensory impairment usually affecting at least the musculoskeletal system and the central nervous system.[4] In most clinical chronic pain syndromes, two kinds of impairment can be identified: (1) a primary impairment caused by a documented pathologic condition affecting an organic system and (2) a secondary impairment resulting from the consequences of a painful experience, such as inactivity, disuse, drug misuse, and learned helplessness.[5]

THE SO-CALLED CHRONIC DISABILITY SYNDROME

Strang[6] proposed the term *chronic disability syndrome* and discussed some of the characteristics of patients who are capable of working but choose to remain disabled. They lack motivation to recover and return to productivity. The impairment is often the result of a fairly minor injury, but actually it represents an inability to cope with problems. Carron[7] showed that the three most striking features in

Portions of this chapter adapted from Brena S. Systemic assessment of impairment and rehabilitation. *J Back Musculoskel Rehab* 1992. Reprinted with permission.

chronic pain-disabled patients are: (1) 78.7 percent of their subjective complaints are not supported by physical findings, (2) 60 percent are receiving dependence-inducing drugs, and (3) 49.3 percent had a previous back injury. He also noticed a high incidence of previous compensable injuries, obesity, low income, and low self-esteem. Leavitt and colleagues[8] found that 70 percent of workers receiving compensation for back pain reported a specific activity or event that triggered the pain or the alleged injury, but only 35 percent of workers with back pain and not receiving compensation reported such a clear-cut work-related event. Workers' compensation statistics suggest that the disability rate from back pain alone is increasing at 14 times the population growth; 25 percent of low back pain cases account for nearly 90 percent of the total cost.[9]

The chronic disability epidemic seems to be a peculiar feature of American patients with back pain. Using the Sickness Impact Profile,[10] Brena and associates[11] studied responses to chronic low back pain in patients from different cultures. They documented that, given cross-matched physical findings, American patients with back pain report a higher rating of work impairment than those in any other culture.

THE DISABILITY PROCESS

Before discussing disability evaluation, it might be interesting to understand in more detail how the disability process evolved.[12]

1. *Premorbid Stage*. At this stage, multiple risk factors can be identified that increase the possibility of accidental injuries and impairments through certain behavioral patterns (such as repeated violations of safety rules, sloppiness in performing different chores, feelings of helplessness, pessimism, dependent life style, the inability to cope with stress or tension, history of frequent unemployment, job dissatisfaction, recent divorce, or death in the family).
2. *The Accident*. The accident itself is the official starting point of a disability process. With tissue damage, nociceptive stimulation is triggered along with the perception of pain. Even a trivial injury, through activation of the sympathetic nervous system and soft tissue damage may cause much acute postaccident pain.
3. *Medical Intervention*. Medical treatment always should start immediately after the injury to allow the damaged tissue to heal. It should be followed by an intense rehabilitation program in an attempt to restore the injured person to a normal state of health and functioning as soon as possible. At the end of the rehabilitation phase, functional capabilities must be assessed to guide the injured person quickly back to productivity. The information obtained from the physical examination and pertinent diagnostic procedures should allow us to determine the patient's capabilities to function at their work place. If the initial rehabilitation process is not successful in restoring the patient to normal function, then a more sophisticated comprehensive interdisciplinary evaluation of the prob-

lem should be done as soon as possible. This can be achieved best by a comprehensive pain rehabilitation program.
4. *Stabilization of Chronicity*. Failure to improve and return to a productive life despite treatment, along with prolonged inactivity and disuse, leads to progressive neurophysiologic and psychosocial malfunction. Excessive reliance on drugs, anxiety, depression, and socioeconomic factors move the patient further into a maladaptive life style.
5. *Legal Intervention*. Lack of widely accepted standards for systematized documentation to support proof of disability and the adversary system in the United States further foster attitudes of passivity, exaggerated illness behavior, and possibly exaggeration of complaints. Unknowingly, the physician may rubber-stamp the patient's dramatized claim to be disabled by chronic pain. After this unfortunate event occurs, it automatically opens a file, eventually leading to litigation or costly settlement.
6. *Learned Helplessness*. As the unresolved medicolegal problems continue, the sick role tends to solidify, with loss of hope for health recovery. Competent coping with daily problems breaks down and a general state of helplessness, which is often irreversible, may be induced.

SYSTEMIC DISABILITY EVALUATION

To be effective in helping to resolve a disability claim, the disability evaluation process should include the following steps (Fig. 38-1)

1. Evaluation of medical pathologic condition that could lead to functional limitations.
2. Determination of health impairment based on pathologic findings and done at the stage of maximum medical improvement.
3. Assessment of residual functional capacity (this should guide the proper vocational management).
4. Vocational evaluation and planning of successful outcome.

Evaluation of Medical Pathologic Condition

Physical examination and the appropriate diagnostic procedures are used routinely to clarify the medical diagnosis and document the existing pathologic findings. Deyo[13] reported that physical and laboratory findings are useful when they correlate with symptoms and functional ability. Similarly Wiesel and associates[14] reviewed CT scans from asymptomatic subjects and observed that, in those older than 40 years of age, 50 percent had abnormal findings. Using the Medical Examination and Diagnostic Information Coding System,[15] Brena and Sanders[16] documented that the most common positive findings in patients with chronic pain across medical diagnoses are abnormalities in soft tissues (94 percent of patients), spine range of motion (76 percent), in gait and posture (63 percent), and in muscular function (63 percent). Spektor[17] emphasized the usefulness of neurophysiologic testing to detect malfunctioning in patients with no evidence of anatomic or structural disease.

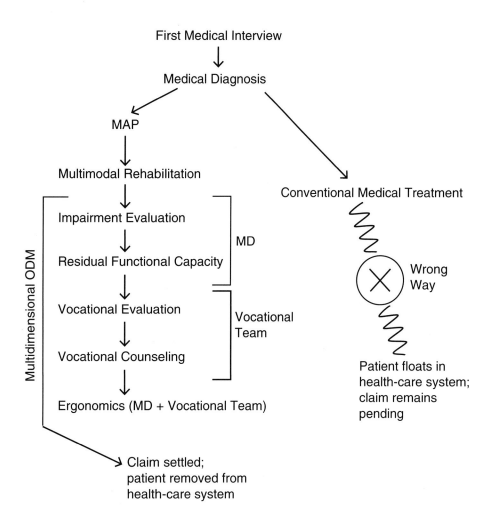

FIGURE 38-1. Occupational disability management for pain-disabled patients. MAP = multi-axial assessment of pain; ODM = occupational disability management.

These tests include: thermography (which assesses the function of the autonomic nervous system and detects the evidence of soft tissue abnormalities); somatosensory-evoked potentials (which determine the function of afferent sensory pathways), and EMG (which detects and documents the function of the motor system). The neurophysiologic evaluation of patients with chronic pain, according to this author, is crucial in achieving several objectives: (1) to document a possible malfunctioning at a nonstructural physiologic level, (2) to reassure the patient that the pain has a physiologic basis; and (3) to provide useful information in the overall disability evaluation process.

Determination of Health Impairment

Several methods have been proposed to quantify impairment.[18–21] From a practical and medicolegal standpoint, the AMA *Guide to the Evaluation of Permanent Impairment*[3] is the most useful instrument to assess impairment. It allows the clinician to translate information obtained by physical examination and various diagnostic procedures into a whole-body impairment percentage. Evaluation of impairment must be done after rehabilitation of the patient to the stage of maximum medical improvement, when no further gains in physical function are ex-

pected. Such impairment is considered permanent and is valid in a court of law for a claim settlement.

Sanders[22] studied the relationship between the Sickness Impact Profile and the impairment rating as determined using the AMA guidelines. The former[10] is a multidimensional instrument composed of 136 items assessing self-reported impairments in 12 areas: ambulation, mobility, body care and movement, social interaction, communication, alertness, emotional behavior, sleep and rest, eating, work, home management, recreation, and pastime activities. Each item includes a statement describing a specific dysfunctional behavior; patients are requested to indicate whether each item describes a dysfunction they experience at the time in which they take the test. This profile yields a total score and three subscores: physical, psychosocial, and "other" (vocational and avocational items). In his study, Sanders[22] documented a highly significant positive relationship between the total score and the physical subscore of the Sickness Impact Profile and the AMA-based impairment ratings for each patient.

Assessment of Residual Functional Capacity

A key point in a systematic method for evaluating disability is the assessment of a patient's capability to function despite impairment. Residual functional capacity is expressed through restrictions or limitations imposed by medical findings. These pertain to specific tasks (such as lifting, carrying, and standing), as they are described in the *Dictionary of Occupational Titles* by the Department of Labor. The assessment of residual functional capacity leads to a mediolegal judgment as to the outcome of the patient's problem which could mean:

1. Capability to return to a previous job.
2. Necessity of vocational retraining for an alternative gainful employment.
3. A decision of nonemployability and, therefore, possible qualification for Social Security disability benefits.

Table 38-1 depicts a comprehensive system to reach a fair assessment of impairment and residual functional capacity in patients with chronic pain consistently that was developed in the Pain Control and Rehabilitation Institute of Georgia. Four different parameters are considered in this assessment grid:

1. History of chronic pain development and its severity.
2. Physical examination.
3. Results of medical diagnostic procedures.
4. Data obtained through neurophysiologic evaluation.

According to the presence or absence of findings in these parameters, an impairment rating is determined on the basis of the AMA guidelines, ranging from 0 to 100. Residual functional capacity is assessed as the inverse of impairment and expressed in terms of general physical work capacity according to the Department of Labor standards. From left to right, Table 38-1 reflects an increase in pathologic findings and subjective and objective worsening of the patient's condition; this results in an increased percentage of impairment and decreased residual functional capacity. A special case is presented in Table 38-1 for patients with chronic pain and positive thermograms where all other parameters are negative. These patients have no permanent impairment according to AMA guidelines, but their functional capacity probably will be decreased from documented sympathetically maintained pain and/or soft tissue abnormalities. If medical restrictions are not imposed on these patients, they might be allowed to return to nonrestricted heavy-duty work. This would significantly increase the chances of repeated flare-ups and reinjury, leading to an inability to sustain gainful employment, lengthy litigation, and eventually a state of learned helplessness.

Table 38-1 has no direct representation of the patient's psychological condition. Currently, data from the Sander's[22] study are being integrated into the overall grid depicted in this table.

Vocational Intervention

In our society, work is an important contributor to positive self-esteem; the structure provided by the daily work routine is often a positive factor of mental health. Loss of this role and structure may push the patient toward the stage of helplessness. The functional limitations imposed by the medical findings usually provide a useful guide to correct development and planning for vocational outcome whenever a patient is unable to meet the physical demands of a previous job. Various vocational rehabilitation services may be used to help the worker find suitable alternative work,

Table 38-1
Medical Data Presence (+) or Absence (–) of Abnormality

History Trauma Disease	Chronic Pain	–	+	+	+	+	+	Intolerable Pain
Physical Examination	ROM	–	–	+	+	+	+	+ +
	Muscle Strength	–	–	–	+/–	+	+	+ +
	Sensory Exam	–	–	–	+/–	+	+	+ +
Anatomic Tests	MRI	–	–	+/–	+	+	+	+ +
	CT	–	–	+/–	+/–	+	+	+ +
	Myelogram	–	–	–	+/–	+/–	+	+ +
	X-ray	–	–	–	+/–	+/–	+	+ +
Neurophysiologic Tests	TG	–	+	+	+	+	+	+ +
	SEP	–	–	+/–	+/–	+/–	+	+ +
	EMG	–	–	+/–	+/–	+/–	+	+ +
Impairment		0%	0%	0 < 10%	<15%	<25%	>25%	100%
Residual Functional Capacity		100% vs. heavy heavy (>110 lb)	heavy medium (100–50)	medium (50)	medium light (50–20)	light sedentary (20–10)	sedentary (10)	Totally Disabled

ROM: range of motion, MRI: magnetic resonance imaging, CT: computed tomography, TG: thermography, SEP: somatosensory-evoked potentials, EMG: electromyography.

Reprinted with the permission of the American Academy of Disability Evaluating Physicians. *Journal of Disability* 1991; 1(2):98–102.

that is, work within the patient's residual functional capacity that fits the worker's pattern of interests and aptitudes, while offering wages comparable to previous earnings. Vocational counseling may be used to help the worker adjust to this condition, learn about alternatives, and prepare for a suitable occupation. A job analysis may be required to assess whether a specific job and work site is within the physical capacity of the worker. A labor market survey may be used to research the availability of potential occupational goals. Whenever the patient's interests and abilities are unclear, a vocational evaluation may be required. Vocational evaluation, therefore, is the analysis of the factors that make a person employable.

Although the specifics depend on the patient and the questions to be addressed, some characteristics are typical of most evaluations. Among these are assessment of (1) academic ability (reading, spelling, mathematics, and vocabulary), (2) vocational interests, and (3) aptitudes. A transferability of skills analysis also may be done when retraining for different employment. Likewise, a job-site analysis may allow the patient to return to a previous job if certain physical changes in the work site can be accomplished.

MALINGERING

One major task facing disability evaluators is to separate those who have a legitimate claim from those who may be providing inaccurate self-reported data consciously. The prevalence of conscious distortion of self-reported data and the characteristics of those who provide such distortions have received scant clinical and empiric attention. Most related research has addressed malingering; this appears to be a specific type of such a distortion. Malingering has been defined generally as "deliberately faking symptoms for the sole purpose of obtaining an extrinsic goal."[23] Estimates of the scope of malingering vary widely. The Commission on the Evaluation of Pain by the Social Security Administration[24] reached a consensus that malingering is not a significant problem among disability claimants with complaints about pain. However, Leavitt and Sweet,[23] after obtaining questionnaire data from 99 orthopedists, reported that 38 percent of them estimated the incidence of malingering to be approximately 2 percent in their practice, 75 percent believed that the magnitude was 10 percent, and 10 percent thought that the magnitude was more than 30 percent. A major reason for these different interpretations could be that orthopedists may have had difficulties in interpreting psychogenic conditions that may precipitate pain complaints. Currently, there is no good marker that correlates closely with subjective pain reports. Leavitt and Sweet[23] asked the orthopedists who responded to the questionnaire to identify the most important clinical markers for malingering. There was a consensus that the symptoms defined as most important can be categorized along two basic dimensions: exaggeration and inconsistency, including such items as "weakness to manual testing not seen in any other activities" and "overreacting during the examination." Many symptoms they described were similar to those reported by Waddell and colleagues.[25] These authors described so-called nonorganic signs; these represent discrepancies between medical findings observed during a routine physical examination and documented medical pathologic conditions. Physiologically based indicators, including differential nerve blocks, are only marginally adequate to identify the simulators.[26,27]

Various inconsistencies have been proposed to assess possible malingering among pain-disabled patients.[23,28] These have included evidence of submaximum efforts on testing, pain behaviors that vary depending on the setting in which they are observed, evidence of a lack of participation or interest in treatment, inconsistencies between verbal reports and actual behaviors, and lack of reliability of such reports. The diagnosis of malingering should not be reached lightly nor be based on a few inconsistencies or attributes. Such a diagnosis can be made only when it is supported by a significant body of confirmatory evidence and has gained the consensus of an interdisciplinary team of pain experts.

CONCLUSION

A recent article in the magazine *Fortune* (March 23, 1992) provides some shocking figures showing that the United States health care system, "like a swelling malignancy," consumes 13.4 percent of the gross national product, up from 7.3 percent in 1970. The same article provides evidence that, unless current trends are changed, by the year 2000, health care will consume 16.4 percent of the gross national product. All indicators seem to agree that chronic pain is a major contributor to the growing cost of health care and that long-standing unresolved problems of pain and litigation are probably one of the most costly factors. The imperative need for cost effectiveness in health care, and specifically in pain management, demands accurate and accountable outcome studies. A systematic disability evaluation process, as outlined in this chapter, is crucial for cost-effective settlements of sometimes prolonged litigations. Timely resolution of a legal case increases the chance for a reduction in the consumption of health care and a return to gainful employment. However, it must be recognized that the process of evaluating cases of compensatable disability is complex and has no easy solution. As Chapman and Brena[12] remarked, it often requires a careful deductive approach. All pertinent data must be assembled, analyzed, and put into perspective. Table 38-1 shows one way to accomplish this goal. We believe that the resolution of disability claims is a major responsibility in managing pain-impaired patients. Failure to provide this kind of structured information is a disservice to the patient and to all parties that are involved in disputed disability claims. Unfortunately, many physicians, often frustrated by the difficulty of providing accurate determinations of disability, prefer to avoid the disability issue and leave it to the lawyers. Moreover, through the easy accessibility of technologic gadgets, devices, and drugs, they often keep pain-impaired patients in a position of forced dependence on the health-care system. In doing so, they do not realize the human, social, and economic waste caused by fostering disability instead of ability, idleness instead of productivity, and dependency instead of self-reliance, all of which are negative characteristics of learned helplessness, the last and often irreversible stage of the disability process.

References

1. Cailliet R. Disability evaluation. *South Med J* 1969; 62:1380–1382.
2. Turk DC. Evaluation of pain and dysfunction. *J Disab* 1991; 2(1):24–43.
3. *Guide to the Evaluation of Permanent Impairment.* 3rd ed. Chicago: American Medical Association; 1988.
4. Brena SF, Turk DC. Vocational disability: a challenge to pain rehabilitation programs. In: Aronoff GM, ed. *Pain Centers: A Revolution in Health Care.* New York: Raven Press; 1988:167–180.
5. Seligman MEP. *Helplessness.* San Francisco: Freeman; 1975.
6. Strang JP. The chronic disability syndrome. In: Aronoff GM, ed. *Evaluation and Treatment of Chronic Pain.* Baltimore: Urban Schwarzenberg; 1985:603–623.
7. Carron H. Compensation aspects of low back claims. In: Carron H, McLaughlin RE, eds. *Management of Low Back Pain.* Bristol, UK: Wright; 1982:17–26.
8. Leavitt SS, Beyer RD, Johnston TL. Monitoring the recovery process: pilot results of a systematic approach to case management. *Indiana Med Surg* 1972; 41:25–30.
9. Aronoff GM. Chronic pain and the disability epidemic. *Clin J Pain* 1991; 7:330–338.
10. Bergner M, Bobbitt RA, Carter WB, et al. The sickness impact profile: development and final revision of health status measure. *Med Care* 1981; 19:787–805.
11. Brena SF, Sanders SH. The need for more studies to assess the similarities and differences among chronic pain patients from different cultures. *Am Pain Soc Bull* 1991; 1(4):9–10.
12. Chapman SL, Brena SF. Pain and litigation. In: Wall P, Melzak R, eds. *Textbook of Pain,* 2nd ed. London: Churchill-Livingston; 1989:1032–1041.
13. Deyo RA. Measuring the functional status of patients with low back pain. *Arch Phys Med Rehabil* 1988; 64:1044–1053.
14. Wiesel SW, Tsourmas M, Feffer HL, et al. A study of computer assisted thermography. The incident of positive CAT scans in a symptomatic group of patients. *Spine* 1984; 9:549–551.
15. Rudy TE, Turk DC, Brena SF, et al. Quantification of biomedical findings of chronic pain patients: development of an index of pathology. *Pain* 1990; 42:167–182.
16. Brena SF, Sanders SH. Opioids in non-malignant pain: questions in search of answers. *Clin J Pain* 1991; 7:342–345.
17. Spektor S. Chronic pain and pain-related disabilities. *J Disab* 1990; 1(2):98–102.
18. Clayer JR, Bookless-Pratz CL, Ross MW. The evaluation of illness behavior and exaggeration of disability. *Br J Psychol* 1986; 148:296–299.
19. Feinstein AR, Josephy BR, Wells S. Scientific and clinical problems in indexes of functional disability. *Ann Intern Med* 1986; 105:413–420.
20. Mayer TG, Smith SS, Keeley J, et al. Quantification of lumbar function. Part II: Sagittal plain trunk strength in chronic low back pain patients. *Spine* 1985; 10(8):765–772.
21. Keith RA. Functional assessment measures in medical rehabilitation. Current status. *Arch Phys Med Rehabil* 1984; 65:74–78.
22. Sanders SH. Relationship between the sickness impact profile and impairment ratings. Presentation to the Annual Meeting of the American Pain Society, New Orleans, 1991.
23. Leavitt F, Sweet JJ. Characteristics and frequency of malingering among patients with low back pain. *Pain* 1986; 25:357–364.
24. Department of Health and Human Services. *Report of the Commission on the Evaluation of Pain and Disability.* Washington, DC: US Government Printing Office; 1987.
25. Waddell G, McCulloch JA, Kummel E, et al. Non-organic physical science in low back pain. *Spine* 1980; 5:117–125.
26. Rogers R. Current status of clinical methods. In: Rogers R, ed. *Clinical Assessment of Malingering and Deception.* New York: Guilford Press; 1988:293–308.
27. Boris RA, Cousins MJ. Diagnostic neural blockade. In: Cousins MJ, Bridenbaugh PO, eds. *Neural Blockade in Clinical Anesthesia and Management of Pain,* 2nd ed. Philadelphia: Lippincott; 1988:885–898.
28. Chapman SL, Brena SF. Patterns of conscious failure to provide accurate self-reported data in patients with low back pain. *Clin J Pain* 1990; 6:178–190.

CHAPTER 39

Medical–Legal Considerations in Pain Management

John H. Eichhorn and Elizabeth A. Bowyer Malacoff

Many factors have an impact on the medical–legal aspect of a physician's involvement in pain management. Many patients who present to pain management centers are involved in litigation or compensation cases. Patients with pain often are (correctly or incorrectly) labeled "difficult" because of their responses to the stress of their pain. Furthermore, there is a widespread perception that anesthesiologists working in pain management centers are at great risk of being sued for malpractice. There is little published data on this point, but available information does not support this suggestion. For example, during the period 1971 to 1982 in Washington State, of 192 malpractice claims against anesthesiologists, 56 involved regional anesthesia, but only one (for a pneumothorax during stellate ganglion block) involved pain management.[1] Of more than 500 malpractice claims to the St. Paul Fire and Marine Insurance Co. involving anesthesiologists during a recent 5-year period, there was only one case clearly related to pain management. Data from the claims files of the Risk Management Foundation of the Harvard Medical Institutions, which manages claims for the Harvard affiliated institutional shareholders of the Controlled Risk Insurance Company, Ltd., shows only one anesthesia pain management claim, a minor one, during a recent 10-year period. In this claim, a young man received a corticosteroid injection for meralgia paresthetica. Shortly after leaving the hospital, approximately 50 min after receiving the injection, he became dizzy. He turned to return to the pain clinic and fell, allegedly sustaining a back injury that caused permanent residual pain. The claimant alleged a failure to obtain informed consent and that the physician did not advise him to remain for observation for adverse reactions. The claim was resolved without a lawsuit.

Major complications during pain treatment do occur, however. Nerve block injections for relief of pain can cause various unanticipated unexpected outcomes, and these have been discussed thoroughly.[2–5] A comprehensive British review[6] stressed that malpractice claims can arise from long-term complications of neurolytic ablative nerve blocks administered for the relief of chronic pain.

Exposure to the risk of a malpractice claim will vary with the type and degree of a physician's involvement with pain management. The greatest risk for major claims appears to be associated with the administration of ablative nerve blocks. One moderate-sized pain management center in a university teaching hospital doing approximately 1000 procedures (nearly all injections) annually had the following distribution of case mix for 1985 to 1990: lumbar epidural steroids, 66 percent; trigger points, 19 percent; intercostal, 2 percent; epidural narcotic catheters, 1 percent; TENS, 2 percent; stellate ganglion, 6 percent; facet, 3 percent; and blood patch, 1 percent. Only a few blocks done during this period were neurolytic. Therefore, this pain center and others with similar types of cases may be at relatively low risk for major claims from complications of procedures. However, this is only one factor, and one which in no other way should diminish attention to the fundamental principles of pain management practice or its medical–legal aspects detailed in this chapter.

STANDARDS OF CARE

Pain management practitioners must remember that they are practicing medicine. Anesthesiologists engaged in pain management are not technicians who do procedures for referring physicians. It is inappropriate for an orthopedic surgeon, neurosurgeon, or neurologist to "order" an epidural corticosteroid injection or stellate ganglion block. It is equally inappropriate (and legally inadvisable) for the anesthesiologist to follow blindly such an "order".

Many pain management units will accept patients only on referral from other physicians. This procedure functions as a screening to avoid overwhelming the units with direct calls from potential patients. Also, there has been at least one evaluation that suggests the patient may benefit from pain management consultation. The pain management physician thus will receive a referral letter giving the patient's history, findings, past diagnostic tests, and past therapy as background information.

However, it is critical to emphasize that, after the patient

Portions of this chapter reprinted with permission from Danner D. *Medical Malpractice: A Primer for Physicians.* Rochester, NY: The Lawyers Co-operative; 1986:4–7.

is accepted, the pain management physician becomes a fully responsible provider, with all the attendant requirements. As an independent practitioner, the pain management physician takes note of the information accompanying the patient but, functionally, must start from the beginning as any physician does with a new patient. A thorough comprehensive medical history and a complete physical examination are absolutely necessary. When indicated, appropriate diagnostic tests must be done. It is insufficient to focus only on the pain problem. Doing so might cause failure to diagnose some previously undiscovered causal or associated condition that is a threat to the patient. Overlooking this underlying problem (such as a pathologic fracture from a metastatic lesion) represents poor quality medical care and exposes the pain management physician to a potential malpractice claim when the overlooked condition is discovered later; this is likely to occur at a more advanced stage.

Other sections of this book discuss diagnosis and treatment of pain states. Briefly, a patient referred by an orthopedic surgeon for possible epidural corticosteroid injection for suspected or proven disk disease should have compatible symptoms and history obtained by the pain management physician. Furthermore, this patient should have the requisite gait and postural abnormalities, muscle spasm, and/or positive straight leg raising findings verified by the pain management physician, who then may decide that it is appropriate to consider an epidural steroid injection as treatment. It is inadequate to rely on an examination done by someone else. Patients referred by surgeons for neurolytic blocks need the most thorough workups to ensure that the pain is genuinely intractable and would be alleviated by the proposed permanent ablation. Establishing this may take a series of visits and various diagnostic and therapeutic maneuvers.

To repeat, no matter how reliable the referring physician, pain management physicians become independent providers and completely responsible for their own actions. In the event of a complication or unfortunate result, it is no protection to state that one was acting on the suggestion or even "orders" of another physician. The pain management physician must thoroughly evaluate the patient and only then can the most appropriate treatment be recommended.

THE PHYSICIAN–PATIENT RELATIONSHIP

A physician must have a *duty* to the patient that is created by the existence of a physician–patient relationship before a physician can be found liable for medical malpractice. The physician–patient relationship is a consensual agreement, rarely taking the form of an express or written contractual agreement. However, the relationship is implied readily when the physician begins treating a patient, and the patient accepts the physician's services and advice.

After a physician has undertaken the care and treatment of a patient, this does not imply an unlimited right to terminate the relationship at will. The relationship may be terminated in one of the following ways: (1) the patient no longer requires the physician's services, (2) the patient terminates the relationship, or (3) the physician terminates the relationship by giving the patient a reasonable period of notice of termination so that the patient may arrange for alternative services. However, the physician must remain available for consultation until an alternate provider is obtained.

Failure to provide reasonable and timely notice may expose the physician to an action for abandonment. This occurs when the physician does not meet the obligation to provide medical services. Physicians withdrawing from a physician–patient relationship without proper notice while a need for medical services exists also may be found liable for breach of contract and, if a patient suffers harm from the abandonment, malpractice as well.

When the physician wishes to withdraw from the care of a patient, the patient should be notified in writing, preferably by registered mail, of the intent to terminate the relationship. The physician should indicate willingness to provide medical records to subsequent treating physicians and to see the patient for urgent problems that may arise before services of another physician are secured. The reasonableness of the period of time between notice and termination depends on factors including the patient's condition, availability of alternative providers, and the patient's resources.

Although a physician has obligations after a relationship with a patient is established, the physician is not obliged to see every patient seeking an appointment. Some patients proposed for treatment in a pain management unit will be involved in workmen's compensation cases or malpractice suits against other physicians. Some pain management physicians, citing a belief that these patients "do not do well" or stating a preference simply not to be involved, choose not to see such patients. This is permissible as long as there has not been the prior clear establishment of a physician–patient relationship. In the latter case, patients may charge abandonment by the physician who refuses to see them. It is acceptable but it may not be the best public relations to ask the patient at the first visit whether any proceeding to win compensation is at issue. The prescreening process is the more appropriate time to exercise this judgment if desired. An appointment request from a patient's attorney or a compensation board is clear. Frequently, the referral letter from another physician will contain information relative to this point. If there is a question or concern, an inquiry can be made to the referring physician. The use of a medical history questionnaire to be completed by the potential patient before the first appointment is common. Included, if desired, can be the question, "Are you involved in a compensation case or medical malpractice suit related to your pain condition?" When this questionnaire should be completed raises the question of exactly when a physician–patient relationship is established. Traditionally, this is when each of the two "assumes the expected role." It is not clear from case law whether making an appointment (such as with a pain management unit) constitutes a relationship or whether the patient actually must be seen by the physician. For those sufficiently concerned on this point, having the patient complete and return a questionnaire before being given an appointment would seem the most logical course.

There are two types of physician witnesses in medical malpractice cases: fact witnesses and expert witnesses. Any physician involved in a patient's care can be subpoenaed or deposed and thus forced to testify by either the plaintiff or defense. Such testimony would be related only to the facts (history, diagnosis, and treatment) of the witness's involvement with the patient. A fact witness generally is not asked to provide an expert opinion; however, any qualified witness can be asked to render an opinion on a set of facts (such as the cause of the patient's pain). Voluntarily becoming an expert witness involves an agreement with one side or the other in a case to review the facts, usually examine (but not treat) the patient, and render an opinion (usually for a fee) supporting the contention of the client on that side of the case. The medical record of any treating physician is "discoverable" (eligible to be subpoenaed by one or both sides in a legal case involving the patient). Therefore, it is mandatory to keep speculation, especially potentially inflammatory speculation, out of the written record. It is extremely unwise to write, for example, "Patient X comes in with back pain after botched laminectomy by Dr. Y." Such a statement could deepen the involvement of a pain management physician in an unwanted manner. For example,[7] a family physician saw a patient who recently had undergone a prostatectomy and suffered an ulnar nerve palsy. Subsequently, the patient was seen by an orthopedist at the request of the primary care physician who noted in his office record that the ". . . patient is informed that this is an unfortunate complication of his surgery from lying on the table with his arm in the wrong position and should not have happened." When the patient sued the surgeon and anesthesiologist, the patient called the family practitioner as a witness to testify to the cause of the injury. The family practitioner had made his medical record entry after receiving the consultation report. He testified that the entry was not his opinion of how the injury occurred but rather was based totally on the opthopedic surgeon's consultation. An unfortunately ambiguous private office record entry resulted in a time-consuming ordeal for this family practitioner. Assuming no such inappropriate written speculation, when pain management physicians are subpoenaed as routine fact witnesses, they do not need their own attorneys. An attorney would be required if the physician wanted to resist such a subpoena, but the likelihood of successful resistance is small.

RECORD KEEPING (See Appendix B)

After the patient is accepted and a relationship established, it is critical, particularly in pain management, that a complete medical record be kept. Clinics or units that are part of a larger facility (such as a hospital or medical center) usually keep separate charts in the individual unit rather than trust intermittent entries in the large master medical record of the institution. Units using computerized record-keeping systems should back up new entries daily. Many malpractice attorneys claim that the medical record is the single most important factor in determining the outcome of a medical malpractice case. A thorough, objective, concise, unaltered record frequently can deter a plaintiff attorney from filing a suit.

All patient interactions (including telephone calls) should be recorded on the physician's clinic or office record. A particular problem arises when there are questions about undocumented telephone conversations in which treatment recommendations are made to the patient.

All procedures should be documented with a procedure note or, better, on a preprinted graphic record designed for pain treatment. This record should include patient background data and, for blocks, patient position, technique used, preparation, needle and syringe used, paresthesias, solution injected over what period, responses, vital signs throughout, and patient condition and disposition at the end of the procedure. The recovery period needs a similarly complete record. All follow-up telephone calls and visits to the patient should be recorded. Even the smallest details of care can take on great importance in a malpractice suit. In one case,[8] a patient with chronic left shoulder and back pain received an injection of 10 ml of a solution of hydrocortisone, lidocaine, and tetracaine. She immediately complained of chest pain and was advised to lie down because she was "probably just upset about the injection." She did not feel better but was sent home with a prescription for diazepam to calm her. The patient later was admitted to the hospital with a diagnosis of iatrogenic pneumothorax. Her suit alleged that the injection caused the pneumothorax. The defendant's physician said he gave the injection with a ⅝-in 25-gauge needle, which all experts agreed probably would not have caused a pneumothorax. However, the plaintiff expert testified that, because the solution would not flow through a 25-gauge needle, a 19-, 20-, or 21-gauge needle was needed that would be able to penetrate to the pleura. The defendant physician did not remember the details of the injection given and had not recorded the size of the needle used. He could testify only to what he thought he would have done. Both plaintiff and defense expert testimony tended to discount the possibility of spontaneous pneumothorax. Therefore, because the defendant could not remember with certainty the size of the needle and had not documented the procedure thoroughly, the question of causation became simply a competition among various expert witnesses.

An inadequate medical record can render a malpractice case difficult to defend. The medical record and memory of the witnesses are all that can be used to counter the plaintiff's recollection of care rendered. A good medical record can refresh the physician's memory of a particular case and provide precise details of the history, findings, treatment plans, consent process, procedures done, outcome, and follow-up. Even if the medical record is inadequate, incomplete, or misleading, it is absolutely vital that physicians (or anyone) never alter a record after it has been created. If there is need to amend or explain something in the record, this must be done in a later separate entry that is dated and timed appropriately. Any suggestion that the record has been falsified or tampered with makes a case essentially indefensible, even if the facts are legitimately in question and there was no malpractice. Any problem or uncertainty about the record can cloud the issue. In one case,[9] the defendant physician did a disk injection. The plaintiff subsequently complained of numbness; this progressed to paraplegia. One available hospital record stated that an injection of betamethasone and bupivacaine was done under x-ray control. However, the circulating nurse's operative record, on which the drugs were recorded, was missing from the chart. The physician later testified during two depositions that he believed he used betamethasone and bupivacaine. Four years later, the plaintiff's counsel discovered that, instead of these drugs, the defendant mistakenly had injected colchicine, a potentially neurotoxic medication that may have caused the paraplegia. After this discovery of discrepancies in the records and independent of the medical issues, the claim was settled for $1 million.

Finally, hospital records and private office records frequently are requested by patients and plaintiff attorneys. Generally, hospital records are accessible to patients and their authorized representatives when written authorization from the patient is obtained. The laws regarding patient requests for physician office records vary from state to state. In all cases, patient medical information should not be released without the express written authorization of the patient. When medical records are requested properly by the patient, the patient's attorney, or by subpoena, copies of the records should be given to the requesting party. The original files should be retained by the responsible physician or institution.

A subpoena is a legal document which, in effect, is an order to disclose information (in this context, the medical record). Patient authorization may not be necessary.[10] A valid subpoena requires a response, either production of the requested records or a suitable motion to limit the scope of the subpoena. A motion to quash or a protective order is appropriate when the records requested concern a patient who is not a party to the legal proceeding (such as when a plaintiff's attorney is looking for other cases similar to his client's), when the records relate to treatment of alcohol or drug abuse, or when the records would disclose embarrassing information about the patient (e.g., a history of sexually transmitted disease or psychiatric treatment). When a subpoena is received, it should be forwarded immediately to the health-care facility's risk manager or counsel to determine whether it is valid and to initiate appropriate responses. Failure to respond can subject the physician to fines or imprisonment.

INFORMED CONSENT

One of the most important aspects of pain management, especially when nerve block injections are involved, is obtaining genuine informed consent for the proposed treatment. The doctrine of informed consent is based on the recognition of the individual's right to self-determination. This right was stated many years ago by Justice Cardozo who wrote "(e)very human being of adult years and sound mind has a right to determine what shall be done with his own body."[11] For a patient, a nonmedically trained individual, to make an informed decision about whether or not to undergo a proposed course of therapy, the physician must explain and disclose to inform the patient fully in language that can be understood. After the patient is informed fully, consent can be given that will help protect the physician from liability exposure for failing to advise the patient fully of potential risks and benefits of treatment.

Complete informed consent generally requires disclosure of the following elements:

1. Explanation of the diagnosis or condition that requires treatment.
2. Nature and purpose of the treatment.
3. Probable outcome without treatment.
4. Known risks and benefits of proposed treatment.
5. Explanation of reasonable alternative treatments, including the risks and benefits.
6. The probability of success of the treatment.

What disclosure of possible risks is required in obtaining true informed consent is changing. In earlier times, there was a so-called professional standard[12] that required disclosure of risks in a manner customarily used by physicians in the local community. However, this standard now has been replaced largely by the concept of *materiality*.[13] A material risk "is one which the physician knows or ought to know [what] would be significant to a reasonable person in the patient's position of deciding whether or not to submit to a particular medical treatment or procedure."[14] The important *Harnish v. Children's Hospital Medical Center* decision[15] followed other cases[13] and stressed that all material risks must be disclosed or the consent is not informed fully. This created many questions, and an equally important later decision[16] qualified the original materiality requirement by stating that it is not necessary to disclose every incredibly rare complication for which the chances are "negligible." There was emphasis on the idea of balancing full disclosure with fairness for those doing the disclosing, thus avoiding "unrealistic and unnecessary burdens on practitioners."

There is no case law defining how rare a complication has to be for it to be negligible. In one suit alleging failure to obtain informed consent,[17] a patient claimed the permanent partial denervation of the deltoid muscle of his dominant arm was a complication of the brachial plexus injection he received and that this possibility had never been mentioned before the injection. The court ruled against the plaintiff, stating that such a complication was so rare as to not be a material risk that must be disclosed before the procedure. Until there are more precedents of this type, published guidelines, state statutes, or consensus documents created by groups of physicians in a given locality, individual pain management physicians must evaluate which risks are negligible and which are material and then decide on a case-by-case basis exactly what to disclose in obtaining informed consent. Whether all patients receiving blocks should be told there are remote risks of permanent neurologic damage, other injury, or even death still remains an individual decision.

Neurolytic blocks demand the most scrupulous attention to consent. Independent of associated factors (such as advanced metastatic cancer with a bleak short-term prognosis), the gravity and permanence of this type of intervention must be made clear to the patient. Careful explanation of the maximum deficit possible is required. It should be stated clearly that, after the needle is positioned, a local anesthetic will be injected first to demonstrate the desired effect on the chronic pain. Only then will the neurolytic agent be introduced, but it must be made clear explicitly and before the procedure that, despite the most careful planning and technique, the permanent effect may not necessarily be the same as the initial effect of the local anesthetic. It may be more or less and may not fulfill the expectations of either the patient or the pain management physician.

In all cases, careful thought must go into the risk disclosure process.[18] It is difficult to decide what information will be most material to an individual patient. It is especially hard when a jury, looking in retrospect at an injured plaintiff, sees a particular undisclosed risk as material to a supposed informed-consent decision that may have occurred years before.

The informed-consent process must be documented carefully, and it is important to distinguish between obtaining the consent and documenting it. Although asking a patient to sign a preprinted form with a long list of potential complications can be one way to document obtaining the consent, the signing per se is not informed consent. Informed consent is an ongoing process that depends on *discussion* and *understanding* between patient and physician.[19] After this is achieved and the patient gives consent for treatment, then the consent must be documented. Having the patient sign a form or even countersign the physician's note in the medical record is useful to show the contents of the discussion that occurred and that the patient consented. It is valuable to explain to the patient that signing does not constitute a release from liability (which it does not under any circumstance) and does not limit the patient's rights, but it does serve as a memorial of the conversation that took place. It is desirable that the patient receive a copy of the form to reinforce the information disclosed.

A printed form for neurolytic blocks in general should contain basic information on potential complications of any anesthetic or related procedure. Then, in addition, the form could list the following risks: increased pain; hyperesthesia; paresthesias; temporary or permanent paralysis of the affected area or a greater area; temporary or permanent loss of sensation in the affected or greater area; temporary or permanent impairment of autonomic function; bladder, bowel, or sexual dysfunction; loss of skin at the injection site; organ or tissue injury from the needle; and for certain central blocks, blindness, seizures, or coma. Such a comprehensive list is not meant to scare the patient. Patients can be told that it is expected that none of these untoward things will happen and that the printed form is intended to encourage discussion and the disclosure of information.

USE OF APPROVED DRUGS FOR OTHER THAN PUBLISHED INDICATIONS

The Federal law known as the amended Food, Drug, and Cosmetic Act mandates that the Food and Drug Administration (FDA) determine the safety, efficacy, and truthfulness of labeling of drugs available for prescription by American physicians. Drug manufacturers submit data from clinical trials to support their claims for new drugs or existing drugs for new applications (e.g., that an antibiotic cures the target bacterial infection). When requirements are met, the FDA approves new drugs for the indications the manufacturer specified and for which data were provided. New drug X may be approved for indications A and B. This makes drug X available for prescription. The relevance of indications A and B is that these are the only indications the manufacturer can publish in the labeling (on the package, in the package insert, and in the *Physicians' Desk Reference*), and use in marketing and advertising.

It is important to understand that, although the manufacturer is limited to promoting the drug X for the published indications A and B only, physicians are not necessarily limited to using X for A and B only.[20,21] A physician may prescribe any drug that is "consistent with good medical practice." The FDA does not attempt to regulate the practice of medicine, except in instances where prescription of a drug is found to be unsafe. Only in this circumstance would the FDA mandate a label warning that a specific drug was contraindicated for a given condition. Then persistent use of the drug in this circumstance would not be seen as consistent with good practice and could lead to legal liability for the consequences.

After drugs are approved and in use, often new uses for them are discovered by prescribing physicians. When β-adrenergic blockers were introduced, their published indications included only certain cardiac arrhythmias. Many other uses for this class of drugs since have been found. Physicians were using these drugs regularly to treat other conditions for some time before the drug manufacturers assembled the data on safety and efficacy for these conditions and submitted data to the FDA seeking approval for the new indications. Once given, these approvals extended the published indications to include angina, myocardial infarction, hypertension, and migraine.

Most physicians are aware of the current use of approved drugs for other-than-published indications. This is certainly true in pain therapy. Back pain and/or sciatica with or without associated proven or suspected disk disease is not a published indication for injectable corticosteroid preparations, and there is no mention among the published indications of administration of these drugs into the epidural space. However, epidural steroid injections accounted for more than one-half of the procedures in the pain management unit example cited at the beginning of this chapter. The physicians in this unit, like those in many others, decided that the use of these drugs in this manner is safe and effective and thus consistent with good medical practice. Furthermore, current textbooks[22] (including this one) provide extensive discussions of this technique. It is possible that, at some future time, the manufacturers will submit data leading to FDA approval of epidural steroid injection for back pain or sciatica as a published indication. However, to reiterate, the absence of this approval per se should not create liability exposure for physicians doing such injections (that is, for appropriate patients, using proper technique, and consistent with published reports). (Note that steroid medications have a long list of potential side effects; however unreasonable, appearance of any of these could be associated with the steroids used. Even greater attention to informed consent may be necessary.) There are less common examples of the same principle of other-than-published indications. Fentanyl is injected into the epidural space, and tricyclic antidepressants are prescribed for chronic pain. It is important to note that, however, none of this discussion applies to acknowledged experimental drugs that are not approved for any use. These are significantly different and are discussed in the next section.

USE OF EXPERIMENTAL DRUGS: CLINICAL STUDIES

Drugs that are not approved by the FDA for marketing in the United States or chemicals that are not marketed as drugs can be used in therapy by physicians in certain special circumstances. This is covered in the Federal Food, Drug, and Cosmetic Act 21 USCA Section 35S; 21 CFR Section 130.3. One example is their use by an investigator who is part of an experimental clinical trial organized and sponsored by a drug company seeking data for an application for FDA approval. These always are directed by the company's clinical pharmacologists. There could be involvement in Phase I trials (establishing the safety, toxicity, dose, and

pharmacokinetics/dynamics) or Phase II trials (establishing the efficacy of the drug), but more likely, there would be involvement in Phase III trials (widespread clinical use to verify the impressions of Phases I and II and provide statistically significant quantities of data before approval). In each case, there would be extensively detailed protocols and requirements for consent and data collection from the manufacturer, all of which must be approved by the institutional review board (IRB or sometimes called the human studies or human experimentation committee) of the investigator's facility.

Alternatively, individual physicians may use experimental drugs (or chemicals) in trials or projects of their own initiation or even as routine therapy. To do so, the physician (called the investigator or the sponsor) must file an Investigational New Drug (IND) application with the FDA. This extensive form requires information about the drug, the investigator(s), the drug labeling to be used, preclinical (animal) and any prior clinical pharmacologic studies, the exact protocol to be used, consent to be obtained, IRB approval, and the records to be kept. FDA approval of the application will provide the investigator with an IND permit number for the use of that particular drug in the specified situation. The investigator is responsible for all aspects (as listed), but particular attention must be paid to IRB approval and consent. The FDA specifies certain features of the mix of members of the IRB and the need for their absolute objectivity and their ability to judge the acceptability of the proposal. (In the case of an independent practitioner proposing use of a drug outside any institution, the FDA will assume the IRB role.) Consent is a principal issue. Potential recipients of the experimental drug must be informed fully of the unproven nature of the proposed treatment and the fact that there may be unknown side effects or complications (and that there is a mechanism to compensate victims of untoward results of human experimentation). All potential risks must be detailed on a consent form approved by the IRB; the signing of this form by the patient must be witnessed by a disinterested third party who is expected to verify that the patient knew for what they were providing consent. Finally, progress and final reports on the use of the drug are required by the FDA.

Intravenous regional blocks using reserpine or guanethidine occasionally are administered in certain cases of intractable extremity pain; an IND number is necessary because, currently, neither drug is approved for intravenous use in this country.

Many patients with chronic pain syndromes will consent readily to any proposed treatment that offers them even a remote hope of relief from suffering. The need for thorough, complete, well-documented disclosures in the informed consent process is especially important with this vulnerable patient population.

In all cases of experimental drug use, there are strict rules about reporting "alarming adverse drug reactions, including drug-related deaths." All such events (even if questionably related to the drug) must be communicated immediately to the FDA. Failure to do so could increase significantly the potential liability exposure of the involved investigator.

Questions arise as to exactly what constitutes a clinical study. Specifically, if a physician uses only approved drugs and accepted techniques but alternates two different modes of therapy for every other patient with a given condition to see if the therapeutic results differ, is informed consent required from the patients? This is a gray area. However, in the current medical–legal climate, it seems only prudent if there is going to be some organized assignment of different therapies (such as random number table, odd or even patient number, and different days of the week), the process should be considered a study rather than a series of observations. Therefore, IRB approval would be necessary, and fully informed consent for participation in the study should be obtained from the patients.

PAIN MANAGEMENT IN TERMINALLY ILL PATIENTS

Some terminally ill patients, typically with cancer, have severe intractable pain. In certain of these patients, the pain may be reduced or eliminated by neurolytic blocks or epidural or intrathecal narcotics. When requested to provide this pain therapy, some physicians may be reluctant to become involved. There can be a concern that the patient may die during or after a pain management procedure or be compromised by factors that could hasten death, such as respiratory depression from epidural or intrathecal narcotics. The physician may fear that such circumstances could lead to a malpractice suit by the patient's family. Although these concerns might be valid, proper management of the relationship with the patient and family, scrupulously complete disclosure, and careful documentation should prevent any misunderstandings and subsequent problems for the pain management physician.

The pain management physician needs an especially thorough knowledge of the condition of the terminally ill patient proposed for pain therapy. There must be close cooperation and communication with the primary physician(s). For example, if the patient also has pulmonary disease, the potential for respiratory depression by epidural or intrathecal narcotics could be increased, and this must be considered. After the pain management physician studies the case and formulates recommendations for therapy, the potential side effects and complications first should be discussed with the primary physician (who presumably knows the patient and family well). If the primary physician agrees with the suggested therapy, it is probably wise for both physicians to discuss the options and their respective risks and benefits with the patient and the family. Potential complications (such as respiratory depression or, from blocks, loss of limb function or impairment of autonomic function) must be identified clearly to all involved. If the patient and family appear to understand and accept these risks, the discussion must proceed, when appropriate, to include the "what ifs." If the patient does experience respiratory depression from narcotics, is this to be reversed with narcotic antagonists? The answer to this and any similar questions must be clear before the necessity for treatment. Confusion during an emergency situation can cause problems and misunderstanding. Priorities must be established. Some patients may desire pain relief at all costs, including the risk of an accelerated death. Others may want to live out their time but might try therapy that could diminish their constant pain. To repeat, in all cases, these issues must be clear to all involved. After these are established, the understandings on these points must be noted completely in the patient's record. It may be helpful to discuss the note with the primary physician before writing it. After it is written, the note should be shown or read to the patient and the family, and the patient should countersign it in the presence of the family if possible. There may be an institutional ethics committee involved. It may be wise to advise the risk manager and/or counsel. With this degree of care taken, it is unlikely that later misunderstanding would lead to questions about the pain management.

The usual contraindications may not apply in terminally ill patients. For example, it may be permissible to place an epidural or intrathecal catheter in an infected patient or even through an infected back if the risks are outweighed by the potential benefits in the minds of all concerned and this is documented carefully in the record. The same concept may apply to the dose, schedule, and route of administration of narcotics or to doing a block injection through or around a tumor. In any such case, full disclosure of the risks and benefits will help prevent later questions and facilitate achieving optimal pain management.

POINTS OF LAW: NEGLIGENCE

There are extensive discussions of the law and how it applies to medicine and charges of medical malpractice in particular.[10,14] One major recurrent theme that often is misunderstood by physicians is that of negligence. Virtually all malpractice actions against physicians allege negligence. This term generally is understood to mean failure to exercise reasonable care. However, the legal elements of negligence are specific. For an act to be negligent, four elements must be established: duty, breach, causation, and damage.

Duty

The element of duty has two aspects. It first must be proved that the physician owed a duty to the person who was harmed. Second, the scope of the duty owed must be established. Generally, the physician owes a duty of reasonable care to those with whom a physician–patient relationship has been established.

Breach

The plaintiff must prove that the physician breached the duty owed to the patient. That is, that the physician did not meet the standard of care ordinarily exercised by practitioners of the same or similar training in the same or similar circumstances. The claimant must establish (almost always by expert testimony) what the owed standard of care is and then prove that the defendant physician deviated from that standard by omission (that is, by not doing a required act) or commission (that is, doing something that should not have been done).

Causation

The plaintiff must prove that there was a reasonably close causal relation between the breach of duty (or deviation from the standard of care) and the harm suffered by the plaintiff. This can be the most difficult element of negligence to establish.

Damage

Finally, the plaintiff must prove that an actual loss or damage was suffered. The harm alleged can be physical, financial, or emotional.

IF YOU ARE SUED

Good medical practice (including many of the points outlined) and strong patient–physician relationships should help prevent claims of medical malpractice. However, malpractice suits cannot be prevented completely. There are many things to be remembered if you are sued. A noted medical malpractice defense attorney[23] offered many of the following suggestions. Unless instructed otherwise by your defense attorney and/or insurance company representative,

1. Do not panic when served a summons. Notify your institution (if any), insurance company, and attorney immediately.
2. Do not alter your records in any way.
3. Do not transfer your assets.
4. Do not discuss the case with anyone except your claims representative and defense attorney.
5. Do not talk to the plaintiff, their family, and their friends, or the plaintiff's attorney.
6. Do not talk to the media about the suit.
7. In your frustration, do not be hostile to your insurance claims representative and defense attorney. They are on your side.
8. Do not expect that a counterclaim against the plaintiff will get the suit dropped or be successful.
9. Do keep the suit in perspective compared with the entirety of your professional and personal life.
10. Do cooperate fully and quickly with the insurance claims representative and defense attorney.
11. Do gather all relevant records regarding the plaintiff. This includes office records, hospital records, correspondence with the patient, financial records, and results of diagnostic tests.
12. Dictate or write as soon as possible a summary of all that you know about the incidents and parties involved and share it with your claims representative and defense attorney.
13. Be prepared to educate your defense attorney and claims representative about the medical aspects of the case.
14. If a suit has not been brought yet and the patient requests a meeting, consult with your claims representative before discussing the case with the patient.
15. If the patient's lawyer requests medical records, supply a copy or written summary of your care and treatment after notifying your insurer and attorney. Do not send original records. Also be sure you have received authorization to release the patient's records.

Soon after you notify your insurer, your claims representative and defense attorney will be in contact with you to discuss your case and advise you further.

SUMMARY

Even the most experienced pain management physician (using proven techniques and drugs with maximum skill) will encounter some problems and complications. In a large busy pain management unit during a recent year, there were four cases with potential for malpractice litigation. A patient claimed emotional difficulties after several trigger-point injections. Long after an epidural corticosteroid injection for low back pain, a patient claimed bladder difficulty though he previously denied this during follow-up visits to the clinic. A pneumothorax requiring a chest tube developed after a trapezius trigger-point injection. Local muscle twitching developed in the area of a repeat block injection. Little, if anything, can be done to prevent complications such as these completely. It is likely that no genuine negligence was involved. A great deal can be done, however, to prevent these occurrences and others like them from developing into malpractice suits. Sound practice as outlined throughout this book and adherence to the principles outlined in this chapter should help prevent major medical–legal problems significantly. This will lead to continuation of the pattern, mentioned at the outset, of relatively few medical malpractice cases arising from pain management.

References

1. Solazzi RW, Ward RJ. The spectrum of medical liability cases. In: Pierce EC, Cooper JB, eds. *Analysis of Anesthetic Mishaps*. Boston: Little, Brown; 1984:43–59.
2. Swerdlow M. Complications of local anesthetic neural blockade. In: Cousins MJ, Bridenbaugh PO, eds. *Neural Blockade*. Philadelphia: Lippincott; 1980:526–542.
3. Murphy TM. Complications of diagnostic and therapeutic nerve blocks. In: Orkin FK, Cooperman LH, eds. *Complications in Anesthesiology*. Philadelphia: Lippincott; 1983:106–116.
4. Swerdlow M. Complications of neurolytic neural blockade.

In: Cousins MJ, Bridenbaugh PO, eds. *Neural Blockade.* Philadelphia: Lippincott; 1980:543–553.

5. Abram SE, Hogan QH. Complications of nerve blocks. In: Benumof JL, Saidman LJ, eds. *Anesthesia and Perioperative Complications.* St. Louis: Mosby Year Book; 1992:52–76.

6. Swerdlow M. Medical–legal aspects of complications following pain relieving blocks. *Pain* 1982; 13:321–331.

7. *Wiik v Rathmore,* 21 Mass App Ct 399 (1986).

8. *Earlin v Cravetz,* 399 A2d 783 (Pa Super 1979).

9. *Henman v DeLuca,* Harris County (Tex) No. 83-14149 reported in North Carolina Hospital Association Trust Fund Risk Review 4(6):8 (June 1986).

10. MacDonald MG, Meyer KC, Essig B. *Health Care Law: A Practical Guide.* New York: Bender; 1985.

11. *Schloendorff v Society of N.Y. Hosp,* 211 NY 125, 129, 105 NE 92, 93 (1914).

12. *Natanson v Kline,* 168 Kan 393, 350 P2d 1093, 1106 (1960).

13. *Canterbury v Spence,* 464 F2d 772 (DC Cir), *cert denied,* 409 US 1064 (1972).

14. Peters JD, Feinberg KS, Kroll DA, Colins V. *Anesthesiology and the Law.* Ann Arbor: Health Administration Press; 1983:23.

15. *Harnish v Children's Hospital Medical Center,* 387 Mass 152 (1982).

16. Curran WJ. Informed consent in malpractice cases: a turn towards reality. *N Engl J Med* 1986; 314:429–430.

17. *Martin v Stratton,* 515 P2d 1366 (Okla 1973).

18. President' Commission for the Study of Ethical Problems in Medicine and Biomedical and Behavioral Research. In: *Making Health Care Decisions: The Ethical and Legal Implications of Informed Consent in the Patient–Practitioner Relationship.* Washington, DC: US Government Printing Office; 1982.

19. Gutheil TG, Bursztajn H, Brodsky A. Malpractice prevention through the sharing of uncertainty: informed consent and the therapeutic alliance. *N Engl J Med* 1984; 311:49–51.

20. US Department of Health and Human Services. (1982) Use of approved drugs for unlabelled indications. *FDA Bull* 1982; 12(1):4–5.

21. Adriani J. Letter to the editor. *ASA Newsletter* May 1986; 50(5):5.

22. Benzon H. Epidural steroids. In: Raj PP, ed. *Practical Management of Pain.* 2nd ed. St. Louis: Mosby Year Book; 1992:199, 818–828.

23. Danner D. *Medical Malpractice: A Primer for Physicians.* Rochester, NY: Lawyer's Co-operative; 1986:4–7.

Glossary

Accommodation   The property of a nerve by which it adjusts to a slowly increasing strength of stimulus so that the strength at which excitation occurs is greater than it would be were the strength to have risen more gradually

Acroparesthesia   Paresthesia of an extremity or an extreme degree of paresthesia

Adynamia   Weakness

Afferent   Bringing to or into as in nerves transmitting information to the spinal cord

Alexithymia   A state of restricted cognitive and affective characteristics that are common in patients with psychosomatic disorders

Algesia   A state of increased sensitivity to pain

Algodystrophy   Sympathetic dystrophy

Allesthesia (Allaesthesia)   A form of allochesthesia in which the sensation of a stimulus in one limb is referred to the opposite limb

Allocheiria (Allochiria)   Allesthesia

Allochesthesia   A condition in which a sensation is referred to a point other than that to which the stimulus is applied

Allodynia   Any stimulus that results in pain

Alloesthesia (Alloaesthesia)   Allesthesia

Analgesia   Loss of sensibility to pain

Analgesia Algera   Anesthesia dolorosa

Anesthesia (Anaesthesia)   Total loss of all forms of sensation

Anesthesia Dolorosa   Spontaneous pain in a part, associated with loss of sensibility

Antidromic   Propagation of an impulse along a nerve in a direction the reverse of normal

Arthrodesis   The stiffening of a joint by operative means

Arthrosis   A trophic degeneration of a joint

Asymbolia   Loss of the power of appreciation by touch of the form and nature of an object

Auriculotherapy   A form of acupuncture in which points in the ear are stimulated

Axonotmesis   Interruption of the axons of a nerve without severance of the supporting structure

Biofeedback   A training technique used to gain voluntary control over autonomic functions

Blepharospasm   Spasmodic winking of the orbicularis muscle

Bruxism   Grinding together of the teeth

Capsaicin   A pungent alkaloid found in red peppers

Causalgia   Sustained burning pain after a traumatic nerve lesion combined with vasomotor or sudomotor dysfunction and late trophic changes

Central pain   Spontaneous pain and painful overreaction to objective stimulation resulting from lesions confined to the substance of the central nervous system

Cholecystokinin   A peptide first described as a gastrointestinal hormone. It is also a potent analgesic

Coccydynia (Coccygodynia) (Coccygalgia) (Coccyodynia)   Pain in the coccygeal region often caused by a disorder of the sacrococcygeal joint

Commissural Fibers   A bundle of nerve fibers passing from one side to the other in the brain or spinal cord

Cordectomy   Excision of a part of the spinal cord

Cordotomy (Chordotomy)   Division of tracts of the spinal cord by various techniques

Cortectomy   Excision of part of the cortex

Cryalgesia   Pain caused by cold

Cryesthesia   Sensitiveness to cold

Cryoanalgesia   Pain relief by cold, commonly by freezing nerves with a probe

Deafferentation   A loss of sensory nerve fibers from a portion of the body

Dermatome   The area of skin supplied by a single afferent nerve fiber from a single dorsal root

Dynorphin   One of three classes of opioid peptides. The others are β-endorphin and enkephalins

Dysesthesia   A condition in which a disagreeable sensation is produced by ordinary stimuli

Dysnosognosia   A psychopathologic state of abnormal illness behavior

Dystonia   A state of abnormal tonicity in any of the tissues

Efferent   Conducting outward

Electrogenesis   A generation of a neural impulse

Endorphin   One of a family of opioid-like polypeptides

Enkephalin   A pentapeptide that binds to some pain-related opiate receptors

Fibromyalgia   An ambiguous term often used to refer to myofascial syndrome

Fibrositis   An ambiguous term often used to refer to myofascial trigger points

Gangliolysis   The dissolution of a ganglion, e.g., by radiofrequency

Ganglionectomy   Excision of a ganglion

Glossodynia (Glossalgia)   Pain in the tongue

Heterotopic Pain   Referred pain

Hypalgesia   Decreased sensitivity to pain

Hyperalgesia (Hyperalgia)   An increased sensitivity to painful stimuli with a lowered threshold to painful stimuli

Hyperesthesia (Hyperaesthesia)   An increased response to pain and tactile and temperature sense with a lowered threshold to painful stimuli

Hyperpathia   Unpleasant long-lasting pain sensation with delay in its appreciation after stimulation and a continued after sensation when the stimulus is ended, usually associated with a raised threshold to stimulation

Hypesthesia (Hypoesthesia)   A diminution of sensation

Hypoesthesia (Hypoaesthesia)   Hypesthesia

Mydriasis   Dilatation of the pupil

Myelotomy   Any incision of the spinal cord

Myofascial Syndrome Pain and/or autonomic phenomena referred from active myofascial trigger points with associated dysfunction

Myofibrositis A term often used to refer to myofascial syndrome

Myosis (Miosis) Contraction of the pupil

Myositis Inflammation of a muscle

Myotome Those muscles innervated by a single spinal segment

Nerve Block Interruption of nerve conduction wholly or in part, temporarily or permanently

Nervus Intermedius A sensory nerve forming the sensory portion of the facial nerve

Neuralgia Pain of a severe, throbbing, or stabbing character in the course or distribution of a nerve

Neurectomy Excision of a portion of a nerve

Neuritis Inflammation of a nerve

Neuroma A neoplasm of a nerve or a proliferative mass (not neoplasm) of Schwann cells and neurites that may develop at the proximal end of a severed or injured nerve

Neuropathy Any disease of the nervous system

Neuropraxia A state of a nerve in which conduction is blocked across a point but is present above and below the lesion

Neurotmesis Complete division of a nerve

Nociceptors A peripheral nerve organ or mechanism for the appreciation and transmission of painful stimuli

Odontalgia Toothache

Operant Conditioning A technique of increasing the frequency of a specific desired response by pairing it with a reinforcer

Oxyesthesia Hyperesthesia

Pacinian Corpuscles Pressure-sensitive neural structures in the fingers, mesentery, tendons, and elsewhere

Panalgesia Pain in the entire body

Paresthesia Crawling, burning, tingling, or pins-and-needles feelings that arise spontaneously

Percutaneous Through unbroken skin

Pes Cavus An exaggeration of the normal arch

Pes Valgus Eversion of the foot

Pes Varus Inversion of the foot

Proenkephalin Precursor of an opioid peptide

Radiculitis Inflammation of a spinal nerve root

Radiculopathy Disease of the spinal nerve root

Radiofrequency Radiant energy of a certain frequency; often used to create a heat lesion

Referred Pain Pain perceived as coming from an area remote from its actual origin

Reflex Sympathetic Dystrophy A painful syndrome associated with autonomic dysfunction but not preceded by major nerve trauma

Rhizidiotomy A selective microsurgical technique of rhizotomy that spares the large diameter proprioceptive afferents

Rhizotomy Sectioning of the spinal nerve roots

Sciatica Neuralgia of the sciatic nerve usually caused by a herniated lumbar vertebral disk but occasionally by sciatic neuritis

Sclerotome All tissues of embryonic mesodermal origin (muscle, fascia, and connective tissue) innervated by a single spinal segment

Somatic Parietal; relating to the wall of the body cavity

Somatization The conversion of anxiety into physical symptoms

Somatostatin A peptide that inhibits the release of growth hormone but also seems to have effects similar to opiates

Spondylolisthesis Forward movement of the body of one lower lumbar vertebra on the vertebrae below it

Spondylolysis Breaking down or dissolution of the body of a vertebra

Spondylosis Vertebral ankylosis; this term also is applied often nonspecifically to any lesion of the spine of a degenerative nature

Substance P A polypeptide in brain and intestine that may be a neurotransmitter of nociceptive sensory afferents

Substantia Gelatinosa Area of the posterior horn of the spinal cord with large amounts of opiate

Sudek Atrophy Bony atrophy associated with sympathetic dystrophy

Sympathalgia Pain occurring after sympathectomy

Sympathetic Dystrophy Group of autonomic dystrophies that includes causalgia and reflex sympathetic dystrophy

Synesthesalgia (Synaesthesialgia) Painful synesthesia

Synesthesia A condition in which a stimulus, in addition to exciting its usual sensation, gives rise to a subjective sensation of different character or localization

Telalgia Referred pain

Thigmanesthesia Loss of light touch

Topoanesthesia Loss of tactile localization

Tractotomy The operation of severing or incising a nerve tract

Transcutaneous Percutaneous

Trichoanesthesia Loss of sensation on stimulation or movement of the hairs

Trigger point A focus of hyperirritability in a tissue that, when compressed, causes referred pain

William's Exercises A group of exercises aimed at strengthening back and abdominal muscles and used in the treatment of low back pain

Xerostomia Dryness of the mouth

Abbreviations

AIB   Abnormal illness behavior
AIP   Acute inflammatory polyneuropathy
CIBPS   Chronic intractable benign pain syndrome
CT   Computed tomography
DJD   Degenerative joint disease
DREZ   Dorsal root entry zone
DRG   Dorsal root ganglion
ECG   Electrocardiography
EEG   Electroencephalography
EHL   Extensor hallucis longus
EMAS   Endorphin-mediated analgesia system
EMG   Electromyography
ES   Epidural steroid
GABA γ-Aminobutyric acid
IBQ   Illness behavior questionnaire
IVR   Intravenous regional
LLD   Leg length discrepancy
MMPI   Minnesota Multiphasic Personality Inventory
MPQ   McGill Pain Questionnaire

MRI   Magnetic resonance imaging
NSAIDs   Nonsteroidal anti-inflammatory drugs
OA   Osteoarthritis
PCA   Patient-controlled analgesia
PID   Pelvic inflammatory disease
PRI   Pain rating index
PSPI   Psychosocial pain inventory
RSD   Reflex sympathetic dystrophy
SCL   System check list
SG   Substantia gelatinosa
SI   Sacroiliac
SLR   Straight leg raising
SPA   Stimulation-produced analgesia
TCAD   Tricyclic antidepressant
TENS   Transcutaneous electrical nerve stimulation
TMJ   Temporomandibular joint
TP   Trigger-point injection
VAS   Visual analog scales
WHO   World Health Organization

Nerve Blocking Techniques

The following is a guide to the performance of some common techniques used in a pain management practice. For other blocks, the reader is referred to any standard textbook of regional anesthesia. Although not specifically mentioned, the anesthesiologist should use their own discretion regarding such details as whether intravenous placement before the block is necessary, whether the patient should be maintained with an empty stomach for several hours before the injection, and whether resuscitative equipment is needed at the bedside.

The complications and side effects mentioned are those specific to the particular nerve block discussed. Other potential complications inherent in any injection technique include intravascular injection, hematoma formation, and infection, the seriousness of which will be determined by the particular site of injection. The anesthesiologist is advised to keep these potential complications in mind when attempting to perform any block.

I. Stellate Ganglion Block

Technique

The patient lies supine with the neck hyperextended and a thin pillow under the shoulders. The carotid artery is palpated, the trachea identified, and using two fingers, the transverse body of C6 (Chassaignac tubercle) is palpated (block at C7 is associated with a higher incidence of pheumothorax). This is the most prominent of the cervical transverse processes and lies at the level of the cricoid cartilage. A skin wheal is raised and a 22-gauge 1½-inch needle is advanced between the carotid and cricoid perpendicular to the skin until it contacts the transverse process. The needle then is pulled approximately 2 mm back, the syringe is aspirated, and a 1-ml test dose is given. Assuming there is no untoward reaction, the remaining solution is injected. This volume will spread along the fascial plane, typically from the middle cervical ganglion to T4 or T5 ganglion, thus affecting the sympathetic supply to structures of the head and neck, upper extremity, and chest.

Drugs

Use 8 to 20 ml of lidocaine 0.5% to 1%, or bupivacaine 0.25% to 0.5%, or procaine 1%.

Tips

1. Patient should be informed to expect a Horner syndrome, hoarseness, and warmth.
2. Success of block is confirmed by a Horner syndrome (miosis, ptosis, and anhidrosis) and more importantly, a skin temperature of the arm of at least 2°F greater than the contralateral arm.
3. The patient should be cautioned not to swallow or talk during the procedure but should be instructed to communicate paresthesias by raising a hand.
4. Avoid bilateral blocks.
5. Meticulous aspiration for blood or cerebrospinal fluid should be done before and during the procedure.
6. After the block is completed, the patient should be instructed to sit up to avoid undue edema of the airway and promote caudad spread of the drug to the nerve of Kuntz.

Complications and Side Effects

1. Vertebral or carotid artery injection with central nervous system toxicity.
2. High spinal or epidural injection.
3. Pneumothorax.
4. Vocal cord paralysis.
5. Vasovagal syncope.
6. Orthostatic hypotension.

519

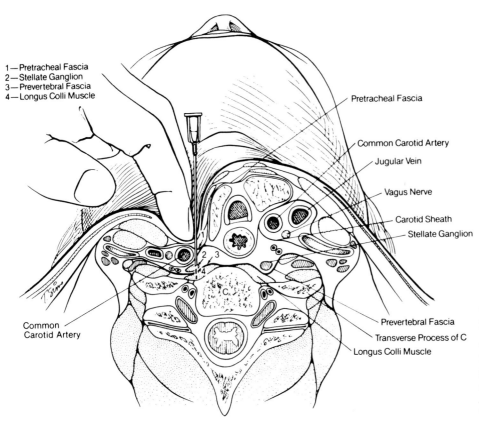

1—Pretracheal Fascia
2—Stellate Ganglion
3—Prevertebral Fascia
4—Longus Colli Muscle

Pretracheal Fascia

Common Carotid Artery

Jugular Vein

Vagus Nerve

Carotid Sheath

Stellate Ganglion

Common
Carotid Artery

Prevertebral Fascia

Transverse Process of C

Longus Colli Muscle

FIGURE A-1. Stellate ganglion block, paratracheal approach. Transverse section at the level of C6, showing the needle medial to the finger retracting the carotid vessel laterally. (Reproduced with permission from Raj PP, ed. *Handbook of Regional Anesthesia.* New York: Churchill Livingstone; 1985.)

II.   Lumbar Sympathetic Block

Technique

The patient is positioned prone with a pillow under the hips. At the lateral edge of the paravertebral muscle opposite to the L2 spinous process, a skin wheal is made and the deeper tissues are infiltrated with a local anesthetic. A 20-gauge 6-inch needle is directed medially at a 45° angle under x-ray control. The vertebral body generally is encountered at a depth of approximately 4 in. The anteroposterior and lateral view of the L2 vertebra is important in verifying the depth and location of the needle tip. The position of the needle tip will be satisfactory if it is close to the anterior aspect of the L2 vertebral body. To determine if the needle is still in the psoas sheath, a small 2 to 3-ml injection of normal saline or local anesthetic is attempted. As long as the needle is in muscle, there will be some resistance to injection. The needle then is advanced slowly until it pierces the fascia when a sudden loss of resistance will be felt. (If a needle smaller than 20 gauge is used, this loss of resistance may be missed.) The correct placement of the tip of the needle is verified repeatedly by aspirating with a dry syringe for the presence of blood or spinal fluid. If a permanent chemical sympathectomy is planned, 1 to 2 ml of contrast media is injected, and radiographic evidence of the spread is verified by taking an x-ray to localize the position of the tip of the needle.

For routine diagnostic or therapeutic lumbar sympathetic blocks, radiologic facilities are helpful but not required. The block can be done safely only with the anatomic landmarks described. If the transverse process is encountered (usually at a depth of approximately 2 in, the needle should be redirected caudad to about twice this depth. After correct placement of the needle and after aspiration with a syringe, a 2-ml test dose of local anesthetic solution is injected. After waiting a few minutes to observe for untoward effects, 15 to 20 ml of local anesthetic is injected.

Drugs

1. Local anesthetic of 12 to 20 ml of lidocaine 1% or bupivacaine 0.25%.
2. Neurolytic of 10 to 15 ml of phenol in saline 6%.

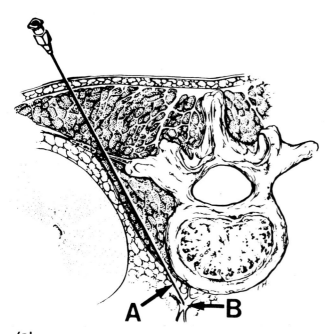

(a)

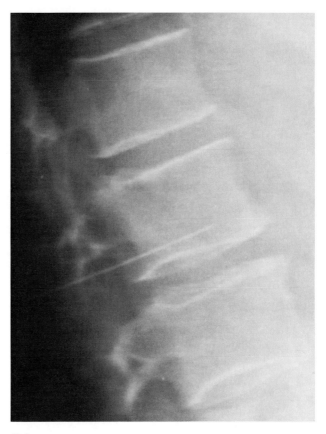

(b)

FIGURE A-2. *(a)* Lumbar sympathetic block. Anatomic drawing showing the relationship of the needle (A) to the sympathetic chain (B) at the L2 level. (Reproduced with permission from Carron H, Korbon GA, Rowlingson JC. *Regional Anesthesia: Techniques and Clinical Applications.* Orlando, FL: Grune and Stratton; 1984.) *(b)* Lumbar sympathetic block. Lateral x-ray view. (Courtesy of S. Jain, M.D.)

Tips

1. Block at L2 alone is usually sufficient to provide sympathectomy to the entire leg; may alternatively be performed at L3. Some prefer individual blocks at L2, L3, and L4, especially for neurolysis since a smaller volume can be used.
2. If a neurolytic procedure is done, a permanent copy of the x-ray confirming correct needle position should be retained.

Complications and Side Effects

1. Orthostatic hypotension.
2. Spinal or epidural injection.
3. Injury to kidney, ureter, or renal pelvis.
4. Genitofemoral block.

III. Celiac Plexus Block

Technique

With the patient in the prone position and a pillow under the abdomen, the T12 and L1 spinous processes and the 12th rib are palpated and marked. The position is confirmed by fluoroscopy if possible. A triangle is drawn using the inferior portion of each spinous process and the third point 7 to 8 cm lateral at the inferior edge of the 12th rib. A skin wheal of local anesthetic is raised at the lateral apex of the triangle, and deeper infiltration along the path is done.

Using a 6-in 20- or 22-gauge needle, the needle is advanced at approximately a 45° angle from the apex, under the inferior edge of the 12th rib toward the body of L1. In an average-sized person, this will approach a depth of approximately 10 to 12 cm. After bony contact is made, the position can be confirmed by fluoroscopy. After this is done and a note is made of the angle and depth of the needle, the needle is redirected so that it ultimately lies 1 to 2 cm beyond the anterolateral edge of the body of L1. Fluoroscopic examination can confirm the position, and aspiration should be done to exclude the possibility of blood, cerebrospinal fluid, or urine aspirate. At this point, a small test dose is given before injection of the usual 20 ml of solution. The same procedure then may be done on the contralateral side.

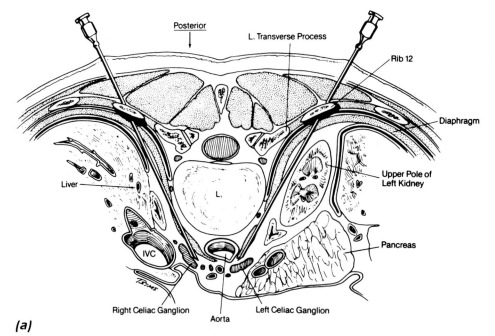

(a)

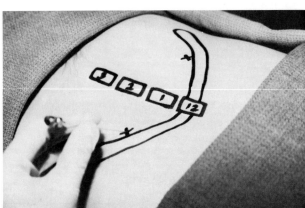

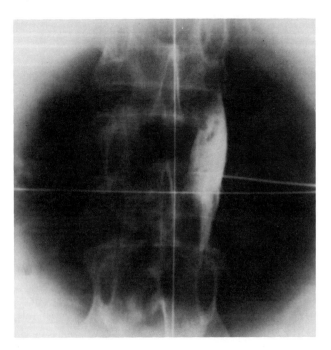

(b)

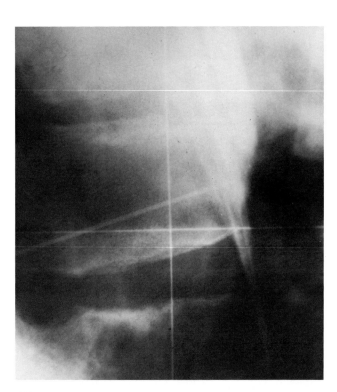

(d)

FIGURE A-3. *(a)* Transverse section at the level of L1 showing entry of 6-in 20-gauge needles bilaterally to the celiac plexus. (Reproduced with permission from Raj PP, ed. *Handbook of Regional Anesthesia.* New York: Churchill Livingstone; 1985.) *(b)* X marks point of entry of needle for celiac plexus block. *(c and d)* AP *(c)* and lateral *(d)* views of needle in position for left celiac plexus block. Contrast dye further confirms position.

(c)

Drugs

1. Local anesthetic of 15 to 20 ml of lidocaine 1% or bupivacaine 0.5%. (A unilateral block with a large volume (50 ml) should provide bilateral anesthesia.)
2. Neurolytic of 15 to 20 ml of alcohol 50% to 95% or phenol 6% (phenol 10% in Renografin 76 is useful for observing dispersion of the injection).

Tips

1. Patient should be well hydrated before the block.
2. Because the left ganglion is usually lower than the right, needle placement on the left should be two-thirds of the way down L1 and, on the right, 1 cm above L1.
3. Fluoroscopy with a permanent spot film to confirm needle placement may be desirable for a neurolytic procedure.

Complications and Side Effects

1. Orthostatic hypotension.
2. Aortic or venacaval puncture with retroperitoneal hematoma.
3. Pneumothorax.
4. Puncture of liver, spleen, kidney, pancreas, or ureter.
5. Neurolytic blocks may result in neuritis, sensory and motor loss, skin sloughing, and alcohol intoxication.

IV. Intravenous Regional Vasodilators

Technique

A 20-gauge intravenous line is started in the affected extremity with a heparin lock. A double-cuff tourniquet is applied at either the upper arm or thigh level, and the affected extremity is elevated and exsanguinated by means of an Esmarch bandage. The tourniquet is inflated above arterial pressure (200 to 250 mmHg). After injection of the solution, the tourniquet remains inflated for 20 to 30 min and then is deflated slowly over 3 min.

Drugs

Use guanethidine in the arm at a dose of 10 to 20 mg in 25 ml of lidocaine 0.5% or in the leg at a dose of 20 to 40 mg in 50 ml of lidocaine 0.5%. (Currently available in the United States only as an investigational drug.)

Tips

1. Heparin (500 IU for the arm or 1000 IU for the leg) often is added to the solution to prevent venous thrombosis.
2. In a patient with sympathetic dystrophy, intravenous access to the affected extremity may be limited severely. Use of warm packs, topical nitroglycerin ointment, and blind intravenous techniques may be needed.

Complications and Side Effects

1. Hypotension.
2. Facial flushing.
3. Diarrhea.
4. Vertigo.
5. Nausea.
6. Vomiting.
7. Somnolence.

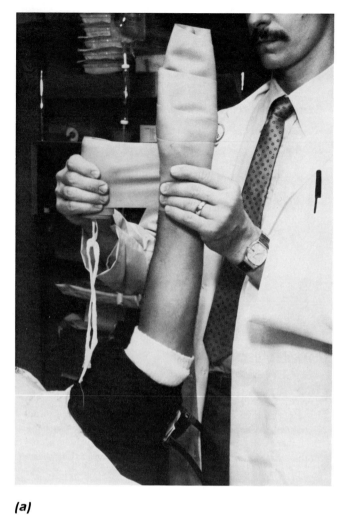

(a)

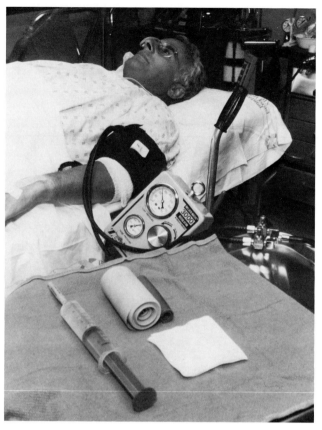

(c)

FIGURE A-4. *(a)* Esmarch bandage is used to exsanguinate the limb. *(b)* After the tourniquet is inflated, the solution is injected. *(c)* Tourniquet remains inflated for 20 to 30 min.

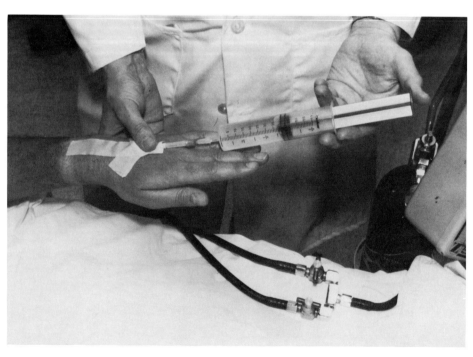

(b)

V.   Epidural Corticosteroid Injection

Technique

The patient is positioned in the lateral decubitus position with the painful side down. Standard sterile precautions are observed, and local anesthesia of the injection site is obtained by infiltration. A 17- to 20-gauge Tuohy needle is used, and the epidural space is identified with loss of resistance to air or saline. After the solution is injected slowly, the needle is cleared with 1 ml of a local anesthetic or saline. The patient should remain in the lateral decubitus position for 15 min.

Drugs

1. 50 to 100 mg of triamcinolone diacetate in 5 to 10 ml of lidocaine 1% or bupivacaine 0.5%.
2. 80 to 120 mg of methylprednisolone acetate also has been used.

Tips

1. Injection should be made at the involved level.
2. A paramedian approach may be useful for patients who cannot flex and is mandatory for patients with previous posterior spinal fusion.

Complications and Side Effects

1. Immediate: high spinal injection.
2. Late: spinal headache, exacerbation of symptoms for 24 to 48 h, epidural hematoma, arachnoiditis, adrenal suppression, Cushing syndrome, and neurologic deficit.

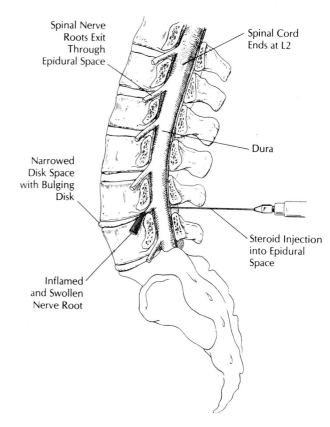

FIGURE A-5. Because root compression in diskogenic disease occurs most commonly in the epidural space, epidural injection of corticosteroids is the preferred procedure. Injection is given at the level of the affected nerve root. (Reproduced with permission from *Hosp Pract* 1985; 20:32k. Illustration by Pauline Thomas.)

VI.   Facet Joint Injection

Technique

The patient is positioned prone on a radiolucent table with a pillow under the hips. Under fluoroscopic control, the appropriate vertebral level is located in the anteroposterior direction. The image intensifier (or patient) then is rotated until the facet joint space is seen clearly. A skin wheal is raised where an imaginary line from the center of the image intensifier intersects the skin. A 22-gauge 3½-in needle is advanced at right angles to the image intensified under fluoroscopic guidance until it enters the joint.

Drugs

Use 1 to 2 ml of lidocaine 1% or bupivacaine 0.5% followed by 20 to 25 mg of triamcinolone diacetate.

Tips

To confirm needle placement, rotate the patient or image intensifier after the needle is in the joint. The needle should continue to appear to be in the joint regardless of the angle of view.

Complications and Side Effects

1. Spinal anesthesia.
2. Neurologic deficit.

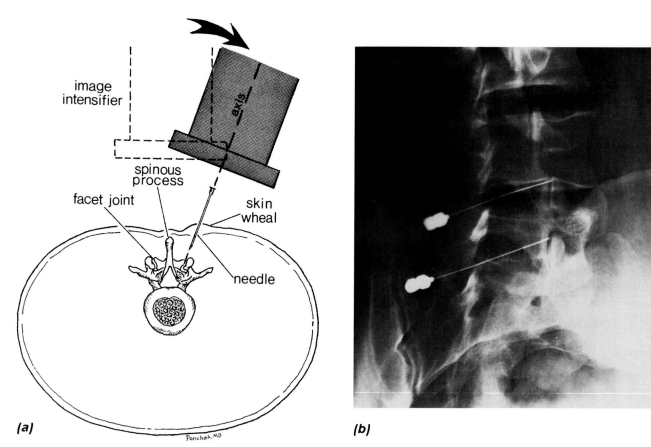

(a)

(b)

FIGURE A-6. *(a)* The image intensifier (or patient) is rotated until the joint space is seen clearly. A skin weal is raised where an imaginary line from the center of the image intensifier intersects the skin. Under fluoroscopic control, a 22-gauge, 3-in needle is advanced into the facet joint along this axis. (Illustration by Steven Ponchak, M.D.) *(b)* X-ray indicating correct needle position in the L4,5 and L5S1 facet joints.

VII.   Paravertebral Somatic Block

Technique

With the patient in the prone position, a skin wheal is raised, and a 22-gauge 3½-in needle is inserted 3 cm lateral to the cephalad end of the dorsal spinous process of the vertebral level to be blocked. It is directed perpendicular to the skin to meet the corresponding transverse process. The needle then is redirected so that it lies approximately 3 cm medial and caudad to the transverse process. The aim is to have the tip of the needle close to the intervertebral foramen, where the corresponding nerve emerges. Paresthesias may or may not be elicited.

Drugs

Use 10 ml of lidocaine 1%, bupivacaine 0.5%, or procaine 1%.

Tips

When a paresthesia is elicited, less local anesthetic (6 to 8 ml) will be needed.

Complications and Side Effects

1. Subdural, epidural, and subarachnoid block.
2. Pneumothorax.
3. Hypotension from sympathetic block.

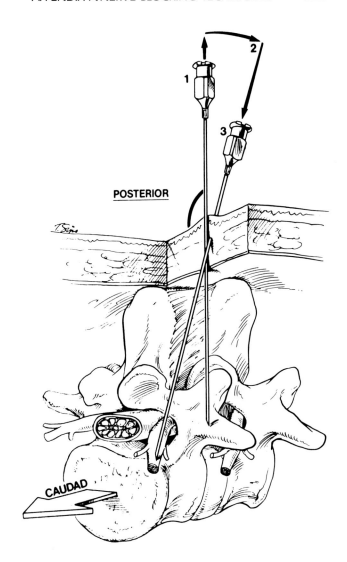

POSTERIOR

CAUDAD

FIGURE A-7. Lateral view of the lumbar nerve roots, showing point of entry and direction of the needle for lumbar somatic block. (Reproduced with permission from Raj PP, ed. *Handbook of Regional Anesthesia.* New York: Churchill Livingston; 1985.)

VIII.   Permanent Intraspinal Catheter Implantation

Technique

The following implantation technique for permanent intraspinal narcotic catheters has been used successfully at the Beth Israel Hospital in Boston:

"After informed consent is obtained, the patient is given a dose of an anti-staph antibiotic, is positioned in the lateral decubitus position and the back, flank and lower lateral abdominal wall are prepped and draped. After infiltration with local anesthetic a three centimeter paraspinous incision is made at the appropriate lumbar level. A Tuohy needle is introduced through the incision and the epidural space identified via a paraspinous approach with a loss of resistance technique. The epidural catheter is then threaded six to eight centimeters past the tip of the needle. The needle is removed, the catheter is aspirated and a test dose of local anesthetic is injected to rule out entry into the subarachnoid space or vessel. Local anesthetic is then injected through the catheter in a dose and volume adequate to not only confirm positioning within the epidural space but also to provide anesthesia for the tunneling procedure (20cc 3% chlorprocaine, for example). The catheter is secured with a purse string suture. The catheter is then tunneled subcutaneously around the flank to the lower abdominal wall and is connected either to an externalized catheter, a subcutaneous injection port, or a subcutaneous continuous infusion device. The wounds are then closed."

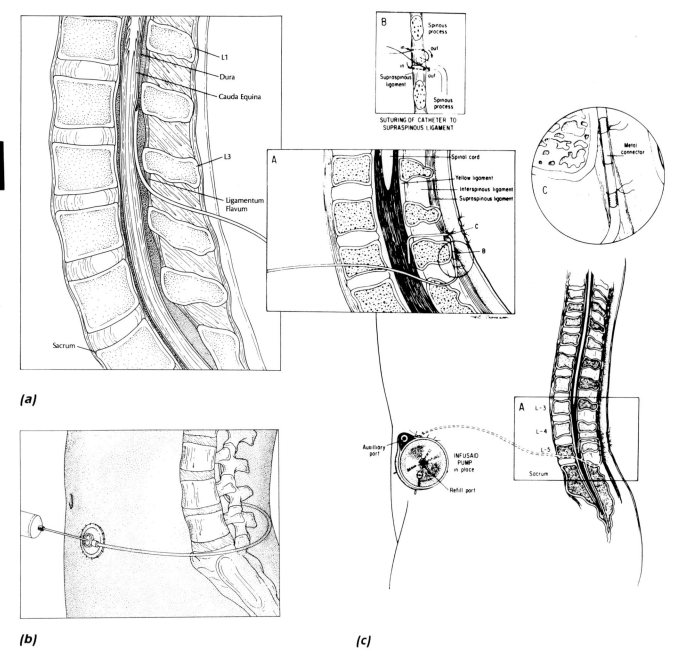

FIGURE A-8. *(a)* Position of the epidural catheter after it has been tunneled subcutaneously through the lower abdominal wall for long-term use. *(b)* Narcotics can be injected through a subcutaneous port as shown or infused continuously. *(c)* Continuous-infusion pump is located in a subcutaneous pocket on the abdominal wall and anchored to the underlying fascia with heavy nonabsorbable sutures at four quadrants. Either an intrathecal or epidural catheter placement can be selected; only the former is shown to emphasize the spinal anchoring technique. The joined catheters wrap around the flank in a subcutaneous tunnel. (A) Close-up perspective of the catheter entrance into the spine. (B) Close-up of the suture technique used to anchor the catheter firmly to the supraspinous ligament to discourage dislodgement. A figure eight is placed before introducing the Tuohy epidural needle, thus eliminating the risk of needle injury to the spinal catheter. When snugged down, the figure eight will reduce the leakage of cerebrospinal fluid along the catheter and forestall hygroma formation. (C) Close-up of the fixation technique to bond the two catheters together over a straight metal connector. (Figures *(a)* and *(b)* reproduced with permission from *Hosp Pract* 1989; 24:44–48, illustrations by Susan Tilberry. Figure *(c)* reproduced with permission from Coombs D. *Continuous Intraspinal Morphine Analgesia for Relief of Cancer Pain.* Norwood, MA: Intermedics Infusaid; 1981:5.)

IX. Intercostal Block

Technique

The injection may be made at the angle of the ribs; at the lateral border of the sacrospinalis muscle; or at the posterior, mid, or anterior axillary line as indicated. With the patient in the lateral or prone position with the arms abducted overhead, the rib is palpated and the skin retracted slightly upward. A 25-gauge 1½-in needle is introduced through a skin wheal until it contacts the rib. It then is "walked off" the inferior edge of the rib and advanced approximately 2 mm. After a negative aspiration, 3 to 5 ml of local anesthetic are injected, and the needle is removed. This procedure is repeated at each of the levels to be blocked. Control of the needle at all times is of the utmost importance in this procedure, and the hand must at all times stabilize its position.

Drugs

Use 3 to 5 ml of lidocaine 1%, bupivacaine 0.5%, or procaine 1%.

Tips

1. A 25-gauge needle is associated with a low incidence of pneumothorax, but breath sounds should be checked and documented after the block.

2. A large dose of local anesthetic may provide a block of several interspaces.

Complications and Side Effects

1. Local anesthetic toxicity from rapid intravascular absorption.
2. Pneumothorax.
3. Epidural or spinal block.

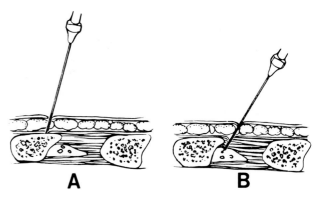

FIGURE A-9. Intercostal nerve block. Anatomic drawing showing (A) step I and (B) step II. (Reproduced with permission from Carron H, Korbon G, Rowlingson J. *Regional Anesthesia.* Orlando, FL: Grune and Stratton; 1984.)

X. Lateral Femoral Cutaneous Block

Technique

With the patient lying supine, a skin wheal is raised 2 to 3 cm medial to and 2 to 3 cm caudad to the anterior superior iliac spine. A 22-gauge 3½-in needle is inserted at right angles to the skin until a "pop" is felt when it passes through the fascia. Then 10 to 15 ml of a local anesthetic is injected as the needle is moved in and out of the fascia in a lateral and medial fan-like direction.

Drugs

Use 10 to 15 ml of lidocaine 1%. (When this block is used to treat meralgia paresthetica, 40 mg of methylprednisolone acetate or triamcinolone often are added to the local anesthetic.)

Tips

Because this is actually a field block, the fanning motion during injection is critical.

Complications and Side Effects

Femoral nerve block with resultant temporary motor loss may occur.

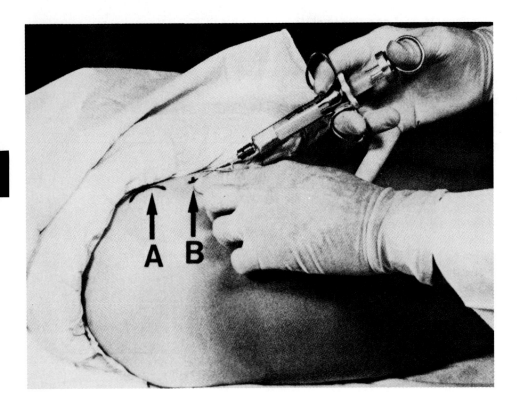

(a)

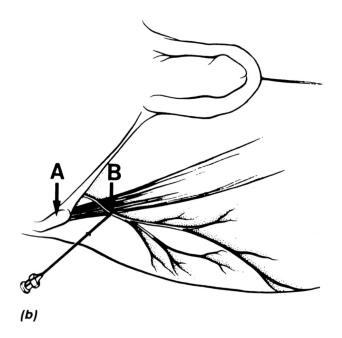

(b)

FIGURE A-10. *(a)* Lateral femoral cutaneous nerve block. Landmarks: (A) indicates the anterior superior iliac spine. Needle entry point (B) is 2 cm medial and 2 cm caudad to point (A). *(b)* Lateral femoral cutaneous nerve block. Anatomic drawing showing relationship of the anterosuperior iliac spine (A) to the nerve (B). (Reproduced with permission from Carron H, Korbon G, Rowlingson J. *Regional Anesthesia.* Orlando, FL: Grune and Stratton, 1984.)

XI.   Greater Occipital Nerve Block

Technique

With the patient seated and their head flexed, a skin wheal is raised just caudad to the superior nuchal line at the lateral edge of the insertion of the trapezius muscle. This point is midway between the mastoid and the midline. A 22- to 25-gauge 1½-in needle then is inserted in a cephalad direction until bone is contacted. After negative aspiration, 3 to 5 ml of a local anesthetic is injected.

Drugs

Use 3 to 5 ml of lidocaine 1% or bupivacaine 0.5%. (Methylprednisolone or triamcinolone 20 to 40 mg sometimes are added to the local anesthetic in the treatment of occipital neuralgia.)

Tips

In a patient with occipital neuralgia, the greater occipital nerve often is tender, and therefore, the most tender spot along the superior nuchal ridge will provide the location for injection.

Complications and Side Effects

1. Accidental occipital artery injection may produce seizures.
2. Injection into the foramen magnum may produce a cisternal block or damage to the brainstem.

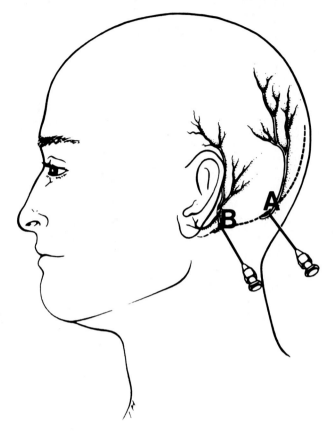

FIGURE A-11. Occipital nerve block. Anatomic drawing showing relationships and distribution of the greater (A) and lesser (B) occipital nerves. (Reproduced with permission from Carron H. *Relieving Pain with Nerve Blocks*. Cleveland, OH: Modern Medicine Publications; 1978:50.)

XII.   Intrathecal Neurolysis

Technique

The patient is positioned at a 45° angle with the painful side uppermost for alcohol and downward for phenol. Under fluoroscopic control, a 22-gauge spinal needle for alcohol, or 20-gauge for phenol, then is inserted into the subarachnoid space at the level of the most painful segment. The needle is withdrawn until cerebrospinal fluid just flows. Then 0.2 ml of solution is injected, and pain relief is assessed. The table is tilted as necessary to confine the flow, and additional 0.1-ml increments of solution are injected at 3-min intervals as needed. The patient's position is maintained for 45 min.

Drugs

1. 0.2 to 0.5 ml of phenol 5% in glycerin or
2. 0.2 to 0.5 ml of alcohol 95% ± 0.1 to 0.2 ml of absorbable contrast medium.

Tips

1. Bilateral block should not be done at the same time because it is associated with a higher incidence of paresis.
2. A permanent spot film should be obtained for later confirmation of needle position.

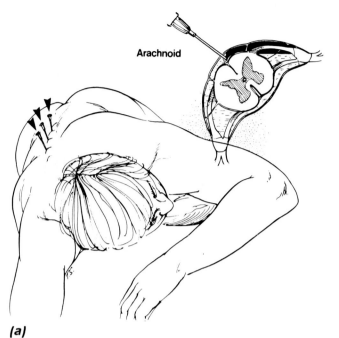

(a)

FIGURE A-12. *(a)* Technique of alcohol neurolysis in the sub-arachnoid space. The painful part is uppermost, and the angle is 45° to position the posterior nerve roots uppermost. *(b)* Phenol neurolysis in the subarachnoid space. The painful part is lowermost, and the angle is 45° to position the posterior nerve roots lowermost. (Reproduced with permission from Raj PP, ed. *Handbook of Regional Anesthesia.* New York: Churchill Livingstone; 1985.)

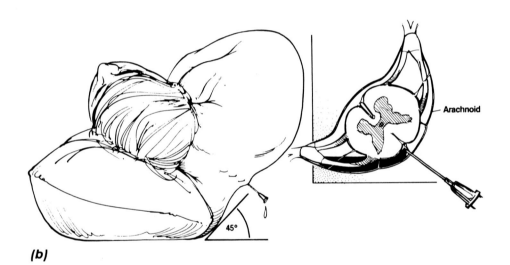

(b)

3. The injection is made at the level corresponding with the spinal cord segment involved; this may be above the level corresponding with root exit.
4. Alcohol is more painful on injection than phenol, and the patient must be warned of this. Some practitioners use local anesthetic to ablate the pain and confirm positioning before neurolysis. Others believes this interferes with the patient's feedback regarding pain relief.
5. Saddle block for rectal pain may be performed with the patient sitting and a 20-gauge spinal needle placed at L5S1. Phenol 5%

in .5 ml increments is injected. Bowel and bladder dysfunction are possible.

Complications and Side Effects

1. Motor weakness.
2. Neuritis.
3. Tissue necrosis.
4. Bowel and bladder dysfunction.

Pain Clinic Record

730-05Y 2/85

BETH ISRAEL HOSPITAL
BOSTON
PAIN MANAGEMENT UNIT

PRE-OP
DIAGNOSIS—

POST-OP
DIAGNOSIS—

ANESTHESIOLOGIST—

PROCEDURE—

| AGE | HT | WT | CONSENT SIGNED? |
| | | | YES ☐ NO ☐ |

MEDICATIONS—

ANESTHESIA   TIME   TO   KNOWN ALLERGIES—

| AM / PM | | TOTALS |

HX; PE; ASSESSMENT; PLAN—

AGENTS

FLUIDS

ANESTHESIA LEVEL

LEFT	MOTOR
	SENS.
	SYMP.
RIGHT	MOTOR
	SENS.
	SYMP.

PAIN LEVEL   0-10

USUAL VALUES	PRE-ANES			TEMP ° C
		180		40
		160		38
		140		36
		120		34
		100		32
		80		30
		60		28
		40		26
		20		

RECOVERY ROOM NURSE COMMENTS—   DISCHARGE TO—

SIGNED _____ R.N.   SIGNED _____ M.D.

MEDICAL RECORDS

Local Anesthetics

Drugs	Latency	Duration	Concentration (%)					Maximum Dose [mg]	
			Infiltration	Peripheral Nerve	Epidural	Spinal	Topical	with Epi	without Epi
Esters									
Procaine (Novocain)	Immediate	Short (30–45 min)	1	—	2	2	—	800	500
Chloroprocaine (Nesacaine)	Fast	Short (45–60 min)	1	—	2	2	—	700	600
Tetracaine (Pontocaine)	Slow	Long (2–3 h)	0.1–0.2	0.1–0.2	—	1	0.5–1	100	75
Cocaine	Slow	Intermediate (60–120 min)	—	—	—	—	4–10	—	150
Amides									
Lydocaine (Xylocaine)	Fast	Intermediate (60–120 min)	0.5–1	1–1.5	1–2	5	4	500	200
Mepivacaine (Carbocaine)	Fast	Intermediate (60–120 min)	1	1–1.5	1.5–2	—	—	500	200
Dibucaine (Nupercainal)	Slow	Very long (3–4 h)	—	—	—	0.5	—	—	50
Bupivacaine (Marcaine)	Intermediate	Very long (4–8 h)	0.25–0.5	0.25–0.5	0.5–0.75	0.5	—	250	150
Prilocaine (Citanest)	Slow	Intermediate (60–120 min)	0.5–1	1	2–3	—	—	600	400
Etidocaine (Duranest)	Fast	Very long (4–8 h)	0.5	0.5–1	1–1.5	—	—	400	300

Note: Page numbers in *italics* indicate figures; page numbers followed by t indicate tables.